MILITARY PREVENTIVE MEDICINE: MOBILIZATION AND DEPLOYMENT VOLUME 2

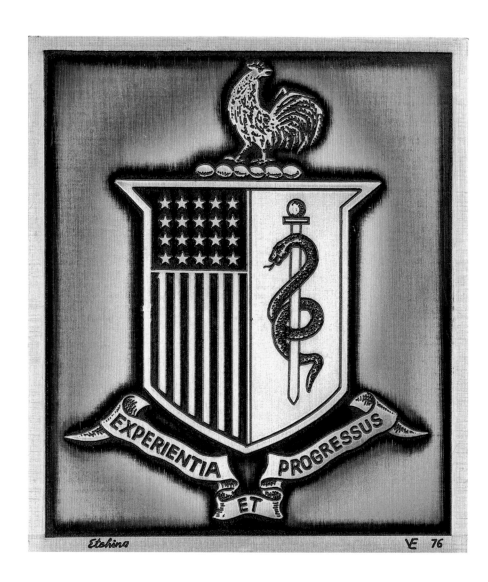

The Coat of Arms
1818
Medical Department of the Army

A 1976 etching by Vassil Ekimov of an
original color print that appeared in
The Military Surgeon, Vol XLI, No 2, 1917

The first line of medical defense in wartime is the combat medic. Although in ancient times medics carried the caduceus into battle to signify the neutral, humanitarian nature of their tasks, they have never been immune to the perils of war. They have made the highest sacrifices to save the lives of others, and their dedication to the wounded soldier is the foundation of military medical care.

Textbooks of Military Medicine

Published by the

Office of The Surgeon General
Department of the Army, United States of America

Editor in Chief and Director
Dave E. Lounsbury, MD, FACP
Colonel, MC, US Army
Borden Institute
Assistant Professor of Medicine
F. Edward Hébert School of Medicine
Uniformed Services University of the Health Sciences

Military Medical Editor
Ronald F. Bellamy, MD
Colonel, US Army, Retired
Borden Institute
Associate Professor of Military Medicine
Associate Professor of Surgery
F. Edward Hébert School of Medicine
Uniformed Services University of the Health Sciences

For sale by the Superintendent of Documents, U.S. Government Printing Office
Internet: bookstore.gpo.gov Phone: toll free (866) 512-1800; DC area (202) 512-1800
Fax: (202) 512-2250 Mail: Stop SSOP, Washington, DC 20402-0001

ISBN 0-16-072923-8

ISBN 0-16-072923-8

90000

9 780160 729232

The *TMM* Series

Published Textbooks

Medical Consequences of Nuclear Warfare (1989)

Conventional Warfare: Ballistic, Blast, and Burn Injuries (1991)

Occupational Health: The Soldier and the Industrial Base (1993)

Military Dermatology (1994)

Military Psychiatry: Preparing in Peace for War (1994)

Anesthesia and Perioperative Care of the Combat Casualty (1995)

War Psychiatry (1995)

Medical Aspects of Chemical and Biological Warfare (1997)

Rehabilitation of the Injured Soldier, Volume 1 (1998)

Rehabilitation of the Injured Soldier, Volume 2 (1999)

Medical Aspects of Harsh Environments, Volume 1 (2002)

Medical Aspects of Harsh Environments, Volume 2 (2002)

Ophthalmic Care of the Combat Casualty (2003)

Military Medical Ethics, Volume 1 (2003)

Military Medical Ethics, Volume 2 (2003)

Military Preventive Medicine: Mobilization and Deployment, Volume 1 (2003)

Military Preventive Medicine: Mobilization and Deployment, Volume 2 (2005)

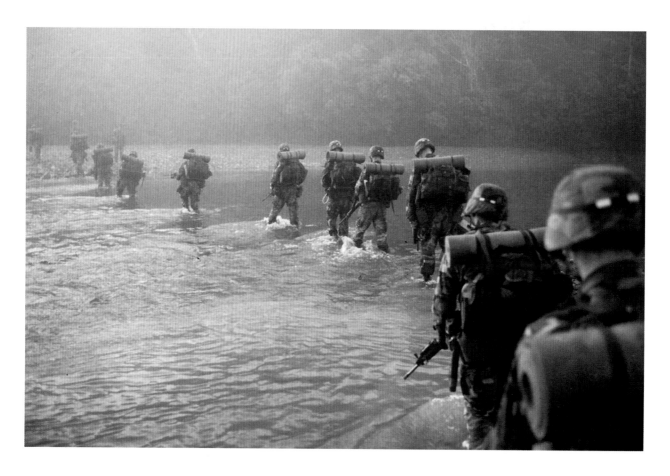

Deploying a healthy force at any time to any part of the world requires comprehensive and coordinated preventive medicine services. The challenges and the achievements of military preventive medicine in the US Armed Forces are embodied by these soldiers crossing a river in Haiti in 1995. They represent a carefully screened cadre of young Americans who enter military service and benefit from a scientifically sound program to reduce the threat of infectious diseases and injuries during basic training and deployment. When deployed to a harsh environment such as this one, they are prepared for potential hazardous exposures—infectious diseases, climatic extremes, chemical and nuclear exposures, and mental stressors—by military preventive medicine professionals. Military medical research and development provides their commanders with effective countermeasures. Their health is monitored to detect events that threaten individual health and operational effectiveness both in the field and in garrison. Military preventive medicine has always been a fundamental factor for ensuring operational success, but as US military doctrine shifts to emphasize rapid and relatively smaller deployments of forces accompanied by small medical elements, the preventive medicine mission takes on a new urgency.

Department of Defense photograph. DoD Joint Combat Camera Center Reference Number -SPT-95-000922. Photographer: SPC Kyle Davis, US Army

MILITARY PREVENTIVE MEDICINE
MOBILIZATION AND DEPLOYMENT
Volume 2

Specialty Editor

PATRICK W. KELLEY
Colonel, Medical Corps, U.S. Army (Retired)

Borden Institute
Walter Reed Army Medical Center
Washington, D. C.

Office of The Surgeon General
United States Army
Falls Church, Virginia

United States Army Medical Department Center and School
Fort Sam Houston, Texas

United States Army Medical Research and Materiel Command
Fort Detrick, Frederick, Maryland

Uniformed Services University of the Health Sciences
Bethesda, Maryland

2005

Editorial Staff: Lorraine B. Davis
Senior Production Manager

Douglas A. Wise
Senior Layout Editor

Bruce G. Maston
Desktop Publishing Editor

Andy C. Szul
Desktop Publishing Editor

Kathleen A. Huycke
Technical Editor

This volume was prepared for military medical educational use. The focus of the information is to foster discussion that may form the basis of doctrine and policy. The opinions or assertions contained herein are the private views of the authors and are not to be construed as official or as reflecting the views of the Department of the Army or the Department of Defense.

Dosage Selection:

The authors and publisher have made every effort to ensure the accuracy of dosages cited herein. However, it is the responsibility of every practitioner to consult appropriate information sources to ascertain correct dosages for each clinical situation, especially for new or unfamiliar drugs and procedures. The authors, editors, publisher, and the Department of Defense cannot be held responsible for any errors found in this book.

Use of Trade or Brand Names:

Use of trade or brand names in this publication is for illustrative purposes only and does not imply endorsement by the Department of Defense.

Neutral Language:

Unless this publication states otherwise, masculine nouns and pronouns do not refer exclusively to men.

Published by the Office of The Surgeon General at TMM Publications
Borden Institute
Walter Reed Army Medical Center
Washington, DC 20307-5001

Library of Congress Cataloging-in-Publication Data

Military preventive medicine : mobilization and deployment / specialty editor, Patrick W. Kelley.
    p. ; cm. -- (Textbooks of military medicine)
  Includes bibliographical references and index.
    1. Medicine, Military. 2. Medicine, Preventive. 3. Military hygiene. I. Kelley, Patrick
W. II. United States. Dept. of the Army. Office of the Surgeon General. III. Series.
  [DNLM: 1. Military Medicine. 2. Preventive Medicine. UH 600 M6444 2003]
  RC971.M64 2003
  616.9'8023--dc21

                                                                    2003048099

PRINTED IN THE UNITED STATES OF AMERICA

10, 09, 08, 07, 06, 05, 04, 03   5 4 3 2 1

Contents

Contributors

DAVID ARDAY, MD, MPH
Medical Epidemiologist, Office of Clinical Standards and Quality, Health Care Financing Administration, 7500 Security Boulevard, Baltimore, MD 21244

NAOMI E. ARONSON, MD
Colonel, Medical Corps, US Army; Director, Infectious Diseases Division, Room A3058, Uniformed Services University of the Health Sciences, 4301 Jones Bridge Road, Bethesda, MD 20814

THOMAS J. BALKIN, PhD
Research Psychologist, Chief, Department of Neurobiology and Behavior, Division of Neuropsychiatry, Walter Reed Army Institute of Research, Silver Spring, MD 20910–7500

PAUL L. BARROWS, DVM, PhD
Colonel, Veterinary Corps, US Army (Ret); l56 Crazy Cross Road, Wimberly, TX 78676

GREGORY BELENKY, MD
Colonel, Medical Corps, US Army; Director, Division of Neuropsychiatry, Walter Reed Army Institute of Research, Silver Spring, MD 20910–7500

S. WILLIAM BERG, MD, MPH
Captain, Medical Corps, US Navy (Retired); Director, Hampton Health District, 3130 Victoria Boulevard, Hampton, VA 23661-1588

LEONARD N. BINN, PhD
Supervisory Research Microbiologist, Department of Virus Diseases, Division of Communicable Diseases and Immunology, Walter Reed Army Institute of Research, Silver Spring, MD 20910-7500

KENT BRADLEY, MD, MPH
Lieutenant Colonel, Medical Corps, US Army; 7th Infantry Division Surgeon, Fort Carson, CO 80913

RICHARD J. BRENNAN, MBBS, MPH
Director, Health Unit, International Rescue Committee, 122 East 42nd Street, New York, NY 10168, (212) 551-3019; Formerly, Visiting Scientist, National Center for Environmental Health, Centers for Disease Control and Prevention, Atlanta, Georgia

LAUREL BROADHURST, MD, MPH
Staff Physician, Weaverville Family Medicine Associates, 117 Hillcrest Drive, Weaverville, NC 28782

RICHARD BROADHURST, MD, MPH
Colonel, Medical Corps, North Carolina Army Guard, Commander, Company C, 161st Area Support Medical Battalion, Weaverville, NC 28782

STEPHANIE BRODINE, MD
Captain, Medical Corps, US Navy (Ret); Professor and Head, Division of Epidemiology and Biostatistics, Graduate School of Public Health, San Diego State University, San Diego, CA 92184

ARTHUR E. BROWN, MD, MPH
Lieutenant Colonel, Medical Corps, US Army; Department of Retrovirology, Armed Forces Research Institute of Medical Sciences, Bangkok, Thailand, APO AP 96546

JOANNE BROWN, DVM
Colonel, Veterinary Corps, US Army (Ret); Rt 2, Box 152B, Monticello, FL 32344

DORIS BROWNE, MD, MPH
Colonel, Medical Corps, US Army (Ret); President and Chief Executive Officer, Browne and Associates, Inc. Washington, DC 21702

JOHN F. BRUNDAGE, MD
Colonel, Medical Corps US Army (Ret); Epidemiologist, Henry M. Jackson Foundation for the Advancement of Military Medicine, Army Medical Surveillance Activity, US Army Center for Health Promotion and Preventive Medicine, Aberdeen Proving Ground, MD

A.P.C.C. HOPPERUS BUMA, MD
Commander, Medical Branch, Royal Netherlands Army; Head of Naval Medical Training; PO Box 1010 (MCP 24D), 1201 DA Hilversum, The Netherlands

FREDERICK BURKLE, MD, MPH
Captain, Medical Corps, US Naval Reserve; Deputy Assistant Administrator, Bureau for Global Health, US Agency for International Development, Washington, DC 20523

ROBERT E. BURR, MD
Director of Endocrine Education, Division of Endocrinology, Bayside Medical Center, 3300 Main Street, Suite 3A, Springfield, MA 01199

WILLIAM R. BYRNE, MD
Colonel, Medical Corps US Army; Infectious Disease Officer, Infectious Disease Service, Walter Reed rmy Medical Center, Washinton, DC 2307-5001

W. PATRICK CARNEY, MPH, PhD
Captain, MSC, US Navy (Ret.); Professor, Department of Preventive Medicine and Biometrics, Uniformed Services University of the Health Sciences, 4301 Jones Bridge Road, Bethesda, MD 20814-4799

DALE A. CARROLL, MD, MPH
Colonel, Medical Corps, US Army (ret); Senior Vice President, Medical Affairs and Performance Improvement, Rockingham Memorial Hospital, 235 Cantrell, Harrisburg, VA 22801

LESTER C. CAUDLE III, MD, MTMH
Lieutenant Colonel, Medical Corps, US Army; Office of The Surgeon General, 5111 Leesburg Pike, Falls Church, VA 22041–3206

KATHRYN L. CLARK, MD, MPH
Infectious Disease Analyst, Armed Forces Medical Intelligence center, 1607 Porter Street, Fort Detrick, Frederick MD 21702-5004

EDWARD T. CLAYSON, PhD
Lieutenant Colonel, MS, US Army; Product Manager, Joint Vaccine Acquisition Program, 64 Thomas Jefferson Dr., Frederick, MD 21702

BRIAN J. COMMONS, MSPH
Colonel, Medical Service, US Army; US Army Center for Health Promotion and Preventive Medicine, Europe, CMR 402, APO AP 09180

CARLOS A. COMPERATORE, PhD
Research Psychologist, US Coast Guard Research and Development Center, Niantic, CT 06357

WILLIAM P. CORR, MD, MPH
Lieutenant Colonel, Medical Corps, US Army; Deputy Commander, Clinical Services, Martin Army Community Hospital, 7950 Martin Loop, Fort Benning, GA 31905-5637

DAVID N. COWAN, PhD, MPH
Lieutenant Colonel, Medical Service, US Army; Special Projects Officer, Division of Preventive Medicine, Walter Reed Army Institute of Research, Silver Spring, MD 20910–7500

STEPHEN C. CRAIG, DO, MTMH
Colonel, Medical Corps, US Army; Chief, Preventive Medicine Service, Keller Army Community Hospital, West Point, NY 10996

JOHN H. CROSS, PhD
Professor of Tropical Public Health, Uniformed Services University of the Health Sciences, 4301 Jones Bridge Road, Bethesda MD 20814-4799

PATRICIA A. DEUSTER, PhD, MPH
Human Performance Laboratory, Department of Military and Emergency Medicine, Uniformed Services University of the Health Sciences, 4301 Jones Bridge Road, Bethesda, MD 20814

EDWARD M. EITZEN, Jr., MD, MPH
Colonel, Medical Corps, US Army; Commander, US Army Medical Research Institute of Infectious Diseases, Fort Detrick, Frederick, MD 21702–5011

TIMOTHY P. ENDY, MD, MPH
Colonel, Medical Corps, US Army; Director, Division of Communicable Diseases and Immunology, Walter Reed Army Institute of Research, 503 Robert Grant Avenue, Silver Spring, MD 20910-7500

RALPH L. ERICKSON, MD, PhD
Lieutenant Colonel, Medical Corps, US Army; Chief, Preventive Medicine Service, Landstuhl Regional Medical Center, APO AE 09180

BRIAN FEIGHNER, MD, MPH
Colonel, Medical Corps, US Army; Interim Chair, Department of Military and Emergency Medicine, Uniformed Services University of the Health Sciences, 4301 Jones Bridge Road, Bethesda, MD 20814-4799

JAMES FLECKENSTEIN, MD
Assistant Professor of Medicine, Departments of Medicine and Molecular Sciences, Infectious Disease Division, University of Tennessee Health Science Center and Veterans Affairs, 1030 Jefferson Avenue, Memphis, TN 38104

VICKY L. FOGELMAN, DVM
Colonel, Biomedical Science, US Air Force; Academic Director, International Health Program, US Air Force Radiobiology Research Institute, 8901 Wisconsin Avenue, Bethesda, MD 20889–5603

ARTHUR M. FRIEDLANDER, MD
Colonel, Medical Corps, US Army (Retired); Senior Military Scientist, US Army Medical Research Institute of Infectious Diseases, Fort Detrick, MD 21702-5011; Adjunct Professor of Medicine, Uniformed Services University of the Health Sciences, 4301 Jones Bridge Road, Bethesda, Maryland 20814-4799

JEFFREY M. GAMBEL, MD, MPH, MSW
Lieutenant Colonel, Medical Corps, US Army; Staff Physiatrist, Walter Reed Army Medical Center, Washington, DC 20307-5001

DAVID GOLDMAN, MD, MPH
Director, Rappahannock Area Health District, Virginia Department of Health, 608 Jackson Street, Fredericksburg, VA 22401; Formerly, Major, Medical Corps, US Army; Command Surgeon, On-site Inspection Agency, Washington, DC 20041-0498

W. DAVID GOOLSBY, DVM, MPH
Lieutenant, Veterinary Corps, US Army (Ret); 1247 Shadowwood Drive, Spartanburg, SC 29301

GREGORY C. GRAY, MD
Captain, Medical Corps, US Navy, (Retired); Professor, Department of Epidemiology, University of Iowa College of Public Health, 200 Hawkins Drive, Iowa City, IA 52242

HARRY GREER, MD
Captain, Medical Corps, US Navy; Instructor, Defense Medical Readiness Training Institute, Fort Sam Houston, TX

THOMAS A. GRIEGER, MD
Captain, Medical Corps, US Navy; Associate Professor, Department of Psychiatry, Uniformed Services University of the Health Sciences, 4301 Jones Bridge Road, Bethesda, MD 20814-4799

JEFFREY D. GUNZENHAUSER, MD, MPH
Colonel, Medical Corps, US Army; Preventive Medicine Staff Officer, Office of The Surgeon General, 5109 Leesburg Pike, Suite 684, Falls Church, VA 22041

RAJ K. GUPTA, PhD
Colonel, Medical Service, US Army; Research Area Director, Research Plans and Programs, US Army Medical Research and Development Command, Fort Detrick, Frederick, MD 21702–5012

PAUL S. HAMMER, MD
Commander, Medical Corps, US Navy; Staff Psychiatrist, Mental Health Department, Naval Medical Center, San Diego, CA 92136

KEVIN HANSON, MD, MPH
Captain, Medical Corps, US Navy; Uniformed Services University of the Health Science, 4301 Jones Bridge Road, Bethesda, MD 20814-4799

CLIFTON A. HAWKES, MD
Colonel, Medical Corps, US Army; Chief, Infectious Disease Service, Walter Reed Army Medical Center, Washington, DC 20307-5001

ROSE MARIE HENDRIX, DO, MPH
Medical Director, Santa Cruz County Health Clinic, 1080 Emeline, Santa Cruz, CA 95060

WILLIAM C. HEWITSON, MD, MPH
Lieutenant Colonel, Medical Corps, US Army; Department of
Preventive Health Services, Community Health Practices
Branch, AMEDD Center and School, ATTN: MCCS-HPC, Fort
Sam Houston, TX 78234-6124

KENNETH J. HOFFMAN, MD, MPH
Colonel, Medical Corps, US Army; Medical Director, Population
Health Programs, Office of the Assistant Secretary of Defense
(Health Affairs)/TRICARE Management Actiity, 5111 Leesburg
Pike, Falls Church, VA 22041

CHARLES W. HOGE, MD
Colonel, Medical Corps, US Army; Chief, Department of
Psychiatry and Behavioral Sciences, Division of Neuropsychiatry, Walter Reed Army Institute of Research, Silver Spring, MD
20910-7500

HARRY C. HOLLOWAY, MD
Colonel (Retired), Medical Corps, US Army; Professor of
Psychiatry, Department of Psychiatry, Uniformed Services
University of the Health Sciences, 4301 Jones Bridge Road,
Bethesda, MD 20814-4799

DAVID HOOVER, MD
Colonel, Medical Corps, US Army; Infectious Disease Officer,
Department of Bacterial Diseases, Division of Communicable
Diseases and Immunology, Walter Reed Army Institute of
Research, Silver Spring, MD 20910-7500

STEVE HOROSKO III, PhD
Lieutenant Colonel, Medical Service Corps, US Army; Preven-
tive Medicine Staff Officer, Office of the Surgeon, XVIII ABN
Corps, Fort Bragg, NC 28310

DUANE R. HOSPENTHAL, MD, PhD
Lieutenant Colonel, Medical Corps, US Army; Chief, Infectious
Disease Service, Brooke Army Medical Center, 3851 Roger
Brooke Drive, Fort Sam Houston, TX 78234-6200

CHARLES R. HOWSARE, MD
Medical Director, Healthforce, 210 W. Holmes Avenue, Altoona,
PA 16602

BRUCE L. INNIS, MD
Colonel, Medical Corps, US Army (Retired); Group Director,
New Vaccines, GlaxoSMithKline Pharmaceuticals, 1250 S.
Collegeville Rd (mailcode UP 4330), Collegeville, PA 19426

BRUCE H. JONES, MD, MPH
Colonel, Medical Corps, US Army (Ret); Division of Uninten-
tional Injury Prevention/National Center for Injury Prevention
and Control, Centers for Disease Control and Prevention, 4770
Buford Highway, Atlanta, GA 30341–3724

PEGGY P. JONES, MS, RD, LD
Major, Medical Service, US Army; Nutrition Care Division,
General Leonard Wood Army Community Hospital, Fort
Leonard Wood, MO 65473

NIRANJAN KANESA-THASAN, MD, MTM&H
Lieutenant Colonel, Medical Corps, US Army; Chief, Clinical
Studies Department, Medical Division, US Army Medical
Research Institute of Infectious Diseась, 1425 Porter Street, Fort
Detrick, Frederick, MD 21702-5011

JEROME J. KARWACKI, MD, MPH
Colonel, Medical Corps, US Army (Retired). JUSMAGTHAI, PO
Box R3081, APO AP 96546

LISA KEEP, MD, MPH
Lieutenant Colonel, Medical Corps, US Army; Residency
Director, General Preventive Medicine Residency, Walter Reed
Army Institute of Research, Silver Spring, MD 20190–7500

PATRICK W. KELLEY, MD, DRPH
Colonel, Medical Corps, US Army (Retired); Director, Board on
Global Health, Institute of Medicine, 500 Fifth Street, NW,
Washington, DC 20001

DARYL J. KELLY, PhD
Lieutenant Colonel, Medical Service, US Army (Retired);
Research Associate, Department of Evolution, Ecology, and
Organismal Biology, The Ohio State University, 388 Aronoff
Laboratory, 318 West 12th Avenue, Columbus, Ohio, 43210

KENT E. KESTER, MD
Lieutenant Colonel, Medical Corps, US Army; Chief, Depart-
ment of Clinical Trials, Division of Communicable Diseases and
Immunology, Walter Reed Army Institute of Research, Silver
Spring, MD 20910-7500

MARK G. KORTEPETER, MD, MPH
Lieutenant Colonel, Medical Corps, US Army; Chief,Medicine
Division, US Army Medical Research Institute of Infectious
Diseases, 1425 Porter Street, Fort Detrick, Frederick, MD 21702-
5011

MARGOT R. KRAUSS, MD, MPH
Colonel, Medical Corps, US Army; Deputy Director, Division of
Preventive Medicine, Walter Reed Army Institute of Research,
Silver Spring, MD 20910–7500

DAVID M. LAM, MD
Colonel, Medical Corps, US Army (Ret); Associate Professor,
University of Maryland School of Medicine, National Study
Center for Trauma and Emergency Medical Systems, and US
Army Telemedicine and Advanced Technology Research Center,
PSC 79, Box 145, APO AE 09714

ROBERT LANDRY, MS
Colonel, Medical Service, US Army; Headquarters and Head-
quarters Company, 18th Medical Command, Unit 15281, APO
AP 96205–0054

PHILLIP G. LAWYER, PhD
Colonel, Medical Service, US Army; Department of Preventive
Medicine and Biometrics, Division of Tropical Public Health,
Uniformed Services University of the Health Sciences, 4301
Jones Bridge Road, Bethesda, MD 20814

MAY-ANN LEE, PhD
Programme Head, Defence Medical and Environmental
Research Institute, @DSO National Laboratories, 27 Medical
Drive, Singapore 119597

HEE-CHOON S. LEE, MD, MPH
Lieutenant Colonel, Medical Corps, US Army; Preventive
Medicine Consultant, Preventive Services Directorate, 18th
Medical Command, APO AP 96205

LYNN I. LEVIN, PhD, MPH
Division of Preventive Medicine, Walter Reed Army Institute of Research, Silver Spring, MD, 20910-7500

SCOTT R. LILLIBRIDGE, MD
Director, Center for Biosecurity and Public Health Preparedness, University of Texas Health Science Center at Houston School of Public Health, PO Box 20186, Houston, TX 77225

CRAIG H. LLEWELLYN, MD
Colonel, Medical Corps, US Army (Ret); Professor of Military Medicine, Professor of Preventive Medicine and Biometrics, Professor of Surgery, Director, Center for Disaster and Humanitarian Assistance Medicine (CDHAM), Uniformed Services University of the Health Sciences, 4301 Jones Bridge Road, Bethesda, MD 20814–4799

CHARLES F. LONGER, MD
Colonel, Medical Corps, US Army (Retired); Chief, Division of Hospital Medicine, Department of Medicine, University of Tennessee College of Medicine, Chattanooga Unit, 975 East 3rd Street, Chattanooga, TN 37403

JENICE N. LONGFIELD, MD, MPH
Colonel, Medical Corps, US Army; Chief, Department of Clinical Investigation, Brooke Army Medical Center, San Antonio, TX 78234-6200

GEORGE V. LUDWIG, PhD
Chief, Diagnostic Systems Division, US Army Medical Research Institute of Infectious Diseases, 1425 Porter Street, Fort Detrick, Frederick MD 21702–5011

SHARON L. LUDWIG, MD, MPH
Commander, US Public Health Service, Operational Preventive Medicine/Epidemiology Staff Officer, US Coast Guard Commandant (G-WKH-1), 2100 Second Street SW, Washington DC 20593

ALAN J. MAGILL, MD, MPH
Colonel, Medical Corps, US Army; Science Director, Walter Reed Army Institute of Research, Silver Spring, MD 20910-7500

RAMY A. MAHMOUD, MD, MPH
Lieutenant Colonel, Medical Corps, US Army Reserve; Group Director, Janssen Research Foundation, 1125 Trenton–Harbourton Road, PO Box 200, Room A11010, Titusville, NJ 08560–0200

CARL J. MASON, MD, MPH
Colonel, Medical Corps, US Army; Commander, USAMC-AFRIMS, APO AP 96546-5000

LAUREL A. MAY, MD
Commander, Medical Corps, US Navy; Epidemiologist, Naval Medical Clinic, 480 Central Avenue, Pearl Harbor, HI 96860–4908

JAMES E. McCARROLL, PhD, MPH
Colonel (Retired), MS, US Army; Research Professor, Department of Psychiatry, Uniformed Services University of the Health Sciences, 4301 Jones Bridge Road, Bethesda, MD 20814-4799

DAVID J. McCLAIN, MD
Asheville Infectious Disease, 445 Biltmore Center, Suite 500, Asheville NC 28801

KELLY T. McKEE, JR., MD, MPH
Colonel, Medical Corps US Army (Retired); Director of Extramural Clinical Research, USArmy Medical Research Institute of Infectious Diseases,1425 Porter Street, Fort Detrick, MD 21702

K. MILLS McNEILL, MD, PhD
Colonel, Medical Corps, US Army (Ret); Medical Director for Bioterrorism Preparedness, Office of Epidemiology, Mississippi State Department of Health, 570 E. Woodrow Wilson, PO Box 1700, Jackson, MS 39215-1700

KEVIN MICHAELS, MD, MPH
Lieutenant Colonel, Medical Corps, US Army; Chief, Department of Preventive Medicine, Eisenhower Army Medical Center, Fort Gordon, GA 30905

ROY D. MILLER, PhD
Department of Preventive Medicine and Biometrics, Uniformed Services University of the Health Sciences; 4301 Jones Bridge Road, Bethesda, MD 20814–4799

GEORGE E. MOORE, DVM
Colonel, Veterinary Corps, US Army; Chief, Department of Veterinary Sciences, Army Medical Department Center and School, Building 2840, Suite 248, 2250 Stanley Road, Fort Sam Houston, TX 78234–6145

LELAND JED MORRISON, MD
Captain, Medical Corps, US Navy (Ret); Chief Physician Naval Forces, United Arab Forces

ANDREW S. NATSIOS, MPA
Lieutenant Colonel, US Army Reserve (Retired); Administrator, US Agency for International Development, Ronald Reagan Building, Washington, DC 20523-1000

CHRISTIAN F. OCKENHOUSE, MD, PhD
Colonel, Medical Corps, US Army; Infectious Disease Officer, Department of Immunology, Division of Communicable Diseases and Immunology, Walter Reed Army Institute of Research, Silver Spring, Maryland 20910-7500

DOUG OHLIN, PhD
Hearing Conservation Program, Occupational and Environmental Medicine, US Army Center for Health Promotion and Preventive Medicine, 5158 Blackhawk Road, Aberdeen Proving Ground, MD 21010

RELFORD E. PATTERSON, MD
Colonel, Medical Corps, US Army (Ret); Medical Director, General Motors Corporation Truck Group Assembly Plant, 2122 Broenig Highway, Baltimore, MD 21224

LISA A. PEARSE, MD, MPH
Major, Medical Corps, US Army; Chief, Mortality Surveillance Division, Armed Forces Institute of Pathology, 1413 Research Boulevard, Building 102, Rockville, MD 20850

BRUNO P. PETRUCCELLI, MD, MPH
Lieutenant Colonel, Medical Corps, US Army; Director, Epidemiology and Disease Surveillance, US Army Center for Health Promotion and Preventive Medicine, 5158 Blackhawk Road, Aberdeen Proving Ground, MD 21010–5403

JULIE A. PAVIN, MD, MPH
Lieutenant Colonel, Medical Corps, US Army; Chief, Department of Field Studies, Division of Preventive Medicine, Walter Reed Army Institute of Research, Silver Spring, MD 20910–7500

WILLIAM A. PETRI, JR., MD, PhD
Professor of Medicine, Microbiology, and Pathology, Division of Infectious Diseases, Room 2115, MR4 Building, University of Virginia Health Sciences Center, Charlottesville VA 22908

WILLIAM A. RICE, MD, MPH
Lieutenant Colonel, Medical Corps, US Army; currently, Division Surgeon, 1st Armored Division, Germany

LEON L. ROBERT Jr., PhD
Lieutenant Colonel, Medical Service, US Army; Department of Preventive Medicine and Biometrics, Division of Tropical Public Health, Uniformed Services University of the Health Sciences, 4301 Jones Bridge Road, Bethesda, MD 20814

WELFORD C. ROBERTS, PhD
Department of Preventive Medicine and Biometrics, Uniformed Services University of the Health Sciences, 4301 Jones Bridge Road, Bethesda, MD 20814–4799

ANDREW F. ROCCA, MD
Lieutenant Commander, Medical Corps, US Navy; Senior Resident, Department of Orthopedics, National Naval Medical Center, Bethesda, MD 20889-5600

BRENDA ROUP, RN, PhD
Lieutenant Colonel, Nurse Corps, US Army (Retired); Nurse Consultant in Infection Control, Maryland Department of Health and Mental Hygiene, Baltimore, Maryland 21201

JOSE L. SANCHEZ, MD, MPH
Colonel, Medical Corps, US Army; Medical Epidemiologist and Military Chief, Department of Global Epidemiology and Threat Assessment, US Military HIV Research Program, 13 Taft Ct. Suite 200, Rockville, MD 20850

JOANNA M. SCHAENMAN, PhD
Chief Resident, Department of Internal Medicine, Stanford University School of Medicine, 300 Pasteur Drive, Stanford, CA 94305

BERNARD A. SCHIEFER, MS
Colonel, Medical Service, US Army (Ret); 7238 Ford Street, Mission, TX 78572–8946

RICHARD A. SHAFFER, PhD, MPH
Lieutenant Commander, Medical Service Corps, US Navy; Head, Operational Readiness Research Program, Naval Health Research Center, PO Box 85122, San Diego, CA 92186–5122

G. DENNIS SHANKS, MD, MPH-TM
Colonel, Medical Corps, US Army; Program Manager, DOEM, US Army Center for Health Promotion and Preventive Medicine, 5158 Blackhawk Road, Aberdeen Proving Ground, MD 21010-5403

TRUEMAN W. SHARP, MD, MPH
Commander, Medical Corps, US Navy; Officer in Charge, US Navy Medical Research Unit No. 3, PSC 452, Box 5000, FPO AE 09835-0007

STERLING S. SHERMAN, MD, MPH
Commander, Medical Corps, US Navy; Head, Threat Assessment Department, Naval Environmental and Preventive Medicine Unit No. 5, 3235 Albacore Alley, San Diego, CA 92136

FREDERICK R. SIDELL, MD
Chemical Casualty Consultant, Bel Air, MD 21014

ANITA SINGH, PhD
Food and Nutrition Service, US Department of Agriculture, 3101 Park Center Drive, Alexandria, VA 22302

RICHARD W. SMERZ, MD, MPH
Colonel, Medical Corps, US Army (Ret)

PAUL D. SMITH, DO, MPH
Lieutenant Colonel, Medical Corps, US Army; Occupational Environmental Medicine Staff Officer, Proponency Officer for Preventive Medicine, Office of The Surgeon General, 5109 Leesburg Pike, Falls Church, VA 22041–3258

STEVE SMITH, MD, MPH
Site Medical Director, Umatilla Chemical Agent Demilitarization Facility, Umatilla Chemical Depot, 78068 Ordnance Road, Hermiston, OR 97838

BONNIE L. SMOAK, MD, PhD, MPH
Colonel, Medical Corps, US Army; Director, Division of Tropical Public Health, Department of Preventive Medicine and Biometrics, Uniformed Services University of the Health Sciences, 4301 Jones Bridge Road, Bethesda, MD 20814–4799

VICTORIA B. SOLBERG, MS
Department of Entomology, Division of Communicable Diseases and Immunology, Walter Reed Army Institute of Research, Silver Spring, MD 20910-7500

HENRY P. STIKES, MD, MPH
Colonel, Medical Corps, US Army (Ret); Commander, Lawrence Joel US Army Health Clinic, 1701 Hardee Avenue, SW, Fort McPherson, GA 30330–1062

JAMES W. STOKES, MD
Colonel, Medical Corps, US Army; Combat Stress Control Program Officer, Behavioral Health Division, Health Policy and Services, US Army Medical Command, 2050 Worth Road, Fort Sam Houston, TX 78234–6010

DANIEL A. STRICKMAN, PhD
Colonel, Medical Service, US Army (Retired); Santa Clara County Vector Control District, 976 Lenzen Avenue, San Jose, CA 95126

WELLINGTON SUN, MD
Colonel, Medical Corps, US Army; Chief, Department of Virus Diseases, Division of Communicable Diseases and Immunology, Walter Reed Army Institute of Research, Silver Spring, MD 20910-7500

DAVID N. TAYLOR, MD
Colonel, Medical Corps, US Army (Retired); Department of International Health, Johns Hopkins University Bloomberg School of Public Health, 624 North Broadway, Baltimore, MD 21205

RICHARD THOMAS, MD, MPH
Captain, Medical Corps, US Navy; Naval Environmental Health Center, 2510 Walmer Avenue, Norfolk, VA 23513–2617

RANDALL THOMPSON, DVM
Major, Veterinary Corps, US Army; 18th Medical Command, Unit 15252, APO AP 96205–0025

DAVID H. TRUMP, MD, MPH
Captain, Medical Corps, US Navy; Associate Professor and Director, Medical Student Education Programs,, Department of Preventive Medicine and Biometrics, Uniformed Services University of the Health Sciences, 4301 Jones Bridge Road, Bethesda, MD 20814-4799

PAULA K. UNDERWOOD, MD, MPH
Colonel, Medical Corps, US Army; Preventive Medicine Staff Officer, Proponency Office for Preventive Medicine at the office of The Surgeon General, 5111 Leesburg Pike, Falls Church, VA 22041

DAVID W. VAUGHN, MD, MPH
Colonel, Medical Corps, US Army; Director, Military Infectious Diseases Research Program, US Army Medical Research and Materiel Command, 504 Scott Street, Fort Detrick, Frederick, MD 21702-5012

COLEEN WEESE, MD, MPH
Program Manager, Occupational and Environmental Medicine Program, US Army Center for Health Promotion and Preventive Medicine, Aberdeen Proving Ground, MD 21010-5422

NANCY JO WESENSTEIN, PhD
Research Psychologist; Department of Neurobiology and Behavior, Division of Neuropsychiatry, Walter Reed Army Institute of Research, Silver Spring, MD 20910–7500

RICHARD WILLIAMS, MD
Captain, Medical Corps, US Navy; Chief Clinical Consultant, Armed Forces Medical Intelligence Center, Fort Detrick, Frederick, MD 21702–7581

BENJAMIN G. WITHERS
Colonel, Medical Corps, US Army; Command Surgeon, US Army Materiel Command, 5001 Eisenhower Avenue, Alexandria VA 22333–0001

JAMES WRIGHT, MD
Colonel, Medical Corps, US Air Force (Ret); Occupational Medicine Physician, Concentra Medical Centers, 400 East Quincy, San Antonio, TX 78235

JAMES V. WRITER, MPH
Environmental Monitoring Team, US Department of Agriculture Animal and Plant Health Inspection Service, 4700 River Road, Riverdale, MD 20737

ERIC P. H. YAP, MBBS, DPHIL
Programme Head, Defence Medical and Environmental Research Institute, @DSO National Laboratories, 27 Medical Drive, Singapore 119597

KEVIN S. YESKEY, MD, FACEP
Captain, US Public Health Service; Director, Office of Emergency Preparedness and Response, US Department of Homeland Security, Washington, DC 20528

STEVEN YEVICH, MD, MPH
Colonel, Medical Corps, US Army (Ret); Director, VA National Center for Health Promotion and Disease Prevention, 3000 Croasdaile Drive, Durham, NC 27707

MARGAN J. ZAJDOWICZ, MD
Captain, Medical Corps, US Navy; Directorate for Medical Affairs, Naval Medical Center, Portsmouth, VA 23708

THADDEUS R. ZAJDOWICZ, MD
Captain, Medical Corps, US Navy; Command Surgeon, Joint Task Force Civil Support, US Joint Forces Command, Fort Monroe, VA 23551

Foreword

It has been over 60 years since George Dunham wrote the last major US textbook on military preventive medicine. Both then and now, the mission of military preventive medicine has been to preserve the fighting strength through population-based methods of disease and injury avoidance. A comparison, however, of the tables of contents of Dunham's textbook and this one, *Military Preventive Medicine: Mobilization and Deployment*, illustrates that the scope of military preventive medicine has grown tremendously. This reflects changes in US warfighting doctrine, the expansion of the US military's role in operations other than war, the emergence of new disease and injury threats, and the changing demographics of our warfighters.

US military doctrine is increasingly focused on rapid deployment of lighter units that (1) are more widely dispersed on the battle space and (2) achieve advantages through information, tactical, and strategic dominance. Future military engagements will often evolve rapidly and put a premium on conserving scarce, highly trained, human resources. Central to the conservation of human resources are the needs for knowledgeable leadership, an understanding of the lessons of past conflicts, and systematic estimates of the medical threat prior to exposure; this new volume in the *Textbooks of Military Medicine* series reflects these needs. In a force drawn from a finite pool of volunteers, it is critical to have balanced accession standards and to do minimal damage while realistically training recruits. The growing interest of women in military service has not only increased the pool of much-needed talent but has also necessitated that approaches to prevention of training injuries and health maintenance be reevaluated to ensure that they reflect the needs of all service members.

Unlike 50 years ago, our forces are now expected to be able to move within hours from the US to the battlefield and arrive ready to fight. Although warfare is obviously dangerous, the risk of disease and nonbattle injury on the battlefield has often been underappreciated—along with the potential of countermeasures to mitigate that risk. This morbidity is appreciated increasingly as not just physical but also psychological. In Dunham's era, war-associated syndromes, nuclear and biological warfare, and emerging infections such as drug-resistant malaria, hepatitis C, and acquired immunodeficiency syndrome were not the threats that they are today. The requirement to conduct continuous surveillance for disease and nonbattle injury before, during, and after deployment speaks to the high investment that our military has in each service member and of their individual importance to military success.

In the post–Cold War era, the US military has been called on increasingly to assist with operations other than war including not only peacekeeping operations but also humanitarian assistance operations. In many of these operations, military preventive medicine is at the tip of the spear. Thus it is critical that all military medical personnel have an appreciation for the challenges posed by natural and manmade disasters, by large numbers of displaced persons, and for the different roles we may be called on to fill.

Military Preventive Medicine: Mobilization and Deployment reflects the evolution of preventive medicine in the military from its traditional focus on field hygiene and infectious disease control to encompassing the wide range of threats and scenarios associated with modern military service. There are many lessons to be learned from the textbook's emphasis on history and the military relevance of the conditions covered. However, the essence of this volume, like the practice of military preventive medicine, is timeless: our nation's greatness is reflected in our comprehensive care of those who serve. Preventive medicine of the highest quality is just recognition for their sacrifices and those of their families and communities. It is also a cornerstone to our military readiness. I hope that this textbook will help illuminate the path for those dedicated to pursuing that vision.

Lieutenant General Kevin C. Kiley, M.D.
The Surgeon General
US Army

Washington, DC
September 2005

Preface

Force health protection, although often a loosely defined focus of military medical departments in the past, has in the aftermath of the Persian Gulf War received especially explicit, thorough, and vigorous emphasis within the US Department of Defense. The overall US national military strategy at the turn of the millennium is to "shape, prepare, and respond" to potential national security threats around the world. As is noted in the Department of Defense's *Doctrine for Health Service Support in Joint Operations*, force health protection has three corresponding functions: to shape a healthy and fit force, to prevent casualties through proper preparation of personnel, and to respond to casualties when they occur. Preventive Medicine is inherently central to developing a healthy and fit force and in keeping the force healthy through mobilization and deployment—even into the postdeployment phase. This is more critical than ever in light of a shrinking medical footprint and the need to provide immediate casualty care on the modern, rapidly mobile battlefield. Even once casualties occur, Preventive Medicine has an important tertiary prevention role that must be vigorously pursued if service members are to be successfully rehabilitated and avoid having their relatively manageable physical or mental problems evolve into long-term disabilities.

Force health protection is not only beneficial to the individual but also essential to unit readiness and performance. Contemporary military operations, whether in training, on the battlefield, or in the conduct of operations other than war, place units under the threat of an ever-widening array of biological, physical, and mental stressors. The mitigation of these requires military Preventive Medicine professionals to be familiar with a broad array of disciplines and to provide cohesive leadership and sound advice up and down the chain of command. This textbook aims to provide enabling insights with respect to these scientific, administrative, and leadership challenges.

The challenges of military Preventive Medicine are becoming ever more complex but are also very old. The solutions in many cases are well documented but often forgotten. In 1827, John Macculloch wrote prophetically that

> it would seem, as if fatal, that the wisdom and experience of one generation should be forgotten by the next, that peace should extirpate the knowledge that had been gained in war.[1]

In 2003, *Preventive Medicine: Mobilization and Deployment* emphasizes these often-forgotten lessons of the past and it also provides a comprehensive approach to protecting the force in the current context of the US military's global security mission. We, as military medical professionals, must understand this approach to be well prepared for responding to this mission in a focused, competent, and compassionate manner. Our great nation and its sons and daughters who volunteer to take on its most arduous burdens have ever-rising expectations of military Preventive Medicine. At their peril, we ignore the lessons at our fingertips.

Patrick W. Kelley
Colonel, Medical Corps, U.S. Army (Retired)
Director, Board on Global Health
Institute of Medicine
National Academy of Sciences

Washington, DC
September 2005

1. Macculloch J. *Malaria: An essay on the production and propagation of this poison and on the nature and localities of the places by which it is produced: With an enumeration of the diseases caused by it, and to the means of preventing or diminishing them, both at home and in the naval and military service.* London, England: Longman & Co; 1827.

The current medical system to support the U.S. Army at war is a continuum from the forward line of troops through the continental United States; it serves as a primary source of trained replacements during the early stages of a major conflict. The system is designed to optimize the return to duty of the maximum number of trained combat soldiers at the lowest possible echelon. Far-forward stabilization helps to maintain the physiology of injured soldiers who are unlikely to return to duty and allows for their rapid evacuation from the battlefield without needless sacrifice of life or function.

MILITARY PREVENTIVE MEDICINE: MOBILIZATION AND DEPLOYMENT
Volume 2

Section 5: Epidemiology in the Field

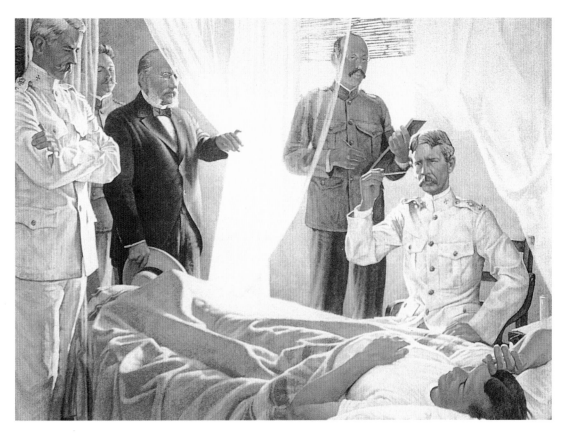

Robert Thom   *The Conquest of Yellow Fever*   *1963*

The US Army Yellow Fever Board was established to discover the etiology of yellow fever. In Cuba in 1900, the Board completed a series of classic experiments that showed the role of the mosquito in yellow fever transmission. Attending Private John Kissinger, who volunteered to be infected with yellow fever, are (from left) Major William C. Gorgas, the sanitation officer for Havana who would go on to rid Havana of yellow fever; Contract Surgeon Dr. Aristides Agramonte; Dr. Carlos J. Finlay, a Cuban physician and an early believer in the mosquito's role in yellow fever; Contract Surgeon Dr. James Carroll; and Major Walter Reed, the president of the Yellow Fever Board. Missing from this painting is Dr. Jesse Lazear, also a member of the Board, who contracted yellow fever while conducting experiments and died.

Art: Courtesy of Pfizer Inc.; 235 E 42nd St.; New York, NY 10017-5755

Chapter 31

DISEASE AND NONBATTLE INJURY SURVEILLANCE: OUTCOME MEASURE FOR FORCE HEALTH PROTECTION

KEVIN HANSON, MD, MPH

K. Hanson; Captain, Medical Corps, US Navy; Uniformed Services University of the Health Sciences, 4301 Jones Bridge Road, Bethesda, Maryland 20814-4799

INTRODUCTION

In recent years, a great deal of emphasis has been placed on the concept of Force Health Protection (FHP).[1,2] Under current doctrine, commanders at all levels are expected to maximize readiness by taking every reasonable measure to protect their personnel from health threats. This includes protection not only from hostile fire, but also from disease and nonbattle injury (DNBI). Whether in combat situations or in routine training, losses from DNBI have often had a tremendous impact on unit effectiveness. Ironically, most DNBIs are preventable through basic measures such as immunization, field sanitation, protection of food and water sources, personal protection measures, and an emphasis on safety. Although these measures are not new, command failure to implement them has become increasingly unacceptable under FHP.

Operational medical personnel have traditionally been responsible for providing line commanders with recommendations for preventive measures. In effect, medical personnel establish the blueprint for much of FHP. In addition to this advice, medical personnel also provide technical assistance in implementing specific FHP measures. This might include such things as designing and engineering appropriate field latrines, inspecting field dining facilities, and training personnel to use protective measures against biting insects.

Beyond these traditional roles of advising and assisting, operational medical personnel are in a unique position to provide commanders with a tremendously powerful tool in FHP—an outcome measure. By collecting and analyzing key data on DNBI, medical personnel can objectively determine how well the FHP program is working. If DNBI rates are high, this may indicate a breakdown in preventive measures. High rates may also be the first clue to an unanticipated disease threat for which no countermeasures were mounted. The ability to rapidly troubleshoot the FHP program, identify deficiencies, and take corrective action can make the difference between mission success and failure.

This type of health outcomes monitoring is known as surveillance and has long been a cornerstone of public health. The Centers for Disease Control and Prevention defines surveillance as the ongoing, systematic collection, analysis, and interpretation of health data essential to the planning, implementation, and evaluation of public health practice, closely integrated with the timely dissemination of these data to those who need to know. The final link of the surveillance chain is the application of these data to prevention and control.[3]

Surveillance has been described as a cycle consisting of 4 steps: data collection, analysis, feedback, and action (Figure 31-1).[4] The whole point of surveillance is taking corrective action to control disease or injury. In a military context, controlling disease and injury is the essence of preserving the fighting strength—the primary focus of military medicine. DNBI surveillance is therefore an essential component of military medicine and central to an effective FHP program. A formalized, unit-level DNBI surveillance system has recently been mandated for deployed military units.[1,2,5]

DNBI rates in a unit are the military medical equivalent of vital signs for an individual patient. For the clinician, vital signs provide a quick initial assessment of the patient's overall condition. Abnormal vital signs do not, by themselves, lead to specific diagnoses, but they may be an important clue pointing to a serious problem. Recognizing this clue may stimulate and focus a more detailed clinical evaluation, leading ultimately to specific interventions.

In military medicine, the "patient" is an entire population, typically an operational unit. DNBI rates (eg, diarrhea or heat injury rates) are key indicators of unit health, and abnormally high rates indicate a threat to a unit's readiness. When DNBI rates are collected, analyzed, disseminated, and acted on, threats can be identified and countered early and the health of the force can be better protected. Continued monitoring of rates will indicate whether the corrective action has been effective, just as a patient's vital signs indicate changes in his or her condition.

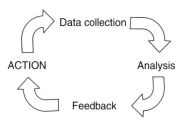

Fig. 31-1. Surveillance is actually a continuous cycle beginning with data collection. Data are continuously analyzed to identify problems. Feedback from this analysis must be given to decision makers and to the collectors of the data so that appropriate action can be taken to correct the problem—action is the focus of the entire system. Data are then collected to measure the effectiveness of the remedying actions.

DNBI SURVEILLANCE AND COMMAND EMPHASIS

One of the fundamental precepts of operational medicine is that the commanding officer prevents most DNBI. As General Slim observed during World War II after his force was almost decimated by malaria in Southeast Asia, "Good doctors are of no use without good discipline. More than half the battle against disease is fought not by medical officers, but by regimental officers."[6p180] Medical recommendations, no matter how sound, do not keep unit personnel from becoming sick. Successful DNBI prevention requires unit leaders who enforce the implementation of specific measures. Command emphasis is the key factor, one that General Slim recognized.

Command emphasis can be dramatically influenced by objective data. In the world of military operations, where resources are often highly constrained, preventive medicine (PM) recommendations must compete with many other priorities for command attention. Before supporting or emphasizing a specific measure, commanders must be persuaded with convincing evidence that it will directly contribute to FHP and operational effectiveness. DNBI surveillance provides exactly this type of evidence. If sound PM recommendations are not being followed, due to lack of command emphasis or any other reason, excessively high DNBI rates will be the measurable result. When they are backed by hard, objective surveillance data on the outcome, PM recommendations are far more convincing to a commander and are likely to receive the necessary command emphasis.

PRACTICAL ASPECTS OF AN OPERATIONAL DNBI SURVEILLANCE SYSTEM

The currently mandated operational DNBI surveillance system is a powerful tool for FHP. It provides simplified, uniform data collection and organization at all units, basic unit-level analysis, rapid transfer of information up the chain of command to appropriate PM organizations, focused PM investigation and intervention, and usable feedback from PM down the chain of command. It is the first line of defense against DNBI. Figure 31-2 summarizes the key features of optimal surveillance information flow.

Background—The Medical Infrastructure in an Operational Environment

The need for DNBI prevention is most pronounced when units are facing significant medical threats, usually during deployment or field opera-

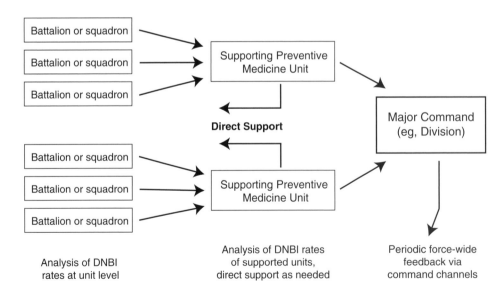

Fig. 31-2. Surveillance information flows up the chain of command and feedback flows back down that chain. The information is gathered at the battalion or squadron level and sent to the supporting preventive medicine unit, which sends information up to the major command level and also supplies feedback to the battalion or squadron. Analysis of the rates of disease and nonbattle injury take place at all three levels.
DNBI: disease nonbattle injury

tions. The medical infrastructure of deployable military units is particularly well-suited for conducting DNBI surveillance. A brief general description of this infrastructure is necessary for a discussion of the practical aspects of DNBI surveillance.

Although field medical treatment capabilities are constantly evolving, operational units such as ships, squadrons, or battalions usually provide their own primary medical care (ie, sick call) within the unit. Typically, units have a cadre of corpsmen or medics led by a medical officer or senior enlisted medical technician. Virtually all of the medical complaints arising in a particular unit will be evaluated locally, and most patients can be returned directly to duty. Diagnoses are generally recorded in a log of some type. It is important to note that the unit's senior medical representative also acts as a special adviser to the commander on all medical matters, including FHP.

Patients requiring care beyond the primary unit level are referred to supporting medical treatment facilities. Most serious illness or injury will require referral. Depending on their specific configurations, these supporting facilities can provide necessary outpatient specialty consultation, laboratory diagnostics, roentgenograms, and inpatient treatment. Patients who can be returned to duty are treated and sent back to the unit primary care provider with a consultation in their health records. Those who cannot be returned directly to duty are admitted or evacuated for the necessary medical or surgical treatment. Records are kept of the patient's unit and diagnosis for all outpatient visits and admissions.

Within this field medical structure, it is possible to capture virtually all of the illness and injury that is treated in specific units and, by extension, the entire deployed population. From a surveillance standpoint, this represents an ideal data collection mechanism. Military units have an additional advantage for surveillance: a known population or denominator. This makes it possible to calculate reasonably precise DNBI rates for individual units, as well as for larger organizations composed of individual units (eg, divisions, wings). The essential first step of the surveillance cycle, data collection, is therefore greatly facilitated.

In addition to primary care providers, operational units frequently have PM personnel assigned to them. Corpsmen, medics or PM technicians within the unit perform basic PM functions, such as testing water chlorine levels, advising on field sanitation and personal protection measures, and monitoring heat conditions. Higher-level PM support, such as disease vector identification, pesticide application, bacteriological testing of water, and food service inspections, is provided by specialized PM support units. These units, which vary in the different military services, may be staffed by PM technicians, entomologists, environmental health or environmental science officers, and PM physicians. Typically, these units are also responsible for investigating disease outbreaks. In some settings, epidemiologic investigation teams may also be assigned. Thus, there is capability within the operational medical infrastructure to conduct the analysis required in surveillance and, in many cases, to take necessary corrective action. Unlike many civilian settings, where medical treatment and public health are separated, deployed military units combine these functions into a single organization. This greatly facilitates transfer of information and feedback, essential to successful surveillance.

Perhaps the most important feature of the operational medical infrastructure from a surveillance perspective is the relationship between the commander and the senior medical representative. The senior medical representative in an individual unit serves as a special advisor to the commander. This unique relationship enables the medical representative to provide direct and immediate feedback on the unit's health to the single person who can take the necessary action. A senior medical officer is also assigned at higher levels of the organization, providing direct input and recommendations to senior commanders.

DNBI Surveillance at the Outpatient Level

In the operational setting, many of the most significant medical problems are first recognized at the outpatient level, usually at a unit's sick call. Examples include a diarrhea outbreak or a cluster of heat casualties, which might not be serious enough to require referral. A surveillance system that focuses only on hospitalizations would not recognize this significant event and would not stimulate the actions required to contain the problem. Outpatient surveillance at the unit level is therefore the first line of defense in DNBI prevention.

Organization of Data

There are many illnesses and injuries that are significant from an operational public health perspective, but attempting to individually track a large number of specific diagnoses would be complex and cumbersome. A more manageable approach is to combine related diagnoses into logical categories.

There are, for example, many different viruses, bacteria, and parasites that cause diarrhea. Since all these distinct etiologies generally represent some variation of enteric transmission, it is logical to group them into a single reporting category. From a practical disease control perspective, all require similar preventive measures. The same is true for the many types of respiratory disease and for dermatological problems. In surveillance, the precision of knowing which specific pathogens are causing a problem is less important than knowing that a certain type of transmission is occurring. Table 31-1 lists the DNBI surveillance categories for outpatient surveillance currently mandated by the Joint Staff. This framework is intended to capture those medical problems with the most significant potential impact on readiness. Diagnoses that have no operational public health significance (eg, peptic ulcer, appendicitis) are not specifically monitored and are combined into a miscellaneous category labeled "all other."

Several categories in this system are noteworthy. Injuries are classified according to the setting in which they occurred (ie, training, recreation, motor vehicle, or other), rather than by specific anatomic diagnosis. This reflects a conscious link to the preventive measures, which differ depending on the setting. For psychiatric problems, a separate category exists for those problems related to operational or combat stress. This represents a focus on recognizing and countering the significant mental health effects that have, in previous operations, jeopardized readiness.

This system also includes a category of "unexplained fever." This reflects the reality that many significant infectious diseases, such as malaria, dengue, and hemorrhagic fever with renal syndrome, present initially as a nonspecific fever. A precise diagnosis may be unobtainable at the primary care level. This surveillance category is designed to recognize patterns of unexplained fevers, which may be essential clues to their etiology and ultimate control. A cluster of fevers (or even a single case) is a significant sentinel event, which should rapidly trigger an in-depth investigation and evaluation.

Figure 31-3 is the Weekly DNBI report format used in the currently mandated DNBI surveillance system. This report is a tally of all cases seen in an individual unit during a week. This form is designed to be filled out by medical personnel at each unit. The information is ideally shared with unit-level PM personnel immediately; in some cases, PM personnel may do the actual collection and compilation of the data. The form is designed to be simple

and requires no specialized epidemiologic knowledge, complex calculations, or computer databases to complete. This DNBI system is designed to focus on new complaints only. Follow-up visits for an initial complaint are not recorded because this would count a case twice. It is possible, though, for a single patient to have multiple unrelated diagnoses recorded in more than one category (eg, fungal skin infection and diarrhea). When diagnoses are closely related (eg, a patient who becomes a heat casualty due to dehydrating diarrhea), only the main underlying problem should be recorded in the appropriate category, as defined in Table 31-1.

Calculation of Rates

For each DNBI category, rates are calculated, using the average unit strength as the denominator. Rates are most conveniently expressed as percent of the unit treated per week, using this formula:

$$\frac{\text{Number of } \textit{new} \text{ cases in the unit per week} \times 100}{\text{Size of population in the unit (average for the week)}} = \text{Percentage treated per week.}$$

This relatively straightforward rate enables the medical personnel to quantify and report the magnitude of the DNBI problem in the unit in a way that is easily understood by commanders and medical personnel. Rates are also absolutely essential for comparing different units within a larger DNBI surveillance system, as will be discussed later. The 1-week reporting interval for DNBI rates represents a workable compromise between timeliness of analysis and the stability of rates. The interval is short enough to recognize an abnormality within the typical window of opportunity for intervention but long enough to provide relatively stable rates despite the normal, minor, day-to-day fluctuations of sick call visits.

Initial Unit-level Analysis

The Weekly DNBI Report also provides reference DNBI rates for direct comparison with unit rates. These were derived from surveillance data on previous deployments, as well as from garrison-based surveillance. They are intended to provide a unit with its own internal yardstick to help determine whether its DNBI rates are abnormal for a given week. They can be used to set action thresholds that when reached prompt more detailed investigation. Space is also provided to record the number of servicemembers who are placed on light duty, placed

TABLE 31-1

CURRENTLY MANDATED DISEASE NONBATTLE INJURY CATEGORIES

Category	What is Included
Combat/Operational Stress Reactions	Acute reaction to stress and transient disorders that occur without any apparent mental disorder in response to exceptional physical and mental stress; also includes post-traumatic stress disorder, which arises as a delayed or protracted response to a stressful event or situation of an exceptionally threatening or catastrophic nature
Dermatological	Diseases of the skin and subcutaneous tissue, including heat rash, fungal infection, cellulitis, impetigo, contact dermatitis, blisters, ingrown toenails, unspecified dermatitis, and sunburn
Gastrointestinal, infectious	All diagnoses consistent with infection of the intestinal tract; includes any type of diarrhea, gastroenteritis, "stomach flu," nausea/vomiting, hepatitis, etc; does NOT include noninfectious intestinal diagnoses such as hemorrhoids and ulcers
Gynecological	Menstrual abnormalities, vaginitis, pelvic inflammatory disease, or other conditions related to the female reproductive system
Heat/Cold Injuries	Climatic injuries, including heat stroke, heat exhaustion, heat cramps, dehydration, hypothermia, frostbite, trench foot, immersion foot, and chilblain
Injury, Recreational/ Sports	Any injury occurring as a direct consequence of the pursuit of personal or group fitness, excluding formal training
Injury, Motor Vehicle Accidents	Any injury occurring as a direct consequence of a motor vehicle accident
Injury, Work/Training	Any injury occurring as a direct consequence of military operations/duties or of an activity carried out as part of formal military training, to include organized runs and physical fitness programs
Injury, Other	Any injury not included in the previously defined injury categories
Ophthalmologic	Any acute diagnosis involving the eye, including pink-eye, conjunctivitis, sty, corneal abrasion, foreign body, vision problems, etc; does not include routine referral for glasses (nonacute)
Psychiatric, Mental Disorders	Any conventionally defined psychiatric disorder, as well as behavioral changes and disturbance of normal conduct, which is out of normal character or is coupled with unusual physical symptoms such as paralysis
Respiratory	Any diagnosis of the (*a*) lower respiratory tract, such as bronchitis, pneumonia, emphysema, reactive airway disease, and pleurisy or (*b*) the upper respiratory tract, such as "common cold," laryngitis, tonsillitis, tracheitis, otitis, and sinusitis
Sexually Transmitted Diseases	All sexually transmitted infections, including chlamydia, human immunodeficiency virus infection, gonorrhea, syphilis, herpes, chancroid, and venereal warts
Fever, Unexplained	Temperature of 100.5°F or greater for 24 hours or history of chills and fever without a clear diagnosis (this is a screening category for many tropical diseases such as malaria, dengue fever, and typhoid); such fever cannot be explained by other inflammatory or infectious processes such as respiratory infections, heat, and overexertion
All Other, Medical/ Surgical	Any medical or surgical condition not fitting into any category above
Dental	Any disease of the teeth and oral cavity, such as periodontal and gingival disorders, caries, and mandible abnormalities
Miscellaneous/ Administrative/ Follow-up	All other visits to the treatment facility not fitting one of the above categories, such as profile renewals, pregnancy, immunizations, prescription refills, and physical exams or laboratory tests for administrative purposes
Definable	An additional category established for a specific deployment, based upon public health concerns (eg, malaria, dengue, airborne/HALO* injuries)

*high altitude, low opening (type of parachute jump)
Source: Chairman of the Joint Chiefs of Staff. *Deployment Health Surveillance and Readiness*. Washington, DC: Dept of Defense; 1998. Joint Staff Memorandum MCM-251-98, 4 Dec 1998.

Weekly DNBI Report

Unit/Command: _____ Troop Strength: _____

Dates Covered: _____ (Sunday 0001) Through: _____ (Saturday 2359)

Individual Preparing Report: _____

Phone: _____ E-Mail: _____

CATEGORY	INITIAL VISITS	RATE	SUGGESTED REFERENCE RATE (%)		DAYS OF LIGHT DUTY	LOST WORK DAYS	ADMITS
Combat/Operational Stress Reactions			0.1				
Dermatologic			0.5				
GI, Infectious			0.5				
Gynecologic			0.5				
Heat/Cold Injuries			0.5				
Injury, Recreational/Sports			1.0				
Injury, MVA			1.0				
Injury, Work/Training			1.0				
Injury, Other			1.0				
Ophthalmologic			0.1				
Psychiatric, Mental Disorders			0.1				
Respiratory			0.4				
STDs			0.5				
Fever, Unexplained			0.0				
All Other, Medical/Surgical							
TOTAL DNBI			4.0				

Dental		XXXXXX					
Misc/Admin/Follow-up		XXXXXX					
Definable							
Definable							

Problems Identified: **Corrective Actions:**

_____   _____

_____   _____

Fig. 31-3. This is the Weekly Disease Nonbattle Injury (DNBI) Report format used in the currently mandated DNBI surveillance system. It is a summary of a unit's rates during the week, prepared by unit medical personnel. The data are analyzed at the unit (usually by corpsmen or medics) and sent up the chain to supporting preventive medicine personnel.

on "sick in quarters status," or admitted during the week. These serve as an additional indicator of the magnitude of a problem within a unit.

The weekly DNBI report also contains an important section for specific comments on problems identified and corrective actions taken. This section is intended to prompt and document the evaluation and analysis process at the local level. For example, heat casualty rates 10 times the action threshold would be identified as a problem. Simple unit-level analysis might reveal that an extended march was conducted during excessively hot conditions in a remote training area, and that the "black flag" heat index was not posted. Based on this unit-level investigation and analysis of the problem, the action taken might have been to recommend improvements in communicating hot weather "flag" conditions throughout the training area. This recommendation, supported by the data, could have been given directly to the unit commander by the medical officer. This example is representative of a local analysis that results in an action taken at the unit level. In cases where a problem requires more detailed investigation, assistance from a supporting PM unit may be needed. To be of any benefit, though, analysis must take place in a timely fashion. If the problem is not recognized until days or weeks later, the opportunity for intervention may be lost.

It is useful for each unit to monitor its own DNBI trends from week to week. This enables a unit to customize its own baseline for a given set of conditions, rather than compare with a fixed reference, which may not apply. In addition, small increases from one week to the next may be an early indication of a developing problem. A trend of relatively small but cumulative increases may stimulate an investigation that identifies a problem before it becomes critical.

Centralized Analysis of Force-wide Data

A mechanism to assemble and centrally analyze data from all unit treatment facilities must exist to recognize significant DNBI patterns above the unit level. Actual rates (rather than simple case counts) are needed for this type of comparison. This is often the only way to recognize problems affecting multiple units or to pinpoint a specific problem at an individual unit. For example, the commander of an infantry battalion with consistently high heat injury rates (eg, 3% per week) might believe that heat casualties are unavoidable under the operational circumstances. This conclusion might be reached even with full knowledge that unit rates are above the reference level. The unit commander and medical officer may adjust their

expectations and consider 3% per week "normal." However, division-wide data showing significantly lower rates (eg, 0.5% per week) in similar units engaged in similar operations may convince them that many of the casualties can be prevented through practical command measures without compromising the mission. Expectations can be adjusted based on objective, real-time data.

The weekly rates and denominator information contained in Figure 31-3 must be transferred up the appropriate chain of command to a location where it can be analyzed and acted on. Most often, this will be a PM unit with area-wide or command-wide responsibility, such as a division PM section, a PM support unit, or a designated disease surveillance team. The specific means of transferring information may vary with circumstances but can include fax, computer networks, message, radio transmission, or hand delivery. Timeliness is again a critical factor. Periodic visits to units by PM personnel may help speed up information transfer.

Although it is not essential for surveillance data to be computerized at the individual unit level, some type of computer database is needed at the central level, where reports from many units must be assimilated and analyzed. Ideally this database would be maintained by the PM section responsible for supporting a large unit, typically a division-sized element. As information technology evolves in deployed forces, the entire system could be electronic, with automated analysis algorithms and prompts to action.

Centralized Feedback

Providing general feedback to all individual commanders and medical personnel on DNBI patterns throughout a large organization or theater is a key element of an operational surveillance system. Such feedback may be the only means by which some units can develop and maintain a "DNBI situational awareness" for the area of operations and be alerted to actual disease threats. Units in a certain location, for example, may have no way of knowing that a neighboring unit has had an outbreak of malaria. With feedback from the system indicating that malaria is being transmitted nearby, all units can maximize command emphasis on protective measures before additional cases occur.

Surveillance feedback can take the form of a weekly DNBI situation report, issued by PM personnel at the division level or higher. This report can provide a valuable review of current patterns, current problems, and other relevant information derived from the surveillance system. Such information should be disseminated to individual commanders and medical personnel by whatever means are available, including message, fax, computer networks, or personal visits. This information should also be reported up the chain of command to the joint or theater level, so that theater-wide DNBI patterns can be assessed. In some situations, this information may need to be treated as confidential or classified.

INPATIENT SURVEILLANCE SYSTEMS IN MILITARY OPERATIONS

Although no specific inpatient DNBI surveillance system has been mandated for deployed forces as of this writing, it is nonetheless an important FHP tool. Those illnesses or injuries that are serious enough to warrant hospitalization in the field or evacuation out of theater merit special attention, since they are obviously the source of significant lost person-days. Inpatient surveillance can be more complex than outpatient surveillance and usually requires the skill and judgment of an epidemiologist to organize and interpret the data. Different situations may require specifically tailored approaches. Inpatient surveillance can be viewed as the second line of defense in DNBI prevention. Although usually very few patients in an operational setting require hospitalization, it is absolutely essential to have the capacity to recognize systematically those conditions severe enough to require hospitalization. This may be the only way that some of the most serious disease threats can be identified. Take, for example, a patient with an unexplained fever who is seen in an outlying unit's sick call. Since it is impossible to accurately diagnose or care for the patient in the unit, he is referred for hospitalization and specialty care. Patterns might become evident in outpatient surveillance if multiple cases of unexplained fever occur, but this single case would probably not significantly alter overall disease rates. After hospitalization and further evaluation, this patient is diagnosed with Japanese encephalitis. Without a system of inpatient surveillance, this highly significant event may have gone unrecognized, and the opportunity to institute immediate countermeasures to prevent additional cases might have been missed.

There are a number of highly significant diseases that typically require an inpatient setting for diagnosis and treatment; they include hepatitis A and E, hemorrhagic fever with renal syndrome, dengue fever, leptospirosis, and scrub typhus. There must be a system in place to recognize these illnesses even in small or sporadic numbers, investigate them immediately, and react to them quickly.

Inpatient surveillance adds a higher level of clarity to the overall DNBI surveillance picture. It is indispensable to an FHP program that effectively counters the serious disease threats the military faces. The combination of inpatient and outpatient surveillance gives a comprehensive picture that greatly increases the chances that DNBI will be recognized and dealt with before it can seriously degrade combat effectiveness. This is the goal of surveillance.

Data Sources

An accurate final diagnosis is needed for optimal inpatient surveillance. There are several sources that can provide these data or a useful surrogate. Hospital admission logs or databases usually record a presumptive diagnosis, which may change significantly during the course of hospitalization. The presumptive diagnosis can be a valuable piece of information, however, because it focuses interest on a particular patient and raises an appropriate index of suspicion. Hospital discharge logs or databases are more likely to contain the final diagnosis, and they may be the only practical way to capture accurate data routinely on the diagnoses of all patients who were admitted. Unfortunately, this information may only be available relatively long after the patient became ill; the resulting lag time may mean that the window of opportunity for intervention to prevent others from developing the same illness has closed.

PM personnel should be alerted to the final diagnosis as soon as possible after it is made. This may require direct contact between epidemiologists and key clinicians in the hospital to keep updated on particular patients. A system of immediate reporting between hospital physicians and an epidemiologist for selected diagnoses or presumptive diagnoses may also serve this purpose. Since laboratory tests are often the means by which diagnoses are made, laboratory logs are another potential source of important data on diagnoses. A system of immediate reporting of selected laboratory diagnoses to the epidemiologist may be effective. Whatever the specifics of the system, direct proactive involvement of a PM physician with all inpatient treatment facilities is the most effective way to capture and interpret appropriate data. Diagnoses of infectious diseases are of greatest interest, especially for those diseases with epidemic potential. The index of suspicion should be high for the specific diseases thought to be present in the local area of operations.

Inpatient DNBI Rates

Inpatient surveillance can also detect patterns of illness or injury, similar to the outpatient system. A general organization of categories similar to the outpatient system can be developed by an epidemiologist to summarize the rates and pattern of admissions, with the level of subclassification varying to meet the needs. For example, the outpatient category of respiratory disease might be expanded so bronchitis, viral pneumonia, bacterial pneumonia, and reactive airway disease can be monitored separately. The size of the entire population being supported by a facility should be used to calculate weekly or monthly rates, as determined by the epidemiologist.

Surveillance can also be conducted at the referral facilities in theater where patients initially seen at unit sick calls receive specialized outpatient consultation. In some situations, this may provide an important early warning mechanism to augment the outpatient unit-level DNBI surveillance. A reporting system for specific diagnoses can be tailored to a given set of operational circumstances.

Individual Epidemiologic Investigations

Cases admitted for a potentially high-impact disease such as malaria will usually require further epidemiologic investigation. This might include an interview with the patient to determine exposure location, protective measures used, chemoprophylaxis taken, and so on. Other members of the patient's unit might be interviewed using standardized questionnaires and relevant surveillance data examined to identify patterns. Unit-specific attack rates can be calculated from inpatient data if needed. Sophisticated outbreak investigation techniques may be necessary to fully appreciate patterns of certain diseases. This type of investigation is an important component of surveillance triggered by inpatient disease surveillance and is best accomplished by trained epidemiologists. Depending on the situation, this function may be performed by a surveillance and epidemiology team or by the epidemiologist who reviews inpatient data. The key is a capacity to recognize significant diseases systematically at the earliest possible point and respond appropriately.

Specialized Public Health Diagnostic Laboratories

Unexplained fevers in a tropical environment present a huge challenge to the clinician. Malaria, dengue fever, typhoid fever, hemorrhagic fever with renal syndrome, Japanese encephalitis, and many other infectious diseases initially present with very nonspecific symptom complexes that include fever and offer few other definite clinical diagnostic features. Effective treatment depends on an accurate diagnosis, and this usually requires a very capable laboratory that can provide rapid, on-site diagnosis.

The public health value of a rapid and accurate diagnosis goes far beyond an individual patient or clinician. The diagnosis may identify a threat facing an entire population at risk for the same disease. Dengue fever and typhoid fever have very different exposure mechanisms and therefore different approaches to prevention. Disease control efforts cannot be effectively targeted unless it is known whether the problem is enterically transmitted or vector-borne.

The capabilities of such a laboratory should be tailored to the anticipated medical threat in the area of operations, with emphasis on rapidity of results. Laboratory officers with highly specific diagnostic expertise may be required, as might highly specialized reagents. Sophisticated techniques, such as polymerase chain reaction and plasmid identification, are often required for the rapid identification of tropical infectious diseases. The equipment, reagents, and expertise may be available only within the military medical research community, particularly in the Army and Navy overseas laboratories located in or near the area of operations. On-site deployment of a specialized public health diagnostic laboratory with this extremely high level of capability is an invaluable addition to DNBI surveillance. Both the Army and the Navy[7] have recently developed and fielded such laboratories.

Feedback from Inpatient Surveillance

As with outpatient surveillance, the information derived from inpatient surveillance is of limited value unless it is rapidly communicated back to those responsible for preventive measures throughout the organization. If, for example, hemorrhagic fever with renal syndrome was diagnosed in a patient in a certain unit, that unit and all others in the area must be made aware of the diagnosis as quickly as possible. Knowledge of the diagnosis is the clearest possible indication of the threat and should lead to the implementation of appropriate counter-

EXHIBIT 31-1

SAMPLE WEEKLY DISEASE NONBATTLE INJURY (DNBI) SITUATION REPORT

From: Division Commanding General

To: All Division Battalion Commanders and Medical Officers

Subj: Weekly DNBI Situation Report for Operation Strong Endeavor—East Africa

1. DNBI surveillance information was available for 23 of the 25 Division units for the week of 18 August, covering 18,590 of the 19,780 personnel in theater (94%). Overall rates of DNBI continue to be low, with the exception of dermatological conditions, which continue to affect 2-3% of the force per week:

	4 Aug	11 Aug	18 Aug
Total reporting	18,980	18,640	18,590
Heat injury	0.2	0.2	0.1
Diarrhea/GI	0.7	0.6	0.7
Dermatologic	1.9	2.8	2.5
Respiratory	0.3	0.5	0.4
Injury (upper)	0.2	0.5	0.5
Injury (lower)	1.0	1.1	0.9
Injury (back)	0.4	0.2	0.5
Injury (other)	0.9	1.2	1.2
Unexplained fever	0.0	0.3	0.0
Sexually trans	0.1	0.0	0.1
Ophthalmologic	0.1	0.0	0.2
Psychiatric	0.0	0.1	0.1
All other	1.4	1.5	1.2
Totals	6.0	6.8	6.4

2. Significant events during the week of 18 August:

   A.   Dermatological complaints continue to occur at relatively high levels. Most cases are heat rash, impetigo, and fungal infection. Lack of shower facilities and opportunity for optimal personal hygiene throughout most units appears to be the main contributing factor. As logistics permit, additional shower units are being established. Commands should continue to emphasize basic hygiene, including frequent changes of socks.

   B.   Three shigella cases were diagnosed from a single unit this week. Overall diarrhea rates in the unit have been higher than average (2% per week). Investigations of food/water sources have failed to reveal a deficiency. A severe fly problem in the area appears to account for at least some of the diarrhea cases. Fly control and field sanitation measures continue to receive increased emphasis.

   C.   Four unexplained fever cases from a single unit during the week of 11 August were subsequently diagnosed as viral syndrome after inpatient evaluation. Malaria, hepatitis, and dengue have been ruled out. Though the threat is high, vector-borne disease continues to be rare, with a total of 6 malaria cases and 10 dengue cases scattered throughout the division in the past month. Continued emphasis on personal protective measures and chemoprophylaxis appears to be effective.

   D.   An artillery battalion experienced 3 gonorrhea and 2 NGU cases during the week, attributable to recent 3-day liberty outside the area of operations in Kenya. Additional briefs on the HIV threat throughout Africa have been given. STD acquired in the immediate area of operations continues to be very low.

3. There were 52 admissions during the week of 18 August, representing 0.26% of the 19,780 division personnel in theater. Approximately 60% of hospitalizations were for injuries, including 6 from a motor vehicle accident, and a variety of fractures, sprains, and lacerations scattered throughout the division. No significant disease patterns have been identified.

measures, which may not have otherwise been considered a high priority. In addition, it will alert medical personnel to be especially vigilant for the early signs of additional cases. A summary analysis of inpatient data and relevant outbreak investigations should be included in a widely distributed communication such as a weekly DNBI situation report (Exhibit 31-1).

SURVEILLANCE IN ACTION—US MARINE CORPS FORCES IN THE PERSIAN GULF WAR

During Operations Desert Shield and Desert Storm (1990-1991), a simple weekly unit-level surveillance system was instituted for Marine Corps forces operating ashore. Selected data from this system illustrate how surveillance can quickly identify a disease problem and facilitate corrective action.

Figure 31-4 shows diarrhea rates from a Marine Air Group, which initially occupied a host-nation airbase. Although Marines lived under field conditions in tent camps, they were fed in a host-nation military dining facility that was modern, air-conditioned, and operated and managed entirely by local nationals and contract personnel from other nations. Ordinarily, military PM personnel recommend strongly against relinquishing control of food service to outside organizations unless they have been previously certified and are known to meet US standards. However, under the difficult circumstances

early in Desert Shield, there were distinct advantages to accepting the food service support offered by the host nation, especially since the facilities appeared to be very clean and modern. Aside from the positive impact on morale, receiving this food service assistance from a military ally reduced the logistical burden of providing rations or a field mess facility for several thousand Marines.

While it was expedient to use this host-nation dining facility, the surveillance data showed an almost immediate increase in diarrhea rates, rapidly exceeding 5% per week in a rising trend. In analyzing the problem at the airbase, Marine PM personnel on-site had already established the potability of the water supply and eliminated water as a possible source of disease. Furthermore, military personnel had no access to food on the local economy. Rates were clearly consistent with a food-related outbreak

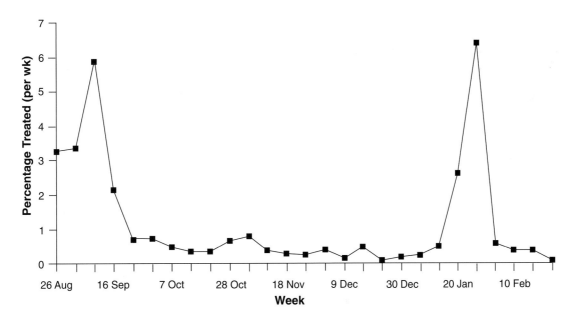

Fig. 31-4. This graph shows the rates of diarrhea in a Marine Air Group (Fixed Wing) serving in the Persian Gulf War. The first outbreak occurred early and was caused by problems in a host-nation dining facility. The diarrhea rates declined once dining facilities were brought under Marine control. The second outbreak was tied to lapses in food handling procedures during a time of heightened operational tempo. Any breakdowns in basic public health procedures were very quickly reflected in increased rates of diarrheal disease.

and followed an alarming upward trend, making the dining facility the most likely source. This definitive assessment was based solely on the surveillance data gathered from this unit, without knowing disease rates from any other unit in the operation.

Medical recommendations citing these data prompted and facilitated the decision to quickly introduce Marine food service and PM personnel into the host-nation facility, initially in a supervisory and monitoring role. PM inspections identified numerous significant deviations from US standards of food handling practices by the local staff. Within a relatively short period of time, commanders made the necessary arrangements and committed the assets required for Marine personnel to gain complete control of food service. Diarrhea rates subsided dramatically and remained at acceptable levels through the next several months. The impact of diarrhea certainly could have been far greater, compounded as it was by the extreme heat and relatively austere field living conditions.

Figure 31-4 shows a second sudden peak in diarrhea rates occurring in January 1991. This outbreak was related to a single meal served by a Marine field mess facility near the flight line. (This field facility largely replaced the host-nation facility mentioned previously.) Several food service problems had been identified by Marine PM personnel, but correcting

them was considered a low priority by food service personnel, especially as operational tempo increased markedly during the intense air campaign. Deficiencies were quickly corrected after this self-limited outbreak, which was clearly captured with objective data. This episode served to illustrate the significant risk of complacency or cutting corners in a military food service operation.

The value of central analysis of surveillance data from multiple units was also demonstrated during Desert Shield. Early in the operation, the logistical constraints of moving materiel to the theater were enormous. Sealift and airlift assets were committed heavily to the movement of combat personnel and equipment. Since on-site stockpiles of Meals Ready to Eat rations were limited, commanders placed strong emphasis on getting fresh meals to the troops at the earliest possible juncture. Marine food service personnel were deployed, along with equipment and supplies, to set up field mess facilities. In some cases, Marines took over existing kitchen facilities in industrial complexes made available by the host nation.

Due to the severe logistical constraints, the host nation provided significant contracting assistance. Items such as fruits, meats, poultry, eggs, and vegetables were obtained from sources outside the network of contractors officially approved by the US

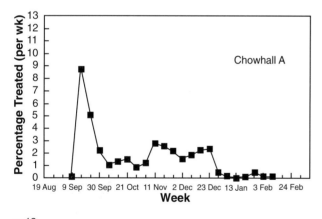

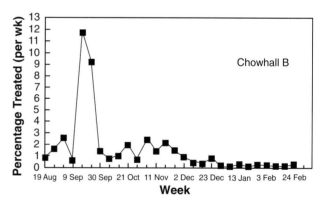

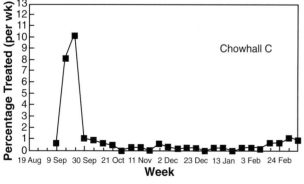

Fig. 31-5. These three graphs show simultaneous diarrhea outbreaks in Marine units during Operation Desert Shield in September and early October of 1990. The Marine units affected ate at three different chowhalls. This pattern indicates problems in centralized food procurement procedures. It turned out that nonapproved food sources were the source of the outbreaks.

military. These foodstuffs were provided in large quantities to a centralized Marine food service warehouse for distribution to a network of Marine field mess halls serving the majority of Marines throughout a large geographic area.

Figure 31-5 shows diarrhea rates at three different units served by three different field mess halls. Other units had similar rates. The epidemiologic pattern of concurrent outbreaks in several different areas strongly suggested a common factor. Marine PM personnel had already assured that the water was potable, and eating on the local economy was forbidden. It was unlikely that this force-wide outbreak was caused by individual food service facilities simultaneously experiencing unrelated difficulties. The remaining common factor was the fresh food being distributed centrally from unap-

proved sources. Lettuce was of particular concern due to its susceptibility to fecal contamination, and subsequent PM investigation implicated this item as a source of at least some of the diarrhea.[8]

Based on the surveillance data and subsequent investigation, a force-wide policy was issued that discontinued the use of lettuce in Marine Corps mess facilities. Diarrhea rates very rapidly declined to approximately 1% per week or less in virtually all units. Without the capacity to look at the overall patterns across several units, it probably would have taken considerably longer to pinpoint or prove the source of the problem and prompt the necessary policy shift. Individual units looking at their own diarrhea rates would have had no way of knowing the exact source of the problem and may not have been able to correct it as quickly.

FUTURE DIRECTIONS

Technological improvements in the flow of information may make surveillance much easier in the future. Advancing technology may enable physicians, corpsmen, and medics to enter diagnoses into a hand-held computer as they treat patients. Such a device might be capable of continuously assimilating and analyzing a unit's rates of disease and injury and transmitting data to a central system. Through advanced data gathering and information management, it may be possible to link outpatient data with inpatient data to describe instantaneously the exact pattern of all disease and injury in a force.

Although surveillance is most critical during deployments where the medical threat is increased, it is also a useful tool during routine training in

garrison. Exotic infectious diseases are not a significant threat on most US training bases, but other problems, such as heat injury, musculoskeletal injuries, sexually transmitted diseases, and psychiatric conditions, can also affect a unit. An emphasis on FHP is still needed, and specific PM strategies must be applied to keep servicemembers healthy. Outcome measures are no less important. Monitoring diseases and injuries in the unit should be a part of the everyday routine of any operational military medical department. Commanders should come to expect that outcome measures of command preventive programs are being monitored and should be familiar with how the information can be used.

SUMMARY

DNBI surveillance is a simple but powerful tool in the military setting. It can cut through the medical equivalent of the "fog of war" and bring specific problems into sharp focus at an early stage. Surveillance is a critical part of maintaining the medical situational awareness needed to stay ahead of problems and drive an effective FHP program. The military medical sys-

tem is very well suited to capturing the right data, translating it into attack rates, analyzing it, and getting sound recommendations into the hands of those who can act decisively on the problems identified. Medical personnel and commanders can quickly target their efforts to protect the force from disease and injuries and preserve the fighting strength.

REFERENCES

1. US Department of Defense. *Joint Medical Surveillance*. Washington, DC: DoD; 1997. DoD Directive 6490.2.

2. US Department of Defense. *Implementation and Application of Joint Medical Surveillance for Deployments*. Washington, DC: DoD; 1997. DoD Instruction 6490.3.

3. Centers for Disease Control. Guidelines for evaluating surveillance systems. *MMWR*. 1988;37(Suppl 5):1–18.

4. Wallace RB, ed. *Maxcy-Rosenau-Last Public Health and Preventive Medicine.* 14th ed. Stamford, Conn: Appleton & Lange; 1998: 10.

5. Chairman of the Joint Chiefs of Staff. *Deployment Health Surveillance and Readiness.* Washington, DC: Dept of Defense; 1998. Joint Staff Memorandum MCM-251-98, 4 Dec 1998.

6. Slim W. *Defeat Into Victory.* London: Cassell and Company, Ltd; 1956.

7. Dept of the Navy. *Forward Deployable Laboratory.* Washington, DC: DN; 1995. Naval Warfare Publication 4-02.4 Part C.

8. Hyams KC, Bourgeois AL, Merrell BR, et al. Diarrheal disease during Operation Desert Shield. *N Engl J Med.* 1991;325:1423–1428.

Chapter 32

OUTBREAK INVESTIGATION

JENICE N. LONGFIELD, MD, MPH

J.N. Longfield; Colonel, Medical Corps, US Army; Chief, Department of Clinical Investigation, Brooke Army Medical Center, San Antonio, TX 78234-6200

INTRODUCTION

The use of the epidemiologic method to identify and control an acute disease problem in a population represents the most dramatic application of the science of epidemiology. Knowledge gained from a well-conducted outbreak investigation can enable the investigator to intervene and control an epidemic. The relatively quick tempo of this scientific endeavor also contributes to its unique place in research. The literature is replete with classic examples of outbreaks occurring in military populations.[1–3] Carrying out the military mission is associated with living, working, eating, and playing in a group environment under harsh conditions. This togetherness, coupled with potentially unique occupational and environmental exposures, can result in outbreaks in deployed service members. Vaccines or effective chemoprophylaxis do not exist for many endemic diseases. Recognition of new pathogens and the reemergence of known pathogens with new drug resistance patterns have contributed to a resurgence of infectious diseases as a threat to the military force in the field.[4–9]

The Epidemic Intelligence Service program for public health officers at the Centers for Disease Control and Prevention (CDC) grew out of the fear of biological warfare during the Korean War.[10] As the 21st century opens, the potential for governments or individual terrorists to use biological or chemical agents against a population has not lessened and may indeed be greater than it was in the 1950s. The 1995 terrorist attack on a Japanese subway train using the nerve gas sarin resulted in more than 5,000 people injured and 11 deaths.[11] Biological warfare and biological terrorist events by definition seek to create epidemics and so the need remains for a cadre of capable epidemiologists to respond to domestic or military public health emergencies of this nature.[12]

This chapter is intended to provide a practical, detailed discussion of the specific steps to use in conducting the investigation of an outbreak in the field (Exhibit 32-1). The initial purpose of the investigation is to determine the population at risk and identify the specific cause or exposure risk factors of disease. As the description of the outbreak becomes clearer, explicit objectives can be formulated for the planned field work to develop and test hypotheses proposed to explain the outbreak. This permits effective intervention, which in turn will end the crisis.

EXHIBIT 32-1

OUTBREAK INVESTIGATION METHODOLOGY

Verify the diagnosis or define the problem
  Establish a case definition
  Ascertain cases

Verify the existence of an epidemic

Organize a multidisciplinary team

Identify disease control measures

Describe the outbreak by person, time, and place

Identify risk factors and mechanisms

Develop tentative hypotheses and a plan
  Determine type of outbreak and critical exposure
  Hypothesize about mechanism of transmission
  Develop survey instruments
  Plan for administrative and logistical considerations
  Identify medical treatment resources
  Reevaluate control measures in place

Test hypotheses
  Collect data and specimens
  Determine the need for additional studies and analysis
  Evaluate the adequacy of the case definition
  Establish criteria for deciding outbreak is under control

Compare results to those of the published literature

Finalize report with control recommendations
  Write an executive summary and prepare a complete report
  Evaluate effectiveness of control recommendations

VERIFY THE DIAGNOSIS OR DEFINE THE PROBLEM

An outbreak investigation is an iterative process that passes through distinct phases. An outbreak investigation begins with the recognition of a problem, usually cases with similar symptoms clustered in space and time. An alert observer must then call on the services of the public health system. The appointed investigator needs to obtain as much detailed information as possible from the initial report. Cases of clinical illness should be fully described, to include the type of symptoms, frequency of symptoms, onset time, and duration of the illness. In some instances, the actual diagnosis is already known. On other occasions, only a collection of signs and symptoms is apparent. When the etiology is unclear, the differential diagnosis for the clinical presentation of symptoms and physical exam findings must be considered. Clinical clues and timing of onset can help narrow the possibilities. For example, the presence of blood and fecal leukocytes in diarrheal stools indicates an inflammatory process and limits the number of pathogens to be considered. The presence of paresthesias or other neurological symptoms immediately suggests the possibility of a chemical intoxication from ciguatoxin, scombrotoxin, paralytic shellfish poisoning, or mushroom poisoning. It is very important at this early stage to determine the type of studies (eg, smears, cultures, serologies, radiographs) necessary to verify the diagnosis. Appropriate laboratories should be made aware of the possible organisms, toxins, or other agents being considered because some will require special media or special testing.

Following this initial notification of a problem, two equally important determinations must take place: (1) verification of the diagnosis or at least definition of the problem and (2) verification of the existence of an epidemic. Often these two fundamental steps will occur simultaneously. The order in which these two steps are listed in the investigation process will vary, depending on the leader's preferences. Part of the complexity of launching and conducting an investigation of this type is the necessity to organize and take action in multiple directions simultaneously. Delay in taking action could result in loss of important data.

Establish a Case Definition

After gathering the initial impressions, the investigators must develop a workable case definition and begin case finding efforts. Simple, objective criteria are best. The type, magnitude, and frequency of symptoms, as well as their duration, must be quantified. Categorization of cases as possible, probable, or confirmed using type and number of symptoms, culture results, and other pertinent information will sometimes be useful in further refining the case definition. Case definitions for known diagnoses have been published by the CDC,[13] and the use of standard definitions allows for better comparisons between outbreaks. The case definition criteria must be applied consistently to all persons studied. A broad case definition may be refined later but a very narrow initial definition may miss cases. Consider the clinical spectrum of apparent illnesses being seen and whether this is a disease or condition in which a large number of asymptomatic cases are likely. Arriving at a clear case definition may sometimes be extremely problematic, as is best exemplified by the attempts to establish a case definition of "Gulf War syndrome."[14] An accurate and sensitive case definition is essential to reduce misclassification and confounding when investigating potential exposure risk factors.[15] Epidemiologic investigation of outbreaks usually begins with identification of a distinct disease syndrome and proceeds to evaluation of risk factors using epidemiologic methods. This is successful even with newly recognized diseases such as toxic shock syndrome.[16] Studies of Persian Gulf War veterans have been complicated because neither a distinct clinical picture nor distinct exposure risks are clear.[17]

Ascertain Cases

Case finding efforts begin using the case definition or definitions established. Investigators must start and maintain a line listing or log of all presumed cases. This log should include name, social security number, unit, sex, age, and other relevant information (eg, pending culture results). It is important to include a phone number or contact location for each presumed case on the list. Other possible sources of information for finding cases with the condition of interest should be considered. These sources might include medical records, emergency room logs, specific clinic logs, or laboratory records. A check on relevant quality control or quality assurance procedures in the laboratory, clinic, or other facilities should be done to rule out artifactual increases in numbers. On military installations, the surrounding civilian community should be checked for additional cases through queries to local physicians, clinics, or public health departments. Because of the mobility of the military population, cases may have been exposed in one location and have traveled elsewhere, even across continents, during the incubation period. Cases of coccidioidomycosis, in a classic example, occurred as the result of exposure on military bases in endemic areas in California but did not present until personnel traveled elsewhere.[18] In situations such as these, distant locations may need to be contacted. The need for a thorough travel history and an elevated level of diagnostic suspicion is key to case recognition. The case finding efforts may need to be broadened to the Offices of the Surgeons General in the Department of Defense and to the CDC. Patients may even self refer once news of the outbreak and the investigation becomes known. The media can assist health authorities in informing the public and in directing the referral of possible cases for evaluation through its public service announcements. In military settings, cases may sometimes be found by using questionnaires to screen units. Follow-up interviews and evaluations may be required to determine actual case status. For communicable diseases, finding the contacts of known cases may identify additional cases and provide other relevant information. Unrecognized cases, those with mild illness or who are asymptomatic, may provide additional clues or supporting data concerning the presumed disease or hypothesized etiology.

VERIFY THE EXISTENCE OF AN EPIDEMIC

After describing, defining, and finding cases, then the question is whether the number of cases found constitutes an epidemic. Last defines an epidemic as the "occurrence in a community or region of cases of an illness... [or] health-related behavior or...event clearly in excess of normal expectancy.[19p54] A single case of an extremely rare or exotic disease, such as botulism poisoning, pulmonary anthrax, or Ebola infection, also constitutes an epidemic (and may indicate a biological terrorist event). To determine the usual level of disease occurrence, investigators must examine available historical data, such as medical records, clinic logs, and laboratory logs. Personally visiting sites such as the records department or the laboratory may lead to other useful data sources (eg, culture logs by body site of specimen source). Site visits will also provide a better understanding of the type and quality of the data available. To conclude that the current level of disease is excessive, investigators must first define the event and then compare the current rate with that of the past. Comparing the routine surveillance rates for skin disorder consultations for British troops in Bosnia disproved media reports of a serious outbreak.[20] The significance of possible differences can be depicted graphically and assessed statistically by testing differences of proportions or calculating confidence intervals.

The limitations of the data or the data source affect the interpretation of the data. The ideal or preferred morbidity measures for disease ascertainment should also be identified. The profound changes in the practice of medicine precipitated by the managed care movement make comparisons with historical rates problematic. Changes in access to care, referral patterns, test-ordering practices, hospitalization decisions, utilization management mandates, and other health management procedures can all affect the apparent incidence of disease.[21] These changes in practice patterns decrease the utility of historical data, such as hospitalization rates, for assessing secular trends and identifying outbreaks. Investigators must judiciously determine if the epidemic is real or artifactual after assessing the situation, data sources, and practice patterns.

Pseudoepidemics can also occur because of false-positive results of laboratory tests or from changes in personnel or administrative processes affecting the sensitivity of diagnosis. In the 1980s, an apparent outbreak of skin cancer occurred at Letterman Army Medical Center, as determined by inpatient admission statistics. However, it was an administrative policy change directing that all patients with skin cancer be admitted for biopsy and excision that led to this artifactual epidemic (Kadlec RK. Walter Reed Army Institute of Research, 1989. Unpublished data). Specimen contamination in the microbiology laboratory has also been implicated in a number of "clusters" of multidrug-resistant tuberculosis. Newer techniques of molecular biology, such as pulsed-field gel electrophoresis (PFGE), may be used to detect these pseudo-outbreaks and document their extent and resolution.[22,23] The risk also exists of cross contamination in the molecular laboratory from contamination of polymerase chain reaction assays. The most serious dangers are contamination of specimens with postamplification products from previous analyses or contamination of negative specimens with controls or positive specimens.[24] Emphasis on new and expanded surveillance programs for emerging infectious diseases has already been demonstrated to increase the potential for identifying pseudo-outbreaks, as occurred with cyclosporiasis in Florida and cryptosporidiosis in New York.[25] It is advisable to get confirmation by an appropriate reference laboratory early in any investigation of apparent clusters of emerging pathogens (see chapter 34, Laboratory Support for Infectious Disease Investigations in the Field).

ORGANIZE A MULTIDISCIPLINARY INVESTIGATIVE TEAM

After the initial assessment has verified the diagnosis (or at least delineated the problem) and verified the existence of an epidemic, a multidisciplinary investigative team should be organized. The team may be organized from the staff available locally or may be a consultant team of experts invited to travel to the location of the epidemic. The following guidance can be applied to either a small local group of public health workers or to a large, experienced consultant team.

Composition of the Team

The optimal composition of the team by type of expertise is key. Epidemiologists do not work alone, and cooperation between disciplines is essential to the success of the investigation. Physicians and nurses trained in preventive medicine need the expertise of statisticians and scientists in sanitary engineering, environmental science, industrial hygiene, health physics, entomology, microbiology, or toxicology, as the situation dictates. Clinical expertise in such areas as infectious diseases and neurology may be added, depending on the problem being investigated. Veterinary public health experts are critical to any investigation of possible foodborne disease outbreaks or zoonotic outbreaks. Appropriate laboratory expertise must be present from the outset to ensure the correct specimens are obtained and properly processed and that appropriate diagnostic testing is used. New techniques in molecular biology may be incorporated into the laboratory investigation, often at an off-site reference laboratory. Addition of someone with medical informatics expertise will facilitate the proper planning for data entry, computer programming, and automated analysis of investigation results. Software packages designed for outbreak investigation (eg, Epi Info, CDC, Atlanta, Ga) may expedite data management and analysis. Frequently, the programming and analysis phase of the investigation will continue long after the field portion is completed. Logistic or supply experts may be needed for large, complicated operations, especially those conducted outside the United States. A public affairs representative or a media spokesman should be identified and made an integral part of the investigation team. For teams of outside experts, assignment of a key local staff member to be a liaison with the investigation team should help ensure command access and support.

The team leader, who is responsible for organizing and conducting the investigation, should be specified. The nature of the problem, the complexity and sensitivity of the situation, and the expertise, experience, and availability of potential leaders will determine who is given this responsibility. An additional senior person with experience in outbreak investigation may be identified to serve as an off-site consultant to the operation. The team leader should report daily to this consultant, and the consultant can help update other consultants, agencies, and commands outside of the local jurisdiction. This will decrease demands on the time of the team leader. The senior consultant is also vital to obtaining any additional support (eg, personnel, equipment, supplies, references) required for the investigation, but this should not occur independently of the normal chain of command.

Logistical Plans and Management

The supplies needed by both local and outside investigative teams are similar, but logistical support planning is more complicated for a nonlocal team. This section will discuss some of the logistical issues that outside teams face. Documents required in preparation for team travel may include government orders, country clearances, passports, international driver's licenses, immunization records, powers of attorney, credit cards, and property passes. Specific arrangements must be made for transportation of equipment and personnel on-site and lodging of the team. Members of the group may need additional immunizations and chemoprophylactic medicines, as well as supplies of their personal medications. Diagnostic, laboratory, and automation equipment are usually essential. Supplies for human specimen collection and environmental specimen collection may be available locally; if they are not, they must be brought in by the team. Published references that discuss collection of laboratory specimens in specific types of outbreaks should be consulted.[26] Questionnaires, blank rosters, preprinted labels, key phone numbers, cellular telephones, beepers, laptop computers, software programs, scanners, portable photocopy machines, digital cameras, and any other relevant specialized equipment should be included. Statistical references and disease-specific reference material are also important. Exhibit 32-2 lists a basic supply package designed for the Army's Problem Definition and Assessment team, which must be able to deploy to the site of a public health crisis within 24 hours. The supply chain to be used for any future require-

EXHIBIT 32-2

CONTENTS OF PROBLEM DEFINITION AND ASSESSMENT TEAM KIT

Bag No. 1:   Medical Equipment

Stethoscope, sphygnomanometer, otoscope/ophthalmoscope (1 each)

Extra bulbs for otoscope/ophthalmoscope

Extra batteries for othoscope/ophthalmoscope (4 large)

Tongue depressors (50)

Tempa dots (box of 100)

Penlight (1)

McArthur microscope and attachments (1)

McArthur microscope instructions (1 set)

Extra batteries for McArthur, size AA (8)

Microscope slides, frosted end (300)

Cover slips for slides (300)

Immersion oil, 1 bottle

Lens paper

Slide holding box (2)

Calculator, solar powered and case (1)

Bag No. 2:   Blood or Stool Specimen Collection Supplies

Vacutainers, 13 cc red top with silicone separator (100)

Vacutainers, 7 cc green top (50)

Vacutainer holders and tourniquets (6 each)

Multidraw vacutainer needles, 20 g (125)

Syringes, 20 cc (5) and hub needles, 21 g (10)

Alcohol swabs and 2x2s (200 each)

Band-Aids (100)

Plastic Serum transport vials, 5cc (200)

White labels, silk-type, marked PDA (200)

Labels, silk-type, marked PDA (200)

Polyethylene specimen bags, ziplock type (25)

Perma markers for labeling specimens and plastic vials (6)

Stool cups, carton-type (20)

Sterile urine cups, plastic-type (20)

Culturette, throat swabs (20)

Biohazard bags (10)

Gloves, 7 1/2" & 8 1/2" (10 each)

Ammonia inhalant capsules (10)

Parafilm sealant paper (1 roll)

Filter paper for PCR of blood samples

Sharps disposal boxes

Centrifuge

Transfer pipettes

Freezer boxes

Boxes to store and ship plastic vials

Bag No. 3:   Bacteriology and Parasitology Supplies

Cary-Blair media in REMEL plastic tubes (50)

Buffered glycerol saline in REMEL plastic tubes (50)

PVA fixative in REMEL plastic tubes (50)

3 cc syringe with 24 g (or 25 g) needle for leish aspiration (25)

Blades, scalpel type for scraping of lesions

NNN culture media in slants (20)

Schneider's media in slants (20)

Gram stain kit (1)

CAMCO giemsa quick stain (1 bottle)

Diff quick stain set (1)

Methylene blue stain (1 box of squeeze type)

Stain jars (3), forceps (1) and paper towels (1 small roll)

Distilled water, 100 cc (1 bottle)

Sterile saline, 5 cc (10 glass vials) for leish aspiration (*without* Na Azide)

Normal saline in dropper bottle (1)

Methanol, 100 cc (1 bottle)

Plastic squeeze type bottles for use in washing slides, 100 cc (2)

Na Azide, 15%, preservative for serum preservation (1 bottle)

One set of Gram stain and Diff quick staining instructions

One set of REMEL kit instructions

One set of leishmania aspirate/smear instructions

Bag No. 4:   Forms and Administrative Supplies

Rubber bands (1 bag)

Notebook and notepad (1 each)

Pencils, sharpened (20)

Questionnaires, postdeployment type (400)

Questionnaires, febrile illness type (100)

Clinical flow chart and lab sheets (20 each)

Medical surveillance report forms, two-sided (200)

Daily and weekly medical surveillance summary forms (200 daily, 50 weekly)

Medical surveillance instruction sheets (50)

PDA team booklet (1 copy)

Laptop Computer (1) with Case

Portable printer (1) with printer paper

ments should be determined. Local administrative support for generating rosters, typing, photocopying, or just answering the phone should be requested before the team arrives. The local laboratory should be consulted about the team's need for work space, laboratory space, centrifuges, freezer space for specimens, dry ice, liquid nitrogen, and shipping assistance. Any local staff support needed for key tasks such as venipuncture and aliquotting should also be discussed. The extent of local support available may affect the size and composition of the team and the need for off-site laboratory support. The team leader should determine which reference laboratory will be used for more sophisticated requirements.

Leadership and management skills are key to the success of the scientific investigation. It is critical for the team leader and team members to conduct the investigation in a calm, methodical manner even though decisions may need to be made quickly and actions taken promptly. Team members must resist the impulse to jump to premature conclusions in response to the intense pressure to solve the problem immediately. The possibility of a second wave of cases should be kept in mind before the team quickly declares the outbreak over. If new cases do continue to occur, the pressure on the team to find the cause and end the outbreak will dramatically increase. Departure dates should not be set until it becomes apparent how both the epidemic and the investigation will unfold.

The leader must assign areas of responsibility to team members in accordance with their expertise and identify locations for work space. A list of phone numbers and beeper numbers for team members and work sites should be established and exchanged. A time and location for team meetings should be determined. These should be held at least daily and probably twice daily initially. The leaders should make a task list with assignments for follow-up and track status reports at subsequent meetings. All decisions made at these meetings, such as case definitions to be used or source and type of controls needed, should be recorded.

The investigation should be organized both with the big picture in mind and with very close attention to the details—the details may provide important ideas. It is also essential to be tactful when obtaining detailed information because the existence of an epidemic is a source of potential embarrassment. Some epidemics will have major economic and political ramifications. Careful judgement about the release of preliminary results is thus vital. Diplomacy will be needed to establish and maintain cooperation from the many groups within the community.

A local staff member must be put in charge of media relations and determine what information has already been given to the press. The team leader should not be the spokesperson. The public affairs director should attend team meetings and ensure all press releases are cleared by the team leader and local command authorities. Likewise all news releases and statements to the press should be given to each member of the investigative team. Only objective, factual information should be released; the release of preliminary information should be avoided. The rationale for any emergency control measures should be explained. Some situations may warrant setting up an emergency hot line to answer questions. Hot line operator staff must be trained to provide consistent information to all callers.

The military chain of command and the responsible public health authorities do not change when an outbreak occurs. Authority to ban food sources and to close dining facilities, swimming pools, operating rooms, and other such facilities remains with the local commander acting on the guidance of the local preventive medicine officer. The investigation team serves as a consultant and makes recommendations to the local commander. Investigation team members are subordinate to the designated team leader. Local preventive medicine staff should be integrated functionally with the investigation team to conduct the investigation. The team leader should have an initial in-briefing with the local commander, provide interim updates as the situation dictates, and provide an out-briefing before the team leaves.

IDENTIFY DISEASE CONTROL MEASURES

When feasible, disease control measures should be implemented immediately after determining the nature of the problem and that an epidemic is ongoing. The initial control measures are intended to keep the outbreak from spreading and to limit its impact on the population. Examples of control measures prescribed to individual susceptible persons

at risk would include the use of immune globulin during hepatitis A outbreaks, use of rifampin as chemoprophylaxis for meningococcal meningitis, use of penicillin to prevent streptococcal disease, and initiation of case isolation or contact notification. Examples of general control measures include reinforcing handwashing recommendations and changing food preparation processes. In some situations, seizing raw materials (eg, drugs, food), closing an establishment (eg, restaurant, pool), or issuing an advisory to boil water may be warranted. Environmental interventions, such as mosquito or rodent control, may also be indicated. Control measures should be tailored to the situation and may be as simple as restricting movements of the population at risk or temporarily discontinuing new trainee arrivals, as was required by varicella outbreaks in at the Defense Language Institute at Lackland Air

Force Base in San Antonio, Tex.[27] Implementation of control measures will often require coordination with other agencies, such as major commands, civilian health departments, or the Food and Drug Administration (to hold or recall commercial items). The effectiveness of any disease control measures implemented by local health authorities or recommended by the investigation team will need to be evaluated as the investigation proceeds. Control measures should then be added or the existing ones altered, as indicated by the evaluation.

DESCRIBE THE OUTBREAK BY PERSON, TIME, AND PLACE

Studying the distribution of the disease or condition in the affected population begins with a detailed description of the outbreak in terms of person, time, and place. Hippocrates was among the first to note the importance of this triad in his paper *Air, Waters, Places.*[28]

Orient the Outbreak to Person

The first task is to identify the population at risk. This is done by characterizing the population members by age, race, sex, occupation, military unit, or other demographic grouping. If the outbreak appears to be associated with a special event, rosters of attendees must be obtained from the event organizers. Within this population, the nature of the risk may be seen in the presumed intensity of exposure. The likelihood of transmission should be considered both within and beyond this population. Noting who has been spared often provides important clues for formulating a hypothesis on the cause of the outbreak. Factors affecting the population at risk to be considered include the extent of migration into and out of the group.

Subjects for evaluation must be selected from within the population at risk. These should include both cases of the disease under investigation and controls or persons with no symptoms of disease. Both cases and controls should have had the opportunity for exposure to suspected risk factors. Controls should also be susceptible to the condition of interest. The team must decide if it will study all of the targeted population or just a particular subset or sample. A method will have to be decided on to choose an appropriate sample, depending on the circumstances of the outbreak and the population (see chapter 33, Epidemiologic Measurement: Basic Concepts and Methods). Alternatively, investigators could select one or more matched or unmatched controls for each case.

Although it is not the job of the team to provide clinical care for cases, it is of the utmost importance for clinician team members to conduct a personal interview and evaluation of at least a few cases in the early phase of the investigation. This will assist in verifying the diagnosis and in subsequent planning of specific objectives for data collection and analysis. Team members should ask those being interviewed what they think caused the outbreak, since they may have surprising insight and will frequently provide additional, pertinent information.

Attack rates of disease in the population at risk should be estimated based on the interview data from cases, providers, and others. Rates of disease by substrata are also very useful. Investigators should always examine attack rates by militarily relevant groupings, such as unit, barracks, training site, military job specialty, and rank (eg, officer versus enlisted). In foodborne outbreaks, attack rates for those who did and did not eat specific food items will be used for formal hypothesis testing.

Orient the Outbreak in Time

Viewing graphic displays of epidemic curves or flow charts may yield important conclusions about the outbreak, such as whether it is a common source event or whether transmission is ongoing. Correlating both time and place on spot maps can show secular trends of waves of illness moving across a community. The epidemic curve should be plotted using a histogram to quantify the number of cases; this will graphically display the outbreak. Cases meeting the previously determined case definition are plotted by date of symptom onset, with the X axis depicting time and the Y axis showing number of cases. The first case recognized is sometimes referred to as the index case if this case is thought to have introduced the organism into the population. From this curve, the incubation period of known diseases can be used to determine a range estimate for the time of exposure. Alternatively, the incubation period of an unidentified disease may be calculated from the time of symptom onset and a time of known probable exposure from a unit event. Other important characteristics of cases can be annotated on a histogram of the epidemic curve by designating specific symbol notations to indicate cases who are asymptomatic, work as food handlers, have positive cultures, or have died. Arrows may be used to note on the graph the arrival of the investigation team and the application of any control measures. A frequency polygon is sometimes used instead of a histogram to depict distribution of data from two or more categories.

Investigators must assess evidence for transmission patterns from the time distribution of cases. Certain patterns indicate a specific type or mode of transmission. Figure 32-1 depicts a common source outbreak of *Shigella dysenteriae* infection among hospital staff members.[29] Common source epidemics occur when a population is exposed to a patho-gen spread by a vehicle such as food or water at a single event or within a short period of time. Cases occur rapidly after the first onset, reach a peak, and then decline because of the relative uniformity of the incubation period. The rapid rise with a tight temporal clustering of cases and subsequent fall of the epidemic curve is compatible with a point source. The epidemic curve of a common source epidemic follows a log-normal distribution. The median incubation period for a common-source, single-event epidemic can be determined by finding on the histogram the time at which 50% of the cases have occurred. The approximate time of infection can be determined by subtracting the average incubation period in hours or days from the time at which the median case is located on the epidemic curve.

In some outbreaks, the common source may continually or intermittently expose the population, resulting in an epidemic curve from multiple exposures at different times. The distribution of cases will continue over a protracted period of time, and interpreting the curve will be more complex. These outbreaks may be referred to as a common-source, multiple-event epidemic. Epidemics resulting from person-to-person transmission will be reflected in an epidemic extended over a number of incubation periods. The curve will show a clustering of cases but with a relatively gentle upslope, and, after several generations of cases, an eventual decline in cases will occur. Figure 32-2 depicts a person-to-person outbreak of respiratory disease at Fort Leonard Wood, Mo, with seasonal variation and the effect of bicillin applied as a control measure.[30] An epidemic curve can have a mixed pattern if the initial transmission occurs via exposure to a common source but subsequent transmission is person-to-person.

Creating flow charts is useful to trace a chain of infection associated with the cases. Concentrating on the earliest cases may help pinpoint the precipitating event. Determining who the earliest cases were may help explain how the disease was introduced into the setting. Also, evaluation of unusual or atypical cases may provide additional clues. But investigators must beware of red herrings. In the shigella outbreak depicted in Figure 32-1, a hospital staff dining facility was implicated as the source. However, case ascertainment identified one culture-positive case with the same uncommon strain who had no exposure to the staff facility but had eaten at a small cafe in the same institution. No other cases were traced to that cafe. On additional questioning, the cafe staff remembered borrowing lettuce and tomatoes at the end of the day from the implicated

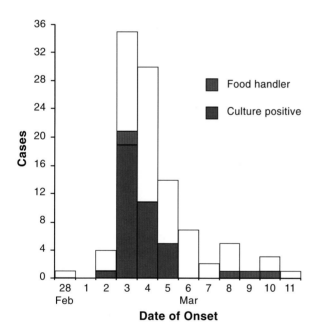

Figure 32-1. This is a graph showing the cases of hospital-associated infection with *Shigella dysenteriae* by date of onset and culture result. (Four cases with unknown date of onset have been excluded.) These cases occurred in the Bethesda Naval Hospital, Maryland. No index case was identified. Five food handlers with illnesses meeting the case definition had onset of symptoms concurrent with other cases.
Source: Centers for Disease Control. Hospital-associated outbreak of *Shigella dysenteriae* type 2—Maryland. *MMWR*. 1983;32:250–252.

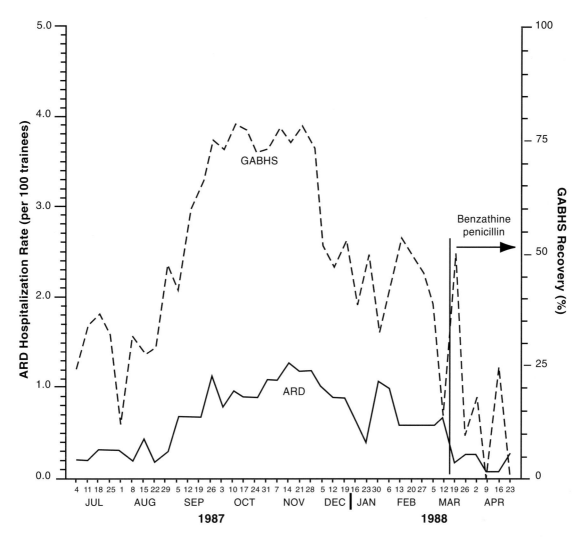

Figure 32-2. This graph shows the rates of hospitalization for acute respiratory diseases for Army trainees at Fort Leonard Wood, Mo, from July 1987 through April 1988. The dashed line represents the percent of recovery of group A β-hemolytic streptococcus (GABHS) from the trainees. Prophylaxis with benzathine penicillin was started in March 1988 as a response to the outbreak and is noted on the graph. GABHS recovery rapidly declined following initiation of benzathine penicillin prophylaxis, which effectively controlled the outbreak. The acute respiratory disease rate also declined following initiation of penicillin prophylaxis.
Source: Centers for Disease Control. Acute rheumatic fever among Army trainees—Fort Leonard Wood, Missouri, 1987–1988. *MMWR*. 1988;37:519–522.

dining facility. Further analyses implicated salad served at the dining facility as the vehicle of transmission. Exhibit 32-3 lists possible reasons for exposed persons not becoming ill and for nonexposed persons who appear ill.[31]

Evidence must be assessed for chronological distribution of disease. Recurrent cycles of epidemics allow investigators to calculate the generation time. Seasonality may affect rates of certain diseases such as influenza. Investigators must be careful interpreting secular trends, however, because small numbers may affect data analysis. Disease rates characterized by time may also vary with the provider's en-

thusiasm or the resources available to help detect and report disease. Changes in personnel, clinical practices, reporting procedures, data collection forms, or case definitions may all alter the apparent rates of disease.

Orient the Outbreak to Place

The pattern of disease should be described by determining the location of quarters, work, and recreation and noting geographic distribution of cases by creating a spot map. The dimension of time can be added to place with the use of colored pins. Biological,

EXHIBIT 32-3

POSSIBLE EXPLANATIONS
FOR INACCURATE MEASURES
OF ASSOCIATION

Endemic background cases

Errors in case definition

Individual susceptibility and immune status

Exposure to insufficient dose and inoculum

Cross contamination between potential vehicles

Exposure to vehicle contaminated in another way

Misclassification of exposures

Technical errors

Untruthful or inaccurate responses

Secondary person-to-person transmission

Adapted with permission from *Guidelines for the Establishment of Systems for the Epidemiological Surveillance of Food-borne Diseases and the Investigation of Outbreaks of Food Poisoning.* Pan American Health Organization. Division of Communicable Diseases Prevention and Control. 1993.

chemical, physical, or climatic factors affecting the environment should be included. Geographic information software may help plot space-time characteristics. Preparing and maintaining an outbreak investigation kit with supply items routinely needed for most environmental investigations will assist investigators in performing timely on-site evaluations.

Investigators should consider case clustering by source of food, water, milk, ice, or shellfish. If foodborne disease is under consideration, an on-site inspection of all facilities potentially associated with the outbreak is appropriate. Any problems in air quality, food sanitation, water sanitation, or hygiene practices should be identified. Utensils, equipment, filters, and surfaces used in preparing the food or other suspect vectors should be cultured. Leftover foods should be set aside for possible laboratory analysis.[32] Water should also be considered as a possible etiologic agent at the outset. Too often water and ice are only considered as a potential source of contamination after food has been ruled out as the cause. The time factor is crucial to ensure rapid collection and culture of food, water, ice, and other environmental samples before food or ice have been consumed or thrown away or water lines have been superchlorinated. In a large outbreak of campylobacteriosis in 1990 at Fort Knox, Ky, the investigation team hypothesized that sludge and dead birds found in a water storage tower were associated with infection. The tank was disinfected and refilled before culturing of the suspect water and sludge could be accomplished.[33] Investigators always look for inadequate health practices, such as improper handwashing or food handling practices and recent procedure changes; the adequacy of training and supervision of workers should also be evaluated. Microbiological or chemical contamination can occur at numerous points, and investigators may need to examine multiple sequences of events or look for a unique order of events to find the cause. Correlation of time and temperature at each stage of food processing should help identify the critical point.

Samples of water should be collected directly from the source, from storage tanks, and from high and low points of the distribution system, in accordance with standard methods.[34] Characteristics to be measured include temperature; pH; turbidity; and free, combined, and total residual chlorine. Bacterial examinations for potable water should include total organisms of the coliform group, indicative of fecal contamination, and a standard plate count (heterotrophic plate count) because large bacterial populations may suppress the growth of coliforms. Turbid waters may contain particles with embedded bacteria protected from contact with chlorine. This may also contribute to coliform masking. The absence of coliforms does not ensure the absence of viruses, protozoa, or helminths, which may be more resistant to chlorine treatment than fecal bacteria. Norwalk virus and the related small round structured viruses, which are very resistant to chlorine, are a major cause of acute nonbacterial gastroenteritis in adults.[35] Protozoa such as *Giardia lamblia, Entamoeba histolytica*, and *Cryptosporidium* species have also been implicated in waterborne outbreaks.[36] Plumbing cross connections between potable water and contaminated water, loss of positive line pressure, line breaks, and line repairs may allow bacterial contamination. Spot maps of water distribution lines and points may provide insight on potential areas for contamination.

The on-site inspection is vital to the environmental evaluation of any outbreak associated with a military field setting. A broad knowledge of military food technology and field water supply options is essential for preventive medicine staff. Investigators must carefully identify all local sources of food and all types of rations served in the field: A, B, T, or Meals Ready to Eat (MREs). Food purchased from the local market in foreign countries may require specific washing and disinfection before consumption. MREs, a foil-wrapped ration packaged in a laminate pouch, have been the main operational ration used by the Department of Defense since they replaced the C-ration in 1983. Although MREs have been found to be extremely safe, contamination could occur at the manufacturing and processing plants or if a break in package integrity occurs. Investigators must determine the lot number, storage temperature, and transport history for all meals consumed in the field. The time of storage should be evaluated in relation to safety recommendations. An outbreak of disease caused by *Staphylococcus aureus* in a reserve unit, which was caused by ham that had been stored for more than 4 hours in mermite transport containers, is a typical example (JNL, unpublished data, 1993). Investigators must obtain samples from all points of the field water distribution system: the supply pipe line, water trailers, water buffaloes, and individual canteens. They must also document in detail the exact decontamination, disinfection, and chlorination procedures used for the water. Then they must assess the availability of soaps, brushes, and handwashing sites for personal hygiene. It is also critical to review trash management and waste disposal practices and note any unusual aspects of the location altitude and topography. The distance should be measured between field kitchens, water sources, sanitation centers, laundry lines, soakage pits, and garbage pits.

Depending on the outcome of the environmental evaluation, additional clinical specimens may be required for testing, for ova and parasite examinations, or for heavy metals or toxin analysis. Environmental samples must be obtained, transported, and labeled properly. If airborne transmission is of concern, measurement of ventilation rates, adequacy of fresh make up air, and space per occupant should be considered. Air tracer studies with smoke or oil of wintergreen may be useful. Presence of fungal growth could be significant. The limitations of environmental testing methods by sensitivity and specificity, as well as reliability, need to be noted.

An interview and clinical evaluation of workers is frequently a key part of the environmental evaluation of foodborne or waterborne outbreaks, nosocomial epidemics, or other occupational cluster outbreaks. Food handlers, health care staff, or other workers may be case victims as well as vectors. History of recent illnesses with symptoms comparable to the outbreak cases should be carefully obtained because workers are often the earliest cases and may or may not be vectors. Investigators should examine workers for skin lesions on the hands, arms, face, and neck and evaluate them for infection of the respiratory or gastrointestinal tract. Appropriate laboratory specimens, as determined by the presumptive diagnosis, should be obtained from the nasopharynx, throat, hands, or rectum of workers. Interviews should determine in detail the chronological handling of the food, ice, medicine, and other pertinent materials from time of entry until exit from the facility. Food handlers should also be queried concerning their consumption of food and drink.

Team members must identify any potentially critical events occurring in the environment before and during the outbreak. Examples include picnics, parties, sewage spills, field training exercises, construction, floods and heavy rains, and by-passes of the water filtration system. Obtaining detailed information on seemingly irrelevant details, such as recent replacement of pipes in sewage lines or pressure changes due to testing of boilers, may provide the crucial details for unraveling the mechanism of transmission. Six years of drought followed by unusually heavy rains and snows in the spring of 1993 are thought to have contributed to an abundant food supply for the deer-mouse that was ultimately linked to the recognition of hantavirus pulmonary syndrome in North America.[37]

IDENTIFY RISK FACTORS AND MECHANISMS

Frequency Measures and Severity Assessment

After completion of initial assessments, a few cases can be described clinically, incorporating quantitative details obtained by interviewers characterizing symptoms. Organizing frequency of signs and symptoms by percentage of cases may help clarify the disease causing the outbreak. The clinical picture, laboratory results, or estimate of the incubation period from the epidemic curve should help to identify the disease. See Tables 32-1 through 32-3 for a chart of etiological agents in foodborne diseases with their known incubation periods and their associated clinical syndromes. Diagnosis of the disease, number of symptomatic cases, and laboratory results help investigators estimate the symptomatic-to-asymptomatic ratio. Even asymptomatic cases are relevant because they help accurately discriminate cases from susceptible noncases, thus assisting in the rapid development of a tentative hypothesis. Epidemiologists use morbidity measures, such as incidence, prevalence, and attack rates, to quantitatively

TABLE 32-1

CDC GUIDELINES FOR CONFIRMATION OF FOODBORNE DISEASE OUTBREAKS: BACTERIAL

Etiological Agent	Incubation Period	Clinical Syndrome	Confirmation
1. *Bacillus cerus*			
a. Vomiting toxin	1-6 h	Vomiting, some patients with diarrhea; fever uncommon	Isolation of organism from stool of two or more ill persons and not from stool of controls OR Isolation of ≥10^5 organisms/g from epidemiologically implicated food, provided specimen properly handled
b. Diarrheal toxin	6-24 h	Diarrhea, abdominal cramps, and vomiting in some patients; fever uncommon	Isolation of organism from stool of two or more ill persons and not from stool of controls OR Isolation of ≥10^5 organisms/g from epidemiologically implicated food, provided specimen properly handled
2. *Brucella*	Several days to several mo, usually >30 d	Weakness, fever, headache, sweats, chills, arthralgia, weight loss, splenomegaly	Two or more ill persons and isolation of organism in culture of blood or bone marrow, greater than 4-fold increase in SAT over several wk, or single SAT titer ≥1:160 in person who has compatible clinical symptoms and history of exposure
3. *Campylobacter*	2-10 d, usually 2-5 d	Diarrhea (often bloody), abdominal pain, fever	Isolation of organism from clinical specimens from two or more ill persons OR Isolation of organism from epidemiologically implicated food
4. *Clostridium botulinum*	2 h-8 d, usually 12-48 h	Illness of variable severity; common symptoms are diplopia, blurred vision, and bulbar weakness; paralysis, which is usually descending and bilateral, may progress rapidly	Detection of botulinal toxin in serum, stool, gastric contents, or implicated food OR Isolation of organism from stool or intestine
5. *Clostridium perfringens*	6-24 h	Diarrhea, abdominal cramps; vomiting and fever are uncommon	Isolation of ≥10^6 organisms/g in stool of two or more ill persons, provided specimen properly handled OR Demonstration of enterotoxin in the stool of two or more ill persons OR Isolation of ≥10^5 organisms/g from epidemiologically implicated food, provided specimen properly handled
6. *Escherichia coli*			
a. Enterohemorrhagic (*E coli* O157:H7 and others)	1-10 d, usually 3-4 d	Diarrhea (often bloody), abdominal cramps (often severe), little or no fever	Isolation of *E coli* O157:H7 or other Shiga-like toxin-producing *E coli* from clinical specimen of two or more ill persons OR Isolation of *E coli* O157 or other Shiga-like toxin-producing *E coli* from epidemiologically implicated food
b. Enterotoxigenic (ETEC)	6-48 h	Diarrhea, abdominal cramps, nausea vomiting and fever are less common	Isolation of organisms of same serotype, which are demonstrated to produce heat-stable and/or heat-labile enterotoxin, from stool of two or more ill persons
c. Enteropathogenic (EPEC)	Variable	Diarrhea, fever, abdominal cramps	Isolation of same enteropathogenic serotype from stool of two or more ill persons
d. Enteroinvasive (EIEC)	Variable	Diarrhea (may be bloody), fever, abdominal cramps	Isolation of same enteroinvasive serotype from stool of two or more ill persons

Organism/Disease	Incubation period	Clinical syndrome	Confirmation
7. *Listeria monocytogenes*			
a. Invasive disease	2-6 wk	Meningitis, neonatal sepsis, fever	Isolation of organism from normally sterile site
b. Diarrheal disease	Unknown	Diarrhea, abdominal cramps, fever	Isolation of organism of same serotype from stool of two or more ill persons exposed to food that is epidemiologically implicated or from which organism of same serotype has been isolated
8. Nontyphoidal *Salmonella*	6 h-10 d, usually 6-48 h	Diarrhea, often with fever and abdominal cramps	Isolation of organism of same serotype from clinical specimens from two or more ill persons OR Isolation of organism from epidemiologically implicated food
9. *Salmonella typhi*	3-60 d, usually 7-14 d	Fever, anorexia, malaise, headache, and myalgia; sometimes diarrhea or constipation	Isolation of organism from clinical specimens of two or more ill persons OR Isolation of organism from epidemiologically implicated food
10. *Shigella*	12 h-6 d, usually 2-4 d	Diarrhea (often bloody), frequently accompanied by fever and abdominal cramps	Isolation of organism of same serotype from clinical specimens from two or more ill persons OR Isolation of organism from epidemiologically implicated food
11. *Staphylococcus aureus*	30 min-8 h, usually 2-4 h	Vomiting, diarrhea	Isolation of organism of same phage type from stool or vomitus of two or more ill persons OR Detection of enterotoxin in epidemiologically implicated food OR Isolation of $\geq 10^5$ organisms/g from epidemiologically implicated food, provided specimen properly handled
12. *Streptococcus* Group A	1-4 d	Fever, pharyngitis, scarlet fever, upper respiratory infection	Isolation of organism of same M- or T-type from throats of two or more ill persons OR Isolation of organism of same M- or T-type from epidemiologically implicated food
13. *Vibrio cholerae*			
a. O1 or O139	1-5 d	Watery diarrhea, often accompanied by vomiting	Isolation of toxigenic organism from stool or vomitus of two or more ill persons OR Significant rise in vibriocidal, bacterial-agglutinating, or antitoxin antibodies in acute-phase and early convalescent-phase sera among persons not recently immunized OR Isolation of toxigenic organism from epidemiologically implicated food
b. non-O1 and non-O139	1-5 d	Watery diarrhea	Isolation of organism of same serotype from stool of two or more ill persons
14. *Vibrio parahaemolyticus*	4-30 h	Diarrhea	Isolation of Kanagawa-positive organism from stool of two or more ill persons OR Isolation of $\geq 10^5$ Kanagawa-positive organisms/g from epidemiologically implicated food, provided specimen properly handled
15. *Yersinia enterocolitica*	1-10 d, usually 4-6 d	Diarrhea, abdominal pain (often severe)	Isolation of organism from clinical specimen of two or more ill persons OR Isolation of pathogenic strain or organism from epidemiologically implicated food

TABLE 32-2

CDC GUIDELINES FOR CONFIRMATION OF FOODBORNE DISEASE OUTBREAKS: CHEMICAL

Etiological Agent	Incubation Period	Clinical Syndrome	Confirmation
1. Marine toxins			
a. Ciguatoxin	1–48 h, usually 2–8 h	Usually gastrointestinal symptoms followed by neurologic symptoms (eg, paresthesia of lips, tongue, throat, or extremities) and reversal of hot and cold sensation	Demonstration of ciguatoxin in epidemiologically implicated fish OR Clinical syndrome among persons who have eaten a type of fish previously associated with ciguatera fish poisoning (eg, snapper, grouper, barracuda)
b. Scombroid toxin (histamine)	1 min–1 h, usually <1 h	Flushing, dizziness, burning of mouth and throat, headache, gastrointestinal symptoms, urticaria, and generalized pruritus	Demonstration of histamine in epidemiologically implicated food OR Clinical syndrome among persons who have eaten type of fish previously associated with histamine fish poisoning (eg, mahi-mahi or fish of order Scomboidei)
c. Paralytic or neurotoxic shellfish poison	30 min–3 h	Paresthesia of lips, mouth or face, and extremities; intestinal symptoms; generalized weakness; respiratory difficulty	Detection of toxin in epidemiologically implicated food OR Detection of large numbers of shellfish-poisoning–associated species of dinoflagellates in water from which epidemiologically implicated mollusks are gathered
d. Puffer fish, tetrodotoxin	10 min–3 h, usually 10–45 min	Paresthesia of lips, tongue, face, or extremities, often following numbness; loss of proprioception or "floating" sensations	Demonstration of tetrodotoxin in epidemiologically implicated fish OR Clinical syndrome among persons who have eaten puffer fish
2. Heavy metals (antimony, cadmium, copper, iron, tin, zinc)	5 min–8 h, usually <1 h	Vomiting, often metallic taste	Demonstration of high concentration of metal in epidemiologically implicated food
3. Monosodium glutamate (MSG)	3 min–2 h, usually <1 h	Burning sensation in chest, neck, abdomen, or extremities; sensation of lightness and pressure over face or heavy feeling in chest	Clinical syndrome among persons who have eaten food containing MSG (ie, usually ≥1.5 g MSG)
4. Mushroom toxins			
a. Shorter-acting toxins: Muscimol Muscarine Psilocybin *Coprinus artrementaris* Ibotenic acid	≤2 h	Usually vomiting and diarrhea, other symptoms differ with toxin: Confusion, visual disturbance Salivation, diaphoresis Hallucinations Disulfiram-like reaction Confusion, visual disturbance	Clinical syndrome among persons who have eaten mushroom identified as toxic type OR Demonstration of toxin in epidemiologically implicated mushroom or mushroom-containing food
b. Longer-acting toxin (eg, *Amanita* spp)	6–24 h	Diarrhea and abdominal cramps for 24 h followed by hepatic and renal failure	Clinical syndrome among persons who have eaten mushroom identified as toxic type OR Demonstration of toxin in epidemiologically implicated mushroom or mushroom-containing food

TABLE 32-3

CDC GUIDELINES FOR CONFIRMATION OF FOODBORNE DISEASE OUTBREAKS: PARASITIC AND VIRAL

Etiological Agent	Incubation Period	Clinical Syndrome	Confirmation
Parasitic			
1. *Cryptosporidium parvum*	2-28 d, median: 7 d	Diarrhea, nausea, vomiting, fever	Demonstration of organism or antigen in stool or in small-bowel biopsy of two or more ill persons OR Demonstration of organism in epidemiologically implicated food
2. *Cyclospora cayetanensis*	1-11 d, median: 7 d	Fatigue, protracted diarrhea, often relapsing	Demonstration of organism in stool of two or more ill persons
3. *Giardia lamblia*	3-25 d, median: 7 d	Diarrhea, gas, cramps, nausea, fatigue	Two or more ill persons and detection of antigen in stool; or demonstration of organism in stool, duodenal contents, or small-bowel biopsy specimen
4. *Trichinella* spp	1-2 d for intestinal phase; 2-4 wk for systemic phase	Fever, myalgia, periorbital edema, high eosinophil count	Two or more ill persons and positive serologic test or demonstration of larvae in muscle biopsy OR Demonstration of larvae in epidemiologically implicated meat
Viral			
1. Hepatitis A	15-50 d, median: 28 d	Jaundice, dark urine, fatigue, anorexia, nausea	Detection of IgM anti-hepatitis A virus in serum from two or more persons who consumed epidemiologically implicated food
2. Norwalk family of viruses (SRSVs)	15-77 h, usually 24-48 h	Vomiting, cramps, diarrhea, headache	More than 4-fold rise in antibody titer to Norwalk virus or Norwalk-like virus in acute and convalescent sera in most serum pairs OR Visualization of SRSVs that react with patient's convalescent sera but not acute sera—by immune-electron microscopy; assays based on molecular diagnostic (eg, polymerase chain reaction, probes, assays for antigen and antibodies from expressed antigen) are available in reference laboratories
3. Astrovirus, calicivirus, others	15-77 h, usually 24-48 h	Vomiting, cramps, diarrhea, headache	Visualization of SRSVs that react with patient's convalescent sera but not acute sera—by immune-electron microscopy; assays based on molecular diagnostics (eg, PCR, probes, or assays for antigen and antibodies from expressed antigen) are available in reference laboratories

SAT: standard agglutination titer
SRSV: small round-structured viruses
Source: Centers for Disease Control and Prevention. Guidelines for confirmation of bloodborne-disease outbreaks. *MMWR*. 1996;45(SS-5):59–66.

describe disease or injury among a population. Attack rates by sex, military unit, residence, or other factors may provide helpful clues. Ideally all members of a denominator should be eligible to enter the numerator in a rate calculation. For example, only persons susceptible to hepatitis A should be in the denominator of a hepatitis A attack rate. The investigators must calculate secondary attack rates in unit members, family members, or contacts of ill service members who had no exposure to the presumed primary event or source. Attack rates by history of food and drink consumption play a key role in the investigation of foodborne and waterborne outbreaks.

Severity can be assessed by calculating the days lost from training, work, or duty as disability days or by the duration of hospitalization. In severe disease or injury clusters, case fatality rates and mortality rates will also be used and should be compared with those in the literature for the specified condition. In all rates, the definition of a case and the limitations of the data source must be specified. This is especially critical when using medical records to identify quantitative measures.

Epidemiologic Measures of Risk

To establish risk factors, a variety of epidemiologic measures of risk are available. Either chi-square or Fisher's exact test is used to test the association between categorical variables. Relative risk calculated for a cohort is the critical measure for assessing the etiological role of a factor in a disease. The relative risk reflects the excess risk in the exposed

group when compared with the unexposed group. The risk or attack rate in an acute outbreak setting in the exposed group is divided by the risk or attack rate in the unexposed group. Case-control studies are often used in outbreak investigations as a means to identify significant risk factors. For case-control studies, the excess risk cannot be measured directly because the exact denominator population (needed to calculate attack rates) is not known. The odds ratio is the most commonly used measure of risk for case-control studies. The odds ratio calculated from a standard 2 x 2 table is ad/bc and from a matched case-control study is b/c. Fisher's exact test is used when any of the expected values for a 2 x 2 contingency table is less than five.[38] Chi-square or Fisher's exact test can be used to assess the significance of observed effects against the null hypothesis. Confidence intervals can also be calculated for relative risk or odds ratios to determine if the measure includes or excludes 1.0.

Attributable risk examines the contribution of an exposure to the frequency of a disease in a population. In an epidemic, it is expected that most of the cases become ill because of an exposure to the imputed risk factor. The population attributable risk percentage represents the proportion of disease in a population attributable to an exposure. It reflects both the relative risk and the frequency of the factor in the population. It can be calculated by subtracting the risk in the unexposed from the risk in the exposed and then dividing by the risk in the exposed. This fraction, called the etiologic fraction, would then be multiplied by 100 and reported as a percentage.

DEVELOP TENTATIVE HYPOTHESES AND A PLAN

The information gathered to this point by the investigation team should be sufficient to allow them to formulate a tentative hypothesis and further refine the investigation plan.

Determine Type of Outbreak and Critical Exposure

The type of outbreak—point or continuing common source, person-to-person propagation, or mixed—should be evident from the epidemic curve. Initial case interviews and the environmental investigation may have identified a presumed critical exposure at an event or from a particular source. Synthesizing facts on the epidemiology and clinical characteristics of a disease, host factors, role of vectors, and importance of reservoirs should lead to a presumed mechanism of transmission. A tentative theory (or theories) that explains the observed

pattern of disease in a given environmental situation should have surfaced. Initially several broad hypotheses may be under consideration.

Hypothesize About Mechanism of Transmission

The complexity of our global community will make identification of risk factors and mechanisms of transmission extremely difficult. The shifting epidemiology of foodborne diseases in the United States during recent years caused by changes in food production and distribution methods warrants additional discussion.[39] The traceback of an *Escherichia coli* O157H outbreak implicating meat is an example. The traceback might take investigators from a dining facility to a distribution center to a meat processing plant to a boning and packaging plant to a slaughter plant to feed lot auctions to individual ranchers.[40] Along the way, meats from multiple sources are mixed, and contamination could occur at many points in this complex chain. The largest (224,000 cases) common-vehicle outbreak of salmonellosis ever recognized in the United States implicated a nationally distributed brand of ice cream by a company that provided home delivery. Investigators found that cross-contamination of pasteurized ice cream premix occurred during transport in tanker trailers that had previously hauled nonpasteurized liquid eggs containing *Salmonella enteritidis*.[41] Extensive tracebacks to identify the source of a pathogen are most useful when the implicated vehicle is either novel or has a long shelf life. The increase in foreign travel and the internationalization of the market for food supplies and other commerce also vastly complicates investigations.[42] Implicated in a 1997 outbreak of hepatitis A were contaminated strawberries imported from Mexico that were distributed to at least six states.[43] Military investigators must be prepared to deal with multinational outbreaks and should not be surprised to identify novel vehicles, new mechanisms, or an unusual chain of events contributing to the occurrence of outbreaks.

The possibility of sabotage or purposeful contamination should always be considered. A single act of terrorism that contaminates a water supply can place an entire force at risk. Identification of unusual diseases or rare strains may be the first indication of an unnatural event. A gastroenteritis outbreak of *Shigella dysenteriae* type 2, which is rare in the United States, occurred in 1996 following the removal of a stock culture of the organism from a medical center's laboratory. Health care workers at the medical center became ill after eating food that had been maliciously contaminated.[44] If the terrorists do not make demands or claim responsibility, as was the case in this outbreak, it may be extremely difficult to recognize that the contamination of food or water did not occur naturally. Another example of sabotage that was initially unrecognized was the largest foodborne outbreak reported in the United States in 1984.[45] Evidence obtained in an independent criminal investigation was essential to determining that members of a religious commune had intentionally contaminated restaurant salad bars with *Salmonella typhimurium*. Good laboratory work helped demonstrate that the *Salmonella* type was one found in a reference type collection rather than a strain more typically found in general circulation. This outbreak also demonstrates the vulnerability of self service foods to intentional contamination. Although recognition of an outbreak caused by a biological warfare attack can be quite challenging, a number of indicators listed in Exhibit 32-4 should

---

EXHIBIT 32-4

INDICATIONS OF POSSIBLE BIOLOGICAL WARFARE ATTACK

A disease entity (sometimes even a single case) that is unusual or that does not occur naturally in a given geographic area, or combinations of unusual disease entities in the same patient population

Multiple disease entities in the same patients, indicating that mixed agents have been used in the attack

Large numbers of both military and civilian casualties when such populations inhabit the same area

Data suggesting a massive point-source outbreak

Apparent aerosol route of infection

High morbidity and mortality relative to the number of personnel at risk

Illness limited to fairly localized or circumscribed geographical areas

Low attack rates in personnel who work in areas with filtered air supplies or closed ventilation systems

Sentinel dead animals of multiple species

Absence of competent natural vector in the area of outbreak (for a biological agent that is vector-borne in nature)

Source: Wiener SL, Barratt J. Biological warfare defense. In: *Trauma Management for Civilian and Military Physicians*. Philadelphia: WB Saunders; 1986.

suggest the possibility.[46] The disease pattern is an important factor in differentiating between a naturally occurring outbreak and a terrorist attack.[47] Terrorist objectives may include inducing a large number of cases, so health care workers may see many cases presenting simultaneously. This compressed epidemic curve with a very high case-to-exposure rate contrasts with the more gradual rise in disease incidence expected in most naturally occurring epidemics. Animals may also be affected by biological or chemical warfare attacks. Disease may appear in unexpected geographic areas that lack the normal vector for transmission. Unusual clinical presentations may occur because of a combination of agents or altered routes of transmission induced by the saboteur. The accidental release of aerosolized anthrax from a Russian biological weapons facility in 1979 resulted in respiratory instead of cutaneous disease, and the location of cases followed a distinctive downwind pattern from the site of release.[48] Anthrax continues to be considered as a biological warfare agent. The Aum Shinrikyo cult members arrested following the sarin attack in a Tokyo subway were also conducting research on anthrax and botulinum toxin.[12] Drone aircraft equipped with spray tanks found in the cult's arsenal made the potential for aerosolization of these agents a real threat. Some terrorist actions may be recognized only when first responders become secondary cases from toxic gas exposure. Thirteen of fifteen emergency room doctors treating victims of the sarin attack in Japan noted onset of their own symptoms while they were resuscitating victims.[49] Simultaneous outbreaks of multiple agents should also raise suspicion of biological terrorist etiology.

Identification of risk factors for the formulated hypothesis should determine the need for more specialized tests or for outside expert consultation in the appropriate field, be it medicine, engineering, entomology, or other fields. The differential diagnosis should be further narrowed, and the collection of the optimal source and type of specimens should be started, if not already underway. See chapter 34 for collection, transport, and processing considerations. Laboratory and field instruments must be calibrated. The specific laboratory designated to support the investigation should be fully aware of the tentative hypotheses of the team.

Develop Survey Instruments

Investigators should incorporate standard methods for designing questionnaires used for detailed risk factor interviews.[50] The instrument must achieve the specific objectives of the investigation. Items should be simple and unambiguous. Included should be exposure information and demographic factors, as well as clinical history and host factors that may affect risk. Any potentially relevant history, including such factors as chronic disease, nutrition, housing conditions, crowding, work locations, job, stress, pets, source of food, and source of water, should be obtained. The possibility of exotic house pets (eg, iguanas, snakes, hedgehogs, ferrets) or stray animals adopted in the field may be important. A site visit and some preliminary interviewing in the early designing of the questionnaire will improve the sensitivity and specificity of the instrument. Leading questions and lengthy surveys should be avoided. Survey design must take into account the coding scheme for entering the data into a database and whether data entry will occur in the field as it is collected or at a later time. Forms that can be optically scanned may be useful to facilitate data entry. Investigators must consider the data analysis methods planned to accomplish specific study objectives and construct empty tables for variables of interest in which data can be inserted after collection. Validation and quality control checks of the data should be planned. On-site scanning equipment can help with this. Figure 32-3 is a questionnaire designed by the CDC for use in a foodborne disease outbreak.

Cases and controls from the population under study should be interviewed in a consistent fashion using the survey tools developed. Interviewers must strive to create a nonthreatening environment in which those being questioned feel free to share all possible information without punishment. Initial questions should be simple and designed to put the subject at ease. For large, complex, or unusual outbreaks, interviewers should be trained first in both interviewing technique and the subject matter under investigation.[51] Time used to pretest the proposed questionnaire adequately is time well spent because pretesting can identify unclear or problem questions. The questionnaire and plans for its administration should be revised in accordance with the results of the pilot testing. As a quality control measure, each survey should be reviewed for legibility and completeness as it is returned. The same principles of developing forms, training interviewers, and pretesting forms and procedures apply to the process of abstracting data from medical records.

Most field outbreak investigations are the "emergencies" of the specialty of preventive medicine. Thus the time-sensitive investigation of this acute public health problem is considered operational and

CDC USE ONLY ☐☐☐☐
(1-4)

FORM APPROVED
OMB NO. 0920-0004

INVESTIGATION OF A FOODBORNE OUTBREAK

1. Where did the outbreak occur ?

State _____ (5-6) City or Town _____ County _____

2. Date of outbreak: (Date of onset 1st case)

MO / DA / YR   (7-12)

3. Indicate actual(a) or estimated (e) numbers:

Persons exposed _____ (13-17)

Persons ill _____ (18-22)

Hospitalized _____ (23-27)

Fatal case _____ (28-31)

4. History of Exposed Persons;

No. histories obtained _____ (32-35)

No. persons with symptoms _____ (36-39)

Nausea _____ (40-43) Diarrhea _____ (44-47)

Vomiting _____ (48-51) Fever _____ (52-55)

Cramps _____ (56-59) Other, specify _____

_____ (60-79)

5. Incubation period (hours):

Shortest _____ Longest _____
(80-83)   (84-87)

Approx. for majority _____ (88-91)

6. Duration of illness (hours):

Shortest _____ Longest _____
(92-95)   (96-99)

Approx. for majority _____ (101-104)

7. Food - specific attack rates:

Food Items Served	Number of persons who ATE specified food				Number who did NOT eat specified food			
	Ill	Not Ill	Total	Percent Ill	Ill	Not Ill	Total	Percent Ill

8. Vehicle responsible (food item incriminated by epidemiological evidence):   (105-106)

9. Manner in which incriminated food was marketed: (Check all Applicable)

Yes No
1   2

(a) Food Industry
 Raw .... ☐☐ (107)
 Processed .... ☐☐ (108)
Home Produced
 Raw .... ☐☐ (109)
 Processed .... ☐☐ (110)

(b) Vending Machine ... ☐☐ (111)

Yes No
1   2

(c) Not Wrapped .... ☐☐ (112)
 Ordinary Wrapping .... ☐☐ (113)
 Canned .... ☐☐ (114)
 Canned —Vacuum Sealed ☐☐ (115)
 Other (specify) .... ☐☐ (116)
                        (117-129)

(d) Room Temperature ..... ☐☐ (130)
 Refrigerator .... ☐☐ (131)
 Frozen .... ☐☐ (132)
 Heated .... ☐☐ (133)

If a commerical product, indicate brand name and lot number

_____ (134-150)

10. Place of Preparation of Contaminated Item: (151)

Restaurant .... ☐ 1
Delicatessen .... ☐ 2
Cafeteria .... ☐ 3
Private Home ..... ☐ 4
Caterer .... ☐ 5
Institution:
School .... ☐ 6
Church .... ☐ 7
Camp .... ☐ 8
Other, specify ..... ☐ 9

_____ (152-171)

11. Place where eaten: (172)

Restaurant .... ☐ 1
Delicatessen .... ☐ 2
Cafeteria .... ☐ 3
Private Home ...... ☐ 4
Picnic .... ☐ 5
Institution:
School .... ☐ 6
Church .... ☐ 7
Camp .... ☐ 8
Other, specify .... ☐ 9

_____ (173-192)

DEPARTMENT OF HEALTH AND HUMAN SERVICES
PUBLIC HEALTH SERVICE
CENTERS FOR DISEASE CONTROL
ATLANTA, GEORGIA 30333

CDC 52.13   REV. 9/83   (over)

(**Fig.32-3** *continues*)

LABORATORY FINDINGS (Include Negative Results)

12. Food specimens examined: (193)
Specify by "X" whether food examined was original (eaten at time of outbreak) or check-up (prepared in similar manner but not involved in outbreak).

Item	Orig.	Check up	Findings Qualitative	Quantitative
Example: beef	X		C. perfringens Hobbs type 10	2×10^6/gm

13. Enviromental specimens examined: (194)

Item	Findings
Example: meat grinder	C. perfringens, Hobbs Type 10

14. Specimens from patients examined (stool, vomitus, etc.): (195)

Item	No. Persons	Findings
Example: stool	11	C. perfringens, Hobbs Type 10

15. Specimens from food handlers (stool, lesions, etc.): (196)

Item	Findings
Example: lesion	C. perfringens, Hobbs Type 10

16. Factors contributing to outbreak (check all applicable):

	Yes 1	No 2	Unk.
1. Improper storage or holding temperature	☐	☐	☐ (197)
2. Inadequate cooking	☐	☐	☐ (198)
3. Contaminated equipment or working surfaces	☐	☐	☐ (199)
4. Food obtained from unsafe source	☐	☐	☐ (200)
5. Poor personal hygiene of food handler	☐	☐	☐ (201)
6. Other, specify	☐	☐	☐ (202)

17. Etiology: (203-204)

Pathogen _____ Suspected · · · · · · · · · · · · · · · · · · · ☐ 1 (205)
Chemical _____ Confirmed · · · · · · · · · · · · · · · · · · · ☐ 2
Other _____ Unknown · · · · · · · · · · · · · · · · · · · ☐ 3

18. Remarks: Briefly describe aspects of the investigation not covered above, such as unusual age or sex distribution: unusal circumstances leading to contamination of food, water, epidemic curve; etc. (Attach additional page if necessary)

(206-225)

Name of reporting agency: (226)

Investigating offical: Date of Investigation:

NOTE: Epidemic and Laboratory Assistance for the investigation of a foodborne outbreak is available upon request by the State Health Department to the Centers for Disease control, Atlanta, Georgia 30333

To improve national surveillance, please send a copy of this report to: **Enteric Diseases Branch**
Bacterial Diseases Division
Center for Infectious Diseases
Centers for Disease Control
Atlanta, Georgia 30333

Submitted copies should include as much information as possible, but the completion of every item is not required.

CDC 52.13 (back)
REV. 9/83

Fig. 32-3. This is an example of a questionnaire developed by the Centers for Disease Control and Prevention to be used in foodborne disease outbreaks.
Source: Reference: Centers for Disease Control and Prevention. Guidelines for confirmation of bloodborne-disease outbreaks: appendix A. *MMWR.* 1996;45(SS-5):56–57.

does not require a preapproved protocol in most circumstances. However, human experimental testing consisting of invasive procedures or procedures having risks greater than that encountered in daily life would require a research protocol approved by an Institutional Review Board.[52] Investigations using surveys containing questions on sensitive subjects (eg, sexual history, drug or alcohol consumption, illegal activities) also are subject to the federal policy for protection of human subjects and may require voluntary informed consent. Title 45 of the Code of Federal Regulations Part 46 Subpart A-D establishes Institutional Review Boards as the approval authority for research conducted by federal agencies or other institutions conducting research supported by federal funds. Current military regulations and service clinical investigation consultants should be consulted to ensure compliance with both regulatory and ethical standards.

Plan for Administrative and Logistical Considerations

Following the initial in-brief, the investigation team needs to provide the local chain of command with regular updates on the progress of the investigation. A local command liaison should attend all team meetings and can expedite obtaining additional supplies or other administrative support. This should obviate the need for daily meetings of the team with the local commander, who will be kept informed by his or her liaison. Periodic meetings with the commander can then occur as dictated by progress in the investigation. The team leader will determine the specific type and magnitude of additional help needed based on the level of expertise available locally. The specific number of personnel needed by discipline (eg, lab technician, data entry clerk, nurse interviewers) should be assessed. Resources can include both military and civilian public health officials. The Army has the Epidemiologic Consultant Service (EPICON), the US Public Health Service has investigation teams from the CDC using Epidemic Intelligence Service officers, and states have various capabilities within state and local health departments. Reporting of diseases to military health authorities and to state health departments as required by law must also not be forgotten.

The team leader must establish clear operational priorities and then ensure a systematic and orderly progress of the investigation in all areas: clinical, laboratory, environmental, and epidemiologic. Tracking the status and progress of the simultaneous actions taking place is one of the biggest challenges for the leader. Logging all decisions and delegating specific taskings at team meetings are tools the leader can use to help keep the investigation team on track. The team cannot afford the time to follow each phase of the investigation sequentially to completion before beginning to pursue knowledge in another area. The purpose of the multidisciplinary consultant team is to allow each expert to concentrate on those factors within his or her discipline that may have contributed to the event under investigation. Reference materials and experts should be consulted as new facts emerge. Working as a team adds the necessary intellectual synergy to the complex investigation process. At each team meeting, investigators assimilate new data resulting from the efforts of their colleagues. The ensuing discussion should result in productive, thoughtful analysis. But many decisions will still have to be made with inconclusive or inadequate data. Laboratory analysis is frequently still incomplete when critical decisions have to be made. The team leader's fund of clinical and epidemiologic knowledge and his or her experience in making judgement calls in these high-pressure public health emergencies will be of the utmost value. The team leader must continually synthesize new data as they accrue, keep all phases on track, and direct the future lines of inquiry of the investigation. The team leader should seek advice from the off-site consultant on a daily basis, but the team leader on-site must have ultimate decision-making authority for the team.

Suspicion of a biological warfare attack mandates additional immediate responses: reporting to local military police and to the Federal Bureau of Investigation.[47] Rapidity of communicating this suspicion up the military chain of command is especially critical in a theater of operation. The Federal Bureau of Investigation is responsible for crisis management, which includes actions taken before an incident to avert it. The Federal Emergency Management Agency is in charge of consequence management or actions taken after the incident to mitigate its effects.[53] Department of Defense staff are key players in both phases of operations precipitated by such incidents. Because terrorism generates panic in a population, coordination to establish an emergency operations center and to enhance security must be one of the initial steps taken. Ongoing communication between law enforcement officials and health authorities is critical to the optimal investigation and management of such incidents. Rapid transport of specimens to the US Army Research Institute of Infectious Diseases, US Navy Medical Research Center, and the CDC is vital to obtain an accurate, rapid diagnosis where biological attack is a consideration.

Identify Medical Treatment Resources

Field triage sites, outpatient clinics, emergency rooms, and hospitals that can receive and treat potential cases should be identified and a list of them provided to the team public affairs officer for distribution to the media. This will allow the investigation team to focus on conducting the investigation and making appropriate prevention and control recommendations. Clinicians should be notified when to expect cases and briefed on presumed condition, appropriate diagnostic evaluation, treatment regimens, and any recommended isolation precautions. Education of medical staff may be needed to update them on rare conditions or to explain occupational risks and precautions warranted. Guidelines for transfer or evacuation of patients to the next echelon of care should be established and the referral center identified. If the saboteur used a biological agent, there will probably be an immediate clamor for large quantities of medical supplies, such as antibiotics or vaccines, for which only limited quantities exist.[12] The priority of use and specific distribution plans for these limited resources should be addressed.

Reevaluate Controls Measures in Place

This periodic reassessment of preventive medicine controls should include degree of compliance and adequacy of the initial guidelines in view of the latest information. The team must determine the need for additional strategies and resources, whether personnel or supplies. The need to open an additional unit or an entire field hospital should be assessed. The need for any product recall should also be assessed. The initiation and timing of such actions require considerable judgement to weigh the preponderance of the evidence, the strength of the hypothesized association, and the severity of the risk to individuals if a recall is delayed. Such decisions may have great economic impact on an industry. Epidemiologists must balance the need to warn the public against the damage of falsely accusing an industry or other postulated source. Unfounded allegations could result in unnecessary economic losses, such as occurred to the California strawberry industry during the cyclosporiasis outbreaks.[54] Mistakes in identifying etiological agents may also lead to the loss of public confidence in future public health warnings.

TEST THE HYPOTHESIS

At this point in the investigation, investigators have postulated risk factors and developed a hypothesis that explains the source, mode of transmission, and duration of the epidemic. Hypotheses are now tested by determining whether or not a statistical association exists between two categories: exposure (eg, to a specific food or chemical) and clinical outcome (eg, illness or injury). The analysis of the results collected to date and the statistical testing of these results will determine the accuracy of the hypothesis specifying a risk factor to be the cause of the epidemic.

Collect Data and Specimens

Follow-up of the clues provided from the description of the epidemic by person, time, and place, and laboratory analysis should result in confirmation of the diagnosis. All possible cases should be identified. Both cases and appropriate controls should be interviewed and given the survey tool to obtain data that will establish risk factors. From these data and the environmental evaluation, the mechanisms of transmission are determined. The cross-sectional or case-control data collected must be analyzed. Investigators should calculate attack rates of symptomatic disease from the suspected risk factors. If food is the suspected exposure and a suspected dining facility serves multiple meals, meal-specific attack rates should be calculated first. To do this, investigators must know the number of cases and controls who did and did not eat the specific meals being compared. When a single suspect meal is obvious (eg, a banquet), investigators can initially calculate the food-specific attack rates. Similarly they must determine the number of cases and the number of controls who did and did not eat the specific food item in question. Investigators compare the rates of illness for those who were and were not exposed via consumption of a particular food or drink item by calculating the differences between the disease attack rate for those who did eat the food item and those who did not. The food item that shows the greatest percentage difference is the most likely source. Combining attack rates is often useful (eg, potatoes and gravy, ice cream and chocolate sauce, ice and water). The highest attack rates will be observed in all combinations involving the suspected food. Cumulative food attack rates may be calculated when a specific food is served on more than one occasion to the same population of people. Next is the calculation of the difference between cumu-

TABLE 32-4

SHIGELLA DYSENTERIAE TYPE 2 OUTBREAK, CHI SQUARE AND P VALUES FOR COMMON FOOD ITEMS

Food	Cases		Controls		Chi Square	*p* Value
	Ate	Did Not Eat	Ate	Did Not Eat		
Salad	80	9	35	26	21.38	0.0001[*]
Grilled sandwich	27	62	28	33	3.78	0.0520
Fruit cocktail	11	78	8	53	0.02	0.8913
Ice	56	33	33	28	1.17	0.2799
Water	27	62	12	49	2.14	0.1435
Soft Drink	41	48	30	31	0.14	0.7076
Punch	19	70	9	52	1.04	0.3086
Lemonade	9	80	10	51	1.29	0.2559
Iced tea	6	83	2	59	0.86	0.3538
Milk	52	37	20	41	9.53	0.0020[*]
Coffee/tea	17	72	15	46	0.65	0.4202
Hot chocolate	4	85	2	59	0.14	0.7090
French fries	31	58	20	41	0.07	0.7951
Ice cream	50	39	24	37	4.10	0.0428[*]

[*]*p* Value < .05
Source: Centers for Disease Control. Hospital-associated outbreak of *Shigella dysenteriae* type 2—Maryland. *MMWR.* 1983;32:250–252.

lative attack rates for each specific food between cases and controls. Then a statistical test is applied to determine if there are significant differences between foods as a risk factor for the illness. Tests used for these purposes include chi-square and Fischer's Exact Test for individual food comparisons as shown in Table 32-4. Other risk measures investigators may apply are odds ratios with confidence intervals for univariate and stratified Mantel-Haenszel analyses. In a case-control design, investigators can study the discordant exposures of cases. Testing a hypothesis using data from a case-control design can be an extremely powerful tool to identify a contaminated vehicle when dealing with mega-outbreaks. A single case-control study of 15 matched pairs provided the evidence implicating the ice cream in the massive salmonellosis outbreak referred to previously. This association was demonstrated 10 days before the isolation of the organism from the ice cream.[41] Control measures were taken based on this statistical association before laboratory confirmation, thus preventing many additional cases.

Because factors other than the etiological risk factor may affect outcome, a stratified analysis is sometimes required. This involves examining the exposure–disease association within different categories of a third factor. The third factor is referred to as the confounder. This is an effective method for looking at the effects of two different exposures on the disease, and it is one way to tease apart association with multiple factors, such as two foods. The most common method used to control for confounding is to stratify the data and then compute measures that represent weighted averages of the stratum-specific data using methods such as the Mantel-Haenszel formula.[55] The Mantel-Haenszel formula was used to analyze the data from the shigella outbreak to differentiate among salad, milk, and ice cream as the etiological agent (Table 32-5).

Stratification is also used to assess effect modification or interaction. Effect modification refers to the situation in which the degree of association between an exposure and an outcome differs in different subgroups of the population. Evaluation for effect modification is accomplished by determining whether the stratum-specific odds ratios differ from one another. There are more complete discussions of analysis strategies for outbreak investigations elsewhere.[56]

TABLE 32-5

SHIGELLA DYSENTERIAE **AND CONSUMPTION OF SALAD, MILK, AND ICE CREAM**

Rate	Salad	Milk	Ice Cream
Crude odds ratio	6.60	2.89	1.98
MH OR adjusted for salad, 95% (CL)	—	2.29 (1.10-4.77)	1.65 (0.80-3.41)
MH OR adjusted for milk, 95% (CL)	5.87	—	—
MH OR adjusted for ice cream, 95%(CL)	5.99 (2.49-14.42)	—	—

MH: Mantel-Haenszel
OR: odds ratio
CL: confidence limits
Source: Centers for Disease Control. Hospital-associated outbreak of *Shigella dysenteriae* type 2—Maryland. *MMWR.* 1983;32:250–252.

Determine the Need for Additional Studies and Analysis

If the results of the investigation thus far have not yielded a definitive diagnosis and a presumed mechanism of disease transmission, then additional investigation is indicated. A more detailed questionnaire may be needed to elucidate new details. More sensitive or sophisticated laboratory testing or additional environmental consultation may be necessary. Investigators should consider whether the initiation of carriage studies in controls or other populations at risk would be helpful. Successful outbreak investigations will frequently depend on the critical integration of epidemiologic and laboratory sciences. The application of molecular techniques to analyze epidemiologic interrelationships has led to the use of the term molecular epidemiology. Traditional laboratory methods to characterize epidemic strains have relied on the measurement of phenotypes, such as antibiotic resistance, phage typing, or serotyping. Plasmid profile analysis was the first molecular tool to fingerprint bacteria. The newer techniques can potentially type any strain by using the chromosomal DNA present in all bacteria and fungi. Genomic (chromosomal) digests, restriction fragment length polymorphisms (RFLPs), and PFGE analyze differences in chromosomal DNA organization.[57] The PFGE is increasingly being viewed as a new gold standard for the epidemiologic analysis of nosocomial infection,[58] and applications to disease outbreaks caused by bacterial contamina-

tion of food will become routine in the future. Molecular biology will often be key to identifying previously unknown infectious disease agents, as in the case of human ehrlichiosis.[59] Molecular biological methods may be used to determine early in the investigation whether a single strain or type of microorganism is responsible for the majority of cases. Linkage to a single strain suggests that patients were exposed to a common source or reservoir. Molecular analysis of dengue viruses was a useful adjunct to the epidemiologic investigation of virus distribution over distance and time in US personnel in Somalia.[60] Molecular techniques can be applied to the study of reservoirs of infection and to trace the modes of transmission.

Epidemiologists must be willing to reject early theories if initial hypothesis testing is not statistically significant. Examination of alternative hypotheses to explain investigation findings is the next step. The process is iterative in nature, as a hypothesis is tested and rejected and then followed by new planning to explore alternative explanations for the event under study.[61] Subsequent studies may involve additional data collection before testing the next hypothesis under consideration. Subsequent iterations of this process should accurately determine the true risk factors or etiology. Initial investigations of three outbreaks of infection with *Cyclospora* attributed the risk to consumption of strawberries at special events. However, this was inconsistent with the observation that while cases occurred primarily in the eastern United States, most strawberries are grown in the western United States. Further investigation showed that raspberries from Guatemala (sometimes served with strawberries) were the actual vehicle.[62] Even if the data collected are sufficient, a more sophisticated analysis method, such as logistic regression, may be required to identify the underlying association.

Evaluate the Adequacy of the Case Definition

Case confirmation by laboratory testing permits evaluation of the sensitivity and specificity of the definition used during the outbreak investigation. Additional systematic studies may attempt to find more cases, obtain more data, (clinical, laboratory, or epidemiologic), or both. Use of serologic data and clinical history may improve the case definition and clarify the population at risk for disease. Repeat interviews of confirmed cases may reveal quantitative data on exposure dose. If multiple working case definitions were used, the sensitivity of each case definition can now be compared (eg, definite versus probable, primary versus secondary).

Establish Criteria for Deciding the Outbreak Is Under Control

Surveillance to find new cases as they occur should be ongoing. The investigators should have established numerical criteria for determining that the outbreak is under control. They must consider whether this is a complete return to preoutbreak levels or whether it is the expected small numbers of cases that will occur as the final contacts of cases in a propagated epidemic pass through the incubation period window. In almost all cases of infectious disease outbreaks and in selected occupational clusters, some type of surveillance sys-

tem should be established to monitor the situation for a specified period following the outbreak. Ascertaining cases of gastroenteritis appearing at sick call in a field unit following a foodborne epidemic or monitoring wound infections by surgeon or operating room in certain nosocomial outbreaks are typical examples.

To ensure a smooth transition from the consultant team to local health workers, special care should be taken to hand off responsibilities and follow-on investigation taskings (eg, laboratory results follow-up, new surveillance activities). Timing and details of the transition should be clearly delineated before the team departs.

COMPARE RESULTS TO THOSE OF THE PUBLISHED LITERATURE

After the field investigation and the subsequent analysis are complete, it is important to thoughtfully compare the findings with those conducted previously and recorded in the medical literature. Frequently the introduction of new diagnostic

methods or technological advances in the interim will have allowed a new understanding of pathophysiological mechanisms that can help explain associations. New insights or the validation of new approaches should be published.

FINALIZE A REPORT WITH RECOMMENDATIONS TO CONTROL FURTHER SPREAD

Write an Executive Summary and Prepare a Complete Report

Updating local health officials and local command authorities on the investigation results is essential before the team's departure. This out-briefing should include diagnosis, risk factors, presumed etiology, treatment, environmental controls, surveillance plan, diagnostic improvements, and additional preventive measures for the future. This preliminary report may be oral but must be followed by a written summary. A final executive report summary written in language appropriate for nonmedical commanders should be provided to the local commanders of the site and unit involved. A more detailed final report should be prepared after all the analyses are completed. This final report should define the problem, describe the methods used in the field investigation, display the epidemiologic analysis, discuss the results, and present the final conclusions and recommendations. It should be submitted to the appropriate medical authorities.

This documentation of the epidemic and the investigation findings is important for possible future use to support or justify changes in public health decisions. In certain situations, rapid publication of preliminary results in the *Morbidity and Mortality Weekly Report* or internal organizational publications is important to alert health care providers or health authorities of apparent new risks or diseases. Rapid initial disease report summaries may also serve to alert civilian physicians to potential problems, such as malaria, in redeploying service members.[63]

Evaluate the Effectiveness of Recommendations

An assessment plan to evaluate the effectiveness of control procedures and recommendations should be part of the final report. Specific surveillance for the disease or condition of interest following the departure of the team is critical. Active surveillance is preferred over passive surveillance to detect any subsequent outbreaks, as well as to evaluate the effect of the control measures.

SUMMARY

Epidemiology is the fundamental science of public health, and outbreak investigation is the most visible example of applied field epidemiology. Results from field studies are critical to finding effective interventions for disease control. The great epidemiologic challenge of today is the development of

new tools, such as molecular epidemiology, to apply to the investigation of emerging infections. Thoughtful, careful investigation will continue to be necessary to identify new pathogens, find their natural reservoirs, and determine their routes of transmission. This will not be easy. For example, despite the occurrence of outbreaks of Ebola hemorrhagic fever in the past few decades, the virus's natural reservoir remains unknown, and concern about the possibility of airborne transmission remains.[64]

Reductions in public health infrastructure and the complexities associated with outsourcing of clinical care and certain public health functions all compound the problem of outbreak detection and control. Military preventive medicine specialists affected by military medical downsizing will be challenged to meet the need for rapid-response, multidisciplinary teams to direct investigations of highly dynamic events. These challenges call for the rapid adoption of new technology for team communication, field laboratory analysis, specimen holding and processing, and further automation of data analysis. As the scope of potential problems increases, major new prevention modalities (eg,

food irradiation) will be adopted and will need to be evaluated. Vital partnerships between the Department of Defense, the CDC, the National Institutes of Health, the Food and Drug Administration, the Department of Agriculture, the Environmental Protection Agency, and the World Health Organization will have to be productive, cooperative relationships with clearly delineated roles and responsibilities to achieve maximum efficiency and effectiveness. Telecommunication, telemedicine, and computer modeling need to be evaluated as potential additions to the suitcase of the shoeleather epidemiologist, who is now working on outbreaks that can spread over continents. Ultimately, the outcome of these futuristic investigations should be the same as those of today: new health policies for prevention based on supportive data proven valid by rigorous hypothesis testing.

REFERENCES

1. Rammelkamp CH, Wannamaker LW, Denny FW. The epidemiology and prevention of rheumatic fever. *Bull NY Acad Med*. 1952;28:321–334.

2. Joseph PR, Millar JD, Henderson DA. An outbreak of hepatitis traced to food contamination. *N Engl J Med*. 1965;273:188–194.

3. Wallace MR, Garst PD, Papadimos TJ, Oldfield EC. The return of acute rheumatic fever in young adults JAMA. 1989;262:2557–2561.

4. Duchin JS, Koster FT, Peters CJ, et al. Hantavirus pulmonary syndrome: a clinical description of 17 patients with a newly recognized disease. *N Engl J Med*. 1994;330:950–955.

5. Bell BP, Goldoft M, Griffin PM, et al. A multistate outbreak of *Escherichia coli* O157:H7-associated bloody diarrhea and hemolytic uremic syndrome from hamburgers: the Washington experience. *JAMA*. 1994;272:1349–1353.

6. Centers for Disease Control and Prevention. Update: outbreaks of *Cyclospora cayetanensis* infections—United States and Canada, 1996. *MMWR*. 1996;45:611–612.

7. Feighner BH, Pak SI, Novakoski WL, Kelsey LL, Strickman D. Reemergence of *Plasmodium vivax* malaria in the Republic of Korea. *Emerg Infect Dis*. 1998;4:295–297.

8. Bjorkman A, Phillips-Howard PA. The epidemiology of drug-resistant malaria. *Trans R Soc Trop Med Hyg*. 1990;84:177–180.

9. Frieden TR, Sterling T, Pablos-Mendez A, Kilburn JO, Cauthen GM, Dooley SW. The emergence of drug-resistant tuberculosis in New York City. *N Engl J Med*. 1993;328:521–526.

10. Foege WH. Alexander D. Langmuir—his impact on public health. *Am J Epidemiol*. 1996;144(8):S11–S15.

11. Okumura T, Takasu N, Ishimatsu S, et al. Report on 640 victims of the Tokyo subway sarin attack. *Ann Emerg Med*. 1996;28:129–135.

12. Henderson DA. Bioterrorism as a public health threat. *Emerg Infect Dis*. 1998;4:488–492.

13. Centers for Disease Control. Case definitions for infectious conditions under public health surveillance. *MMWR*. 1997;46(RR-10):1–58.

14. Wegman DH, Woods NF, Bailar JC. Invited commentary: how would we know a Gulf War syndrome if we saw one? *Am J Epidemiol*. 1997;146:704–711.

15. Hyams KC, Roswell RH. Resolving the Gulf War syndrome question. *Am J Epidemiol*. 1998;148:339–342.

16. Davis JP, Chesney PJ, Wand PJ, LaVenture M. Toxic-shock syndrome: epidemiologic features, recurrence, risk factors, and prevention. *N Engl J Med*. 1980;303:1429–1435.

17. Gray GC, Knoke JD, Berg SW, Wignall FS, Barrett-Connor E. Counterpoint: responding to suppositions and misunderstandings. *Am J Epidemiol*. 1998;148:328–333.

18. Olson PE, Bone WD, LaBarre RC, et al. Coccidioidomycosis in California: regional outbreak, global diagnostic challenge. *Mil Med*. 1995;160:304–308.

19. Last JM, ed. *A Dictionary of Epidemiology*. 3rd ed. New York: Oxford University Press, 1995.

20. Croft A, Smith H, Creamer I. A pseudo-outbreak of skin disease in British troops. *J R Soc Med*. 1996;89:552–556.

21. Dunn D. Health care 1999: a national bellwether. *J Health Care Finance*. 1996;22(3):23–27.

22. Burki DR, Bernasconi C, Bodmer T, Telenti A. Evaluation of the relatedness of strains of *Mycobacterium avium* using pulsed-field gel electrophoresis. *Eur J Clin Microbiol Infect Dis*. 1995;14:212–217.

23. Wurtz R, Demarais P, Trainor W, et al. Specimen contamination in mycobacteriology laboratory detected by pseudo-outbreak of multidrug-resistant tuberculosis: analysis by routine epidemiology and confirmation by molecular technique. *J Clin Microbiol*. 1996;34:1017–1019.

24. Whelen AC, Persing DH. The role of nucleic acid amplification and detection in the clinical microbiology laboratory. *Annu Rev Microbiol*. 1996;50:349–373.

25. Centers for Disease Control and Prevention. Outbreaks of pseudo-infection with Cyclospora and Cryptosporidium—Florida and New York City, 1995. *MMWR*. 1997;46:354–358.

26. Centers for Disease Control. Recommendations for collection of laboratory specimens associated with outbreaks of gastroenteritis. *MMWR*. 1990;39(RR-14):1–13.

27. Longfield JN, Winn RE, Gibson RL, Juchau SV, Hoffman PV. Varicella outbreaks in Army recruits from Puerto Rico: varicella susceptibility in a population from the tropics. *Arch Intern Med*. 1990;150:970–973.

28. Jones WHS, ed. *Hippocrates: Airs, Waters, Places*. Cambridge, Mass: Harvard University Press; 1948.

29. Centers for Disease Control. Hospital-associated outbreak of *Shigella dysenteriae* type 2—Maryland. *MMWR*. 1983;32:250–252.

30. Centers for Disease Control. Acute rheumatic fever among Army trainees—Fort Leonard Wood, Missouri, 1987–1988. *MMWR*. 1988;37:519–522.

31. Pan American Health Organization. *Guidelines for the Establishment of Systems for the Epidemiological Surveillance of Food-borne Diseases and the Investigation of Outbreaks of Food Poisoning*. PAHO, Division of Communicable Diseases Prevention and Control; 1993.

32. *Laboratory Sample Submission Guide*. Ft. Sam Houston, Tex: Dept of Defense Veterinary Laboratory; 1998.

33. DeFraites RF. *Preliminary Report of* Campylobacter enteritis *Outbreak*. Washington, DC: Walter Reed Army Institute of Research; 1990. Memorandum, 14 June 1990.

34. International Association of Milk, Food and Environmental Sanitarians. *Procedures to Investigate Waterborne Illness*. 2nd ed. Des Moines, Iowa: IAMFES; 1996.

35. Blacklow NR, Greenberg HB. Viral gastroenteritis. *N Engl J Med*. 1991;325:252–264.

36. Centers for Disease Control and Prevention. Surveillance for waterborne-disease outbreaks—United States, 1993–1994. *MMWR*. 1996;45(SS-1):1–33.

37. Wenzel RP. A new hantavirus infection in north America. *N Engl J Med*. 1994;330:1004–1005.

38. Kahn HA, Sempos CT. *Statistical Methods in Epidemiology*. New York: Oxford University Press; 1989.

39. MacDonald KL, Osterholm MT. The emergence of *Escherichia coli* O157:H7 infection in the United States: the changing epidemiology of foodborne disease. *JAMA*. 1993;269:2264–2266.

40. Tauxe RV. Emerging foodborne diseases: an evolving public health challenge. *Emerg Infect Dis*. 1997;3:425–434.

41. Hennessy TW, Hedberg CW, Stutsker L, et al. A national outbreak of *Salmonella enteriditis* infections from ice cream. *N Engl J Med*. 1996;334:1281–1286.

42. Blaser MJ. How safe is our food? Lessons from an outbreak of salmonellosis. *N Engl J Med*. 1996;334:1281–1286.

43. Centers for Disease Control and Prevention. Hepatitis A associated with consumption of frozen strawberries—Michigan, March 1997. *MMWR*. 1997;46:288,295.

44. Kolavic SA, Kimura A, Simons SL, Slutsker L, Barth S, Haley CE. An outbreak of *Shigella dysenteriae* type 2 among laboratory workers due to intentional food contamination. *JAMA*. 1997;278:396–398.

45. Torok TJ, Tauxe RV, Wise RP, et al. A large community outbreak of salmonellosis caused by intentional contamination of restaurant salad bars. *JAMA*. 1997;278:389–395.

46. Wiener SL, Barratt J. Biological warfare defense. In: *Trauma Management for Civilian and Military Physicians*. Philadelphia: WB Saunders; 1986: 508–509.

47. McDade JE, Franz D. Bioterrorism as a public health threat. *Emerg Infect Dis*. 1998;4:493–494.

48. Meselson M, Guillemin V, Hugh-Jones M, et al. The Sverdlovsk anthrax outbreak of 1979. *Science*. 1994;266:1202–1208.

49. Nozaki H, Hori S, Shinozawa Y, et al. Secondary exposure of medical staff to sarin vapor in the emergency room. *Intensive Care Med*. 1995;21:1032–1035.

50. Aiken LR. *Questionnaires and Inventories: Surveying Opinions and Assessing Personality*. New York: John Wiley & Sons; 1997.

51. Aday L. *Designing and Conducting Health Surveys*. 2nd ed. San Francisco: Jossey-Bass Publishers; 1996.

52. Levine RJ. *Ethics and Regulation of Clinical Research*. 2nd ed. Baltimore: Urban & Schwarzenberg Publishers; 1986.

53. Presidential Decision Directive 39; 1996.

54. Osterholm MT. Cyclosporiasis and raspberries—lessons for the future. *N Engl J Med*. 1997;336:1597–1599.

55. Schlesselman JJ. *Case Control Studies: Design, Conduct, Analysis*. New York: Oxford University Press; 1982.

56. Gregg MB. *Field Epidemiology*. New York: Oxford University Press; 1996.

57. Barg NL. An introduction to molecular hospital epidemiology. *Infect Control Hosp Epidemiol*. 1993;14:395–396.

58. Goering RV. Molecular epidemiology of nosocomial infection: analysis of chromosomal restriction fragment patterns by pulsed-field gel electrophoresis. *Infect Control Hosp Epidemiol*. 1993;14:595–600.

59. Tompkins LS. The use of molecular methods in infectious diseases. *N Engl J Med*. 1992;327:1290–1297.

60. Kanesa-thasan N, Chang GJ, Smoak BL, Magill A, Burrous MJ, Hoke CH Jr. Molecular and epidemiologic analysis of dengue virus isolates from Somalia. *Emerg Infect Dis*. 1998;4:299–303.

61. Reingold AL. Outbreak investigations—a perspective. *Emerg Infect Dis*. 1998;4:21–27.

62. Herwaldt BL, Ackers ML, et al. An outbreak in 1996 of cyclosporiasis associated with imported raspberries. *N Engl J Med*. 1997;336:1548–1556.

63. Centers for Disease Control and Prevention. Malaria among U.S. military personnel returning from Somalia, 1993. *MMWR*. 1993;42:524–526.

64. Breman JG, van der Groen G, Peters CJ, Heymann DL. International Colloquium on Ebola Virus Research: summary report. *J Infect Dis*. 1997;176:1058–1063.

Chapter 33

EPIDEMIOLOGIC MEASUREMENT: BASIC CONCEPTS AND METHODS

LYNN I. LEVIN, PhD, MPH

L.I. Levin; Division of Preventive Medicine, Walter Reed Army Institute of Research, Silver Spring, MD 20910-7500

INTRODUCTION

This chapter will provide the public health professional with the basic tools and concepts of epidemiology. The target audience is the military practitioner of public health who may be deployed or working in a public health setting where surveillance activities or rudimentary research studies are needed. The epidemiologic methods covered in this chapter are at the elementary level and are presented from the more simple concepts to the more complex. Other chapters in this volume specifically address outbreak investigations and surveillance activities (see chapters 31, Disease and Nonbattle Injury Surveillance: Outcome Measures for Force Health Protection, and 32, Outbreak Investigation). The epidemiologic tools that are used to conduct these activities are presented here. The focus is on data collection methods that are necessary to run programs, assess outbreaks, allocate resources, or perform other activities that are related to the formulation of public health policy and practice.

DEFINITION OF EPIDEMIOLOGY

Epidemiology is the study of the distribution and determinants of disease, injury, or health-related factors in human populations.[1] In contrast to clinical medicine, which focuses on the individual, epidemiology evaluates groups of people or populations. A basic premise of this discipline is that diseases, injuries, or other medical conditions are not randomly distributed across populations but rather vary according to factors such as environmental exposures (eg, deployment history) or personal characteristics (eg, smoking status). As early as the 5th century BC, Hippocrates hypothesized that the development of human diseases may be associated with the environment.[2] The goal of the epidemiologist is to determine who becomes ill and why, and this is accomplished by comparing groups with differing characteristics.

BASIC MEASURES OF DISEASE FREQUENCY

Epidemiology is a quantitative science. One of the fundamental measures used by epidemiologists is the rate of disease. By computing rates, it is possible to compare two populations or groups. A rate requires consideration of the population from which the cases are derived:

$$\text{Rate} = \frac{\text{Number of Events}}{\text{Population at Risk of Event}}$$

Typically, the denominator is the total population at risk of disease, and the numerator is the number of people with disease. The rate is usually expressed in some conventional base, such as events per 1,000 individuals. There are several types of rates used in epidemiology to describe morbidity and mortality.

Prevalence

A commonly used measure in epidemiology is the prevalence rate. Although it has historically been called a rate, prevalence is a proportion representing the fraction of the population that has a disease at a single point in time. It is a snapshot of the burden of disease in a defined population and includes both new and existing cases. Thus, prevalence depends on both the incidence of new cases of disease and the duration of disease in those cases. This measure typically is used to assess the need for and costs of health services.

$$\text{Prevalence} = \frac{\text{Number of Existing Cases of Disease at a Given Time}}{\text{Total Population at a Given Time}}$$

For example, a 15% prevalence of rash-associated illness in units of an Army support battalion in Operation Joint Endeavor, Bosnia, was determined in this way[3]:

$$\text{Prevalence} = \frac{69 \text{ Cases of Rash-associated Illness}}{466 \text{ Deployed Unit Members}}$$
$$= 0.148 = 15\%$$

Incidence Rate

Incidence describes the rate of development of a disease or a medical condition in a population over a period of time, that is, the occurrence of new events in a specified time period. This measure is used to evaluate the causal or etiologic role of risk factors and the development of disease.

$$\text{Cumulative Incidence Rate} = \frac{\text{Number of New Cases During a Specified Period}}{\text{Total Population at Risk of the Disease During that Period}}$$

This measure is called the cumulative incidence rate because it accumulates the number of cases over time that derive from the population at risk determined at the beginning of the time period (ie, fixed population with the assumption that no individuals are lost to follow-up). The denominator contains the count of people. Cumulative incidence is a proportion that ranges from 0 to 1 (assuming only one possible occurrence of the disease per person). When reporting a cumulative incidence, the time frame must be specified. Attack rates are a measure of cumulative incidence.

For example, in a study among US Army soldiers in infantry basic training, 303 individuals were followed for 12 weeks of training to determine the incidence of training-related injuries. Of the 303 soldiers, 112 developed one or more lower extremity musculoskeletal injuries.[4]

Cumulative Incidence Over a 12-week Period

$$= \frac{112 \text{ Soldiers Injured}}{303 \text{ Soldiers in Basic Training}}$$
$$= 0.369 = 37\%$$

Another measure of incidence is the incidence density rate. This is a measure of the instantaneous rate of development of a disease in a population.

Incidence Density Rate

$$= \frac{\text{Number of New Cases of a Disease During a Specified Period}}{\text{Total Person-time of Observation During the Given Time Period}}$$

The numerator of the incidence density is the number of new cases occurring in the population (the same as in the cumulative incidence). The denominator, however, is the sum of each person's time at risk or the sum of the time that each person was under observation and susceptible to the disease rather than the count of individuals at the beginning of the follow-up period. Thus, this measure can incorporate data from a dynamic population: individuals who are followed for various periods of time or who are lost to follow-up. An incidence density rate must include the relevant time units in the denominator, such as person-days or person-

years. In calculating person-time, following 10 individuals for 3 years (30 person-years) is equivalent to following one individual for 30 years. Incidence density can range from zero to infinity.

For example, in a study of the incidence of HIV-1 infection in the US Army during the period 1 November 1985 to 31 October 1993, a total of 1,061,768 active-duty soldiers were followed for a total of 3,629,688 person-years of follow-up. During the period of the study, 978 soldiers with HIV-1 seroconversion were identified.[5]

Incidence Density Rate

$$= \frac{978 \text{ HIV-1 Soldiers}}{3,629,688 \text{ Person-years}}$$
$$= 2.7/10,000 \text{ Person-years}$$

Prevalence and incidence measures are interrelated. When the incidence rate has been constant over time (a "steady state" situation), the duration of disease has remained unchanged, and the prevalence of disease overall is low, then the prevalence (P) equals the product of the incidence density (I) and the average duration ($\overline{D}$):

$$P = I \bullet \overline{D}$$

If two of these measures are known, the third can be calculated.

Incidence density rates, like other rates, can be calculated for subpopulations, such as different age, sex, or race-ethnic groups. The following is an age-specific incidence rate:

Age-specific Incidence Rate

$$= \frac{\text{Number of New Cases in a Specified Age Group}}{\text{Total Person-years of Observation for the Age Group}}$$

For example, the incidence rate of HIV-1 infection among 20- to 24-year-olds in the study[5] cited above was determined in this way:

Age-specific Incidence Rate for Ages 20 to 24

$$= \frac{405 \text{ HIV-1 Soldiers}}{1,216,125 \text{ Person-years Among Soldiers Aged 20 to 24}}$$
$$= 3.3/10,000 \text{ Person-years}$$

Mortality Rate

Incidence rates describe the incidence of disease in a population, whereas mortality rates describe the incidence of death in a population. The crude mortality rate can be determined using this equation:

Crude Mortality Rate

$$= \frac{\text{All Deaths in a Calendar Year}}{\text{Total Population at Risk of Death During Year}}$$

$$\bullet \ 10^n$$

For example, the following is the crude non–battle-related mortality rate among deployed servicemembers to the Persian Gulf region, 1 August 1990 to 31 July 1991.[6]

Crude Mortality Rate

$$= \frac{\text{225 Nonbattle-related Deaths}}{\text{264,868 Person-years in the Persian Gulf Region}}$$

$$= 85/100{,}000 \text{ Person-years}$$

The cause-specific mortality rate is determined in a similar fashion:

Cause-specific Mortality Rate

$$= \frac{\text{Number of Deaths from a Specific Cause in a Year}}{\text{Total Population During the Year}}$$

A cause-specific mortality rate was determined for motor vehicle mortality among deployed servicemembers to the Persian Gulf region for the period 1 August 1990 to 31 July 1991[6]:

Cause-specific Mortality Rate

$$= \frac{\text{62 Deaths Due To Motor Vehicle Accidents}}{\text{264,868 Person-years in the Persian Gulf Region}}$$

$$= \frac{23}{100{,}000 \text{ Person-years}}$$

All of these measures of morbidity and mortality are used to monitor disease trends in surveillance activities, identify outbreaks, and plan and evaluate health services.

DIRECT METHOD OF RATE ADJUSTMENT

Rate adjustment allows the public health officer to compare rates of disease or injury in two communities that have different demographic characteristics, such as different age distributions or race-ethnic compositions. Because incidence rates or mortality rates typically vary by age and race, it is necessary to adjust or standardize these rates by these factors so that the rates can be compared on equal terms. Adjusted rates are artificial in that they are only used for comparison purposes and do not describe a particular

population. The process of adjusting rates requires the use of a standard population with which both communities are compared and data on the factor-specific rates of disease in both communities. If, for example, injury rates in the Army are to be compared with injury rates in the Navy, these rates would have to be adjusted for age and sex, because the composition of the two services differs in these factors. Texts such as Kahn and Sempos[7] or Selvin[8] have examples on how to perform a direct age adjustment.

TYPES OF VARIABLES

Categorical Variables

In addition to obtaining information on rates of disease, epidemiologic studies can also collect information on many variables about individuals.

Variables that are divided into categories or are assigned codes are called categorical variables. Each category is defined and there are a limited number of values that can be measured. Dichotomous variables are categorical variables that assume only two values, such as male and female or inducted into military services and not inducted. Polychomotous variables can be divided into more than two categories,

such as race and cause of death. Some discrete variables can be ordered or ranked. Examples of ordered variables are severity of pain (eg, mild, moderate, intense) and military rank.

Continuous Variables

Variables that can be measured on a continuous scale, such as height or 1-mile run times, are considered continuous variables. The values that these variables can assume are only limited by the level of accuracy of the scale on which they are measured.

SUMMARY STATISTICS FOR CATEGORICAL AND CONTINUOUS VARIABLES

Categorical Variables

Discrete data can be summarized by calculating frequencies, proportions, or percentages. A proportion is the number of people with a characteristic divided by the total number of people. The percentage is a proportion multiplied by 100.

Continuous Variables

Measures of Central Tendency

There are three main measures of central tendency to describe the distribution of a continuous variable. The arithmetic mean, is calculated as the sum (Σ) of all of the observed values (x_i) divided by the total number of observations (n):

$$\overline{x} = \frac{\sum_{i=1}^{n} x_i}{n}$$

The mode is the most frequently observed value. The third measure, the median, is the midway point of a series of numbers such that 50% of the numbers are above the value and 50% are below. For an odd number of entries, the median is the middle number. For an even number of entries, it is the average of the two middle numbers. If the distribution is fairly symmetric, then the median value will be close to the mean value. If the distribution is skewed, then the median value is a better measure of central tendency than the mean.

Measures of Variation or Dispersion

The range is the difference between the highest and lowest values. The standard deviation estimates the amount of variability in a set of numbers. It is defined as the square root of the sum of the squared deviations from the mean, divided by the number of observations minus 1.

$$\text{Standard Deviation} = s = \sqrt{\frac{\sum_{i=1}^{n} \left(x_i - \overline{x}\right)^2}{n-1}}$$

The larger the standard deviation, the more variable or nonhomogenous the distribution. Statistical theory states that a population with a normal distribution of values will have a characteristic bell-shaped curve. Since the shape of this frequency distribution is symmetrical, the mean, median, and mode are the same. With normally distributed data, the standard deviation describes the width of the curve. The range of values one standard deviation above and below the mean will include 68% of the observations. The range of values two standard deviations above and below the mean will include 95% of the observations. The range of values three standard deviations above and below the mean will encompass over 99% of the observations. Exhibit 33-1 contains an example illustrating how to calculate a standard deviation.

METHODS FOR DISPLAYING DATA

Tables

A concise way to summarize data is to present the data in a table. Tables typically contain frequency data on a range of values for discrete variables or summary statistics for continuous variables. A contingency table is used to summarize counts of people or observations. The number of rows and columns in the table represent the various levels of two variables. A particular type of contingency table, the 2 x 2 table or 4-fold table, is used for dichotomous variables such as exposed or nonexposed and diseased or nondiseased. Examples of 2 x 2 tables are presented later in this chapter.

The title of the table should be clear and contain enough information on the who, when, and where of the study that the reader does not have to refer to the text to understand the table. Rows and columns should be clearly labeled. Footnotes are often used to clarify headings or abbreviations.

Graphs

Displaying data graphically is another effective way to summarize information. The type of data dictates the type of graph that should be used. The x-axis, also known as the horizontal axis or abscissa, typically represents the values of the variable of interest. The y-axis, also known as the vertical axis or ordinate, displays the number of cases, the rate of disease, or some other measure of the frequency of occurrence. As with a table, a graph should be clearly labeled (including a legend if it displays more than one factor) so that the reader does not have to read the accompanying text to interpret the graph.

EXHIBIT 33-1

A HYPOTHETICAL EXAMPLE TO CALCULATE MEASURES OF VARIATION OR DISPERSION

To determine the age as well as other demographic characteristics of female applicants to military service, a survey was conducted at a Military Entrance Processing Station. The ages of the first seven women chosen for the sample were 18, 19, 19, 20, 21, 22, and 24 years. For this example:

Mean = $\bar{x}$ = (18 + 19 + 19 + 20 + 21 + 22 + 24) / 7 = 20.4

Mode = 19

Median = 20

Range is 18 to 24 (6 years)

The standard deviation is calculated in the following way:

x_i	$\bar{x}$	$x_i - \bar{x}$	$(x_i - \bar{x})^2$
18	20.4	−2.4	5.76
19	20.4	−1.4	1.96
19	20.4	−1.4	1.96
20	20.4	−0.4	0.16
21	20.4	0.6	0.36
22	20.4	1.6	2.56
24	20.4	3.6	12.96
			25.72

$$s = \sqrt{\frac{\sum_{i=1}^{n}\left(x_i - \bar{x}\right)^2}{n-1}} = \sqrt{\frac{25.72}{6}} = 2.1$$

Pie Graph

A pie graph or chart displays data in a circular fashion, comparing parts or segments of the data to the whole. Data are converted into percentages, adding up to 100%. The percentages are converted to degrees by multiplying the percentage by 3.6 (Figure 33-1).

Bar Graph

Discrete data can be displayed in a bar graph. An important feature of a bar graph is that the bars do not touch. The data are noncontinuous and the only possible values are the ones that are noted by each bar (Figure 33-2).

Histogram

Continuous data can be displayed in a histogram. The bars in a histogram touch because the data on the x-axis are continuous and each bar represents an interval of values and not just one value. If all bars represent intervals of the same width, then the height of each bar represents the relative frequency of each interval. The histogram provides a visual picture of the shape of the frequency distribution (Figure 33-3).

Arithmetic Scale Line Graph

A line graph is typically used when the x-axis represents time and the y-axis represents rates of disease. Each axis is measured in arithmetic units, with equal distances between the units (Figure 33-4).

Semilogarithmic Scale Line Graph

In a semilogarithmic scale line graph, the y-axis is based on a logarithmic scale and the x-axis on an arithmetic scale. When displaying rates of disease, it is useful to use semilogarithmic graphs because a straight line indicates a constant rate of change,

the slope of the line indicates the rate of increase or decrease, and parallel lines represent identical rates of increase or decrease (Figure 33-5).

SAMPLING

A critical component of any study design is the method used for selecting the study population. The target population is that group of individuals from which inferences about disease patterns are to be drawn. Typically, it is not possible or efficient to obtain data on all members of the target population. Instead, sampling procedures are used to select a suitable sample or subset of the target population.

In a probability sample, every individual has a known (usually equal) probability of being included in the sample. Therefore, generalizations to the target population can be made with a measurable amount of precision and confidence. In a nonprobability sample, probability theory may not apply and there is more opportunity for bias in selection of subjects.

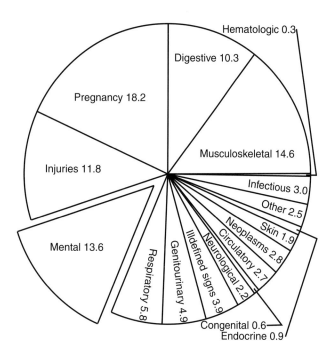

Fig. 33-1. Each wedge in this example of a pie graph represents percent of hospitalizations by 17 major diagnostic categories for active duty soldiers in 1997.
Source: Trends in hospitalizations due to mental disorders, US Army active duty soldiers. *Medical Surveillance Monthly Report.* 1998;4(5):15.

Nonprobability Sampling Designs

Consecutive Sampling

With this design, every individual in a given setting who meets the selection criteria is chosen over a specified time period. A consecutive sample can be drawn, for example, by using every recruit in-processing at a basic training post in a defined time period. If all individuals are studied in a given time period, the sample may be a good representation of the overall population, but there is no known probability of any given individual being included in the sample.

Convenience Sampling

Individuals from a population who are readily available are included in a convenience sample. Examples of convenience samples include sailors in a clinic waiting room or soldiers entering the post exchange. Selecting such a sample is inexpensive and easy. Results from this type of survey may be biased, however, as there is no assurance that individuals in this sample reflect the characteristics of the target population. At times, this method is used to obtain preliminary data or to generate hypotheses for future studies.

Judgmental Sampling

With this technique, individuals are handpicked to be in the study. Specific individuals are chosen for the sample because they are considered to be representative of the population of interest or possess specific selection criteria. The dangers of bias using this method can easily go unrecognized.

Quota Sampling

The composition of the survey population in this method is determined in advance. Then quotas are determined for individuals from various demographic categories, such as age and race. The only requirement is that the specified number of individuals in a given category be recruited. The basis for the quotas and the method of recruitment often

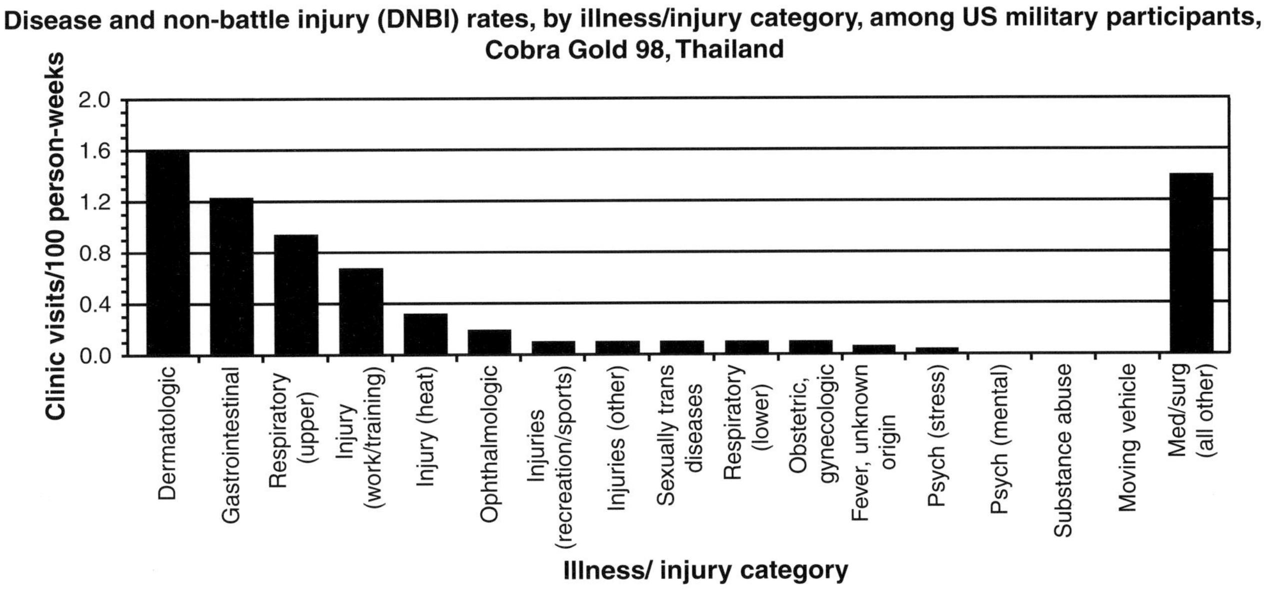

Disease and non-battle injury (DNBI) rates, by illness/injury category, among US military participants, Cobra Gold 98, Thailand

Fig. 33-2. This example of a bar graph shows the disease and nonbattle injury rates for US military participants in the Cobra Gold 98 exercise (Thailand). The data have been divided by illness and injury category.
Source: Morbidity surveillance during a joint multinational field training exercise (Operation Cobra Gold 98), Thailand. *Medical Surveillance Monthly Report.* 1998;4(6):3.

leads to bias since people are excluded from the study because of convenience factors in finding the designated number of subjects.

Probability Sampling Designs

Simple Random Sampling

The most elementary type of probability sample is the simple random sample. In this design, each person has an equal chance of being selected for the sample from the population under study. To select a random sample, the first step is obtaining a list of all individuals in the population. Each individual (or household or other basic unit) is called a sampling unit. A sampling frame is the list of all the sampling units in the study population. At times, it may be very difficult to generate such a list. Telephone directories or personnel lists are examples of lists that may be used. It is important to consider possible inaccuracies in a given list. If the list is incomplete or not updated regularly, then a biased sample may be drawn. Once the list is obtained, each person is assigned a number and the numbers are then selected at random, usually using a table of random numbers. The sample then consists of the sampling units that are selected. By chance, even a simple random sample may not adequately represent the underlying target population.

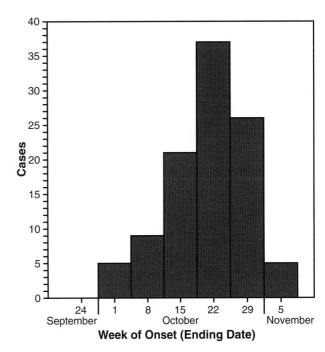

Fig. 33-3. This example of a histogram shows cases of febrile illness among US military personnel in Haiti from September 18, 1994, to November 5, 1994. The height of each bar represents the frequency. (The graph excludes three cases for which dates on onset were unknown.)
Source: Centers for Disease Control and Prevention. Dengue fever among U.S. military personnel—Haiti, September-November, 1994. *MMWR.* 1994;43:845–848.

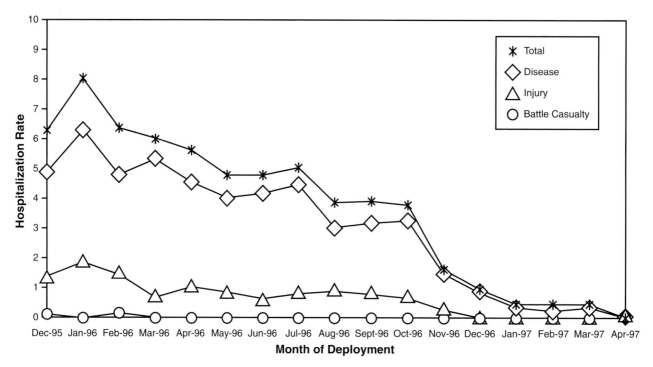

Fig. 33-4. This example of an arithmetic line graph shows monthly active duty hospitalization rates for disease, injury, battle casualty, and the total rates in Operation Joint Endeavor (Bosnia) from December 1995 to April 1997. Source: *Medical Surveillance Monthly Report.* 1997;3(2):8.

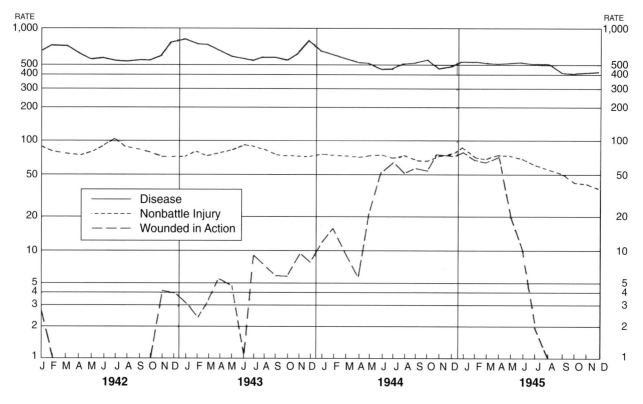

Fig. 33-5. This example of a semi-logarithmic scale line graph shows monthly admission rates for disease, nonbattle injury and wounded in action worldwide from 1942 to 1945 among US Army troops. Source: Lada J, Reister FA, eds. *Medical Statistics in World War II.* Washington, DC: Office of the Surgeon General, Department of the Army; 1975: frontispiece.

Systematic Sampling

This technique is more widely used than simple random sampling because it does not require a complete listing of the study population or sampling frame. For a systematic sample, a fraction of the population to be studied is chosen. Instead of using a table of random numbers, the investigator chooses every k^{th} individual. If one-tenth of the population is to be surveyed, then every tenth person in a sequence will make up the study population. To begin the selection, a random starting point is chosen. For example, a systematic sample of pregnant soldiers who deliver in a medical treatment facility could be selected such that every 5th woman admitted to the maternity ward over a specified time period is included. Knowledge about all women who are admitted over a given time period is not necessary. In fact, it would be impossible to generate such a listing of these women before the study begins. To obtain an unbiased sample with this method, there must not be any periodic ordering of the sampling units.

Stratified Sampling

In a stratified random sample, the population is divided into distinct subgroups or strata based on important characteristics, such as age or race, and then a simple random sample or systematic sample is selected within each stratum. An individual only appears in one stratum, and each stratum is designed to be homogeneous with respect to the characteristic being studied. This technique is frequently used to increase the numbers of persons from a specific stratum of the population and therefore may improve the efficiency of the sampling design.

Cluster Sampling

In cluster sampling, the population is divided into large subgroups or clusters that are not homogeneous in composition. The clusters then become the sampling unit and a random sample of clusters is obtained. All persons in the cluster are in the study or a random sample of individuals from the cluster may be drawn. The entire population does not have to be enumerated in advance. For example, logistically it may be too difficult to obtain a random sample of soldiers engaged in a field operation. However, it may be possible to select a random sample of Army units and then randomly select soldiers from those units. This technique is used for conducting immunization surveys in developing countries.

Multistage Sampling

Multistage sampling is more complicated than other sampling methods and involves randomly choosing, in stages, a series of clusters or subunits of a population. For example, multistage sampling would be useful when conducting a survey in an Army division on the use of personal protective measures. The first stage in this sampling scheme, or the primary sampling unit, may be a simple random sample of the battalions in the division. Then, the second stage, or the secondary sampling unit, would consist of a simple random sample of the companies within the selected battalions (a smaller cluster). The tertiary sampling unit would be a random sample of the platoons within the chosen companies. Then, within the platoon selected, a random sample of soldiers would be taken. An advantage of this scheme is that complete enumeration is necessary only for each chosen platoon.

Standard Error

A standard deviation is the spread of individual observations around the mean in a single sample. The standard error is the standard deviation of the means of repeated samples randomly drawn from the same population. The standard error (SE) of a mean of the simple random sample is calculated as follows:

$$\text{Standard Error of the Sample Mean} = \text{SE} = \frac{s}{\sqrt{n}}$$

where s is the estimated standard deviation from the sample and n is the sample size.

When a sample is chosen in an unbiased fashion, then the only source of error is random variation. The size of the sample and the heterogeneity of the population influence this variation. In an unbiased sample, as the sample gets larger, it is more likely that the sample estimate will be close to the value obtained for the target population. In other words, the larger the sample, the more precise the estimate will be. A precise estimate gives a value that is likely to be repeated if the sampling were done again and again. A smaller standard error implies greater precision and results from a larger sample.

Sampling can become quite involved and may require expert assistance in the planning stages of a study. The calculation of the standard error for the other probability sampling techniques becomes quite complex. With each technique, the investigator must be aware of biases that may be introduced in the selection of a study population. A large sample size will not correct for a biased sample, and the standard error reflects only random variation and does not address bias.

The costs involved in obtaining a sample may limit the investigator's choice of sampling method. These costs must be balanced against the efficiency of the design. In general, the method that produces a smaller standard error for a given cost should be used. Further discussion of sampling techniques can be found elsewhere.[7]

MAJOR TYPES OF STUDY DESIGNS AND MEASURES OF ASSOCIATION USED IN EPIDEMIOLOGY

Much of epidemiology assesses the relationship between exposures or risk factors and disease or injury occurrence. In experimental studies, the investigator has control over some factor or exposure that can be altered. This variation in an exposure can then be associated with different outcomes. A specialized form of the experimental approach is the randomized clinical trial. Such studies rarely are feasible during a combat deployment. In contrast, training exercises commonly present opportunities to conduct clinical trials, as noted in a study to determine the efficacy of new treatments for diarrhea.[9]

The vast majority of epidemiologic investigations rely on the observational approach. With this approach, there is no manipulation of a risk factor, but rather the risk factors are evaluated as they vary naturally from one individual to another. Different outcomes are then observed under natural conditions. Control of extraneous variables is accomplished in the design of the study or in data analysis. Observational studies can be descriptive or analytic. Descriptive studies characterize the distribution of disease in terms of attributes of person, place, and time. Analytic studies attempt to evaluate disease associations with specific factors. An important component of these designs is the availability of a comparison or control group.

Case Series

Case series, also known as case reports, are collections of notable cases, which, for example, may present at a medical clinic during deployment. Case series also can result from medical surveillance activities. They do not constitute an analytic study as there is no comparison or control group, nor are they good as descriptive studies since they do not report disease rates. They can, however, provide insight into potentially important characteristics of the disease. For example, several soldiers with acute respiratory disease (ARD) were discovered at Fort Dix in 1976, one of whom subsequently died. Further investigations determined that a new type of influenza, swine influenza A, was the cause of this morbidity and mortality.[10]

Ecological Studies

In a study with an ecological design, data are not collected on specific individuals, but rather aggregate data are collected on groups of individuals. These studies also are known as correlational studies because a characteristic of a group usually is plotted against a characteristic of another group. An international comparison of risk factors and disease based on country-level data is an example of the type of data used for ecological analyses. Such analyses are usually done as a first step in assessing whether a public health problem may exist. Interpreting these data can be difficult as an undefined factor, on which data were not collected, may explain the observed association. Moreover, because the data are grouped, it is not known whether the individuals with the disease are the same individuals exposed to the risk factor. For example, an ecologic study was conducted to evaluate the relationship between alcohol consumption levels and mission readiness indicators among shipboard sailors. Data on alcohol consumption and various medical and legal indicators of mission readiness were not obtained on the same individual. Rather aggregate data based on the platforms ships were used in the analysis.[11]

Descriptive Studies

Descriptive studies describe the prevalence, incidence rate, or mortality rate of disease in a population according to characteristics of person (Who gets the disease?), place (Where do they live or work or travel?), and time (When does the disease occur?). Who gets a disease can be described by factors such as age, sex, rank, military occupational specialty, unit, or immunization status. Where disease is found can be addressed by information on international, national, or local comparisons; urban and rural differences; travel history; and altitude or climate. Information on how the pattern of disease changes with time (secular trends) or the impact of seasonal fluctuations describe when the illness occurs. Results from descriptive studies are used to assess the need for health services and to generate hypotheses about factors that may cause disease. The etiologic importance of these factors can be further evaluated using other study designs. For example, a medical surveillance system was used to track weekly incidence rates of disease and non-battle injuries among multinational peacekeepers deployed to Haiti in 1995. Results from the surveillance system were used to direct health care resources to prevent and treat casualties.[12]

Cross-Sectional Studies

Cross-sectional studies, also known as prevalence surveys, examine the relationship at one point in time between risk factors, such as environmental exposures or demographic factors, and existing disease. A problem with the interpretation of findings from a cross-sectional study is that it can be difficult to determine the sequence of events. For example, if results from a cross-sectional survey showed that a measure of stress was associated with duodenal ulcers, it cannot be assumed that the stress preceded the onset of ulcers since both the risk factor and the disease were evaluated at the same time. Conceivably, the ulcers might have been responsible for the stress rather than the reverse. For some exposures that do not vary with time, such as genetic factors, a cross-sectional study can provide meaningful information on an exposure–disease relationship. This study design is also useful for studying chronic conditions, such as arthritis or chronic respiratory disease, where the onset of disease is difficult to determine. A cross-sectional study is the only one that estimates the prevalence of disease, an important measure for health care planning purposes. Because these studies determine prevalence rather than incidence of disease, they can provide only limited information on etiologic factors. Individuals who are surviving with disease are included in cross-sectional studies and individuals who have a rapid recovery or die quickly from the disease are often not included and thus are underrepresented. Results from these studies, however, can be further evaluated in cohort and case-control studies.

In 1990, Smoak and colleagues[13] conducted a cross-sectional study of healthy young adults (404 females and 534 males) at induction into the US Army at Fort Jackson, SC. Serum collected on all individuals was used to determine the seroprevalence of *Helicobacter pylori* infection. Demographic data were abstracted from accession records. The associations between antibody levels and several demographic factors were then assessed.

Case-Control Studies

The defining feature of a case-control study is that study subjects are selected as individuals with disease (cases) and without disease (controls), then data on past exposures that pertain to etiologic factors are collected in both groups. Cases can be ascertained from several sources, including hospitals, outpatient clinics, and disease surveillance activities. Possible sources of controls include hospital patients who do not have the disease of interest, friends or relatives of the case, and a random sample of a population such as servicemembers living in the same barracks or assigned to the same unit.

There are several methodological concerns and potential biases that must be considered when conducting a case-control study. It is assumed that the cases are representative of or include all cases that come from the source population and the controls are representative of all people without disease in the same source population. The definition of a case must be clearly specified with criteria for who is eligible to be included in the study. It is preferable to include only incident cases rather than prevalent cases, so that factors that are associated with the occurrence of disease can be evaluated rather than factors that are associated with surviving with the disease. Because exposure is determined after the identification of disease, there is the potential bias that cases may recall events differently than controls or that an interviewer may query cases differently than controls. To obtain better comparability of cases and controls and to control for potential confounding, cases and controls may be "matched" on characteristics such as age or sex that are already known to be associated with both exposure and disease. Confounding and potential biases are discussed in greater detail later in this chapter.

Although exposure is ascertained after the onset of disease in case-control studies, there are several reasons why case-control studies are desirable. These studies generally require fewer resources, fewer study subjects, and less time to collect data compared with cohort studies, which are described later in the chapter. They also are more feasible for the study of rare diseases (Exhibit 33-2).

Calculation of the Odds Ratio

When the exposure information and disease status are coded as dichotomous variables, the data from a case-control study can be arrayed in a 4-fold or 2 x 2 contingency table. The table in Exhibit 33-3 summarizes the essential data obtained in a case-control

EXHIBIT 33-2

ADVANTAGES AND DISADVANTAGES OF A CASE-CONTROL STUDY

Advantages

- Smaller number of study subjects required compared to cohort studies

- Relatively inexpensive

- Relatively quick results

- Several exposures can be evaluated

- Efficient for studying rare diseases

- Efficient for studying diseases with long latency

Disadvantages

- Temporal relationship between exposure and disease may be difficult to establish

- Possible bias in the selection of cases and controls

- Possible bias in ascertainment of exposure (recall bias)

- Cannot calculate incidence rates individually for exposed and unexposed groups (estimates only the ratio)

study. A relative risk (RR), also known as a rate ratio, is defined as the risk of disease in the exposed divided by the risk of disease in the nonexposed and cannot be directly calculated using data from a case-control study because the incidence of disease cannot be determined. In fact, during the design of a case-control study, the investigator arbitrarily determines the estimated number of cases to be studied.

An estimate of the RR, known as the odds ratio (OR), can be calculated.[14] An odds is defined as the likelihood of an event happening versus the likelihood of the event not happening. According to the notation in Exhibit 33-3, the odds of exposure in cases is given by this formula: $(a/a + c)/(c/a + c) = a/c$. Similarly, the odds of exposure in controls is b/d. Therefore, an odds ratio is defined in this way:

$$OR = \frac{\text{Odds of Exposure Among the Diseased}}{\text{Odds of Exposure Among the Nondiseased}}$$
$$= (a/c)/(b/d) = ad/bc$$

An RR and an OR are known as "measures of association" as they measure the association between an exposure and disease. An RR and an OR of greater than one implies a positive association of the disease with exposure to the factor (ie, exposure leads to an increased risk of disease). An RR and an OR of less than one implies a negative asso-

EXHIBIT 33-3

HOW TO CALCULATE AN ODDS RATIO

Risk Factor	Disease		
	Cases	Controls	
Exposed	a	b	a + b
Nonexposed	c	d	c + d
	a + c	b + d	

a = the number of individuals who are exposed and have the disease

b = the number of individuals who are exposed and do not have the disease

c = the number of individuals who are nonexposed and have the disease

d = the number of individuals who are nonexposed and do not have the disease

EXHIBIT 33-4

AN EXAMPLE OF THE CALCULATION OF AN ODDS RATIO

	Cases	Controls
Ever in Vietnam	45	145
Never in Vietnam	172	454

Odds ratio = ad/bc

= (45 x 454)/(145 x 172)

= 20,430/24,940

= 0.82

Source: Kang H, Enzinger FM, Breslin P, Feil M, Lee Y, Shepard B. Soft tissue sarcoma and military service in Vietnam: a case-control study. *J Natl Cancer Inst.* 1987;79:693–699. Published erratum: *J Natl Cancer Inst* 1987;79:1173.

ciation of the disease with exposure to the factor
(ie, exposure leads to a decreased risk of disease or
has a protective effect against disease). Finally, an
RR and an OR of one implies no association between
disease and exposure to the factor. Thus, the RR
indicates the strength of the association between a
factor and a disease and is an important measure
in studies of disease etiology.

For example, a case-control study was conducted
to examine the association of soft tissue sarcomas
with military service in Vietnam by interviewing
217 men with soft tissue sarcoma and 599 controls.[15]
The data collected and the odd ratio that can be
calculated from them are shown in Exhibit 33-4.

Based on these data, Vietnam veterans had a
lower risk of soft tissue sarcomas than those men
who had never served in Vietnam, as the OR is less
than one. These data can also be interpreted by stating that there was an 18% lower risk of sarcoma in
men who served in Vietnam compared with men
who did not serve in Vietnam.

Cohort Studies

Cohort studies also have been referred to as incidence, prospective, follow-up, or longitudinal
studies. Typically a group of individuals (a cohort)
that is free of the disease under investigation is assembled, evaluated to determine exposure history
and other risk factors, and then followed forward
in time to determine the occurrence of disease. Some
designs provide for repeated examinations of study
subjects over the course of the follow-up period. The
development of disease is then observed in the various exposure groups. Incidence of disease can be
calculated for those who have been exposed to a
risk factor and for those who have not. If the entire
cohort has been exposed, then the cohort can be
compared with the general population or some
other nonexposed comparison group or well-studied cohort. A critical feature of this design is the
comparison between a group of individuals defined
as exposed and a group defined as nonexposed. A
major strength of cohort studies is that the exposure is ascertained before the onset of disease. Other
advantages of the cohort design include the ability
to calculate incidence rates directly in the exposed
and nonexposed populations and to evaluate several disease outcomes in relation to the defined exposures. These studies, however, are often costly,
require large numbers of subjects, may require a
long follow-up period, and are subject to attrition
problems (known as "lost to follow-up") that can bias

EXHIBIT 33-5

ADVANTAGES AND DISADVANTAGES OF A COHORT STUDY

Advantages

- Ideal time sequence (exposure precedes disease)
- Lack of bias in the measurement of exposure
- Several disease outcomes can be evaluated
- Efficient for studying rare exposures
- Yields incidence rates in the exposed and unexposed populations

Disadvantages

- Often impractical for studying rare diseases
- Long follow-up period may be required for outcomes with long latency
- Relatively expensive
- Problem of loss of subjects to follow-up
- Exposure levels may change over time, requiring sophisticated follow-up and analysis

---

the generalizability of results (see Exhibit 33-5).

Cohort studies also can rely on historical records.
This design is sometimes referred to as a noncon-
current follow-up study or a historical cohort study.
For example, a cohort of Navy shipyard workers in
the 1940s could be assembled based on personnel
records and then divided into asbestos exposure
groups based on job title. These workers could then
be followed to the present for outcomes such as lung
cancer. An important limitation in this design might
be the absence of data on smoking exposure since
this information might not have been captured in
the historical records.

Calculation of the Risk Ratio and Rate Ratio

In a cohort study, the ratio of two proportions
(based on cumulative incidence data) is called a risk
ratio (Exhibits 33-6a and 33-6b), while the ratio of
two rates (based on incidence density sampling) is

EXHIBIT 33-6a

HOW TO CALCULATE A RISK RATIO

The RR based on cumulative incidence data from a cohort study can be readily calculated using a 2 x 2 table:

Risk Factor	Disease		
	Yes	No	
Exposed	a	b	$a+b=N_1$
Nonexposed	c	d	$c+d=N_0$
	$a+c=M_1$	$b+d=M_0$	

Risk Ratio = $[a/(a + b)]/[c/(c + d)]$

EXHIBIT 33-6b

HOW TO CALCULATE A RATE RATIO

The RR for data based on incidence density rates is displayed in the following way (where PT stands for person-time):

Risk Factor	Disease	
	Yes	
Exposed	a	PT_1
Nonexposed	c	PT_0

Rate Ratio = $(a/PT_1)/(c/PT_0)$

called an incidence rate ratio (IRR). The RR and IRR do not measure the probability that someone with a risk factor will develop disease; they compare the risk or rate of disease in an exposed group with the risk or rate of disease in a nonexposed group. The calculation of the IRR is illustrated in Exhibit 33-7. In a historical cohort study at four Army training centers during a 47-month period, incidence rates of febrile acute respiratory disease (ARD) were compared between basic trainees in modern, energy-efficient barracks and those in old barracks. These data were collected at Fort Jackson, South Carolina. These data show that the crude rate of ARD among basic trainees at Fort Jackson who lived in the modern barracks is 1.45 times greater than the rate of ARD among basic trainees who lived in the old barracks.

Attributable Risk in the Exposed Group

In addition to the RR, the attributable risk in the exposed group (AR_e) also can be calculated from a cohort study. The AR_e, also known as the risk difference or excess risk, is defined as the rate of disease in the exposed group minus the rate in the nonexposed

EXHIBIT 33-7

AN EXAMPLE OF THE CALCULATION OF A RATE RATIO

Risk Factors	Admissions for Acute Respiratory Disease at Fort Jackson, 1982-1986		
	Yes		Person-time
Modern Barracks	3,355		451,294 trainee-weeks
Old Barracks	3,312		647,056 trainee-weeks
Total	6,667		1,098,350 trainee-weeks

$$\frac{\text{Rate of Disease in Modern Barracks}}{\text{Rate of Disease in Old Barracks}} = \frac{3,355/451,294}{3,312/647,056} = \frac{.00743}{.0051} = 1.45$$

Source: Brundage JF, Scott RM, Lednar WM, Smith DW, Miller RN. Building-associated risk of febrile acute respiratory diseases in army trainees. *JAMA.* 1988;259:2108–2112.

group. From the example shown in Exhibit 33-7, the rate difference was calculated in this way:

AR_e = Incidence Rate in Exposed − Incidence Rate in Nonexposed

$$= 3,355/451,294 - 3,312/647,056$$

$$= .00743 - .00512 = 0.0023$$

$$= .23 \text{ admissions}/100 \text{ trainee-weeks at Fort Jackson}$$

This is the excess amount of disease over baseline (estimated by using the nonexposed rate) that is attributed to the exposure. Thus, this measure answers the question, "In Army trainees who live in modern barracks, how many of the admissions for ARD are attributed to living in modern barracks?" If this exposure is eliminated, then the attributable risk is the amount of decrease in the disease rate that is expected.

The attributable risk proportion is the proportion of the incidence in the exposed population that is attributed to the exposure. It also can be presented as a percent ($AR_e\%$). This measure defines the percentage of disease in an exposed population that would be prevented by eliminating the exposure.

$$AR_e\% = \left(\frac{\text{Incidence Rate in Exposed Group} - \text{Incidence Rate in Nonexposed Group}}{\text{Incidence Rate in Exposed Group}} \right) \bullet 100$$

Using the data presented above,

$$AR_e\% = \left(\frac{.00743 - .00512}{.00743} \right) \bullet 100 = 31\%$$

This formula can also be calculated using the RR:

$$AR_e\% = ([RR-1]/RR) \bullet 100 = [(1.45-1)/1.45] \bullet 100 = 31\%$$

The attributable risk percent (but not the attributable risk itself) also can be calculated using the OR generated from a case-control study.

Attributable Risk in the Total Population

The population attributable risk (PAR) is the incidence of disease in the total population that is attributed to the exposure. Since this measure is based on the total population, it takes into account both exposed and nonexposed individuals. Using the data obtained from Fort Jackson, the PAR is calculated in this way:

PAR = Incidence in the Total Population − Incidence in the Nonexposed Group

$$= 6,667/1,098,350 - 3,312/647,056$$

$$= .00607 - .00512$$

$$= .00095$$

$$= .95 \text{ admissions per } 1,000 \text{ trainee-weeks}$$

The incidence in the total population must be known to use this formula. The population attributable risk percent (PAR%) is the percent of the incidence in the total population that is attributed to the exposure and can be calculated by the formula:

$$PAR\% = \left(\frac{\text{Incidence in the Total Population} - \text{Incidence in Nonexposed Group}}{\text{Incidence in the Total Population}} \right) \bullet 100$$

From the above example,

$$PAR\% = \left(\frac{.00005}{.00607} \right) \bullet 100 = 16\%$$

It can also be calculated using the RR and an estimate of the proportion of the population that has the exposure (p_e):

$$PAR\% = p_e(RR-1)/[p_e(RR-1) + 1]$$

$$p_e = \frac{451,294}{1,098,350} = 0.41$$

$$\frac{.41(1.45-1)}{.41(1.45-1) + 1} = \frac{.185}{1.185} \bullet 100 = 16\%$$

If the OR is used, then the proportion exposed in the control group is substituted for the proportion exposed in the population at large. Other terms that are used to describe this measure are the attributable fraction in the population or etiologic fraction in the population. This measure answers the question, "What proportion of ARD admissions at Fort Jackson can be attributed to living in modern barracks?"

Measures of attributable risk assume that there is a causal relationship between exposure and disease and, therefore, should be calculated only when there is sufficient evidence to imply causality.

Experimental Studies and Randomized Clinical Trials

The major type of experimental study in medicine is the clinical trial. In a controlled clinical trial, the investigator manipulates or intervenes with one group (the treatment group) and withholds intervention or gives a placebo to another group. Random allocation of patients to various treatment or nontreatment groups is the central tenet of randomized clinical trials. The randomization of patients attempts to make the groups comparable at the onset of the study, so any differences noted between the two groups can be ascribed to the intervention. This design is commonly used for testing drugs or vaccines, but it can be used to test any intervention against a control. Examples of studies done during US military deployments include the treatment of traveler's diarrhea with ciprofloxin and loperamide[9] and the efficacy trial of doxycycline chemoprophylaxis against leptospirosis.[16] The reader is referred to other texts[17] for further discussion of this study design.

BIAS

Definition

Bias is manifest in a study when study results differ systematically from the true values. It is also known as systematic error, as opposed to random error or chance. Bias can be introduced at any stage of an investigation, including the design, the conduct, or the inferences drawn from the results. Because of this systematic error, the strength of an association can be underestimated or overestimated. Types of bias in epidemiologic studies can be broadly classified into selection bias, information bias, and confounding. As the field of epidemiology has evolved and study designs have become more elaborate, new types of bias have been described.[18] The following is a listing of some of the more common types of selection bias and information bias that can be found in epidemiologic studies.

Types of Selection Bias

Ascertainment Bias

This bias is the systematic error that arises from the method used to identify individuals for a study. In cohort studies, selection bias occurs if individuals are included in the study based on their disease status. In case-control studies, selection bias occurs if the likelihood an individual is selected for study is based on exposure status. For example, an outbreak investigation may base conclusions on cases that are not very ill, as these patients may be more willing to participate and be available for an interview. These milder cases of disease may differ from more serious cases with respect to exposure factors.

Healthy Worker Effect

Individuals who are employed or are inducted into military service are more physically fit and healthier than the general population, resulting in lower disease rates when compared with the total population.

Volunteer Bias

This error is the result of systematic differences between study subjects who volunteer to participate in a study or who return a questionnaire and those who do not.

Types of Information Bias

Detection Bias

This is a systematic error due to methods of diagnosis or verification of cases. For example, a pathologist may make the diagnosis for some cases, while the diagnosis of other cases is based solely on medical records.

Interviewer Bias

This systematic error is the result of interviewers not questioning study subjects in a uniform manner.

Measurement Bias

This bias arises from inaccurate quantification or classification of exposures or outcomes. It can result from the subjectivity of the measurement scale.

Recall Bias

This error is the result of differences in either the truthfulness, accuracy, or completeness of participants' recall of events. Recall bias is due to systematic differences in recall between the groups being compared and often reflects the greater thought a sick person will have given to possible explanations for his or her plight.

Avoiding or Reducing Bias

There are no statistical methods to control for selection or information bias that is introduced into a study. If a bias is present, the results of the study are very difficult to interpret. There are study design features, however, that can help reduce or avoid some biases. These include blinding the interviewers to the participant's diagnosis; blinding the volunteers in a randomized clinical trial so that they are unaware of their treatment assignment; blinding study staff who review or code data so that they are unaware of the diagnosis or treatment; achieving high response rates in studies (over 80%); comparing the characteristics of individuals who are lost to follow-up with those who remain in the study; establishing explicit criteria for assessing exposures and outcomes; obtaining information about exposures from independent sources that are unaffected by memory; and recognizing potential confounding variables and controlling for them in the design or analysis of the study (as described below). If there is concern that bias is present in a study, it is often possible to estimate the direction of the bias (ie, whether the bias results in an apparent association towards the null value of 1.0 or away from the null). In a case-control study, for example, if some cases do not recall their smoking history with the same completeness as the controls, then the smoking histories of the two groups may appear to be more similar than they are. This problem with recall would result in a bias toward the null.

Confounding

Definition

Confounding bias occurs when the observed relation between the risk factor and the outcome is distorted by the influence of a third variable, the confounder. A confounding variable must be associated with both the risk factor of interest and the outcome. Confounding can be introduced into a study because of the complex relationship between several exposures or demographic factors and the outcome. Thus, as a result of confounding, an apparent association between a specific exposure and disease may be noted when no real association exists. Confounding can also lead to an overestimate or underestimate of the true measure of association between the risk factor and the disease. Statistical tests are not used to assess whether confounding is present in a study; several other techniques (described below) are available to the investigator to assess and control confounding.

A hypothetical example adapted from a study of injury in male and female Army trainees based on cumulative incidence rates will demonstrate these concepts more clearly. Results from a cohort study

showed that female trainees were two times more likely to develop a stress fracture as compared with male trainees. The data are presented in Exhibit 33-8.

To evaluate the association between sex and training injury, factors that might confound the relationship need to be assessed. Physical fitness and various anthropometric measurements are possible confounders because these factors are known to be associated with both sex (the exposure) and stress fractures (the disease). To consider the possible confounding effect of fitness, the data shown above are stratified into tables according to the aerobic fitness of the trainee (1-mile run times). For this example, the data are divided into two tables, based on those trainees who had fast 1-mile run times and those who had slow 1-mile run times (Exhibit 33-8). The overall

---

EXHIBIT 33-8

ASSOCIATION BETWEEN SEX AND THE RISK OF STRESS FRACTURES AMONG ARMY TRAINEES

Crude

Sex	Stress Fracture		
	Yes	No	Total
Women	66	434	500
Men	52	748	800
Total	118	1,182	1,300

RR = (66/500)/(52/800) = .132/.065 = 2.0

Stratified

Trainees with fast 1-mile run times

Sex	Stress Fracture		
	Yes	No	Total
Women	6	94	100
Men	30	570	600
Total	36	664	700

RR = (6/100)/(30/600) = .06/.05 = 1.2

Trainees with slow 1-mile run times

Sex	Stress Fracture		
	Yes	No	Total
Women	60	340	400
Men	22	178	200
Total	82	518	600

RR = (60/400)/(22/200) = .15/.11 = 1.4

or crude RR is 2.0. The RRs within each stratum are both less than the crude RR and are similar to each other. Therefore, the association is uniform between the strata. If the stratum-specific RRs are averaged, then the effect of fitness level is removed (ie, controlled for). As noted above, fitness met the definition of a confounder because it was related to both sex (the exposure) and stress fractures (the disease). Among those without stress fractures, 14% (94/664) of fit trainees were women while 66% (340/518) of nonfit trainees were women. Moreover, men who were fit had a lower rate of stress fractures compared with men who were not fit [5% (30/600) versus 11% (22/200)]. These data are used later in this chapter to illustrate a common method to control for confounding in the analysis of data.

Controlling for Confounding in the Design of a Study

Randomization

Randomization is a method of allocating individuals to groups based on a predetermined plan, such as one based on a table of random numbers. The goal is to make comparison groups similar at the start of an investigation. This technique is used in clinical trials to randomly distribute study subjects between the treatment and placebo group. A major advantage of randomization is that it can control for both known and unknown confounders. The disadvantages include the difficulty in maintaining the randomization scheme once it is established.

Restriction

To control for confounding in the design of a study, participants can be restricted to a particular category of the confounding variable. For example, if smoking is a proposed confounder, then the study participants can be restricted to nonsmokers. Some problems with this approach include a reduction in the number of eligible subjects and a decrease in the generalizability of the results.

Matching

Study participants can be matched or "balanced" with respect to potential confounding variables, thereby removing the effect of confounding. This approach is frequently used in outbreak investigations and case-control studies. If a factor such as

age is already known to be related to both exposure and disease, then the cases and controls can be matched on age. Matching in this context controls for the effects of age only if the analysis stratifies on the matching factor. Once a factor is used for matching purposes, its role as an etiologic factor cannot be evaluated because the cases and controls have been chosen to be similar with respect to this factor.

In pair matching, each identified case has a corresponding control chosen from the pool of eligible controls such that the case and control pair will be similar with respect to the matching variables. During the analysis, the pair matches must be maintained. For outcome exposure variables, the McNemar's chi-square test statistic is computed. For continuous outcome variables, the paired t-test is used. Matched pair analysis may increase the statistical power of a study. As noted above, however, once a factor becomes a matching variable, the effect of this variable on disease cannot be analyzed. At times, it is difficult to find matches, and this problem can greatly increase the cost of the study. There also is the danger of overmatching, which occurs when several factors are controlled for, and differences between cases and controls are, therefore, minimized.

Frequency matching refers to matching groups on the basis of the prevalence of confounders. For example, if 25% of the cases are in the age group 20 to 24 years, then controls will be chosen such that 25% of the controls fall in this category. With frequency matching, the data must be stratified by these matching variables during the analysis. The reader is referred to Kahn and Sempos[7] or Selvin[8] for a more-detailed discussion on matching.

Controlling for Confounding in the Analysis of the Study

Stratified Analysis

Controlling for confounding during the analysis of a study can be accomplished using many different techniques. The data are divided into strata based on the confounding variable, and the analysis is done separately for each stratum. As shown in Exhibit 33-8, to assess the relationship between sex and stress fractures, the data were divided into strata based on fitness level, the confounding variable. In this example, there were two strata—fast 1-mile run times and slow 1-mile run times.

Mantel-Haenszel Summary Odds Ratio

The Mantel-Haenszel summary OR (OR_{MH}) can be used to obtain a uniform OR that takes into account the effect of the confounding. To calculate an OR_{MH}, several 2 x 2 tables (*i* tables) are constructed according to the number of levels of the stratified variable. It is assumed that the true OR in each of the tables is uniform and that the variability in the OR that is observed in each stratum-specific table is due entirely to random error. The following is the formula for OR_{MH} with the weight for each table equal to $b_i c_i / T_i$:

$$OR_{MH} = \frac{\sum a_i d_i / T_i}{\sum b_i c_i / T_i}$$

where a_i, b_i, c_i, and d_i are cell counts for the ith stratum, T_i is the total in the ith stratum and the sum is across the strata of the confounder. For cohort studies with count denominators, the RR_{MH} is calculated in this way[19]:

$$RR_{MH} = \frac{\sum a_i(c_i + d_i) / T_i}{\sum c_i(a_i + b_i) / T_i}$$

For cohort studies with person-year denominators, the IRR_{MH} is calculated in this fashion[19]:

$$IRR_{MH} = \frac{\sum a_i(PT_{0i}) / T_i}{\sum c_i(PT_{1i}) / T_i}$$

In Exhibit 33-8, where the data were stratified into two tables based on fitness level, the RR_{MH} is computed as follows:

$$RR_{MH} = \frac{[6(30 + 570)/700] + [60(22 + 178)/600]}{[30(6 + 94)/700] + [22(60 + 340)/600]} = 1.3$$

To assess the role of confounding on the relation between sex and stress fractures, the adjusted RR_{MH} of 1.3 is then compared with the unadjusted RR of 2.0. The investigator must use his or her judgment to determine if the unadjusted or adjusted RR should be reported. As a rule, if there is more than a 10% change in the RR_{MH} compared with the crude RR, then the RR_{MH} should be presented; in this example, the RR_{MH} would be reported as it is the best estimate of the association between sex and stress fractures.

Of note, if the RRs are not similar across the strata, then it is not appropriate to present a summary RR. Rather, RRs for each stratum are reported separately. This phenomenon is called interaction or effect modification. Statistical tests can be performed to determine the heterogeneity of the stratum-specific RRs. See the text by Kahn and Sempos[7] or Selvin[8] for further discussion of these methods.

Multivariate Analysis

Multiple logistic regression is another technique used to control for confounding variables. In addition to controlling for multiple confounders, this approach is also used for predictive modeling of epidemiologic data. The reader is referred to software packages such as EGRET (Statistics and Epidemiology Research Corporation, Seattle, Wash) or SAS (SAS Institute, Inc, Cary, NC) and to texts[7,8] for further discussion of these techniques.

HYPOTHESIS TESTING

Elements of Hypothesis Testing

There are several possible explanations to account for an observed increased (or decreased) RR or OR. The association could have been observed by chance. The findings could be the result of bias or confounding or both. Finally, the association could represent a cause-and-effect relationship.

The purpose of statistical hypothesis testing is to determine the role random variation or chance plays in interpreting the results of a study. Hypothesis testing is a structured process. Before a study begins, an epidemiologic question or hypothesis is formulated. The hypothesis is stated in two forms: the null hypothesis (H_0) and the alternative hypoth-

esis (H_1). The null hypothesis always states that there is no association between the risk factor and disease in the population or no difference in outcomes between the two groups compared. An example of a null hypothesis is that there is no difference in malaria risk between servicemembers who use bednets and those who do not. The alternative hypothesis always states that there is an association between the risk factor and disease in the population: that there is a difference in the risk of malaria between bednet users and nonusers. A two-sided alternative hypothesis implies that the difference may go in either direction. A one-sided alternative hypothesis states that the difference can only be in one direction, (eg, there is an increased risk of ma-

EXHIBIT 33-9

HYPOTHESIS TESTING

Conclusion from hypothesis test using the sample data	True situation in the population	
	Difference Exists (H_1)	No Difference Exists (H_0)
Difference exists (reject H_0)	Correct, Power ($1-\beta$)	Type I error, α error
No difference (do not reject H_0)	Type II error, β error	Correct

the significance level chosen for the test. For example, if the null hypothesis is rejected at the 5% level, this means that there is a 5% chance of rejecting the null hypothesis when it is true.

Type 1 error occurs when the H_0 is rejected when it is actually true. This is signified by α. An α level of 0.05 or 0.01 is often used in studies. A type II error (or β error) occurs when the study results fail to reject H_0 when it is actually false. The levels set for β typically are 0.10 or 0.20. Power, a statistical term defined as $1-\beta$, is the ability to detect a difference when a difference exists. Thus, if the β error is 0.20, then the power of a study is 80%. Generally speaking, the larger the sample size, the greater the power of a study. Exhibit 33-9 summarizes the relationship between α level and β level. Exhibit 33-10 summarizes the necessary steps in hypothesis testing.

p **Value**

The *p* value is based on the assumption that the null hypothesis is true. It reflects the probability of obtaining a measure of association such as a RR or OR as large as (or larger than) the one observed in the study if the null hypothesis is correct. A very small *p* value means that the measure of association that is observed is very unlikely if the null hypothesis is true. For example, if a statistical test is significant at a *p* value of less than 0.05, this means that under the null hypothesis less than 5% of the time a difference of the observed magnitude or greater would occur by random variation alone. It should be noted that 5% is an arbitrary cut-off point used to reject the H_0 and many epidemiologists do not place much value on $p < .05$. If the exact *p* value is reported, then the level of significance can be better assessed.

laria associated with nonuse of bednets). One-sided alternative hypotheses should be used when there is prior evidence that the difference is in only one direction and a finding in the opposite direction would not be believed.

Statistical tests are based on a null hypothesis under which any observed difference between two groups would be attributed to chance in the data. The purpose of statistical testing is to determine whether the null hypothesis can be confidently rejected. Thus, these tests determine the probability that an association as strong or stronger than the one observed could have occurred by chance alone if no association really existed. There is some probability that the null hypothesis will be rejected when, in fact, it is true. This risk is determined by

EXHIBIT 33-10

STEPS IN STATISTICAL SIGNIFICANCE TESTING

- State the hypothesis: an association exists between the factor and disease
- Formulate the null hypothesis: no association exists between the factor and disease
- Choose α and β levels
- Collect data
- Choose and apply the correct statistical test
- Determine the probability of obtaining the observed or more extreme data if null hypothesis is true
- Reject or fail to reject the null hypothesis based on observed *p* value

Confidence Interval

A confidence interval is a range of values of a measure of association, such as the RR or OR, that has a defined probability of containing the true measure. Thus, a 95% confidence interval implies that if a study is repeated 100 times, 95 times the true value of a measure such as a RR will fall within the confidence interval. Confidence intervals of 90% and 95% are commonly used. The upper and lower bounds of a confidence interval define the limits of the interval. When the 95% confidence interval does not include 1.0 (eg, the null value for a RR), then the association is considered statistically significant and has similar meaning to rejecting the null hypothesis at the p-value less than 0.05 level. In addition to providing information on the statistical significance of a test, a confidence interval conveys information on the precision of the point estimate as noted by the width of the confidence interval. The width of a confidence interval is determined both by the size of the study and the level of confidence that the investigator chooses. The larger the sample size, the more precision in the study findings. As a sample size increases, the confidence interval becomes narrower.

Confidence Interval Based on a Proportion

A prevalence can be expressed as a proportion or a percentage. The standard error for a proportion is calculated in the following way:

$$SE(p) = \sqrt{\frac{p(1-p)}{n}}$$

and the 100(1-α)% confidence interval (CI) is calculated using this formula:

$$100(1-\alpha)\% = p \pm Z_{\frac{\alpha}{2}} \bullet SE(p)$$

where p is the proportion and n is the sample size. When the sample size is large [np is ≥ 5 and n(1 – p) is ≥ 5], then p approximates a normal distribution. The critical value of the standard normal distribution associated with a specified level of confidence is z. Tables of critical values of the standard normal distribution that correspond to desired levels of confidence can be found in standard statistic textbooks. For a 95% CI, $\alpha = 0.05_{\alpha/2} = 0.025$, and $z_{.025}$ corresponds to the critical value of 1.96.

The following example illustrates how to calculate a 95% CI using prevalence data. A serologic survey of vaccine-preventable infections conducted in 1,504 US Army recruits without prior service found that 17.2% lacked measles antibody.[20] The 95% CI for this percentage was calculated in this way:

p = 0.172
n = 1,504
z = 1.96

$$SE(p) = \sqrt{\frac{p(1-p)}{n}} = SE(.172) = \sqrt{\frac{.172(1-.172)}{1,504}} = .0097$$

$$95\% \text{ CI} = p \pm 1.96 \bullet SE(p) = 172 \pm 1.96 \bullet .0097$$
$$= (.153, .192) = (15.2\%, 19.2\%)$$

Confidence Interval Based on Rate Ratio

Consider the study of building-associated risk of febrile ARD in Army trainees.[21] The IRR based on the incidence rate of ARD in trainees living in modern barracks versus old barracks in Fort Jackson was 1.45. A 95% CI for IRR can be constructed using the method shown in Exhibit 33-11 based on Woolf's[22] estimate of the standard error of the natural log (ln) of the IRR. This is interpreted to mean that there is a 95% chance that the interval (1.38, 1.52) includes the true value of the IRR in the population. Because the interval does not include the null value 1.0, the result is statistically significant.

Confidence Interval Based on an Odds Ratio

Constructing a CI based on an OR can also be best understood by working through an example. Consider the case-control study of soft tissue sarcoma and military service in Vietnam.[15] The OR

EXHIBIT 33-11

AN EXAMPLE FOR THE CALCULATION OF A 95% CONFIDENCE INTERVAL FOR A RATE RATIO

$$IRR = 95\% CI = \exp\left[\ln(IRR) \pm 1.96 \sqrt{\left(\frac{1}{a} + \frac{1}{c}\right)}\right]$$
$$= \exp\left[\ln(1.45) \pm 1.96 \sqrt{\left(\frac{1}{3,355} + \frac{1}{3,312}\right)}\right]$$
$$= (1.38, 1.52)$$

Source: Brundage JF, Scott RM, Lednar WM, Smith DW, Miller RN. Building-associated risk of febrile acute respiratory diseases in army trainees. *JAMA*. 1988;259:2108–2112.

comparing men who never served in Vietnam to those who ever served in Vietnam was 0.82 (see Exhibit 33-4). A 95% CI for the OR in the population can be constructed using the following method based on Woolf's[22] estimate of the standard error based on the OR:

$$95\% \text{ CI} = \exp\left[\ln(\hat{\text{OR}}) \pm 1.96 \sqrt{\left(\frac{1}{a} + \frac{1}{b} + \frac{1}{c} + \frac{1}{d}\right)}\right]$$

$$= \exp\left[\ln(0.82) \pm 1.96 \sqrt{\left(\frac{1}{45} + \frac{1}{145} + \frac{1}{172} + \frac{1}{454}\right)}\right]$$

$$= (0.56, 1.20)$$

This means that there is a 95% chance that the interval (0.56, 1.20) includes the true value of the OR in the population. Because this interval includes the null value (1.0), the result is not statistically significant.

In addition to the method proposed by Woolf, there are other formulas to construct confidence intervals around a RR or OR, and they are discussed elsewhere.[7,8]

Calculation of the Mantel-Haenszel Chi-square Test Statistic

If study participants are classified by the presence or absence of an exposure and the presence or absence of disease (ie, a 2 x 2 table), then the chi-square (χ^2) test is an appropriate test statistic. In epidemiologic studies, the Mantel-Haenszel summary chi-square (χ^2_{MH}) is often used as it combines information from each table in a stratified analysis resulting in a test statistic that measures the overall association between a risk factor and disease.

For a series of 2 x 2 tables or i tables (as shown above for the Mantel-Haenszel summary RR), the Mantel-Haenszel chi-square is calculated in this way:

$$\chi^2_{MH} = \frac{\left(\sum_{i=1}^{N} a_i - \sum_{i=1}^{N} \frac{N_{1i}M_{1i}}{T_i}\right)^2}{\sum_{i=1}^{N} \frac{N_{1i}N_{0i}M_{1i}M_{0i}}{T_i^2(T_i - 1)}}$$

The chi-square value obtained from the study is then compared with a table of chi-square distributions with one degree of freedom, or its square root can be looked up in a normal distribution table. These tables are usually included in statistic books. The chi-square test statistic corresponds to a p value (explained below). The chi-square test statistic is

more likely to be statistically significant as the sample size gets larger or as the difference between the two groups gets bigger.

For example, to test the hypothesis that sex is related to the risk of stress fractures in trainees, the Mantel-Haenszel chi-square would be the appropriate test statistic as it is designed to incorporate data from a stratified analysis. First the hypothesis is posed in terms of the null: there is no difference in the risk of stress fractures among male and female trainees. An alternative hypothesis is then formulated stating that there is a difference in the proportion of male versus female trainees who develop stress fractures during basic training. A Mantel-Haenszel chi-square is always a two-sided test. From the data that were collected (see Exhibit 33-8), the Mantel-Haenszel chi-square would be calculated as follows:

$$\chi^2_{MH} = \frac{[66 - (100 \bullet 36/700 + 400 \bullet 82/600)]^2}{\begin{array}{c} 100 \bullet 600 \bullet 36 \bullet 664/(700^2 \bullet 699) \\ + \ 400 \bullet 200 \bullet 82 \bullet 520/(600^2 \bullet 599) \end{array}}$$

$$= 1.92$$

This Mantel-Haenszel chi-square corresponds to a p value of 0.17. Exact probabilities for a given chi-square value can be obtained from software packages such as Epi Info and SAS. Exhibit 33-12 presents a partial table of critical values of the chi-square with one degree of freedom. From this table, the chi-square of 1.92 falls between the p values of 0.20 and 0.10. In these data, no statistically significant association exists between sex and the risk of stress fractures once the effect of aerobic fitness has been controlled since the p value is greater than the arbitrary cut-off level of 0.05.

Of note, there are many other types of test statistics that can be used for hypothesis testing, depend-

---

EXHIBIT 33-12

CHI-SQUARE CRITICAL VALUES FOR VARIOUS PROBABILITIES (ONE DEGREE OF FREEDOM)

p^*	0.50	0.20	0.10	0.05	0.02	0.01	0.005	0.001
χ^2	0.455	1.642	2.706	3.841	5.412	6.635	7.879	10.827

*Probability of obtaining an observed value as large as or larger than the one observed in the study under the null hypothesis ing on the type of variables in a study and whether certain assumptions are made about the underlying distribution of the data. These inferential procedures are called nonparametric statistics or distribution-free statistics. The reader is referred to several texts for a discussion of the use of other test statistics.[7,8,23]

Sample Size and Power

The calculation of a sample size depends on the study design and the measure of outcome variables. For example, to calculate a minimum sample size needed for a case-control study, the investigator determines the following parameters: the α level (eg, 0.05), the β level (eg, 0.20), the minimum size of the OR that will be significant at the 0.05 level (eg, OR = 2.0), and the proportion of subjects exposed versus nonexposed (Exhibit 33-13).

The power of a test is the probability of rejecting H_0 if in fact it is false (a correct decision). Power calculations are important in planning a study, as the larger the study population, the greater the probability of detecting a difference if a difference really exists. Power calculations are also important in the evaluation of a negative study. The conclusion that no association was found may be the result of a small sample size or a true lack of association. In a case-control study, multiple controls are commonly obtained for each case to increase the sample size and therefore the power of the study. This is usually done if the cost of accruing controls is low. In calculating the power $(I-\beta)$ for a case control study, four basic parameters are required: α (Type I error), difference or effect size, the proportion of the population exposed to the risk factor, and sample size.

There are several computer programs now available to determine sample sizes when planning a study and to solve for power in evaluating the con-

---

> **EXHIBIT 33-13**
>
> **COMMON ELEMENTS IN CALCULATING SAMPLE SIZE FOR A STUDY**
>
> ---
>
> - Determine the type of study design
> - State the null hypothesis
> - State the alternative hypothesis and determine if a 1- or 2-sided test is needed
> - Determine the appropriate measure of association
> - Determine type I error (α) and power (I-β)
> - Determine the proportion of the population exposed to risk factors
> - Determine the magnitude of measures of association

---

clusions of a negative study. Epi Info is one such program that is useful for epidemiologists in the field.

Statistical Significance Versus Clinical Significance

The word *significant* in the expression statistically significant is often misinterpreted as representing the medical or biological significance of an association. For example, a small difference in the mean diastolic blood pressure between two groups may be statistically significant if the groups are very large, but this finding may or may not be of clinical or biological significance. In addition, statistical significance addresses only random error, not bias or confounding. Thus, an incorrect result due to bias may show statistical significance.

STATISTICAL ASSOCIATIONS AND CAUSE-AND-EFFECT RELATIONSHIPS

Statistical associations from well-controlled experimental studies may represent cause-and-effect relationships. In epidemiology, however, most studies are observational (ie, the investigator does not determine who is exposed and who is nonexposed), and important decisions affecting preventive medicine and public health activities must be made on the basis of observational data. Since statistical tests do not provide proof of a causal relationship between an exposure and disease, guidelines have been established over the years to aid epidemiologists in deciding whether a statistical association obtained from an observational study design is "causal."[24]

One important criterion is the strength of the association or the size of the RR. In general, the larger the RR, the greater the likelihood that the association is causal. Even if some uncontrolled or unknown confounding is present, it is unlikely that controlling for this confounder could decrease the RR sufficiently to make the association unimportant. However, uncontrolled confounding plays a more important role when the RR is close to 1.0 and could account for the magnitude of the risk that is reported. Another important criterion to determine if an association is causal is that the exposure must precede the disease. This temporal relationship is not always clear in a cross-sectional or case-control study and is one reason why these studies are not conclusive. A strength of the cohort design is that the exposure always precedes the disease. Another criterion is biological plausibility. If the relationship between the exposure and disease outcome makes sense in terms of known biological facts and mechanisms, then it is more plausible that the exposure could cause the disease. Although a threshold effect is found for some biological phenomena, in general, a dose-response relationship between exposure and disease is another criterion that may help establish a cause-and-effect relationship. A spurious association, however, may also exhibit a dose-response relationship. Finally, although the design of any given study may have unique features or may introduce bias, findings that are consistent across studies, especially studies with different designs or conducted in different populations, suggest a cause-and-effect relationship. This is one of the most important tenets used by epidemiologists.

SUMMARY

This chapter was written to provide military preventive medicine personnel with a better understanding of the fundamental epidemiologic methods and tools used during outbreak investigations and medical surveillance during deployments. The public health officer on deployment often is faced with assessing whether a public health problem exists among servicemembers; proposing a plan; implementing an appropriate intervention; and then evaluating the impact of an intervention. Using appropriate epidemiologic methods to collect data, to interpret data, and to present data in an understandable format will greatly aid in this mission.

Acknowledgment

The author would like to acknowledge Colonel John W. Gardner and Dr. Yuanzhang Li for their help in the preparation of this chapter.

REFERENCES

1. MacMahon B, Pugh TF. *Epidemiology: Principles and Methods.* Boston: Little, Brown; 1970.

2. Jones WHS, ed. *Hippocrates: Airs, Waters, Places.* Cambridge, Mass: Harvard University Press; 1948.

3. US Army Medical Surveillance Activity. Injury incidence in soldiers attending medical specialist (MOS91B) AIT, Fort Sam Houston, Texas. *Med Surv Month Rep.* 1997;3(Dec):10–11.

4. Jones BH, Cowan DN, Tomlinson JP, Robinson JR, Polly DW, Frykman PN. Epidemiology of injuries associated with physical training among young men in the Army. *Med Sci Sports Exerc.* 1993;25:197–203.

5. Renzullo PO, McNeil JG, Wann ZF, Burke DS, Brundage JF, the United States Military Consortium for Applied Retroviral Research. Human immunodeficiency virus type-1 seroconversion trends among young adults serving in the United States Army, 1985–1993. *J Acquir Immune Defic Syndr Hum Retrovirol.* 1995;10:177–185.

6. Writer JV, DeFraites RF, Brundage JF. Comparative mortality among US military personnel in the Persian Gulf region and worldwide during Operations Desert Shield and Desert Storm. *JAMA.* 1996;275:118–121.

7. Kahn HA, Sempos CT. *Statistical Methods in Epidemiology.* New York: Oxford University Press; 1997.

8. Selvin S. Statistical Analysis of Epidemiologic Data. 2nd ed. New York: Oxford University Press; 1996.

9. Petruccelli BP, Murphy GS, Sanchez JL, et al. Treatment of traveler's diarrhea with ciprofloxacin and loperamide. *J Infect Dis.* 1992;165:557–560.

10. Gaydos JC, Hodder RA, Top FH Jr, et al. Swine influenza at Fort Dix, New Jersey, Jan–Feb 1976: Case finding and clinical study of cases. *J Infect Dis.* 1977;Suppl 13:S356–S362.

11. LCDR Tanis Batsel, Walter Reed Army Institute of Research. Personal Communication, 2000.

12. Gambel JM, Drabick JJ, Martinez-Lopez L. Medical surveillance of multinational peacekeepers deployed in support of the United Nations Mission in Haiti, June–October 1995. *Int J Epidemiol.* 199;28:312–318.

13. Smoak BL, Kelley PW, Taylor DN. Seroprevalence of *Helicobacter pylori* infections in a cohort of US Army recruits. *Am J Epidemiol.* 1994;139:513–519.

14. Cornfield J. A method of estimating comparative rates from clinical data: applications to cancer of the lung, breast, and cervix. *J Natl Cancer Inst.* 1951;11:1269.

15. Kang H, Enzinger FM, Breslin P, Feil M, Lee Y, Shepard B. Soft tissue sarcoma and military service in Vietnam: a case-control study. *J Natl Cancer Inst.* 1987;79:693–699. Published erratum: *J Natl Cancer Inst* 1987;79:1173.

16. Takafuji ET, Kirkpatrick JW, Miller RN, et al. An efficacy trial of doxycycline chemoprophylaxis against leptospirosis. *N Engl J Med.* 1984;310:497–500.

17. Friedman LM, DeMets DL, Furberg CD. *Fundamentals of Clinical Trials.* New York: Springer-Verlag New York, Inc; 1998

18. Sackett DL. Bias in analytic research. *J Chronic Dis.* 1979;32:51–63.

19. Rothman KS. Greenland S. *Modern Epidemiology.* 2nd e. Philadelphia: Lippincott Williams & Wilkins; 1998

20. Kelley PW, Petruccelli BP, Stehr-Green P, Erickson RL, Mason CJ. The susceptibility of young adult Americans to vaccine-preventable infections: A national serosurvey of US Army recruits. *JAMA.* 1991;266:2724–2729.

21. Brundage JF, Scott RM, Lednar WM, Smith DW, Miller RN. Building-associated risk of febrile acute respiratory diseases in army trainees. *JAMA.* 1988;259:2108–2112.

22. Woolf B. On estimating the relation between blood groups and disease. *Ann Hum Genet.* 1954;19:251–253.

23. Siegel S. *Nonparametric Statistics for the Behavioral Sciences.* New York: McGraw Hill Book Company; 1956.

24. Hill AB. The environment and disease: association or causation? *Proc R Soc Med.* 1965;58:295–300.

Chapter 34

LABORATORY SUPPORT FOR INFECTIOUS DISEASE INVESTIGATIONS IN THE FIELD

EDWARD T. CLAYSON, PhD AND CARL J. MASON, MD, MPH

E.T. CLAYSON; Lieutenant Colonel, MS, US Army; Product Manager, Joint Vaccine Acquisition Program, 64 Thomas Jefferson Dr., Frederick, MD 21702

C.J. MASON; Colonel, Medical Corps, US Army; Commander, USAMC-AFRIMS, APO AP 96546-5000

INTRODUCTION

Infectious disease surveillance and outbreak investigations in a field environment differ significantly from those conducted in a hospital, clinic, or laboratory and require special planning and coordination. Microbiology laboratory support may be hundreds or even thousands of miles away from a theater of military operations. Methods of specimen collection, storage, and transportation routinely used in a clinical setting are often not appropriate in a field setting. This chapter describes some of the special laboratory considerations needed to conduct infectious disease surveillance and outbreak investigations in a field environment. It was written for the military specimen collector and is not meant to be a laboratory guide for microbiologists. Considerations are discussed below for planning investigations, such as study purpose, study design, and laboratory support. Brief descriptions of common microbiological diagnostic methods are provided to aid in the selection of proper specimens for examination. Special considerations for specimen collection, handling, and storage are described. And finally, issues relating to specimen shipping are discussed. This information provides the medical investigator with the knowledge necessary to ensure that an investigation yields results that are useful to both the health care provider and the military commander.

STUDY CONSIDERATIONS

The usefulness of the information to be gained from a field study depends greatly on careful planning and coordination before the study begins. Issues such as study purpose and design must be addressed before the start of the study (see Chapter 32, Outbreak Investigation). Laboratory support is also an issue that needs to be addressed early. Preventive medicine personnel need to understand the available laboratory resources; this will aid in coordination and facilitate testing and reporting. Deployable military medical facilities are not usually equipped with microbiology laboratory capabilities, so organic microbiology laboratory capabilities are often lacking in the theater. However, during some large-scale operations, the Theater Area Medical Laboratory or the Navy Forward Laboratory may be deployed to provide some diagnostic capabilities to the theater of operations.[1]

These laboratories are staffed with selected personnel and equipped with relevant but limited diagnostic capabilities. Often permanent (nondeployable) laboratories must be solicited for support. Army and Navy infectious disease research laboratories can serve as both reference and support centers (Exhibit 34-1). Because these laboratories have been given a formal mission of surveillance for emerging infectious diseases and provided with a budget to conduct surveillance and outbreak investigations, they can be considered for laboratory support for an infectious disease outbreak or surveillance investigation. If support from the military medical system is not available for the disease of interest, support from an international reference laboratory may be obtained. A partial list of international laboratories is shown in Exhibit 34-2.

LABORATORY DIAGNOSIS OF INFECTION

A principal role of a clinical microbiology laboratory is to provide accurate information about the presence or absence of microorganisms that may be involved in a patient's disease process. In a military environment, the identification of causative organisms is important for two reasons: first, therapeutic intervention is now possible for many infectious diseases, thus allowing for earlier return to duty of infected personnel, and second, combat commanders need to be informed of the medical threats facing their units.

A fundamental step in any diagnosis is the choice of an appropriate specimen, which ultimately depends on an understanding of the pathogenesis of infectious diseases. Awareness of the types of diagnostic tests available and their complexity will facili-
tate choosing the appropriate specimen (Table 34-1). Microbiological tests fall into four main categories: (1) identification of microorganisms by microscopic examination, (2) identification of microorganisms by isolation and culture, (3) detection of a specific microbial component or product, and (4) detection of specific antibodies to a microorganism.[2] General principles and applicability of various diagnostic assays in each of these four categories will be discussed below and are shown in Table 34-2. The information provided is not meant to be a "cookbook" description of each assay for use by a microbiologist. Rather, information is provided to aid medical investigators in the field in identifying and collecting appropriate specimens for transport to supporting laboratories.

EXHIBIT 34-1

LIST OF US DEPARTMENT OF DEFENSE MEDIAL RESEARCH LABORATORIES FOR INFECTIOUS DISEASES[*]

Army CONUS Laboratories

Walter Reed Army Institute of Research
  503 Robert Grant Avenue
  Silver Spring, MD 20910-7500
  Phone: (301) 319-9100
  Fax: (301) 319-9227

US Army Medical Research Institute of Infectious
  Diseases
  1425 Porter Street
  Fort Detrick, MD 21702-5011
  Phone: (301) 619-2833
  Fax: (301) 619-4625

Army OCONUS Laboratories

Armed Forces Research Institute of Medical
  Sciences
  US Army Medical Component—Thailand
  APO AP 96546
  Phone: 66-2-644-4888
  Fax: 66-2-247-6030

US Army Medical Research Unit—Kenya
  Unit 64109 Box 401
  APO AE 09831-4109
  Phone: 254-2-729-303
  Fax: 254-2-714-592

Navy CONUS Laboratory

Naval Medical Research Command
  503 Robert Grant Ave
  Silver Spring, MD 20910-7500
  Phone: (301) 319-9208
  Fax: (301) 319-7410

Navy OCONUS Laboratories

Naval Medical Research Institute Detachment
  (Peru)
  American Embassy, Unit 3800
  APO AA 34031
  Phone: 51-1-561-2733
  Fax: 51-1-561-3042

US Naval Medical Research Unit No. 2 (Indonesia)
  Box 3, Unit 8132
  APO AP 96520-8132
  Phone: 62-21-421-4457
  Fax: 62-21-424-4507

US Naval Medical Research Unit No. 3 (Egypt)
  PSC 452, Box 5000
  FPO AE 09835-0007
  Phone: 20-2-684-1375
  Fax: 20-2-684-7139

[*]Telephone and fax numbers may have changed.
CONUS: continental United States
OCONUS: outside the continental United States

Identification of Microorganisms by Microscopic Examination

Direct microscopic inspection of clinical specimens is usually the fastest and most economical method available for the detection of microorganisms. Some infectious agents can be reliably identified with only a few simple stains and a basic microscope—without the need for time-consuming and expensive cultivation techniques. In addition, microscopic methods sometimes permit diagnosis of infections when microorganisms cannot be cultivated and in specimens where the microorganism is no longer viable. Numerous methods for microscopic examination exist, including bright field, dark field, phase-contrast, fluorescence, and electron microscopy. The best method to use in a given situation depends on the equipment and reagents available in the support laboratory. A description of the principles and applicability of the various microscopy methods is beyond the scope of this chapter but can be found in common microbiological laboratory texts.[3–5]

Identification of Microorganisms by Isolation and Culture

In general, rapid diagnostic methods, which today exist for a broad range of microorganisms, are preferred over the time-consuming and labor-intensive methods of isolation and cultivation. Cultivation of microorganisms requires a day to several weeks, but many of today's rapid diagnostic methods require only a few minutes to a few hours. Nevertheless, cultivation is still the gold standard for diagnosis of infectious diseases, and it is likely to remain one

EXHIBIT 34-2

PARTIAL LIST OF INTERNATIONAL REFERENCE LABORATORIES FOR COMMUNICABLE DISEASES[*]

Center for Applied Microbiology Research
Porton Down
Salisbury Wiltshire SP4 0JG
United Kingdom
Phone: 44-1980-612100
Fax: 44-1980-611096
www.camr.org.uk

Centers for Disease Control and Prevention
National Center for Infectious Diseases
1600 Clifton Road, N.E.
Atlanta, Georgia 30333
USA
Phone: 1-800-311-3435
Fax: 1-404-639-2334
www.cdc.gov

Epicentre
8 Rue St Sabin
75011 Paris
France
Phone: 33-1-40-212850
Fax: 33-1-40-212803

Institut de Medicine Tropicale Prince Leopold
Nationalestraat 155
B-2000 Antwerp
Belgium
Phone: 32-3-247-6666
Fax: 32-3-216-1431
www.itg.be

National Institute of Infectious Disease, Japan
1-23-1 Toyama
Tokyo 162-8640
Japan
Phone: 81-3-5285-1111
Fax: 81-3-5282-1150
www.nih.go.jp

Public Health Laboratory Service
61 Colindale Ave
Colindale, London NW9 5HT
United Kingdom
Phone: 44-181-2004400
Fax: 44-181-2007874
www.phls.co.uk

South African Medical Research Council
PO Box 9070
7505 Tygerberg
Republic of South Africa
Phone: 27-21-9380911
Fax: 27-21-9380200
www.mrc.ac.za

Statens Seruminstitut
Artillerivej 5
2300 Kobenhavn S
Denmark
Phone: 45-32-683268
Fax: 45-32-683868
www.serum.dk

[*]Specimens should be forwarded to these or other laboratories only after consultation. Proper shipping containers must be used, and all regulations for shipping hazardous, high-risk specimens must be observed. Telephone and fax numbers may have changed.

of the more important microbiological methods in the laboratory for some time. Cultivation of microorganisms isolated from patient specimens is often necessary before laboratory technicians can carry out the multitude of assays needed to identify or differentiate the agent from among various disease-causing agents or determine the susceptibility of isolated microorganisms to various antimicrobial agents.

Unfortunately, there is no universal method for the cultivation of all microorganisms. Each microorganism has its own optimum conditions for growth, which vary widely. The determination of the optimum cultivation conditions for various microorganisms has taken years of experimentation, and the optimum conditions for many microorgan-

isms remain unknown. However, the various methods available for the cultivation of a broad range of microorganisms can be divided into three main categories: cultivation using artificial media, cultivation using cell culture, and cultivation using experimental animals. Descriptions of these methods can be found in common microbiological laboratory texts.[2,6]

Detection of Microbial Components or Products

Clinical microbiologists now have many new techniques to aid them in the laboratory diagnosis of infectious diseases. These new methods may involve the detection of structural components of the microorganism, detection of microbial products (eg, toxins), or

TABLE 34-1

LABORATORY SPECIMENS REQUIRED FOR TESTS FOR PARTICULAR CAUSATIVE AGENTS

Suspected Agent or Disease	Specimen	Test
Arbovirus	Blood or brain (-70°C)	Isolation
	Blood or serum (4°C)	Serology
Cholera	Rectal swabs or stool specimens in transport medium, as recommended by the laboratory	Culture
Gastroenteritis	Stool	Culture (bacterial,viral), electron microscopy, ELISA
	Blood or serum (4°C)	Serology
Hepatitis	Serum (4°C)	ELISA
Legionella	Sputum in enrichment broth, blood	Culture; FA
Malaria	Blood (thick and thin smears)	Staining
Meningococcal meningitis	Spinal fluid, blood, pharyngeal swabs (all on transport media)	Culture, counter-immunoelectrophoresis
Plague	Bubo fluid, blood (in broth or on blood agar slants)	Culture, FA
Rabies	Brain (-70°C)	FA and isolation
Salmonella typhi	Blood (early in disease) in enrichment broth	Culture
Shigella	Rectal swabs in enrichment broth or fecal specimens	Culture
Typhus	Blood	Inoculation
	Serum (4°C)	Serology
Varicella and Suspected Smallpox	Lesion fluid, crusts	Electron microscopy, cell culture

ELISA: Enzyme-linked immunosorbent assay
FA: Fluorescent antibody test
Source: Reprinted with permission from Brès P. *Public Health Action in Emergencies Caused by Epidemics.* Geneva: World Health Organization; 1986: 238.

detection of specific gene sequences. Since these methods do not depend on the growth and multiplication of microorganisms, they are potentially more rapid than culture methods. In addition, these methods permit diagnosis of uncultivatable agents and are more specific than direct microscopic examination. They are potentially applicable to all microorganisms, as long as specific antibodies or probes are available. A brief explanation of the principles of several of the more common techniques is provided below.

Detection of Microbial Antigens or Products

Methods for the detection of microbial antigens or products rely on the ability of microorganism-specific antibodies to bind microbial antigens or products. Monoclonal antibodies, which are increasingly being used in microbiology, are highly specific and allow for distinction among different species and among strains of the same species. As more antigen-specific monoclonal antibodies become commercially available, the detection of microorganisms will be accomplished with a higher degree of sensitivity and specificity than was ever possible before. However, these methods are limited by the availability of specific antibody probes. Detection of the antibody–antigen reaction is facilitated by the use of labeled antibodies. Antibodies can be labeled with fluorescent markers, particles (eg, latex), enzymes that permit colorimetric analysis, or radioisotopes. Available

TABLE 34-2

USE OF VISUALIZATION AND OTHER TECHNIQUES FOR LABORATORY EXAMINATIONS

Agent	Techniques					
	Direct Microscopy			EIA and ELISA	Histopathological and Cytological	Biochemical
	Gram Stain	Geimsa Stain	IF			
Parasitic		+	+	+	+	+
Mycotic		+	+	+	+	+
Bacterial	+	+	+	+	+	+
Mycoplasmal		+	+	+		+
Rickettsial		+	+	+	+	+
Chlamydial		+	+	+	+	+
Viral			+	+	+*	+

*Electron microscopy in certain diseases
IF: immunofluorescence
EIA: enzyme immunoassay
ELISA: enzyme-linked immunosorbent assay
Source: Reprinted with permission from Brès P. *Public Health Action in Emergencies Caused by Epidemics*. Geneva: World Health Organization; 1986: 101.

detection methods include immunofluorescence, latex agglutination, enzyme-linked immunosorbent assay (ELISA), and radioimmunoassay.

Detection of Microbial Genes

An alternative approach to using antibodies to detect microbial antigens is to use specific nucleic acid probes to detect microbial gene sequences. Nucleic acid–based detection methods were first described in the mid 1970s, but they have only recently been accepted in the clinical laboratory. The early procedures were not widely adopted in clinical laboratories because they were more expensive, more labor-intensive, more time-consuming, less sensitive, and potentially more hazardous than prevailing antibody-based methods. Recent improvements in nucleic acid amplification and nonradioactive detection systems, however, have greatly improved the sensitivity and specificity of nucleic acid–based detection systems and have made these methods more acceptable for the clinical laboratory. In addition, these methods are useful in detecting nonviable microorganisms or those that are difficult or dangerous to cultivate.

The key to nucleic acid–based methods is the gene probe, a nucleic acid molecule (usually DNA) with a sequence complementary to the gene to be detected. Polynucleotide probes can be synthesized from scratch if the genomic sequence of the microorganism is known or can be obtained from naturally occurring DNA by cloning DNA fragments into appropriate vectors and isolating the cloned DNA. Nucleic acid probes can be labeled with a radioisotope (usually phosphorus-32P [^{32}P]) with biotin, a specific enzyme or a fluorescent marker, or with digoxigenin, a chemiluminescent marker. Biotinylated probes using streptavidin detection systems have been used in some laboratories, but these methods are not as sensitive as radioactive methods. A commonly used label today is the chemiluminescent marker because of the long shelf-life of the assay components, the marker's sensitivity, which approaches that of radioactivity, and the elimination of hazards associated with the use of radioactivity. Increasingly, nucleic acid probes for a wide variety of microorganisms are becoming commercially available.

Gene detection methods rely on the ability of one or more nucleic acid probes to hybridize with the genome of the microorganism. In some methods, the nucleic acid of a tissue or of a culture of a patient specimen is first extracted and then hybridized with one or more microbe-specific probes. Alternatively, hybridization can occur in situ in patient tissues or laboratory cultures. Specific infected cells containing intracellular parasites (eg, viruses, rickettsia, chlamydia) may be identified by the in situ technique. Nucleic acid–based detection methods include blot assay, in situ hybridization, and polymerase chain reaction. Descriptions of these methods can be found elsewhere.[7–10]

Detection of Antibodies to Microorganisms

During the early stages of an infection, the immune system is exposed to a rise in the amount of microbial antigen as the infecting microorganism replicates. The initial host response is nonspecific, directed at infectious processes in general, until the host can generate a more efficient, specific immune response. For assay purposes, the specific immune response is divided into cellular and humoral response mechanisms. These two response mechanisms are closely related and interdependent. The cellular mechanism is more difficult to measure and is not used as the basis of any routinely performed assays.

Early in infection, there is a surge in available antigen (the microorganism itself or one of its products) in patient serum. Culture, antigen detection, and genomic detection techniques are most likely to be useful during this period. A transient rise in specific IgM antibodies and a subsequent, more persistent rise in specific IgG antibodies follow the surge in antigen. For microorganisms that invade mucosal surfaces, there will also be an accompanying rise in specific IgA antibodies at the mucosal surface. The rise in IgA antibodies may not be detectable in serum or plasma.

Detection of antibodies specific for the infecting microorganism will be most successful following the rise in IgM antibodies. Evidence for infection by a given microorganism may be provided by detection of high levels of specific IgM antibodies or

by detection of a 4-fold or greater rise in specific antibodies in paired serum or plasma samples (Table 34-3). The finding of a high titer of agent-specific IgG in a single specimen is not considered indicative of recent infection, but a rise in agent-specific IgG as detected in paired specimens suggests recent infection. In addition, a serum with high levels of agent-specific IgM strongly suggests recent infection. Ideally, the paired samples should consist of one sample collected at the onset of infection (when antibody production is minimal) and a second sample collected at least 7 to 14 days later, when antibody is maximal (or longer for some rickettsial infections). This provides strong evidence of recent infection with the given microorganism. Unfortunately, the initial acute sample is not always collected. For US military personnel, a predeployment sample from the Department of Defense Serum Repository in Rockville, Md, may sometimes be substituted for the initial acute specimen.

In parallel to the rapid developments in nucleic acid techniques, advances have been made in the detection of antibodies specific for microorganisms. Two of these techniques, ELISA and agglutination, have been widely adapted for use in assays in both clinical and research settings and serve as the basis of most commercially available antibody assays. Three other techniques—complement fixation, hemagglutination, and precipitation—although important in the past are used less frequently today.

Diagnostic and Reporting Issues

Understanding the various diagnostic assays described above is not enough. There are other issues that must be understood to interpret test results properly. The sensitivity and specificity of the diagnostic test must be known to determine the reliabil-

TABLE 34-3

SEROLOGICAL EVIDENCE OF RECENT INFECTION

Specimen	Result
Single Serum	Presence of IgM specific for the suspected agent (non-specific reactions must be eliminated)
	High titer of specific undifferentiated (IgM + IgG) antibody, if higher than the long-lasting immunity level for the disease concerned
Paired Sera[*]	4-fold increase in titer (IgM + IgG) with specific antigen

[*]The first sample should be collected soon after disease onset, the second ideally 10 to 14 days later for most diseases.
Adapted with permission from Brès P. *Public Health Action in Emergencies Caused by Epidemics.* Geneva: World Health Organization; 1986: 103.

ity of test results. An understanding of the incidence of the specific disease among the population examined is also required to determine the predictive value of the test.

Sensitivity and Specificity

Sensitivity and specificity are terms used to describe the performance of a given test or assay compared with one or more widely accepted standards. A widely accepted standard is often referred to as the gold standard. Sensitivity is a measure of the capability of the test or assay to detect all true positive cases in a given population. It is usually expressed as a percent and given by this formula:

$$\text{Sensitivity (\%)} = 100 \text{ (Assay True Positives)} / [\text{(Assay True Positives)} + \text{(Assay False Negatives)}]$$
$$= 100 \text{ (Assay True Positives)} / \text{(True Positives)}$$

For example, a test with a stated sensitivity of 99% is expected to detect 99 of 100 positive cases when correctly performed (and interpreted) on properly collected specimens from a population similar to that used originally to determine the sensitivity.

Specificity is a measure of the capability of the test or assay to detect all true negative cases. It is also usually expressed as a percent and given by the formula:

$$\text{Specificity (\%)} = 100 \text{ (Assay True Negatives)} / [\text{(Assay True Negatives)} + \text{(Assay False Positives)}]$$
$$= 100 \text{ (Assay True Positives)} / \text{(True Positives)}$$

For example, a test with a stated specificity of 99% is expected to detect 99 of 100 negative cases when correctly performed (and interpreted) on properly collected specimens from a population similar to that originally used to determine the sensitivity.

Positive Predictive Value

The positive predictive value is a measure of the meaning of a positive test or assay result. It depends on the prevalence of the disease or condition in the population from which the specimens being tested were collected. The positive predictive value is usually expressed as a percent and given by the formula:

$$\text{Positive Predictive Value (\%)} = \frac{100 \text{ (Assay True Positives)} / [\text{Assay Positives (True + False)}]}{}$$

For example, given a population with a prevalence of disease markers of 20% and an assay with a stated sensitivity and specificity of 99%, the positive predictive value of the assay will be 96%. This implies that a positive result on this assay in this population will predict the presence of disease markers 96% of the time. Given a different population with a prevalence of disease markers of 1% and the same assay with a stated sensitivity and specificity of 99%, the positive predictive value of the assay will be 50%, which implies that a positive result in this population will correctly predict the presence of disease markers only 50% of the time. Therefore, the use of tests (even highly sensitive and specific tests) to screen for diseases of low prevalence is problematic.

The positive predictive value can be improved by combining two or more tests in series. For example, a positive test result on an ELISA test for human immunodeficiency virus-1 (HIV-1) is usually followed by a Western blot assay for HIV-1; this improves the positive predictive value of the screening program in the United States, where the prevalence of antibodies to HIV-1 is extremely low.

Interpretation

Laboratory results should always be interpreted in combination with epidemiologic data, historical information, and other clinical and laboratory findings. Several reasons for test error are included in Table 34-4. Inappropriate sample collection, sample storage, and sample shipping are major sources of laboratory error. Steps to minimize these problems are covered elsewhere in this chapter.

The selection of appropriate laboratory tests and assays must be a coordinated effort with the laboratory to ensure that the results obtained are meaningful and useful. Many of the assays that are approved by the Food and Drug Administration (FDA) and are commercially available have been standardized on Western European or North American populations. They can thus be expected to perform as stated when applied to specimens collected from US military personnel or civilians in the United States. But FDA-approved tests and well-characterized assays are not available for many of the agents from areas of the world that are of potential interest and importance to deploying US forces.

Within the United States, unapproved medical devices (including diagnostic assays) may not be used in clinical care settings without an FDA Investigational Device Exemption (IDE). By custom, the US Department of Defense attempts to comply

TABLE 34-4

CAUSES OF ERROR IN THE INTERPRETATION OF LABORATORY TESTS

False Positive Results	False Negative Results
Microscopic Methods	
Saprophyte present	Inappropriate sampling
Nonspecific staining	Inappropriate dye
	Need for electron microscopy
	Inappropriate specimen
	Inexperience of microscopist
Isolation Methods	
Concurrent agent in specimen is easier to detect than causative agent or withstands storage conditions better	Inappropriate sampling: specimen inadequate or taken at wrong time
Concurrent chronic infections (eg, malaria, schistosomiasis)	Damage to agent by shipping or storage conditions
	Inappropriate laboratory techniques
Concurrent pathogen in an outbreak primarily caused by a toxic agent	"New" agent requiring unusual conditions for isolation
	Presence of immune complexes
Contamination of specimens or reagents	Bacterial or contaminant overgrowth
Antibody Detection Methods	
Presence of antibodies (IgG) to endemic disease	Sample taken at wrong time
Cross reaction of antibodies among antigenically-related agents	Damage to specimen during shipping and storage
	Inappropriate laboratory techniques
Nonspecific reactions	Inappropriate antigen battery
Previous immunization or skin test	Presence of immune complexes
Presence of excess IgG or rheumatoid factors when detecting IgM	Immunosuppression

Adapted with permission from Brès P. *Public Health Action in Emergencies Caused by Epidemics.* Geneva: World Health Organization. 1986: 104.

with FDA requirements in the diagnosis and treatment of US military personnel and dependents overseas, but procedures exist for emergency use of an unapproved medical device for medical care. These procedures require the user to notify the Institutional Review Board within 5 days of use of the device or assay and to submit an application for an IDE if future use is likely. If clinical use of an unapproved diagnostic assay is being considered, every effort should be made to seek guidance. For the US Army, guidance may be obtained from the Human Subjects Protection Division at the US Army Medical Research and Materiel Command, Fort Detrick, Md.

SPECIMEN COLLECTION, HANDLING, AND STORAGE

All too often, the importance of collecting the proper specimens and transporting them to the laboratory is neglected or not emphasized. Perhaps the most common reason for failure to establish a diagnosis (or suggesting a wrong one) is the collection of an inappropriate specimen. To obtain a test result that correctly identifies the etiology of the infection, it is important to collect an appropriate specimen, use appropriate transport, and deliver specimens to the laboratory rapidly. No matter how sophisticated the laboratory or how expert its personnel, if the specimen is inappropriately chosen,

TABLE 34-5

METHODS TO BE EMPLOYED IN COLLECTING RESPIRATORY TRACT SPECIMENS

Purpose	Procedure
Bacteriology, mycology or parasitology	Direct examination of sputum: thin smear on a slide for Gram staining
	Cultivation: make a cough swab. Fragile bacteria require special media and particular precautions (ask laboratory for guidance)
Virology	Direct examination by immunofluorescence: cough swab transported in Hanks' medium at 4°C, or preferably nasopharyngeal aspirate obtained with a suction apparatus
	Cultivation: same specimens. Fragile viruses require special media and particular precautions (ask laboratory for guidance)

Source: Reprinted with permission from Brès P. *Public Health Action in Emergencies Caused by Epidemics.* Geneva: World Health Organization; 1986: 241.

collected, or transported, results will be less than optimal and will often be misleading. Early communication between the investigator and the laboratory is extremely important. Laboratory personnel can advise the investigator on the collection of optimum specimens and will be better able to guide the processing of these specimens if potential problems have been discussed. Some specific methods are listed in Table 34-5, Table 34-6, Table 34-7, and Table 34-8. This section discusses some general issues regarding specimen collection in the field and provides specific guidance in the collection of specimens for microscopic examination, isolation and culture, detection of microbial components or products, and detection of antibodies to infectious agents.

Practical Issues

All clinical specimens (including serum samples for antibody detection) should be handled as if they are infectious. Universal precautions as outlined by the Occupational Safety and Health Act should be followed during collection and transport to the laboratory.[11] In particular, appropriate barriers should be used during specimen collection to prevent exposure of skin and mucous membranes to specimens. Gloves must be worn at all times, and masks, goggles, and gowns or aprons must be worn in situations in which there is a risk of splashes or droplet formation. After specimen containers are sealed, they should not be opened until they reach the laboratory, where they can be opened safely in

TABLE 34-6

METHODS TO BE EMPLOYED IN COLLECTING SPECIMENS OF FECES

Purpose	Procedure
All examinations	3 mL (or equivalent in solid) in screw-cap "bijou" bottle (capacity 7 mL). Store at 4°C or normal refrigerator temperature
Parasitology	3 parts of 10% formaldehyde solution are added to 1 part of stool
Bacteriology	Use special transport medium for cholera, other vibrios, *Salmonella*, *Shigella*, etc; store at room temperature in shade, not in refrigerator. If medium not available, consult laboratory
Virology	A suitable virus transport medium may be provided by the laboratory

Source: Reprinted with permission from Brès P. *Public Health Action in Emergencies Caused by Epidemics.* Geneva: World Health Organization; 1986: 241.

TABLE 34-7

METHODS OF COLLECTING SPECIMENS OF FOOD AND OTHER MATERIALS

Type of Specimen	Method
Liquid food	Shake, pour 200 mL into sterile container, refrigerate but do not freeze
Solid or mixed food	Separate portions with sterile knife, transfer to a sterile glass jar (eg, jam jar); take samples from periphery to central laboratory; refrigerate
Meat and poultry	Cut portion of meat or skin aseptically from different parts of carcass; alternatively, wipe large portions of carcass with sterile gauze squares or swabs; place in transport medium
Water	See Table 34-8
Other	Collect any fabric (eg, sheets or towels) known or suspected to contain poison, vomit, urine, or feces

Source: Reprinted with permission from Brès P. *Public Health Action in Emergencies Caused by Epidemics*. Geneva: World Health Organization; 1986: 245.

a biological safety cabinet.[12]

Whenever possible, specimens should be collected before antimicrobial agents have been given. Collection of specimens after initiation of antimicrobial therapy may drastically affect recovery of bacteria and parasites and lead to misdiagnosis. Likewise, fecal specimens to be examined for parasites should be collected before barium is used for radiological examination.[13] Specimens should be obtained from the site of infection with minimal contamination from adjacent tissues and organ secretions. Knowledge of the stage of the infection (eg, acute vs. chronic, time of onset) is helpful in the selection of appropriate specimens. The type of specimen and stage of infection when a culture is taken may determine whether or not the etiological agent will be isolated. Specimens should be large enough to allow thorough examination. Many microbiological techniques are relatively insensitive, so it is important to collect large enough samples and to maintain viable organisms in the samples while they are in transit to the laboratory. However, due to regulations regarding the shipment of clinical specimens, 50 mL per specimen should be considered the upper limit.[14] Specimens should be collected in appropriate, safe, and sterile containers with tight-fitting lids. In general, the quicker the specimen is delivered to the laboratory, the better the laboratory results will be. Quick delivery, though, is not usually possible in a field setting.

Each specimen should be labeled with the name or

TABLE 34-8

COLLECTION OF WATER SAMPLES*

Type of Water	Method of Collection
Tap water	1. Disinfect the mouth of the tap with a burning cotton wool swab soaked in alcohol
	2. Let the water flow for 2 m
	3. Fill the bottle
Well-water	Weight a bottle with a sterile stone attached with sterile string and dip into well
Open water†	Plunge the bottle neck down into the water and then turn it upwards with the mouth facing the current

*Water should be collected in sterile bottles (1–5 L)
†Water from springs, streams, rivers, and lakes
Source: Reprinted with permission from Brès P. *Public Health Action in Emergencies Caused by Epidemics*. Geneva: World Health Organization; 1986: 249.

identification number of the person from whom the specimen was collected, the source or type of specimen, and the date and time of collection. Labeling of specimens is especially important in surveillance and outbreak investigations. These investigations often generate hundreds or thousands of specimens that can easily be misidentified if improperly labeled. Unfortunately, errors in specimen labeling are too common and often lead to faulty results. Maintaining correct specimen identification during the specimen's passage through the laboratory is critical.

Sufficient clinical information should be provided to guide the microbiologist in proper, optimal processing of the specimen. A list of the tests desired by the investigator is helpful. Age and sex of the patient are important with respect to some infections, and the patient's clinical features must be included. Relevant geographic and travel details are also important to indicate possible exposure to pathogens in endemic areas. Finally, the date and time of specimen collection and of arrival in the laboratory indicate how much time has elapsed since the specimen was collected.

Specimens for Microscopic Examination

Microscopy plays a fundamental role in microbiology and is an important first step in the examination of all diagnostic specimens, especially when a parasite is suspected as the etiological agent. Preferably, slides for microscopy are prepared with fresh specimens, but in a field setting this is not always possible. If blood is to be examined for parasites, then it should be collected using an anticoagulant ([EDTA] is preferred).[13] Thick or thin films for parasite identification may be prepared on slides in the field and sent to the laboratory; alternately, tubes

of blood containing an anticoagulant may be sent to the laboratory and slides prepared there. If examination of a sputum specimen is to be delayed for any reason, then a portion of the sputum should be fixed in 5% or 10% formalin so that helminth eggs or larvae may be preserved. The remainder of the specimen should be saved for bacterial and viral cultivation. Wet mount slides may be prepared in the field (preferably) or in the laboratory. If examination of a fecal specimen is to be delayed (more than 30 minutes for liquid specimens, 1 hour for soft specimens, and 1 day for formed specimens), then the specimen should be fixed in one of several available fixatives. A series of at least three specimens collected 48 hours apart is preferred for the diagnosis of intestinal parasites. Slides of fecal material should be prepared in the laboratory.[13] Other aspects of collecting fecal samples are listed in Table 34-6.

Slides and specimens prepared for microscopic examination can be stored at room temperature or in a refrigerator (4°C). Care should be taken to prevent overheating specimens intended for microscopic examination (Table 34-9).

Specimens for Culture

A fluid specimen (including exudate and excreta) collected early in the acute phase of illness is the most desirable specimen for isolation and culture. In a typical clinical setting, a sterile swab is commonly used to collect fluid specimens.[2] In a field environment, however, swab collection usually fails to provide suitable specimens for analysis. Swabs absorb only a small quantity of sample and provide an arid, unfriendly environment for transport to the laboratory. Therefore actual fluid should be collected whenever possible to ensure that a large

TABLE 34-9

GENERAL GUIDELINES FOR STORAGE AND SHIPPING TEMPERATURES OF BIOLOGICAL SPECIMENS

Type of Specimen	Storage Conditions	Shipping Conditions
Specimens for microscopic examination	Room temperature or refrigerator temperature (4°C)	Ambient temperature or wet ice
Specimens for culture and isolation	Refrigerator temperature (4°C) if for less than 24 h; < –70°C otherwise	Dry ice or liquid nitrogen
Specimens for detection of microbial components or products	Refrigerator temperature (4°C) if for less than 24 h; < -70°C otherwise	Dry ice or liquid nitrogen
Specimens for detection of antibodies	Freezer temperature (-20°C)	Wet ice

enough volume of sample is collected.

Maintaining viable organisms in the sample until the specimen reaches the laboratory is critical. Specimens for culture should be collected in sterile containers and should not be put into fixatives or preservatives, which are lethal to microorganisms. In cases when a virus is suspected as the etiological agent, placing the specimen in a viral transport medium is preferred. A virus transport medium should preserve the virus in the specimen, prevent loss of the specimen due to bacterial or fungal contamination, be nontoxic to cell cultures, and not interfere with direct tests to detect and identify virus antigens (eg, immunofluorescence, enzyme immunoassays). Several transport media are commercially available. Antibiotics can be added to specimens for the isolation of viruses, fungi, and algae to reduce bacterial contamination, but specimens containing antibiotics cannot be used for the isolation of bacteria.

Specimens for culture may be stored in a refrigerator or on ice (0°C–4°C) if less than a 5-day delay is expected. Specimens expected to be stored or in transit longer than 5 days should be frozen at or below -70°C initially and shipped on dry ice or liquid nitrogen. Specimens for culture should not be stored or transported at room temperature, in normal kitchen freezers (-20°C), or in incubators (30°C–38°C) because many microorganisms degrade quickly at these temperatures. Care should be taken to prevent thawing of specimens, as multiple freezing and thawing of specimens is known to reduce recovery of microorganisms.

Specimens for Detection of Microbial Components or Products

Specimens suitable for culture are also suitable for the detection of microbial components or products, but the detection of microbial components or products does not depend on the presence of living organisms. Therefore, samples containing fixatives, preservatives, or sometimes antibiotics are acceptable. However, minimizing contamination by extraneous organisms is very important, so sterile containers should be used. Specimens should be stored and shipped at the coldest temperature achievable under field conditions or at temperatures equal to or lower than -70°C in the laboratory.

Specimens for Detection of Antibodies

Samples of sera and sometimes cerebrospinal fluid are used to detect antibody responses. Specimens should be collected in a sterile manner. Paired sera, collected in the acute and convalescent phases of the disease (ideally 10 to 14 days or more apart), should be tested at the same time. Whenever possible, whole blood should not be sent to the laboratory. Serum should be separated from the cells in the blood and the serum sent to the laboratory. Serum samples can be stored at normal scientific freezer temperatures (-20°C to -25°C) for months or years without loss of antibody titer. The thermal cycling associated with residential-type frost-free freezers can, however, reduce antibody levels.

SPECIMEN SHIPPING

The job of the field investigator is not over when the specimens have been collected. The specimens must be sent to the laboratory for examination. Care should be taken to get the specimens to the laboratory as soon as possible and in a condition useful for examination. In addition, certain regulatory guidelines must be followed so that persons handling potentially infectious material are not exposed to it.

Timely Delivery

Specimens should be transported to the laboratory as quickly as possible. By their very nature, many clinical specimens provide a good medium for the growth of bacteria and fungi. Microorganisms may multiply during the time between collection and cultivation in the laboratory. With time, the hardy species may overgrow the fastidious, giving a false impression of the balance between species; in some cases, this will make it impossible to isolate and identify the less-hardy species. Bacteria or fungi may render specimens for the detection of viruses useless if allowed to grow unchecked. The addition of antibiotics in viral transport media may be necessary to preserve these specimens. Some specimens are naturally prone to drying (eg, specimens collected with swabs), which will complicate or make impossible the isolation and cultivation of microorganisms. Rapid transport to the laboratory will help prevent many of these problems.

Regulatory Issues

Packages of clinical or laboratory specimens prepared for mailing or shipping must conform to US postal regulations and those of the US Department of Transportation and the US Public Health Service.[14-17] Packages shipped between overseas locations must conform to these regulations as well as the Dangerous Goods Regulations of the International Air Transport Association (Figure 34-1). The regulations, which govern package containers, volume limitations, and labeling requirements, were designed to protect all who may come in contact with the package. Compliance with these regulations is the responsibility of the sender, and large financial penalties may be levied on senders of improperly packaged and labeled shipments.

Containers

In general, diagnostic specimens or infectious substances must be mailed in double containers. Each specimen is contained in a primary container (eg, tube, vial). The cap of the primary container should be sealed with waterproof tape. One or more primary containers may be packed together in a secondary container filled with cotton or other absorbent material that is capable of absorbing the entire contents of all the primary containers. The secondary container must be sealable and break-resistant, and its lid should be taped to prevent loss of contents during shipment. The secondary container should be placed in a shipping container. Wet or dry ice to be included with the shipment, if any, should be placed between the secondary container and the shipping container.

Microscope slides containing specimens do not require double containers for shipment. They may be packed in boxes, cardboard slide holders, or any other suitable container that will prevent damage or breakage. Slides should be completely dry before packing and should be individually wrapped in soft tissue. If more than one slide is to be shipped or mailed, the slides can be wrapped together in tissue as follows: a slide is placed on the tissue and wrapped several times, and then the next slide is placed on top of the first and both are wrapped several times. The series of slides wrapped this way will be padded and can be easily unwrapped on arrival. Slides packed in flat cardboard containers need additional protection. Plastic slide containers with snap tops work well for shipping slides.[13]

Volume Limitations

Various regulations limit the amount or volume of specimen that may be shipped in any one package.[14–16] The limit depends on whether the specimen is categorized as a diagnostic specimen or an infectious substance. In general, a diagnostic specimen is defined as any human or animal material, including but not limited to excreta, secreta, blood and its components, tissue, and tissue fluids, being shipped for purposes of diagnosis. It is not known at the

time of shipment whether a diagnostic specimen contains microorganisms or toxins that may cause human disease. For diagnostic specimens, primary containers must not exceed 1L. The maximum volume that may be shipped in a secondary container is 4 L. Likewise, the maximum volume that may be shipped in a shipping container is 4 L. An infectious substance is defined as any substance that is known to contain a viable microorganism or its toxin that is known or suspected to cause disease in animals or humans. The etiological agent is known at the time of shipment. The maximum volume of infectious substance that may be shipped in a shipping container is 50 mL.

Temperature

Specimens should be shipped at the same or similar temperatures as that recommended for storage. In general, specimens prepared for microscopic examination or for detection of antibodies should be shipped on wet ice but not be frozen; they may be shipped at ambient temperature ($< 24°C$) if necessary. Prepared slides may also be shipped at ambient temperature. Specimens for culture or for detection of microbial components should be shipped on dry ice or liquid nitrogen (see Table 34-9). Properly collected sera for antibody testing can usually be transported, if necessary, at ambient temperature for a day or so without substantial loss of antibody.

Finding dry ice or liquid nitrogen in developing countries can be challenging. In some developing countries, ice cream makers and distributors produce dry ice and may be willing to sell sufficient quantities to support the temporary storage and shipment of clinical specimens. In some countries where cattle breeding is conducted, local veterinary centers often produce liquid nitrogen for the storage of bull sperm. These centers may be willing to sell excess liquid nitrogen for the right price. In large urban areas in developing countries, larger medical centers may have access to either dry ice or liquid nitrogen. However, many developing countries do not have the capability to produce either dry ice or liquid nitrogen locally, so dry ice or liquid nitrogen must be imported. Arrangements can be made with a supporting laboratory to ship sufficient quantities of dry ice or liquid nitrogen to support specimen storage and return shipment.

Labeling

All packages prepared for shipping should contain complete information sheets about the specimens. The information sheets should be placed between the sec-

a

SHIPPER'S DECLARATION FOR DANGEROUS GOODS   **(Provide at least two copies to the airline)**

Shipper	Air Waybill No.
	Page of Pages
	Shipper's Reference Number
	(optional)

Consignes	

Two completed and signed copies of this Declaration must be handed to the operator

WARNING

Failure to comply in all respects with the applicable Dangerous Goods Regulations may be in breach of the applicable law, subject to legal penalties. This Declaration must not, in any circumstances, be completed and/or signed by a consolidator, a forwarder of an IATA cargo agent.

TRANSPORT DETAILS

This shipment is within the limitations prescribed for: *(delete non-applicable)*	Airport of Departure
PASSENGER AND CARGO AIRCRAFT CARGO AIRCRAFT ONLY	

Airport of Destination:

Shipment type: *(delete non-applicable)*
NON-RADIOACTIVE | RADIOACTIVE

NATURE AND QUANTITY OF DANGEROUS GOODS

Dangerous Goods identification

Proper Shipping Name	Class or Division	UN or ID No.	Packing Group	Subsidiary Risk	Quantity and Type of packing	Packing inst.	Authorization

Additional Handling Information

24 hr. Emergency Contact Tel. No.

I hereby declare that the contents of this consignment are fully and accurately described above by the proper shipping name and are classified, packaged, marked and labelled/placarded, and are in all respects in proper condition for transport according to applicable international and national governmental regulations.

Name/Title of Signatory

Place and Dete

Signature
(see warning above)

(**Fig 34-1** continues)

b

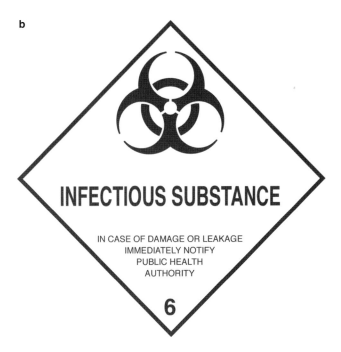

INFECTIOUS SUBSTANCE

IN CASE OF DAMAGE OR LEAKAGE
IMMEDIATELY NOTIFY
PUBLIC HEALTH
AUTHORITY

6

Fig. 34-1. The form (**a**) and label (**b**) that must be fixed to packages containing infectious substances before they are mailed. These are required by US and international postal regulations.

ondary and shipping containers. Labels should have names, addresses, and telephone numbers of both the sender and the recipient and should be inside the package on the secondary container, as well as on the outside of the shipping container. If the package contains known infectious substances (not likely in the context of this chapter), then an "Etiological Agents" label must be displayed on the outside of the shipping container.[14–17] Likewise, if the shipment contains dry ice (officially declared a hazardous material), then the shipping container must be marked "Dry Ice, Frozen Medical Specimens."[17]

Inventory and Clinical Information

If more than one specimen is contained in a shipment, then a complete inventory should accompany the shipment. Sufficient clinical information should also be provided to the laboratory to guide the microbiologist in the selection of suitable diagnostic assays. The inventory and clinical information should be placed between the secondary and shipping containers. When the package is opened, the recipient should reconcile the specimens with the inventory list. A notice should be sent back to the sender that the shipment was received, along with a report of any discrepancies between the inventory list and the specimens received.

SUMMARY

Surveillance and outbreak investigations in a field environment require additional planning and coordination beyond that required for similar investigations in a hospital or clinical setting. In particular, laboratory support must be coordinated before the investigation begins. Plans for specimen collection, handling, storage, and shipment must be made early and potential problems addressed. Successful laboratory results depend on the selection of a proper specimen that will survive storage and transport. A general knowledge of the types of diagnostic assays available for infectious diseases will aid the investigator in the proper selection of patient specimens. For purposes of specimen storage and transport, specimens may be divided into four categories, and storage and transport conditions vary between these specimen categories. In addition, federal regulations must be observed when shipping biological specimens, even between two locations outside the United States. When done with the proper coordination, field medical investigations can be an important tool for the commander to identify medical threats facing US forces.

REFERENCES

1. US Dept of the Army. *Planning for Health Service Support*. Washington, DC: DA; 1994. Field Manual 8-55.

2. Mims CA, Playfair JHL, Roitt IM, Wakelin D, Williams R. *Medical Microbiology*. Hong Kong: Mosby-Year Book Europe; 1993: Chap 17, 18.

3. Hoeprich PD, Jordan MC, Ronald AR, eds. *Infectious Diseases*. Philadelphia: J.B. Lippincott; 1994.

4. Lennette EH, ed. *Laboratory Diagnosis of Viral Infections*. 2nd ed. New York: Marcel Dekker; 1992.

5. Galasso GJ, Whitley RJ, Merigan TC, eds. *Practical Diagnosis of Viral Infections.* New York: Ravin Press; 1993.

6. Baron EJ, Peterson LR, Finegold SM. *Bailey & Scott's Diagnostic Microbiology.* 9th ed. St. Louis: Mosby-Year Book; 1994.

7. Southern EM. Detection of specific sequences among DNA fragments separated by gel electrophoresis. *J Mol Biol.* 1975;98:503–517.

8. Alwine JC, Kemp DJ, Stark GR. Method for detection of specific RNAs in agarose gels by transfer to diazobenzyloxymethyl-paper and hybridization with DNA probes. *Proc Natl Acad Sci USA.* 1977;74:5350–5354.

9. Kafatos FC, Jones CW, Efstratiadis A. Determination of nucleic acid sequence homologies and relative concentrations by a dot hybridization procedure. *Nucleic Acids Res.* 1979;7:1541–1552.

10. Saiki RK, Scharf S, Faloona F, et al. Enzymatic amplification of beta-globin genomic sequences and restriction site analysis for diagnosis of sickle cell anemia. *Science.* 1985;230:1350–1354.

11. US Dept of Labor, Occupational Safety and Health Administration. Occupational exposure to bloodborne pathogens: final rule. *Fed Regist.* 1991;56:64175–64182. 29 CFR Part 1910.1030.

12. Woods GL, Gutierrez Y. *Diagnostic Pathology of Infectious Diseases.* Philadelphia: Lea & Febiger; 1993: Chap 54.

13. Garcia LS, Bruckner DA. *Diagnostic Medical Parasitology.* 2nd ed. Washington, DC: American Society for Microbiology; 1993: Chap 25, 29, 30.

14. Public Health Service. Interstate shipment of etiologic agents. *Fed Regist.* 1980;45:28–29. 42 CFR part 72.

15. US Postal Service. Nonmailability of etiologic agents. *Fed Regist.* 1988;53:23775–23776. 39 CFR part II.

16. US Postal Service. Mailability of etiologic agents. *Fed Regist.* 1989;54:11970–11972. 39 CFR part III.

17. US Dept of Transportation. Hazardous materials regulations. *Fed Regist.* 1998;63:52843–52851. 49 CFR part 173.

MILITARY PREVENTIVE MEDICINE: MOBILIZATION AND DEPLOYMENT
Volume 2

Section 6: Infectious Diseases of Concern

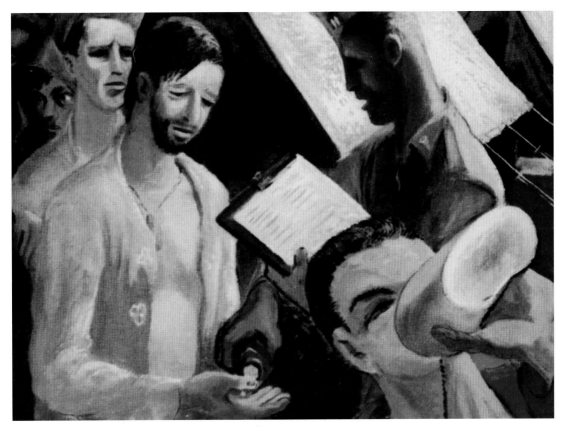

Franklin Boggs   *Pill Call*

Soldiers in the South Pacific theater during World War II get their daily dose of atabrine, described by the artist as "the famous new malaria medicine." Atabrine was used by the allies because Japan controlled the sources of quinine, the main malaria treatment of the pre-atabrine era. The artist also mentioned that "these pills turn you about the color of a lemon." It was the control of malaria that gave General MacArthur of the US Army and General Slim of the British Army an edge in their battles with the Japanese.

Art: Courtesy of US Center of Military History, Washington, DC.

Chapter 35

DISEASES TRANSMITTED PRIMARILY BY ARTHROPOD VECTORS

G. Dennis Shanks, MD, MPH-TM
Jerome J. Karwacki, MD, MPH
Niranjan Kanesa-thasan, MD, MTM&H
Wellington Sun, MD
Bruce L. Innis, MD
Timothy P. Endy, MD, MPH
Charles F. Longer, MD
David W. Vaughn, MD, MPH
George V. Ludwig, PhD
David J. McClain, MD
Kevin Michaels, MD, MPH

Hee-Choon S. Lee, MD, MPH
Victoria B. Solberg, MS
Kathryn L. Clark, MD, MPH
Arthur E. Brown, MD, MPH
Daniel A. Strickman, PhD
Daryl J. Kelly, PhD
Mark G. Kortepeter, MD, MPH
William P. Corr, MD, MPH
Alan J. Magill, MD
William C. Hewitson, MD, MPH

MALARIA

DENGUE VIRUS INFECTIONS

DENGUE-LIKE SYNDROMES

YELLOW FEVER

JAPANESE ENCEPHALITIS

THE EQUINE ENCEPHALITIDES

TICKBORNE ENCEPHALITIS

SANDFLY FEVER

LYME DISEASE

EHRLICHIOSIS

TYPHUS

PLAGUE

FILARIASIS

THE LEISHMANIASES

TRYPANOSOMIASIS

G.D. Shanks; Colonel, Medical Corps, US Army; Program Manager, DOEM, US Army Center for Health Promotion and Preventive Medicine, 5158 Blackhawk Road, Aberdeen Proving Ground, MD 21010-5403

J.J. Karwacki; Colonel, Medical Corps, US Army (Retired). JUSMAGTHAI, PO Box R3081, APO AP 96546; Formerly, Preventive Medicine Officer, US Army Medical Component, Armed Forces Research Institute of Medical Science, APO AP 96546-5000

N. Kanesa-thasan; Lieutenant Colonel, Medical Corps, US Army; Chief, Clinical Studies Department, Medical Division, US Army Medical Research Institute of Infectious Diseass, 1425 Porter Street, Fort Detrick, Frederick, MD 21702-5011

W. Sun; Colonel, Medical Corps, US Army; Chief, Department of Virus Diseases, Division of Communicable Diseases and Immunology, Walter Reed Army Institute of Research, Silver Spring, MD 20910-7500

B.L. Innis; Colonel, Medical Corps, US Army (Retired); Group Director, New Vaccines, GlaxoSMithKline Pharmaceuticals, 1250 S. Collegeville Rd (mailcode UP 4330), Collegeville, PA 19426; Formerly, Chief, Department of Virus Diseases, Division of Communicable Diseases and Immunology, Walter Reed Army Institute of Research, Silver Spring, MD 20910-7500

T.P. Endy; Colonel, Medical Corps, US Army; Director, Division of Communicable Diseases and Immunology, Walter Reed Army Institute of Research, 503 Robert Grant Avenue, Silver Spring, MD 20910-7500

C.F. Longer; Colonel, Medical Corps, US Army (Retired); Chief, Division of Hospital Medicine, Department of Medicine, University of Tennessee College of Medicine, Chattanooga Unit, 975 East 3rd Street, Chattanooga, TN 37403; Formerly, Assistant Chief, Department of Virus Diseases, Division of Communicable Diseases and Immunology, Walter Reed Army Institute of Research, Washington, DC 20307-5100

D.W. Vaughn; Colonel, Medical Corps, US Army; Director, Military Infectious Diseases Research Program, US Army Medical Research and Materiel Command, 504 Scott Street, Fort Detrick, Frederick, MD 21702-5012

G.V. Ludwig; Chief, Diagnostic Systems Division, US Army Medical Research Institute of Infectious Diseases, 1425 Porter Street, Fort Detrick, Frederick MD 21702–5011

D.J. McClain; Asheville Infectious Disease, 445 Biltmore Center, Suite 500, Asheville NC 28801; Formerly, Research Medical Officer, Division of Virology, US Army Medical Research Institute of Infectious Diseases, 1425 Porter Street, Fort Detrick, Frederick MD 21702–5011

K. Michaels; Lieutenant Colonel, Medical Corps, US Army; Chief, Department of Preventive Medicine, Eisenhower Army Medical Center, Fort Gordon, GA 30905

H.S. Lee; Lieutenant Colonel, Medical Corps, US Army; Preventive Medicine Consultant, Preventive Services Directorate, 18th Medical Command, APO AP 96205

V.B. Solberg; Department of Entomology, Division of Communicable Diseases and Immunology, Walter Reed Army Institute of Research, Silver Spring, MD 20910-7500

K.L. Clark; Infectious Disease Analyst, Armed Forces Medical Intelligence center, 1607 Porter Street, Fort Detrick, Frederick MD 21702-5004; Formerly, Major, Medical Corps, US Army; Coordinator, Accession Medical Standards Analysis and Research Activity, Division of Preventive Medicine, Walter Reed Army Institute of Research, Washington, DC 20307–5100

A.E. Brown; Lieutenant Colonel, Medical Corps, US Army; Department of Retrovirology, Armed Forces Research Institute of Medical Sciences, Bangkok, Thailand, APO AP 96546

D.A. Strickman; Colonel, Medical Service, US Army (Retired); Santa Clara County Vector Control District, 976 Lenzen Avenue, San Jose, CA 95126; Formerly, Chief, Department of Entomology, Walter Reed Army Institute of Research, Silver Spring MD 20910-7500

D.J. Kelly; Lieutenant Colonel, Medical Service, US Army (Retired); Research Associate, Department of Evolution, Ecology, and Organismal Biology, The Ohio State University, 388 Aronoff Laboratory, 318 West 12th Avenue, Columbus, Ohio, 43210; Formerly, Department of Rickettsial Disease, Division of Retrovirology, Walter Reed Army Institute of Research, Silver Spring MD 20910-7500

M.G. Kortepeter; Lieutenant Colonel, Medical Corps, US Army; Chief,Medicine Division, US Army Medical Research Institute of Infectious Diseases, 1425 Porter Street, Fort Detrick, Frederick, MD 21702-5011

W.P. Corr; Lieutenant Colonel, Medical Corps, US Army; Deputy Commander, Clinical Services, Martin Army Community Hospital, 7950 Martin Loop, Fort Benning, GA 31905-5637

A.J. Magill; Colonel, Medical Corps, US Army; Science Director, Walter Reed Army Institute of Research, Silver Spring, MD 20910-7500

W.C. Hewitson; Lieutenant Colonel, Medical Corps, US Army; Department of Preventive Health Services, Community Health Practices Branch, AMEDD Center and School, ATTN: MCCS-HPC, Fort Sam Houston, TX 78234-6124

MALARIA

Introduction and Military Relevance

Malaria is perhaps the most potentially devastating vector-borne disease for the military. This is because of its ability to appear in a military unit suddenly and cause near universal infection, its ability to incapacitate and kill nonimmune personnel within a few days, and the practical difficulty of controlling infections in tropical garrison units. Service members with even mild cases of malaria often have poor stamina and fitness for any military duties. Malaria is especially a threat for operations in sub-Saharan Africa, the Amazon River basin, Central America, Hispaniola, and much of Southeast Asia and Oceania.

The role of the mosquito in malaria was unknown until 1897 when MAJ Ronald Ross of the Indian Army Medical Department discovered that mosquitoes transmit malaria. Despite this knowledge, personnel deployed to the tropics continue to be plagued by malaria.[1] The age of chemotherapy, using at first the old specific febrifuge quinine and later synthetic antimalarials from the dye industry, offered great promise. Ever-present logistical and discipline problems, however, have been compounded by drug resistance such that the casualty-producing potential of malaria is little different today than it was more than a century ago (Figure 35-1).

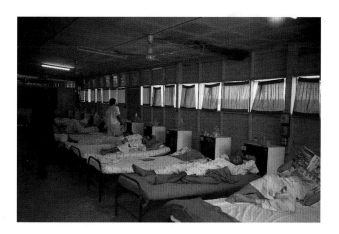

Fig. 35-1. This photograph shows a hospital ward in eastern Thailand filled with Thai Marines, all with drug-resistant falciparum malaria. Multidrug resistant malaria can cause mass casualties in service members deployed in the tropics.
Photograph: Courtesy of Colonel G. Dennis Shanks, Medical Corps, US Army.

Burma Campaign, World War II

General William Slim of the British Army had several problems with illness in his troops in 1943 during the Burma Campaign. Nearly a thousand men became ill everyday, and the ratio of sick to combat wounded was 120 to 1, with malaria causing 840 cases per 1,000 men per year. In General Slim's words, "A simple calculation showed me that in a matter of months at this rate my army would have melted away. Indeed, it was doing so under my eyes."[2p177] Several measures turned this unacceptable situation around, and not one of them was primarily medical. Malaria treatment units were moved up into the combat zone so failure to take prophylactic medication only earned a soldier a trip to a field treatment camp and a rapid return to his combat unit. Discipline in taking prophylactic atabrine medication was stepped up, and orders were issued to relieve any commander whose units did not achieve 95% drug positivity measured by unannounced urine testing. Again using General Slim's words: "I only had to sack three; by then the rest had got my meaning."[2p180] Medical support was not enough to win against malaria; command emphasis and discipline were key elements in the victory in Burma (See chapter 2, The Historical Impact of Preventive Medicine in War).

Vietnam War

Malaria was a leading cause of illness in the Vietnam War, with more than 40,000 cases in the US Army alone.[3] In spite of very sophisticated medical care, malaria killed on average one US service member during each month of the Vietnam War. Malaria's impact on combat effectiveness was magnified by two facts: (1) the concentration of cases in the frontline infantry operating in the jungle and (2) drug resistance leading to extended hospital stays. During 1965, entire battalions of the 1st Cavalry (Airmobile) Division were pulled out of the Ia Drang Valley because of malaria casualties exceeding 1% per day.

Somalia

Operation Restore Hope in Somalia (1992-1993) resulted in the largest epidemic of malaria in US military forces since the Vietnam War. Mostly due to noncompliance with the malaria chemoprophylaxis regimens (either daily doxycycline or weekly mefloquine), 48 US soldiers and Marines became infected with malaria while in Somalia.[4] Following the redeployment of US Marines to southern California and the 10th Mountain Division to upstate New York, epidemics were noted in both areas consisting primarily of vivax malaria from liver-stage relapses.[5] The risk of vivax malaria was underestimated because of the expectation that Somalia's malaria risk would resemble that of other areas in sub-Saharan Africa. Somalis have Duffy blood group antigen, unlike most Bantu peoples of Africa, and are thus susceptible to vivax malaria. The post-Somalia epidemic of relapsing malaria demonstrated the great need for an easily administered postdeployment medication to eliminate liver-relapse forms of malaria.[6] Despite the importation of malaria into the United States, the risk of resultant locally transmitted cases is small. Malaria, however, remains a very current medical threat to US forces deployed to the tropics.

Description of the Pathogen

Malaria is caused by a genus of parasite known as *Plasmodium*, of which four species are known to commonly infect humans. *P falciparum* is the most important, in terms of the numbers of symptomatic disease and deaths. Both *P vivax* and *P ovale*

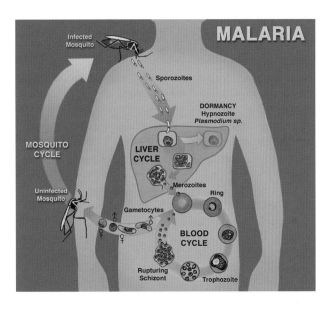

Fig. 35-2. The malaria life cycle.
Art by Annabelle Wright, Walter Reed Army Institute of Research; research by Amelia Pousson.

cause relapsing malaria through their ability to live in the liver in a quiescent form for long periods of time. Relapsing malaria rarely kills. *P malariae* (and *P vivax* less commonly) can cause very long-term bloodstream infections that can be inapparent and are a problem for blood banks because of the possibility of transfusion malaria. All four species are capable of causing human disease noted by fever, chills, headache, sweats, and malaise. The malaria parasite's three separate but interdependent cycles of development take place in the mosquito, the human liver, and the human bloodstream (Figure 35-2). All three cycles are required for the parasite to grow and spread successfully.

Mosquito Cycle

The mosquito is not a passive means of transferring infection; the infection must develop inside the mosquito under very precise conditions. Other conditions determine whether a female anopheline mosquito will actually survive long enough to pass malaria to another human. Malaria parasite development in the mosquito ceases entirely when mean temperatures remain lower than 18°C. Those limits determine the season, geography, and altitude that can support malaria transmission. Gametocytes taken from human blood by the mosquito undergo sexual reproduction and eventually become the infective form known as sporozoites in the insect's salivary glands.

Liver Cycle

Sporozoites, the first stage of the parasite, are injected into a human from the mosquito. The sporozoites are rapidly cleared from the bloodstream. Those sporozoites taken up by the reticuloendothelial system are destroyed and do not result in further infection. Sporozoites that make it to a liver cell, however, invade and set up the exoerythrocytic (or liver) cycle. Merozoites develop in the liver and are released into the bloodstream, initiating the blood cycle. When blood parasites seeded from the liver reach sufficient density, symptoms of malaria are induced. The time from mosquito bite to symptoms, called the incubation period, is about 10 to 14 days. Some liver parasites (*P vivax*, *P ovale*) appear to stop their development early in the cycle and thus form a hypnozoite, which appears to serve as the source of malaria relapses months to years later without further infective mosquito bites.

Blood Cycle

The merozoites enter and infect red blood cells and develop into trophozoites (ring forms). These consume hemoglobin and reproduce in the human bloodstream. This cycle of infection is often relatively synchronous and results in regular phases of symptoms, such as chills, fever, and sweats. The diagnosis of malaria is made by microscopic examination of stained blood smears and the detection of the blood forms of the parasite. The rupture of the infected erythrocyte releases factors that can induce symptoms of illness and new parasites (schizonts), which then infect new erythrocytes. Erythrocytes infected with later stages of the parasite (schizonts of *P falciparum*) can bind to the walls of small blood vessels in the brain, lung, and kidney and thus produce lethal infections such as cerebral malaria. Some blood-stage parasites develop into the sexual forms of the parasite in the blood (gametocytes), which serve to reinfect a biting mosquito, thus completing the cycle.

Epidemiology

Transmission

Malaria transmission requires three things: an infected person with gametocytes in his or her bloodstream, an anopheline mosquito to support the development of the gametocytes taken in a human blood meal into the infective form known as sporozoites, and a susceptible person who is bitten by a sporozoite-containing mosquito. Malaria transmission is actually a fragile chain that can be disrupted at several points.[7] In areas of the world with anopheline mosquitoes but without malaria-infected persons, there is no malaria transmission; however, the potential for transmission remains should malaria-infected persons enter the area. This situation currently exists in many parts of the continental United States and in Australia north of about 19° South longitude.

The mosquito itself is usually the weak link in the chain of transmission. Adequately controlling anopheline mosquitoes stops malaria transmission. This worked dramatically well during the malaria eradication campaign of the 1950s and 1960s in marginal areas of transmission using DDT (dichloro-diphenyl-trichloroethane) insecticide. Control of anopheline mosquitoes in the tropics is usually feasible only under special circumstances of limited geographic area and unlimited resources. Protec-

tion of the uninfected person is the military's usual method of malaria control. This can take the form of personal protection from mosquito bites (eg, screens, bed nets, repellents) or prophylactic drugs, which suppress the development of malaria infection and symptoms in the service member. Transmission potential in an area can vary widely over time depending on a variety of meterologic and sociologic factors. When efficient transmission occurs, however, infection rates approaching 1% a day have been seen in unprotected personnel participating in night jungle operations.[8]

Malaria can also be spread by blood transfusion and from mother to fetus.

Geographic Distribution

Malaria has a certain expected geographic range which can be predicted from historical records. A quick guide to a country's malaria risk can be found in the Centers for Disease Control and Prevention's annual publication *Health Information for International Travel.*[9] Areas of intense, year-round transmission, often near the equator, are marked by constant warm temperatures and humidity. The vast majority of clinical cases of malaria, especially falciparum malaria, occur in sub-Saharan Africa, the Amazon River basin, and parts of Southeast Asia. Tropical areas free of malaria tend to be urban areas in Southeast Asia and the Americas—areas where effective health services or environmental factors have eliminated the human infection reservoir or areas where deforestation or desertification have eliminated mosquito vectors. Local mosquito information on areas of military interest is often limited and should always be interpreted cautiously because developing countries have inadequate data for military planning, and civil strife usually increases the potential for malaria transmission.

There have been epidemics of malaria recorded as far north as Siberia in the former Soviet Union when summer temperatures allowed transmission to occur, so no fixed latitude lines for malaria transmission can be drawn. Cold temperatures usually limit malaria to altitudes below 1,500 m, but in some areas with population or ecological shifts, malaria transmission can be found in some parts of Africa at heights of greater than 2,000 m.[10] Malaria does not occur in deserts because mosquitoes require a certain amount of water to breed. This water may not be readily apparent, however, and oases in the Arabian Desert are small foci of malaria transmission in a great sea of sand.

Imported malaria refers to cases of malaria in which infection was acquired in another country. In the United States and Europe, most malaria is imported from tropical areas. For physicians treating service members, this presents a particular diagnostic problem if an accurate travel history is not obtained. Imported malaria cases in military personnel represent an extremely small chance of malaria reintroduction to formerly malarious areas because an infection must last at least 2 weeks to have a realistic chance to produce enough gametocytes to infect mosquitoes. This is likely only in an immune individual or one with no access to health care. Most autochthonous cases of malaria in the United States and Europe have been traced to transfusion malaria, relapsing malaria in travelers carrying gametocytes, or "airport malaria" (transmitted by mosquitoes transported in baggage or aircraft from a malarious country).

The most recent example of a military operation causing the reintroduction of malaria from an endemic area into an area that had eradicated the disease is the Afghan War in the 1980s.[11] Large numbers of Soviet military personnel were infected with falciparum malaria. Many of the soldiers were subsequently demobilized and returned to areas of the former Soviet Union, such as Azerbaijan and Tajikistan, that were still potentially malarious despite earlier near-elimination of the disease. At least some secondary spread occurred from the military-associated cases introduced from Afghanistan. A similar incident with vivax malaria was reported in the United States following the Korean War.[12]

Evidence for importation of falciparum malaria via returned military personnel during the Vietnam War is sparse, but veterans did manage to cause a small focal epidemic of falciparum malaria in California by sharing needles to inject illicit drugs. Imported malaria was directly related to military personnel with malaria in 1942 when large numbers of evacuated soldiers from New Guinea caused an epidemic of malaria in Cairns in northern Queensland, Australia.[13]

Incidence

In some locations, the actual risk of new malaria infections varies considerably within fairly small areas. Thai border-guard units stationed only a few kilometers apart on the Thai-Cambodian border had nearly no malaria or attack rates in excess of 1% a day.[14] This example points out the difficulties in making any generalized statements about malaria incidence except that malaria can be very focal.

Malaria incidence can be endemic or epidemic.

Endemic malaria is seen in areas of intense transmission, where most of the local population is infected early in life and develop protective immunity to malaria by the time they reach adulthood. Children bear the brunt of malaria disease and deaths, whereas adults usually show low parasitemias with few symptoms. Endemic malaria is usually very stable, and the population shows little disease on superficial inspection. The risk to nonimmune personnel in endemic malaria areas such as sub-Saharan Africa is very high, and particular efforts are necessary to prevent malaria. Missions involving humanitarian support to local populations in areas with endemic malaria require pediatric suspensions for malaria treatment and relatively fewer supplies for adult patients.

Epidemic malaria produces more adult disease than endemic malaria. In areas where malaria transmission is usually low and depends on a conjunction of weather and population factors, most local adults do not have effective immunity to malaria. When malaria transmission occurs, it is unstable and large numbers of adults may die. The Punjab in India is known to have periodic malaria epidemics when the monsoon rains are heavy.[15] Epidemic malaria can also be produced without any climatic changes by population shifts. Large movements of nonimmune service members during military operations or civilians during humanitarian emergencies may introduce a susceptible population into an endemic area, thus producing an epidemic in the newcomers. Epidemic malaria is particularly dangerous in civilian populations because of its ability to overwhelm health care services and confound physicians inexperienced with malaria who confuse it with other febrile illnesses.

In areas that benefited from the global effort to eradicate malaria by spraying dwellings with DDT more than a generation ago, malaria has often resurged following the discontinuation of malaria control efforts.[16] This decay of the public health infrastructure has been widespread and has also hindered malaria surveillance. Sri Lanka nearly eradicated malaria, only to experience its resurgence secondary to the consequences of civil war. Social disruption in North Korean rural areas has lead to some cases of vivax malaria being seen in South Korea. This includes at least 40 cases of vivax malaria seen in US soldiers stationed on the demilitarized zone from 1994 through 1997.[17] Moving semi-immune infected persons from one tropical area to another may spread drug-resistant strains of malaria across the world rapidly.

Pathogenesis and Clinical Findings

Malaria requires a certain incubation period, both in the mosquito before it is infective and in the human until an infection becomes apparent in the blood. The later period, the intrinsic incubation period, is about 10 days for most species of *Plasmodium*. The practical import of this is that very short military operations may not be directly affected by malaria; those sick within the first week of a tropical deployment do not have malaria. The reverse side of this issue is that service members may develop the first symptoms of malaria after returning to areas where the awareness of the disease is often low.

Nonimmune individuals may develop prodromal symptoms of malaria before parasites can be located in a blood smear. The usual clinical findings of malaria include fever, headache, chills, sweats, dysphoria, and mylagia; they have sometimes been described as being similar to a particularly bad case of influenza. In nonimmune persons, this may rapidly progress to severe malaria and death within hours to days. Any service member with a fever who has a travel history within the past year that includes a possible exposure to malaria should promptly have serial malaria blood smears to rule out this very treatable and potentially lethal infection. Although other laboratory signs, such as mild leucopenia, anemia, and thrombocytopenia, are consistent with acute malaria, direct evidence of the parasite must be sought.

Fever

Fever is almost always present when malaria exists in a nonimmune person. Many adults who have become tolerant to malaria through long exposure will have parasitemia without fever, but this situation could serve as an operational definition of malarial immunity. The fever is typically seen in conjunction with the classical triad of the malaria paroxysm: chills, fever, and sweats. The periodicity of malarial fevers is not often noticed if the diagnosis is made and treatment instituted in an expeditious manner. Antipyretics are useful to make the patient feel better because temperatures of up to 40°C are not uncommon. Distinguishing the delirium of high fever due to malaria from early cerebral malaria is nearly impossible and usually unnecessary as both require the same urgent antimalarial treatment.

Anemia

Malaria parasites destroy host erythrocytes, but usually this is not enough to induce anemia unless the infection becomes chronic. Severe anemia, however, is a fairly common finding in young children living in intensely malarious areas. Hyperparasitemia (>100,000 parasites/mm^3) has been treated with exchange blood transfusion to lower the parasitemia, but this approach has not reduced mortality.[18] When frank anemia is seen during acute malaria in a service member, antimalarial drug reactions, such as glucose 6–phosphate dehydrogenase (G6PD) deficiency–induced hemolysis, should be ruled out.

Severe Malaria

Most deaths from malaria within the military are due to failure to consider the diagnosis until the disease has progressed to a severe form. Nonimmune personnel have died after only a few days' illness when adequate treatment was not given quickly. Severe malaria is nearly always caused by *P falciparum* as the parasitized cells attach to small blood vessels in various internal organs.[19] Cerebral malaria appears as a parasite-induced metabolic coma. When treated promptly, patients generally recover full neurologic function, but cerebral malaria is a medical emergency. Analogous forms of severe malaria are seen with renal involvement producing acute renal failure and with pulmonary involvement producing a form of adult respiratory distress syndrome. Both are treated with appropriate physiologic support in an intensive care unit while attempting to kill the parasites as quickly as possible. Parental drugs, such as intravenous quinine (in the United States intravenous quinidine is used), are the keystone of severe malaria treatment.[19] The presence of malaria parasitemia and severe end organ damage does not mean that the two are causally related when dealing with immune adult patients with low parasitemias.

Diagnostic Approaches

The Standard

Thin and thick blood smears are currently the standard for diagnosing malaria. Failure to consider malaria as a diagnosis and to examine microscopically serial thick and thin blood smears is a frequent error noted in the treatment of patients who died of severe malaria in the United States. Small malaria parasites are more concentrated in thick blood smears, where the parasites can look like platelets or other forms of cellular debris. Coloration of stain and patience are important issues when examining blood films. Besides missing actual parasites due to an inadequate blood examination, false positive results are very common when inexperienced persons examine blood smears for malaria. Pseudo-epidemics of malaria have also been caused from over-interpreting normal cellular elements in an effort not to miss a serious treatable disease. Experience in reading blood slides and knowledge of when to obtain a smear are valuable in medical personnel deploying to the tropics.

Newer Diagnostic Tools

In an effort to eliminate some of the subjectivity from the reading of malaria blood films, several new tests to measure parasites in the blood have been developed. They have not yet replaced blood smears, and any military medical unit deploying to the tropics should have the capacity to examine blood films until more experience is gained with the newer antigenic or nucleic acid detection methods. Microscopic examination can be speeded through the use of fluorescent dye in a capillary tube, but this method still requires the ability to interpret microscopically visible parasites.[20] Fixed antigen detection methods using either the histidine-rich protein II or parasite lactate acid dehydrogenase of *P falciparum* have shown promising results and give an answer that is relatively easy to interpret.[21] The usefulness of such techniques in the field remains to be proven. The polymerase chain reaction holds promise as a diagnostic method for a multitude of infectious agents including malaria, but it is still a research tool and is not soon expected to be useful in the field because of the level of technology required for accurate analysis.[22] Rapid diagnostic methods are most likely to be useful in situations where large numbers of samples need to be tested quickly. Until the technology greatly improves, microscopic examination of stained blood films remains the best way to determine if any single service member has malaria.

Recommendations for Prophylaxis, Therapy, and Control

Prophylaxis

Chemoprophylaxis can kill or suppress the parasites, but a continuous concentration of drug must be maintained. Prophylactic and treatment regimens recommended vary over time because of evolving resistance patterns and other factors; it is critical that medical officers consult with command medical authorities to ensure regimens are current

(Figure 35-3). The *Health Information for International Travel*[9] and the package inserts of antimalarial medications are also important sources of information regarding issues such as dosage, adverse effects, and contraindications.

Any US deployment into an area with significant malaria transmission requires chemoprophylaxis (Table 35-1). There have been two traditional approaches to chemoprophylaxis during exposure: weekly medication or daily medication. Currently drug possibilities for weekly administration include chloroquine (300 mg base) or mefloquine (228 mg

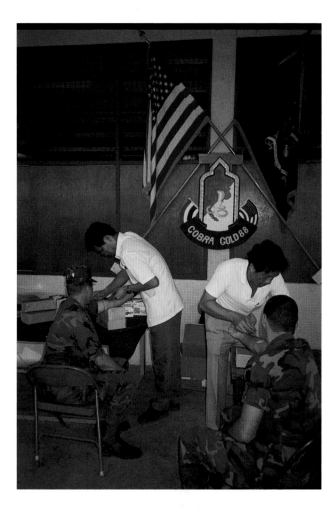

Fig. 35-3. Two technicians from the Armed Forces Research Institute of Military Science, Bangkok, Thailand, are drawing blood from US Army soldiers of the 25th Infantry Division during the 1988 Cobra Gold exercise in Thailand. The soldiers were enrolled in a malaria chemoprophylaxis trial using mefloquine and doxycycline. Both the Thai and US Armies have been involved in important collaborative work on malaria chemoprophylaxis.
Photograph: Courtesy of Colonel G. Dennis Shanks, Medical Corps, US Army.

TABLE 35-1

DRUGS USED IN THE PROPHYLAXIS OF MALARIA

Drug (Proprietary Name)	Usage	Adult Dose	Pediatric Dose	Comments
Mefloquine (Lariam)	In areas with chloroquine-resistant *Plasmodium falciparum*	228 mg base (250 mg salt) orally, once/wk	<15 kg: 4.6 mg/kg base (5 mg/kg [salt]) once/wk; 10–19 kg: 1/4 tab/wk 20–29 kg: 1/2 tab/wk 30–45 kg: 3/4 tab/wk >45 kg: 1 tab/wk	Contraindicated in persons allergic to mefloquine. Not recommended for persons with epilepsy and other seizure disorders, with severe psychiatric disorders, or with cardiac conduction abnormalities
Doxycycline	An alternative to mefloquine	100 mg orally, once daily	> 8 years of age: 2 mg/kg of body weight orally daily up to adult dose of 100 mg/d	Contraindicated in children < 8 y of age, pregnant women, and lactating women
Atovaquone/ Proguanil (Malarone)	In areas of multidrug-resistant *Plasmodium falciparum*	1 adult tablet daily 250 mg/100 mg orally	11-20 kg: 1 pediatric tablet[*] 21-30 kg: 2 pediatric tablets[*] 31-40 kg: 3 pediatric tablets[*] >40 kg: 1 adult tablet All given once daily	Very well tolerated with some gastrointestinal distress, best given with food
Chloroquine phosphate (Aralen)	In areas with chloroquine-sensitive *P falciparum*	300 mg base (500 mg salt) orally, once/wk	5 mg/kg base (8.3 mg/kg [salt]) orally, once/wk, up to maximum adult dose of 300 mg base	
Hydroxy-chloroquine sulfate (Plaquenil)	An alternative to chloroquine	310 mg base (400 mg salt) orally, once/wk	5 mg/kg base (6.5 mg/kg [salt]) orally, once/wk, up to adult dose of 310 mg base	
Chloroquine + proguanil	A less-effective alternative for use in Africa only if mefloquine or doxycycline cannot be used	Weekly chloroquine dose as above, plus daily proguanil dose 200 mg orally, once daily	Weekly chloroquine dose as above, plus for proguanil: <2 y: 50 mg/d 2–6 y: 100 mg/d 7–10 y: 150 mg/d >10 y: 200 mg/d	Proguanil is not sold in the United States but is widely available in Canada, Europe, and many African countries

[*] The pediatric tablet is 62.5 mg atovaquone and 25 mg proguanil
Adapted from: Centers for Disease Control and Prevention. Information for health care providers: Prescription drugs for preventing malaria. www.cdc.gov/travel/malariadrugs2.htm. Accessed on May 25, 2001.

base in the United States), and daily possibilities include proguanil (200 mg) alone or in combinations with other drugs or doxycycline (100 mg).[23] Recently daily atovaquone/proguanil (Malarone) has been licensed for daily malaria chemoprophylaxis (Table 35-2). Choice depends on parasite susceptibility in particular regions and other factors.

Weekly prophylactic regimens generally require less effort from the service members. Daily regimens require an enforced administration system, with the drugs typically being given out by squad leaders and supervised by medics. Different armies have favored different drugs for historical and other reasons.[24] Daily administration regimens fail quickly when the drugs are not taken every day because the drugs are eliminated from the circulation in a matter of hours. Weekly administration provides more leeway, but missing a weekly medication dose means that the individual may have a suboptimal drug concentration in his or her blood for several days. Both daily and weekly regimens are usually effective when the appropriate drugs are taken on schedule.

TABLE 35-2

PRESUMPTIVE TREATMENT OF MALARIA

Drug	Adult Dose	Pediatric Dosage	Comment
Pyrimethamine-sulfadoxine (Fansidar) Self-treatment drug to be used if professional medical care is not available within 24 hours. **Seek medical care immediately after self-treatment.**	3 tablets (75 mg pyrimethamine and 1,500 mg sulfadoxine) orally as a single dose	5–10 kg: 1/2 tablet 11–20 kg: 1 tablet 21–30 kg: 1 1/2 tablets 31–45 kg: 2 tablets > 45 kg: 3 tablets	Contraindicated in persons with sulfa allergy
Atovaquone/proguanil (Malarone)	4 tablets taken once daily for 3 days (1000 mg atovaquone/ 400 mg proguanil)	Daily dose for 3 days: 11-20 kg: 1 adult tablet 21-30 kg: 2 adult tablets 31-40 kg: 3 adult tablets >40 kg: 4 adult tablets	Best taken with food, may cause gastro-intestinal distress

Adapted from: Centers for Disease Control and Prevention. Information for health care providers: Prescription drugs for preventing malaria. www.cdc.gov/travel/malariadrugs2.htm. Accessed on May 25, 2001.

Side effects remain a key issue when giving medication to large numbers of healthy personnel. Even minor objectionable drug effects will seriously decrease compliance with the preventive regimen. It is good policy to brief all the medical personnel in depth and inform the service members about side effects and how to counter them. This will also help suppress rumors that occur whenever personnel are placed on mass medication. Doxycycline can cause many gastrointestinal problems, such as stomach upset, when taken on an empty stomach and needs to be taken with food. Women developing vaginitis and light-skinned personnel developing severe sunburn are other problems of doxycycline. Mefloquine can rarely produce serious central nervous system effects, such as psychosis and seizures.[25] Mefloquine is not given to personnel with a history of seizures or serious neuropsychiatric disorders. Flight crews do not take mefloquine because they need to avoid even minor mental problems. More commonly, patients taking mefloquine complain of vague dysphoria. During recent military deployments, there has been a tendency to blame all physical and psychological problems regardless of etiology on prophylactic drugs. The best way to avoid having service members feel that they are being harmed by chemoprophylaxis is to circulate adequate information before starting any mandated medication. This is especially true with primaquine or other postexposure regimens because service members often feel that their risk ends

when they leave the endemic area and discontinue taking their medication.

New drugs are under development and can be expected to take their place in the chemoprophylactic universe soon. Azithromycin is a long-acting antibiotic related to erythromycin that may be a substitute for doxycycline. Atovaquone/proguanil has been shown to prevent malaria in Africa and Asia.[26] A long-acting primaquine analog known as tafenoquine is under development and may provide a postdeployment treatment that is easier to use than primaquine. Although used for prophylaxis in some areas of China, the qinghaosu derivatives, such as artemenisin, cannot be recommended for long-term administration.

Treatment

When a nonimmune service member develops malaria, the goal is to bring the parasite count down rapidly to levels where severe malaria is not a consideration and then eliminate the last parasites to effect a cure. Before the development of widespread drug resistance in malaria, one drug (eg, chloroquine) could often perform both functions. Now in many countries, it is often necessary to use one drug to lower the parasitemia rapidly and other, longer-acting drugs to eliminate the last parasites. For severe infections, aggressive treatment in an intensive care unit is indicated. Quinine, or the closely related quinidine, is often used to reduce parasitemia rapidly. Quinidine is the only licensed drug available to Western physicians for severe malaria.[27] Quinine has a narrow therapeutic ratio and should always be given orally if the patient is able to tolerate oral medication. If oral medications are not tolerated, then quinine is administered via slow intravenous infusion over several hours. Quinine causes a number of objectionable side effects (eg, tinnitus) when given in an adequate dosage and usually causes more problems to the patient than the malaria does by about the third day of treatment. Almost no one will take a 7-day course of quinine unless forced to do so. It is possible that qinghaosu derivatives, such as artesunate, may replace quinine in Southeast Asia, but as of 2000, none of them are licensed compounds in the United States.

Because of the relatively short half-life of quinine and qinghaosu derivatives, it is important to give other drugs to eliminate the last parasites and so effect a parasitological cure. Doxycycline or tetracycline given over the course of 1 week will eliminate residual falciparum parasites. A single dose of mefloquine has been used for the same purpose following a course of artesunate. In some areas where drug resistance has not reached extreme levels, treatment with single-dose drugs such as pyrimethamine/sulfadoxine or mefloquine is still effective. It is unclear how long this situation will last, and all medical officers who treat malaria patients need to be aware that drug resistance is a growing problem that may necessitate longer courses of drugs or combination therapy to obtain cures. If a service member with a previous malaria infection returns within 1 to 3 months of an apparently successful treatment, any reoccurrence may actually be a return of the old infection (recrudescence), which was suppressed but not completely cured. Blood film examinations should be repeated on any individual treated for malaria to ensure that the parasitemia does actually resolve completely.

Postdeployment Malaria

Malaria often occurs in service members after redeployment to nonmalarious areas. This can happen with recrudescence of suppressed infections once prophylactic drugs are stopped or when residual liver stages (hypnozites) cause malaria to relapse long after the initial mosquito bite. The former can be avoided by continuing antimalarial prophylaxis after leaving the malarious area. When using either doxycycline daily or mefloquine weekly, it is recommended that medication be continued for 4 weeks after leaving the malarious area. This is a challenge as personnel often go on leave following major deployments and medication compliance falls accordingly.

Relapsing malaria presents a different problem. Where service members have been heavily exposed to relapsing malaria species (*P ovale* or *P vivax*), it is currently recommended that primaquine (15 mg base daily for 2 weeks) be given to eliminate hypnozites and thus prevent relapses. There is evidence from Papua New Guinea[28] and Somalia[6] that some forms of *P vivax* may be relatively tolerant to primaquine and thus require longer courses using more total primaquine. Primaquine can cause severe hemolysis in some individuals with G6PD deficiency, typically those with ancestors from the southern Mediterranean region and some areas of Southeast Asia and Africa. About 12% of blacks in the US military are G6PD deficient, although their deficiency is usually relatively less severe than that found in other ethnic groups. Testing service members for G6PD deficiency will eliminate most of this risk but involves predeployment testing and accurate recordkeeping. Testing for G6PD deficiency is not done by all military services (as of 2000 the US Army does not), and this must be considered when giving primaquine to large groups.

Much of the primaquine that is dispensed is not taken. Some compliance difficulties may be solved by a new long-acting drug related to primaquine (tafenoquine) under development. Primaquine should be taken with food, as doxycycline is, because this seems to minimize the gastrointestinal intolerance. Blood donors who have had malaria are deferred for 3 years after becoming asymptomatic, donors from countries on the Centers for Disease Control and Prevention's malaria-endemic list are allowed to donate 3 years after leaving the malarious area if they have had no unexplained symptoms suggestive of malaria, and donors who have visited a malarious area are allowed to donate 12 months after leaving the malarious area if they have had no unexplained symptoms suggestive of malaria regardless of their history of antimalarial prophylaxis.[29]

Emergence of Drug Resistance

Prophylaxis and treatment have been severely compromised by the rise of drug-resistant strains of *P falciparum*. When large numbers of persons living in malaria-endemic areas are taking long-acting drugs, such as chloroquine or mefloquine, resistant strains have a significant evolutionary advantage and gradually spread through the population. Since multidrug resistance has now evolved, the situation on the Thai-Cambodian and Thai-Burmese borders is approaching the point where incurable infections can be anticipated.[30] The current situation in Africa and South America is not so severe, but resistance to both chloroquine and pyrimethamine/sulfadoxine is widespread. Improved access to antimalarial drugs in these areas will inevitably result in further drug resistance. As newer drugs are circulated more widely, more difficult issues of drug resistance can be anticipated. In well-supplied military units, most problems of drug resistance can currently be handled with alternative drugs. This is not the case in many armies from poorer nations, which are now making up an increasing proportion of United Nations peacekeeping missions in malarious areas. A well thought out plan is important to engendering confidence in and compliance with the assigned drug regimens from military personnel.

Some of the islands of Melanesia and Indonesia and some areas of northern South America have chloroquine-resistant vivax malaria. There is no obvious replacement drug for chloroquine in treating relapsing malaria. Relative resistance to primaquine may exist in Melanesia[28] and Somalia based on reports of difficulty eliminating relapses in individuals returning from these areas.[6] Noncompliance, confused orders, inactive or expired drugs, malabsorption, and failure to complete a drug course after returning home are also potential explanations for high malaria attack rates. In vitro analysis of parasite isolates can aid determination of drug resistance evolution, and efforts should be made to obtain blood from problem cases. Most antimalarial drug concentrations can be determined from plasma samples that have been frozen for later analysis to confirm compliance or drug resistance.

Control

Personal Protective Measures. Antimalarial drugs form a vital but not exclusive part of the means of preventing malarial illness. As noted in chapter 22 (Personal Protection Measures Against Arthropods), personal and unit level protective measures are vital to reduce the number of bites from infected mosquitoes and deserve great command emphasis.

Vaccines. Hope that a malaria vaccine might give a simple, durable solution to the problem of malaria prevention in service members became widespread once the molecular nature of malaria antigens began to be uncovered. Unfortunately, no simple fix is in sight.[31,32] Malaria is a protozoan parasite of great complexity that has defied simple immunologic solutions. If and when a practical malaria vaccine comes into use, it will likely include multiple antigens presented with new adjuvants to induce immunity capable of handling the genetic plasticity of plasmodia. Traditional tools of military preventive medicine, including antimosquito measures, chemoprophylaxis, and military discipline, will be needed for the foreseeable future to protect those deployed into tropical regions.

[G. Dennis Shanks, Jerome J. Karwacki]

DENGUE VIRUS INFECTIONS

Introduction and Military Relevance

Dengue viruses are mosquito-borne flaviviruses related to the yellow fever virus. They are responsible for an estimated 20 million to 100 million new infections annually, making them the most common arthropod-borne virus infection of humans.[33] Infection with dengue virus is a prominent cause of febrile illness in tropical areas, where it is known as dengue or breakbone fever. Dengue viruses can cause abrupt epidemics, in which cases of dengue may affect more than 50% of susceptible persons. Since the 1970s, the incidence of new infections has increased in parallel with an exponential rise in abundance of the principal mosquito vector, *Aedes aegypti*.[34] The mosquito species has spread into regions where previously it had been well controlled, most notably in Latin America and the Caribbean region. Increased mobility of human populations has also contributed to the introduction and spread of dengue viruses into many areas of the tropics and subtropics.[35]

Dengue viruses and mosquito vectors pose significant hazards to nonimmune persons when they enter endemic areas.[36] US military populations in particular become exposed to dengue viruses while deployed in tropical regions. Often, sporadic cases occur in service members operating in these environments, but large numbers of personnel may be affected by epidemic dengue if there are favorable entomological circumstances. The continuous prominence of dengue as a common arthropod-borne disease encountered by service members in the tropics has prompted much research, resulting in diagnostic tests and stimulating vaccine development.

The first recorded observation of dengue among US forces was during the Spanish-American War, when troops were stationed in Cuba. During an 8-month period in 1898, 249 cases of clinical dengue were noted, with a case fatality rate of 8 per 1,000 troops.[37] In comparison, yellow fever was observed to be the most prominent disease, with 1,169 cases and a case fatality rate of 123 per 1,000. Dengue was of no importance during World War I as the major American Expeditionary Force campaigns were waged in temperate regions. During the postwar period, classic studies[38,39] in the transmission and pathogenesis of dengue were conducted by Siler and Simmons with personnel garrisoned in the Philippines, where dengue was an immense military health problem. These studies helped identify the arthropod vectors for dengue infection and unequivocally characterized the clinical and hematologic features of the disease.

Dengue was the second most common arthropod-borne infection (after malaria) during World War II, causing an estimated 91,000 cases among US Army forces.[40] Dengue was a particular problem throughout the Pacific, the China-Burma-India theater, and the Mediterranean theaters of operation, where average rates of infection from 1942 to 1945 ranged from 18 to 32 cases per year per 1,000 average strength. Dengue epidemics affecting tens of thousands of service members occurred in New Guinea, Saipan, Hawaii, and other areas (Figure 35-4). Continuous movement of personnel and materiel associated with military operations may also have been related to huge outbreaks of dengue that occurred in ports in Japan, Hawaii, Australia, and many of the Pacific islands.[41]

The major impact of dengue on operations was its propensity to cause epidemics of disease among nonimmune populations taking inadequate preventive measures. Incapacitation of military personnel by

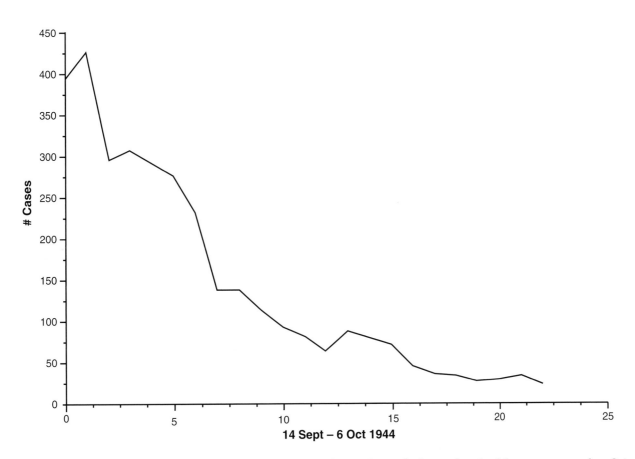

14 Sept – 6 Oct 1944

Fig. 35-4. Daily report of new cases of dengue, Saipan epidemic. An explosive outbreak of dengue occurred on Saipan following the assault on the Marianas Islands in June 1944. It was estimated that over 20,000 cases occurred in the most extensive epidemic of dengue during World War II. Rates exceeding 400 new cases per day only decreased after introduction of aerial DDT spraying on 12 September.
Data source: McCoy OR, Sabin AB. Dengue. Coates JB Jr, Hoff EC, Hoff PM, eds. *Communicable Diseases: Arthropodborne Diseases Other than Malaria*. Vol 7. In: *Preventive Medicine in World War II*. Washington, DC: Office of the Surgeon General, Department of the Army; 1964: 39.

dengue during the first weeks of exposure while facing an entrenched and usually immune enemy force was of great concern to commanders. Outbreaks of disease during World War II often were related to combat operations, which complicated mosquito control measures. It was quickly realized that the incidence of dengue was inversely correlated with the effectiveness of the preventive measures imposed by commanders. Epidemics of dengue subsided as rapidly as they arose, generally following institution of vigorous control measures. These included intensification of vector control (eg, destruction of larvae, pesticide spraying, sweeps every 10 days to eliminate containers breeding mosquitoes) and enforced preventive measures (eg, use of personal protection, mandatory use of screened quarters for patients, restricted contact between civilian and military populations). These prevention measures were credited, at least in part, with keeping the rates as low as they were.[37] These policies were pursued to great effect in many regions, and declines in the incidence of dengue in the US Army were seen in all theaters (Figure 35-5).

Many advances in dengue virus research occurred during World War II, primarily due to a team led by LTC Albert Sabin, who later developed oral poliovirus vaccine. Using the Dengue Research Unit at Princeton, NJ, established by the Army Epidemiology Board, Dr. Sabin and colleagues isolated and propagated two serotypes (types 1 and 2) of dengue virus in human volunteers and adapted the viruses to grow in suckling mouse brains.[42] They developed diagnostic tests for each and, using these unique reagents, they characterized immunity to dengue, identified the existence of neutralizing antibodies after infection, and prepared an attenuated dengue virus vaccine.[43] The dengue vaccine was

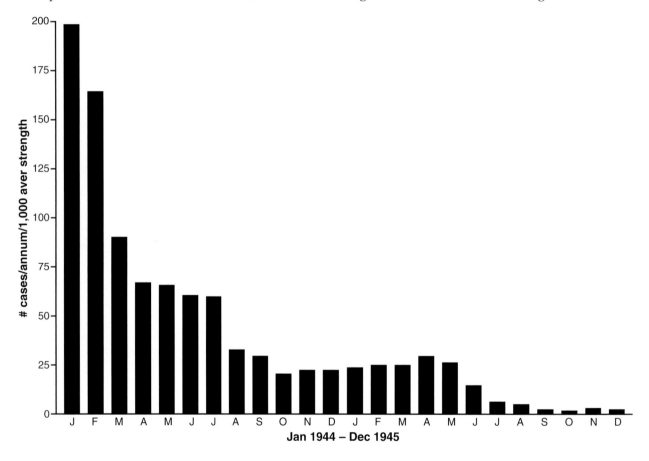

Fig. 35-5. Incidence of dengue in US Army personnel, New Guinea and adjacent islands, January 1944 through December 1945. Epidemic dengue was observed in troops deployed to New Guinea during the rainy season (January-February) 1944. Rates of dengue often exceeded that for malaria in some units. However, introduction of intensive mosquito control and preventive measures, and possibly immunity from the previous epidemic, resulted in lower incidence of dengue in 1945.
Data source: McCoy OR, Sabin AB. Dengue. Coates JB Jr, Hoff EC, Hoff PM, eds. *Communicable Diseases: Arthropodborne Diseases Other than Malaria*. Vol 7. In: *Preventive Medicine in World War II*. Washington, DC: Office of the Surgeon General, Department of the Army; 1964: 37.

tested in volunteers but never administered to personnel in the field, as the war's end interrupted vaccine development.

Subsequent personnel deployments overseas benefited from the lessons of World War II. Increased attention to preventive measures reduced the rate of medical casualties from arthropod-borne illnesses. But as sanitary and personal hygiene were dramatically improved, fevers of undetermined origin (FUOs, febrile illnesses not specifically diagnosed during the 3 days following admission to a military hospital) assumed greater importance as causes of combat ineffectiveness.[44] While dengue did not have a significant role during the war in Korea, the experience of US forces in Vietnam underscored the importance of dengue as a military infectious disease.

Fever of undetermined origin was "perhaps one of the greatest diagnostic dilemmas for military physicians in Vietnam."[45p75–76] It was common—the average incidence rate was 58 FUO cases per 1,000 average troop strength per year (range: 35-100/1,000 per year). Several comprehensive studies documented the etiologies of tropical fevers in personnel deployed to Vietnam; they showed that dengue was the cause of 4% to 28% of all FUOs (Table 35-3). On the other hand, US service members in Vietnam did not suffer major epidemics of dengue "undoubtedly because of the high level of environ-

mental sanitation and the resulting absence of *A aegypti* on most US Army bases in Vietnam. Dengue was contracted mainly by support forces who had contact with civilian populations, as most mosquito transmission occurred in local communities."[41p97] No preventive measures are totally effective in the control of sporadic occurrences of dengue among service members entering an urbanized civilian area.

No dengue occurred during the Persian Gulf War (1990-1991). This may have been due to the exclusion of Coalition personnel from urban areas, the war's occurrence in winter (which decreased vector abundance), and strict preventive measures, including early establishment of disease monitoring and diagnostic laboratory support.[46]

The next major movements of personnel and materiel through the tropics occurred during Operation Restore Hope (Somalia, 1992-1993) and Operation Uphold Democracy (Haiti, 1994-1997). During Operation Restore Hope, more than 25,000 US military personnel were deployed and concerted efforts were made to adopt the preventive medicine lessons learned from the Persian Gulf War.[47] Rates of disease were low, perhaps because of limited contact with the local population. Nevertheless, dengue was responsible for 20% of all febrile illnesses in US military personnel.[48]

Twenty thousand US military personnel were deployed during Operation Uphold Democracy to

TABLE 35-3

DENGUE AS A CAUSE OF FEVER OF UNDETERMINED ORIGIN CASES IN US FORCES IN VIETNAM, 1966-1969

	Study 1	Study 2	Study 3	Study 4	Study 5	Study 6[*]
Location	93rd Evacuation Hospital	8th Field Hospital	Dong Tam	I Corps (Navy)	12th USAF	9th Medical Laboratory
Dates	4/66 - 8/66	10/66 - 2/67	6/67 - 12/67	2/67 - 9/67	7/67 - 6/68	1/69 - 12/69
# cases	110	94	87	295	306	1,256
% specific diagnosis						
Malaria	7.0	6.4	12.6	†	70.0	†
Dengue	28.0	10.6	11.0	3.4	5.0	10.4
Japanese encephalitis	1.0	0	1.0	8.1	0	3.9
Undetermined	26.0	38.0	54.0	51.0	12.0	†

[*] Records of LTC Andre J. Ognibene, from data collected at the 9th Medical Laboratory, Long Binh, Vietnam.
† excluded by study design
Adapted from: Deller JJ Jr. Fever of undetermined origin. Ognibene AJ, Barrett O Jr, eds. *General Medicine and Infectious Diseases*. Vol 2. In: *Internal Medicine in Vietnam*. Washington, DC: Office of the Surgeon General and Center of Military History, US Army; 1982.

Haiti, a known high-risk area for dengue and malaria. In the first weeks of deployment, personnel were located in an urban area close to the local population and to high densities of mosquito vectors. In recognition of the threat of vector-borne disease, service members were given malaria chemoprophylaxis, bednets, and insect repellents. Despite these measures, an outbreak of dengue resulted in significant morbidity and consumption of medical resources.[49] In the first weeks of the operation (from 27 September to 5 November 1994), 112 patients, or approximately 0.1% of US personnel, were evaluated for nonspecific febrile illness. Of a series of 103 consecutive patients admitted to the combat support hospital (25% of all hospital admissions during the period), 30 had confirmed dengue infection.[50] After this initial cluster of cases among personnel centered in the major urban areas, sporadic cases continued to occur. In a 1995-1996 survey of 61 consecutive febrile admissions to a US Army field hospital in Haiti, 25 soldiers were confirmed to have dengue (Sun W. Unpublished data, 1997).

Dengue remains a common cause of sporadic febrile illness in service members deployed to the tropics. However, the explosive spread of dengue virus and vectors throughout the tropics worldwide suggests that the medical threat of dengue may increase in the future, especially when forces are deployed under less-controlled field conditions. Vigilance and adherence to vector control and personal preventive measures will be necessary. Until vaccination becomes possible, sporadic dengue will continue to occur when military individuals must move during daylight hours among civilian populations in endemic areas.

Description of the Pathogen

Dengue viruses are a group of four related viruses, which are distinguished serologically as types 1, 2, 3, and 4.[51] The virus serotypes share 60% to 80% homology at the nucleotide level. All are pathogenic, causing clinically indistinguishable infections in a susceptible human host. Dengue viruses are enveloped 40-50 nm virions that contain single-stranded 11 kilobase RNA enclosed by nucleocapsid proteins.

Epidemiology

Transmission

The vectors of dengue virus are principally urban-dwelling, day-biting, anthropophilic *Aedes* species

mosquitoes. The one of greatest importance is *Aedes aegypti*. The vector status of *Aedes albopictus*, the tiger mosquito, remains to be comprehensively established.

Following a 10- to 14-day extrinsic incubation period within an infected mosquito that has fed on an infected person, the mosquito can inoculate virus intradermally whenever it probes into a new host. Dengue virus then infects skin Langerhan cells and migrates to lymphoid organs such as the draining lymph nodes, liver, and spleen.[52] After several cycles of replication, generally within 5 to 7 days after the mosquito bite, dengue virus is detectable circulating in the blood (Figure 35-6). The period of viremia is typically brief (less than 3 to 5 days) and usually coincides with onset of fever and symptoms.

Geographic Distribution

A aegypti is found worldwide and is established in the continental United States. Though *A aegypti* was eradicated from large portions of the Americas, the mosquito returned as control programs waned.

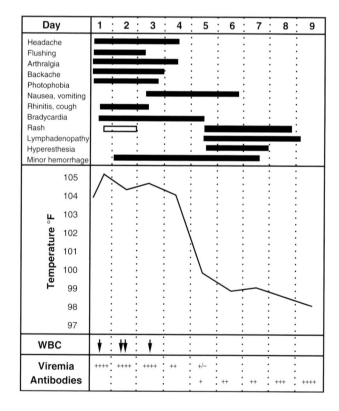

Fig. 35-6. The typical clinical course of dengue fever. Reprinted with permission from: Monath TP, Tsai TF. Flavivirusus. In: Richman DD, Whitley RJ, Hayden FG, eds. *Clinical Virology*. New York: Churchill Livingstone; 1997.

Dengue poses a particular threat to forces deployed in the densely populated urban centers of the tropics, where the disease is often hyperendemic and underrecognized among the local populace. The incidence of dengue virus infections worldwide may be expected to increase in the near future as dengue viruses are introduced into new areas, perhaps even including the southern United States. The increasing pace of short-term deployments to tropical areas may also contribute to increased exposure to dengue.

Dengue hemorrhagic fever (DHF) occurs in areas where three or more dengue serotype viruses circulate simultaneously or sequentially. The disease was first recognized in Asia, but since the 1980s, it has emerged and intensified in Latin America and the Caribbean region.[53] No DHF has been observed yet in Africa.

Incidence

In dengue-endemic areas, infections usually occur in children of preschool and school-age years (peak ages 2 to 9 years) but rarely result in prominent symptoms.

Some infected individuals develop more severe disease with varying degrees of circulatory collapse and hemorrhage (dengue hemorrhagic fever/dengue shock syndrome or DHF/DSS). This occurs in one of several hundred or thousand cases of dengue virus infection.[54] DHF principally affects children younger than 15 years old but may also occur in adults. In all regions where it is found, DHF occurs more frequently, but not exclusively, in individuals with secondary infections with dengue virus.[55] The risk of DHF is increased 100-fold in secondary compared to primary infections in Thailand.[56] Infants with circulating maternal antibodies to dengue virus are susceptible to severe primary infection. The presence of prior immunity to dengue virus poses only part of the explanation for DHF, as severe dengue occurs only in approximately 1 in 200 secondarily infected children.[57]

Dengue-naïve adults traveling to endemic areas are at risk for developing dengue, but their risk for developing DHF appears remote. Despite thousands of cases of dengue in US service members since the 1960s, no case of DHF has been observed. However, if military personnel sustain sequential dengue infections over several years, as children do in areas where DHF is endemic, their risk of developing DHF may increase. Only speculation is possible until the pathogenesis of DHF is fully understood and all risk factors are identified.

Pathogenesis and Clinical Findings

Pathogenesis

Dengue viruses replicate within the cytoplasm of infected cells after receptor-mediated entry. The native receptor on the dengue target cell has not been determined. The known sites of viral replication in vivo are leukocytes, especially circulating B cells, Kupffer cells, and tissue macrophages outside of the neuroaxis. Dengue antigen has been detected by immunofluorescence within tissue macrophages in affected target organs, such as the liver, spleen, kidney, and skin.[58]

Monocytes and macrophages are critical target cells for dengue virus because their infection may be enhanced by cross-reactive nonneutralizing antibody, a phenomenon known as antibody-dependent enhancement (ADE).[59] In ADE, dengue virus binds available group-specific antibody from previous dengue infection and enters the cell through membrane F_c receptors. There is increasing evidence that ADE is important in the causation of dengue hemorrhagic fever.

Coincident with occurrence of fever is a characteristic depression of circulating neutrophil and platelet counts.[60] Infection of dendritic cells by dengue viruses may play an important role in disease pathogenesis.[61] Viremia and fever cease with the appearance of IgM and IgG antibodies to dengue virus (see Figure 35-6). In general, symptoms become most profound as the immune response clears extracellular and intracellular virus. Uncomplicated dengue resolves uneventfully, although some patients experience weeks of convalescent lassitude and asthenia. Rash, pruritis, and acral desquamation can occur up to 2 weeks after defervescence.

Infection with one dengue virus type appears to confer lifelong homologous immunity but little to no heterologous immunity.[62] In many areas of the tropics, three or more dengue type viruses may simultaneously circulate, prompting the occurrence of sequential infections, also termed secondary infections. Secondary infection with a dengue virus has been identified as the major risk factor for DHF/DSS, the most severe manifestations of dengue infection.[57]

The hallmark of DHF is a transient increase in vascular permeability, resulting in a shift of plasma from the intravascular space to the interstitium.[63] When plasma leakage is profound, hypovolemic shock results. It is heralded by hemoconcentration and thrombocytopenia, usually after 3 to 5 days of illness as fever remits.

The body of evidence suggests that monocyte/ macrophage interactions with dengue virus are central to the pathogenesis of DHF. Virus entry and replication is probably enhanced by cross-reactive antibody; subsequently, these cells produce cytokines.[64] Complement is activated, generating vasoactive cleavage products C3a and C5a. Immune activation and the resulting cytokine and complement cascade appear to account for the plasma leakage and hemostatic defects that occur in DHF. Conversely, less immune activation in dengue fever accounts for the absence of overt plasma leakage and less severe hemorrhage.

The relative importance of viral virulence in the pathogenesis of DHF is still unclear. Two studies suggest that viruses derived from Southeast Asian genotypes were associated with DHF, in contrast to viruses originating from the Americas.[65,66] Recent data indicate a possible role for viral determinants in severe dengue.[67] As more genetic data becomes available, it is probable that viral factors, and associated host responses, may be key to pathogenesis of DHF.

TABLE 35-4

DENGUE FEVER IN US SERVICE MEMBERS (HAITI, N =55)

Symptoms		
Fever	55	(100%)
Chills or rigors	51	(93%)
Headache/retro-orbital pain	48	(87%)
Nausea or vomiting	36	(65%)
Malaise	35	(64%)
Myalgia	34	(62%)
Diarrhea	21	(38%)
Signs		
Conjunctival injection	29	(53%)
Rash	23	(42%)
Cervical lymphadenopathy	20	(36%)
Laboratory (N = 25)		
Leukopenia (leukocyte count < 3,000/ mm³)	14	(56%)
Thrombocytopenia (plt<100,000/mm³)	10	(40%)
Elevated serum transaminases	9	(36%)

Plt: platelet count

Clinical Findings

Adults with dengue have a more overt and characteristic illness than children, prompting some authorities to speak of dengue in adults as "classic" dengue fever. The incubation period is 2 to 8 days. The most common symptoms include abrupt onset of fever (39.5°C-40.5°C), generalized myalgias, arthralgias, malaise, headache frequently accompanied by retro-orbital pain or pain on eye movement, and rash (Table 35-4). Prostration from diffuse bone and muscle pains can be severe (hence the name breakbone fever). Not uncommonly, the patient will experience gastrointestinal symptoms such as nausea, vomiting, bloating, and loose stools. Upper respiratory symptoms are uncommon. An exanthem during the febrile phase is a characteristic yet not pathognomonic finding. It is usually a diffuse, blanching, erythematous macular rash over the trunk and extremities, sparing the palms and soles (Figure 35-7). Less commonly, the rash may be pruritic and evolve to become petechial, morbilliform, or papular and to become associated with desquamation in the digits during convalescence. Symptoms remain intense for 3 to 5 days, then subside rapidly, usually within a week. The patient will occasionally manifest a "saddle-back" fever pattern. The majority of individuals recover and are able to return quickly to normal activity. A few patients, however, may experience prolonged convalescent asthenia. In contrast to this typical adult course, one of the most common presentations in school-aged

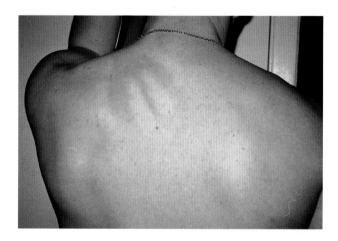

Fig. 35-7. A photograph of a generalized, blanching, erythematous macular rash in a US soldier with dengue fever. The soldier was ill for 2 weeks and took 50 days to return to normal.
Photograph: Courtesy of Amy L. Wyatt.

children in endemic areas is mild fever without localizing signs; many others present with abdominal pain or an upper respiratory syndrome with pharyngitis and rhinorrhea.

Laboratory findings in dengue include transient leukopenia and thrombocytopenia. The drop in white blood cell count is principally due to depletion of mature neutrophils. Occasionally, atypical large lymphocyte forms are also detectable on the blood smear. Elevated transaminases (up to 400 U/L) without rise in bilirubin are seen in about a third of cases; rarely (0.01% to 0.1% of cases), more profound increases in asparate aminotransferase and alanine aminotransferase may be associated with severe liver injury or even liver failure, as is seen in yellow fever.

Diagnostic Approaches

An increase in sporadic cases of fever may be the first indication that dengue transmission has begun in a unit or encampment. The virus has the potential to cause epidemics among exposed personnel. The challenge to the clinician in the acute phase of the illness is to differentiate dengue from other treatable febrile illnesses. Differential diagnosis is complicated by the lack of widely available diagnostic tests and the inability to clinically distinguish dengue from other tropical fevers. It is imperative to exclude malaria, as individuals may be ill with either or both infections. Falciparum malaria is potentially fatal and eminently treatable. Other treatable entities to be considered are rickettsioses and leptospirosis.[68] The hemorrhagic manifestations of dengue may be indistinguishable from yellow fever. It is important to make the distinction because there is an effective vaccine for yellow fever, a disease with 10% to 20% mortality.

The diagnosis of dengue requires laboratory confirmation but should be entertained in any febrile patient having possible exposure who lacks localizing signs and has a normal or depressed leukocyte count. Confirmation of a clinical diagnosis of dengue can be made by identification of virus in blood or by serology. Cross-reactive responses among different flaviviruses complicate definitive serologic diagnosis, though.[69] There are assays currently in use to detect recent or past infection, including hemagglutination-inhibition and plaque reduction neutralizing antibody assays, but these tests are generally unavailable. The most useful diagnostic test is a enzyme-immunoassay for dengue-specific IgM and IgG antibodies.[70]

The presence of detectable dengue-specific IgM or 4-fold rises in IgG titer confirm dengue virus infection. This diagnosis is ideally confirmed by virus isolation and identification with reference antisera. The viruses are best isolated from sera collected from febrile individuals and stored at -70°C prior to shipping on dry ice. Definitive diagnosis of dengue virus infection is most easily achieved from paired sera specimens, one drawn during the acute phase of illness and another drawn at least 2 days after defervescence. Recent experience of deployed US Army personnel in Haiti has shown the limitation of serologic diagnosis.[71] Of 224 serum specimens collected from patients at first evaluation, 58% had no dengue IgM but had positive dengue virus isolation. In the future, nucleic acid detection methods may enable rapid diagnosis even under field conditions.

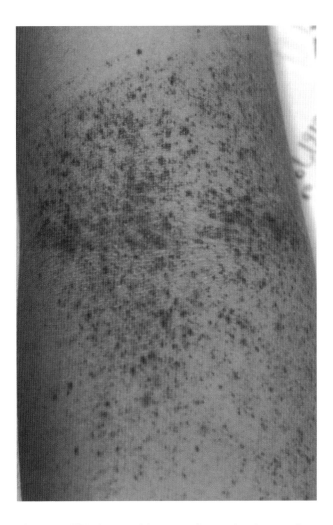

Fig. 35-8. This is a positive tourniquet sign in a patient with dengue hemorrhagic fever from Thailand.
Photograph: Courtesy of Dr. Siripan Kalayanrooj, Thailand.

For the present, a tourniquet test should be performed, as experience in children in Thailand suggests that a negative tourniquet test excludes the diagnosis of dengue infection with greater than 75% certainty after two days of fever.[72] However, a positive tourniquet test is not specific for DHF. The test is done by inflating the blood pressure cuff to midpoint between the systolic and diastolic pressures for 5 minutes and then releasing the cuff. Increased capillary fragility is marked by a shower of petechiae below the cuff. If 20 or more petechiae per square inch are observed, the tourniquet test is positive (Figure 35-8).

The clinician should also be alert to the development of DHF/DSS during the period in which fever remits. The disease starts similarly to dengue but may progress to shock and hemorrhage, usually in the gastrointestinal tract. Warning signs are a falling platelet count (less than 100,000/mm³) and rising hematocrit. The loss of intravascular volume results in narrowed pulse pressure with tachycardia, hemoconcentration, and evidence of interstitial fluid collection (eg, pleural effusions, ascites). Circulating complement and clotting factors are depleted. In the Cuban outbreak in 1981, the first large outbreak of DHF/DSS in the Americas, the disease in adults was characterized by fever (100%), constitutional symptoms (100%), gastrointestinal symptoms (90%), purpura (66%), and upper gastrointestinal bleeding (40%).[73] Hepatomegaly (35%) and hematemesis (35%) were poor prognostic signs. Laboratory abnormalities of thrombocytopenia and hemoconcentration were seen in 71% and 92%, respectively. Ninety-eight percent of the cases of DHF/DSS in this Cuban outbreak exhibited a secondary antibody response.

There is a continuing need for clinical and laboratory expertise to recognize and treat these infections early, particularly if DHF should occur among previously exposed personnel. Future efforts should concentrate on ways to expedite diagnosis of dengue virus infection and on the development of dengue virus vaccines that offer solid immunity.

TABLE 35-5

TREATMENT AND CLASSIFICATION OF DENGUE AND DENGUE HEMORRHAGIC FEVER

Grade	Symptoms	Signs	Treatment
Dengue fever	Headache, retro-orbital pain, myalgia	Fever (39°C-41°C), rash (blanching, erythematous)	-Treat symptoms -Use anti-inflammatory agents (not aspirin) -Monitor clinical status daily -Determine hematocrit & platelet count
DHF Grade I	Same as above	Hemoconcentration (≥20% rise in hematocrit), thrombocytopenia (<100,000/mm³), positive tourniquet test	Same as above, plus: -Monitor vital signs q 2h, then q 6h -Determine hematocrit, platelet count -Provide oral hydration
DHF Grade II	Same as above	Hemoconcentration and thrombocytopenia, spontaneous bleeding	Same as above, plus: -Type and cross match -Determine PT and PTT
DHF Grade III	Restlessness, confusion, lethargy	Hemoconcentration and thrombocytopenia, rapid weak pulse, narrowed pulse pressure (<20 mm Hg), hypotension, cold clammy skin	Same as above, plus: -Administer isotonic intravenous fluids (rapid 20 mL/kg bolus) -Obtain electrolytes, ALT/AST -Monitor vital signs more frequently (q 30 min or less) -Follow urine output
DHF Grade IV	Depressed sensorium, stupor	Hemoconcentration and thrombocytopenia, undetectable pulse and blood pressure	Same as above, plus: -Administer intravenous colloid or plasma 10-20 mL/kg -Provide critical care support as needed

PT: prothrombin time; PTT: partial thromboplastin time; ALT: alanine aminotransferase test; AST: aspartate aminotransferase test
Reprinted with permission from Kanesa-thasan N, Hoke CH Jr. Dengue and related syndromes. In: Schlossberg D, ed. *Current Therapy of Infectious Disease*. 2nd ed. Chicago: Mosby-Year Book; 2000: 617.

Recommendations for Therapy and Control

Therapy

Dengue is a self-limited illness, and symptoms generally resolve with judicious use of nonsalicylate analgesics and fluids. There is no specific treatment.[74] The treatment of both DHF and DSS is principally supportive, along with close monitoring of hematocrit and blood pressure (Table 35-5). DHF should be suspected in individuals who manifest sudden onset of restlessness, confusion, or lethargy after a dengue-like syndrome. Hospital admission is required for individuals who are at risk for shock, that is, for those who have bleeding, hemoconcentration, narrowed pulse pressure, oliguria, significant prostration, thrombocytopenia of less than $100,000/mm^3$, or clinical deterioration. Hospitalization should be considered for other patients who cannot be adequately monitored. Aggressive fluid support can be lifesaving. These measures when used effectively decrease mortality of DHF/DSS to less than 1%.[75]

Control

Efforts to eradicate dengue mosquito vectors have failed, and the vectors resist most conventional control efforts, including ultra-low-volume spraying of insecticides outside homes. Community prevention programs involving removal of fresh water receptacles where the vector may breed and education regarding the habits of the mosquito vectors in the area and the mosquito transmission cycle have had some success. Other available methods for preventing infection involve personal protection using long-acting insect repellents and elimination of local breeding sites. During dengue epidemics, there may be a limited role for insecticide spraying to reduce the density of infected mosquitoes, but traditionally this measure has had little immediate impact. Effective vector control and personal protection measures should be emphasized to military personnel deploying to endemic areas.

The US Army has been a leader in dengue vaccine development, with the goal being a tetravalent vaccine that confers protection against all four dengue serotypes. Since the 1960s, efforts have been made to develop safe, live, attenuated vaccines that would infect and immunize recipients.[76] The pace of vaccine development accelerated in the early 1990s.

[Niranjan Kanesa-thasan, Wellington Sun, Bruce L. Innis]

DENGUE-LIKE SYNDROMES

Introduction and Military Relevance

It is of utmost importance to the clinician and preventive medicine officer to be able to generate a clinical differential diagnosis of diseases that may present like dengue does. This differential will guide the clinician in obtaining the proper sera for a definitive diagnosis and in direct clinical management of potential serious complications such as coagulopathy or shock in the case of the hemorrhagic fevers. This differential will also guide the preventive medicine officer in expanding case definitions of reportable diseases in a theater of operations, as well as the list of potential vectors that may be targeted for vector control. This section will discuss several dengue-like diseases to emphasize the wide diversity of these viruses and their vectors. Since dengue is currently occurring as a worldwide pandemic of the tropical and subtropical regions, the simultaneous occurrence of the viral pathogens discussed in this section and dengue is a very real and valid concern for US service members and their health care providers.

Dengue fever can manifest itself in a broad range of clinical presentations ranging from an asymptomatic infection to a viral syndrome to classical dengue to its severest form—dengue hemorrhagic fever with or without shock syndrome. The differential for a dengue-like disease will change with the nature of presenting clinical symptoms, which themselves depend on factors such as the day of illness, host immunity, and variables that affect immunity (eg, combat fatigue and stress, preexisting immunity, host genetic factors, viral virulence). These factors will generate a continuum of possible etiologies as the disease manifests and progresses in the patient (Figure 35-9).

Oropouche Fever

Introduction and Military Relevance

Oropouche virus was first isolated in Trinidad in 1955 from the blood of a charcoal worker with a febrile illness.[77] A series of epidemics of this disease involving approximately 263,000 persons occurred from 1961 to 1981 primarily in the Amazon River basin but also in the Brazilian states of Manaus, Barcelos, Amazonas, and Amapa.[78] The estimated incidence of oropouche fever during these epidemics ranged from 17 to 60 per 100 persons. From 1961 to 1992, there have been 23 documented outbreaks of

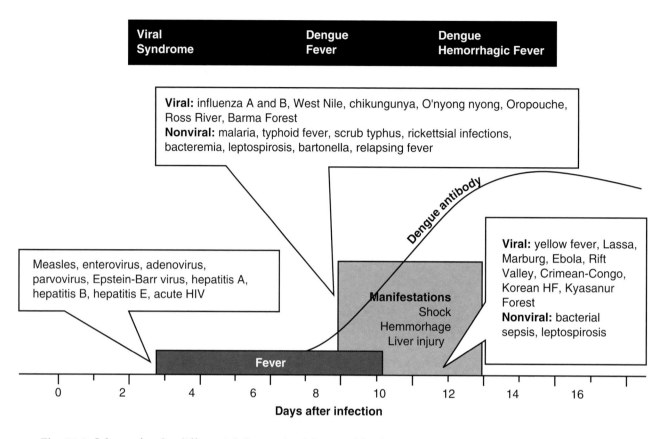

Fig. 35-9. Schema for the differential diagnosis of dengue-like diseases based on clinical dengue illness day.

Oropouche fever in Brazil, 2 outbreaks in Panama, and 1 outbreak in Peru.[79] The wide range of occurrence of this virus throughout the Central and South America, its ability to produce high attack rates among immune-naives, and its high morbidity rate makes this virus militarily relevant for US military personnel deploying into potentially endemic areas.

Description of the Pathogen

Oropouche virus is in the family *Bunyaviridae* and the genus *Bunyavirus;* antigenically it is a member of the Simbu serogroup of RNA viruses.[78]

Epidemiology

It is postulated that Oropouche fever has two cycles of transmission: (1) an epidemic urban cycle in which humans are the primary host and the biting midge *Culicoides paraensis* is the vector and (2) a silent maintenance cycle in which forest animals, primarily sloths, are the primary hosts but the vector is unknown. Recent studies of febrile patients in Panama indicate that Oropouche virus was a common cause of fever and suggests that the virus may be maintained

endemically in communities over long periods of time.[79] The endemicity of this disease was confirmed in a cross-sectional serosurvey of a rural community near Iquitos, Peru.[80] The overall seroprevalence of antibody in adults to Oropouche virus in this community was 33.7%; the risk factors for seropositivity were travel to forest communities and travel to Iquitos.

Oropouche fever has been largely reported in the tropics of South America and primarily in northern Brazil. The biting midge *C paraensis* was confirmed to be a potential vector in laboratory studies.[78] The midge, which also is found in Central and North America, feeds readily on humans, breeds in garbage and rotting organic material, and feeds diurnally, with peak blood feeding occurring just before sunset.

Pathogenesis and Clinical Findings

Serosurveys provide an estimate that 63% of persons infected with Oropouche virus will develop clinical manifestations of Oropouche fever.[78] Human disease appears after an incubation period of 4 to 8 days. Viremia occurs during the first two days of illness and is manifested clinically by the sudden onset of fever, headache, muscle ache, joint pains, and photophobia. Leukopenia associated with neutropenia is a common laboratory finding, although some individuals may have a leukocytosis.[77] Rash is observed infrequently, and other manifestations may be gastrointestinal in nature (eg, nausea, vomiting, diarrhea). Central nervous system involvement can occur primarily as an aseptic meningitis. Infection with Oropouche virus may be teratogenic, based on the teratogenic potential of other related Simbu group bunyaviruses. The illness lasts from 2 to 7 days, and immunity may be life-long.

Diagnostic Approaches

Diagnosis of Oropouche infection can be achieved serologically by standard enzyme-linked immunosorbent assay measuring IgG or plaque reduction neutralization titers. Virus can be isolated during the first days of illness but sera must be stored at -70°C. Oropouche fever in the early stages of disease is clinically indistinguishable from dengue. The absence of rash, hemorrhage, or shock in Oropouche fever are key clinical observations that may distinguish it from dengue.

Recommendations for Therapy and Control

The treatment is supportive, and there is no vaccine for Oropouche fever. Prevention and control of epidemics involve vector control and personal protection measures (see Chapter 22, Personal Protection Measures Against Arthropods).

Rift Valley Fever

Rift Valley fever was first clinically described in 1912 and 1913 in the Great Rift Valley in Kenya. From 1930 to 1931, extensive studies of Rift Valley fever established it as a viral disease that produces illness primarily in domestic animals (especially sheep) but that could produce illness in humans.[81] Further studies elucidated its wide geographic range and demonstrated its potential for fatal outcomes in humans.

Description of the Pathogen

Rift Valley fever virus is in the family *Bunyaviridae* and the genus *Phlebovirus*. Serologic characterization of its antigenic make-up subclasses this virus into the sandfly fever serogroup of the phleboviruses.[82]

Epidemiology

Rift Valley fever virus has been isolated in a large number of blood-feeding arthropods, such as *Aedes,*

Anopheles, and *Culex* mosquitoes, *Culicoides* midges, *Simulium* flies, and *Rhipicephalus* ticks.[81,83] Transovarial and venereal transmission of the virus has been documented in male and female *Aedes liniatopennis* mosquitoes and may be the mechanism for the maintenance of the virus in the environment. It is postulated that during periods of heavy rainfall, the numbers of infected mosquitoes increase by transovarial amplification, and they spread the virus to susceptible vertebrate hosts, including domestic animals. Rift Valley fever virus can occur naturally in a wide number of animal species, including all domestic animals and such small mammals as mice, rodents, and hedgehogs. In experiments, dogs, cats, rabbits, and monkeys have been infected as well. Animals become a source to infect arthropods, which in turn become vectors, resulting in the escalation of this disease into humans. Risk factors for infection include occupations that demand close contact with animals (eg, veterinarians, butchers, abattoir workers).

Current theory suggests two different types of epidemiologic patterns for Rift Valley fever: (1) epizootics and epidemics occurring in eastern and southern Africa and (2) enzootic and endemic disease in western Africa.[84]

There has been Rift Valley fever activity in 24 African nations. From 1960 to 1978, there have been several isolated outbreaks of Rift Valley fever in Angola, Egypt, Kenya, Namibia, South Africa, Zambia, and Zimbabwe.[81] An outbreak of Rift Valley fever occurred i n Kenya from 1997 to 1998, resulting in more than 80,000 cases.[85] This outbreak is estimated to be the largest reported outbreak in eastern Africa. Phylogenetic analysis of isolates from this outbreak revealed their genealogy to be related to an isolate obtained during the 1990 outbreak in Madagascar. Outbreaks of Rift Valley fever have been characterized by high attack rates in domestic animals, with 30% mortality and an abortion rate of 80% to 100%.[81]

In a study conducted in the northern province of Sudan, 23% of 185 individuals demonstrated antibody to Rift Valley fever virus.[86] In the Nile River delta of Egypt, a seroprevalence of 15% was documented.[87] Cases of Rift Valley fever were not detected in combat troops deployed in during the Persian Gulf War nor was there evidence of infection by postdeployment antibody serosurveys for virus.[88]

Pathogenesis and Clinical Findings

Rift Valley fever in humans is characterized by the onset of fever (which can be saddleback in nature), severe "back-breaking" myalgia, headache, and anorexia.[81] The illness lasts approximately 4 to 7 days, with viremia occurring in the first 2 days of illness, followed by complete recovery in the majority of patients in 2 weeks. A more severe form of Rift Valley fever can occur and produces ocular hemorrhage with diminished visual acuity, encephalitis, hemorrhagic illness, and death.[84] Ocular Rift Valley fever occurred during an outbreak in Egypt and was characterized by the onset of diminished visual acuity 7 to 20 days after initial symptoms, retinal hemorrhage, and vasculitis. Meningoencephalitis was reported during the South African outbreak in 1975, with the onset of encephalitis 5 to 10 days after the development of fever.[81] Hemorrhagic Rift Valley fever occurs 2 to 4 days after the onset of fever and was the cause of 598 human deaths (case-fatality rates between 0.2% and 14%) during a 1977 outbreak in Egypt and was a feature of the Zimbabwe outbreak in 1978.[81] Outbreaks of Rift Valley fever followed no seasonal pattern but occur after periods of excessive rain or during the development of irrigation projects.[89]

Diagnostic Approaches

Diagnosis of Rift Valley fever can be accomplished by standard viral isolation or molecularly by polymerase chain reaction. Rising antibody titers or seroconversion as detected by enzyme immunoassay or plaque reduction neutralization titers can establish a serologic diagnosis. The clinical distinction between Rift Valley fever and dengue may be difficult, especially if the presentation is a hemorrhagic fever. However, clinically distinct features of Rift Valley fever, such as ocular involvement or encephalitis, and concomitant reports of illness and abortions among local livestock will distinguish Rift Valley fever from dengue.

Recommendations for Therapy and Control

Prevention and control of this disease rely on an active disease surveillance program in domestic animals (as well as humans), immunization of livestock with currently available killed or attenuated veterinary vaccines, and vector control. The effectiveness of antiviral therapy in humans has not been established; however, interferon-alpha and ribavirin have been shown to have protective efficacy in nonhuman primates infected with Rift Valley fever virus.[90] A formalin-inactivated Rift Valley fever vaccine, currently not licensed, has been developed and demonstrated to be highly effective in domestic livestock and in humans.[91] The immunogenicity of the inactivated Rift Valley fever vaccine in humans

was recently reviewed.[92] The TSI-GSD-200 inactivated RV vaccine was administered to 540 vaccinees from 1986 to 1997 using three subcutaneous doses at 0, 7, and 28 days. Approximately 90% of vaccinees developed titers of greater than 1:40 of which 98% retained high titers after successful boosting by the vaccines. Of the 10% who were nonresponders, 75% developed antibody titers on boosting with the vaccine. The vaccine was safe and immunogenic, with good long-term immunity after a primary series and one booster dose vaccine. It is available at the US Army Medical Research Institute for Infectious Disease, Fort Detrick, Md. Human vaccination may be indicated for persons at high-risk, such as laboratory or veterinary staff working with the virus or those in areas that are endemic for Rift Valley fever.

Chikungunya

Introduction and Military Relevance

Historically, it has been difficult to distinguish mosquito-borne chikungunya from dengue fever. A number of large outbreaks of "dengue fever" during the 1800s in Egypt, the East African coast, and India were clinically more closely related to chikungunya infection than dengue. The Tanzanian word *chikungunya* was used to designate the severe joint and muscle pains associated with this disease during a large outbreak of clinical disease in that country in 1952 to 1953.[93]

Description of the Pathogen

Chikungunya virus is a positive-sense, single-stranded RNA virus in the family *Togaviridae* and the genus *Alphavirus*. It is antigenically closely related to O'nyong nyong virus.[94,95] Chikungunya virus is genetically highly conserved within Asian and African countries, with parsimony analysis revealing two distinct lineages, one from isolates occurring in western Africa and the other from southern and east Africa and Asia.[96]

Epidemiology

Aedes aegypti mosquitoes in India, Thailand, and Nigeria and *Ae africanus* mosquitoes in Africa transmit chikungunya virus. It has been demonstrated experimentally that these other mosquitoes can carry the virus: *Ae albopictus, Ae calceatus, Ae pseudoscutellaris, Anopheles albimanus,* and *Eretmapodites chrysogaster*.[97] Disease occurs in areas where *Ae aegypti* and *Ae africanus* are present, suggesting that these are the principle vectors for transmission into humans. Serosurveys of primates have demonstrated chikungunya virus antibody in monkeys, baboons, and chimpanzees, suggesting a possible means of environmental maintenance of this virus.

Chikungunya virus is distributed worldwide. It has produced pandemics in the African nations of Uganda, Tanzania, Zimbabwe, South Africa, Angola, the Democratic Republic of the Congo (formerly Zaire), Nigeria, and Senegal and is endemic throughout sub-Saharan Africa.[98] Chikungunya virus has produced pandemics, and it has become endemic in India and has extended into Southeast Asia including Thailand, Cambodia, and Vietnam. Epidemics of chikungunya fever occurred in the Philippines in 1954, 1956, and 1968; cases of chikungunya fever were diagnosed among US Peace Corps volunteers in the Philippines in 1986.[99] Two large epidemics have been documented in Thailand in 1988 and 1995.[100]

Serosurveys for chikungunya virus in Ibadan, Nigeria, from 1970 to 1974 indicated a seroprevalence of less than 10% in children younger than 1 year of age that increased to 75% by the time the children were 10 to 15 years old. There was an overall seroprevalence of 50% for all ages.[101,102] In Burma, seroprevalence of chikungunya virus antibody ranged from 38.4% in the state of Magwe to 97.7% in Rangoon.[103]

Pathogenesis and Clinical Findings

Human illness from chikungunya occurs after an incubation period of 2 to 4 days, heralded by the abrupt onset of fever and followed in 3 to 5 days by a lymphadenopathy and a generalized maculopapular rash affecting the trunk, limbs, palms, and soles of the feet.[104] A biphasic, saddleback fever can occur and be followed by the development of arthralgia, which becomes a prominent symptom that distinguishes chikungunya fever clinically from dengue fever. Other symptoms include headache, backache, conjunctivitis, and retro-orbital pain. The mortality rate from chikungunya is low, and long-term complications rare. In a study of 107 patients diagnosed with chikungunya 3 years previously, 87.9% fully recovered, 3.7% experienced occasional stiffness, 2.8% had persistent residual joint stiffness, and 5.6% had persistent joint pain and stiffness with effusion.[105]

Diagnostic Approaches

Chikungunya has a higher frequency of rash, conjunctival injection, and arthralgias than dengue fever, and chikungunya's fever ends 2 days earlier than dengue's.[98,104] Chikungunya can manifest hemorrhagic signs (eg, a positive tourniquet test, petechiae, epistaxis) but not the coagulopathy and shock syndrome typical of dengue hemorrhagic fever and shock syndrome. Diagnosis of chikungunya is by viral isolation or serology with complement fixation or neutralization assays. An enzyme-linked immunosorbent assay to immunoglobulin M has been developed that has a high degree of sensitivity and specificity.[106]

Recommendations for Therapy and Control

Treatment of this disease is primarily supportive, and convalescence can be prolonged. A live, attenuated vaccine for chikungunya virus that produces viral-neutralizing antibodies has been shown to be safe.[97] Currently not licensed, it is available at the US Army Medical Research Institute for Infectious Disease. Vector control of this disease involves eliminating the breeding sites for the mosquito and active spraying, as well as personal protective measures.

O'nyong-nyong

Introduction and Military Relevance

O'nyong-nyong was first described in a large epidemic occurring between 1959 and 1962 that started in northwestern Uganda and spread to Kenya, Tanzania, and Zaire; an estimated 2 million people were infected.[98,107] Cases also occurred in the Central African Republic in 1964 and 1965.[98] In June 1996, a disease suspected to be o'nyong-nyong fever was recognized in the Rakai district of southwestern Uganda that spread into the neighboring Mbarara and Masaka districts and in the bordering Bukoba district of northern Tanzania. This was confirmed as o'nyong-nyong virus and documented the first major outbreak of o'nyong-nyong in southwestern Uganda after an absence of 35 years.[108]

Description of the Pathogen

O'nyong-nyong virus is in the family *Togaviridae*, genus *Alphavirus*, and closely related to the chikungunya virus.

Epidemiology

O'nyong-nyong virus has been isolated from the mosquitoes *An funestus* and *An gambiae*, suggesting these as the principle vector for transmission to humans.[109] O'nyong-nyong is widely distributed throughout Africa; serosurveys demonstrate antibody prevalence to o'nyong-nyong virus in Malawi, Mozambique, and Senegal.[98]

Pathogenesis and Clinical Findings

Clinical illness from o'nyong-nyong occurs after an incubation period of more than 8 days and is characterized by the sudden onset of fever (which can be saddleback in character), headache, and severe arthralgia.[98] A viral exanthem can occur, which can be papular or maculopapular. Lymphadenopathy, conjunctivitis, photophobia, myalagias, aphthous stomatitis, anorexia, and epistaxis are other clinical features of this disease. Fever can last for up to 5 days and arthralgia, weakness, and mental depression can be prolonged. No fatalities from this disease have been documented.

Diagnostic Approaches

Laboratory diagnosis is by viral isolation. Serologic confirmation can be made with standard methods; neutralization assays have the greatest specificity. Clinical differentiation from dengue may be made on the basis of joint involvement and absence of hemorrhage or shock syndrome.

Recommendations for Therapy and Control

Similar to chikungunya, treatment of this disease is primarily supportive, and convalescence can be prolonged. Vector control and personal protective measures are the principle means of controlling disease transmission.

Sindbis and Sindbis-like Viral Infections

Introduction and Military Relevance

Sindbis virus was isolated from *Culex* mosquitoes in 1952 in the village of Sindbis, Egypt. Sindbis and viruses similar to Sindbis, termed Sindbis-like, were later reported in parts of Europe, Asia, Africa, and Australia. The potential for causing epidemics in humans was documented during large outbreaks of Sindbis and Sindbis-like viral infections in South Africa in 1974, as well as outbreaks in Sweden, Finland, and the Soviet Union from 1981 to 1984.[110]

Description of the Pathogen

Sindbis and Sindbis-like viruses are RNA viruses in the *Togaviridae* family of the genus *Alphavirus;* antigenically, they are in the western equine encephalitis complex of viruses.[81]

Epidemiology

Sindbis virus has been isolated from a number of mosquito genera, including *Culex, Anopheles,* and *Aedes.*[81,111] Virus has been isolated from a number of different birds, suggesting the environmental maintenance of this virus in avian species, with transmission by mosquitoes into humans.

Sindbis-like infection in Sweden, Finland, and the former Soviet Union occurs between the 60th and 64th parallels, with human infection occurring from late July into September and peak incidence in August. It is known by a variety of names (eg, Ockelbo disease, Pogosta disease, Karelian fever).[112] In South Africa, the virus occurs throughout the country, and high infection rates are seen after greater-than-normal rainfall or flooding.[113] In other parts of Africa, antibody prevalence is associated with regions attracting migratory bird populations.

Human infection as described in previous outbreaks occurs primarily in adults between the ages of 30 to 60 years; males are equally at risk for infection as females. Forest exposure is a risk factor for infection.

Pathogenesis and Clinical Findings

The symptoms of Sindbis and Sindbis-like viral infection occur after an incubation period of less than 1 week and include fever, headache, malaise, joint pain, and a maculopapular rash over the trunk and limbs with occasional vesicles.[112] Severe debilitating arthralgias can occur involving, in descending frequency, ankles, wrist, knees, hips, and fingers. The arthralgias can last for up to 3 years. Nonpruritic rash and fever can occur for up to 2 to 3 weeks. No deaths from this infection have been reported.

Diagnostic Approaches

Diagnosis is made by viral isolation and serology (eg, enzyme immunoassay, neutralization titers).

Recommendations for Therapy and Control

Similar to other viruses presented here, treatment of this disease is primarily supportive and convalescence can be prolonged. Clinical distinction of this disease from dengue can be made on the degree of joint involvement, the production of skin vesicles in Sindbis infection but not dengue, and the absence of hemorrhage or shock as can be seen in dengue hemorrhagic fever. Vector control and personal protective measures are the principle means of controlling disease transmission.

Ross River Disease

Introduction and Military Relevance

Ross River disease, clinically known as epidemic polyarthritis, can produce large outbreaks of rash, fever, and severe polyarthritis. The first report of epidemic polyarthritis was made in 1928 at Narrandera in New South Wales, Australia. The virus was subsequently isolated from a pool of *Ae vigilax* mosquitoes in 1963 near the Ross River at Townsville, Australia. Ross River virus infection is endemic in Queensland, where approximately 300 to 600 cases are diagnosed each year. It has potential to produce large epidemics in other parts of Australia, such as southwest Western Australia and the Murray-Darling River basin. Epidemics have been reported outside of Australia in Papua New Guinea, the Solomon Islands, American Samoa, Cook Island, Fiji, and New Caledonia.[114]

Description of the Pathogen

Ross River virus is in the family *Togaviridae*, genus *Alphavirus*. It is in the antigenic complex of the Semliki Forest viruses, Getah serogroup.[115]

Epidemiology

Ross River virus is endemic in Australia and causes periodic epidemics. The yearly incidence of epidemic polyarthritis in Queensland is 23.6 cases per 100,000 residents. Clinical manifestations of polyarthritis after infection vary between areas that are endemic for disease versus areas that experience epidemics. The incidence of clinical to subclinical infection is estimated to be 1:80 in an endemic area and 1:0.4 in an epidemic area. Ross River virus occurs year-round in central and northern Queensland and during March to June following the summer rains throughout the rest of Australia. The disease occurs most commonly in adults aged 20 to 50 years. Urban-dwelling housewives are more commonly diagnosed with epidemic polyarthritis. There is a positive association between clinical infection and the haplotype HLA-DR7, though no particular ethnic group is at higher risk for infection.[115]

Ross River virus has been isolated from a number of different genera of mosquitoes during the times of outbreaks, suggesting that the mosquito is the major vector of this disease. The virus has been isolated in Australia from *Cx annulirostris, Ae vigilax, Ae normanensis, Ae notoscriptus, An amictus, Mansonia uniformis,* and *Cx liniealis* and in the Cook Islands from *Ae polynesiensis*.[115] During the 1994 outbreak in suburban Brisbane, Ross River virus was isolated from *Cx annulirostris, Cx sitiens, Ae notoscriptus, Ae procax, Ae funereus, Ae vigilax,* and *Ae alternans*. These are peridomestic mosquitoes that breed in fresh and brackish water and may be important during suburban outbreaks.[116] A large number of vertebrate hosts have antibody to Ross River virus, including cattle, horses, sheep, kangaroos, and wallabies, as well as domestic and native birds. None of these vertebrate hosts develop clinical disease nor have any been implicated as a zoonotic reservoir for this virus. This suggests that humans are the principle reservoir during outbreaks, and overwintering of the virus within mosquitoes is the cause for subsequent seasonal disease.[115]

Within the past decade, there have been several large outbreaks of Ross River disease in Australia, raising concerns that the epidemiology of this disease might be changing. From July 1990 to June 1991, there were 368 cases of epidemic polyarthritis in the Northern Territory of Australia.[117] The epidemic started in September and peaked in January, with the highest attack rates occurring in the rural areas and among those 30 to 34 years old. The cause of the outbreak was attributed to higher-than-normal rainfalls and the resultant increase in the mosquito vector. In 1995 to 1996, 540 serologically confirmed cases of Ross River disease were reported in the southwest region of Western Australia.[118] The areas affected were coastal towns and communities in semirural areas and suburbs close to major cities. The changing epidemiology of Ross River virus was examined in a longitudinal questionnaire-based survey of notified cases.[119] The distribution of the disease has changed over time and new areas identified, including the lower Yorke Peninsula, the Flinders Ranges, and metropolitan Adelaide. Symptom severity and duration has increased with recent outbreaks; clinical cases have had a higher frequency of lethargy, tiredness, and arthritis than in past outbreaks and symptoms have persisted 15 months after infection.

Pathogenesis and Clinical Findings

Clinical infection from Ross River virus occurs 7 to 9 days after the bite of an infected mosquito, though a period of up to 21 days has been reported.[120] Arthralgia, arthritis, myalgia, fatigue, and fever characterize Ross River virus disease. Headache, photophobia, lymphadenopathy, and sore throat may occur as well. Rash occurs in over half of clinically ill patients and can occur 11 to 15 days after the onset of arthritis. The rash occurs mainly on the limbs and trunk and is maculopapular but not vesicular in character. Joint involvement is the most common clinical feature and can occur in up to 98% of clinically ill patients; more than half have joint pain lasting greater than 6 months, with some patients experiencing arthritis up to 15 months after infection.[119,120] The rash associated with Ross River virus disease is the result of a cell-mediated immune response to viral antigen within the skin,[115] and laboratory evidence suggests that antibody-dependent enhancement and persistence of virus within macrophages may be a cause of the arthritis.[121]

Diagnostic Approaches

Ross River virus infection can be diagnosed by viral isolation or through molecular techniques such as polymerase chain reaction. Documenting a 4-fold rise in antibody titer by hemagglutination inhibition assay, neutralization titers, or enzyme immunoassay will establish a case of acute Ross River virus infection. An IgM enzyme immunoassay can detect acute cases, though IgM to Ross River virus may persist for months to years.[120] Individuals may develop secondary Ross River viral infection as detected by rising antibodies, but this is not associated with clinical disease.[115] The clinical differentiation of Ross River virus disease from dengue can be made on the basis of the occurrence and persistence of arthritis and the absence of hemorrhage or shock.

Recommendations for Therapy and Control

Therapy for Ross River disease is supportive, with antiinflammatory drugs providing relief from the joint pain.[120] The utility of steroids in relieving joint pain has not been established. Prevention and control of epidemics involve vector control of the mosquito and personal protective measures. A candidate killed-virus vaccine against Ross River virus infection is being developed that has shown immunogenicity in mice.[122] Human efficacy studies have not been performed with this vaccine.

West Nile Fever

Introduction and Military Relevance

West Nile virus was first isolated in the West Nile province of Uganda in 1937. Outbreaks of West Nile disease described in Israel in 1950 involved more than 500 hospitalized patients. Outbreaks recurred each year in Israel from 1951 to 1954 and in 1957.[123] The largest recorded epidemic of West Nile disease, involving several thousands of cases, occurred in the Karoo and southern Cape Province of South Africa in 1974. A subsequent South African epidemic in the Witwatersrand-Pretoria region occurred from 1993 to 1994, with cocirculation of Sindbis virus as a cause of encephalitis.[124]

Description of the Pathogen

West Nile virus is in the family *Flaviviridae*, genus *Flavivirus*. West Nile virus is in the antigenic complex that includes these viruses: Japanese encephalitis virus, St. Louis encephalitis virus, Murray Valley encephalitis virus, Kunjin, Usutu, Kokobera, Stratford, Alfuy, and Koutango.[123]

Epidemiology

Clinical disease from West Nile virus has been reported from countries within Europe, the former Soviet Union, Africa, Southwest Asia, and most recently the eastern United States.[123,125] A serologic survey of West Nile virus in Ibadan, Nigeria, revealed an overall seroprevalence rate of 40% in 304 human sera tested.[126] Both sexes were equally likely to be positive, and there was a higher prevalence in adults as compared to children. In 1990, a serosurvey in Madagascar of 3,177 children between the ages 5 to 20 years revealed an overall seroprevalence rate of 30% to West Nile virus.[127] Seroprevalence rates of West Nile antibody have been reported to be 55% in Karachi, Pakistan,[128] and 32.8% from residents of the Chiniot and Changa Manga National Forest areas of Punjab Province, Pakistan.[129] The cocirculation of Japanese encephalitis and West Nile viruses in fatal cases of encephalitis was observed in the Kolar district of Karnataka, India.[130] The first major West Nile virus epidemic in Romania occurred in 1996 and was characterized by high rates of neurologic complications.[131] During this epidemic, the highest incidence of disease occurred in Bucharest (12.4/100,000), followed by the surrounding districts near Bucharest (1.1-10/100,000). In 835 patients admitted to hospitals with suspected central nervous system infections, 92% met the case's definition for West Nile viral infection, and serologic confirmation was obtained in 352 (80%).

The recent introduction of West Nile virus into

the United States is an example of the continued spread and emergence of the virus into areas previously not thought to be at risk. Since its initial introduction into the New York City area in August 1999, the geographic range of West Nile virus had increased by the end of 1999 to include Connecticut, Maryland, New Jersey, and upstate New York and there were over 60 cases of clinical encephalitis.[132] By the end of the year 2000, West Nile virus was detected in the northeastern United States extending into Maryland and the District of Columbia.

West Nile virus has been isolated only from mosquitoes and ticks.[123] Mosquito species include *Cx antennatus*, *Cx pipiens*, *Cx univittatus*, *Cx perexiguus*, *Ae caballus*, *Ae circulateolus*, *Ae africanus*, *An coustani*, and *An maculipennis*. Tick species include *Argas hermanni*, *Hyalomma asiaticum asiaticum*, and *Ornithodoros capensis*. *Cx univittatus* was the primary arthropod source of West Nile virus isolation during clinical disease in Egypt and South Africa. In southwest Asia, *Cx vishnui* complex mosquitoes, which include *Cx tritaeniorhynchus*, *Cx vishnui*, and *Cx psuedovishnui*, were the primary sources of vector viral isolation.[115] Mosquito surveys and viral isolation during the 1996 Romanian outbreak revealed *Cx pipiens* as the predominant mosquito species in Bucharest. West Nile viral isolation from mosquito pools were all from *Cx pipiens* at a minimum infection rate of 0.3/1,000 mosquitoes.[131] Ticks have not been associated with human disease transmission, and the tick's role in the maintenance or spread of diseases has not been elucidated.[115] Transmission in the New York city area and the eastern United States is thought to be primarily by *Cx pipiens* mosquitoes.[133]

Many vertebrate species have been found to carry antibody to West Nile virus, but only wild birds have been consistently implicated as important hosts in its transmission cycle. Antibody rates of 40% among domestic and wild birds were found in Egypt and 12% in South Africa.[115] In Romania, antibody seroprevalence was 41% in domestic fowl and 8% in wild birds.[131]

The transmission of West Nile virus occurs in two cycles, a sylvatic cycle and an urban cycle. The virus is spread and maintained by migratory birds from Africa and the Middle East. Infected migratory birds then establish a sylvatic cycle, in which virus is maintained and spread by *Cx modestus*, a bird mosquito. Eventually the urban bird population becomes infected, and *Cx pipiens* becomes the primary arthropod vector. An urban cycle is then established, resulting in an epidemic of human clinical disease with humans as the dead-end host and urban birds as the reservoir of the virus.[131] Based on the US experience, black crows have been particularly susceptible to the effects of West Nile virus and have demonstrated a high mortality on infection.[134] Gross hemorrhage of the brain, splenomegaly, meningoencephalitis, and myocarditis were the most prominent lesions.

Because of the migration of infected birds and the mosquito breeding cycle, West Nile viral infection follows a seasonal pattern, with highest transmission activity during the summer months in temperate areas. In Egypt, the highest monthly activity occurred from June to September. In Israel, peak numbers of cases occurred in August to September. In South Africa, outbreaks of human disease occurred during the summer months of December through April.[115] The Romanian outbreak demonstrated a peak incidence of clinical disease between August and September.[131]

Pathogenesis and Clinical Findings

Age does not appear to be important for acquiring infection from West Nile virus, but age is an important determinant of clinical manifestation. Most cases of infection in children are asymptomatic.[115] Symptomatic West Nile viral infection is characterized by the rapid onset of fever that lasts for 5 to 6 days. Other symptoms include malaise, frontal headache, muscle pain, lymph node enlargement, and a maculopapular rash. Convalescence may last 1 to 2 weeks. Neurologic involvement is the most severe manifestation of West Nile viral infection, and the age of the patient correlates to the severity of neurologic disease. During the Romanian outbreak, there was a large proportion of neurologic cases: 40% had a diagnosis of meningitis, 44% had meningoencephalitis, and 16% had encephalitis. The onset of disease was abrupt in these cases, with 91% having fever, 77% acute headache, 57% neck stiffness, 53% vomiting, and 34% confusion. The predominant signs in patients with encephalitis were disorientation, disturbed consciousness, and generalized weakness.[131] Other neurologic manifestations include ataxia, hyptonia, hyperreflexia, extrapyramidal signs, cranial nerve palsies, and seizures. Coma developed in 13% of cases. Case fatality increased with increasing age. No fatalities were observed in patients younger than 50 years, a 3.4% case-fatality rate in those 50 to 59 years old, a 4.3% rate in those 60 to 69 years old, and a 14.7% rate in those older than 70. Among cases of West Nile virus encephalitis in the United States, a mean age of 81.5 years was observed, with common clinical manifestations of fever and muscle weakness.[135]

Diagnostic Approaches

The clinical differentiation of West Nile virus infection from dengue can be made on the basis of the neurologic manifestations and absence of hemorrhage or shock. The differentiation will be difficult for milder cases of West Nile infection and for dengue cases that may manifest neurologic involvement. Diagnosis of West Nile infection may be made using viral isolation during the acute period or viral detection by polymerase chain reaction.[136] Serologic diagnosis can be made by demonstrating a high antibody titer on convalescence or a 4-fold rise in antibody titer by hemagglutination inhibition assay or neutralization titer. Detection of IgM or IgG by enzyme immunoassay can also be performed. Antibody to West Nile virus can cross-react to any of the other flaviviruses, including Japanese encephalitis virus, St. Louis encephalitis virus, and dengue virus. Attempts to confirm clinical cases by viral isolation or polymerase chain reaction should be made in areas that are also endemic for other flaviviruses.

Recommendations for Therapy and Control

Therapy for West Nile viral disease, including encephalitis, is supportive. There is no literature to support the use of steroids in the encephalitis associated with West Nile infection. Control of this disease is similar to other previously discussed arboviruses—vector control through the use of spraying and personal protective measures.

[Timothy P. Endy]

YELLOW FEVER

Introduction and Military Relevance

Yellow fever is a viral zoonosis maintained in nature in monkeys. Humans are an incidental host. The disease was named for the icterus that is frequently present during the illness. Yellow fever occurs in a sylvan, or jungle, pattern and in an urban pattern. Jungle yellow fever is transmitted by arboreal mosquitoes among forest-dwelling monkeys. Human cases occur through incidental contact in the forest with these infected mosquitoes. Urban outbreaks occur when urban-breeding mosquitoes transmit the disease from one infected human to another.

Much of the information here on yellow fever is contained in several excellent reviews on the disease (Exhibit 35-1). Yellow fever was first described as a specific entity in the 1700s. This "bilious fever" was confused with malaria, leptospirosis, and typhoid fever and was thought to be a contagious disease transmitted by miasmas or fomites. Dr. Carlos Findlay proposed the theory of mosquito transmission in 1881.[137] During the Spanish-American War (April–December 1898), the US Army recorded 1,169 cases of yellow fever, and in 1899 the mortality rate was recorded at 21%.[37] US Army Major Walter Reed, working in Cuba in 1900 as president of the Yellow Fever Commission,

---

EXHIBIT 35-1

RECOMMENDED REVIEWS OF YELLOW FEVER

- Meegan JM. Yellow fever. In: Beran GW, Steele JH, eds. *Handbook of Zoonoses, Section B: Viral.* 2nd ed. Boca Raton, Fla: CRC Press; 1994:111–124. An excellent review article.

- Monath TP. Yellow fever. In: Monath TP, ed. *The Arboviruses: Epidemiology and Ecology.* Vol 5. Boca Raton, Fla: CRC Press; 1989: Chap 51. A fine treatment of the epidemiology of the disease.

- Monath TP. Yellow fever: A medically neglected disease; report on a seminar. *Rev Infect Dis.* 1987;9:165–175. A thorough treatment of current clinical and therapeutic matters.

- Monath TP. Yellow fever: Victor, Victoria? Conqueror, conquest? Epidemics and research in the last forty years and prospects for the future. *Am J Trop Med Hyg.* 1991;45:1–43. A detailed monograph of the history of yellow fever from 1951.

- Monath TP, Heinz FX. Yellow fever virus. In: Fields BN, Knipe DM, Howley PM, eds. *Virology.* 3rd ed. Philadelphia: Lippincott-Raven; 1995: 1009–1016. An excellent review article.

- Strode GK, ed. *Yellow Fever.* New York: McGraw-Hill; 1951. The definitive book on the history of yellow fever and state of knowledge up to 1951.

observed the absence of person-to-person transmission between patients and the nurses caring for them. He disproved the popular theory of fomite transmission by housing nonimmune volunteers in a closed room with soiled linens and clothes from yellow fever patients. None of the volunteers became ill. Reed then demonstrated mosquito transmission by allowing *Aedes aegypti* mosquitoes that had fed on yellow fever patients to feed on nonimmune volunteers. Of 12 volunteers, 10 developed yellow fever. Two volunteers in the same room but separated by a wire screen from the infected mosquitoes did not develop yellow fever.

Reed determined the extrinsic incubation period of yellow fever when he observed that a mosquito could not transmit the disease until 12 days after it fed on a yellow fever patient. Reed later showed that yellow fever was caused by a "filterable" agent in the serum of patients.[138] When volunteers were injected subcutaneously with blood obtained from yellow fever patients, 6 of 7 individuals developed the disease. Filtered, bacteria-free serum from a patient, when inoculated into a volunteer, produced yellow fever. Blood from this second patient, when inoculated into a third volunteer, again produced yellow fever. Reed documented the period between exposure to infected mosquitoes or blood inoculation to the onset of symptoms, the intrinsic incubation period, to be 2 to 6 days.

In February 1901, US Army Major William Gorgas, chief sanitary officer in Havana, instituted measures to control yellow fever based on the findings of Reed's Yellow Fever Commission. By September 1901, yellow fever was eradicated in Havana (See Figure 2-16 in Volume 1).

Yellow fever was originally thought to be an urban disease of humans transmitted only by *A aegypti*, an urban-breeding mosquito. However, in South America rural epidemics were reported where *A aegypti* was not present. In 1932, jungle yellow fever transmitted by forest-breeding mosquitoes was documented. Dynamic mosquito-primate enzootic transmission, composed of wandering epizootic foci in susceptible monkey populations in South America, was finally documented in the early 1940s. A similar jungle cycle was described in Africa during the same period.[139]

Yellow fever epidemics were common in Africa and the Americas through the 17th, 18th, and 19th centuries. Because the disease was thought to be contagious, fear intensified the social disruption caused by the epidemics. During the summer, epidemics occurred along the eastern US seacoast as far north as Boston. Philadelphia had 20 reported epidemics. In 1878, an epidemic in the Mississippi Valley caused an esti-

mated 13,000 deaths. The last US epidemic was in 1905 in New Orleans with 5,000 cases and 1,000 deaths. In Central and South America, vaccination and *A aegypti* control in the 1940s eliminated urban yellow fever, and since then yellow fever incidence has depended on fluctuations in the jungle cycle.[140] Long-term control has been less successful in Africa. In the 1940s in French West Africa, a mandatory yellow fever immunization program was initiated, resulting in control of the disease. The program was abandoned in 1960 and yellow fever reemerged in the area. In English-speaking African countries, control attempts were limited to mass local vaccination campaigns in response to epidemics, and epidemics have continued to occur.[139]

Description of the Pathogen

The yellow fever virus is a single-strand, positive sense RNA virus. It is the first virus characterized of the family later named after it—*Flaviviridae* (from *flavus*, Latin for yellow). This family includes the viruses that cause dengue fever, Japanese encephalitis, St. Louis encephalitis, and tickborne encephalitis. Nucleotide sequencing has identified three geographic topotypes: West Africa (E-genotype IA), America (E-genotype IB), and Central/East Africa (E-genotype II).[141,142] No difference in human pathological response has been noted between yellow fever from South America or Africa.

Antigenic differences exist among yellow fever virus isolates, and some geographic distinctions have been made.[141] Virus isolates from different sources in the same geographic region appear genetically homogeneous and stable over time.[143] All yellow fever strains have been cross-reactive in neutralization tests.[144] There is a close antigenic relationship between yellow fever virus and other flaviviruses found in Africa; some cross-protection is apparent. In monkeys, previous infection with some group B arboviruses was partially protective against subsequent experimental yellow fever virus infection.[145,146] In a yellow fever outbreak in the Gambia, the ratio of inapparent to apparent yellow fever infections was 10 times greater in patients with serologic evidence of a prior flavivirus infection than in the patients with no prior flavivirus infection (22:1 vs. 2:1).[147]

Epidemiology

Transmission

Yellow fever is transmitted only by mosquitoes, not by contact or fomite. In the Americas and in Africa, person-to-person yellow fever is transmit-

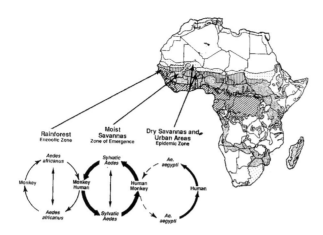

Fig. 35-10. Yellow fever transmission cycles in Africa. Reprinted from: Monath TP. Yellow fever: Victor, Victoria? Conqueror, conquest? Epidemics and research in the last forty years and prospects for the future. *Am J Trop Med Hyg*. 1991;45:30. With permission of the *American Journal of Tropical Medicine and Hygiene*.

ted primarily by *A aegypti* mosquitoes. In South and Central America, jungle yellow fever is transmitted by *Haemagogus* species mosquitoes. In Africa, jungle yellow fever is transmitted by *A africanus* and five other *Aedes* species.[139] In addition, *A africanus* can sustain human epidemics.[148] These transmission cycles are shown in Figure 35-10. A mosquito found in Asia but introduced into the Americas in the 1980s, *A albopictus*, has been shown in experiments to be capable of transmitting yellow fever and is a potential vector for epidemic transmission.[149] There is no evidence for transmission by *Culex* species mosquitoes. *Amblyomma* ticks in Africa have been shown to harbor yellow fever virus, but their role in transmission has not been defined.[140,141]

Blood from a yellow fever patient is infective for a mosquito shortly before the onset of the human's fever and up to 5 days afterward. The virus incubates in the mosquito for 9 to 12 days (the extrinsic incubation period), after which the mosquito remains infected for life. There is evidence that yellow fever virus can be transmitted transovarially in mosquitoes in Africa.[150] This, along with the prolonged survival of adult mosquitoes, may account for maintenance of the virus during the dry season.

In the rain forest, vector mosquitoes (*A africanus* in Africa, *Haemagogus* species in South America) remain high in the tree canopy. Humans do not often come in contact with these mosquitoes unless the trees are being or have recently been cleared. In less-dense forests in climates with dry seasons, these mosquitoes are more active at ground level.

Biting intensity is high during the wet season and nearly absent during the dry season. *A aegypti* mosquitoes breed in areas of human habitation and bite during the day. As a result, human contact with these mosquitoes is almost constant.

In Africa, yellow fever patterns depend on vegetation and rainfall patterns, which influence the population of mosquitoes and primate hosts. The equatorial rain forest of West Africa is a zone of low-level enzootic transmission. The surrounding zone of forest and savannah with cyclic rainy and dry seasons can sustain high transmission rates because of its abundant vector and primate populations. A high level of jungle transmission may occur without human cases if the human population is small or there is a high prevalence of vaccine-induced immunity. The junction of mixed savannah-forest and savannah is the "emergence zone" that allows the annual sylvatic amplification of the virus during the rainy season and repetitive infections in the human population living in the area.[141] Most outbreaks in sub-Saharan Africa occur during the late rainy season and the early dry season (September to December), although an urban outbreak occurred in 1987 in western Nigeria during the late dry season (April to May). This outbreak was thought to be due to high concentrations of domestic *A aegypti* mosquitoes and an earlier sylvatic outbreak nearby.[148] In the tropics of the Americas, the incidence of jungle yellow fever is highest during the months with the greatest rainfall: January to March.[141]

In urban areas or the savannah areas with a prolonged dry season, sylvatic mosquito populations are too low to sustain a sylvatic maintenance cycle. Therefore transmission to humans is absent and the prevalence of immunity in humans is low. These regions have the highest risk for epidemic (urban) yellow fever.

Sylvatic yellow fever transmission may be a "wandering epizootic" because the monkeys that survive infection are immune for life. In South American primates, several species develop fatal infection and several years are necessary for the population to redevelop. In Brazil, yellow fever appeared in monkeys every 7 to 10 years, an interval similar to that found for human yellow fever in that country. Few African primate species develop fatal infection. Because the primate population is not decimated, a larger population of susceptible individuals can accumulate in a shorter time and may account for the shorter interval between periods of yellow fever typical in Africa.[140]

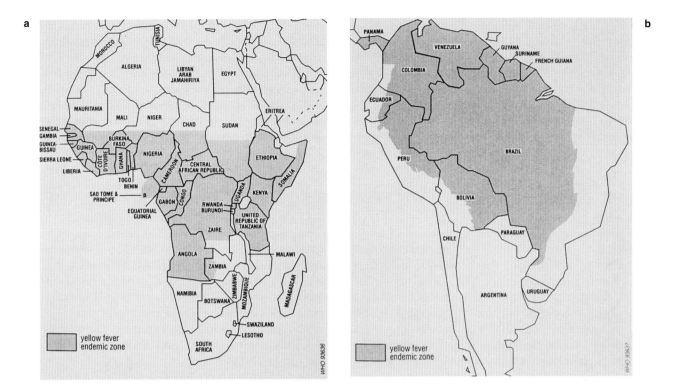

Fig. 35-11. The Yellow Fever Endemic Zones in Africa (*a*) and the Americas (*b*).
Reprinted with permission from: World Health Organization. *International Travel and Health: Vaccination Requirements and Health Advice*. Geneva: WHO; 1996; 14, 15.

Geographic Distribution

Yellow fever occurs in tropical areas of Central and South America and from 15° North latitude to 10° South latitude in Africa (Figure 35-11). In South America, 95% of yellow fever cases occur in the rain forests of Peru, Bolivia, Colombia, and Brazil. Since the last urban case of yellow fever occurred in Trinidad in 1954, all this transmission had been forest-related.[140] *A aegypti* populations have expanded in South and Central America since the early 1980s, creating potential for the recurrence of urban epidemics, and urban cases have recently been reported in Bolivia.[151] For reasons that are not clear, yellow fever is absent in Asia, despite the widespread distribution of *A aegypti* mosquitoes there.

Incidence

The age distribution of yellow fever patients depends on the prevalence of immunity in the population from prior epidemics and vaccination campaigns. In urban yellow fever in endemic areas the greatest incidence is in children; they account for up to 73% of cases. Jungle yellow fever in the Americas is most common in young adults, due to occupational exposures. Yellow fever incidence from 1986 to 1990 was the highest reported to the World Health Organization (WHO) since official reporting began in 1948, with 17,728 cases worldwide and 4,710 deaths; 16,782 of the cases were in Africa.[139]

Pathogenesis and Clinical Findings

Most of the knowledge of the pathogenesis of yellow fever is based on findings in experimentally infected rhesus monkeys.[152] Virus in the saliva of the infected mosquito replicates in cutaneous tissues of the animal at the site of inoculation and in local lymph nodes. The virus then spreads hematogenously to the liver, spleen, bone marrow, and cardiac and skeletal muscle. The liver is the primary organ affected, and hepatocellular injury is due to the direct effect of the replicating virus. Replication is in the cytoplasm, with release of particles by cell lysis. Inflammation is minimal or absent. Hepatic histopathology shows swelling and coagulative necrosis of hepatocytes but inflammatory cellular infiltrates are minimal. Histopathologic findings are not specific for yellow fever, and liver biopsy is contraindicated because of the high risk of hemorrhage. After recovery from yellow fever, there is no evidence of residual damage.[153] Renal glomerular changes are mild and the cause is unclear. Renal injury appears to be due to prerenal impairment with subsequent acute tubular necrosis.[152,154,155] The virus appears to injure the myocardium directly, but there is no evidence of direct viral injury to the brain[155] or the lung.[153] Subsequent clinical complications result from liver, renal, and cardiac dysfunction and may include acute renal failure, acidosis and shock, myocarditis, disseminated intravascular coagulation (DIC) and hemorrhage, and encephalopathy.

Yellow fever is an illness of acute onset, short duration, and variable severity. The clinical course has been divided into three phases: infection, remission, and intoxication. The onset of yellow fever, the period of infection, is characteristic but not specific for yellow fever. Symptoms appear after an incubation period of 3 to 6 days, and a prodrome is usually absent. Usual manifestations include the abrupt onset of fever, headache, myalgia, lumbosacral pain, nausea, malaise, and weakness. During this phase, the patient is viremic and infectious to mosquitoes. Associated findings include apprehension, an initial rapid, bounding pulse followed by a relative bradycardia (Faget's sign), conjunctival suffusion, flushing of the head and neck, reddening of the edges of the tongue, minor gingival hemorrhage, and occasional epistaxis. This first phase lasts approximately 3 days. In abortive infections, these symptoms resolve and the patient recovers. In the mildest infections, the patient may have nothing more than a transient fever and headache, which resolves in hours.

In more severe cases, the period of infection is followed by a brief period of remission. This lasts up to a day, during which the patient's symptoms improve, but then the blood pressure falls and there is a return of fever, vomiting, and prostration. These events mark the onset of the period of intoxication, during which the patient may develop severe yellow fever's classic triad of findings of jaundice, hemorrhage, and intense albuminuria.[156] In this phase, there is no viremia and antibodies appear. Some patients may recover in 3 to 4 days, but 50% of patients who enter this phase die, usually at 7 to 10 days, with hemorrhage, shock, encephalopathy, and renal failure. Jaundice is of variable severity and often not prominent. Hypothermia and delirium progressing to coma are terminal findings. Findings that indicate a fatal outcome include rapid progression to the period of intoxication and rapid rise in the serum bilirubin, severe hemorrhagic diathesis and DIC, acute tubular necrosis, early hy-

potension, shock, coma and convulsions, and intractable hiccoughs.[155] Signs of a good prognosis include diuresis and normal mental status.[156]

Laboratory findings include early leukopenia with neutropenia, thrombocytopenia, liver transaminase and bilirubin elevations; proteinuria; azotemia; and coagulation defects (prolonged prothrombin time and partial thromboplastin time) suggesting DIC. Electrocardiogram findings are nonspecific and may show prolonged PR and QT intervals and ST abnormalities. Hepatic transaminase levels rise on the second or third day, peak 2 to 5 days later, and decline over the next 2 weeks, although mild elevations may persist for 2 months. The degree of transaminase elevation indicates the severity of the disease and the prognosis.[155] Alkaline phosphatase levels remain near normal. Cerebrospinal fluid has increased pressure, elevated protein, a normal cell count, and normal glucose levels.

Complications include suppurative parotitis, bacterial pneumonia, sepsis, and acute tubular necrosis. Atypical fulminant cases may cause death in 3 days, occasionally without hepatic or renal signs. Convalescence may take 1 to 2 weeks. Late deaths may occur after weeks and are attributed to myocardial dysfunction or dysrhythmias. Recovery is usually complete, but jaundice can persist for months.

The differential diagnosis in the early period of infection is broad and must include other arboviral diseases, malaria, rickettsial infections, leptospirosis, typhoid fever, and viral hemorrhagic fevers. During the period of intoxication, the appearance of jaundice makes the diagnostic considerations viral hepatitis, leptospirosis, malaria, typhoid fever, and other viral hemorrhagic fevers. The high case fatality rate in yellow fever, often more than 30% in hospitalized cases (compared to viral hepatitis where the case fatality rate is usually less than 1%) can be valuable in the differential diagnosis.

Yellow fever has characteristic findings, but they are nonspecific and nondiagnostic. Therefore, a clinical diagnosis of yellow fever is not indicated except in the setting of a documented outbreak. In an outbreak, fever and jaundice are often used for case identification.[147] Other diagnoses must remain in consideration until the laboratory diagnosis of yellow fever is made. In a patient with hemorrhagic manifestations, viral hemorrhagic fever must be considered and appropriate infection control precautions taken until a definitive diagnosis is made. Because treatment for yellow fever is supportive only, severe diseases that can be treated, such as malaria and typhoid fever, should be considered first and if diagnostic tests cannot be performed, empiric and possibly lifesaving therapy should be considered.

Subclinical, or inapparent, infection is common. The ratio of infections to clinical cases ranges from 2:1 to 20:1. In a Gambian epidemic in 1978, 33% of the population showed serologic evidence of infection, and the overall clinical-to-subclinical infection ratio was 1:12.[147] Antibody appears within the first week, and recovery confers lifelong immunity. In infants, passive immunity persists up to 6 months after birth.

Diagnostic Approaches

Yellow fever can be diagnosed by detecting the virus in blood or liver biopsy specimens or by detecting serum antibody specific for the yellow fever virus. Because of the danger of hemorrhage, liver biopsy is absolutely contraindicated in the living patient. Detection of the virus or viral antigen in the blood is the most specific diagnostic method. Viremia is greatest 3 to 6 days after the onset of the illness but has been detected as late as day 17. The virus can be isolated by inoculating the patient's blood into suckling mice, mosquitoes, or mammalian or mosquito cell culture. Viral antigen can be detected in blood by enzyme immunoassay (EIA)[157] and in tissue by labeled antibody binding. Viral genome can be detected by polymerase chain reaction (PCR) amplification.

Acute yellow fever can be diagnosed by detecting IgM specific for the yellow fever virus in a patient with a compatible illness or during an outbreak. IgM develops within the first week of the infection, persists for months, and is the target of the serologic test of choice to diagnose acute infection. Acute infection cannot be diagnosed by detecting IgG in a patient with possible previous yellow fever infection or in a person vaccinated against yellow fever, except when a significant rise in the IgG titer in convalescent serum compared to acute serum indicates acute infection. Cross-reacting antibodies due to other flavivirus infections are difficult to distinguish from antibody due to acute infection. This distinction can sometimes be made using a yellow fever type-specific antigen EIA and other serologic tests, such as hemagglutination and complement fixation.

For laboratory detection of yellow fever virus, blood specimens must be obtained from the patient during the first 3 to 4 days of the illness and a postmortem liver biopsy specimen must be obtained within 12 days after the onset of the illness. Specimens for virus detection, such as blood or liver tissue, should be kept at 4°C or on wet ice if they can be delivered to a laboratory within 48 hours. If they must be held longer, they should be frozen on dry ice or in liquid nitrogen. Standard refrigerator freezer temperatures will cause deterioration of the virus. If refrigeration or freezing is not possible, the specimen should be placed in a 50% glycerol solution and shipped at ambient temperature.[158] Virus can be detected in cell culture after 3 to 4 days, while EIA and PCR results take less than a day.

Recommendations for Therapy and Control

Therapy

Therapy consists of symptom control and support only. Ribavirin has some antiviral effect but showed no clinical benefit in experimentally infected monkeys.[141] Interferon gamma showed some benefit if initiated before organ injury occurred.[154] Hypotension and hypoxemia should be managed aggressively. The PTT (partial thromboplastin time) should be kept under 30 seconds using fresh frozen plasma. The value of heparin for DIC is unclear. Nonaspirin antipyretics should be used. Prerenal azotemia should be managed aggressively. Sepsis and bacterial pneumonia must be diagnosed early and treated promptly. There is no evidence to support use of corticosteroids. Immune serum may be protective if given immediately at the time of infection, but it has no effect after the disease appears.[144] Routine blood and body fluid precautions should be used, and the patient must be protected from mosquito access for at least 5 days after the onset of symptoms.

Control

Suspected yellow fever patients should stay inside bed nets or screened rooms to avoid further transmission. The patient's house and nearby houses should be sprayed with an insecticide, and family and other contacts should be immediately immunized. Possible sites where the patient acquired the infection and possible contacts should be investigated. In outbreaks, mass vaccination and vector control must be initiated immediately.[140] A case definition and case finding and confirmatory methods must be established, including clinical facility visits and house-to-house surveys. Mass vaccination during the early phase of an outbreak is difficult because of the delay in recognition of the epidemic and the 5- to 7-day lag between vaccination and appearance of antibody.[148]

Quarantine

Entomologic investigation of an epidemic is necessary to identify the vector, mode of contact with humans, breeding sites, and methods of control. *Aedes* mosquito breeding places must be eliminated. No quarantine is required for individual cases, but quarantine measures apply to all transportation coming into and out of affected areas. WHO International Health Regulations state that every port and airport be kept free of *A aegypti* in an area extending 400 m outside the perimeter of the facility.[158] Specimens must be sent to reference laboratory testing facilities, and once yellow fever is confirmed, testing should be established in a local facility or even in the field.

The International Health Regulations of 1969 mandate the reporting of yellow fever cases to WHO and neighboring countries. Travelers coming from "infected local areas" into "yellow fever receptive areas" may be required to possess a valid international certificate of vaccination or spend 6 days in quarantine.[62p553–558] This vaccination certificate is valid for 10 years, starting 10 days after the vaccination date. Exposure should be avoided until 5 days after vaccination.

Vaccine. In 1928 in Dakar, West Africa (now Senegal), Mathais infected rhesus monkeys with the blood from a yellow fever patient. This yellow fever virus, which became known as the "French strain,"[159] was used to infect mouse brains and so to produce the first effective yellow fever vaccine. It was named the French Neurotropic Vaccine (FNV). It was used for mass immunization in French West Africa from the early 1940s until 1965 and nearly eliminated yellow fever there. However, encephalitis occurred in some children who received the vaccine. One investigator reported 3 cases per 1,000 vaccinees, with a fatality rate of 38%.[154] Routine use of the vaccine in children in West Africa was stopped in 1961.

In 1937, Thieler at the Rockefeller Institute developed an attenuated live virus vaccine, strain 17D, which led to the substrains (17D-204 and 17DD) used for current vaccines. The 17D strain originated from blood of a 28-year-old West African man named Asibi who had mild yellow fever.[137] The original Asibi strain was passed many times in mouse embryonic cell culture, eventually producing an attenuated mutant. The attenuated strain was designated 17D and in 1937 was used for human immunization. The US Army approved use of the 17D vaccine on 30 January 1941. From February to December 1942, however, 49,111 cases of hepatitis, with 81 deaths, were caused by the 0.04 mL of human serum in each dose of vaccine.[160] A serum-free vaccine was formulated, and no further hepatitis cases occurred.

The 17D strain yellow fever vaccine is one of the safest and most effective live, attenuated vaccines. The vaccine induces an antibody response in more than 95% of vaccinees within 10 days, and neutralizing antibodies persist 30 to 35 years after vaccination. Since 1965, more than 250 million doses of 17D vaccine have been administered.[161] Less than 5% of vaccinees develop mild headache or fever. Encephalitis has been noted in 20 recipients, 14 of whom were under 6 months old. One recipient died, but the encephalitis resolved without sequelae in the other cases. As a result, the vaccine is contraindicated in children under 4 months of age, and children between 4 and 9 months should be vaccinated only when the risk of yellow fever exposure warrants it. Preventive immunization is extremely effective, but the program must continue to immunize individuals born or immigrating into the population. Currently, 17 African countries use routine yellow fever immunization, most in infants at 9 months of age.[62] This approach is recommended by the WHO in yellow fever–endemic countries.

Vaccination during pregnancy has been relatively contraindicated because of the theoretical risk of transplacental infection and postvaccinal encephalitis in the fetus.[155] During an epidemic, however, the maternal risk from natural infection is much greater than the risk from the vaccine. Only one study on the use of the vaccine by pregnant women has been reported, and no effect on the fetus was found.[162] However, one case has been reported of congenital yellow fever infection without malformation in the child; the woman was immunized during pregnancy.[163] The vaccine is not recommended when live-virus vaccines are contraindicated, such as in immunodeficient individuals or those on immunosuppressive drugs. The vaccine is recommended for asymptomatic individuals who are seropositive for human immunodeficiency virus; the risk in symptomatic seropositive individuals is unknown.[62]

Factors that may decrease the efficacy of the vaccine include poor nutritional status, simultaneous administration of the cholera vaccine, and pregnancy. Cholera vaccine given with or up to 3 weeks before yellow fever vaccine causes a temporary reduction in antibody response. In pregnant women, seroconversion rates were found to be only 39%.[162] Prior yellow fever vaccination or concomitant administration of other vaccines, such as those for tuberculosis (bacille Calmette-Guérin [BCG]), diphtheria, pertussis, tetanus, measles, polio, hepatitis A, hepatitis B, and typhoid fever (injectable), or immunoglobulin does not interfere with the antibody response to the vaccine.[164–166] At usual antimalarial doses, chloroquine does not decrease the immune response.[167] Presence of antibodies against other group B arboviruses does not interfere with the immunogenicity of yellow fever vaccine. Presence of antibodies against other group B arboviruses, including Japanese encephalitis virus, does not interfere with the immunogenicity of yellow fever vaccine.[168] The vaccine must be handled carefully under field conditions.[140] A cold chain must be maintained, keeping the vaccine frozen or at 4°C. Reconstituted vaccine should be used within 1 hour and any residual discarded.

Allergic reactions to the vaccine occur rarely (1 in 1 million recipients) and primarily in persons with an allergy to eggs.[141] One patient with a history of egg allergy was skin tested with a skin prick test of the yellow fever vaccine diluted 1:10 and then an intradermal test of yellow fever vaccine diluted 1:100. There was no reaction, and the yellow fever vaccine was administered without complication.[169]

[Charles F. Longer]

JAPANESE ENCEPHALITIS

Introduction and Military History

Worldwide, Japanese encephalitis (JE) is the most important mosquito-borne viral encephalitis. Within Asia, JE is a major cause of encephalitis, accounting for more than 35,000 cases and 10,000 deaths each year.[170] In Japan, epidemics of "summer encephalitis" were recorded yearly from 1873 until changes were made in agricultural practices and the advent of universal immunization against JE in the 1960s.[171] At the beginning of World War II, the military anticipated possible epidemics among US forces in the Pacific. To address this, the Commission on Neurotropic Virus Diseases of the Board for the Investigation and Control of Influenza and Other Epidemic Diseases in the Army (later reorganized as the Army Epidemiological Board) assigned MAJ Albert Sabin to develop a vaccine against JE and then to stockpile it. Sabin built on earlier work of Japanese investigators[172] to grow Japanese encephalitis virus (JEV) (Nakayama strain) to high concentrations in the brains of sucking mice, make a 10% suspension of the brains, and inactivate the virus with formalin. By 1942, lyophilized vaccine had been produced and shown to be safe in volunteer medical students and laboratory staff in Cincinnati, Ohio. Neutralizing antibodies were elicited in just over 50% of recipients.[173] In July 1945, an epidemic of summer encephalitis occurred among the native and US military populations of Okinawa and nearby islands. Within 10 days of the first case reports, vaccine was administered to US military personnel in the high-risk areas. As many as 70,000 personnel received two doses of vaccine, which was generally well tolerated. Among the 55,000 for which follow-up data were available, however, there were 19 systemic, immediate-type allergic reactions and four instances of "infectious polyneuritis" (Guillain-Barré syndrome).[174] In 1946, 250,000 military personnel in the Far East received this vaccine and the decision was made to vaccinate all Occupation troops.[172]

Starting in 1946, mouse brain–derived vaccine, which lost its potency during storage, was replaced with a more stable, inactivated vaccine derived from chick embryo.[175] JE vaccine was routinely administered to all US military personnel in the Far East Command between 1946 and 1951 and to tens of thousands of Japanese children, in whom its protective efficacy was estimated to be nearly 80%.[176,177] In 1950 despite the vaccination policy, 299 cases of proven or suspected JE occurred among US soldiers in Korea.[178] In 1952, the Army stopped the routine use of JE vaccines.[179] With the availability of more recent vaccines described below, including a more highly purified version of the mouse brain vaccine, JE has been less of a problem for military units in endemic areas, although there were cases among US and Australian troops during the Vietnam War[180,181] and more recently among military personnel stationed in Okinawa.[182] JEV remains a threat throughout Asia.

Description of the Pathogen

JEV was first isolated in Japan in 1935 from the brain of a patient dying from summer encephalitis.[183] This "Japanese" encephalitis was also called type B encephalitis to differentiate it from the type A encephalitis (von Economo encephalitis or encephalitis lethargica), which occurred during winter months and had a different clinical course. Encephalitis epidemics in 1933 and 1937 in the United States were initially thought to be caused by the same virus (type B). Cross-challenge and cross-neutralization studies in mice demonstrated that the St. Louis type B encephalitis virus was distinct from the Japanese type B encephalitis virus.[184] The designation "type B" is no longer used.

JEV belongs to the virus family *Flaviviridae* and genus *Flavivirus*.[185] It is a small, enveloped, positive-stranded RNA virus, 40 to 50 nm in diameter. The genome is approximately 11 kilobases in length, coding for a single open reading frame that translates into three structural proteins (C, M, E) and seven nonstructural proteins (NS1, NS2a, NS2b, NS3, NS4a, NS4b, NS5).[186,187] There is only one serotype of JEV, although two immunotypes of JEV (Nakayama and JaGAr) have been suggested.[188] Several genotypes have been identified (those having more than 12% divergence), but associations between virus genotypes and disease severity remain uncertain.[189]

Epidemiology

Transmission

The principle vector for JEV in Asia is the *Culex tritaeniorhynchus* mosquito, which is zoophilic.[190] Humans are considered to be a dead-end host for this virus because of the preference of vector mosquitoes for animals over humans.[191] Also, virus is only rarely isolated from blood in patients, suggesting that the duration and titer of viremia may be too low to support transmission. Pigs and birds are the most important animals for virus maintenance, amplification, and spread. Most mosquitoes and animals infected with JEV remain well, but fatal encephalitis occurs in horses and fetal wastage may occur in infected sows.[170] Animal vaccines for pigs and horses are available.[192,193]

While *C tritaeniorhynchus* is the principle vector, many other species of mosquitoes have been infected with JEV in the laboratory and have been found infected in field collections; this suggests that they serve as vectors to a certain degree.[194] In most endemic regions, *C tritaeniorhynchus* mosquitoes are present in large numbers following seasonal periods of heavy rain. This mosquito breeds in swamps, marshes, and rice fields away from human housing but can fly up to a kilometer and a half and has been found in tree tops 15 m (50 ft) off the ground seeking blood meals.[190,195] The mosquito is most active during the hour following sunset.[196]

Geographic Distribution and Incidence

Countries or areas that have had proven epidemics of JE are Australia (Torres Strait[197]), Bangladesh, Burma, Cambodia, China, India, Indonesia, Japan, the Korean peninsula, Laos, Malaysia, Nepal, Philippines, Saipan, maritime Siberia, Singapore, Sri Lanka, Thailand, and Vietnam[194,198] (Figure 35-12). A single case diagnosed by polymerase chain reaction (PCR) has been reported from Pakistan.[199] Epidemiologic data are limited because most countries report only total numbers of encephalitis without more specific diagnoses.

In endemic areas, the highest age-specific attack rates occur in children 3 to 6 years of age. Fewer cases in younger children may be due to protection from maternal antibody in the first year and avoidance of vector mosquitoes. With increasing age, children tend to play more outside, especially after dusk, which increases exposure.[200] In some areas (eg, Nepal, northern India, Sri Lanka), all age groups are affected, suggesting recent introduction of the virus into these relatively nonimmune populations.[201] Adult travelers to endemic areas are susceptible to JEV infections.[198]

JEV transmission in the tropics may occur year round. Seasonal epidemics generally begin during the rainy seasons, when mosquito populations are maximal.[201] JEV transmission is not static and may increase due to the construction of dams, use of irrigation, and changes in pig-raising practices and similar activities.

Pathogenesis and Clinical Findings

Infection with JEV may be asymptomatic or manifest as a mild febrile illness, aseptic meningitis, or classic severe meningomyeloencephalitis.

Asymptomatic Infection

Between 25 and 300 JEV infections occur for each identified clinical case of JE.[202–205] Why some infections progress and others remain subclinical is not clear. Viral factors may be important, such as route of inoculation, virus titer in mosquito saliva, and

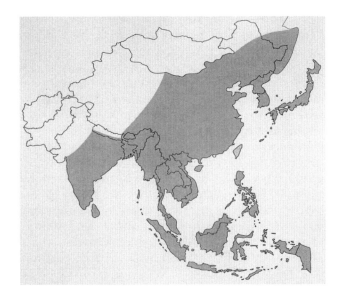

Fig. 35-12. Geographical distribution of confirmed or suspected cases of Japanese encephalitis.

neurovirulence of the inoculum. Host factors, such as age, genetic makeup, general health, and preexisting immunity, may play a key role in disease severity. Virus inoculated directly into a blood vessel by the infecting mosquito may be transported more rapidly to the central nervous system; virus inoculated subcutaneously may proliferate harmlessly for several life cycles of the organism before entering the circulatory system, allowing time for an immune response.[194]

Encephalitis

Following an incubation period of 1 to 2 weeks, patients typically present following 1 to 3 days of fever and headache, often accompanied by nausea or vomiting; they may also be stuporous or comatose. Generalized seizures are common, especially in children. Physical findings include fever, a depressed state of consciousness, and impairment of cranial and motor nerves. Stupor progresses to coma that, in nonfatal cases, may resolve in 1 to 2 weeks. A severely depressed sensorium at the time of presentation is associated with a poor outcome.[206] The mortality rate is approximately 25%; 50% suffer neuropsychiatric sequelae and 25% recover fully.[200,207] Comatose patients may experience respiratory arrest and require ventilatory support. A mild-to-moderate viral pneumonitis is common and may be followed by bacterial pneumonia. Computer tomography and magnetic resonance imaging reveal typical acute and convalescent changes that involve the thalamus, basal ganglia, and other areas.[208–211] Long-term sequelae in survivors include weakness, ataxia, tremor, athetoid movements, paralysis, memory loss, and abnormal emotional behavior.[212,213]

Autopsy of fatal cases has shown the brain to have vascular congestion, mild edema, and minimal overlying cellular exudate.[214] Virus can be isolated from all areas of the brain, but virus is most commonly found in the thalamus and brain stem. The destruction of neurons in the brain stem can explain the profound coma and respiratory failure.[215]

Diagnostic Approaches

An acute febrile illness with changes in mental status and signs of meningeal irritation occurring in endemic areas for JE should prompt the physician to consider JE as the cause. In some areas where diagnostic support is limited, a presumptive diagnosis of JE is made if the cerebrospinal fluid (CSF) is clear. Other conditions that should be considered are shown in Table 35-6.

CSF findings that are consistent with a diagnosis of JE include an opening pressure for the CSF that is normal or moderately increased, a total protein that is slightly increased, and a lymphocyte pleocytosis that is typically 10 to 1,000 mononuclear cells per milliliter.[200] The presence of JEV-specific immunoglobulin M (IgM) in the CSF is thought to be diagnostic of JE, as opposed to infection with JEV without encephalitis which results in increased IgM in the sera but not in the CSF.[216] The presence of infectious virus in the CSF and low levels of JEV-specific IgM in both CSF and serum at presentation are associated with a poor outcome.[206]

Many methods of detecting JEV antibodies have been developed. The most reliable method at present is a carefully standardized enzyme-linked immunosorbent assay (EIA). This approach distinguishes between JE and dengue infections, as well as primary and secondary flavivirus infections, by comparing the number of units of specific IgM versus immunoglobulin G antibody.[217] Hemagglutination inhibition is a simple and reliable approach,[218] but its interpretation may be more difficult than the EIA's. Antibody test results may be confusing because of considerable cross-reactivity with other flaviviruses.[219] In Southeast Asia, where dengue and JEV both circulate, previous exposure to either virus in an individual patient increases the difficulty of virus-specific serological diagnosis. Natural infection or vaccination for yellow fever, West Nile fever, or tick-borne encephalitis may also produce false-positive tests for JEV antibody.

The PCR can be used to detect viral genome.[220] Isolation of JEV may be performed in mosquito or other cell lines. Virus isolation from brain tissue gathered postmortem is usual, but positive cultures from CSF are much less common, and isolations from serum are rare.[221] Because of the low sensitivity of viral detection methods, diagnosis is usually based on the presence of JEV-specific IgM antibodies in the CSF or serum. Commercial assays are just becoming available, although none are currently licensed in the United States. Specimen testing can be coordinated through the Armed Forces Research Institute of Medical Sciences in Bangkok, Thailand; the Centers for Disease Control and Prevention in Fort Collins, Colorado; or the Walter Reed Army Institute of Research in Silver Spring, Md.

Recommendations for Therapy and Control

Therapy

Currently, there is no effective treatment for JE beyond supportive care. Dexamethasone does not reduce mortality nor provide any other benefit but

TABLE 35-6

DIFFERENTIAL DIAGNOSIS OF FEVER AND MENINGISMUS OR ALTERED MENTAL STATE IN AREAS WHERE JAPANESE ENCEPHALITIS IS ENDEMIC

Diagnosis	Specific Therapy Available
Disease states lacking a CSF pleocytosis	
-Metabolic encephalopathy complicating infection or other systemic process	Yes
-Cerebral malaria	Yes
-Dengue encephalopathy	No
-Acute toxic encephalopathy including Reye's syndrome	No
-Sub-arachnoid hemorrhage	No
Disease states with CSF pleocytosis and low CSF glucose	
-Pyogenic meningitis	Yes
-Tuberculous or fungal (cryptococcal) meningitis	Yes
Disease states with CSF pleocytosis and normal glucose	
-Brain abscess	Yes
-Infections associated with immunosuppression: toxoplasmosis, progressive multifocal leukoencephalopathy, etc.	Yes (for some)
-Aseptic meningitis	
Leptospirosis	Yes
Rickettsioses	Yes
-Cerebral vasculitis	Yes
-Acute viral encephalitis	
Herpes simplex encephalitis	Yes
Japanese encephalitis	No
West Nile encephalitis (overlap with JE in western India)	No
Murray Valley encephalitis (overlap with JE at southern limit of JE virus range)	No
Meningoencephalitis due to enteroviruses (eg, Coxsackie, echo, polio viruses)	No
Rabies	No
Encephalitis due to viruses of the California encephalitis virus serogroup (viruses present in Sri Lanka and China by serology; no human cases recognized)	No
-Parainfectious and postvaccinal encephalomyelitis	
Measles encephalitis	No
Varicella-zoster encephalitis	No
Disease following other infections: rubella, mumps, infectious mononucleosis, influenza, parainfluenza, *Mycoplasma* infection	No
Disease following vaccinations: Semple rabies vaccine, measles vaccine	No

CSF: cerebrospinal fluid
JE: Japanese encephalitis
Adapted from: Innis, BL. Japanese encephalitis. In: Porterfield, JS, ed. *Kass Handbook of Infectious Diseases: Exotic Viral Infections.* London: Chapman & Hall Medical, 1995. Reproduced with permission of Edward Arnold Limited.

is still sometimes used despite the lack of evidence of efficacy.[200] Various interferons have shown promise, but definitive trials have not been done.[222,223]

Approaches to the prevention of JE include vector control, vector avoidance, immunization of susceptible persons, and immunization of amplifying hosts.

Vector Control and Personal Protection

Spraying pesticides produces limited reductions of JEV vectors in a limited area for a limited amount of time at great cost. Reasons for this lack of effectiveness include: (*a*) the vector *C tritaeniorhynchus* has a wide flight range, so new mosquitoes quickly replace those killed by local spraying of insecticides in and around human and animal housing areas; (*b*) application of insecticides to rice fields to kill larvae is effective for only 1 to 2 weeks; and (*c*) organophosphorus and carbamate insecticides have become largely ineffective because of the development of insecticide resistance.[224]

Personal precautions should be taken by residents of endemic regions and travelers to these areas to avoid mosquito bites. These precautions include:

- minimizing outdoor exposure at dusk and dawn and on overcast days,
- sleeping in screened quarters or under mosquito netting,
- wearing clothing leaving a minimum of skin bare,
- using insect repellents containing DEET (N,N-diethylmeta-toluamide) appropriately on exposed skin surfaces,[225] and
- keeping farm animals away from housing and avoiding the animals at dusk.[226]

Vaccination

Vaccines that are distributed commercially contain formalin-inactivated virus derived from mouse brain. This type of vaccine was first tested in humans in Japan and Russia in the late 1930s and licensed in Japan in 1954. Partial purification with protamine sulfate was introduced in 1958. The presently available vaccine—JE-VAX, produced by BIKEN (The Research Foundation for Microbial Disease of Osaka University, Japan) and distributed in the United States since 1992 by Pasteur-Adventist, USA—is more highly purified.[227]

Efficacy and Safety. Vaccine efficacy trials have been reviewed,[194,198,227] and efficacy has ranged from 81% to 96%. Among pediatric participants, fever has followed immunization in less than 1% of the vaccinees and local reactions have been seen in approximately 5%. The most definitive trial was performed in Thailand from 1984 to 1985.[228] The highly purified BIKEN vaccine (Nakayama-Yoken strain) and a bivalent vaccine consisting of Nakayama-Yoken and Beijing-1 strains were compared in a placebo-controlled, masked, randomized study. Two doses of vaccine, given a week apart, were administered to approximately 22,000 children in each of the three groups. The efficacy of both monovalent and bivalent vaccines was 91%. There were no major side effects. Minor side effects, such as headache, sore arm, rash, and swelling, were similar to the control group (who received tetanus toxoid) and generally affected less than 1%.

JE vaccine safety and immunogenicity trials began in the United States in 1983. One hundred twenty-six volunteers received two 1.0 mL doses of the vaccine 1 week apart. A three-dose series was recommended after two doses failed to provide an optimal immune response. Adverse reactions included one apparent immediate hypersensitivity reaction to the first dose, manifested by generalized urticaria that responded to subcutaneous epinephrine. Eighteen percent reported tenderness at the injection site, and 9% reported headache lasting an average of 1 day.[229]

In expanded US trials from 1987 to 1989, 4,034 US military volunteers received vaccine without severe adverse reactions. Twenty percent of the volunteers reported mild arm soreness lasting no more than a few hours; 10% reported headache. These studies also suggested the need for a third dose,[230] and subsequent studies have demonstrated that the antibodies produced by a three-dose primary series of JE-VAX persists for at least 3 years in healthy US soldiers.[231]

Although the safety record of JE vaccines used in Japan has been excellent, reports from Denmark, Australia, and Canada in the 1990s have suggested an increased incidence of hypersensitivity reactions.[232-234] In a prospective study of US military personnel and their family members on Okinawa, the hospitalization rate for treatment of refractory urticaria following vaccination was 3 per 10,000. A history of urticaria increased the risk of an adverse reaction 9-fold.[227] Nevertheless, the vaccine is generally felt to be safe for individuals at risk for the disease.[235,236] Due to the risk of hypersensitivity reactions, it is recommended that persons receive the vaccine at least 10 days before departure to assure their access to medical care should the need arise.

Indications for Vaccination. Current recommendations from the Advisory Committee on Immunization Practices (ACIP) for primary and booster vaccination are given in Table 35-7. A three-dose vaccination series is recommended for US inhabitants traveling to areas where they may be at risk of exposure to JEV. Most travelers to Asia will not require JE vaccination. JEV transmission is seasonal and confined to rural areas where animals are present. Consulting with public health officials before travel may clarify the need for immunization. Living for extended periods in endemic areas and

TABLE 35-7

RECOMMENDED SUBCUTANEOUS IMMUNI-
ZATION SCHEDULE FOR BIKEN JAPANESE
ENCEPHALITIS VACCINE

	< 3 y of age	≥ 3 y of age	Schedule
Primary series	0.5 mL	1.0 mL	0, 7, and 30 d*
Booster	0.5 mL	1.0 mL	Dose at 2 y and then at 3-y intervals or as determined by serology

* The primary series may be given at 0, 7, and 14 days, but this
will result in lower neutralizing antibody titers.
Source: Advisory Committee on Immunization Practices. Inactivated Japanese encephalitis virus vaccine: Recommendations
of the Advisory Committee on Immunization Practices (ACIP).
MMWR. 1993;42(RR-1):1–15.

having contact with farm animals, especially in the
evening, will increase risk. Vaccination is not indicated for travel to urban centers in Asia for short
periods. JE incidence figures for the area to be visited may not be helpful if the vaccine is in widespread use. The vaccine may be given with the diphtheria-tetanus-pertussis, measles, and oral polio
vaccines, but its interaction with other vaccines is
unknown.[198] In addition to selected military units
and individuals traveling to high-risk areas, vaccination is recommended for those participating in
Cobra Gold exercises in Thailand and for units on
alert status for possible missions into JE-endemic
areas. Updated country information is available
from the resources listed in Chapter 11, Medical
Threat Assessment.

Contraindications. Contraindications to immunization are as follows. Persons with a history of
significant reaction to JE vaccine should not receive
additional doses. Although no adverse outcomes
have been associated with administration during
pregnancy, it should be avoided unless significant
exposure to JEV cannot be otherwise avoided. There
are no safety data for children younger than 1 year
of age. As mentioned above, persons with a history
of allergic conditions, such as asthma, allergic rhinitis, drug or hymenoptera venom sensitivity, food
allergy, and especially urticaria, seem to be at increased risk. These persons should be advised of
the potential for vaccine-related angioedema and
generalized urticaria.

[David W. Vaughn]

THE EQUINE ENCEPHALITIDES

Introduction and Military Relevance

Venezuelan, western, and eastern equine encephalitis viruses have been recognized as causative
agents of fatal neurologic disease in horses since
the first half of the 20th century. By the 1930s, advances in the field of virology had made isolation
and basic characterization of these disease-causing
agents possible. Western equine encephalitis (WEE)
virus was first isolated from sick horses in 1930.[237]
Eastern equine encephalitis (EEE) virus and Venezuelan equine encephalitis (VEE) virus were similarly isolated and described by the end of the
1930s.[238–240] While these viruses were initially described during the first half of the 20th century, their
presence in the Americas almost certainly predates
the arrival of the Spanish in the New World. There
are anecdotal stories of Spanish invaders entering
Colombia with thousands of horses and leaving
with only a few surviving animals. While not necessarily attributable to the equine encephalitides,
such mortality testifies to the presence of severe
horse disease in that area during the early 16th century. First recognized as horse diseases, the equine
encephalitides became associated with naturally
occurring cases of encephalitis in humans by the
late 1930s,[241,242] and the importance of this group of
viruses in the Americas was firmly established.

Because of their endemicity throughout Central
and South America, the equine encephalitides are
significant health threats to US troops deployed
in these areas. The risk is significant enough that
preventive vaccination has been requested for service members participating in special missions in
these areas. Cases of VEE have been reported in
troops conducting training exercises in Central
America.[243,244]

While VEE, WEE, and EEE viruses were recognized as the etiologic agents of encephalitis in
horses and humans in the 1930s, it was not until
EEE virus was isolated from *Culiseta melanura*[245]
mosquitoes in the 1950s that there was some indication that these viruses were transmitted by mosquitoes. Today these viruses are collectively
grouped, along with several Old World mosquito-
borne viruses, into the genus *Alphavirus* (formerly
known as the group A arboviruses) in the family
Togaviridae.

Description of the Pathogen

While the names given to the equine encephalitis viruses—VEE, WEE, and EEE viruses—suggest that these are individual agents, each represents a complex of serologically related viruses that, together with four additional virus complexes, have been grouped together into the *Alphavirus* genus.[246]

The alphaviruses are spherical particles, typically 60 to 65 nm in diameter. Alphavirus particles are composed of a lipid envelope containing two structural glycoproteins (El and E2) surrounding a protein core. The icosahedral protein core or nucleocapsid contains the viral ribonucleic acid and forms the backbone for the overall shape and structure of the mature virion.[247] The envelope glycoproteins form heterodimers that further associate to form trimers.[248,249] It is these trimers, which form the spikes, that are clearly visible on electron micrographs of alphavirus particles[250] (Figure 35-13). Alphavirus spikes are the major targets of the host's immune response to infection[251] and directly influence important biological characteristics of this group of viruses, such as tissue tropism, host range, and virulence.[252]

Alphavirus replication involves the classic steps of viral replication, including viral attachment, uncoating, transcription, translation, packaging, and escape and has been reviewed in detail.[247]

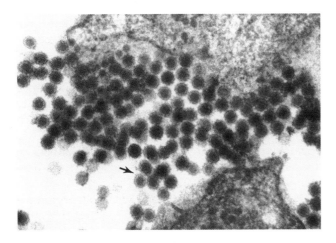

Fig. 35-13. An electron micrograph of Vero cells infected eastern equine encephalitis virus (140,000x magnification). The arrow identifies the viral envelope, which contain heterodimer spikes composed of glycoproteins E1 and E2.
Photograph courtesy of Tom Geisbert, Pathology Division, US Army Medical Research Institute of Infectious Diseases.

TABLE 35-8

CLASSIFICATION OF THE VENEZUELAN EQUINE ENCEPHALITIS VIRUS ANTIGENIC COMPLEX

Subtype	Variety	Epidemiology
I	A/B	Epidemic/epizootic
I	C	Epidemic/epizootic
I	D	Endemic/enzootic
I	E	Endemic/enzootic
I	F	Endemic/enzootic
II	Everglades	Endemic/enzootic
III	A (Mucambo)	Endemic/enzootic
III	B (Tonate)	Endemic/enzootic
III	C (71D-1252)	Endemic/enzootic
IV	Pixuna	Endemic/enzootic
V	Cabassou	Endemic/enzootic
VI	AG80–663	Endemic/enzootic

Epidemiology

The VEE complex consists of six closely related subtypes, each differing in its ecology, epidemiology, and virulence for humans and equines. The IA/B and IC varieties are commonly referred to as epizootic strains (Table 35-8). These strains have been responsible for extensive epidemics in North and South America and are highly pathogenic for both humans and equines.[246] All of the epizootic strains are exotic to the United States and have been the etiologic agent responsible for natural epidemics only twice since 1973.[253] An outbreak of fatal encephalitis caused by epizootic VEE virus between April and October of 1995 in Venezuela and Colombia was the first major outbreak since the 1970s.[254]

The WEE virus complex consists of six viruses: WEE, Sindbis (SIN), Y 6233, Aura, Fort Morgan, and Highlands J. The EEE virus complex consists of a single virus found in two antigenically distinct variants, the North and South American forms. All North American and Caribbean isolates show a high degree of genetic and antigenic homogeneity, whereas South and Central American isolates tend to be much more heterogeneous.[255,256]

Transmission

Understanding the epidemiology of the equine encephalitides in humans requires an appreciation of the factors affecting the mosquito vectors and vertebrate hosts and their interactions in naturally occurring endemic foci. Most commonly, disease in humans follows expansion or intrusion into geographic regions and ecological zones where natural transmission cycles are in progress. Human activities that disrupt or alter natural transmission cycles, such as introduction of alien mosquito vectors or unnatural modifications to the environment, may predispose human populations to disease. Natural changes to the environment or alteration of the viruses themselves through accumulation of genetic mutations may also be contributing factors to human disease.

The epizootic subtypes of VEE virus are more opportunistic, relying on a variety of mosquito species and any susceptible equines that may be present

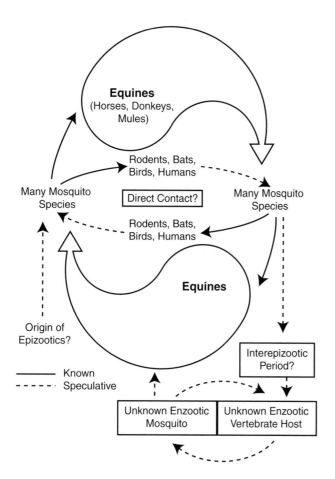

Fig. 35-14. Transmission cycle of epizootic and enzootic subtypes of Venezuelan equine encephalitis virus. Horses, donkeys, and mules are the principle amplifying hosts for the epizootic subtype of the virus, and mosquitoes from at least four genera have been implicated in transmission. For the enzootic subtype, *Culex (Melanoconion) taeniopus, C aikenii,* and *C portesi* are species that have been implicated as important vectors in past outbreaks. Art by Annabelle Wright, Walter Reed Army Institute of Research.

(Figure 35-14). Horses, donkeys, and mules serve as important amplifying hosts because they develop high-titer viremias capable of infecting many mosquito species. Varieties D, E, and F of subtype I and subtypes II, III, IV, V, and VI are referred to as the enzootic strains (see Table 35-8).[246,254] Like the epizootic strains, the enzootic strains may cause disease in humans, but they differ from the epizootic strains in their lack of virulence for horses. Infection of horses with enzootic subtypes leads to an immune response capable of protecting animals from challenge with epizootic strains.[257] Limited data, acquired after accidental laboratory exposures, suggest that similar cross-protection may not occur in humans.[258,259]

Enzootic VEE virus subtypes are maintained quite efficiently in transmission cycles involving mainly mosquitoes belonging to the subgenus *Melanoconion.* The mosquitoes are ground feeders and prefer feeding on mammals rather than birds.[260] In part because their ecology is similar to that of the mosquito vector, ground-dwelling rodents serve as the primary vertebrate host for the enzootic forms of VEE virus. After infection, these animals develop viremias of sufficient magnitude and duration to infect mosquitoes during their blood meals.[261] Other animals, such as bats and certain birds, may play a secondary role.[258,259]

Unlike the enzootic strains, the fate of the epidemic strains during interepidemic periods is unclear. As epidemic forms of VEE virus appear so rarely, the natural ecology of these viruses has been difficult to study. The two most likely theories suggest that either epidemic strains evolve from enzootic strains[264,265] or they are maintained in cryptic foci, remaining undetected for long periods of time.

WEE virus is maintained in transmission cycles involving perching birds and the mosquito *Culex tarsalis.* Humans and horses become involved only tangentially and are considered dead-end hosts.[266] Endemic and epidemic WEE virus activity in California has been extensively studied.[267] Results from these studies suggest that enzootic activity is difficult to control completely.

Enzootic transmission of EEE virus occurs almost exclusively between perching birds and the mosquito *Culiseta melanura.*[268,269] Because of the strict ornithophilic feeding behavior of this mosquito, human and equine disease requires the involvement of more general feeders, such as members of the genera *Aedes* and *Coquillettidia.*[257] Equines are typically dead-end hosts for EEE virus. They may, however, develop viremias of sufficient magnitude following infection to infect vector mosquitoes, but this is not considered an important mechanism of virus dissemination.[253]

In the case of naturally occurring outbreaks of VEE, WEE, and EEE, evidence of infection in equines almost always precedes human disease.[270,271] With EEE and WEE viruses, isolations are also often made from domestic or wild birds before the onset of human involvement, making these hosts useful for detecting potential epidemic activity.[272] With VEE, the magnitude of viremias in infected horses can be extremely high; as a result, these animals can serve as efficient amplifying hosts.

Geographical Distribution

Most subtypes of VEE viruses are enzootic in South and Central America, but subtype II circulates in the Everglades region of Florida. The enzootic viruses are commonly isolated in specific ecological habitats, where they circulate in transmission cycles primarily involving rodents and *Culex* mosquitoes of the *Melanoconion* subgenus.[273–275] These mosquitoes often occur in very humid localities with abundant open spaces, such as sunny, swampy pastures cut by slowly flowing, meandering streams. EEE virus is endemic to focal habitats ranging from southern Canada to northern South America.[253] The virus has been isolated as far west as Minnesota but is most common along the eastern coast of the United States between New England and Florida. Several antigenic subtypes of WEE virus have been identified, but the geographic distributions of the subtypes overlap.[15] Most members of the WEE virus complex are distributed throughout the Americas, but the SIN virus and Y 62–33 subtypes are found only in the Old World.[246]

The largest known outbreak of epidemic VEE occurred in the late 1960s and early 1970s. Epidemic virus first reached Mexico in 1966 and eventually reached the United States in 1971. A study of this virus in Central America, Mexico, and the United States showed that the virus easily invaded territories in which it was formerly unknown.[276] This probably resulted from the availability of large numbers of susceptible equine hosts and the presence of competent mosquito vectors. Immunization of millions of horses throughout North America and unprecedented mosquito abatement efforts eventually stopped the epidemic before it was able to spread north of Texas.[277,278] Epidemic VEE virus has not been isolated in the United States since the 1971 outbreak.

An outbreak of the epidemic IC strain of VEE virus between April and October 1995 occurred in Colombia and Venezuela and involved 75,000 to 100,000 people.[254] Factors contributing to this outbreak included greater than normal rainfall resulting in large increases in vector populations, decreased surveillance for the virus, and accumulation of large numbers of susceptible horses as a result of reduction or elimination of vaccination programs. The epidemiology of disease in humans was typified by its sudden appearance, rapid increase, and brief occurrence in affected communities. In hospitals in Manaure and Riohacha in northern Colombia, admissions of cases consistent with VEE reached 330 per day. Interestingly, 90% of the cases were seen within 2 weeks in September and October.[279]

Incidence

While VEE virus has been quite active in recent years, the median number of cases of EEE and WEE during the same time period in the United States has been less than 5 each annually.[280] In the United States, EEE activity peaks between July and October in the northern part of its range and between May and August in the southern part. Human cases of EEE in Florida have occurred year-round.[281] Humans living in or near endemic foci for VEE have a high seroprevalence rate, often 100%, reflecting their cumulative experience with continuous transmission that occurs in these areas.[246] Epidemic transmission of VEE virus is sporadic, occurring only twice during the last 30 years. During both epidemics, thousands of individuals were involved, resulting in many deaths.[276]

VEE has been a problem in US service members deploying to endemic areas. On at least two occasions, soldiers undergoing jungle operations training in Fort Sherman, Panama, became ill with fever, chills, and headache.[243,244] On both occasions, infections occurred during the last quarter of the year, a time in Panama characterized by increased vector populations brought on by heavy rainfall. While Panama has been the source of all known VEE virus exposures in US soldiers, deployment to any VEE virus–endemic area within South or Central America presents significant risk to military personnel operating where active transmission is occurring.

Pathogenesis and Clinical Findings

Because outbreaks of viral equine encephalitis occur so infrequently and the majority of human cases occur in rural areas of developing countries, detailed studies on the pathogenesis of the viruses that cause these diseases in humans have not been completed. From the information that is available, experimentally infected animals serve as adequate models for pathogenesis of fatal encephalitis in humans. However, systemic disease is highly host specific and is dependent on a variety of other factors, including age, immune status, route of infection, and strain and dose of virus. The lymphoid and central nervous systems appear to be common targets in both experimental animal models and humans.[282–286] The Trinidad donkey (TrD) strain of VEE virus causes moderate but reversible lesions to the lymphoid organs in mice and nonhuman primates but causes marked destruction of those organs in guinea pigs and hamsters.[283,284]

Pathological changes to the central nervous system differ significantly depending on the animal models and the strains of virus tested. Inoculating mice with the TrD strain of VEE virus results in diffuse encephalomyelitis,[283,284] while monkeys develop only mild pathological changes to the thalamus, hypothalamus, and olfactory areas of the brain.[284] However, infection of monkeys by the aerosol route, a common route of accidental exposure in humans, can result in much more severe pathology, including perivascular cuffing and nodular and diffuse gliosis, especially in the cortex and hypothalamus.[287] Aerosol exposure of monkeys to a highly pathogenic strain of VEE virus resulted in significant mortality (35%) and development of severe clinical and pathological changes in all animals.[288] Observations on the severity of aerosol infection of nonhuman primates suggest that encephalitis in humans could be a more common occurrence when infection occurs by this route. Aerosol infection is most likely to occur in a laboratory setting, so technicians attempting to isolate and identify the virus are at greatest risk of aerosol infection.

Clinical disease in humans caused by the equine encephalitides falls into one of two general categories. A systemic febrile illness with occasional encephalitis is observed with viruses in the VEE complex, while a primarily encephalopathic syndrome is observed with EEE and WEE viruses. Disease caused by all three groups of viruses begins in a similar fashion. After a relatively short incubation period (1 to 6 days for VEE, 5 to 10 days for EEE, 5 to 15 days for WEE), patients present with chills, high fever, headache, and malaise. With VEE, these symptoms can be quite severe and may be accompanied by photophobia, sore throat, myalgias, and vomiting.[289] Although the majority of VEE infections are symptomatic, less than 1% of adult cases and 4% of childhood cases progress to encephalitis, and mortality rates are relatively low.[290] While no con-clusive clinical studies have been conducted, there are some laboratory data to suggest that congenital VEE may be an important cause of fetal malformations and spontaneous abortion in endemic areas.[291,292] EEE is the most severe of the equine encephalitides, having case fatality rates as high as 50% to 75%.[293,294]

As with the other equine encephalitides, the severity of neurological disease seen with WEE increases with decreasing age. Of children less than 1 year old with WEE, greater than 90% will exhibit focal or generalized seizures.[295] Neurological symptoms caused by all of the viruses may include lethargy, somnolence, or mild confusion with or with or without nuchal rigidity. More severe signs may include seizures, ataxia, paralysis, or coma.[296] With EEE, children frequently exhibit generalized facial or periorbital edema and disturbances of the autonomic nervous system, such as impaired respiratory regulation or excess salivation. Neurological sequelae, such as seizures, spastic paralysis, cranial neuropathies, and mental retardation, can occur in up to 30% of survivors.[294,297] Neurological sequelae from VEE and WEE virus infection can also occur, but their incidence and severity are generally less pronounced than from EEE. The clinical presentation of patients with one of the equine encephalitides does not provide sufficient information to make a specific diagnosis.

Diagnostic Approaches

Because of the large number of alphaviruses associated with disease throughout the world, selecting diagnostic methods should be based on a thorough understanding of the clinical features and epidemiology of these viruses.[298] Serum and other biosamples should be frozen at -70°C and immediately transported to theater-area diagnostic laboratories or medical laboratories in the United States for testing.

Epidemiologically significant diagnosis of the equine encephalitis viruses requires one or more of the following: (*a*) presence of virus-specific IgM in serum, (*b*) at least a 4-fold increase in virus-specific serological response between acute and convalescent serum samples, and (*c*) isolation and identification of the virus.

Serological tests for these viruses include hemagglutination inhibition, immunofluorescence, complement fixation, neutralization, or IgG or IgM enzyme-linked immunosorbent assay (ELISA). Of these tests, the IgM-capture ELISA is probably the most useful, as the presence of virus-specific IgM in a single serum sample can serve as an indicator of recent infection.[299,300] Identification of virus-specific IgM in the cerebrospinal fluid is an extremely useful method of serodiagnosis, because IgM antibodies do not cross the blood-brain barrier. IgM in cerebrospinal fluid, therefore, implies local antibody synthesis in response to infection of the central nervous system.[299] IgM antibodies to alphaviruses in humans appear to be subtype-specific, so variety typing of VEE or WEE virus infection would not be possible with this technique.[301] Diagnosis by other methods requires testing sequential sera from the same patient taken during different phases of disease. A 4-fold increase in antibody titer between acute and convalescent samples is considered diagnostic. Most serological assays for EEE and VEE viruses tend to be quite specific, but low-level cross-reactivity may be noted between WEE and SIN virus antigens.[298]

Isolation of virus is critical to permit differentiation of viral subtypes within the VEE virus complex. VEE, WEE, and EEE viruses can only be isolated from serum samples taken within the first several days of illness. However, virus may be isolated from throat swabs from individuals infected with VEE virus[302] even after viremias have fallen below detectable levels. Isolation of virus from throat swabs has been used successfully for the identification of VEE virus infections in troops stationed in Panama.[243,244] Isolations can be made in suckling mouse brains or in Vero cell cultures with about equal sensitivity. Isolates can be identified by using a variety of techniques but most commonly by cross-neutralization tests or immunofluorescence. Newer methods of virus identification, including polymerase chain reaction and real-time fluorogenic 5'-nucleases assays, show great promise and are now becoming available outside the research setting.

Recommendations for Therapy and Control

No specific therapy exists for treating the equine encephalitides. Therefore, treatment is aimed at managing specific symptoms. Antipyretics and analgesics will help to relieve the fever, headache, and myalgias. In encephalitic cases, anticonvulsants can be used to control seizures, and intravenous mannitol or corticosteroids may be used to control brain edema.

Control of the equine encephalitides is best accomplished through detailed knowledge of viral activity in deployment areas combined with judicious use of vaccination before deployment into endemic or epidemic areas. The US Army has extensive experience with a live-attenuated vaccine for VEE used as an investigational new drug product in humans; it produces moderate-to-strong virus-specific antibody responses in 80% of recipients. However, this vaccine (TC-83) is reactogenic, causing flu-like symptoms in approximately 20% of recipients. TC-83 should not be administered to pregnant women because of the possibility of teratogenic effects.[303,304] Long-term protection against only subtypes IA/B and IC can be expected. The magnitude or duration of a cross-protective response to heterologous subtypes is unknown.

Formalin-inactivated vaccines for human use exist for VEE, WEE, and EEE viruses. While the inactivated VEE vaccine has been shown to be a strong immunogen, it is currently being used only to boost TC-83 nonresponders. The WEE and EEE vaccines are weakly immunogenic and require multiple injections and regular boosters to develop and maintain protective antibody responses. Because of the problems associated with both the live and killed vaccines, it is doubtful that vaccination of rapidly deploying troops would be possible with any of the currently available vaccines. Like the TC-83 vaccine, these inactivated vaccines are only available as investigational products.

Environmental control of VEE, WEE, and EEE is a viable option under certain conditions. Interruption of secondary transmission cycles involving horses and other secondary vector species is likely to be the most efficient method of preventing or controlling epidemic spread of VEE virus. Because epidemic VEE is amplified by equines, vaccinating these animals with TC-83 has been used effectively to control outbreaks. Similar control of endemic VEE, WEE, and EEE is probably not possible because horses do not serve as major amplifying hosts for the viruses that cause these diseases. Widespread mosquito control through the use of insecticides, biological control, and source reduction is effective during epidemic episodes but is probably ineffective for the control of endemic viruses because of the difficulty in identifying restricted endemic foci. In the absence of vaccination or other environmental control procedures, educational programs that reduce mosquito biting rates and increase use of personal protective measures, such as use of insect repellents, bed nets, appropriate clothing, and window screens, are the most effective means of infection control.

Preventing the equine encephalitides will require prior knowledge of their presence in deployment areas coupled with personal protection and use of insect control measures. Currently available investigational vaccines can be used effectively if they are administered with sufficient time (1 to 2 weeks) for recipients to recover from sometimes deleterious reactions and for administration of booster immunizations when necessary. Vaccination of service members should be considered when they deploy to endemic or epidemic areas. If operational requirements dictate vaccination, the Director of the Research Area Directorate, Medical, Chemical, and

Biological Research Program (RAD 4), Fort Detrick, Maryland, may be contacted for information on how to obtain vaccine. A new, safer, and more effective genetically engineered vaccine for VEE is under development by the US Army and should be available in the future. This new vaccine will resolve many of the problems inherent with TC-83 and may be an effective tool for the control of VEE epidemics.

[George V. Ludwig]

TICK-BORNE ENCEPHALITIS

Introduction and Military Relevance

One of approximately 446 known arboviruses, tick-borne encephalitis (TBE) has a wide geographic distribution. At times, it has been a devastating and socially important epidemic and enzootic disease.[305] The involvement of US military forces in European and Asian regions that are endemic for TBE emphasizes the importance of understanding the disease-specific interactions of host, virus, and vector that result in disease or asymptomatic infection. US military personnel represent an immunologically naive population who may be required to perform in an endemic environment in a manner that maximizes their exposure to the tick vector. The combination of these factors produces the potential for a high rate of morbidity and mortality from TBE. A study[306] of US service members who trained extensively in areas of Central Europe endemic for TBE was conducted in 1985. Although clinical symptoms for TBE had not been recognized in this population, three individuals were seropositive for TBE, for a seroprevalence of 1.5% and an estimated infection rate of 0.9/1,000 person-months of exposure. It should be noted that the risk of TBE is geographically focal, even in areas that are considered endemic, and the rates of infection in this military population may not be widely generalizable.

TBE was not clinically recognized until 1927 when Schneider, in southern Austria, described patients with seasonal encephalitis, which he named "meningitis serosa epidemica." Zilber in 1937 further characterized this disease in eastern Siberia, isolated the virus (Russian spring-summer encephalitis virus, now called the Far Eastern subtype of TBE virus), and suggested that the vector for this virus was the tick *Ixodes persulcatus*. In 1954 the first case of TBE was described in Sweden, and TBE virus was isolated from *I ricinus* ticks (Central European encephalitis virus, now known as European or Western subtype TBE virus).[307] TBE is considered the most important arboviral disease in Central Europe. Cases of TBE have been reported from nu-

merous countries, including Sweden, Finland, Denmark, Norway, France, Greece, the Czech Republic, Slovakia, Hungary, Poland, Romania, Turkey, countries of the former Soviet Union and the former Yugoslavia, and the federal states of Saarland and Rhineland Paltinate in Germany.[308] Other names used for this disease include Central European encephalitis, Russian spring-summer encephalitis, Fruhsommer-meningoenzephalitis (FSME), diphasic meningoencephalitis, biundulant meningoencephalitis, diphasic milk fever, Schneider's disease, Kumlingesjukan, Roslagssjukan, and Ryssjukan.

Description of the Pathogen

TBE viruses are one group of approximately 70 members of the family *Flaviviridae*, genus *Flavivirus* (formerly group B arboviruses of the family *Togaviridae*).[309] Flaviviruses have a positive sense genomic RNA, which is single-stranded and approximately 11 kilobases in length.[310]

The TBE complex is composed of eight major viral subtypes: tick-borne encephalitis Far Eastern subtype, tick-borne encephalitis Western subtype, Kumlinge virus, louping ill virus, Omsk hemorrhagic fever virus, Kyasanur Forest disease virus, Langat virus, and Powassan virus[311–313] (Table 35-9). Studies using hemagglutination-inhibition tests with monoclonal antibodies to TBE virus revealed a close antigenic relationship among all subtypes of the TBE complex except for Powassan virus.[314] Based on hemagglutination-inhibition titers, there is a great deal of antigenic similarity among Far Eastern TBE virus, Western TBE virus, louping-ill virus, and Omsk hemorrhagic fever virus.

Epidemiology

Transmission

TBE infection depends on exposure to the tick vector or ingestion of the virus in contaminated milk or milk products. Peak morbidity occurs between the

TABLE 35-9

SUMMARY OF CLINICALLY IMPORTANT TICK-BORNE ENCEPHALITIS COMPLEX VIRUSES

Far Eastern Tick-borne Encephalitis

Also Known As:	Russian spring-summer encephalitis (RSSE), Taiga encephalitis, Far East Russian encephalitis
Principal Vector:	*Ixodes persulcatus* tick
Principal Hosts:	Small mammals (eg, rodents, squirrels), large vertebrates (eg, deer, elk, domestic animals); bird infection has also been demonstrated
Geographic Distribution:	Far eastern Russia (former USSR provinces of Primorie, Khabarovsk, Krasnojarsk, Altai, Tomsk, Omsk, Kemerovo, Ural, Priural, and western Siberia)
Seasonal Transmission:	May to August
Incubation Period in Humans:	10 to 14 d
Severity of Disease:	Severe
Major Clinical Manifestations:	Fever, headache, nausea, meningeal irritation with aseptic meningitis; flaccid lower motor neuron paralysis of upper extremities and bulbar centers; may be indistinguishable from poliomyeltis
Case Fatality Rate:	8%–54%
Vaccine Available:	Yes

Western Tick-borne Encephalitis

Also Known As:	TBE, Central European TBE (CEE), Czechoslovak TBE, diphasic milk fever, biphasic meningoencephalitis
Principal Vector:	*Ixodes ricinus* tick
Principal Hosts:	Small mammals (eg, rodents), large vertebrates; unique is infection of and transmission of virus in the milk of goats, sheep, and cows
Geographic Distribution:	Czech Republic, Slovakia, Austria, Bulgaria, Romania, former Yugoslavia, Hungary, former USSR, Finland, France, Germany, Greece, Italy, Sweden, Switzerland
Seasonal Transmission:	Spring, summer, autumn
Incubation Period in Humans:	7 to 14 d
Severity of Disease:	Moderate
Major Clinical Manifestations:	A monophasic or biphasic illness characterized by fever, headache, nausea, anorexia, with the development of aseptic meningitis, encephalitis, or encephalomyelitis; remission can occur 4 to 5 d into illness but is followed by neurologic involvement (2nd phase); long-term neurologic complications are infrequent
Case Fatality Rate:	1%–5%
Vaccine Available:	Yes

Powassan Encephalitis

Also Known As:	POW
Principal Vector:	*I marxi, I cookei, I spinipalpus, Dermacentor andersoni* ticks
Principal Hosts:	Squirrels, porcupines, groundhogs
Geographic Distribution:	North America, Russia, Asia
Seasonal Transmission:	Spring, summer
Incubation Period in Humans:	1 or more wks
Major Clinical Manifestations:	Fever, headache, sore throat, somnolence, encephalitis; long-term neurologic complications can occur, including hemiplegia
Severity of Disease:	Severe
Case Fatality Rate:	10.5%
Vaccine Available :	No

Louping Ill

Also Known As:	——
Principal Vector:	*I ricinus* tick
Principal Hosts:	Small mammals, cattle, pigs, deer, sheep
Geographic Distribution:	England, Scotland, Wales
Seasonal Transmission:	Spring, summer
Incubation Period:	1 or more wks
Severity of Disease:	Mild
Major Clinical Manifestations:	Fever, lymphadenopathy, flu-like illness with development of mild meningoencephalitis without neurologic complications
Case Fatality Rate:	Minimal
Vaccine Available:	Yes

Kyasanur Forest Disease

Also Known As:	——
Principal Vector:	*Haemaphysalis spinigera* tick
Principal Hosts:	Small vertebrates
Geographic Distribution:	Karanataka State, India
Seasonal Transmission:	Dry season (January-April)
Incubation Period in Humans:	1 or more wks
Major Clinical Manifestations:	Fever, headache, pulmonary infiltrates, gastrointestinal hemorrhage; biphasic illness may occur with the development of meningoencephalitis
Severity of Disease:	Severe
Case Fatality Rate:	10.5%
Vaccine Available:	No

Omsk Hemorrhagic Fever

Also Known As:	——
Principal Vector:	*D reticulatus, D marginatus,* and Ixodid ticks
Principal Hosts:	Wild muskrats
Geographic Distribution:	North America, Russia, Asia
Seasonal Transmission:	Spring, summer, autumn
Incubation Period in Humans:	3 to 7 d
Major Clinical Manifestations:	Headache, biphasic fever, hemorrhage of the nose and gastrointestinal tract, pneumonia, rash
Severity of Disease:	Moderate
Case Fatality Rate:	0.5%-3%
Vaccine Available :	Yes

Adapted from: Gresíková M, Calisher CH. Tick-borne encephalitis. In: Monath TP, ed. *The Arboviruses: Epidemiology and Ecology.* Vol 4. Boca Raton, Fla: CRC Press; 1989: 177–198.

ages of 15 and 40 years, with females at equal risk to males in populations where tick exposure is not sex biased. People living in rural areas are at higher risk. The most frequently infected individuals are forest workers, farmers, and vacationers traveling into endemic areas. Western subtype TBE can be acquired orally by consuming contaminated milk and milk products. Transmission via the milk of cows, sheep, and goats has been responsible for several outbreaks of this disease. Infection by the oral route presents as a milder form of illness than does infection by ticks.

The principal vector of Far Eastern TBE and Western

TBE are the ticks *I persulcatus* and *I ricinus*, respectively. Seasonal *I persulcatus* activity in far eastern Russia begins at the end of April and lasts until June. Tick infection rates with TBE have ranged from 3.4% to 9.4%.[315] Activity of *I ricinus* in Europe has two peak seasons, April through May and September through October. In certain geographic areas, peak tick activity may occur in June and August, with less activity in July. TBE infection in these ticks ranges from 0.07% to 6%.[316] Western TBE virus has been isolated from other ticks, including *I trianguliceps, I arboricola, Haemaphysalis inermis, H punctata,* and *Dermacentor marginatus.*[312] The life span of these ticks is approximately 3 years. Their principal hosts are small mammals, such as hedgehogs, shrews, and moles.[317] The high level of viremia achieved in these animals after infection maintains an ideal TBE virus reservoir. Large vertebrates, such as domesticated animals and humans, are incidental hosts and contribute little toward maintaining the virus in the environment.

A noninfected tick becomes infected with TBE virus after taking an infected blood meal (Figure 35-15). One to twenty-five days after infection, virus can be found in the gut, salivary glands, and ovaries of the tick.[318] Laboratory studies document prolonged viral persistence up to 9 months after infection. Virus is amplified in the tick population by transovarial transmission, by sexual transmission from infected male ticks to females, and by cofeeding of an uninfected tick with an infected tick on a nonviremic host.[319–321] Transstadial transmission (eg, nymph to larva, larva to adult tick) also occurs. The virus is transmitted to the vertebrate host by infected saliva; the efficiency of viral transmission depends on the length of feeding. Adults are more effective transmitters than nymphs and larvae. Feeding of infected ticks on birds, though documented, is of unknown epidemiologic significance. Under laboratory conditions, bats can be infected with TBE virus and maintain viremia for long periods.[312]

Western TBE virus can be isolated in the milk of infected goats, sheep, and cows 1 to 7 days after acute infection and transmitted to humans by the ingestion of raw infected milk or cheese.[322–326] This virus has been shown to be infectious in milk, as well as sour milk and cheese, for as long as 2 weeks at 4°C and in butter for 60 days at 4°C.[312]

Geographic Distribution

I persulcatus is the principal vector for Far Eastern subtype TBE and occurs in the far eastern part of

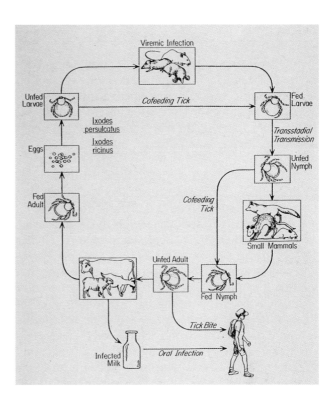

Fig. 35-15. The transmission cycle of tick-borne encephalitis showing the tick larvae becoming infected by feeding on a viremic host or by cofeeding with an infected larvae tick. Virus infection can occur throughout the life cycle of the tick by feeding on an infected host or by vertical transmission to its progeny. Infection and subsequent viremia of larger vertebrates perpetuate the transmission of virus to nymph and adult tick stages and eventually back to the host reservoir. As demonstrated, humans are dead-end hosts and do not contribute to the transmission cycle of TBE and become infected by the bite from an unfed infected adult tick or by drinking infected milk.
Reprinted with permission from: Fields BN, Knipe DM, Howley PM, eds. *Fields Virology.* 3rd ed. Philadelphia: Lippincott-Raven; 1996: 994.

Russia. The distribution of Western subtype TBE correlates to that of its principle tick vector, *I ricinus;* the disease occurs throughout the European part of Russia, Scandinavia, France, Germany, Poland, Austria, Switzerland, Italy, Romania, Hungary, Bulgaria, the Czech Republic, Slovakia, and the countries of the former Yugoslavia.[327] The most frequent occurrence of TBE and its tick vector is associated with humid, marshy, densely wooded areas.

Ixodes tick activity is greatest at an average temperature of 8°C to 11°C and an annual average rainfall of 800 mm.[316]

Incidence

Incidence rates of TBE are dependent on the degree of endemicity of the specific country, as well as geographic and meteorological conditions that affect the tick vector. The highest incidence of TBE is reported to be of the Far Eastern subtype from western Siberia, at an annual incidence of 11.7/100,000. The Ural mountain area has an incidence of 6.6/100,000.[311] An epidemiologic study of TBE performed in the Tribec region of Czechoslovakia (a highly endemic area for TBE) during the years 1953 to 1963 described an 11-year mean incidence of 19.3/100,000 and a peak incidence of 107.9/100,000 during 1955.[328] The highest age-specific incidence occurred in the 10- to 14-year-old age group, with an incidence of 33.2/100,000. Adult farmer and forestry workers were the occupational group at highest risk, with a rate of 21.3/100,000. TBE in this region coincided with the activity of the tick vector, which started in April and peaked during June. Incidence rates declined after June, with no cases seen after September. Of 67 patients infected with TBE during 1960 to 1963, 55.3% reported tick bite exposure only, 8.9% goat milk consumption only, and 22.3% both tick bite exposure and goat milk consumption; 13.5% had an unknown exposure. In 1,037 acute neurological cases observed in Hungary from 1963 to 1965, TBE was serologicaly confirmed in 23% of patients with encephalitis and 10% of patients with aseptic meningitis.[329] Germany, Switzerland, and Yugoslavia reported between 10 and 140 cases per year during the 1980s. Sweden experiences between 50 and 80 cases per year, with cases restricted to the archipelagoes and the coastal areas of the Baltic Sea. Austria experienced 400 to 700 cases per year in the 1980s, which declined to 81 cases per year after an active TBE campaign that vaccinated more than 5 million inhabitants.[307]

Serological surveys suggest that about 50% of TBE infections are subclinical. In endemic areas, seropositivity has been noted to reach 50% to 63% in individuals older than 55 years of age.[312] In a serosurvey conducted in Sweden,[307] clinical disease was estimated to have occurred in 6% against a background seroprevalence of 22%. In subpopulations with no clinically apparent TBE, the seroprevalence rate ranged between 4% and 12%.

Pathogenesis and Clinical Findings

The pathogenesis of this disease and reasons for asymptomatic versus severe disease are not known.

Far Eastern TBE

The Far Eastern subtype of TBE is the more severe clinical form of TBE, which manifests itself with the sudden onset of high fever, severe headache, nausea, vomiting, and photophobia after a 10- to 14-day incubation period.[312] An aseptic meningitis develops, which is manifested by nuchal rigidity and which progresses to changes in mentation and sensorium; this heralds the onset of encephalitis. Long-term neurologic sequelae can occur, such as hemiparesis, hemiplegia, and chronic progressive encephalitis, which may have an onset more than 10 years after primary infection.[330] Other complications of Far Eastern TBE infection include lower motor neuron paralysis, beginning with the upper extremities and progressing to the neck muscles and bulbar centers. Far Eastern TBE can present as a highly fatal (case-fatality rate of 29.2%) poliomyelitis type illness in 20% of cases.[331] Long-term residual complications of this form of TBE are spastic paresis of the lower extremities, epilepsy, and chronic encephalitis.

Western TBE

The Western subtype of TBE is the milder form of TBE and has a relatively low case-fatality rate of 1% to 5%.[312] The incubation period is usually 7 to 14 days, though it may be as long as 28 days. Initial symptoms include headache, nausea, vomiting, anorexia, hyperesthesia, photophobia, and fever. The illness can also be biphasic. The first phase of illness lasts 4 to 6 days, followed by a variable period without symptoms. The second phase, which affects about 35% of cases, begins with spread of the virus to the central nervous system, manifested by a return of fever and the development of aseptic meningitis.[307] Long-term neurologic sequelae are uncommon, but complications of monoplegia and sensorineural deafness have been described.[332]

Powassan Encephalitis

Powassan encephalitis was first clinically described and the virus (POW virus) isolated from the brain of a child from Powassan, northern Ontario, who died of encephalitis in September 1958. Subsequent studies revealed that the virus was a member of the tick-borne flaviviruses closely related to TBE virus. POW virus has been isolated from four species of North American ticks: *I cookei, I marxi, I spiniplapus,* and *D andersoni.*[333] POW virus has also been isolated in Russia from the following ticks: *H neumanii, I persulcatus,* and *D silvarum.* It is found in variety of small, wild vertebrates and in domesticated animals, such as dogs, cats, horses, cattle, and goats. POW virus has also been isolated in several species of birds in Russia and North America. The geographic distribution of POW virus is widespread in North America, with virus having been isolated in animals from Ontario, California, Colorado, Connecticut, Massachusetts, New York, South Dakota, and West Virginia. POW virus has also been demonstrated in Russia, China, and parts of Southeast Asia.[334]

Humans are incidental hosts for the infected ticks, and after an incubation period of 1 or more weeks, the clinical symptoms of fever, sore throat, headache, somnolence, disorientation, and nuchal rigidity occur.[334] Encephalitis, meningoencephalitis, or aseptic meningitis develop, with a case-fatality rate of 10.5%. There may be long-term residual neurologic deficits, including hemiplegia, muscle atrophy, and spasticity. The incidence of Powassan encephalitis is extremely low in North America; there have been 19 confirmed infections and no cases since 1981.[333] Patients vaccinated with TBE virus vaccine had low-titered cross-reactivity to POW virus at a level insufficient for protection.

Louping Ill

Louping ill virus is part of the TBE complex and is primarily a disease of sheep in Great Britain.[335] Infection can also occur in cattle, pigs, and deer. The virus is transmitted by the bite of the tick *I ricinus.*[318] Infection in humans can occur by the bite of infected ticks or by contact with infected tissues of diseased animals. Butchers and veterinarians are at highest risk for acquiring infection. Human disease presents with fever, lymphadenopathy, and flu-like symptoms. A mild meningoencephalitis can occur, but neurologic complications are rare.[334] The case-fatality rate is extremely low. A formalin-inactivated vaccine is available for animals and humans who are at high risk of exposure.

Omsk Hemorrhagic Fever

Omsk hemorrhagic fever is a subtype of the TBE complex described in the Omsk province of the former Soviet Union. The spring–summer pattern of disease depends on the activity of this virus's tick vectors, *D reticulatus* and *D marginatus.*[84] Ixodes ticks are also vectors. There is an incubation period of 3 to 7 days, followed by the onset of headache and a biphasic

fever. Gastrointestinal bleeding and hemorrhage, bronchopneumonia, and rash can occur. Case-fatality rates are 0.5% to 3%. A vaccine for Omsk hemorrhagic fever is available in Russia.

Kyasanur Forest Disease

Kyasanur Forest disease (KFD) virus is a subtype within the TBE complex first described in 1957 in Karnataka State, India.[84] There are approximately 400 to 500 cases per year there. The highest incidence occurred in 1983: 1,555 cases and 150 deaths, producing a case-fatality rate ranging from 5% to 10%.[336] KFD virus and disease are found in the towns of Saga and Sorab in Shimoga District, Karnataka State, India. Serological surveys of this district demonstrated neutralizing antibody to KFD in 2 of 287 individuals tested. Antibodies to KFD have been detected in animals and humans from the semiarid areas of Saurashtra and Kutch, India, which are 700 miles from the KFD focus.[337] The tick vector is *H spinigera.* The virus is maintained in small vertebrates; humans and primates are incidental hosts. Clinical disease in humans is manifested by fever, headache, and severe myalgias, but gastrointestinal hemorrhage and pulmonary involvement can also occur. A biphasic course of illness can be seen with an initial prodromal phase, followed by a 1- to 2-week period of remission, followed by clinical illness. Meningoencephalitis can occur with no long-term residual effects.

Diagnostic Approaches

The differential diagnosis of early TBE is broad and includes a number of etiologies for acute meningitis and early encephalitis, to include *Streptococcus pneumonia, Neisseria meningitidis, Listeria monocytogenes,* herpes simplex 1 and 2, enteroviruses, and adenovirus. As the disease progresses and becomes consistent with a viral encephalitis by clinical and laboratory findings, the differential of potential etiologies narrows but continues to include viral pathogens such as the ones that cause polio, mumps, St. Louis encephalitis, Western equine encephalitis, Venezuelan equine encephalitis, and lymphocytic choriomeningitis and the human immunodeficiency virus. Essential to making an accurate and expedient diagnosis is an awareness of local disease threats and epidemiology, a history of tick bite or exposure or ingestion of unpasteurized milk products, and laboratory support that can test for TBE.

Viral isolation and identification is the gold standard for diagnosis. TBE virus can be isolated in serum during the viremic phase of illness. All specimens should be stored at -70°C. Virus can also be isolated by intracranial inoculation of infected serum or tissue into suckling mice or plaque assay in Vero cells.[84,312] Chick embryo cell cultures may also be used. Viral isolation in ticks can be accomplished by suspending 5 to 10 adult ticks in 1 mL of Eagle's medium with 10% heat-inactivated bovine serum.

Serologic diagnosis is by virus neutralization (the most specific method), complement fixation, hemagglutination inhibition, EIA, or indirect hemagglutination.[84,312] IgM antibody capture EIA of serum is the test of choice for acute infection.[338] A high IgM titer or a 4-fold increase in serum IgG as measured by complement fixation or hemagglutination inhibition between acute and convalescent serum provides convincing evidence for TBE infection. Rapid identification of TBE virus by the fluorescent antibody technique and an enzyme-linked immunosorbent assay have also been described.[339,340] Antibody-based assays can give false-positive results due to the cross-reactivity of TBE with flaviviruses in general and with other flaviviruses within the TBE complex in particular. Individuals previously vaccinated against yellow fever or Japanese encephalitis may also cross-react. Reverse transcription polymerase chain reaction has been developed for the rapid detection of TBE viruses and offers the opportunity for rapid diagnosis with a high degree of sensitivity and specificity in the field.[341]

Recommendations for Therapy and Control

Treatment of TBE infection is supportive, with emphasis on protecting the airway and providing ventilatory support if needed. There is no literature for or against the use of steroids. As with other viral infections, the use of salicylates may be contraindicated in the pediatric population because of the risk of Reye's syndrome. A TBE immune globulin is available in Austria and Germany for passive immunization and preexposure and postexposure prophylaxis of TBE (FSME-Bulin, Baxter Immuno AG, Austria). This is a hyperimmunoglobulin concentrate containing TBE-specific immunoglobulin at a titer of 1:640 as measured by hemagglutination inhibition. It is reported to be 60% to 70% effective when given within 96 hours of exposure; protection is manifest within 24 hours of administration and for 4 weeks thereafter. Four days after exposure, the prophylactic efficacy of TBE immune globulin diminishes, and clinical disease may actu-

ally be exacerbated by its administration.[342] TBE immune globulin should not be administered for 28 days (the maximal TBE incubation period) after the window of potential benefit.

Vaccine

The Far Eastern TBE virus was isolated in 1937 and developed by Zilber into an inactivated mouse brain–derived vaccine used to vaccinate Russian troops. In 1950, a vaccine against the western strain of TBE was developed by Danes and Benda in Czechoslovakia and found to be highly effective in human volunteers, causing few hypersensitivity reactions.[343] TBE was further modified into a highly purified, killed vaccine with few side effects, which resulted in the licensure of an Austrian TBE vaccine named FSME-Immun. Other inactivated whole virus TBE vaccines that are commercially available or are in development are the TicoVAC vaccine (Baxter AG, Vienna, Austria), Enceput (Behringwerke AG, Marburg, Germany), and the Cultural Purified Concentrated Inactivated Freeze-dried Tick-borne Encephalitis Vaccine (Institute of Poliomyelitis and Viral Encephalitides, Moscow, Russia).[344–346]

Trials with FSME-Immun demonstrated antibody production in 93% of vaccine recipients after two vaccinations and 100% after the third dose. Pyrexia occurred in 4% to 10% of recipients, local pain in 23% to 58%, malaise in 19% to 33%, and headache in 14% to 33%.[347] Neutralizing antibodies were achieved after a three-dose schedule in all volunteers; cross-neutralizing antibodies were present for both Far Eastern and Western TBE isolates from 12 geographic regions and for louping ill virus.[348] A multinational phase II study with this vaccine using two dose schedules (an abbreviated schedule with 0.5 mL given intramuscularly [IM] on days 0, 7, and 21 or the conventional schedule on days 0, 28, and 300) showed both to be equally immunogenic.[349] Active TBE immunization in nonimmune volunteers demonstrated an IgG antibody response comparable to that seen after natural infection.[350] Intradermal administration of FSME Immun demonstrated quicker seroconversion and higher antibody levels than achieved by intramuscular injection.[351,352] Serious side effects from FSME Immun are rare. Only 15 cases of mild meningoencephalitis and 1 case of myelitis have been reported.[353]

Side effects with Encepur have been reported and include asthenia, back pain, chills, flu syndrome, fever, lymphadenopathy, arthralgia, headache, and pain at the injection site.[354] Fever following vaccination with this vaccine was a frequent finding though adverse events were less frequently observed following the second dose of vaccination.[355] Adverse reactions have also been observed with the TicoVac vaccine, especially with high fevers in very young children who received the vaccine.[356] This resulted in the recommendation by Germany's Federal Agency for Sera and Vaccinations that this vaccine not be used in children under 3 years of age.

Countries that experience high rates of TBE have pursued widespread immunization campaigns using TBE vaccine.[307] Currently, no TBE vaccine is licensed by the US Food and Drug Administration (FDA). FSME-Immun is available as an investigational new drug with the FDA under a protocol filed by the US Army Medical Research and Materiel Command. Under this protocol, vaccine is available to US military personnel going to TBE-endemic areas and considered to be at high-risk for infection.[357]

The current recommended vaccination schedule of FSME-Immun consists of a 0.5 mL intramuscular (IM) dose at days 0 and 28 and at 1 year. One 0.5 mL dose contains 2 µg of viral antigen, 1 mg of $Al(OH)_3$, less than 0.6 mg of human albumin, less than 0.005 mg of formaldehyde, and less than 0.05 mg of the preservative merthiolate. An abbreviated schedule of 0.5 mL IM at days 0, 7, and 21 may be used with equal efficacy.[342] An accelerated schedule was used in US military deployed in Bosnia using a three-dose schedule delivered at 0, 7, and 28 days with an 80% seroconversion rate.[357] Few side effects were noted with this dosing schedule with a 0.18% rate of self-limited symptoms. Intradermal administration has been demonstrated to be more effective than intramuscular dosing.[351,352] A booster dose of the IM vaccine is recommended every 3 years.[312]

Current contraindications for the administration of TBE vaccine include having an acute febrile illness or having a history of allergies to any of the vaccine components, including egg albumin. A merthiolate-free vaccine is available for patients allergic to this chemical. The vaccine is safe for pregnant and lactating women.

Personal Protection

Personal protection is the mainstay to prevent TBE infection. Insect repellent with DEET (N,N-diethylmeta-toluamide), permethrin-impregnated clothing, long shirts worn with cuffs buttoned, pants worn tucked into boots, and daily tick surveys are all effective measures. Avoidance of unpasteurized milk and milk products is also recommended. Tick control by insecticide spraying of local endemic areas has also been effective in eradicating the tick and the virus.

Preparation of safe milk products requires 30 minutes or more of pasteurization at 65°C, pasteurization at 80°C for 1 minute, or boiling for longer than 1 minute.

[Timothy P. Endy]

SANDFLY FEVER

Introduction and Military Relevance

Sandfly fever is a self-limited, febrile, viral illness transmitted by biting flies of the genus *Phlebotomus*.[358] It occurs in Africa, Europe, and Asia with seasonal incidence peaking between April and October.[359] The military significance of sandfly fever is magnified because its short incubation period makes it capable of rendering large numbers of nonimmune service members ineffective during an operation while the native populace remains largely immune and unaffected.[360,361] Sandfly fever has attacked nonimmune troops in epidemic proportions when they are stationed in an area where the virus is endemic.

Accounts by British military surgeons during the 19th century of epidemic febrile illness among British troops stationed in various locales around the Mediterranean Sea have been cited as accurate clinical descriptions of sandfly fever.[362-364] In 1905, Taussig[365] provided epidemiologic evidence to support the popularly held belief that the midges known as pappataci flies (*Phlebotomus papatasi*) were connected with the 3-day fever that afflicted Austrian troops every summer by the Adriatic Sea. The disease was commonly called pappataci or phlebotomus fever.

In 1909, the etiologic agent of sandfly fever was identified in the classic investigations by the Austrian military commission of Doerr, Franz, and Taussig.[366] These investigators reproduced the disease in humans by inoculating volunteers living in areas free from the disease with blood obtained from patients on the first day of fever. The Austrian commission also established that the infectious agent was filterable and that *P papatasi* was the vector of the illness.

Description of the Pathogen

The agent, Sandfly fever virus, belongs to the family *Bunyaviridae*, genus *Phlebovirus*.[367] Like other viruses in *Bunyaviridae*, Sandfly fever virus possesses negative-sense, single-stranded RNA segments designated as small (S), medium (M), and large (L). It has three major structural proteins: two surface glycoproteins encoded by the M segment that project from the virion's lipid bilayer envelope and a nucleocapsid protein encoded by the S segment.

Sandfly fever virus is recovered most easily in Vero cells, where it demonstrates both cytopathic effect and plaques under agar. Field isolates of Sandfly fever virus have demonstrated poor infectivity in various laboratory animals in previous studies. These studies have failed to demonstrate pathogenicity of the virus for mice, hamsters, rats, rabbits, guinea pigs, or monkeys.[367–370] Although intracerebral injection of Sandfly fever virus is lethal to suckling mice, similar effects in adult mice can be demonstrated only after serial passage and adaptation to mouse brain.

Seminal investigations by Sabin in the 1940s demonstrated that two virus isolates, from Sicily and Naples, were antigenically distinct. Cross-protection experiments[371] demonstrated that immunity is strain-specific (Naples *vs.* Sicilian) and that a single infection gives solid protection against the same antigenic type. That is to say, patients are immune to subsequent intravenous challenge with homologous wild-type Sandfly fever virus. Sabin's challenge experiments also demonstrated the duration of immunity to be at least 9 years. A seroprevalence study[372] demonstrating the longevity of neutralizing antibody following natural infection with a given strain suggests that immunity is probably lifelong.

There are more than 20 viral isolates from phlebotomine flies in both the Eastern and Western hemispheres that are antigenically related to Sandfly fever virus and that cause infrequent cases of human disease.[373–375] Toscana virus represents a *Phlebovirus* strain that is distinct from, albeit related to, Naples serotype[376] and that has been reported as a cause of aseptic meningitis in Portugal,[377,378] Cyprus,[379] and the Tuscany and Marche regions of Italy.[380] Sandfly fever virus Sicilian and Naples, however, are the two most important strains epidemiologically, both having caused recurrent epidemics among military populations.

Epidemiology

Transmission

The deployment of military service members to a foreign country entails their intimate contact with its natural environment, which may include sand flies. The destruction of property and breakdown in public health measures that inevitably accompany warfare are important epidemiologically, as has been shown by the frequent clustering of sandfly fever cases around areas of rubble and debris—good breeding habitats for *Phlebotomus* species.

The sand fly seeks a blood meal in the early evening and is small enough to penetrate mosquito netting. The extrinsic incubation period in the vector is approximately 7 to 10 days. Although the fly will take a blood meal from a variety of species (eg, humans, cattle, canines, equines, birds),[381] the virus and its vector may also persist via autogeny (the ability to lay eggs in the absence of a blood meal). Despite demonstration of infection by Sandfly fever group viruses in some animals,[373] a vertebrate reservoir has yet to be demonstrated. Serosurveys have suggested that small mammals may have antibody to certain viral strains, but the significance of this finding to the maintenance of the disease is uncertain.[382] During epidemics, humans may also serve as viremic vertebrate hosts in a human-*Phlebotomus*-human cycle. The virus is vertically, or transovarially, transmitted in sand flies,[383–385] a phenomenon that is important to the maintenance of endemic disease, but decline of virus infection rates in successive generations suggests that these agents may not be maintained indefinitely in the insect vector by this mechanism.[386]

Sandfly fever occurrence is distinctly seasonal, with the highest incidence occurring during the late spring and summer months, depending on the prevailing temperatures and timing of the rainy season.[387] This distinct seasonality probably accounts for the lack of reported cases during the Persian Gulf War in northern Saudi Arabia and southern Iraq. The virus can overwinter either via transovarial transmission[388] or diapause in the fourth larval stage.[389]

Geographic Distribution

Sandfly fever has a wide geographic distribution in those parts of Europe, Africa, and Asia between 20° and 45° North latitude, reflecting the range of *P papatasi*.[359,390] This vector breeds in dry, sandy areas near rubble or debris and in the nooks and ceiling corners of buildings. The disease persists mainly in the lower altitudes of subtropical and tropical countries in which there are long periods of hot, dry weather.

Studies[373,391–393] have discovered other phlebo-viruses that are serologically related to Naples and Sicilian types and are broadly distributed in Eurasia and the Americas. These viruses have been recovered from phlebotomine flies of the genus *Lutzomyia,* as well as from mosquitoes. Several of these phleboviruses (eg, Chagres, Alenquer, Candiru, Punta Toro viruses) may cause a nonspecific febrile illness in humans similar to sandfly fever.[394–396]

Incidence

The recurrent problem with phlebotomus fever in the earlier half of this century prompted study by several British military commissions.[397] During World War II, there were 19,000 cases of sandfly fever, with the highest incidence reported in the Middle East theater. Attack rates were 3% to 10% of all troops, although in some units the attack rate was greater than 50%. During the Sicily campaign in the summer of 1943, the 7th US Army sustained approximately 8,500 cases of sandfly fever, constituting more than half of the medical battalion's workload once the number of casualties dropped off after the first 10 days of the invasion. In the Persian Gulf Command, the attack rates were 50% higher than those in the Middle East as a whole and reached a peak of 235 cases per 1,000 men in August 1942. These epidemics instigated a US Army investigation in 1943 and 1944 led by Major Albert Sabin.[370]

The disease can also be a problem for hospital personnel, as was illustrated by four hospital-centered outbreaks in the Middle East during World War II.[360,387] In these epidemics, 25% of all doctors and nurses and nearly 100% of other hospital personnel were affected. Twenty percent of the nearly 2,000 patients admitted with other diagnoses contracted sandfly fever while in the hospital.

Outbreaks in the 1980s in United Nations troops in Cyprus[398] and Russian soldiers in Afghanistan[360,399] demonstrate sandfly fever's continued potential for significant morbidity. The fact that both Sicilian and Naples strains are distributed widely in the Middle East, which has been a focal point of American economic and political policy for the past quarter century, reemphasizes this disease's military relevance.

Pathogenesis and Clinical Findings

The clinical manifestations of sandfly fever were extensively documented by Sabin in the 1940s.[369] In the course of experimentally inducing more than 100 cases of sandfly fever, Sabin and his coworkers demonstrated the clinical illness as well defined and self-limited (hence the name "3-day fever"), hav-

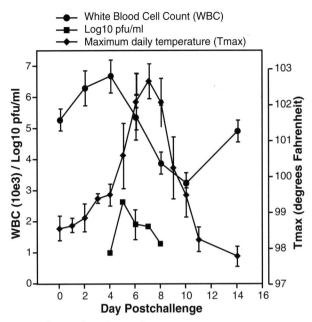

PFU: Plaque-forming units

Fig. 35-16. The temporal correlation of fever (degrees Fahrenheit), neutropenia (granulocytes x 10^3 cells/mm^3), and viremia (PFU/ml) in a typical course of sandfly fever.

ing a very predictable clinical course, and with no mortality or sequelae.[370] Indeed, the relatively uniform nature of the classic febrile syndrome of sandfly fever has made it a model in the study of viral and febrile illnesses.[400] After an incubation period of 2 to 6 days, a fever of 39°C (102°F) or higher develops in two thirds of patients (Figure 35-16). The duration of fever is from 1 to 4 days in 85% of patients and is accompanied by a frontal or retroorbital headache, malaise, myalgias, anorexia, lymphopenia, and viremia. In addition, many will also have low back pain, photophobia, and nausea. A smaller percentage may suffer from arthralgias, odynophagia, or vomiting. Infrequently, a patient may experience abdominal pain lasting 1 to 2 days. On physical examination, persons with sandfly fever appear flushed and often have conjunctival injection (Figure 35-17).

The most distinctive laboratory feature of sandfly fever is leukopenia, which occurs in approximately 90% of patients.[400,401] Characteristically, on the first day of fever there is a normal total white blood cell (WBC) count with an absolute lymphopenia (400-900 cells per milliliter) and a corresponding increase in neutrophils, including immature forms. Within 2 to 3 days of resolution of the fever, a leukopenia averaging 3,000 WBC per milliliter (range 2.5–3.5 x 10^3 WBC per milliliter) develops as neutrophils diminish and lymphocytes

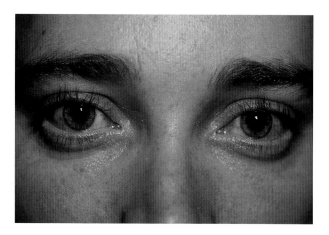

Fig. 35-17. Although neither specific nor universal for sandfly fever, this patient's conjunctival injection illustrates why the disease earned the appellation "Hundskrankeit" (hound fever) when first characterized by Taussig.* This stage of the illness renders the patient bedridden for 2 to 4 days and is accompanied by moderately severe fever, chills, headache, myalgias, and malaise.
Photograph: Courtesy of Dr. David McClain.
*Taussig S. Die Hundskrankheit, endemischer Magankatarrh in der Herzegowina. *Wien Klin Wchnschr.* 1905;18:129–136,163–169.

increase their relative percentages in the differential WBC count. Slight decrements in patients' platelet counts, as well as mild elevations of the liver transaminases and alkaline phosphatase, may also occur during the febrile period and rapidly return to normal after cessation of fever.

Toscana virus has been clearly implicated in summer cases of aseptic meningitis, although it also causes subclinical or asymptomatic infections.[402,403] Both the clinical and cerebrospinal fluid findings in these meningitis cases were those of a viral syndrome with aseptic meningitis, with no specific features to distinguish them from enteroviral or other viral etiologies. Assertions that other serotypes of the Sandfly fever virus group may cause meningitic inflammation remain unproven.[404]

Diagnostic Approaches

Given the relatively nonspecific nature of the clinical illness, sandfly fever must be suspected when patients in an endemic area have a short-lived

(2 to 4 days) viral syndrome with prominent fever, malaise, and headache. Epidemic illness among expatriates that spares most of the native populace is especially suggestive. Viremia is relatively low titer (1-3 $\log_{10}$ plaque-forming units) and runs concurrently with the fever; it is within the sensitivity of classic viral isolation procedures or polymerase chain reaction but not detectable by antigen-capture enzyme-linked immunosorbent assay (ELISA). Serologic diagnosis may be made by detecting a 4-fold rise in neutralization or ELISA titers between acute and convalescent sera or by the demonstration of IgM antibody acutely. Both ELISA and neutralizing antibodies appear within 2 weeks after acute infection.[368]

Recommendations for Therapy and Control

Palliation for the clinical symptoms of sandfly fever may be achieved with antipyretics and analgesics. Despite its in vitro activity against the virus, oral ribavirin failed to prevent the disease (McClain DJ, Summers PL, Byrne R, Huggins JW, unpublished data, 1997).

The most useful countermeasure against sandfly fever at present remains vector control of *Phlebotomus* species. Pesticides were effectively used in Italy after World War II to control the transmission of the virus.[372] The larvae develop in shaded microhabitats that contain their requirements for darkness, humidity, and organic matter.[405] Therefore, pesticide control should target areas such as stables, poultry houses, animal burrows, and crevices in rock and masonry. For example, the spraying of animal burrows and termite mounds with cyfluthrin will provide short-term area control of adult sand flies.[406] The flight range of sand flies is limited to a few hundred meters from their breeding and resting sites, often resulting in a rather focal distribution.[407] Notably, the mesh in mosquito netting is too big to exclude sand flies. Using permethrin-treated screens is only partially effective in reducing sandfly populations within a dwelling.[408]

Although experience with a related *Phlebovirus*-caused disease, Rift Valley fever, indicates that a vaccine that induces neutralizing antibody will protect against disease,[409] at present there is no available sandfly fever vaccine.

[David J. McClain]

LYME DISEASE

Introduction and Military Relevance

Lyme disease is a rapidly emerging infectious

disease (Figure 35-18). Both European and American literature describe a wide array of clinical symptoms associated with those of Lyme disease since

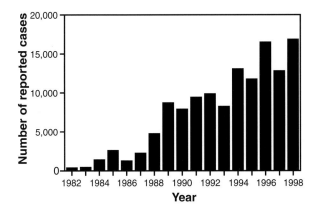

Fig. 35-18. The number of reported cases of Lyme disease by year in the United States, 1982 through 1998. Source: Centers for Disease Control and Prevention. Surveillance for Lyme disease—United States, 1992—1998. *MMWR*. 2000;49(SS03):1–11.

the 1900s.[410,411] Since the initiation of surveillance by the Centers for Disease Control in 1982 and its designation as a nationally notifiable disease in January 1991, Lyme disease has become the most common vector-borne disease in the United States.[412] The relative ease of contracting this tick-borne spirochetal disease, difficulties in its diagnosis, controversies in its management, and occurrence of debilitating manifestations in chronic Lyme disease and post-Lyme syndrome make this disease a significant public health issue for both civilians and the military.

US military personnel are at increased risk for contracting this disease because their training, combat, and humanitarian assistance missions, as well as recreational activities such as hiking, hunting, and camping, bring them in contact with the disease vectors. Several outbreaks of Lyme disease have occurred at military installations and in military personnel. Of 117 persons who acquired Lyme disease in New Jersey from 1978 to 1982, 30 were exposed to ticks at the Naval Weapons Station Earle in Monmouth County.[413] Isolation of the etiologic agent in animal reservoirs and tick vectors established Fort McCoy, Wisconsin, a military field training camp, as a highly endemic area.[414] Among military personnel reported with Lyme disease from North Carolina and Virginia in 1989, the majority of cases were exposed during field operations or training at Camp Lejeune, NC, and Quantico, VA.[415] Other high-risk sites include Fort A.P. Hill, Virginia, and Fort Chaffee, Ark. The mobility of military personnel also increases the chances that they will be exposed in one part of the world and develop illness in another part. Reports of cases have been published from both Germany and the United States in which the infection was acquired in the United States but the patient came down with the disease in Germany and vice versa.[416,417]

Description of the Pathogen

The causative agent, *Borrelia burgdorferi*, was identified as a spirochete in 1982 by Burgdorfer and colleagues.[418] Borreliae are corkscrew-shaped bacteria resembling other members of the family *Spirochaetaceae*. They are best visualized under phase-contrast or darkfield microscopy. They do not live in soil, water, or plants and are not transported by fecal contamination or aerosols.[411] They have complex nutritional requirements, making growth in culture difficult.

Epidemiology

Transmission

Borrelia burgdorferi is transmitted to humans through the bite of infected ticks, specifically certain members of the *Ixodes* species complex of the hard-bodied ticks. Several species of this complex transmit *B burgdorferi* to humans: *I scapularis* (in the northeastern, upper midwestern, and southeastern United States),[419] *I pacificus* (the West Coast of the United States),[420] *I ricinus* (in Europe),[421] and *I persulcatus* (in Asia).[422] The Lone Star tick (*Amblyomma americanum*) also has been found to contain the spirochete, but it is not clear that it can transmit the infection to humans.

Ixodes scapularis, also known as the deer tick, is the most common vector of Lyme disease in the United States. (The name *I dammini*, which was used to describe the deer tick in the northeastern United States, was relegated to a junior synonym of *I scapularis* upon finding that the deer tick of the northeastern and southeastern United States are the same species.) *I scapularis* has a 2-year life cycle, in which environmental cues trigger its host-seeking activity. The larval and nymph stages of deer ticks are parasites of a wide variety of vertebrate species (eg, mice, passerine birds, chipmunks, voles, squirrels, raccoons, foxes, deer, and other mammals). The white-footed mouse (*Peromyscus lecopus*), chipmunks (*Tamais striatus*), and passerine birds—including American robins (*Turdus migratorius*), common grackles (*Quiscalus quiscala*), Carolina and house wrens (*Thryothorus ludovicianus, Troglodytes aedon*), ovenbirds (*Siiurus aurocapillus*), and common yellowthroats (*Geothlypis trichas*)—serve as competent reservoirs of the spirochete in nature, especially when larval and nymphal ticks co-feed in close proximity.[414,423–426] Since many people in the Northeast are exposed to nymphal ticks on their residential lawns, passerine birds are the probable contributing hosts.[424] In some areas, more than 40% to 50% of white-footed mice, chipmunks, and birds are infected with *B burgdorferi*.[425–427] White-tailed deer (*Odocoileus virginianna*) also may be competent hosts for immature stages, though several other researchers disagree.[428–430] Adult ticks show a preference for larger animals, particularly the white-tailed deer. Adult ticks mate while they are feeding on the deer.

In the western United States, *I pacificus*, the Western black-legged tick, is the major vector of *B burgdorferi*.[431] Reservoir hosts include the dusty-footed wood rat (*Neotoma fuscipes*), mice (*Peromyscus*

ssp.), other rodents, and perhaps passerine birds.[431–432] Columbian black-tailed deer (*Odocoileus hemionus columbianus*) and carnivores are the major host for adult *I pacificus*.[433]

Increasing cases of Lyme disease occur as humans increase their contact with nature. Ticks prefer a relatively humid (85%) environment in mixed hardwood woodlands near creeks, river valleys, lakes, and coastal areas.[410] These are the same areas people tend to select for recreational areas and residential communities. During the 18th and 19th centuries, deer were hunted to near extinction, and their forest habitats were turned into farmland. Recent ecological efforts, hunting regulations, and reversions of marginal farms to woodlands have been favorable for deer populations, which have increased from a low of approximately 350,000 at around 1900 to more than 18 million in 1992. The

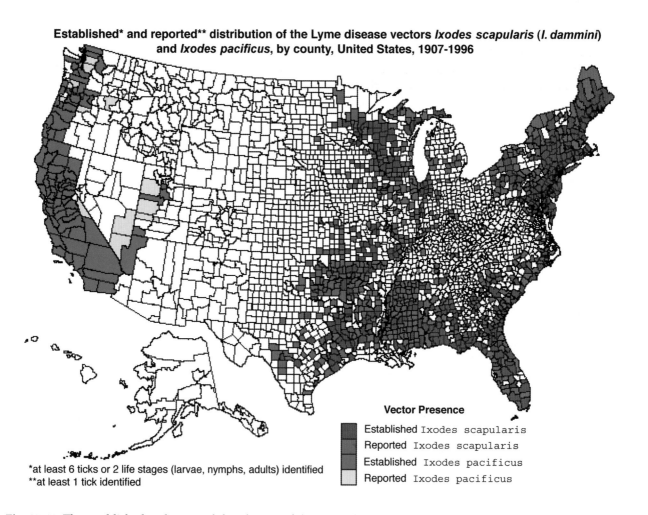

Established* and reported** distribution of the Lyme disease vectors *Ixodes scapularis* (*I. dammini*) and *Ixodes pacificus*, by county, United States, 1907-1996

Vector Presence

Established *Ixodes scapularis*
Reported *Ixodes scapularis*
Established *Ixodes pacificus*
Reported *Ixodes pacificus*

*at least 6 ticks or 2 life stages (larvae, nymphs, adults) identified
**at least 1 tick identified

Fig. 35-19. The established and reported distribution of the Lyme disease vectors *Ixodes scapularis* (*I dammini*) and *Ixodes pacificus*, by county, in the United States from 1907 through 1996. Source: Centers for Disease Control and Prevention. CDC Lyme Disease web page. http://www.cdc.gov/ncidod/dvbid/tickmap.htm. Accessed on 16 Sept 1998.

increase in the deer population has led to an increase in the deer tick population and contributed to the emergence of Lyme disease.[434] A many-fold increase in the population of the immature *I scapularis* ticks was reported from 1984 to 1991.[419]

Experimental studies have suggested that the duration of bite required for transmission of *B burgdorferi* is 24 to 48 hours.[435] The spirochetes, which reside in the tick's midgut, begin to multiply after the tick starts to feed, and they migrate into the salivary glands and enter the host's skin as the tick continues to feed. This process requires about 24 hours. This time lag between onset of the bite and transmission of *B burgdorferi* allows for preventive measures to be taken against Lyme disease.

Geographic Distribution

Lyme disease is reported in most temperate regions, to include North America, Europe, Asia, and South Africa.[436–441] It is reported from all states in United States except Alaska and Montana; the Northeast and upper Midwest are areas of heavy concentration. Moderate risk of Lyme disease is also seen in the Pacific Coast. Lyme disease distribution correlates closely with the white-tailed deer and deer tick populations[442,443] (Figure 35-19).

Incidence

The number of cases of Lyme disease reported to the Centers for Disease Control and Prevention (CDC) has increased since 1982 and exceeded 16,000 cases in 1996.[412] But this number is likely to be grossly underestimating the true incidence of Lyme disease. According to one estimate, only 11% to 16% of Lyme disease cases in their state were reported by Connecticut physicians in 1992.[444] On the other hand, Steere reported that 57% of 788 patients who were referred to a Lyme disease specialty clinic with a diagnosis of Lyme disease did not have the disease.[445] Most of these non–Lyme disease patients had either chronic fatigue syndrome or fibromyalgia. Such underreporting and misdiagnosis due to confusion with similar illnesses interfere in assessing the exact magnitude of the problem caused by Lyme disease.

Pathogenesis and Clinical Findings

The body's immune response to the spirochete may be classified into acute localized disease, acute disseminated disease, chronic disease, and post-Lyme syndrome. The acute disease occurs from 2 days to 2 weeks after a tick bite. The classic finding of erythema migrans (Figure 35-20), an expanding annular erythematous skin lesion with central clearing, develops at the site of the tick bite in 50% to 75% of patients. Additional satellite lesions may occur. The majority of patients with EM also experience systemic symptoms (eg, fever, malaise, headache, stiff neck, fatigue), but these flu-like symptoms may occur without EM.

Hematogenous spread allows dissemination of the spirochete to the rest of the body within the first few weeks of the infection. This acute disseminated disease may manifest as multiple EM, acute meningitis, cranial neuropathies, myocarditis, cardiac conduction abnormalities, hepatitis, myositis, and frank arthritis. Symptoms suggestive of acute meningitis include malaise, fatigue, lethargy, headache, and neck stiffness. Unilateral or bilateral seventh cranial nerve involvement (eg, Bell's palsy) is the most common cranial neuropathy. Only 1% to 2% of patients with acute disseminated disease manifest cardiac abnormalities (eg, myocarditis, pericarditis, varying degrees of reversible atrioventricular block). Arthralgia affecting one or more joints is the most common sign of acute disseminated disease and lasts from hours to days.

Chronic Lyme disease is characterized by localized inflammation primarily of the nervous system, skin, and musculoskeletal system. Prominent focal central nervous system abnormalities, subtle cognitive dysfunction, and peripheral neuropathies

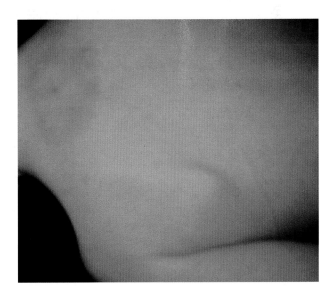

Fig. 35-20. An erythema migrans skin lesion in a patient with Lyme disease.
Photograph: Courtesy of Mary Schmidt, the Armed Forces Institute of Pathology.

presenting as paresthesia and hyperesthesia characterize the chronic involvement of the nervous system.[446] Chronic skin manifestations include Borrelia lymphocytoma and acrodermatitis chronica atrophicans. Chronic arthritis most commonly affects the knee, but this tends to remit spontaneously.

Another manifestation of Lyme disease is post-Lyme syndrome. This is distinct from chronic Lyme disease in that post-Lyme syndrome patients have been treated with antibiotics early in the disease process. Symptoms of severe fatigue, recurrent muscle and joint aches, headaches, mental sluggishness, and difficulty concentrating persist for 6 months or more without response to further antibiotic therapy.[447] These patients are often misdiagnosed as having chronic fatigue syndrome or fibromyalgia. The possibility of *B burgdorferi* persistence in patients with negative serological tests[448] and the presence of *B burgdorferi* DNA in urine of treated patients with symptoms of chronic Lyme disease have been reported.[449] So without a clear-cut definition for Lyme disease, much controversy surrounds the diagnosis and management of this disease. The potential for long-term disability from both chronic Lyme disease and post-Lyme syndrome requires further elucidation of the pathogenesis of this disease.

Diagnostic Approaches

History of exposure is critical to the diagnosis of Lyme disease. A careful history should address issues such as residence in or travel to endemic areas, previous tick exposures, EM lesions, objective or subjective neurologic dysfunction, arthritis, and history of heart disease. Providers may elicit a history of a "summer cold" acquired in an area with endemic Lyme disease. The signs and symptoms of Lyme disease may appear quite specific, but the development of late-stage manifestations may cause diagnostic uncertainty. A careful physical examination, to include a complete skin examination for EM, together with an appropriate exposure history may make the diagnosis. Other skin manifestations, as well as joint, cardiac, and neurological abnormalities, may be detected by physical examination.

Beyond a careful history and physical examination, numerous serologic tests are available to test for antibodies to *B burgdorferi*. An enzyme-linked immunosorbent assay (ELISA) is available to detect IgG and IgM antibodies associated with *B burgdorferi*. The Western immunoblot assay is used to confirm positive and equivocal results from the ELISA, in accordance with the 1999 CDC recom-

mendations.[450] Interpreting these results is not without complications, however; problems include cross-reactivity with normal oral flora and treponema species (eg, *Treponema pallidum*), cross-reactivity with antibodies present in autoimmune diseases such as systemic lupus erythematosus and rheumatoid arthritis, prior exposure to *B burgdorferi*, and the lack of standardization in serologic assays.[434] Serologic tests done at an early stage of Lyme disease may also be negative due to inadequate time for the body to respond with antibodies. Repeat serologic testing is recommended 4 to 6 weeks after the initial test in the early stages of disease. To what extent the availability of new assays (eg, polymerase chain reaction) and genetic sequencing of *Borrelia* species will clarify diagnosis and management of this disease remains to be seen. The diagnosis of Lyme disease still relies on the clinical presentation, the history of exposure, the clinical suspicion of an alert health care provider, and the recognition of the incomplete state of our understanding of this disease.

Recommendations for Therapy and Prevention

Therapy

Prophylactic therapy following a potential bite exposure is not recommended in most circumstances.[451–453] Prompt treatment is indicated for suspected infections.[454,455] For the acute localized illness, doxycycline, amoxicillin, cefuroxime, oral penicillin, and tetracycline have been given for approximately 10 to 20 days with success. The decision of which drug to use is determined by drug allergies, the possibility of co-infection with other tick-borne pathogens, patient compliance, and cost. Misdiagnosis of co-infection with *Babesia microtus*, a malaria-like protozoan, or the *Ehrlichia* species that causes human granulocytic ehrlichiosis may lead to the erroneous diagnosis of treatment-resistant Lyme disease. When co-infections with the human granulocytic ehrlichiosis pathogen are possible, treatment with doxycycline should be considered because it is effective against both infections.[456] Disseminated Lyme disease infection should be treated with intravenous cefotaxime, ceftriaxone, or penicillin for 10 to 30 days[454,455] (Table 35-10).

In patients with continued symptoms following appropriate treatment, use of polymerase chain reaction and culture methods to determine if *B burgdorferi* is present may be considered. Fibromyalgia and chronic fatigue syndrome should also be considered. Other conventional medications may be used

TABLE 35-10

TREATMENT OF LYME DISEASE

Drug	Route	Adult Dose	Child Dose	Duration
Acute Localized				
Amoxicillin	PO	500 mg tid	50 mg/kg/d tid	10-20 d
Cefuroxime	PO	500 mg bid	50 mg/kg/d bid	20 d
Penicillin	PO	250 mg qid	50 mg/kg/d qid	10-20 d
Tetracycline	PO	250 mg qid	Avoid in children	10-20 d
Doxycycline	PO	100 mg bid	Avoid in children	10-20 d
Disseminated and Chronic				
Cefotaxime	IV	2 g qd or q12 h	50 mg/kg/d q12h	10 d
Ceftriaxone	IV	2 g qd or q12 h	50 mg/kg/d	10-14 d
Penicillin	IV	24 million units qd	50,000 units/kg/d	20-30 d

bid twice a day, IV intravenous, po by mouth, q every, qd every day, qid four times a day, tid three times a day
Reprinted with permission from: Gilbert DN, Moellering RC, Sawde MA, eds. *The Sanford Guide to Antimicrobial Therapy*. 31st ed. Hyde Park, Vt: Antimicrobial Therapy, Inc: 2001.

for symptomatic treatment, to include antiinflammatory agents such as aspirin, ibuprofen, hydroxychloroquine, and prednisone. While alternative therapies may be considered, patients should be educated about the dangers of popular remedies such as malariotherapy.[457]

Another complication in the treatment of *B burgdorferi* infection is the Jarisch-Herxheimer reaction, noted in association with antibiotic therapy for spirochetes.[458] After the start of antibiotic treatment, the death of *B burgdorferi* organisms may release large amounts of cytokines and hormones. The minority of patients who experience this reaction feel worse for the first few days, with increased inflammation of EM lesions, fever, and aches, but then improve.

Prevention

Tick populations peak in the spring and summer months, which is when people are outdoors most and opportunities increase for contact between vector and host. The environment surrounding the home is a major determinant of the risk of getting a tick bite; nearly 70% of tick bites are acquired at home,[459] and residences with larger woodlots are more likely to have ticks.[460]

Many environmental controls have been tried to control both the tick and the host populations. Acaricide-impregnated nest material for use by mice has been used to kill the larval stages of the deer

tick on the white-footed mouse with mixed results.[461,462] Use of acaricides has successfully controlled the number of deer ticks.[463–466] Removal of deer from proximity to human populations has been used to decrease the numbers of adult deer ticks. These environmental controls are not always successful, however, so the need for personal preventive measures cannot be overemphasized.[467]

The most effective and obvious means of preventing exposure to hard-bodied ticks is to avoid their known habitats, but this is not always possible for military personnel. The risk of Lyme disease can be minimized greatly by the use of the DoD Repellent System (see Chapter 22, Personal Protection Measures Against Arthropods). This system includes wearing a loose-fitting, permethrin-impregnated uniform with pant legs tucked into boots, sleeves rolled down and fastened, and collar closed. Extended-duration DEET lotion should be applied to exposed skin. No repellent system is 100% effective, though, so service members use the "buddy system" to check each other; it works well for finding ticks crawling on the uniform and feeding on the body. Ticks can be found anywhere on the body, but they prefer moist areas.[468] Service members performing buddy checks must be reminded to look for any rash in an area of a tick bite and that such a rash requires immediate medical attention.

The ability of a feeding tick to infect the host is reduced by prompt removal of the tick. Forceps or tweezers should be used to grab the tick as gently and as close to the skin as possible. The tick should then be slowly and gently pulled away from the bite site until it detaches. Care should be taken not to crush or twist the tick, since this can leave the mouthparts embedded in the skin. Once the tick is removed, it should not be manipulated with bare hands. The tick should be sent in an alcohol-filled container to the US Army Center for Health Promotion and Preventive Medicine, Aberdeen, Maryland, for identification and testing for *B burgdorferi*. The skin should be washed with soap and water, followed by an application of rubbing alcohol. The bite should be observed for at least a month in case a rash or redness develops.[469]

Two vaccines using the outer surface protein of *B burgdorferi* have been developed and tested.[470–472] One that has been approved by the Food and Drug Administration requires a three-shot series (at 0, 1, and 12 months) and has an efficacy of 50% after two doses and 78% after all three doses.[473] While vaccination would decrease the threat that Lyme disease currently presents to military members and their families, personal protective measures still need to be emphasized to prevent Lyme disease if the vaccine fails and to prevent other arthropod-transmitted diseases.

[Kevin Michaels, Hee-Choon S. Lee, Victoria B. Solberg]

EHRLICHIOSIS

Introduction and Military Importance

Ehrlichiae have been known as veterinary pathogens since the 1930s. A serious epizootic of canine ehrlichiosis caused the deaths of 200 to 300 military working dogs in Vietnam in the late 1960s. They died of a hemorrhagic disease caused, it was discovered later, by *Ehrlichia canis*.[474] *E sennetsu* (called *Rickettsia sennetsu* until 1984) was described in Japan in the 1950s and was thought to be the only ehrlichial human pathogen. It targets monocytes and causes an illness that resembles mononucleosis.[475–478] *E sennetsu* has been confined to Japan and Southeast Asia.[477,478] It is presumed to be transmitted by ticks, and tetracycline is the treatment of choice.[478] In the last part of the 20th century, two other distinct human diseases caused by ehrlichiae have emerged. Human monocytic ehrlichiosis (HME) has been found to be caused by *Ehrlichia chaffeensis*, which was characterized in 1991. Human granulocytic ehrlichiosis (HGE) is caused by an organism yet to be definitively identified but one that is very similar to *E equi* and *E phagocytophila*, which cause granulocytic infections in sheep, cattle, and horses.[479,480] HGE may be caused by a different strain of one of these two. Although both diseases are caused by ehrlichiae, they have some different qualities. The military has played a role uncovering these two diseases, and the diseases will continue to affect the military, especially because training is often conducted in tick-infested areas.[481] Although there have been many advances in the study of ehrlichiae, much about the organisms and their epidemiology, diagnostics, and control is still unknown. Future control measures should include a system for notifying public health officials of cases and increasing physician and soldier awareness.[482]

Description of the Pathogen

Ehrlichiae are obligate, intracellular, Gram-negative cocci that infect white blood cells.[483] The bacteria can be found grouped into morulae, which are distinct monocytic or granulocytic intracytoplasmic inclusions.[480] *E chaffeensis*, the causative agent of HME, has two identified strains. The first strain, Arkansas, was isolated from a US Army reservist; the second, 91HE17, was discovered in 1995.[479,483] There may be further diversity among the bacteria infecting humans, and the taxonomy will likely become clearer in the future.

Epidemiology

HME and HGE are transmitted by ticks, with greater than 80% of symptomatic people reporting a tick bite within 3 weeks before illness onset.[475,476] Exact incidence rates and prevalence are unknown. Most reported estimates are biased toward identification of the more serious cases.[484]

Human Monocytic Ehrlichiosis

Transmission. HME is believed to be transmitted by *Amblyomma americanum* (the lone star tick) and *Dermacentor variabilis* (the American dog tick).[481,482,485,486] The organism has been found in the white-tailed deer. The presence of persistent bacteremia in dogs suggests that mammals other than deer may be hosts.[481] Disease occurrence is seasonal, with most cases occurring from March to October, and the majority of those in May, June, and July.[477,478,481,486]

Geographic Distribution. Cases have been confirmed in 30 states and are concentrated in the south and south-central United States.[484,485]

Incidence. HME seroconversion in a large study of military personnel at Fort Chaffee, Ark, to *E canis* and *E chaffeensis* was 1.3% (13 of 15 positive for *E chaffeensis*). The seroconversion rate was higher in those that actually lived and worked at Fort Chaffee (3.3%) than in those there for training (0.7%).[481] A 12% prevalence was reported among samples submitted for Rocky Mountain spotted fever testing to the Oklahoma State Department of Health.[476] Incidence reportedly rises with age, but older people may be more likely to have worse disease and thus seek medical attention and diagnosis. Median incubation periods have been found to be approximately 7 to 9 days.[484]

Human Granulocytic Ehrlichiosis

Transmission. HGE is transmitted by *Ixodes scapularis* ticks and has also been identified in *D variabilis* ticks.[485,487] Possibilities for a reservoir include deer and rodents. There is year-round occurrence, peaking in June and July,[474,480,482] but tick activity has been found in the upper Midwest in all months of the year except February and September.[487] The median incubation period is 8 days.[482]

Geographic Distribution. HGE has been found in 11 states but more often in the Northeast and Midwest. This is in contrast to HME, which is more often found in the South and South-Central.[474,480] There may also be HGE in Sweden and Switzerland.[482]

Incidence. HGE was discovered in the early 1990s. It was found in 11% of a sample of patients presenting with an undiagnosed acute febrile illness in Minnesota and Wisconsin in the summer and fall of 1993. Annual incidence has been estimated to exceed 50 per 100,000 per year in that location.[487]

Pathogenesis and Clinical Findings

Human Monocytic Ehrlichiosis

In HME, *E chaffeensis* enters the skin via a tick bite and spreads hematogenously. Infection is established intracellularly in macrophages in various tissues. The infection can lead to tissue necrosis, perivascular lymphohistiocytic infiltrates, interstitial pneumonitis, and pulmonary hemorrhage. Granulomas and marrow histiocytosis are a result of the macrophage's reaction to the organism.[482] Much of the pathogenesis and the role of the host in this disease remain unknown.

The extent of asymptomatic infected persons has not yet been fully uncovered. In the study of the military at Fort Chaffee, only 33.3% of seroconverters reported characteristic symptoms.[481] In a study of HME in a retirement community bordering a wildlife preserve, asymptomatic infection with *E chaffeensis* was thought to have occurred because many people with serologic evidence of past infection had not reported illness in the 5 months prior to the study.[486]

Symptoms of those getting medical attention or being studied are nonspecific. Systemic symptoms, such as fever, headache, myalgia, anorexia, and nausea, are common without any clinical diagnostic findings. These clinical findings are similar to those found in Rocky Mountain spotted fever but without the characteristic rash of that seasonal tick-borne disease. Complications of HME include serious pulmonary, renal, and cerebral compromise.[477] Hospitalized patients are likely to be older. Laboratory findings, which can be of great assistance in making the diagnosis, include leukopenia, thrombocytopenia, and elevated hepatic transaminases.[477,484] Anemia is common, occurring later in the illness and lasting longer than other hematologic abnormalities.[484] Infiltrates on chest radiographs and cerebrospinal fluid pleocytosis are possible findings amidst complications.[477] A new strain of HME, 91HE77, was isolated from a patient who nearly died and raises the possibility of infection with alternative strains resulting in differential morbidity and mortality.[479]

Human Granulocytic Ehrlichiosis

In HGE, the pathogenesis is unknown after the organism enters via a tick bite. The organism appears to infect myeloid precursors in the marrow instead of mature granulocytes.[482] The corresponding ehrlichiae in animals are believed to somehow impair the host immune response and allow opportunistic infections. Clinical findings in humans include fever, chills, malaise, myalgias, headaches, nausea, vomiting, and rarely a rash.[474,487] The clinical picture is quite similar to infection with *E chaffeensis*, with similar laboratory abnormalities.[474,480]

Diagnostic Approaches

When faced with a patient with possible human ehrlichiosis, serology for both HGE and HME are appropriate because their geographic distributions overlap.[485]

Human Monocytic Ehrlichiosis

E chaffeensis is very rarely isolated from tissue in cases of HME. It is difficult to diagnose early in the course of disease. A high index of suspicion is needed with nonspecific febrile illness, especially when faced with a patient with a history of a tick bite or exposure to ticks.[484] The presence of leukopenia and thrombocytopenia is helpful diagnostically. Diagnosis can be made later after detecting an immune response to *E chaffeensis* antigen or *E canis* antigen. (The *E canis* antigen was used primarily in the early stages of uncovering this organism and is a less-sensitive indicator than finding the *E chaffeensis* antigen.[482]) A 4-fold rise in indirect fluorescent antibody titer of the appropriate level is diagnostic if the clinical picture is consistent.[481,484] Because of the variation in the diagnostic criterion by laboratory, contacting the performing laboratory is useful in determining the minimal peak titer. There is evidence that early treatment and advancing age can result in a decreased serologic antibody response.[481,486] *E chaffeensis*–specific polymerase chain reaction (PCR) is available and can be positive in the absence of antibody criteria for diagnosis. Because of this, PCR is felt to be more sensitive than serologic testing.[482] Unlike the situation with HGE, finding morulae of the organism in the leukocyte in HME is difficult and not a useful diagnostic tool.

Human Granulocytic Ehrlichiosis

The agent in HGE has not yet been isolated, so alternative diagnostic approaches must be used.[480] Peripheral blood smears may be helpful in illustrating neutrophil cytoplasmic morulae of ehrlichiae.[474,480] These morulae are easy to differentiate from other cytoplasmic inclusions.[474] Finding them is the most sensitive and widely available diagnostic tool. Immunofluorescent assay using *E equi* or *E phagocytophila* can be used for serologic diagnosis but not early in the illness.[487] PCR is being refined and is not yet widely available.

Recommendations for Therapy and Control

Therapy

Tetracycline or doxycycline is the treatment for HME and HGE, with typical marked improvement in 48 hours.[474,484,487] Chloramphenicol has been used in some patients who have recovered; the efficacy of chloramphenicol, though, is not clear because some patients respond spontaneously without any treatment, and chloramphenicol is not effective in vitro against *E chaffeensis*. Rifampin is effective in vivo, but clinical experience with this drug is lacking.[488] Improvement with the use of effective therapy can itself be an aid in diagnosis. Treatment must begin before a definitive diagnosis is made because earlier treatment may lower the risk of adverse outcomes.[485] Persistent infection in animals with *E canis* despite treatment has been reported.[478,487] The possibility of persistent infection in humans is still unknown.

Control

People in areas where ticks are common should take precautions. Military personnel should be made aware of the threat of HME and HGE and the fact that they are threats in off-duty environments as well as during field exercises. In endemic areas such as Arkansas, ticks are a threat even for those not engaged in outdoor recreational activities.[477] Precautions include avoiding if possible areas known to be infested with ticks. Routinely using insect repellent and checking for ticks are both important.[485] Tucking trouser legs into boots, blousing trousers, receiving pertinent educational briefings, and using permethrin-impregnated uniforms have been associated with a decreased risk of tickborne infection.[475,481] These control measures are not practical in the civilian community.[484]

[Kathryn L. Clark]

TYPHUS

Scrub Typhus (*Orientia tsutsugamushi*)

Introduction and Military Relevance

Scrub typhus is an infectious disease that spans a clinical spectrum from mild to fatal depending on the strain of organism, the age and immune status of the host, and the quality of health care provided. While "tropical typhus" has long plagued military forces in Asia and on the Pacific islands, it has only been since the 1930s that scrub and endemic typhus have been distinguished. Because effective antibiotic treatment was not available during World War II, both allied and Japanese forces had large numbers of casualties due to scrub typhus. In some areas, it was a cause of medical casualties second only to malaria. Illustrative of the impact of the infection was the experience of the British in northern Burma: during 2 months in 1944, 18% of one battalion's casualties and 5% of its fatalities were from scrub typhus.[489]

Scrub typhus remains a major concern for military forces deployed in endemic regions. Reservoirs of infection will continue to cycle in nature, and military operations will place susceptible individuals in exposure situations. Personal protective measures can be effective in reducing exposure, but they require command emphasis to maintain the necessary discipline. This disease, much like malaria, tends to be forgotten by military health professionals between major deployments to endemic regions. Preventive medicine strategies against scrub typhus are an essential part of deployment to Southeast Asia and other endemic areas.

Description of the Pathogen

The etiologic agent of scrub typhus is *Orientia tsutsugamushi*. It is a member of the rickettsial family, which are Gram-negative, obligate intracellular bacteria that multiply in the cytoplasm of infected cells. Because of distinctive characteristics in its outer membrane and rRNA sequence, the organism was reclassified in 1995 from the genus *Rickettsia* into the new genus *Orientia*.[490] Strain variability is greater than that of the other disease-producing rickettsial species. While eight "prototype" antigenic types were defined in 1967, molecular studies now suggest that there are actually more than 60 genetic and antigenic variants unique to different localities. Strains also vary greatly in virulence for both humans and mice (a useful laboratory model).

Epidemiology

Transmission. Scrub typhus is a zoonosis acquired by the bite of infected larval trombiculid mites (chiggers) when humans intrude into an enzootic focus of infection. The natural cycle consists of (*a*) *O tsutsugamushi,* (*b*) chiggers of the *Leptotrombidium deliense* group (eg, *L deliense, L akamushi, L fletcheri, L arenicola, L pallidum, L pavlovskyi, L chiangraiensis*), and (*c*) small rodents, especially rats of the genus *Rattus*. The mites are both the reservoir and vector of this infection (Figure 35-21). Their larval "chiggers" are the only stage that feeds on humans and rodents (the vertebrate hosts) and usually cause only minimal irritation. The mites ingest lymph and tissue fluids from the subdermis, although their frequently reddish appearance leads to the incorrect impression that they are full of blood. The rickettsial organisms are distributed through all tissues of the mite, including the salivary glands from which

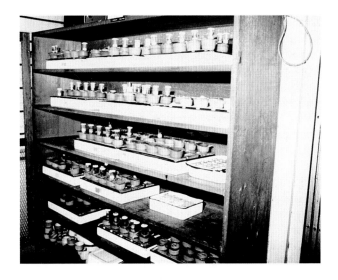

Fig. 35-21. *Orientia tsutsugamushi*–infected mite colony established in 1964 at the US Army Medical Research Unit—Kuala Lumpur, Malaysia. The colony was maintained through 62 generations until closure of the Unit in 1989.
US Army photograph.

they are transmitted during a bite. Transovarial transmission is a necessary part of the maintainence of *O tsutsugamushi* in trombiculid mites. Extensive field observation during World War II indicated that the mites tend to live at ground level rather than on vegetation. Risk of infection to soldiers continuously on the move was associated with their "loitering and resting in contact with the ground en route."[489p186] Certain species of chiggers, though, gather above the ground at the tips of leaves ("lalang" grass) and show that there is diversity in modes of transmission.

Geographic Distribution. The geographic distribution of scrub typhus includes eastern and southern Asia and the islands of the southwestern Pacific. Specifically, scrub typhus occurs in Japan, Korea, Tajikistan, the Maritime Territories of eastern Russia, China, Australia, New Zealand, the Philippines, islands in the South Pacific, Indonesia, India, Pakistan, and all of Southeast Asia. It is distributed from sea level to altitudes as high as 7,000 ft (2,100 m) in the Kumaon Hills of India.[489] Within these endemic areas, scrub typhus infection tends to be localized as either well-established or transient "mite islands." Transovarian transmission of the organism provides the mechanism for maintenance of focal endemicity.

There is no such thing as a typical scrub typhus environment. Infected habitats are quite diverse, varying from semideserts, river banks, and seashores to disrupted rain forests and terrain undergoing secondary vegetative growth. Ecological changes that favor the rodents or other small mammals that are the usual hosts of the chiggers occur when stable vegetation is disturbed and allowed to regrow. Military operations and expanding agricultural efforts often produce these types of ecological changes and lead to exposure of service members and rural people to infectious chiggers.[491] Cases of scrub typhus are seen increasingly in nonendemic regions because of intercontinental travel during the incubation period; the nonrecognition of these cases may lead to life-threatening illness.[492]

Incidence. Incidence of scrub typhus varies with geographic location, occupation, and behavior. In temperate areas such as Japan and Taiwan, disease occurrence is seasonal; in warmer areas, seasonal variation may not be detectable. Surprisingly, the seasonal transmission in South Korea and Japan occurs in fall and winter. Disease in indigenous populations is often underdiagnosed. Systematic study of febrile admissions to a central Malaysian hospital in the late 1970s determined that 20% of cases were due to scrub typhus and that this reached nearly 50% in the subgroup of patients who worked in areas where rain forest had been replaced with oil palm groves.[493] Some scrub typhus antibody prevalences in Southeast Asia are 59% in northern Thailand,[494] 21% near Bangkok,[495] 38% in the Pescadores Islands of Taiwan,[496] and 0.8% in Sabah, East Malaysia.[497]

Military personnel deployed to areas endemic for scrub typhus are at high risk of infection and resulting symptomatic disease. Statistics from World War II indicate that more than 7,000 cases occurred in US forces, nearly as many in British and Indian troops, and more than 3,000 in Australian soldiers. Overall incidence figures are unreliable because of clustering of infections in time and place. Risk to military personnel continues to be a problem, as was documented in the mid-1990s in a study[498] that found incidence as high as 15% in Thai soldiers during 4 months of military exercises. Serologic studies in Malaysia[499] and repeated outbreaks among US Marines deployed to the Mt. Fuji region of Japan[500] (Figure 35-22) confirm the continued risk.

Pathogenesis and Clinical Findings

Rickettsiae bind to cellular receptors, are phagocytosed, escape from phagocytic vacuoles into the cytoplasm, and proliferate by binary fission. The organisms exit the host cell either as a mass following host cell lysis or in discrete packets of rickett-

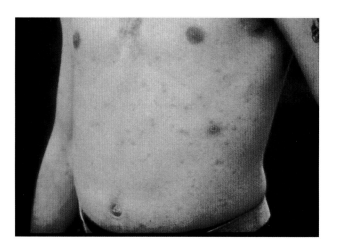

Fig. 35-22. A US Marine with acute scrub typhus acquired while he was deployed to Camp Fuji, Japan, in the autumn of 1983. Note the erythematous (blanching) rash predominately on the trunk and the location of the eschar at the lateral aspect of the right upper quadrant. Photograph: Courtesy of Henry B. Lewandowski, PhD, Savannah, Ga.

siae surrounded by host-cell membrane that buds off from intact cells. Scrub typhus organisms are highly infectious; it is estimated that fewer than 10 viable organisms are an infectious dose for humans. The organisms are transmitted into cutaneous tissues at the site of the chigger's bite. Proliferation in local endothelial cells leads to a visible lesion in about 60% of nonimmune hosts during the 6- to 21-day incubation period. The lesion evolves into an eschar, which is loaded with rickettsiae and highly infectious. Early dissemination via the lymphatic system leads to tender regional lymphadenopathy, which may be augmented by hematogenous spread from infected endothelial cells. Detectable rickettsemia appears late in the incubation period, usually 1 to 2 days before onset of clinical disease.

The wide variation in scrub typhus strains appears to be manifest in its variation in virulence. Symptoms and signs are based on disseminated vasculitis caused by focal infection of the endothelium of small blood vessels. This presents as a maculopapular rash in about one third of patients, which appears late in the first week of illness on the trunk and extremities but may be hard to detect on dark-skinned people. The disease, which may last for weeks, is characterized by fever, headache, and generalized lymphadenopathy. It may be abrupt in onset but is more commonly insidious over several days. Among US Marines in South Vietnam with confirmed diagnoses, the following symptoms and

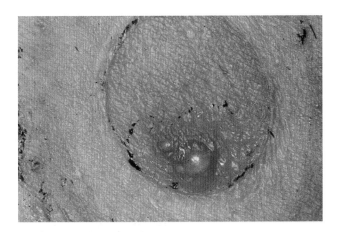

Fig. 35-23. A scrub typhus eschar 1 day after chiggers fed on a US Army volunteer. The chiggers were from the *Leptotrombidium* mite colony shown in Figure 35-21. Photograph: Courtesy of Henry B. Lewandowski, PhD, Savannah, Ga.

signs were observed: eschar (46%), splenomegaly (43%), rash (34%), myalgia (32%), and conjunctivitis (29%)[501] (Figure 35-23). Lung involvement is the most important complication, with adult respiratory distress syndrome the most frequent cause of death. Other complications include deafness, myocarditis, encephalitis, and multiorgan system failure. Mortality rates before the availability of antibiotics ranged from 1% to 55%.[489] Delayed or inappropriate treatment continues to be associated with severe illness and fatality.[492]

Diagnostic Approaches

Clinical. The diagnosis of scrub typhus may be suspected on clinical and epidemiologic grounds. In most parts of Asia, an eschar is pathognomonic of the disease, and a careful search for this lesion in suspected cases is the most important part of the physical exam. Eschars tend to be localized where clothing has been pressed to the skin, as at the ankles and waist. Also helpful diagnostically are rash, conjunctival suffusion, and hearing impairment when associated with onset of illness. Despite these signs, scrub typhus can be easily confused with other febrile illnesses in the endemic area. Prompt, empiric treatment will generally be both diagnostic and curative. Treatment with a tetracycline or chloramphenicol usually leads to clinical improvement and defervescence within 24 to 36 hours.

Laboratory. Rickettsiae may be isolated from the blood of patients, but the techniques are difficult and hazardous. The Weil-Felix test is too insensitive to be useful in diagnosis. Detection of specific antibody is the main tool for proving the diagnosis of scrub typhus. The gold standards for serologic diagnosis are the indirect fluorescent antibody (IFA) and immunoperoxidase (IIP) assays, which use cultured and inactivated organisms as the capture antigen. These antigens have historically been produced and distributed by national research or reference laboratories, but they are now becoming commercially available. Another diagnostic assay in development uses a dot-ELISA (enzyme-linked immunosorbent assay) format. Once validated, such an assay could provide a needed tool for rural clinics and military operations in endemic regions.[502] With any of these serological assays, interpretation of results will differ depending on the population in which it is being used. In adults from endemic areas, acute titers of 1:400 or a 4-fold rise to at least 1:200 may be required to maintain specificity. In contrast, in previously uninfected visitors to an endemic area, a titer of 1:100 would be significant.[503] Molecular assays, under development for scrub typhus and other rickettsial infections, are expected to provide enhanced sensitivity and specificity.

Therapy, Prevention, and Control

Therapy. Tetracyclines and chloramphenicol[504] (Figure 35-24) are specifically effective for the rickettsioses, despite being bacteriostatic (rather than bacteriocidal) agents. Either drug should be given as a loading dose followed by divided daily doses for at least a week and until the patient is afebrile. If treatment is started in the first 3 days of illness, a second course of antibiotics should be given after an interval of 6 days to prevent recrudescence of infection. The responsiveness of scrub typhus to treatment may be changing. In northern Thailand, a high frequency of relapse after treatment associated with relative resistance of *O tsutsugamushi* isolates to both tetracycline and chloramphenicol has been observed.[505] Preliminary studies[506,507] suggest that both azithromycin and rifampin may provide effective alternative therapy for scrub typhus.

Prevention and Control. As general guidance, encampments should not be placed in areas of secondary vegetative growth where agriculture, erosion, or other disturbances favor rodent activity. The best defense for the individual service member against chigger bites is the careful use of treated uniforms and repellents. Three different systems exist for treatment of uniforms with permethrin, which kills chiggers crawling up the uniform be-

a

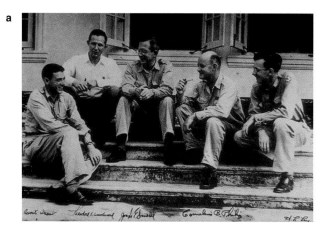

b

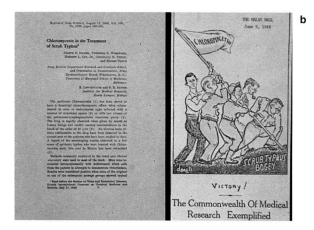

Fig. 35-24. The US Army research team that demonstrated the efficacy of chloramphenicol in the first antibiotic treatment of scrub typhus at the Malayan Institute for Medical Research in Kuala Lumpur in 1948. (a) From left to right, they are: R. Traub, T. Woodward, J. E. Smadel, C. Philip, and H. L. Ley Jr. (b) A cartoon highlighting the accomplishments of the team appeared in the local newspaper, the *Malay Mail.*
(a) Photograph: Courtesy of Dr. Theodore Woodward. (b) The *Malay Mail*

fore they can bite. To be effective, trousers must be bloused inside the boots (not secured with elastic bands) so that the chiggers are forced to crawl up the boot onto the treated uniform before contacting the host.[508] Repellents can be applied directly to exposed skin and, when permethrin-treated uniforms are not available, to boot tops and trouser legs. Two chigger repellents are currently available in the military supply system for topical application to the skin: DEET (N,N-diethylmeta-toluamide) in the standard Army repellent formulation and precipitated sulfur in a specialized formulation for chiggers. When proper permethrin treatment of clothing is not possible, DEET applied from a commercial aerosol can be an effective way of repelling chiggers from boots and trousers. Systemic prophylaxis with weekly doxycycline (200 mg/week) has been demonstrated effective under study conditions,[509] but it has never been used on a routine basis. Weekly administration is necessary so the infected service member develops immunity as the organism multiplies to sufficient levels to induce an immune response. No vaccine is available and development is unlikely because of the diversity of strains.

Old recommendations to treat ground and vegetation with chlorinated hydrocarbons (eg, lindane, dieldrin, chlordane) are no longer appropriate or legal. In fact, no compounds are currently registered for chigger control on an area basis. An alternate approach would be to make an application of a registered insecticide as if for soil pests of turf, though the effectiveness of such treatments is unknown.

Burning vegetation will suppress chigger populations for 30 days, but the regrowth can actually foster an increase in vector numbers. Where personnel find themselves in a more stable situation, general rodent control through sanitation, poison baiting, and trapping can limit chiggers and probably suppress transmission of scrub typhus. The most sensitive way to determine whether control or preventive measures are necessary is to test the local human or rodent population for antibodies. Where scrub typhus is prevalent, the resident human population is constantly boosted and maintains detectable antibody, even though no clinical disease is present. Most infected rodents are only mildly affected by scrub typhus but maintain high levels of antibody.

Murine Typhus Fever (*Rickettsia typhi*)

Introduction and Military Relevance

Murine (endemic, flea-borne) typhus is a rickettsial disease caused by the incidental infection of humans with *Rickettsia typhi* transmitted by infected rat fleas. Occurrence of infection depends on proximity to rats, and estimated incidence rates in military groups are not available. During World War II, there were 786 cases with 15 deaths diagnosed in the US Army[510] despite widespread vaccination against epidemic typhus, which provided some degree of cross-protection. Rodent control has been effective in keeping service member exposure low in US military bases, but new missions, such as assistance to refugee groups (which often occupy rodent-infested temporary camps), increase the risk of exposure. Because plague is dependent on the same host (rats) and vector (fleas), the presence of murine typhus in a given setting provides warning that propagation and transmission of that more serious infection is also possible.

Description of the Pathogen

The etiologic agent of murine typhus is *R typhi,* a Gram-negative, obligate intracellular bacterium that multiplies in the cytoplasm of infected cells. It shares group antigens with *R prowazekii,* the cause of epidemic, or louse-borne, typhus. Both of these typhus-group organisms share membrane antigens with *Proteus* and *Legionella* bacilli, the former being the basis of the Weil-Felix reaction against the OX-19 antigen.[511]

Epidemiology

Transmission. Murine typhus is a zoonosis maintained in nature in a cycle involving rats (and to some extent other small mammals such as the opossum) and their fleas, lice, and mites. The rat serves as the reservoir and amplifying host, while the Oriental rat flea (*Xenopsylla cheopis*) and, to a lesser extent, the cat flea (*Ctenocephalides felis*) serve as vectors for transmission to humans.[512] The flea becomes infected by feeding on rickettsemic rats or other small mammals. *R typhi* is then excreted in the feces for the life of the infected flea. Infection of humans occurs by contamination of a flea bite or skin abrasion by the feces of the vector or through inhalation of dried infective feces. The killing of rats may cause their fleas to transfer to humans at an increased rate.

Geographic Distribution. Murine typhus occurs worldwide, depending on human exposure to rodents and their infected fleas. Most important are rats, in particular *Rattus norvegicus* and *R rattus,* which are prevalent in urban and port areas. Dependent on human food and waste, these rats are found around buildings storing food.[513] Rodent infestation of homes is widespread in the tropics, which leads to domestic exposures.[514] Despite the rodent control measures practiced in the United States, continued endemicity of murine typhus is well documented in the warmer states (where many military training bases are located), with hundreds of cases occurring in Texas in the 1980s.[515] Conditions of refugee camps are also conducive to rodent infestation, and murine typhus occurs in them both sporadically and in outbreak form.[516,517]

Incidence. Murine typhus generally occurs sporadically and few incidence data are available. Estimated annual incidence rates among Khmer refugees in two camps in Thailand were 2.2%[517] and 0.5%.[516] Prevalence of *R typhi*–specific antibody varies greatly; in Africa reports show prevalence in the range of 1% to 20%[518]; in Thailand, 7%[519] and 8%[495]; and in Indonesia, 34%.[520]

Pathogenesis and Clinical Findings

The pathogenesis of murine typhus is very similar to that of scrub typhus, with the endothelial cell as the primary target cell. While the basic lesion causing disease is a vasculitis, disseminated rickettsemia is not preceded by the production of an eschar at the site of inoculation. After a 6- to 14-day incubation period, illness begins as fever and severe headache. A maculopapular rash appears on the trunk and extremities several days later but is difficult to detect in dark-skinned persons. Although the untreated disease can be severe, debilitating, and take months for full recovery, complications are few and the case-fatality rate is less than 5% in untreated cases.

Diagnostic Approaches

Clinical. Murine typhus is a persistent febrile illness that lacks specific clinical signs. Less than a third of patients may recall a preceding flea bite or the presence of rodents in their environment.[515] Medical staff are faced with a wide differential diagnosis, which may include malaria, dengue fever, scrub typhus, and mild cases of epidemic typhus. Persistent fever, retro-orbital headache, and rash in an individual with peri-domestic or urban rodent exposure should lead to consideration of murine typhus. Presumptive treatment with a tetracycline or chloramphenicol leads to a favorable clinical response in most patients within 48 hours.

Laboratory. Diagnosis by isolation of the organism from blood is possible but difficult and hazardous. Thus, in practice, laboratory diagnosis depends on serologic techniques. As with scrub typhus, the IFA test is the serologic gold standard. Antigen slides and control sera are commercially available, but fluorescent microscopes are expensive. The still frequently used Weil-Felix test with *Proteus* OX-19 antigen can have a specificity exceeding 95% when the cut-off value for positivity is defined as greater than or equal to 1:160. Unfortunately, at this cut-off, sensitivity is only 80% overall; the assay does not detect antibody in one third of sera collected during acute infection.[521] A dot-ELISA is commercially available, similar to the one for scrub typhus. This assay is more reproducible than the IFA, has a sensitivity and specificity of about 90%,[521,522] and (similar to the IFA) cannot distinguish murine from epidemic typhus antibodies. The current dot-ELISA requires refrigeration of reagents, but efforts are underway through lyophilization to remove this limitation to field deployability.

Therapy, Prevention, and Control

Treatment regimens are the same as for scrub typhus (see above). The basis of prevention of murine typhus is domestic rodent control directed at the Norway rat (*R norvegicus*) and the roof rat (*R rattus*). Good rodent control can be achieved by preventing access of rodents to buildings, practicing good sanitation, poison baiting, and trapping. Once an infestation of rodents occurs, it is important to protect people from existing flea populations before starting rodent control. The usual recommendation is to dust burrows (Norway rats only) and runs with carbaryl dust, but indoor flea treatments with pyrethroids would also be helpful. For individual service members, DEET in the standard Department of Defense repellent is effective against fleas. Where available, commercial aerosol repellents applied to the trousers and boots are convenient and will prevent flea bites when personnel pass through infested buildings or bunkers. Antibody assay of local domestic rodents would probably be the most sensitive indicator of the presence of murine typhus.

Epidemic Typhus Fever (*Rickettsia prowazekii*)

Introduction and Military Relevance

Epidemic typhus is a louse-borne rickettsial disease with significant mortality that tends to be associated with the poor hygiene frequently accompanying war and civil dislocations. During World War I, epidemic typhus killed 150,000 people in Serbia, including 50,000 prisoners of war and one third of the country's physicians.[510] During World War II, the threat of typhus led the US Secretary of War to establish the Typhus Commission. Because of the Commission's recommendations and research, advances were made in diagnostics, therapeutics, louse-control methods, and vaccine development (Figure 35-25). A military-wide program of vaccination and command enforcement of Commission

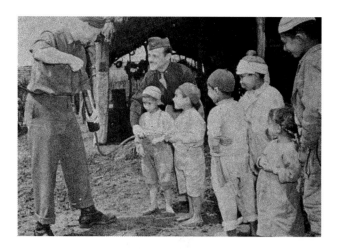

Fig. 35-25. Epidemic typhus prevention during World War II. US Army Medical Service personnel at the Mediterranean Base Section in Algiers treat Arab children with new insecticide powder (DDT) designed to kill typhus lice. Photograph: Courtesy of Dr. Theodore Woodward.

recommendations led to the occurrence of only 104 cases of epidemic typhus in the US Army during World War II, despite epidemic occurrence in other military and civilian populations.[510] There was no significant incidence of epidemic typhus in the US military during either the Korean or Vietnam wars. In contrast, immediately following World War II more than 30,000 cases were reported in Japan and Korea, with a 6% to 10% mortality rate in both countries.[523] Newer missions, including disaster and humanitarian relief efforts that entail medical care of displaced and refugee populations, are likely to place medical units at risk of infection.

Description of the Pathogen

The etiologic agent of epidemic typhus is *R prowazekii,* a Gram-negative, obligate intracellular bacterium that multiplies in the cytoplasm of infected cells. It shares group antigens with *R typhi*. Both typhus group rickettsiae have epitopes also found on the membranes of *Proteus* (OX-19) and *Legionella* bacilli.[511] The epitopes produce cross-reactions.

Epidemiology

Transmission. Humans are infected by *R prowazekii*–containing feces of the body louse (*Pediculus humanus*), which is distinct from the head louse. Body lice actually live and lay eggs in clothing, exiting at least daily to take blood from the host. Infection usually occurs by rubbing the crushed body or feces of the louse into its bite or into skin abrasions but may also occur by inhalation or exposure of mucous membranes. Humans act as the reservoir and maintain the infection between epidemics. Lice may become infected from patients with either acute or recrudescent typhus. *R prowazekii* can remain infectious for months in dried louse feces. In the United States, a zoonosis also exists in flying squirrels and the organism is occasionally spread to humans, most likely via the squirrel flea.

Geographic Distribution. Epidemic typhus occurs in colder climates where people live in conditions of poor hygiene leading to infestation by body lice. Endemic foci exist in the mountainous regions of Mexico and Guatemala, the Andes mountains in South America, the Himalayan countries (eg, Pakistan, Afghanistan), the highland region of Africa (eg, Ethiopia, Burundi, Rwanda, Lesotho) and northern China. The Balkans, Eastern Europe, and Russia continue to experience high rates of recrudescence (Brill-Zinsser disease) because of the millions of people infected during World War II.

Incidence. Epidemic typhus is usually associated with war, famine, and social disruption, which predispose to lousiness and increased population density. An example of this is the major outbreak during the war in Burundi in 1996 and 1997.[524] Endemic patterns of disease occur, such as the sporadic cases seen in the Andes, and are spread at low rates from either acute or recrudescent cases.

Pathogenesis and Clinical Findings

Epidemic typhus occurs after an incubation period of 8 to 12 days following exposure to the organism and is characterized by rickettsemia and systemic infection of endothelial cells. The disease is more severe than scrub or endemic typhus, with fatality rates of 10% to 60% in untreated patients. If the patient does not die in 14 to 18 days, he or she usually recovers, with defervescense over a 2- to 4-day period.

Diagnostic Approaches

Clinical. In the appropriate epidemiologic setting, louse-borne typhus should be suspected in patients with abrupt onset of persistent fever (39°C-41°C), intractable headache, and relative bradycardia. No eschar develops. A rash occurs after 4 to 7 days, starting on the trunk and spreading to the extremities. Multiple systems are involved; death is associated with stupor, renal failure, and hypoten-

sive shock.

Laboratory. The Weil-Felix agglutination test with *Proteus* OX-19 antigen is available and quite specific. IFA can be used to diagnose typhus but requires specific preabsorption to allow differentiation from murine typhus. Differentiation can also be made by species-specific complement fixation or toxin neutralization tests. *R prowazekii* can be isolated from blood or tissue by inoculation of tissue culture or guinea pigs. This is useful to prove etiology but is too slow for use in diagnosis of the individual patient.

Therapy, Prevention, and Control

Therapy. A single dose of doxycycline (100 or 200 mg) is the treatment of choice for epidemic typhus. Temperature usually normalizes in about 60 hours. Recrudescence, which is usually mild, may occur within months of initial infection or many years later (Brill-Zinsser disease); it should be treated with another course of the therapy. Supportive therapy and antibiotics for complicating infections may be required.

Prevention and Control. Medical personnel dealing with lousy prisoners of war or refugees are at considerable risk of infection by inhalation of louse feces and body parts during initial processing of these individuals. A simple particle filter paper mask probably minimizes risk until prisoners or refugees can be bathed and treated for lice. Personnel should also practice good hygiene by bathing after coming in contact with lousy people. The permethrin-treated battle dress uniform should prevent infestation of service members, but this has never been tested. Lice can be eliminated from clothing by boiling or dry cleaning and from individual people by application of pediculicides, but these techniques require a great deal of attention for each lousy person. Formerly, the US military had a system for quickly delousing people using a power duster to inject insecticidal powder into the clothes currently worn by a person. That system depended on an insecticide (lindane) that is no longer considered safe and on equipment that is no longer maintained. There is some possibility that ivermectin could be used as a systemic pediculicide and so eliminate the need for dusting lousy individuals, but this use of the drug has not yet been tested. Long-term control depends on improved hygiene and living conditions. When intensive exposure is anticipated, doxycycline may be used for prophylaxis (100 mg 1 or 2 times per week) although its efficacy has not been proven. Vaccines, consisting of either killed or attenuated organisms or of purified subunit proteins, have been developed and tested but are not currently available except in Russia. Noteworthy is the fact that murine typhus provides cross-immunity against epidemic typhus.[525]

Spotted Fever

Introduction and Military Relevance

Human diseases caused by spotted fever group (SFG) rickettsiae, while having wide geographic distribution, occur infrequently. The diseases and their etiologic agents include the ixodid tick-borne diseases Rocky Mountain spotted fever (RMSF) (*R rickettsii*), Mediterranean spotted fever (MSF) (other names: boutonneuse fever, Kenya tick typhus, Indian tick typhus, Marseilles fever) (*R conorii*), South African tick typhus (*R africae*), North Asian or Siberian tick typhus (*R sibirica*), Japanese spotted fever (*R japonica*), Queensland tick typhus (*R australis*), and Flinders Island agent *(R honei)*. Unlike their status as the reservoir of epidemic typhus–causing *R prowazekii*, humans are incidental hosts of SFG rickettsiae and become infected through the bite of infected ticks or mites that normally feed on a variety of small mammals. RMSF is the most severe of the SFG rickettsial diseases and is the most common fatal tick-borne disease in the United States. RMSF was first recognized in 1873 in the Bitter Root Valley of western Montana. Incidence has declined in that region since the 1930s while increasing in the eastern United States, where it had previously been uncommon.

Studies in military populations have documented the episodic impact of SFG rickettsioses on military training and operations in tick-infested areas.[526] During World War II, the first isolates of *R australis* were recovered from the blood of two soldiers deployed in North Queensland, Australia.[527] In 1989, a cluster of tick-borne infections due to *R rickettsii* or *Ehrlichia* species or both occurred in two military installations in the continental United States.[528] Following a 2-week deployment to Botswana in 1992, 31 of 169 US airborne soldiers based at Vicenza, Italy, were diagnosed with laboratory-confirmed spotted fever rickettsiosis consistent with African tick-bite fever.[529] Later that year, during Operation Restore Hope, MSF was diagnosed in a 36-year-old male soldier following deployment to Somalia.[530] Thus, while SFG rickettsioses continue to occur in service members, the impact of these diseases on military operations and readiness is quite limited.

Description of the Pathogen

The organisms that cause these diseases are Gram-negative, obligate intracellular bacteria that multiply in the cytoplasm of infected cells. In addition to the intracytoplasmic growth common to rickettsiae, the SFG organisms also grow within the nucleus in a small proportion of cells. They have common protein and lipopolysaccharide group antigens and some proteins distinguishable by Western blot. Polymerase chain reaction/restriction fragment length polymorphism (PCR/RFLP) analyses are most useful for identifying and distinguishing species.

Epidemiology

Transmission. Etiologic agents of the rickettsial spotted fevers are enzootic in nature. Several species of ixodid ticks function as reservoir, host, and vector. The agents are transmitted both vertically through transovarial passage and horizontally through vertebrate hosts of the ticks. In the eastern United States, the dog tick (*Dermacentor variabilis*) is the most common vector of *R rickettsii*; in the west it is the wood tick (*D andersoni*). *Amblyomma cajennense* is the common vector in Central and South America. *Rhipicephalus sanguineus* is the most common vector of *R conorii* in Europe, Asia, and northern Africa; in east and southern Africa, *Haemaphysalis* (spreading *R conorii*) and *Amblyomma* (spreading *R africae*) ticks have been implicated. *D nutallii* (spreading *R sibirica*) and *Ixodes holocyclus* (spreading *R australis*) are also vectors.

Geographic Distribution. In the United States, the vast majority of cases of RMSF are reported in the southeastern states, particularly North and South Carolina, but cases are reported in nearly all states.[531] *R rickettsii* is distributed throughout the Western hemisphere; *R conorii* in Africa and the Mediterranean littoral including France, Italy, and Spain; *R australis* in Australia; *R japonica* in Japan; and *R sibirica* in Asia and Eurasia. New distributions are likely to occur; spotted fever was described in both Japan and Thailand for the first time in the 1990s.[532,533]

Incidence. The incidence of RMSF in the United States increased through the 1960s and 1970s to a high of 1,192 cases in 1981, then declined steadily to about half that number in 1995.[534] Recent incidences have been highest in Oklahoma, the Carolinas, and Tennessee, with these states accounting for half of all reported cases.[531] Ninety percent of cases occurred between April and September, with half presenting in May and June. There were 242 cases of RMSF in the United States between 1981 and 1992, 4% of which were fatal; however, in a Brazilian outbreak in 1990-1991, four of six cases were fatal.[535] The fatality rate for MSF has been reported at 2.5%.[536]

Pathogenesis and Clinical Findings

Pathogenesis of the SFG rickettsiae is similar to that of the scrub typhus group and typhus groups, with endothelial cells, including those of capillaries, being the primary target. The bite of the arthropod vector (in the case of ticks, the tick can remain attached for several hours) results in the inoculation of rickettsiae directly into the dermis. Infection by scarification of tick feces and inoculation of conjunctiva by crushed tick juices have been reported. The incubation period for RMSF is 2 to 14 days (mean of 7 days)[531] and about 20% of patients have a small primary lesion. The disease is characterized by fever (in 94% of patients), severe headache (86%), myalgia (82%), rash (80%), malaise, nausea, vomiting, and abdominal pain. The rash appears on about the third day of illness and is pink and maculopapular, localized to the forearms, palms, soles, and legs. In MSF, the frequency of rash is nearly 100% and an initial cutaneous lesion with a necrotic center ("tache noire") at the site of tick bite is frequent[536] (Figure 35-26). The disease course of MSF, Oriental spotted fever, and African, Siberian, and Queensland tick typhus tends to be milder than that of Israeli MSF, which is itself milder than that of RMSF.

Diagnostic Approaches

Clinical. Only about half of confirmed cases of RMSF have the classic triad of rash, fever, and headache.[531] Absence of a rash ("spotless fever") or having G6PD deficiency is associated with increased severity. RMSF should be suspected in patients exposed to wooded areas from April to October or with a specific history of tick bite.

Laboratory. The IFA test remains the standard serological test for the SFG rickettsiae and is highly group specific and group sensitive. Four-fold rises in IgG to greater than 1:64 are considered to be diagnostic, whereas single serum titers greater than 1:128 are suggestive. For MSF, a 4-fold rise or a single titer greater than 1:80 in conjunction with presence of two of the three signs of fever, rash, and eschar is considered diagnostic.[536] Antigen slides for IFA and dipstick assays for detection of *R rickettsii* and *R conorii* are available commercially. The agents can be identified *in situ* by direct fluorescent antibody staining of frozen sections of biopsied lesions. The test is highly specific; however, a sensitivity of about 70% means that a negative test does not rule out infection. Polymerase chain reaction was used to diagnose SFG rickettsiosis in a soldier whose biopsy was negative by direct fluorescent antibody.[530]

Therapy, Prevention, and Control

Therapy. Empiric treatment should be initiated before laboratory confirmation (tetracycline: 25 mg/

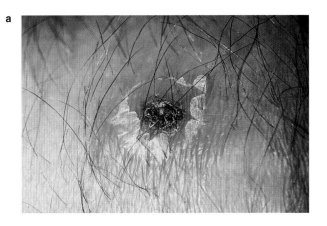 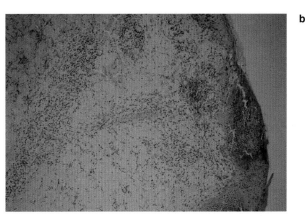

Fig. 35-26. (a) An eschar or "tache noire" on the right calf of a soldier who acquired *Rickettsia conorii* infection in Somalia in 1993. Note the centralized necrosis within the lesion. (b) A hematoxylin and eosin stain of biopsied section (x140) from the eschar in (a). Note the necrosis of the epidermis and the superficial dermis and the perivascular lymphohistiocytic infiltrate with endothelial cell swelling.
Reprinted with permission from: Williams WJ, Radulovic S, Dasch GA, et al. Identification of *Rickettsia conorii* infection by polymerase chain reaction in a soldier returning from Somalia. *Clin Infect Dis.* 1994;19:93–99.

kg per d in four divided doses, doxycycline: 200 mg/d in two divided doses, or chloramphenicol: 50 mg/kg per d in four divided doses).

Prevention and Control. Ticks are often concentrated at the edges of roads, along paths created by large mammals, and near places where animals get water. The permethrin-treated battle dress uniform offers excellent protection from ticks. DEET in the standard DoD repellent discourages tick bites. DEET applied to the trousers and boot tops repels ticks crawling up the outer clothing to find a place to bite. Blousing trousers inside the boots provides more protection than using elastic bands. Area treatment with pesticides for ticks is effective, especially at encampments, fighting positions, and along paths. In infested areas, service members should check themselves for attached ticks at least twice a day, examining all areas including the groin, perineum, and hairline. Whenever possible, ticks should be removed with a forceps, grasping the tick as close to the skin as possible and pulling with a steady, increasing tension. A fully attached tick can sometimes be dislodged more easily if a sterile needle is used to loosen the mouthparts, probing their ventral side while pulling with forceps. All skin contact with the tick should be avoided to prevent exposure to infectious hemolymph (tick blood released from a crushed tick) or coxal fluid (a clear liquid released from glands between the legs during feeding). Where ticks are particularly abundant, it can be useful to keep a small container of alcohol for disposal of ticks. Surveillance of ticks can be accomplished with tick drags (pieces of cloth trailed through the area of interest) or carbon dioxide released from dry ice on a white cloth. No licensed vaccine is presently available.

[Arthur E. Brown, Daniel A. Strickman, Daryl J. Kelly]

PLAGUE

Introduction and Military History

Plague is one of the most deadly infectious diseases in history and has been a "traditional scourge of military operations,"[537p8] often "brought in the train of armies or of commerce."[538p167] The disruption and devastation that occur in the wake of a war lead to a breakdown in sanitary conditions, to crowding, and consequently to favorable conditions for the proliferation of rats and fleas. Despite the expansion of medical knowledge in the 20th century, humans have not been able to eradicate the disease, as is evidenced by a succession of outbreaks and the persistence of natural foci.[538]

In addition to its potential to cause substantial mortality, plague can have a tremendous psychological impact, as is described by Cartwright: "The Black Death must have seemed to be of supernatural origin, a punishment inflicted by a higher power upon unknown sinners for unknown crimes."[539p46] In 1994, an outbreak of pneumonia with a high fatality rate in India was perceived as a global health emergency[540] and caused heightened awareness and increased surveillance internationally.[541] There were press reports at the time describing an exodus of hundreds of thousands of people from the city of Surat, where the outbreak began. The cost of implementing emergency response systems internationally and the losses in Indian tourism were substantial.[542] A few cases were later confirmed as plague but by unvalidated serologic techniques. The devastating psychological and economic consequences of the Indian experience, however, illustrate the importance of using microbiological confirmation and a thorough assessment of risks by a multidisciplinary team before declaring an epidemic emergency.[540,543]

The first documented plague epidemic may have been the Bible's description of illness among the Philistines in 1320 BC.[538,539,544] Since then, there have been three pandemics, all related in part to military operations. The first was the Justinian plague of the 6th century, named after the Byzantine emperor at the time. The outbreak began in Egypt and spread throughout Asia Minor, Africa, and Europe via merchant and military travel. In Constantinople, the epidemic affected the city for 4 months, with 5,000 to 10,000 people dying each day during peak periods. Many of the city's services were disrupted, including the food supply.[545] Warnefried, a German monk and historian from the 8th century, chronicled the devastation made by the disease, which "depopulated towns, turned the country into a desert, and made habitations of men to become the haunts of wild beasts."[544p12] The second, and most well-known, pandemic began its spread to Europe in Caffa, on the Black Sea, in 1346. It has been alleged that the outbreak within the city walls began after Tartar armies besieging the city began catapulting plague-infected corpses into the city. Individuals fleeing the area and merchant ships were suspected of carrying the infection to Europe, beginning a series of epidemics throughout the continent that killed up to one fourth of the population[546] and became known as the "black death."[538] Before devastating Europe, the disease had already killed 250 million Asians.[545] The third pandemic occurred from 1894 to 1920 and may continue today.[540] It began when Chinese troops were sent to the Yunnan Province, a plague-endemic area, to quell a Muslim rebellion. The disease subsequently spread—via a series of outbreaks that followed the military's movements to the coastal cities and beyond—to surrounding Asian countries.[538] During World War II, there were numerous reports of outbreaks in North Africa and the China-Burma-India theater among the civilian population in endemic regions. DDT was used for flea control along with other measures, including rodent trapping, poisoning, and gassing; community sanitation; spraying of ships and aircraft for insect vectors; inspection and quarantining of cases; and restricting access to high-risk areas.[547] During the Vietnam War, although the country was widely known to be endemic for plague and service members were definitely exposed to rat fleas (as was shown by 58 cases of murine typhus), US vaccination efforts may have been the reason there were only eight recognized cases among US forces.[537,548] The US military has not had a severe problem from the disease, largely due to the implementation of effective control measures. Respect for this disease is warranted, though, because an army could be incapacitated quickly by an outbreak of pneumonic plague.

Because of the devastation it can cause, plague is a potential biological warfare agent.[549] During World War II, the Japanese conducted biological warfare experiments on Chinese prisoners, exposing them to plague and other agents. The Japanese also released rice and wheat with plague-infected fleas over Chuhsien and Ningpo in China, killing 21 and 99 people, respectively.[550] During the Korean War, there were unsubstantiated allegations that US planes scattered plague- and cholera-infected insects.[550,551]

Although service members can be at risk for plague when engaged in combat or during operations involving disasters, refugees, or humanitarian assistance, they may also be at risk during routine training exercises in the United States. Plague has been detected in rodents on or around military installations in California, Arizona, Colorado, New Mexico, Washington, Oregon, Texas, and Utah.[552] A case of bubonic plague in a soldier was reported in 1992 after the soldier had been in central California on a military exercise.[553]

Description of the Pathogen

Plague is caused by infection with the Gram-negative, nonspore-forming, nonmotile coccobacillus *Yersinia pseudotuberculosis* subspecies *pestis*, commonly known as *Y pestis* and previously known as *Pasteurella pestis*.[538,554] It was first isolated and described in 1894 by Kitsato and Yersin while both were studying an outbreak of bubonic plague in Hong Kong.[538] Controversy still exists over which one should properly receive credit for discovery of the organism.[546]

Epidemiology

Transmission

Plague is primarily a zoonotic disease of wild rodents[538] and is typically transmitted among them or to other animals (including domestic animals) or humans by the bite of infected fleas infesting the animals. In addition to vector-borne transmission, plague can be transmitted by infected body fluids and tissues through cuts and abrasions. Transmission by ingestion of infected tissues by carnivores has been demonstrated[546] and could theoretically occur in those who ingest uncooked or undercooked rodent meat. Infection can also occur by mechanical spread of airborne organisms through ocular and oropharyngeal mucous membranes. Direct spread to the lungs by infectious droplet nuclei from a human or animal with pneumonic or pharyngeal plague also occurs.[554] Asymptomatic individuals with culture-proven pharyngeal plague have been noted,[546,555] but their role in the transmission of human infections is not known.

Except in the case of pneumonic plague, humans are both accidental and dead-end hosts and do not play a role in the maintenance of *Y pestis* in nature. The risk of transmission to humans corresponds to the presence of the flea vector because plague is generally transmitted to humans by the bite of an infected flea. The largest outbreaks in humans have had the common black and brown rats as reservoirs (*Rattus rattus* and *Rattus norvegicus*, respectively) and the oriental rat flea (*Xenopsylla cheopis*) as the vector.[546] In the United States, only sporadic cases of human plague occur and are generally associated with sylvatic foci and reservoirs such as the ground squirrel, rock squirrel, and prairie dog.[556] Large-scale human outbreaks can occur, however, if humans live in overcrowded, unsanitary urban conditions near a large infected commensal or wild rodent population. Plague is generally felt to occur when humans enter the areas of rodent habitat while an epizootic is ongoing, but infected animals may enter areas of human habitat as well.[557] This includes domestic dogs and cats, which may carry infected fleas into homes.[62p381-387] Since 1977, cats have played an important role in transmitting plague, including pneumonic plague, to humans in the United States.[558]

Geographic Distribution

In recent years, plague has been reported on the major continental areas of North and South America, Africa, and Asia.

Incidence

Data on worldwide incidence are crude and incomplete. In addition, no uniform criteria exist for defining a confirmed or suspected case.[546] For the period 1978 through 1993, there were 16,921 cases and 1,642 (9.7%) deaths reported worldwide (average of 1,057 cases per year, range of 200 to 1,966 per year). During the period 1978 through 1992, the six countries that reported human plague nearly every year were Brazil, Madagascar, Burma, the United Republic of Tanzania, the United States, and Vietnam. China has reported cases annually since 1985. From 1983 through 1992, 61% of cases and 77% of deaths occurred in Africa.[559]

Plague has exhibited a seasonal incidence. In the United States between 1950 and 1975, 84% of cases related to exposure to wild animals and their fleas occurred between May and September. In Brazil, October to December is the peak time. The fluctuations may be related either to seasons when people spend more time outdoors either for leisure or working during the harvest or to variations in reservoir populations. The seasonal variation may also be related to characteristics of the flea vector. The life span of *X cheopis* is 27 days once its feeding tube is blocked by the plague bacillus; however, the fleas will die rapidly if the temperature rises or the humidity falls. In addition, coagulation of the ingested blood in the alimentary tract of the flea is felt to be important in the disease cycle and does not occur at temperatures greater than 25°C.[546]

From 1944 through 1993, there were 362 reported human plague cases in the United States, with the majority occurring in New Mexico, California, Colorado, and Arizona. Human plague has now been reported from all states in the western continental United States, and epizootic plague appears to be spreading eastward and northward.[540,558] In 1993,

there were 10 confirmed cases: seven bubonic, two primary septicemic, and one pneumonic. There was one death. Recent trends include peri-domestic transmission, with cats as a source of human infection[558] and increased risk of human infection because of urban spread into previously wild areas.[552]

Pathogenesis and Clinical Findings

After the flea ingests a blood meal from an animal with *Y pestis* bacteremia, a coagulase from the bacilli clots the blood in the flea's foregut, thus blocking its ability to swallow. The organism multiplies in the clotted blood. During subsequent feeding attempts, thousands of organisms may be regurgitated by the flea into a person's skin. Once in the skin, the bacteria travel through lymphatic channels to regional lymph nodes. Host mononuclear phagocytes and polymorphonuclear leukocytes phagocytize the bacilli, which have a small amount of envelope antigen. The bacilli are not destroyed but may multiply in the mononuclear phagocytes and become relatively resistant to more phagocytosis once the mononuclear cell lyses. Infected lymph nodes are notable for concentrations of extracellular bacilli and polymorphonuclear leukocytes, as well as destruction of the normal lymph node architecture and hemorrhagic necrosis. Explosive multiplication of the organisms occurs with transient bacteria. In the absence of therapy, intense and destructive inflammatory reactions occur in many organs, especially the lymph nodes, liver, and spleen. Explosive bacterial growth generally precedes death.[546,560]

Cases of plague are categorized as bubonic, septicemic, and pneumonic, although other more benign forms have been recognized.

Bubonic Plague

A patient with bubonic plague typically will have the acute onset of fever, malaise, headache, and diffuse aches from 1 to 7 days after being bitten by an infected flea. This may be followed by nausea and vomiting several hours later,[62,538] although vaccination may reduce the incidence and severity of disease.[561] Localized pain and tenderness will occur before palpable adenitis. Buboes are characteristic of the disease but not pathognomonic and usually involve a single lymph node chain in the groin, axilla, or neck. The infecting bite usually occurs on the lower extremity, hence the femoral nodes are the nodes affected up to 90% of the time.[538,553] The bubo can be so tender that patients attempt to avoid any movement of the affected area.[544,556] A striking feature of bubonic plague is the sudden onset of the fever with a bubo, the rapid development of intense inflammation in the bubo, and the fulminant course that can produce death as quickly as 2 to 4 days after the onset of symptoms.[556] The mortality from bubonic plague in treated individuals is 2% but as high as 50% to 60% in the untreated.[562,563]

Patients with bubonic plague may have a variety of dermatologic findings. Up to one fourth of patients in Vietnam had pustules, vesicles, eschars, or papules near the bubo or anatomic area drained by the affected lymph nodes. Rarely, these lesions can progress to cellulitis or abscesses; they may even ulcerate, yielding a large carbuncle.[555,556] A small vesicle (which may go unnoticed) or carbuncles can develop at the primary site of infection, or secondary carbuncles or necrotic ulcers of hematogenous origin may develop on all parts of the body. Generalized pustular eruptions, known as plague pox or plague variola, have been recorded. The dermatologic findings may coincide with or precede the formation of the buboes.[544] Plague meningitis is a complication that can occur when the meninges are hematogenously seeded from a bubo, often after bubonic plague has been inadequately treated.

Septicemic Plague

Septicemic plague can be secondary to untreated bubonic plague or it can be primary, in the absence of adenopathy. Dissemination to any organ can occur, but the most common sites are the lungs, eyes, meninges, joints, and skin. Small vessels can be occluded secondary to vasculitis, leading to purpura and even gangrene of the skin and digits. These obvious physical examination findings probably are responsible for the term "black death."[554] Septicemic plague is rapidly fatal if untreated.

Pneumonic Plague

Plague may affect the lungs in several forms, which exist along a continuum: well-marked foci with consolidation, congestion and edema without consolidation, or a transitory form with a slight pneumonitis.[538,544] The first of these three types is classic pneumonic plague. The patient does not develop a bubo but within 24 hours of the onset of symptoms develops a cough with mucopurulent sputum, which may progress to sanguinopurulent sputum.[538] Although the patient appears acutely ill, it may take 6 to 8 hours for definite signs of clinical pneumonitis to appear. Chest x-ray evidence of pulmonary infiltration can be present despite the initial lack of physical signs of pneumonia.[544,564]

Secondary pneumonic plague occurs in persons with bubonic or septicemic plague when the lungs are seeded by organisms in the bloodstream. In patients with secondary pneumonic plague, average survival time ranges between 2 and 4 days.[553] Primary pneumonic plague occurs from the inhalation of infectious droplet nuclei expelled from a person or animal with pneumonic plague. The average survival time for those with primary pneumonic plague is 1.8 days.[562] The public health consequences of pneumonic plague can be serious[554] because it has a short incubation period of 2 to 4 days, is rapidly fatal, and spreads rapidly to close contacts. An outbreak of pneumonic plague could literally halt an army unit in its tracks.

Plague pharyngitis is a rare form of the disease that may occur as a result of inhalation of organisms from patients with pneumonic plague or from ingestion of plague organisms. Patients with plague pharyngitis may have anterior cervical lymph node swelling and tonsillar exudates, although asymptomatic forms have been noted.[546,555]

Other

More benign forms of plague have been noted. In the type called "ambulant" plague, a vesicle forms at the site of skin inoculation and there is mild local lymphangitis without systemic signs. A second type, called "pestis minor," may have a variable presentation and is difficult to distinguish from cases of bubonic plague without significant bacteria. One or more lymph nodes may be involved, but there is not the significant pain associated with bubonic plague. The patient may have some systemic complaints of fever, headache, and prostration, but the complaints do not last longer than a week and do not include the marked local inflammation of bubonic plague.[544] Pestis minor occurs more commonly at the beginning and end of outbreaks and has been postulated to be related to subinfective doses of *Y pestis*, probably transmitted by flea bites, immunizing the population. Asymptomatic forms of plague exist, since individuals without clinical illness have had plague cultured from the throat despite either antibiotic treatment or vaccination.[555] Whether these "carriers" are contagious is not known.

Diagnostic Approaches

Plague can lead to death in a matter of hours to days in 60% to 90% of patients if they are untreated.[538] Early recognition is key to survival, especially in patients with pneumonic or septicemic plague. Risk for fatality has been linked to a delay in proper diagnosis and treatment.[558] The first step in diagnosis must be a high index of suspicion in a febrile patient who lives in or has recently visited an endemic area. Suspicion should be heightened if the patient recalls contact with fleas or direct contact with wild animals or the physical examination demonstrates a painful bubo, a cough, or meningeal signs (Figure 35-27). Patients are typically febrile with a tachycardia and may be hypotensive secondary to vasodilation. In addition, physical examination may also demonstrate a palpable and tender liver and spleen.[556] The leukocyte count is typically but not necessarily elevated (even up to 50,000/mm³).[538]

Plague may present in an atypical manner, leading to delay in diagnosis and death. Crook and Tempest,[565] in a review of 27 cases seen at an Indian hospital in New Mexico from 1965 through 1989 categorized plague patients into five clinical presentations: (1) classic bubonic plague, (2) fever, sore throat, and headache, (3) nonspecific febrile syndrome, (4) fever with urinary or gastrointestinal symptoms, and (5) fever with meningeal signs. Six out of ten patients in the second and third presentation categories died, mainly because they were given antibiotics (penicillin derivatives) that did not affect plague. Some of the other patients, although not initially considered to have plague, were given antibiotics with activity against plague.

Some of the other diseases that may be considered in the differential diagnosis of plague include tularemia, meningococcemia (because the ecchymoses and purpura seen can occur with plague meningitis), hemorrhagic smallpox, and diphtheria (because pharyngeal or tonsillar plague can have the appearance of a pseudomembrane, and the appearance of the lymph nodes may be similar to that seen in other bacterial infections). If *Y pestis* is used as a biological weapon, the differential diagnosis of an epidemic of pneumonic plague in its early stages might include tularemia, anthrax infection, or staphylococcal enterotoxin B intoxication.[549]

In the field, plague bacilli may be observed in a bubo aspirate or a peripheral blood smear. To aspirate a bubo, one can use a 20 gauge needle with a 10 mL syringe and 1 mL of sterile saline. Saline is first injected with the needle directed toward the periphery of the bubo, then without removing the needle from the skin the syringe is withdrawn a few times until the aspirate becomes blood-tinged. The aspirate can then be used for direct visualization on a slide, using Wayson's or Giemsa stains. The background will appear pink with the Wayson's stain, and the plague bacilli will be appear light blue with dark polar bodies 1 to 2 mm long.[546] They can appear singly or in pairs and can be pleomorphic[538]; they have been described as looking similar to a safety pin.[554]

If more elaborate diagnostic laboratory capabilities exist in the field or in garrison, diagnosis can be confirmed by culture of any involved site on blood and MacConkey agar plates or an infusion broth. Pinpoint colonies may appear on agar after 24 hours at 35°C. The optimal growth rate occurs at 28°C.[546] Serum passive hemagglutination or complement fixation techniques can be used for laboratory confirmation if cultures are unsuccessful.[553] Fluorescent antibody tests on bubo aspirates, sputum, or cerebrospinal fluid can aid in rapid diagnosis if the tests are available.[546]

Recommendations for Therapy and Control

Therapy

According to the World Health Organization expert committee on plague, patients should receive at least 10 days of treatment. Streptomycin is generally considered the drug of choice and is given intramuscularly at a dose of 30 mg/kg daily in two divided doses. Tetracycline 2 to 4 g daily by mouth in four divided doses is an alternative regimen for streptomycin-allergic patients for whom an oral drug is appropriate. Patients who are hypotensive and would have poor intramuscular absorption and those with plague meningitis should receive

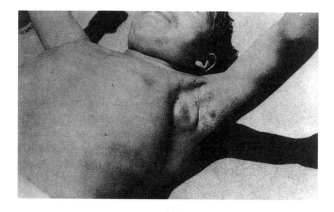

Fig. 35-27. Patient with a bubo. Buboes are extremely tender, and usually involve a lymph node chain draining the site of the infecting flea bite. Although this picture shows a bubo in the armpit, bites are most commonly on the lower extremities, hence femoral nodes are the most common site for buboes.
Photograph: Courtesy of the Armed Forces Institute of Pathology, negative 219900 (7B).

chloramphenicol because it can be given intravenously and has superior penetration of the cerebrospinal fluid. A loading dose of 25 mg/kg can be given intravenously, followed by 60 mg/kg per day in four divided doses. As the patient improves, the dose may be given orally and decreased to 30mg/kg per day to lessen bone marrow suppression.[546,560,566]

Because of plague's high case fatality rate, appropriate treatment must be initiated immediately when plague infection is suspected. Efforts to confirm the diagnosis by culture must not delay the initiation of antibiotic therapy. Patients with pneumonic or pharyngeal plague require droplet isolation precautions for at least 48 hours of therapy or until their sputum or throat cultures are negative. Support staff should use masks, gowns, gloves, and eye protection.[62,538] Drainage and secretion precautions should be used for patients with bubonic plague until 48 hours after beginning antimicrobial treatment; sputum, purulent discharges, and soiled articles need to be disinfected. In outbreaks where fleas are involved, patients, their clothing, and their belongings need to be treated with insecticide to kill the fleas.[62]

Control

Although plague is generally restricted to certain geographic areas worldwide, it has the potential to be imported across international boundaries, so public health authorities should maintain an awareness of the worldwide incidence.[543,546] Plague, cholera, and yellow fever are the three internationally quarantinable diseases.[567] Before departing from a country with an ongoing pneumonic plague epidemic, travelers suspected of significant exposure are required by international regulations to be isolated for 6 days. In addition, those arriving in a country on a vessel suspected to be plague-infested may require disinfecting and surveillance for illness for up to 6 days.[62]

Strategies for control, depending on personnel, resources, and extent of spread, include antibiotic treatment of cases, flea control with insecticides, rodent control by poisoning and trapping, proper garbage disposal, proper food storage, rat-proofing of buildings, antibiotic prophylaxis for potential contacts of pneumonic plague, quarantine of human cases, ship inspection in ports, vaccine administration, and education of the population to avoid contacts with rodents, prevent rodent harborage, and control fleas on pets.[62,546] In a bubonic plague outbreak, it is imperative to institute flea-control measures before killing rodents,[62,538] because fleas will leave a dead rodent and search for a new host, increasing the risk of human infection.[552] Pneumonic plague cases must be isolated, and all household and other close contacts should be given antibiotic prophylaxis with tetracycline (15 to 30 mg/kg) or chloramphenicol (30 mg/kg) daily in four divided doses for 1 week after contact. Close contacts of confirmed bubonic plague cases should be appropriately disinfested with insecticide and put under surveillance for signs of infection.[62]

In the absence of an outbreak situation, ongoing surveillance needs to be added to the measures listed above, especially in endemic areas. The US Army Plague Surveillance Program consists of rodent and flea population characterization through trapping rodents and collecting their fleas, rodent population observation, carnivore blood serum collection, and continuous collaboration with local and state health authorities. These measures should provide baseline information for the early recognition of an epizootic and the need for an epizootic investigation.[552]

The licensed, whole cell, formalin-killed vaccine is no longer manufactured in the United States and is therefore no longer available. Individuals in the past who would have been considered for vaccination included laboratory workers, those who frequently handle field or clinical materials that are potentially infected, those who work in the wilderness with limited access to medical care (eg, Army Special Forces personnel, wildlife and fish workers), and those who work or reside in endemic areas, including Peace Corps workers, journalists, photographers, disaster workers,[554] and certain military personnel (eg, Special Forces). The schedule of the licensed vaccine was three intramuscular doses: 1.0 mL initially, then smaller doses of 0.2 mL at 1 to 3 months after the first dose and 5 to 6 months following the second dose. Then 0.2 mL was given at 6 and 12 months following the completion of the initial series and then every 1 to 2 years, if required.

No randomized field trials exist to substantiate the claim that killed plague vaccines are effective in preventing human disease. Indirect evidence of its efficacy have been cited instead: the fact that there were no cases of plague in World War II among vaccinated US troops and only eight cases during the Vietnam War, despite considerable exposure in both instances.[546] About 7% of vaccinees fail to produce adequate antibody following the initial series. Work is being done to find a more effective plague vaccine. Studies using plague subunit vaccines have demonstrated protection of mice against pneumonic disease.[568,569] Despite prior vaccination, someone with a definite exposure should receive prophylactic antibiotics as previously described.[561] In epidemic situations or when risk of contact with infected rodents or fleas is felt to be high, chemoprophylaxis with tetracycline may be indicated.[570] Also, individuals should understand the importance of personal protective measures, including wearing shoes, wearing clothing that covers the legs, using insect repellent, and wearing gloves when handling potentially infected laboratory specimens and when handling ill or dead animals.[556]

With recent concerns about biological terrorism, plague is at the top of both military and civilian threat lists.[571–575] A recent public health consensus panel has published recommendations for public health management of plague if used as a bioterrorist weapon.[576] Plague will continue to be a concern for the US military as long as plague remains a potential biological warfare agent and military operations take place in plague-endemic regions of the world. As the outbreak in India has shown, the Black Death has periodically gone into hiding, only to resurface with a vengeance.[539] Therefore, the US military and public health community must remain vigilant in their surveillance for this disease to avoid unpleasant surprises in the future.

[Mark G. Kortepeter]

FILARIASIS

Introduction and Military Relevance

Five species of roundworms cause significant human filariasis. Of these, three species cause lymphatic filariasis: *Wuchereria bancrofti*, *Brugia malayi*, and *B timori*. *Onchocerca volvulus* causes river blindness, and *Loa loa* causes dermal afflictions. Three other species can be found in humans but cause little or no morbidity: *Mansonella streptocerca*, *M perstans*, and *M ozzardi*.

Because of their incubation periods of several months, the filarial diseases do not have an immediate tactical impact but may have an operational impact. Filarial fevers, adenitis, and retrograde lymphangitis can be debilitating, especially in the case of brugian filariasis. No effective therapy was available during World War II, and high rates were seen among US servicemen in the Pacific theater. In some units, 30% became infected and symptoms included pain and erythema of the scrotum (56%), arms (38%), and legs (14%).[577]

Bancroftian Filariasis

Description of the Pathogen

Adult *W bancrofti* are creamy white worms measuring 80 to 100 mm long (females) or about 40 mm long (males). Bancroftian microfilaria are speciated by identifying a sheath but no caudal nuclei.

Epidemiology

The larvae of *W bancrofti* are transmitted by a mosquito, typically *Culex quinquifaciatus*, *Anopheles gambiae*, *An funestus*, *Aedes polynesienses*, *Ae scapularis*, or *Ae pseudoscutellaris*.[62p197–201] Humans are the sole reservoir of the disease. *W bancrofti* is the most common and widespread of the filarias infecting humans,[577] affecting populations in sub-Saharan Africa, Asia, the Pacific, the Caribbean region, the eastern coastal plains of South America, and portions of Central America.[578] The World Health Organization estimated in 1994 that 751 million people live in areas endemic for lymphatic filariasis. Of those, 72.8 million were infected with *W bancrofti*.[579]

The incidence of filariasis in immunologically naive arrivals to an endemic area can be quite high. In Indonesia, farmers who moved from nonendemic to endemic areas had microfilarial rates of 6% to 35%.[580] As mentioned above, *W bancrofti* infected servicemen in the Pacific theater during World War II. The major difference between these two natural experiments is that the Indonesian farmers stayed in the infected areas and many of them subsequently developed elephantiasis, as opposed to the World War II soldiers who were evacuated from the region with resolution of their symptoms. Thus, it appears that continued reexposure to the organism leads to the more permanent effects of chronic filariasis.

Pathogenesis and Clinical Findings

When an infected mosquito takes a blood meal, the larvae migrate from its mouthparts onto the person's skin. From there the larvae enter the body through the puncture site, and they typically take up residence in the lymphatic vessels. The females produce microfilariae, which reach the bloodstream 6 to 12 months after infection. The pathogenesis is more commonly due to inflammation and blockage of the lymphatic channels by adult worms, which manifest themselves 3 to 12 months after infection, than to the presence of microfilariae.[581]

The spectrum of disease ranges from infection

without symptoms to the chronic effects of blocked lymphatic vessels. Most filarial infections do not cause symptoms,[581] but the asymptomatically infected still serve as a reservoir. The incubation period varies from 6 to 12 months, but allergic reactions can occur 1 month after infection.

Indigenous and nonindigenous peoples display different clinical features. In populations raised in filarial regions, the disease spectrum ranges from asymptomatic with no detectable microfilaremia to such signs of chronic infection as hydrocele, chylurea, or elephantiasis of limbs, genitalia, or breasts. In those with "expatriate syndrome" (when military personnel or other migrants to endemic areas have acquired these infections), the symptoms typically consist of genital pain (from inflammation of the associated lymphatics), lymphangitis, and lymphandenitis, as well as hives, rashes, eosinophilia, and other allergic manifestations.

Tropical pulmonary eosinophilia is an amicrofilaremic lung condition associated with the lymphatic filariases. It is characterized by a primarily nocturnal paroxysmal cough and wheeze with scanty sputum production, occasional weight loss, adenopathy, low-grade fever, and extreme eosinophilia (greater than $3,000/mm^3$). If not treated with diethylcarbamazine citrate (DEC), tropical pulmonary eosinophilia can progress to a debilitating, chronic, interstitial lung disease.[582]

Diagnostic Approaches

The gold standard for diagnosing bancroftian filariasis (but not brugian filariasis) is detecting circulating filarial antigen (CFA) in the bloodstream.[583] One CFA assay is a semiqualitative ELISA test that requires technical skill and expensive equipment. A simpler CFA assay is the "card test," which yields positive or negative results. The card test has replaced the more cumbersome method of directly demonstrating the parasite by the examination of nocturnally collected blood samples. A colormetric indicator displays a pink line when the test is positive. The test is inexpensive (less than US $1 per card), useable by nonclinicians, and gives immediate results. Its versatility allows the card test to be a diagnostic tool in both the clinical and field setting.

Recommendations for Therapy and Control

Treatment can be either tailored to an individual patient or designed to eliminate filariasis from a community. For individuals, treatment is with DEC, which kills microfilariae and is toxic to adult worms when given at the doses listed in Exhibit 35-2. If no microfilariae can be found in the blood or skin, then full doses (6 mg/kg per day in 3 doses) can be given beginning on day 1. Variations of treatment include a Brazilian treatment protocol that showed efficacy with DEC at 6 mg/kg per day in single, daily doses for 12 days.[584] Additionally, ivermectin, 20 to 200 mg/kg in a single dose, may be effective in clearing microfilariae but does not affect adult worms.[585]

The side effects of DEC are common and can be profound. An inflammatory response marked by fever, nausea, vomiting, arthralgia, chills, and headache is caused by the DEC-induced disintegration of microfilaria. These side effects are reduced by slowly introducing DEC to patients as described in the above dosing schedule. As with many inflammatory and allergic responses, these side effects can be ameliorated by corticosteroids and antihistamines.[585]

Mass treatment by medicated salt or single annual doses combined with vector control are effective ways to control or even eradicate filariasis in a population. DEC-medicated salt can eliminate lym-

---

EXHIBIT 35-2

DOSAGES OF DEC FOR TREATING BANCROFTIAN FILARIASIS

	Adult	Child
Day 1	50 mg, taken orally after a meal	1 mg/kg, taken orally after a meal
Day 2	50 mg, three times a day	1 mg/kg, three times a day
Day 3	100 mg, three times a day	1–2 mg/kg, three times a day
Days 4–21	6 mg/kg per day in three doses	6 mg/kg per day in three doses

Source: Drugs for parasitic infection. *Med Lett Drugs Ther.* 1993;35(911):111–122.

phatic filariasis from a population. Regular table salt fortified with 0.3% DEC has been shown to greatly reduce, and even to eliminate in some areas, the incidence of bancroftian filariasis and, to a lesser extent, *B malayi* filariasis.[586] At such a low dose, DEC has no notable side effects.

Another way to treat populations is annual, single-dose treatment. Annual, single doses of ivermectin (400 mg/kg) with DEC (6 mg/kg) have also been shown to reduce prevalence by 32% and microfilarial levels by 96% 12 months after treatment.[587] Annual, single-dose treatment with DEC alone or ivermectin alone has also been shown to be effective.

Vector control will lower the incidence of filariasis. Vectors can be controlled by pesticides, polystyrene beads dropped in latrines, larvicides, and larvae-eating creatures introduced into mosquito-breeding sites. Ultra-low-volume malathion spraying is effective against adult forms of the mosquito.[580] A major vector of *W bancrofti* in urban areas is *C quinquifaciatus*. This domestic mosquito's larvae develop in organically rich waters such as are found in pit latrines. Tossing a 4- to 6-cm layer of polystyrene beads into pit latrines is effective in reducing the incidence of bancroftian filariasis.[588] The polystyrene beads form a floating layer, which carpets the surface of the water. This inhibits the emergence of new mosquitoes, prevents the larvae from breathing, and inhibits ovipositing (Figure 35-28).

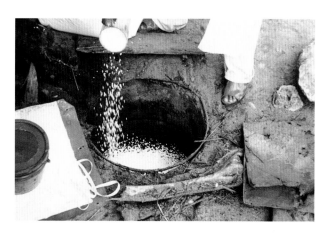

Fig. 35-28. Polystyrene beads being deposited into a pit latrine to reduce the incidence of bancroftian filariasis by interfering with the life cycle of the vector mosquitoes. The floating blanket of beads prevents ovipositing and also serves to asphyxiate larvae and prevent emergence of new mosquitoes.
Photograph: Courtesy of Dr. C. F. Curtis.

Larvicides are also useful in controlling the vector. Attacking the vector larvae is an important way to prevent filariasis. In recent years, antilarval products have become more environmental friendly and specifically designed to destroy mosquito larvae. For larvae control, the pest control industry has discontinued the use of organophosphates sprayed on breeding sites. The leading antilarvae substances are either selective bacillary toxins or insect growth regulators.

A popular larvicide is derived from *Bacillus thurengiensis* var. *israelensis* (typically denoted as "Bt" or "Bti"). Pest control personnel disperse Bt products in a variety of ways, to include tossing Bt time-release briquettes into stagnant pools or spraying Bt pellets or a liquid Bt solution by hand or air. A more persistent toxin is derived from *Bacillus sphaericus*. It is well suited for wetland areas and waters with high organic content, such as waste water and dairy lagoons. *B sphaericus* toxin has also been successfully used to kill *C quinquifaciatus* larvae in pit latrines for up to 10 weeks when applied at 10 mg per liter of sewage.[589]

Methoprene is a stable but nonpersistent compound that inhibits the growth of mosquito larvae. Insect growth regulators prevent insects from maturing to the adult stage. This compound is found in slow release briquettes, pellets, and liquids that are effective from 7 to more than 150 days, depending on the specific way the compound is formulated.[590]

Biocontrol is an environmentally friendlier way to control larvae. Introducing larvae-eating creatures, such certain species of ducks and fish, into mosquito-breeding areas can reduce mosquito larvae.

Individuals should use personal protection measures to prevent transmission from the mosquito (see chapter 22, Personal Protection Measures Against Arthropods). The includes wearing permethrin impregnated outerwear, applying 33% DEET insect repellent to exposed skin, and wearing long-sleeved shirts and long pants. Additionally, sleeping under permethrin-impregnated bed nets should help prevent transmission.

Malayan and Timorian Filariasis

Description of the Pathogen

B timori adult females are approximately 30 mm long; males are 17 mm long. The microfilariae have several distinguishing features: they are longer and have a cephalic space with proportions length to width of about 3:1. In addition, the sheath does not stain pink with Giemsa stain as do those of *B malayi* and *W bancrofti*.

Adult female *B malayi* worms are similar to *W bancrofti* worms except that they are only 43 to 55 mm long. Male worms are 14 to 23 mm long. The microfilariae of *B malayi* are distinguished from those of *W bancrofti* by their two isolated nuclei at the tip of the tail and their absence of nuclei in the cephalic spaces.

Epidemiology

Like bancroftian filariasis, these are also lymphatic filariases transmitted by mosquito bites. *B malayi* is transmitted by species of *Mansonia, Anopheles,* and *Aedes*; *B timori* is transmitted by *An barbirostris*. But as is indicated by their names, their geographic range is much more limited. *B timori* is reported from the Lesser Sunda Islands of Indonesia. They both occur in and around Indonesia, although *B malayi* is also found in Malaysia, the Philippines, Sri Lanka, India, Korea, China, Thailand, and Vietnam. *B malayi* is unique in that animals may also serve as reservoirs for some subperiodic strains, but humans are the primary reservoir.[578] The World Health Organization estimated in 1994 that 5.8 million people were infected with *Brugia malayi* or *Brugia timori*.[579]

Diagnostic Approaches and Recommendations for Therapy and Control

Definitive diagnosis occurs by identifying microfilariae in the blood or adult worms in tissue samples. In most cases, the best time to obtain a blood sample is between 2200 and 0200 hours, when microfilaria reach their maximum concentration in the peripheral blood. This nocturnal emergence coincides with the nighttime feeding patterns of the vectors from the *Culex, Anopheles,* and *Aedes* species. The microfilariae are virtually undetectable in peripheral blood during the day. A notable exception to this nocturnal periodicity occurs in the South Pacific and foci in Southeast Asia, where microfilariae possess a diurnal periodicity and are more concentrated in the peripheral blood during the day. Not surprisingly, this variant is transmitted by a day-biting mosquito of the *Aedes* species. Concentration techniques assist in isolating microfilariae. After centrifuging 2 mL of blood mixed with 10 mL of 2% formalin, a millipore filter (2 to 5 mm pore size) in a Swinney adapter is used to isolate the microfilariae.[62] Giemsa staining of thick and thin smears

allows speciation. A urinalysis may indicate renal abnormalities. More than 50% of microfilaremic patients have microscopic hematuria, proteinuria, or both.[591] The detection of a *B malayi*–specific repetitive DNA sequence by polymerase chain reaction holds promise as an easier way to diagnose malayan filariasis.[592]

Onchocerciasis

Description of the Pathogen

Adult female *Onocerca volvulus* worms are 23 to 70 cm long, whereas the males are 3 to 6 cm long. The microfilariae are unsheathed, possess a sharply pointed tail, and do not have terminal nuclei.

Epidemiology

Onchocerciasis (river blindness) is a chronic, nonfatal disease transmitted by the bite of the female black fly *Simulium damnosum*, which breeds in fast-moving streams and rivers. Humans are the sole reservoir for this disease. Most (95%) of the 17.5 million individuals infected with *O volvulus* live in Africa in a zone between 15° North and 15° South latitude, with one third of global cases living in Nigeria (Figure 35-29). There are small foci in the Western hemisphere, predominantly in Guatemala and Mexico. Smaller foci have been found in Colombia, Venezuela, Brazil, and Ecuador. Cases have also been verified in the southwest tip of the Arabian peninsula in Yemen and Saudi Arabia.[593]

Pathogenesis and Clinical Findings

Like other filarial diseases, onchocerciasis is caused by the direct physical insult of worms in tissues combined with the resultant inflammatory response. The female black fly injects *S damnosum* larvae into the skin, from where they spread to superficial and deep tissues. In those tissues they mature into adult worms, bundled together in characteristic nests. Within 7 to 34 months of the original infection, the females release microfilariae, which commence a grand tour of their human host. The microfilariae migrate to the skin, causing a pruritic rash. Another destination is the ocular tissues, where microfilariae cause blindness in up to 4% of those infected.[594] The disease is characterized by fibrous nodules in subcutaneous tissues, particularly in the head and shoulders (Western hemisphere) or pelvic girdle and lower extremities (Africa).[62] Lichenification and depigmentation can also occur.

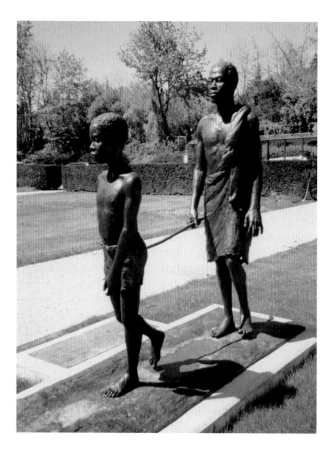

Fig. 35-29. This statue, depicting a blind victim of onchocerciasis being led by a young boy, was dedicated at the World Health Organization headquarters in Geneva, Switzerland, on October 6, 1999. The statue commemorates the 25th anniversary of the World Health Organization's Onchocerciasis Control Programme and its success in combating river blindness in western Africa. Photograph: Courtesy of Colonel Patrick W. Kelley, Medical Corps, US Army.

Diagnostic Approaches

Examination of shave biopsies from the hip or scapula will frequently reveal microfilariae. The specimen must soak overnight in normal saline and then be observed unstained under a microscope for microfilarieae. Slit lamp examination of the anterior chamber of the eye may reveal motile microfilariae or corneal lesions. Examining the blood may reveal eosinophilia but rarely microfilariae.

Recommendations for Therapy and Control

Ivermectin, which is well tolerated, will kill the microfilariae but not the adult forms. The dose is 150 mg/kg given once each year for 5 to 10 years. Occasionally, the treated patient will experience a Mazotti-type reaction, which includes fever, tender lymph nodes, headache, pruritis, and joint and bone pain.[581]

Vectors are controlled by applying larvicides to black-fly breeding areas. Spraying temefos (Abate) 0.05 mg/L for 10 minutes in the wet season and 0.10 mg/L for 10 minutes in the dry season can be effective. The toxin derived from *Bacillus therengensis*, Bt H-14, can also be effective at two and a half times the dose for temefos. Bt H-14 needs to be introduced at more points along the river, though, because it has less spreading ability.[62p363–367]

DEET effectively protects humans from black fly bites. The extended formulation of DEET repelled black flies (*Prosimulium mixtum* and *P fuscum*) bites for up to 9 hours on people in a sedentary setting.[595] DEET is also effective against *Simulium damnosum*. By wearing trousers and hooded jackets impregnated with DEET, subjects experienced 90% fewer bites over a 5-day period as compared to subjects wearing only shorts and short-sleeved shirts.[596] In another experiment, a 10% concentration of DEET protected the subjects for 299 minutes against *S damnosum*.[597] Bites can also be avoided by bivouacking away from *Simulium* species breeding sites.

Loaisis

Description of the Pathogen

Adult *Loa loa* worms are semitransparent and threadlike, growing to 50 to 70 mm in length (females) or 30 to 34 mm (males). The microfilariae are sheathed. The caudal nuclei are not isolated but are a continuation of the main body nuclei. The cephalic space is much shorter than that of *B malayi*.

Epidemiology

The *Loa loa* larvae are transmitted to the human host by the bite of the deer fly of the *Chrysops* species. Loiasis occurs in central African rain forests in Nigeria, Cameroon, Chad, the Central African Republic, the Democratic Republic of the Congo (formerly Zaire), Uganda, Angola, and Zambia. Humans are the only reservoir. The prevalence of *Loa loa* microfilaraemia typically ranges from 25% to 33% in endemic areas. Incidence in immunologically naive individuals seems low, indicated by the fact that only 1.9% of children under 5 years of age in one study had microfilaremia.[598]

Pathogenesis and Clinical Findings

The pathology caused by infection with *L loa* is primarily dermal, with less common changes in the heart, kidneys, and brain. The pathogenesis has not been thoroughly elucidated, but it is probably due to an inflammatory response to the worm.

Like the lymphatic filarial diseases, loiasis has different clinical presentations depending on whether or not the host is native to the area. In natives, infection with adult *L loa* worms causes the characteristic, transient area of erythema and angioedema (Calabar swellings) 5- to 10-cm in diameter, chiefly on the wrists and ankles. Occasionally, a wandering adult worm will move subconjunctivally across the eye. Nonnative visitors manifest prominent signs and symptoms of inflammatory or allergic reactions to the parasites. Frequent Calabar swellings, hives, rashes, and occasionally asthma are the main symptoms.

Diagnostic Approaches

Diagnosis is made by identifying microfilariae in the peripheral blood during the day; the highest density occurs around noon.[598] Nonnative patients often have a greatly elevated eosinophil count (30% to 60% of the total white blood cell count). Elevated filarial antibody titers can also aid in the diagnosis.

Recommendations for Therapy and Control

DEC is the drug of choice and is recommended at the doses listed in Exhibit 35-3. Treatment of heavy infections of *L loa* is sometimes associated with encephalopathy. The risk is reduced by starting with a smaller dose and gradually increasing the dose as indicated above. During treatment, hypersensitivity reactions to the dead and dying parasites are common but can be attenuated with steroids and antihistamines.[62p197–201]

Loiasis can be prevented with a weekly dose of 300 mg of DEC.[62,582] Additionally, personal protection measures and destruction of *Chrysops* breeding areas will reduce the risk of transmission from deer flies.

Streptocerciasis

Streptocerciasis is caused by infection with the filaria *Mansonella streptocerca*. The adult female is 27 mm long and the male is 17 mm long. They are transmitted by the biting midge, *Culicoides grahami*. The disease's distribution is limited to Central and West Africa.

In the same way as other filarial diseases, the organism can induce an intense IgE-mediated allergic reaction. Most of the time, however, there are not symptoms. When present, symptoms are primarily of a dermal nature and include pruritis (the most common), papules, and lichenification.[591]

Streptocerciasis is definitively diagnosed by demonstrating microfilariae in wet mounts prepared from skin snips from the scapula.[599] Adult worms can be identified in tissue sections. Eosinophilia may be present. Microfilariae have not been observed in the blood.

DEC kills both the adult worm and microfilariae. The dose for adults is 2 to 4 mg/kg per day for 21 days.[582] The death of the pathogen causes side effects similar to those seen in other filarial diseases. Most patients experience intense pruritis and papules during treatment.[593]

Others

Mansonella ozzardi causes a typically symptomless filarial infection found only in the New World (eg, southern Mexico, Panama, Brazil, Colombia, Argentina, many Caribbean islands). It is diagnosed by identifying microfilariae in blood or skin snips. DEC is ineffective but a single dose of ivermectin (140 µg/kg) reportedly eliminated microfilariae in a patient.[593]

Mansonella perstans infections are a largely nonpathogenic condition and are found in Africa, the Caribbean region, and Central and South America.

EXHIBIT 35-3

DOSAGES OF DEC FOR TREATING LOIASIS

	Adult	Child
Day 1	50 mg, orally after a meal	1 mg/kg after meal
Day 2	50 mg, three times a day	1 mg/kg three times a day
Day 3	100 mg, three times a day	1-2 mg/kg three times a day
Days 4–21	9 mg/kg per day in three doses	9 mg/kg per day in three doses

Source: Drugs for parasitic infection. *Med Lett Drugs Ther.* 1993;35(911):111–122.

Infection is diagnosed by finding microfilariae in the blood. Unlike other filarial infections, DEC has little effect on *M perstans* infections.[593] The current treatment regimen of 5 to 6 mg/kg per day often must be repeated 8 to 10 times to achieve a cure.[582] However, mebendazole is effective in a dose of 100 mg 2 to 3 times a day for 28 to 45 days.[600]

[William P. Corr]

THE LEISHMANIASES

Introduction and Military Relevance

The leishmaniases are a heterogeneous group of disease syndromes caused by infection with protozoan parasites of the genus *Leishmania*. Worldwide these parasitic infections are responsible for significant morbidity and mortality in civilian populations and are a persistent problem for military forces deployed to endemic areas. Although historically the leishmaniases have never had the major impact on campaigns that malaria has had, they do challenge military physicians with clinical difficulties, including recognition of the different disease syndromes, limitations of diagnostic and treatment options, and activation of latent infection after immunocompromise. The leishmaniases also present challenges for prevention because of the behavior of sand flies; the presence of animal reservoirs; the lack of effective chemoprophylaxis, immunoprophylaxis, or preventive vaccines; and the continual struggle to enforce personal protective measures in military personnel. The risk of leishmaniasis to US service members is directly related to the geographic and seasonal deployment of the force. A potential for hundreds to thousands of cases exists given the right epidemiologic circumstances.

There are three primary clinical syndromes: visceral leishmaniasis (VL), also known as kala-azar; localized cutaneous leishmaniasis (CL), which is usually ulcerative; and mucosal leishmaniasis (ML), also known as espundia. Less commonly seen are other cutaneous syndromes, such as leishmaniasis recidivans (LR), diffuse cutaneous leishmaniasis (DCL), and post–kala-azar dermal leishmaniasis. A variety of nonspecific systemic syndromes—including acute febrile illness, lymphadenopathy (localized, regional, and generalized), and chronic syndromes characterized by malaise, nonspecific gastrointestinal problems, and asthenia—have also been recognized.

It is doubtful if our knowledge of any other tropical parasitic disease owes as much to the activities of military men. A young medical officer in the Indian Army Medical Service, DD Cunningham, wrote the first accurate description of an amastigote from a case of "Delhi Boil" in 1885, although he did not appreciate the protozoan nature of the parasite.[601] A Russian military surgeon, PF Borovsky, provided an accurate description of the parasite in a typical ulcerative lesion (Sart sore) while working in Tashkent in 1898.[602] His work, published in Russian in an obscure military medical journal, went unnoticed until translated into English in 1938.[603] William Boog Leishman, a major in the British Royal Army Medical Corps, was the first to describe amastigotes in the splenic pulp of a young soldier who died after a prolonged febrile illness in London after returning from the station of Dum-Dum near Calcutta, India.[604] Cases of "Dum-Dum fever" had puzzled military physicians for years and were responsible for the morbidity and mortality of hundreds of British soldiers in India. A few months later, Captain Charles Donovan described the same parasites in a splenic smear from a young girl with prolonged fever in Madras, India.[605] Col. H.E. Shortt of the Indian Army Medical Service and his colleagues proved the transmission of *Leishmania donovani* parasites from sand flies to humans in 1942.[606]

World War II

During World War II, approximately 1,000 to 1,500 cases of CL were reported in US forces.[607] Cases were seen in Latin America and North Africa, but the majority of cases occurred in the Persian Gulf Command, mainly in the vicinity of Ahváz, Iran, where an epidemic of 630 cases was reported during one 3-month period in late 1943. Diagnosis and treatment were performed in dispensaries. No military personnel were returned to the United States, failed to perform their usual military duty, or were given a medical discharge because of their infection, but treating these cases still strained medical resources. Over 60% of the local mammalian reservoir hosts, desert gerbils, were found to be infected. Intensive rodent destruction with chloropicrin reduced the incidence of leishmaniasis in the natives in the area from 70% to 0.4%. Cases in American troops declined dramatically as well.

VL occurred in 50 to 75 military personnel, mostly from India, China, and the Mediterranean region.[607] Although not a serious operational problem, individual cases posed significant diagnostic difficulties for physicians. Inexperience of medical corps officers with the disease led to long delays in diagnosis and inappropriate treatments. Although only one death was due to VL, the morbidity was considerable; most of the men lost over 1 year of active duty time and had prolonged hospitalizations. In a well-studied cohort of 30 individuals, 15 cases originated in India and 15 in the Mediterranean.[608] The shortest incubation period was 3 weeks and the longest was 19 months. The average interval from onset of acute symptoms to definitive diagnosis and specific treatment was 10 weeks (range: 2 to 23 weeks), reflecting the unfamiliarity of physicians with the disease. The abrupt onset of fever and chills was seen in 29 of 30 (96%) cases, leading to an initial diagnosis of malaria. Splenomegaly was found in 27 of 30 (90%) patients on first examination and developed later in the other three. In other servicemen stationed in the Mediterranean region, localized lymphadenopathy was described.[609]

The British experience in East Africa during World War II with VL was more sobering. An outbreak occurred in 30 native troops of the King's African Rifles. The troops were from a nonendemic area of Kenya and were training in an endemic area of northern Kenya in 1941.[610] Fourteen soldiers died—specific treatment was not available—and the rest suffered prolonged illness and hospitalization. Similarly, an outbreak of VL was described in 23 native troops raised in a nonendemic area of the Sudan when they trained and fought in endemic areas of Ethiopia.[611] Initially, medical officers suspected malaria, but later the diagnosis of VL was confirmed. It was thought that the stress of battle activated latent VL in these troops.

Leishmaniasis was not a problem in the Korean War or the Vietnam conflict, as the parasite is not endemic to the Korean peninsula or Southeast Asia.

The Middle East

Both CL and VL were reported in British Marines serving in Aden from 1963 to 1965,[612,613] and systemic syndromes with lymphadenopathy have been described in soldiers from Cyprus and Malta.[614] An epidemic of CL occurred in 95 Israeli soldiers while they trained in the Jordan valley for 30 days during the summer of 1967. The incidence of CL was 50%, with an average of 7.4 lesions per soldier.[615] Another outbreak of CL in 60 (20%) of 296 Israeli soldiers occurred during 6 months in the Negev desert.[616] Well over 100 cases of CL have occurred in soldiers of 211 nationalities of the Multinational Force and Observers in the east Sinai since its operations be-

gan in April 1982.[617–620] But the largest recent experience with *Leishmania* and military forces took place during the Iraq-Iran border war (1980-1988). Thousands of cases of zoonotic CL due to *L major* occurred in both armies. CL was such an enormous medical and morale problem in the Iranian Army that 1.2 million soldiers and 240,000 civilians were vaccinated with a live, virulent *L major* parasite in a process called "leishmanization."[621] The Israeli Defense Force also used leishmanization. Unfortunately, leishmanization results in a 5% incidence of active lesions that require drug treatment.

Epidemics of CL have been described in nonimmune soldiers when they are deployed for training or newly based in endemic areas. Deployments to Southwest Asia in 1990 and 1991 during the Persian Gulf War have led to 32 parasitologically confirmed cases of leishmaniasis: 20 cases of CL and 12 cases of atypical "viscerotropic" (VtL) infection. The CL cases were typical in their presentation and response to therapy and were caused by *L major* in those cases where the parasite was characterized. None of the Persian Gulf War patients with VtL had the usual findings of VL but rather had a milder, nonspecific constitutional illness with a wide variety of symptoms.[622,623] The limited number of recognized cases in US service members in Southwest Asia during this time was largely due to the fact that most military personnel were deployed during the winter months (November 1990 to February 1991) when sand fly populations were at their lowest and had returned to the United States by April 1991 before the peak sand fly season (May through September). If the deployment had occurred during the peak months, the number of cases would likely have been much higher.

South America and Panama

In 1978 the British Army established a permanent garrison in Belize of about 1,500 troops who served a 1-year tour of duty. Between 1978 and 1990, there were 306 cases of clinical CL (1.5% of the total personnel deployed), 187 of which were parasitologically confirmed.[624] *L braziliensis* was isolated in 72% and *L mexicana* was isolated in 28% of the 107 samples that were characterized. Most patients presented in Belize during their tour of duty or within 4 months of their return to the United Kingdom. One patient presented 11 months after his return. No cases of ML have been reported.

The Jungle Operations Training Center (JOTC) on the Fort Sherman military reservation in Panama has been the source of the majority of cases of CL for years.[625–630] The cases are sporadic, with a 1% to 2% attack rate in affected units, although outbreaks with much higher site-specific attack rates are well documented.[631] The JOTC is located within Fort Sherman on the Atlantic side of the Canal Zone, although at least two outbreaks at sites on the Pacific side have been documented as well.

A series of 60 cases of CL in US service members was reported in 1988.[632] They were infected in Panama, Brazil, and Colombia. Among 35 soldiers with a 3-week exposure in Panama at the JOTC, the mean maximum incubation period was 33 days (range: 4 to 81 days). Diagnosis was delayed an average of 93 days after onset of skin lesions because of delay by patients in seeking medical attention (mean: 31 days, range: 0 to 365 days), by medical personnel in considering the diagnosis (mean: 45 days, range: 0 to 425 days), and by laboratories in confirming the diagnosis (mean: 17 days, range: 2 to 120 days). Forty-four patients (73%) developed typical ulcerative lesions of CL, while 16 (27%) developed atypical macular, papular, squamous, or verrucous lesions that were confirmed only by culture.

CL also poses a significant problem in the armed forces of several Central and South American countries. In some cases this has led to significant morale problems as soldiers are unwilling to be deployed to areas where they know exposure risks are high. Outbreaks of CL with attack rates of over 50% highlight the potential of leishmaniasis to affect very large numbers of personnel following a short exposure period.

Ninety-six parasitologically confirmed patients treated at the Walter Reed Army Medical Center, Washington, DC, between 1989 and 1996 have included 83 with CL, 3 with VL, and 10 with VtL.[633] The majority of CL patients acquired their infections in Panama at the JOTC, in French Guinea during jungle training, or in Saudi Arabia during the Persian Gulf War. There have also been three cases of VL in young dependent children infected in Sigonella, Sicily, and one adult case infected near Madrid, Spain. Cases of leishmaniasis in the US military from 1954 to 1998 are presented in Figure 35-30. There have been 735 reported cases, for a mean of 16 cases per year.

Epidemiology

Transmission

The vast majority of leishmaniasis transmission occurs through the bite of infected female sand flies; however, other modes of transmission have been described, including intravenous drug abuse and blood transfusions, as well as congenital, sexual, and laboratory acquired transmission.[634] The primary *Leishmania* species that cause disease in humans and their associated clinical syndromes, animal reservoirs, and geographic distribution are presented in Table 35-11. More detailed information can be found elsewhere.[634–639]

Transmission of the leishmaniases often occurs

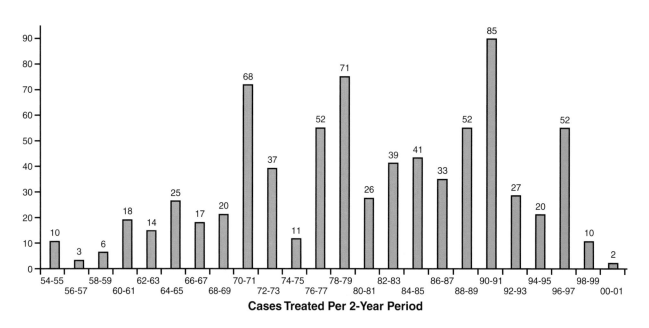

Fig. 35-30. Leishmaniasis in US Military Personnel 1954–1998

TABLE 35-11

PRIMARY LEISHMANIA SPECIES THAT CAUSE DISEASE IN HUMANS, WITH ASSOCIATED ANIMAL RESERVOIRS AND GEOGRAPHIC DISTRIBUTION

Subspecies of *Leishmania*	Primary Clinical Syndrome	Other Clinical Syndromes	Animal Reservoir	Geographic Distribution
Old World				
L donovani	VL	CL, PKDL	Humans?	Epidemic in the Sudan and in the Gangetic plain of India, Nepal, and Bangladesh. Endemic in Iraq, Kenya, and parts of China; sporadic throughout sub-Saharan Africa
L infantum	VL	CL	Dog (and other canines)	Endemic in both the European and African Mediterranean littoral; sporadic in parts of China, SW Asia, and sub-Saharan Africa
L major	CL	ML (uncommon)	Burrowing rodents	Endemic in the Mediterranean littoral of North Africa, the Sahel region of Africa, and most areas of SW and Central Asia
L tropica	CL	VL (India), VtL, LR	Humans?	Focally endemic in North Africa, SW Asia, Central Asia, India, East Africa, Namibia, Turkey, and Greece
L aethiopica	CL	DCL	Hydrax	Ethiopia and Kenya
New World				
L chagasi	VL	CL	Dog	Epidemic in northeast Brazil; focally endemic throughout Central and South America
L mexicana	CL	DCL	Forest rodents	Focally endemic in Texas (USA), Mexico, Dominican Republic, and Central and South America
L amazonensis	CL	ML, DCL, VL	Forest rodents, agouti, opossum	Amazon basin
L braziliensis	CL	ML	Forest rodents?	Focally epidemic and endemic from Mexico to northern Argentina
L guyanensis	CL	ML (uncommon)	Sloth	South America, especially north of the Amazon River
L panamensis	CL	ML (uncommon)	Sloth	Central America, Colombia, Ecuador, Peru, and Venezuela
L peruviana	CL	ML (uncommon)	Rodents, dogs(?)	Peru

CL = cutaneous leishmaniasis, ML = mucosal leishmaniasis ("espundia"), VL = visceral leishmaniasis ("kala-azar"), VtL = viscerotropic leishmaniasis, LR = leishmaniasis recidivans, DCL = diffuse cutaneous leishmaniasis, PKDL = post-kala-azar dermal leishmaniasis

in a very uneven, focal distribution within areas of broad endemicity. This is caused by the behavior and ecology of the anthropophagous species of sand flies (*Phlebotomus* in the Old World and *Lutzomyia* in the New World) and to a lesser extent the density and distribution of the mammalian reservoir animals.[640] Infection risk can vary markedly over just a few hundred meters.

In Panama, sand fly densities are bimodal in distribution, with the highest density at the beginning (May through July) and end (November and December) of the rainy season.[641] Most human infections tend to occur toward the end of the rainy season. *L panamensis* causes over 90% of the *Leishmania* infections in US soldiers who acquire their infections in Panama. The principal reservoir host is the two-toed sloth, *Choloepus hoffmani*, and at least 4 species of sand flies transmit parasites to humans.

Female sand flies transmit motile, flagellated promastigotes to humans and animals when taking a blood meal. Promastigotes attach to mononuclear phagocytes using specific receptors and are engulfed via endocytosis into endosomes. The endosomes then fuse with lysosomes to form a parasitophorous vacuole. The promastigote transforms into a nonmotile oval structure (2 to 5 mm in diameter) with a degenerate flagella, called the amastigote, inside cells of the mononuclear phagocyte system. *Leishmania* amastigotes are distinguished microscopically from other morphologically similar pathogens by the presence of a rod-shaped kinetoplast in their cytoplasm. Amastigotes persist and replicate by binary fission within the parasitophorous vacuole. Eventually the expanding vacuole fills the cell, leading to lysis and cell death. Released daughter amastigotes attach and penetrate nearby mononuclear cells and disseminate throughout the body. The cycle is continued when feeding sand flies ingest infected cells. The ingested amastigotes transform into promastigotes, which live and develop extracellularly in the alimentary tract of the sand fly (Figure 35-31).

Geographical Distribution

CL of the Old World is often distributed in semiarid, rural, savanna and urban areas, while CL and ML of the New World are seen in humid, neotropical forests. VL is associated with a canine reservoir in the Mediterranean region and in Brazil, but no animal reservoir is associated with VL caused by *L donovani* in the Gangetic plain in southern Asia.

Sand flies are rather delicate and do not survive extremes of temperature and humidity. They exist in harsh climates by seeking cool and humid daytime resting sites such as caves, animal burrows, trees, and dark niches in buildings and rubble. They then emerge at night when ambient temperature drops and humidity increases. Sand flies have short, hopping flight and can travel only a few hundred meters in a night. Seasonal variation in population size can also be quite marked depending largely on rainfall in the tropics and both rainfall and ambient temperatures in more temperate climates.

Incidence

Groups at highest risk of disease following infection are nonimmunes such as military personnel, tourists, settlers, and forest or road workers entering endemic areas. Deforestation, irrigation projects, and migration to cities with peri-urban sprawl are all associated with increased rates and epidemics of leishmaniasis.

Pathogenesis and Clinical Findings

CL is the most common form of leishmaniasis. The incubation period usually ranges from several weeks to months following infection but can be as short as 10 days or as long as 5 years. Ulcers usually resolve spontaneously over several months to years with a disfiguring scar. The typical lesion of ulcerative CL starts as a small, erythematous papule at the bite site.[642] The papule enlarges over sev-

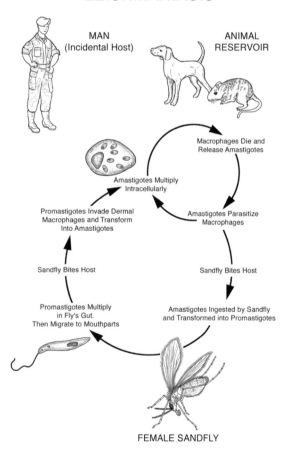

LEISHMANIASIS

MAN
(Incidental Host)

ANIMAL
RESERVOIR

Macrophages Die and
Release Amastigotes

Amastigotes Multiply
Intracellularly

Promastigotes Invade Dermal
Macrophages and Transform
Into Amastigotes

Amastigotes Parasitize
Macrophages

Sandfly Bites Host

Sandfly Bites Host

Promastigotes Multiply
in Fly's Gut.
Then Migrate to Mouthparts

Amastigotes Ingested by Sandfly
and Transformed into Promastigotes

FEMALE SANDFLY

Fig. 35-31. The life cycle of leishmania.
Adapted with permission from: Norton SA, Frankenburg S, Klaus SN. Cutaneous leishmaniasis acquired during military service in the Middle East. *Arch Dermatol.* 1992;128:83

eral weeks, crusts over, and breaks down into a slowly enlarging ulcer. The ulcer can be several centimeters in diameter. It is shallow and well defined and has a raised, erythematous border with central granulation tissue under an exudate. Ulcers may be single or multiple, and surrounding inflammation varies greatly. Ulcers heal with time to give a depressed, hairless, atrophic scar. Involvement of regional draining lymph nodes, the presence of subcutaneous nodules ("sporotrichoid presentations"), and satellite lesions are common. Hyperkeratotic lesions that do not ulcerate can also be seen. A variety of less common presentations have all been reported, including macules; plaques; nodules; and psoriaform, varicelliform, eczematous, and keloidal-like lesions.

ML and LR are chronic, oligoparasitic syndromes associated with persistent and enhanced delayed-type hypersensitivity reactions to leishmanial antigens. ML, most often seen in the New World and associated with *L braziliensis,* is characterized by metastatic involvement of oropharyngeal and nasopharyngeal tissue following a primary ulcerative lesion.[643] Patients may present initially with minor complaints of hoarseness, epistaxis, nasal congestion, and mucopurulent expectoration. The disease progresses slowly over many years and leads to widespread tissue destruction involving the nose, palate, uvula, and hypopharynx. Gross alterations can occur, including septal perforations, irregular vegetative growths, gross swelling, and destruction of the nares, palate, and uvula. Late-stage disease, especially when involving the airway, can be accompanied by persistent cough, hoarseness, or a low muffled voice. Extensive destruction can lead to inspiratory airway compromise and an increase in pulmonary infections because of inability to protect the airway. LR, most often seen in the Old World and associated with *L tropica,* is characterized by recrudescing, brownish-red, lupoid nodules that occur around the periphery of healed primary lesions. These painless lesions may wax and wane for many years.

Diffuse cutaneous leishmaniasis is characterized by disseminated nodules that can be prominent on the head and neck. Lesions appear very similar to those of lepromatous leprosy, but the nodules of lepromatous leprosy are somewhat smaller and are firm to palpation while the nodules of DCL are soft and fleshy to palpation.

Post–kala-azar dermal leishmaniasis is a spectrum of dermatological findings, which includes macules, papules, and nodules following treatment of Indian or African VL with pentavalent antimony. It can occur during, shortly following, or several months after treatment. The initial macules or maculopapular lesions may resolve spontaneously over a few weeks to months or persist and develop into chronic papulonodular lesions. The chronic lesions are rich in parasites, and patients with these lesions are a likely reservoir for anthroponotic (human-sand fly-human) transmission.

Asymptomatic individuals with presumed latent infection can develop localized cutaneous disease at the site of blunt, penetrating, or surgical trauma or disseminated cutaneous lesions if immunosuppressed many years following infection.[644,645]

The classic pentad of clinical findings in VL is fever, wasting, splenomegaly, pancytopenia, and hypergammaglobulinemia. Individuals with culture-proven infection who lack one or more of the classic findings are common in endemic areas. The spectrum of visceralizing infection also includes nonspecific acute and subacute illnesses that can resolve without specific treatment over time.[646–648] These "viscerotropic" infections are poorly documented because of lack of clinical awareness and insensitive parasitologic diagnostic tests. The majority of visceralizing infections have been described as asymptomatic based on skin test surveys of endemic populations. Individuals with a positive reaction to a *Leishmania* skin test antigen without signs or symptoms of disease or a history of classic VL are classified as asymptomatic. It is not possible to determine if these individuals really represent asymptomatic infections or resolved oligosymptomatic disease.

Diagnostic Approaches

The different techniques available to diagnose leishmaniasis are best considered in relation to the concept of parasite burden. Optimal techniques for oligoparasitic syndromes are different from those for polyparasitic syndromes.

Parasitologic diagnosis is defined as any one of these four methods: (1) visualization of amastigotes in Giemsa-stained thin smears, aspirates, impression smears, or histologic sections; (2) isolation of promastigotes in in vitro culture; (3) detection of parasite-specific DNA by hybridization or amplifying parasite-specific DNA with the polymerase chain reaction (PCR); and (4) in vivo culture of parasites (obtaining parasites from tissues of a susceptible animal after inoculation with material from a suspect patient). Giemsa-stained smears are simple and inexpensive but require expert microscopy skills. When amastigotes are unequivocally identified (ie, when the kinetoplast is visualized), the diagnosis is confirmed, but negative Giemsa smears do not exclude the diagnosis of leishmaniasis. In vitro culture is more sensitive than Giemsa-stained smears and should be viewed as a complementary diagnostic technique. For example, 27% of ulcerative CL lesions in Guatemala were smear negative and culture positive, but in the same study 10% of the cases were positive only by smear.[649] Therefore, in vitro culture and Giemsa-stained smears should both be attempted when possible in all clinically suspect cases. Polymerase chain reaction, although not yet available outside research settings, promises to increase the sensitivity of parasitologic diagnosis.

To obtain an optimal sample from a CL lesion for smear and culture, local anesthesia should be administered with 1% lidocaine plus 1:10,000 epinephrine and a typical ulcerative lesion debrided to remove overlying exudate and crusting. Scrapings, aspirates, and biopsies may be obtained from both the center and border of the ulcer. Scrapings and aspirates are more likely to yield a positive result than biopsy. Increasing the number of cultures from the same lesion also appears to improve sensitivity. In Guatemala, a single culture was positive 38% of the time, but increasing the number to five cultures improved the rate to 66%.[649]

Parasitologic diagnosis of visceralizing syndromes requires an invasive procedure to obtain an appropriate sample from the spleen, bone marrow, or liver and an experienced microscopist to identify amastigotes in tissue or smears. Serologic diagnosis is possible for VL. Antibodies to crude promastigote lysate can be detected by immunofluorescence, agglutination, and enzyme-lined immunosorbent assay. However, antibodies to other pathogens cross-react with the crude lysate used as antigen, and none of the assays are standardized. ELISA-based assays detecting antibodies to K39, a recombinant protein, have proven to be very sensitive and specific for the syndrome of VL.[650–653] Antibodies to K39 can also be detected in a rapid immunochromatographic ("dipstick") format, which yields a result in the field in less than 5 minutes using a drop of whole blood obtained by fingerstick.

Unfortunately, there is no sensitive or specific serologic assay for detecting *Leishmania*-specific antibody for any of the cutaneous leishmaniases. Delayed-type hypersensitivity is present at the time of ulcer formation and persists for years, if not for life, so using hypersensitivity skin tests would help detect prior infection with *Leishmania* and corroborate the diagnosis of oligoparasitic syndromes such as ML and LR. Skin tests are commonly used in endemic countries, but there is no licensed or investigational new drug product available in the United States.

In endemic areas, the specificity of a clinical diagnosis for late-stage VL when the spleen is grossly enlarged is likely quite high. The empiric use of pentavalent antimony in this situation often helps confirm the diagnosis if there is a rapid response (3 to 5 days) characterized by a decline in fever and an improved sense of well-being.

Recommendations for Therapy and Control

Pentavalent antimony has been the mainstay of drug treatment for all the leishmaniases since the 1940s. It is available as sodium stibogluconate (Pentostam, Glaxo Wellcome Foundation, London) and meglumine antimoniate (Glucantime, Aventis Pasteur, Paris). Neither of these drugs is licensed in the United States. Pentostam is available from the Centers for Disease Control and Prevention in Atlanta, Georgia, for civilian use, and from the Walter Reed Army Medical Center in Washington, DC, for all branches of the military. Current recommended treatment regimens for pentavalent antimony are 20 mg/kg per day for 20 days for CL and 20 mg/kg per day for 28 days for VL and ML.[654] The current recommended dose for the treatment of CL acquired in the New World was determined in a randomized trial of Pentostam at 10 mg/kg per day versus 20 mg/kg per day in US soldiers.[655] Pentostam is generally considered a safe and effective drug with no long-term or irreversible toxicity. It is, however, poorly tolerated by most individuals and is associated with headache, myalgias, arthralgias, anorexia, and epigastric pain. Elevated serum amylase and lipase is seen in nearly 100% of treated patients, but clinically significant pancreatitis is uncommon.[656] Optimal drug therapy for immunosuppressed patients is unclear, but they generally require a longer duration of primary therapy or maintenance therapy or both. The practical use of Pentostam[657] and other treatment options are discussed elsewhere.[658,659] No drug treatment eradicates the parasite, so there is always risk of reactivation with future immunosuppression.

The individual service member has the responsibility to prevent the bite of sand flies through the use of personal protection measures, which include frequently applying topical repellents containing 33% DEET, applying permethrin to uniforms, wearing the uniform properly, and sleeping under permethrin-impregnated bednets. Failure to use adequate personal protection measures is contributory to the vast majority of leishmaniasis cases.

When easily identified animal reservoirs are implicated (eg, dogs, burrowing rodents), specific measures to eliminate the reservoir can be successful. Barrier spray applications may prove useful, especially for small military encampments.[406] Personnel should receive predeployment education on the transmission, prevention, and typical clinical pre-

sentations of leishmaniasis. Unit commanders and medical personnel should rigorously enforce proper personal protection measures in the field and consider postdeployment surveillance of units with known exposures.

[Alan J. Magill]

TRYPANOSOMIASIS

American Trypanosomiasis (Chagas' Disease)

Introduction

Carlos Chagas discovered the protozoan *Trypanosoma cruzi* in 1909 while studying malaria in Brazil. He found the organism in the intestine of a triatomid and later found the same parasite in the blood of a child suffering from fever, anemia, and lymphadenopathy. Chagas went on to prove that *T cruzi* was indeed the cause of a disease common in certain parts of Brazil. This disease, American trypanosomiasis, or Chagas' disease, is the only disease to be described after its etiologic agent and insect vector were discovered.[660]

Description of the Pathogen

The flagellate protozoan *T cruzi* has a life cycle similar to its *Trypanosomatidae* cousins, *T brucei gambiense* and *T b rhodesiense*, but *T cruzi* has four distinct morphologic forms: an amastigote stage (seen intracellularly in tissue macrophages), a promastigote stage (a transitional stage only), an epimastigote stage (in the midgut of the vector), and a trypomastigote stage (in the feces of the vector). The trypomastigote stage is the infective stage to humans.

The life cycle begins with parasites multiplying (by binary fission) in the midgut of the vector, maturing, and passing as infective forms in the insect's feces. Human infection occurs when insect feces contaminate mucous membranes or breaks in the skin (eg, the puncture wound made by the feeding insect). The parasites then invade host macrophages and other tissue cells, multiply (causing the host cell to rupture), and invade adjacent cells, tissue lymphatics, or the blood stream. The life cycle is complete when an insect vector ingests infected blood.[661]

Epidemiology

Transmission. The insect vector of this disease is a small group of the *Reduviidae* family called the Triatominae or kissing bugs (Figure 35-32). While

there are many species of triatomids that will feed on humans, only a few are efficient vectors for Chagas' disease. The four primary vectors in South and Central America are *Panstrongylus megistus*, *Rhodninus prolixus*, *Triatoma infestans*, and *Tri dimidiata*. Local names for these vectors include the *vinchuca* in Argentina and the *bombero* (fireman) in Brazil. Important North American vectors include *Tri barberi* in Mexico and *Tri gerstaeckeri*, *Tri protracta*, and *Tri sanguisuga* in the United States.[662] All species, both male and female, feed at night and often live in the thatched roofs or cracks in the walls or floors of poorly constructed shacks. In fact, children in some parts of Brazil often awaken with spots on their faces that are actually triatomid feces that "rain" down from the thatched roofs during the night.[663]

In addition to vector transmission, Chagas' disease can be transmitted through blood transfusions, organ transplants, transplacental infection, and laboratory accidents.[62p514–520;664] Other routes of transmission have been described in Mexico, where people in some communities believe that the bugs have aphrodisiac powers or that the bug feces can cure warts. In other communities, the triatomid bugs are eaten with hot sauce by the Huichol Indians.[665]

Humans and more than 150 species of wild and

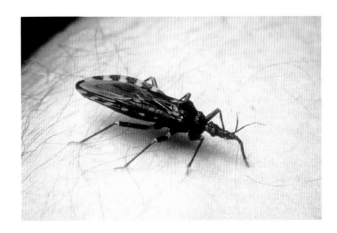

Fig. 35-32. The triatomid vector of American trypanosomiasis, also known as the kissing bug. Photograph: Courtesy of Professor W. Peters, International Institute of Parasitology.

domestic mammals serve as hosts for the parasite. The incubation period is approximately 5 to 14 days after the bite of an infected vector, and the vector becomes infective between 10 and 30 days after biting an infected host. All age groups are susceptible to the parasite, but the young and immunocompromised have the greatest risk for severe disease.[62]

Geographic Distribution. Chagas' disease occurs only in the Western hemisphere, with the vast majority of cases occurring in Latin America. *T cruzi* infection of humans, nonhuman mammals, and reduviid bugs has been found in Mexico and all countries of South and Central America.[661] Although Chagas' disease is found mostly in Latin America, a small number of vector-borne infections acquired in the United States have been reported.[62,661] Additionally, infected triatomids and mammals have been found across the southern part of the United States from Maryland to California.[660] Serological surveys in Washington, DC, demonstrate infection in 4.9% of migrants to that city from Central America.[62]

Incidence. Its prevalence, morbidity, mortality, and incurability make Chagas' disease the most important endemic disease in South America.[666] It is estimated that between 16 million and 18 million people are infected with *T cruzi*[661] and that approximately 50,000 patients die each year from Chagas' disease.[667] Infection can occur at any age but occurs most frequently in infancy. The harmful (often fatal) consequences of infection usually take years to manifest themselves and usually do so in adults. Chagas' disease is the most common cause of myocarditis in South America.[666]

Pathogenesis and Clinical Findings

Three phases of the disease are commonly described: (1) The acute phase can be asymptomatic, can consist of a swelling or "chagoma" at the infection site, or can include fever, malaise, adenopathy, and facial edema (Romana's sign); rarely, acute heart failure or meningoencephalitis can occur. Adults seem more resistant to acute Chagas' disease and usually progress to the next phase of the disease. (2) The indeterminate phase may last for years, in which the infection may be present in tissue without clinical manifestations. (3) The chronic phase may develop into cardiomyopathy, megacolon, or megaesophagus. About 50% of patients with chronic Chagas' disease develop cardiac or gastrointestinal disease. If death occurs during the chronic phase, it is usually due to congestive heart failure, cardiac rupture, or cardiac arrhythmia (eg, ventricular fibrillation, atrioventricular block) secondary to Chagas' cardiomyopathy.[668]

Diagnosis

The diagnosis of acute Chagas' disease is made by detecting parasites in the blood. The parasites can often be seen in wet preparations of buffy coat or anticoagulated blood or in Geimsa-stained smears. If these approaches fail, culturing the parasite in specialized media or by xenodiagnosis (culturing the organism in laboratory-reared insect vectors) may be considered.

The diagnosis of chronic Chagas' disease can be made serologically by detecting IgG specific for *T cruzi* antigen using one or more highly sensitive tests (eg, indirect immunofluorescence, complement fixation, indirect hemagglutination, enzyme-linked immunosorbent assay). A problem with these serologic tests, however, is the false-positive results that occur in patients having diseases such as leishmaniasis, syphilis, malaria, collagen vascular diseases, and other parasitic diseases. Because of this, a definitive diagnosis usually requires a positive result using two or three of the above-mentioned serologic tests.[664]

Recommendations for Therapy and Control

Available drug treatments for *T cruzi* infection are generally unsatisfactory. Two drugs, nifurtimox (available from the Centers for Disease Control and Prevention [CDC], Atlanta, Georgia, on an investigational new drug basis) and benznidazole, are active against both trypomastigotes and amastigotes but are only successful in about 50% of treated patients.[669] Both drugs can cause substantial toxic reactions in treated patients.[670] Though there is no widely accepted treatment for patients with chronic *T cruzi* infection, Gallerano and colleagues have reported that allopurinol is as effective as benznidazole and nifurtimox in suppressing parasitemias.[671] These studies are preliminary, however, and their open and nonrandomized structure makes the interpretation of their findings difficult.

Preventive measures are most important in curbing this disease and include:

- public education on the mode of spread and prevention of the disease,
- effective use of insecticides—especially in poor housing areas where thatched roofs are common,
- use of bednets in infested houses, and

- screening blood and organ donors from endemic areas.[62]

The best way for service members to protect themselves against Chagas' disease is to avoid, if possible, areas and buildings that might harbor the insect vector. If avoidance of these areas is impossible because of mission requirements, service members should practice personal protection measures (eg, the use of deet insect repellent, permethrin-treated uniforms, and permethrin-treated bednets) when operating in high-risk areas.

African Trypanosomiasis (African Sleeping Sickness)

Introduction

Although African trypanosomiasis has probably existed for centuries, it has become a health problem for humans only in the last 150 years. This disease began emerging as a threat to human populations with the colonization of Africa and the spread of the disease from west to east, resulting in its current geographic distribution.[672] An epidemic in Zaire between 1896 and 1906 took approximately 500,000 lives, and another epidemic that occurred along the shores of Lake Victoria around the same time claimed approximately 250,000 lives, two-thirds of the population of the region.[673]

Colonel David Bruce discovered that trypanosomes (*T brucei*) caused a disease in cattle, "nagana," and linked this disease to the tsetse fly in 1895. Forde first saw a trypanosome in the blood of a European in West Africa in 1901; in 1902, Dutton named the parasite *T gambiense*. Castellani then discovered the same parasite in the cerebrospinal fluid of a victim of Ugandan sleeping sickness in 1903. In 1910, Stephens and Fantham discovered a more virulent form of the disease in an English patient in northern Rhodesia who died in just 6 months. They named this form of the disease Rhodesian trypanosomiasis and the parasite *Trypanosoma rhodesiense*. Both parasites were later found to be related to the parasite discovered by Bruce years earlier, *T brucei*.[660,672]

Description of the Pathogen

African trypanosomiasis is caused by the subspecies of the hemoflagellate protozoan, *T brucei*. Gambian, or West African, sleeping sickness is caused by *T brucei gambiense* and is transmitted to humans through the bite of the riverine tsetse fly.

Rhodesian, or East African, sleeping sickness is caused by *T b rhodesiense* and is transmitted by the bite of the savannah tsetse fly. These parasites have two distinct morphologic forms: an epimastigote stage (in the salivary glands of the vector) and a trypomastigote stage (in the proboscis of the vector). The trypomastigote stage is the infective stage to humans.[660]

The life cycle of these trypanosomes, like that of *T cruzi* in American trypanosomiasis, begins with the parasite multiplying in the midgut of the vector. These parasites then migrate to the salivary glands of the fly and form epimastigotes, which in turn form metacyclic trypanosomes (young trypomastigotes) that can infect the bite wound of a new host as the vector feeds.[674]

Epidemiology

Transmission. Humans serve as the primary reservoir for *T b gambiense*, while game animals and domestic cattle act as animal reservoirs for *T b rhodesiense*.[62] *T b gambiense* produces a chronic disease after a 2- to 23-day incubation period, while *T b rhodesiense* produces a more severe, acute infection after an incubation period of 1 to 2 weeks.[660]

Of the more than 22 species of tsetse flies in the genus *Glossina*, only six are important in the transmission of trypanosomiasis (Figure 35-33). The important vectors for *T b gambiense* include *G palpalis*, *G fuscipes*, and *G tachinoides*, and the vectors for *T b rhodesiense* include *G morsitans*, *G swynnertoni*, and *G pallidipes*. Both sexes of the tsetse fly feed on blood and are day feeders. They feed on a wide variety of mammals, particularly cattle and other domestic animals, and some reptiles. Humans are incidental

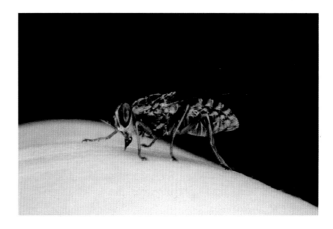

Fig. 35-33. The tsetse fly vector of African trypanosomiasis. Photograph: Courtesy of Colonel Peter Peters, US Army (Retired).

targets for the tsetse fly.[675]

Other modes of disease transmission are possible. Mechanical transmission can occur when a biting fly is interrupted while feeding on an infected host and bites an uninfected host before the blood on the mouth parts has dried (2 to 3 hours).[674] Additionally, congenital transmission has been reported[676] but is rare. Parasite transmission through blood transfusion is also possible but unusual.[674]

Geographic Distribution. African trypanosomiasis is confined to the tropical heart of Africa (between 14° N and 29° S latitude).[677] *T b gambiense* has a much wider-ranging distribution than *T b rhodesiense* and extends from the West Coast of Africa to regions around Lake Victoria. *T b rhodesiense* is confined to the eastern part of the continent and extends from southern Sudan to Mozambique.[660]

Incidence. African sleeping sickness occurs in approximately 200 endemic foci in 36 African countries.[677] There are about 20,000 cases of new human trypanosomiasis reported each year, but experts feel that this is an underestimate due to poor disease surveillance and underreporting.[672,674]

Pathogenesis and Clinical Findings

The pathogenesis of sleeping sickness is thought to be caused by the host's immunological response to the trypanosomes. Initially, there is increased activity in the lymphoid tissue with a proliferation of plasma cells. Large amounts of IgM and autoimmune anti-DNA antibodies are then produced. Next, immune complexes activate physiological cascades resulting in vascular permeability, intravascular coagulopathy, and tissue damage.[672,674]

African trypanosomiasis first manifests as a chancre at the site of the infected tsetse bite 5 to 15 days after the bite. The chancre (which is seldom seen in Africans) appears as a somewhat elevated, painful, and indurated dusky-red papule, approximately 2 to 5 cm in size, which resolves in 2 to 3 weeks.[660,674] Early systemic symptoms include fever, headaches, arthralgias, myalgias, and malaise and are often mistaken for malaria.[672] As the disease progresses, generalized lymphadenopathy follows and often results in enlarged posterior cervical lymph nodes (Winterbottom's sign) in *gambiense* sleeping sickness. Late-stage disease is characterized by central nervous system (CNS) involvement and may occur within weeks to months, depending on the subspecies. CNS manifestations include mood and personality alterations, movement disorders, lassitude, and daytime somnolence. The final stage of the disease consists of pruritis, wasting, and finally coma. Death usually re-

sults from the trypanosomiasis itself, infection, or malnutrition. With acute *rhodesiense* disease, the patient may die before CNS involvement of cardiac failure or cardiac arrhythmia due to pancarditis.[674]

Diagnosis

Diagnoses rely on demonstration of trypanosomes in the blood, the chancre, lymph node aspirates, the cerebrospinal fluid, or any combination of these. Concentration techniques, such as centrifugation of the cerebrospinal fluid or buffy-coat microscopy, may increase the sensitivity of the laboratory diagnosis.[672] Another way to increase diagnostic sensitivity is through culture. Blood, cerebrospinal fluid, or lymph node aspirate can be inoculated into a GLSH culture medium.[674] Current serological tests lack the specificity to be used without demonstration of the organism. A commercially available card agglutination test (CATT) has been developed for *T b gambiense* and has been shown to be useful in screening large populations.[672]

While it is impossible to distinguish morphologically between the two subspecies, they can be differentiated. Perhaps the quickest way to distinguish the two subspecies is by taking a good travel history, because there is very little overlap in their geographic distributions. For travelers who have been in areas endemic for both subspecies, animal inoculation can be performed to make the diagnosis. Rodent inoculation of heparinized blood or cerebrospinal fluid is still the most sensitive method for diagnosing infection with *T b rhodesiense*. *T b gambiense* will usually not infect rodents or only infect them with great difficulty.[674]

Recommendations for Therapy and Control

Once the diagnosis is established, treatment should begin immediately. Identification and proper treatment of early disease usually results in cure; untreated sleeping sickness is fatal. If trypanosomes have been demonstrated and there is still doubt about the subspecies, it is recommended that the patients with rapidly progressing disease be treated as having *T b rhodesiense* sleeping sickness and patients with slowly developing symptoms as having *T b gambiense* sleeping sickness.[678]

Suramin, available from the CDC on an investigational basis, is currently the drug of choice for treatment of early sleeping sickness caused by either subspecies. Since this drug does not cross the blood-brain barrier, however, it will not clear trypanosomes from the CNS. Pentamidine is another drug used in the early treatment of sleeping sickness; it is also used for chemoprophylaxis. Illness caused by *T b rhodesiense* infection, however, often does not respond to pentamidine, so it should be used for the early treatment and prophylaxis of *gambiense* disease only.[678] Melarsoprol (also available from the CDC on an investigational basis) is effective against both subspecies of the parasite and is the drug of choice for treating patients with CNS involvement but is, however, highly toxic and should only be given to patients in a hospital setting. Potential side effects may occur in 5% to 10% of patients and include fever, dermatitis, chest pain, neuropathy, and a fatal toxic encephalopathy.[672,678] If the patient has late-stage disease and *T b gambiense* has been identified as the parasite, eflornithine (available through the World Health Organization, Division of Control of Tropical Diseases) should be used for treatment.[678] Other drugs have been studied for the treatment of African trypanosomiasis (eg, diminazene, nifurtimox, nitrofurazone, melarsonyl potassium), but their toxicity and limited effectiveness curtail their usefulness.[674,678]

Like American trypanosomiasis, African trypanosomiasis is best controlled by preventive measures. They consist of the following:

- education of service members and others on the mode of spread of the disease and how to protect themselves against the tsetse fly,
- use of insecticides and destruction of vector habitats to reduce the fly population,
- disease surveillance in the human host population and prompt treatment for those found to be infected, and
- screening of blood donors from endemic areas.[62]

Chemoprophylaxis with pentamidine (4 mg/kg, to a maximum of 300 mg, intramuscularly every 3 to 6 months) may be indicated for individuals who will have constant, heavy exposure to *T b gambiense*.[672] Service members can best protect themselves from African trypanosomiasis by the same methods used for other vector-borne diseases—vector avoidance and use of personal protective measures (eg, deet, permethrin-treated uniforms, permethrin-treated bednets).

[William C. Hewitson]

REFERENCES

1. Bruce-Chwatt LJ. History of malaria from prehistory to eradication. In: Wernsdorfer WH, McGregor I, eds. *Malaria: Principles and Practice of Malariology*. New York: Churchill Livingstone; 1988.

2. Slim W. *Defeat into Victory*. London: Cassell and Co Ltd; 1956.

3. Ognibene AJ, Conte NF. Malaria: chemotherapy. In: Ognibene AJ, Barrett O eds. Internal Medicine in Vietnam. Vol 2. *General Medicine and Infectious Diseases*. Washington, DC: US Government Printing Office; 1982.

4. Centers for Disease Control and Prevention. Malaria among U.S. military personnel returning from Somalia, 1993. *MMWR*. 1993;42:524–526.

5. Newton JA Jr, Schnepf GA, Wallace MR, Lobel HO, Kennedy CA, Oldfield EC 3rd. Malaria in US Marines returning from Somalia. *JAMA*. 1994;272:397–399.

6. Smoak BL, DeFraites RF, Magill AJ, Kain KC, Wellde BT. *Plasmodium vivax* infections in U.S. Army troops: Failure of primaquine to prevent relapse in studies from Somalia. *Am J Trop Med Hyg*. 1997;56:231–234.

7. Molineaux L. The epidemiology of human malaria as an explanation of its distribution, including some implications for control. In: Wernsdorfer WH, McGregor I, eds. *Malaria: Principles and Practice of Malariology*. New York: Churchill Livingstone; 1988.

8. Nowosiwsky T. The epidemic curve of *Plasmodium falciparum* malaria in a nonimmune population: American troops in Vietnam, 1965 and 1966. *Am J Epidemiol*. 1967;86:461–467.

9. Centers for Disease Control and Prevention. *Health Information for International Travel, 1999-2000*. Atlanta: CDC; 1999.

10. Malakooti MA, Biomndo K, Shanks GD. Reemergence of epidemic malaria in the highlands of western Kenya. *Emerg Infect Dis*. 1998;4:671–676.

11. Sergiev VP, Baranova AM, Orlov VS, et al. Importation of malaria to the USSR from Afghanistan, 1981–89. *Bull World Health Org.* 1993;71:385–388. Published erratum: *Bull World Health Org.* 1994;72(2):321.

12. Schultz MG. Imported malaria. *Bull World Health Org.* 1974;50:329–336.

13. Walker AS. *Clinical Problems of War.* Sydney, Australia: Halstead Press; 1952: 79–80.

14. Shanks GD, Karwacki JJ. Malaria as a military factor in Southeast Asia. *Mil Med.* 1991;156:684–686.

15. Bouma MJ, van der Kaay HJ. Epidemic malaria in India's Thar desert. *Lancet.* 1995;346:1232–1233.

16. Gramiccia G, Beales PF. The recent history of malaria control and eradication. In: Wernsdorfer WH, McGregor I, eds. *Malaria: Principles and Practice of Malariology.* New York: Churchill Livingstone; 1988.

17. Malaria in the Republic of Korea. *18th MEDCOM Med Surv Rep.* 1997;2(5):1–2.

18. Phillips P, Nantel S, Benny WB. Exchange transfusion as an adjunct to the treatment of severe falciparum malaria: Case report and review. *Rev Infect Dis.* 1990;12:1100–1108.

19. Warrell DA, Molyneux ME, Beales PF, eds. Severe and complicated malaria. *Trans R Soc Trop Med Hyg.* 1990;84(suppl 2):1–65.

20. Rickman LS, Long GW, Oberst R, et al. Rapid diagnosis of malaria by acridine orange staining of centrifuged parasites. *Lancet.* 1989;1:68–71.

21. Premji Z, Minjas JN, Shiff CJ. Laboratory diagnosis of malaria by village health workers using the rapid manual Parasight-F test. *Trans R Soc Trop Med.* 1994;88:418.

22. Brown AE, Kain KC, Pipithkul J, Webster HK. Demonstration by the polymerase chain reaction of mixed *Plasmodium falciparum* and *P. vivax* infections undetected by conventional microscopy. *Trans R Soc Trop Med Hyg.* 1992;86:609–612.

23. Shanks GD. Malaria prevention and prophylaxis. In: Pasvol G, ed. *Bailliere's Clinical Infectious Diseases.* Vol 2. London: Bailliere Tindall; 1995.

24. Rieckmann KH, Yeo AE, Davis DR, Hutton DC, Wheatley PF, Simpson R. Recent military experience with malaria chemoprophylaxis. *Med J Aust.* 1993;158:446–449.

25. Boudreau E, Schuster B, Sanchez J, et al. Tolerability of prophylactic Lariam regimens. *Trop Med Parasitol.* 1993;44:257–265.

26. Shanks GD, Gordon DM, Klotz FW, et al. Efficacy and safety of atovaquone/proguanil for suppressive prophylaxis against *Plasmodium falciparum* malaria. *Clin Infect Dis.* 1998;27:494–499.

27. White NJ. The treatment of malaria. *N Engl J Med.* 1996;335:800–806.

28. Krotoski WA. Frequency of relapse and primaquine resistance in Southeast Asian vivax malaria. *New Engl J Med.* 1980;303:587.

29. US Departments of the Army, Navy, and Air Force. *Standard for Blood Banks and Transfusion Services.* 17th ed. Washington, DC: DA, DN, DAF; 1996. Army FM 8-70, Navy NAVMED P-5120, Air Force AFMAN 41-111.

30. Nosten F, ter Kuile F, Chongsuphajaisiddhi T, et al. Mefloquine-resistant falciparum malaria on the Thai-Burmese border. *Lancet.* 1991;337:1140–1143.

31. D'Alessandro U, Leach A, Drakeley CJ, et al. Efficacy trial of malaria vaccine SPf66 in Gambian infants. *Lancet.* 1995;346:462–467.

32. Stoute JA, Slaoui M, Heppner DG, et al. A preliminary evaluation of the recombinant circumporozoite protein vaccine against *Plasmodium falciparum* malaria. *New Engl J Med*. 1997;336:86–91.

33. World Health Organization. *World Health Report*. Geneva: WHO; 1996: 48.

34. Monath TP. Dengue: The risk to developed and developing countries. *Proc Natl Acad Sci USA*. 1994;91:2395–2400.

35. Pan American Health Organization. *Dengue and Dengue Hemorrhagic Fever in the Americas: Guidelines for Prevention and Control*. Washington, DC: PAHO; 1994: 19–21.

36. Horton R. The infected metropolis. *Lancet*. 1996;347:134–135. Published erratum: *Lancet*. 1996;347:482.

37. Fuller HS. Introduction. Coates JB Jr, Hoff EC, Hoff PM, eds. *Communicable Diseases: Arthropodborne Diseases Other than Malaria*. Vol 7. In: *Preventive Medicine in World War II*. Washington, DC: Office of the Surgeon General, Department of the Army; 1964.

38. Siler JF, Hall MW, Hitchens AP. Dengue: Its history, epidemiology, mechanisms of transmission, etiology, clinical manifestations, immunity, and prevention. *Philipp J Sci*. 1926;29:1–304.

39. Simmons JS, St John JH, Reynolds FHK. Experimental studies of dengue. *Philipp J Sci*. 1931;44:1–247.

40. McCoy OR, Sabin AB. Dengue. Coates JB Jr, Hoff EC, Hoff PM, eds. *Communicable Diseases: Arthropodborne Diseases Other than Malaria*. Vol 7. In: *Preventive Medicine in World War II*. Washington, DC: Office of the Surgeon General, Department of the Army; 1964: 29–62.

41. Russell PR. Dengue and dengue shock syndrome. Ognibene AJ, Barrett O Jr, eds. *General Medicine and Infectious Diseases*. Vol 2. In: *Internal Medicine in Vietnam*. Washington, DC: Office of the Surgeon General and Center of Military History, US Army; 1982.

42. Sabin AB. Research on dengue during World War II. *Am J Trop Med Hyg*. 1950;1:30–50.

43. Sabin AB, Schlesinger RW. Production of immunity to dengue with virus modified by propagation in mice. *Science*. 1945; 101:640–642.

44. Heggers JP. Microbial invasion—the major ally of war (natural biological warfare). *Mil Med*. 1978;143:390–394.

45. Deller JJ Jr. Fever of undetermined origin. Ognibene AJ, Barrett O Jr, eds. *General Medicine and Infectious Diseases*. Vol 2. In: *Internal Medicine in Vietnam*. Washington, DC: Office of the Surgeon General and Center of Military History, US Army; 1984.

46. Hyams KC, Bourgeois AL, Escamilla J, Burans J, Woody JN. The Navy Forward Laboratory during Operations Desert Shield/Desert Storm. *Mil Med*. 1993;158;729–732.

47. Gunby P. Extraordinary epidemiologic, environmental health experience emerges from Operation Restore Hope. *JAMA*. 1993;269:2833–2838.

48. Sharp TW, Wallace MR, Hayes CG, et al. Dengue fever in U.S. troops during Operation Restore Hope, Somalia, 1992-1993. *Am J Trop Med Hyg*. 1995;53:89–94.

49. Centers for Disease Control and Prevention. Dengue fever among U.S. military personnel—Haiti, September-November, 1994. *MMWR*. 1994;43:845–848.

50. Trofa AF, DeFraites RF, Smoak BL, et al. Dengue fever in U.S. military personnel in Haiti. *JAMA*. 1997;277:1546–1548.

51. Henchal EA, Putnak JR. The dengue viruses. *Clin Microbiol Rev*. 1990;3:376–396.

52. Wu SJ, Grouard-Vogel G, Sun W, et al. Human skin Langerhans cells are targets of dengue virus infection. *Nature Med*. 2000;6:816–820.

53. Ramirez-Ronda CH, Garcia CD. Dengue in the Western hemisphere. *Infect Dis Clin North Am*. 1994;8:107–128.

54. Burke DS, Nisalak A, Johnson DE, Scott RM. A prospective study of dengue infections in Bangkok. *Am J Trop Med Hyg*. 1988;38:172–180.

55. Halstead SB. Dengue hemorrhagic fever. In: Gear JHS, ed. CRC *Handbook of Viral and Rickettsial Hemorrhagic Fevers*. Boca Raton, Fla: CRC Press: 1988.

56. Sangkawibha N, Rojanasuphot S, Ahandrik S, et al. Risk factors in dengue shock syndrome: a prospective epidemiologic study in Rayong, Thailand, I: The 1980 outbreak. *Am J Epidemiol*. 1984;120:653–669.

57. Halstead SB. Pathogenesis of dengue: Challenges to molecular biology. *Science*. 1988;239:476–481.

58. Yoksan S, Bhamarapravati N. Localization of dengue antigens in tissue specimens from fatal cases of dengue hemorrhagic fever. *Proceedings of the International Conference on Dengue/Dengue Hemorrhagic Fever*. Kuala Lumpur: University of Malaya; 1983: 406–409.

59. Morens DM. Antibody-dependent enhancement of infection and the pathogenesis of viral disease. *Clin Infect Dis*. 1994;19:500–512.

60. Sabin AB. Dengue. In: Rivers TM, Horsfall FL, eds. *Viral and Rickettsial Infections of Man*. Philadelphia: JB Lippincott; 1959: 363–364.

61. Libraty DH, Pichyangkul S, Ajariyakhajorn C, Endy TP, Ennis FA. Human dendritic cells are activated by dengue virus infection: Enhancement by gamma interferon and implications for disease pathogenesis. *J Virol*. 2001;75:3501–3508.

62. Chin J, ed. *Control of Communicable Diseases Manual*. 17th ed. Washington, DC: American Public Health Association; 2000: 142–147.

63. Cohen SN, Halstead SB. Shock associated with dengue infection, I: Clinical and physiologic manifestations of dengue hemorrhagic fever in Thailand, 1964. *J Pediatr*. 1966;68:448–456.

64. Kurane I, Ennis FA. Cytokines in dengue infections: Role of cytokines in the pathogenesis of dengue hemorrhagic fever. *Sem Virol*. 1994;5:443–448.

65. Rico-Hesse R, Harrison LM, Salas RA, et al. Origins of dengue type 2 viruses associated with increased pathogenicity in the Americas. *Virology*. 1997;230:244–251.

66. Watts DM, Porter KR, Putvatana P, et al. Failure of secondary infection with American genotype dengue 2 to cause dengue hemorrhagic fever. *Lancet*. 1999;354:1431–1434.

67. Leitmayer KC, Vaughn DW, Watts DM, et al. Dengue virus structural differences that correlate with pathogenesis. *J Virol*. 1999;73:4738–4747.

68. Innis BL. Dengue and dengue hemorrhagic fever. Porterfield JS, ed. *Exotic Viral Infections*. Chapman & Hall: London; 1995: 103–146.

69. Beaty BJ, Calisher CH, Shope RE. Arboviruses. In: Schmidt NJ, Emmons RW, eds. *Diagnostic Procedures for Viral, Rickettsial, and Chlamydial Infections*. 6th ed. Washington, DC: American Public Health Association; 1989: 828–829.

70. Innis BL, Nisalak A, Nimmannitya S, et al. An enzyme-linked immunosorbent assay to characterize dengue infections where dengue and Japanese encephalitis co-circulate. *Am J Trop Med Hyg*. 1989;40:418–427.

71. Rossi CA, Lewis TE, Drabick J, et al. Laboratory diagnosis of acute dengue fever in military troops during the United Nations Mission in Haiti, 1995-1996. *Am J Trop Med.* 1998;59:275–278.

72. Kalayanarooj S, Vaughn DW, Nimmannitya S, et al. Early clinical and laboratory indicators of acute dengue illness. *J Infect Dis.* 1997;176:313–321.

73. Kouri GP, Guzman MG, Bravo JR, Triana C. Dengue haemorrhagic fever/dengue shock syndrome: Lessons from the Cuban epidemic, 1981. *Bull World Health Organ.* 1989;67:375–380.

74. Kanesa-thasan N, Hoke CH Jr. Dengue and related syndromes. In: Schlossberg D, ed. *Current Therapy of Infectious Disease.* 2nd ed. Chicago: Mosby-Year Book; 2001.

75. World Health Organization. *Dengue Hemorrhagic Fever: Diagnosis, Treatment and Control.* 2nd ed. Geneva: WHO; 1997: 6.

76. Kanesa-thasan N, Putnak JR, Hoke CH Jr. New and improved vaccines for dengue, Japanese encephalitis, and yellow fever viruses. In: Levine MM, Woodrow GC, Kaper JB, Cobon GS eds. *New Generation Vaccines.* 2nd ed. New York: Marcel Dekker; 1997: 587–606.

77. Pinheiro FP, Travassos da Rosa AP, Travassos da Rosa JF, et al. Oropouche virus, I: A review of clinical, epidemiological, and ecological findings. *Am J Trop Med Hyg.* 1981;30:149–160.

78. Leduc JW, Pinheiro FP. Oropouche fever. In: Monath TP, ed. *The Arboviruses: Epidemiology and Ecology.* Vol 4. Boca Raton, Fla: CRC Press; 1989: 1–14.

79. Tesh RB. The emerging epidemiology of Venezuelan hemorrhagic fever and Oropouche fever in tropical South America. *Ann N Y Acad Sci.* 1994;740:129–137.

80. Baisley KJ, Watts DM, Munstermann LE, Wilson ML. Epidemiology of endemic Oropouche virus transmission in upper Amazonian Peru. *Am J Trop Med Hyg.* 1998;59:710–716.

81. Meegan JM, Bailey CL. Rift Valley fever. In: Monath TP, ed. *The Arboviruses: Epidemiology and Ecology.* Vol 4. Boca Raton, Fla: CRC Press; 1989: 51–76.

82. Shope R, Peters CJ, Walker JS. Serological relation between Rift Valley fever virus and viruses of Phlebotomus fever serogroup. *Lancet.* 1980;1:886–887.

83. McIntosh BM, Jupp PG, Dos Santos I, Barnard BJ. Vector studies on Rift Valley Fever virus in South Africa. *S Afr Med J.* 1980;58:127–132.

84. World Health Organization Scientific Group. *Arthropod-borne and Rodent-borne Viral Diseases.* Geneva: World Health Organization; 1985. Technical Report Series 719.

85. Sall AA, Zanotto PM, Vialat P, Sene OK, Bouloy, MB. Origin of 1997–98 Rift Valley fever outbreak in East Africa. *Lancet.* 1998;352:1596–1597.

86. Watts DM, el-Tigani A, Botros BA, et al. Arthropod-borne viral infections associated with a fever outbreak in the northern province of Sudan. *J Trop Med Hyg.* 1994;97:228–230.

87. Corwin A, Habib M, Watts D, et al. Community-based prevalence profile of arboviral, rickettsial, and hantaan-like viral antibody in the Nile River Delta of Egypt. *Am J Trop Med Hyg.* 1993;48:776–783.

88. Richards AL, Malone JD, Sheris S, et al. Arbovirus and rickettsial infections among combat troops during Operation Desert Shield/Desert Storm. *J Infect Dis.* 1993;168:1080–1081.

89. Gordon SW, Tammariello RF, Linthicum KJ, Dohm DJ, Digoutte JP, Calvo-Wilson MA. Arbovirus isolations from mosquitoes collected during 1988 in the Senegal River basin. *Am J Trop Med Hyg.* 1992;47:742–748.

90. Bray M, Huggins J. Antiviral therapy of haemorrhagic fevers and arbovirus infections. *Antiviral Therapy.* 1998;3:53–79.

91. Niklasson B, Peters CJ, Bengtsson E, Norrby E. Rift Valley fever virus vaccine trial: Study of neutralizing antibody response in humans. *Vaccine.* 1985;3:123–127.

92. Pittman PR, Liu CT, Cannon TL, et al. Immunogencity of an inactivated Rift Valley fever vaccine in humans: A 12-year experience. *Vaccine.* 1999;18:181–189.

93. Jupp PG, McIntosh BM. Chikungunya virus disease. In: Monath TP, ed. *The Arboviruses: Epidemiology and Ecology.* Vol 2. Boca Raton, Fla: CRC Press; 1989: 137–157.

94. Blackburn NK, Besselaar TG, Gibson G. Antigenic relationship between chikungunya virus strains and O'nyong nyong virus using monoclonal antibodies. *Res Virol.* 1995;146:69–73.

95. Konishi E, Hotta S. Studies on structural proteins of Chikungunya virus, I: Separation of three species of proteins and their preliminary characterization. *Microbiol Immunol.* 1980;24:419–428.

96. Powers AM, Tesh RB, Weaver SC. Phylogenetic analysis of Chikungunya viruses: Evidence for distinct lineages. *Am J Trop Med Hyg.* 1997;57:225. Abstract 366.

97. Turell MJ, Malinoski FJ. Limited potential for mosquito transmission of a live, attenuated chikungunya virus vaccine. *Am J Trop Med Hyg.* 1992;47:98–103.

98. Halstead SB. Arboviruses of the Pacific and Southeast Asia. In: Feigin RD, Cherry JE, eds. *Textbook of Pediatric Infectious Diseases.* 3rd ed. Philadelphia: WB Saunders; 1992: 1483–1488.

99. Centers for Disease Control. Chikungunya fever among U.S. Peace Corps volunteers—Republic of the Philippines. *MMWR.* 1986;35:573–574.

100. Nisalak A, Thaikruea L, Teeraratku A, Endy TP, Innis BL, Vaughn DW. Chikungunya in Thailand: A reemerging disease? Presented at the International Conference on Emerging Infectious Diseases; March 1998; Atlanta, Ga. Abstract P9.9.

101. Tomori O, Fagbami A, Fabiyi A. The 1974 epidemic of chikungunya fever in children in Ibadan. *Trop Geogr Med.* 1975;27:413–417.

102. Moore DL, Reddy S, Akinkugbe FM, et al. An epidemic of chikungunya fever at Ibadan, Nigeria, 1969. *Ann Trop Med Parasit.* 1974;68:59–67.

103. Thaung U, Ming CK, Swe T, Thein S. Epidemiolgical features of dengue and chikungunya infections in Burma. *Southeast Asian J Trop Med Public Health.* 1975;6:276–283.

104. Kennedy AC, Fleming J, Solomon L. Chikungunya viral arthropathy: A clinical description. *J Rheumatol.* 1980;7:231–236.

105. Brighton SW, Prozesky OW, de la Harpe AL. Chikungunya virus infection: A retrospective study of 107 cases. *S Afr Med J.* 1983;63:313–315.

106. Thein S, La Linn M, Aaskov J, et al. Development of a simple indirect enzyme-linked immunosorbent assay for the detection of immunoglobulin M antibody in serum from patients following an outbreak of Chikungunya virus infection in Yangon, Myanmar. *Trans R Soc Trop Med Hyg.* 1992;86:438–442.

107. Levinson RS, Strauss JH, Strauss EG. Complete sequence of the genomic RNA of O'nyong-nyong virus and its use in the construction of alphavirus phylogenentic tree. *Virology.* 1990;175:110–123.

108. Rwaguma EB, Lutwama JJ, Sempala SD, et al. Emergence of epidemic O'nyong-nyong fever in southwestern Uganda, after an absence of 35 years. *Emerg Infect Dis.* 1997;3:77.

109. Johnson BK, Gichogo A, Gitau G, et al. Recovery of O'nyong-nyong virus from *Anopheles funestus* in western Kenya. *Trans R Soc Trop Med Hyg*. 1981;75:239–241.

110. Niklasson B. Sindbis and Sindbis-like virus diseases. In: Monath TP, ed. *The Arboviruses: Epidemiology and Ecology*. Vol 4. Boca Raton, Fla: CRC Press; 1989: 167–176.

111. Rentier-Delrue F, Young NA. Genomic devergence among Sindbis virus strains. *Virology*. 1980;106:59–70.

112. Espmark A, Niklasson B. Ockelbo disease in Sweden: Epidemiological, clinical, and virological data from the 1982 outbreak. *Am J Trop Med Hyg*. 1984;33:1203–1211.

113. Jupp PG, Blackburn NK, Thompson DL, Meenehan GM. Sinbis and West Nile virus infections in the Witwatesrand-Pretoria region. *S Afr Med J*. 1986;70:218–220.

114. Kay BH, Aaskov JG. Ross River virus (epidemic polyarthritis). In: Monath TP, ed. *The Arboviruses: Epidemiology and Ecology*. Vol 4. Boca Raton, Fla: CRC Press; 1989: 93–112.

115. Calisher CH, Karabatso N. Arbovirus serogroups: Definition and geographic distribution. In: Monath TP, ed. *The Arboviruses: Epidemiology and Ecology*. Vol 1. Boca Raton, Fla: CRC Press; 1989: 19–57.

116. Ritchie SA, Fanning ID, Phillips DA, Standfast HA, Mcginn D, Kay BH. Ross River virus in mosquitoes (Diptera: Culcidae) during the 1994 epidemic around Brisbane, Australia. *J Med Entomol*. 1997;34:156–159.

117. Keat-Song T, Whelan PI, Patel MS, Currie B. An outbreak of epidemic polyarthritis (Ross River virus disease) in the Northern Territory during the 1990-1991 wet season. *Med J Aust*. 1993;158:522–525.

118. Lindsay M, Oliveira N, Jasinska E, et al. An outbreak of Ross River Virus disease in Southwestern Australia. *Emerg Infect Dis*. 1996;2:117–120.

119. Selden SM, Cameron AS. Changing epidemiology of Ross River virus disease in South Australia. *Med J Aust*. 1996;165:313–317.

120. Flexman JP, Smith DW, Mackenzie JS, et al. A comparison of the diseases caused by Ross River virus and Barmah forest virus. *Med J Aust*. 1998;169:159–163.

121. Linn ML, Aaskov JG , Suhrbier A. Antibody-dependent enhancement and persistence in macrophages of an arbovirus associated with arthritis. *J Gen Virol*. 1996;77:407–411.

122. Yu S, Aaskov JG. Development of a candidate vaccine against Ross River virus infection. *Vaccine*. 1994;12:1118–1124.

123. Hayes CG, West Nile fever. In: Monath TP, ed. *The Arboviruses: Epidemiology and Ecology*. Vol 5. Boca Raton, Fla: CRC Press; 1989: 59–82.

124. Jupp PG, Blackburn NK, Thompson DL, Meenehan GM. Sindbis and West Nile virus infections in the Witwatersrand-Pretoria region. *S Afr Med J*. 1986;70:218–220.

125. Asnis DS, Conetta R, Teixeira AA, et al. The West Nile virus outbreak of 1999 in New York: The Flushing Hospital experience. *Clin Infect Dis*. 2000;30:413–418.

126. Olaleye OD, Omilabu SA, Ilomechina EN, Fagbami AH. A survey for haemagglutination-inhibiting antibody to West Nile virus in human and animal sera in Nigeria. *Comp Immun Microbiol Infect Dis*. 1990;13:35–39.

127. Morvan J, Chin LH, Fonetnille D, Rakotoarivony I, Coulanges P. Prevalence of antibodies to West Nile virus in youngsters from 5 to 20 years old in Madagascar. *Bull Soc Pathol Exot*. 1991; 84:225–234.

128. Sugamata M, Ahmed A, Miura T, et al. Seroepidemiological study of infection with West Nile virus in Karachi, Pakistan, in 1983 and 1985. *J Med Virol*. 1988;26:243–247.

129. Hayes CG, Baqar S, Ahmed T, Chowdhry MA, Reisen WK. West Nile virus in Pakistan, 1: Sero-epidemiological Studies in Punjab Province. *Trans R Soc Trop Med Hyg.* 1982;76:431–436.

130. George S, Prsad SR, Rao JA, Yergolkar PN, Setty CV. Isolation of Japanese encephalitis and West Nile viruses from fatal cases of encephalitis in the Kolar district of Karnataka. *Indian J Med Res.* 1987;86:131–134.

131. Tsai TF, Popovici F, Cernescu C, Campbell GL, Nedelcu NI. West Nile encephalitis epidemic in southeastern Romania. *Lancet.* 1998;352:767–771.

132. Update: West Nile Virus activity—Eastern United States, 2000. *MMWR.* 2000;49: 1044–1047

133. Turell MJ, O'Guinn M, Oliver J. Potential for New York mosquitoes to transmit West Nile virus. *Am J Trop Med Hyg.* 2000;62:413–414.

134. Steele KE, Linn MJ, Schoepp RJ, et al. Pathology of fatal West Nile virus infections in native and exotic birds during the 1999 outbreak in New York City, New York. *Vet Pathol.* 2000;37:208–224.

135. Sampson BA, Amrosi C, Charlot A, et al. The pathology of human West Nile virus infection. *Hum Pathol.* 2000;31:527–531.

136. Porter KR, Summers PL, Dubois D, et al. Detection of West Nile virus by the polymerase chain reaction (PCR) and analysis of nucleotide sequence variation. *Am J Trop Med Hyg.* 1993;48:440–446.

137. Warren AJ. Landmarks in the conquest of yellow fever. In: Strode GK, ed. *Yellow Fever.* New York: McGraw Hill; 1951.

138. Reed W. Recent researches concerning the etiology, propagation, and prevention of yellow fever, by the United States Army Commission. *J Hyg.* 1902;2:101–119.

139. Meegan JM. Yellow fever. In: Beran GW, Steele JH, eds. *Handbook of Zoonoses, Section B: Viral.* 2nd ed. Boca Raton, Fla: CRC Press; 1994: 111–124.

140. Monath TP. Yellow fever. In: Monath TP, ed. *The Arboviruses: Epidemiology and Ecology.* Vol 5. Boca Raton, Fla: CRC Press; 1989: Chap 51.

141. Monath TP, Heinz FX. Yellow fever virus. In: Fields BN, Knipe DM, Howley PM, eds. *Virology.* 3rd ed. Philadelphia: Lippincott-Raven; 1995: 1009–1016.

142. Lepiniec L, Dalgarno L, Huong VT, Monath TP, Digoutte JP, Deubel V. Geographic distribution and evolution of yellow fever viruses based on direct sequencing of genomic cDNA fragments. *J Gen Virol.* 1994;75:417–423.

143. Deubel V, Pailliez JP, Cornet M, et al. Homogeneity among Senegalese strains of yellow fever virus. *Am J Trop Med Hyg.* 1985;34:976–983.

144. Smithburn KC. Immunology. In: Strode GK, ed. *Yellow Fever.* New York: McGraw Hill; 1951.

145. Henderson BE, Cheshire PP, Kirya GB, Lule M. Immunologic studies with yellow fever and selected African group B arboviruses in rhesus and vervet monkeys. *Am J Trop Med Hyg.* 1970;19:110–118.

146. Theiler M, Anderson CR. The relative resistance of dengue-immune monkeys to yellow fever virus. *Am J Trop Med Hyg.* 1975;24:115–117.

147. Monath TP, Craven RB, Adjukiewicz A, et al. Yellow fever in the Gambia, 1978–1979: Epidemiologic aspects with observations on the occurrence of orungo virus infections. *Am J Trop Med Hyg.* 1980;29:912–928.

148. Nasidi A, Monath TP, DeCock K, et al. Urban yellow fever epidemic in western Nigeria, 1987. *Trans R Soc Trop Med Hyg.* 1989;83:401–406.

149. Miller BR, Ballinger ME. *Aedes albopictus* mosquitoes introduced into Brazil: Vector competence for yellow fever and dengue viruses. *Trans R Soc Trop Med Hyg.* 1988;82:476–477.

150. Aitken TH, Tesh RB, Beaty BJ, Rosen L. Transovarial transmission of yellow fever virus by mosquitoes (*Aedes aegypti*). *Am J Trop Med Hyg.* 1979;28:119–121.

151. Van der Stuyft P, Gianella A, Pirard M, et al. Urbanization of yellow fever in Santa Cruz, Bolivia. *Lancet.* 1999;353:1558–1562.

152. Monath TP, Brinker KR, Chandler FW, Kemp GE, Cropp CB. Pathophysiologic correlations in a rhesus monkey model of yellow fever with special observations on the acute necrosis of B cell areas of lymphoid tissues. *Am J Trop Med Hyg.* 1981;30:431–443.

153. Bugher JC. The pathology of yellow fever. In: Strode GK, ed. *Yellow Fever.* New York: McGraw Hill; 1951.

154. Monath TP. Yellow fever: Victor, Victoria? Conqueror, conquest? Epidemics and research in the last forty years and prospects for the future. *Am J Trop Med Hyg.* 1991;45:1–43.

155. Monath TP. Yellow fever: A medically neglected disease; report on a seminar. *Rev Infect Dis.* 1987;9:165–175.

156. Kerr JA. The clinical aspects and diagnosis of yellow fever. In: Strode GK, ed. *Yellow Fever.* New York: McGraw Hill; 1951.

157. Monath TP, Nystrom RR. Detection of yellow fever virus in serum by enzyme immunoassay. *Am J Trop Med Hyg.* 1984;33:151–157.

158. World Health Organization. *Viral Hemorrhagic Fevers.* Geneva: WHO; 1985. WHO Technical Report Series 721.

159. Thieler M. The virus. In: Strode GK, ed. *Yellow Fever.* New York: McGraw Hill; 1951.

160. Bayne-Jones S. Yellow fever. In: Coates JB Jr, ed. *Communicable Diseases Arthropodborne Diseases Other than Malaria.* Vol 7. In: *Preventive Medicine in World War II:* Washington, DC: Office of the Surgeon General, US Department of the Army; 1964.

161. Jennings AD, Gibson CA, Miller BR, et al. Analysis of a yellow fever virus isolated from a fatal case of vaccine-associated human encephalitis. *J Infect Dis.* 1994;169:512–518.

162. Nasidi A, Monath TP, Vandenberg J, et al. Yellow fever vaccination and pregnancy: A four-year prospective study. *Trans R Soc Trop Med Hyg.* 1993;87:337–339.

163. Tsai TF, Paul R, Lynberg MC, Letson GW. Congenital yellow fever virus infection after immunization in pregnancy. *J Infect Dis.* 1993;168:1520–1523.

164. Coursaget P, Fritzell B, Blondeau C, Saliou P, Diop-Mar I. Simultaneous infection of plasma-derived or recombinant hepatitis B vaccines with yellow fever and killed polio vaccines. *Vaccine.* 1995;13:109–111.

165. Ambrosch F, Fritzell B, Gregor J, et al. Combined vaccination against yellow fever and typhoid fever: A comparative trial. *Vaccine.* 1994;12:625–628.

166. Robertson SE, Hull BP, Tomori O, Bele O, LeDuc JW, Esteves K. Yellow fever: A decade of reemergence. *JAMA.* 1996;276:1157–1162.

167. Tsai TF, Bolin RA, Lazuick JS, Miller KD. Chloroquine does not adversely affect the antibody response to yellow fever vaccine. *J Infect Dis.* 1986;154:726–727.

168. Wisseman CL Jr, Sweet BH, Kitaoka M, Tamiya T. Immunological studies with Group B arthropod-borne viruses, I: Broadened neutralizing antibody spectrum induced by strain 17 D yellow fever vaccine in human subjects previously infected with Japanese encephalitis virus. *Am J Trop Med Hyg.* 1962;11:550–561.

169. Mosimann B, Stoll B, Francillon C, Pecoud A. Yellow fever vaccine and egg allergy. *J All Clin Immunol.* 1995;95:1064.

170. Burke DS, Leake CJ. Japanese encephalitis. In: Monath TP, ed. *The Arboviruses: Epidemiology and Ecology.* Vol 3. Boca Raton, Fla: CRC; 1988: 63–92.

171. Shiraki H. Encephalitides due to arboviruses: Japanese encephalitis. In: Debre R, Celers J, eds. *Clinical Virology: The Evaluation and Management of Human Viral Infections.* Philadelphia: W.B. Saunders; 1970: 155–175.

172. Sabin AB, Tigertt WD, Ando K, et al. Evaluation of Japanese B encephalitis vaccine, I: General background and methods. *Am J Hyg.* 1956;63:217–249.

173. Sabin AB. The St. Louis and Japanese B types of epidemic encephalitis, development of noninfective vaccines: Report of basic data. *JAMA.* 1943;122:281–293.

174. Sabin AB. Epidemic encephalitis in military personnel: Isolation of Japanese B virus on Okinawa in 1945, serologic diagnosis, clinical manifestations, epidemiologic aspects and use of mouse brain vaccine. *JAMA.* 1947;133:281–293.

175. Smadel JE, Randall CR, Warren J. Preparation of Japanese encephalitis vaccine. *Bull US Army Med Dept.* 1947;November:963–972.

176. Ando K, Satterwhite JP. Evaluation of Japanese B encephalitis vaccine, III: Okayama field trial, 1946-1949. Am J Hyg. 1956;63:230–237.

177. Tigertt WD, Berge TO, Burns KF, Satterwhite JP. Evaluation of Japanese B encephalitis vaccine, IV: Pattern of serologic response to vaccination over a five-year period in an endemic area (Okayama, Japan). Am J Hyg. 1956;63:238–249.

178. Lincoln AF, Siverson SE. Acute phase of Japanese B encephalitis: Two hundred and one cases in American soldiers, Korea, 1950. *JAMA.* 1952;150:268–272.

179. Pond WL, Smadel JE. Neurotropic viral diseases in the far east during the Korean war. *Recent Advances in Medicine and Surgery (19 - 30 April 1954): Based on Professional Medical Experiences in Japan and Korea, 1950–1953.* Vol 2. Washington, DC: Army Medical Service Graduate School, Walter Reed Army Medical Center; 1954: 219–233.

180. Colwell EJ, Brown JD, Russell PK, Boone SC, Legters LJ, Catino D. Investigations on acute febrile illness in American servicemen in the Mekong delta of Vietnam. *Mil Med.* 1969;134:1409–1414.

181. Ognibene AJ. Japanese B encephalitis. In: Ognibene AJ, Barrett O, eds. *General Medicine and Infectious Diseases.* Vol 2. *Internal Medicine in Vietnam.* Washington, DC: US Army Office of Surgeon General and Center for Military History; 1982: 99–107.

182. Berg SW, Mitchell BS, Hanson RK, et al. Systemic reactions in U.S. Marine Corps personnel who received Japanese encephalitis vaccine. *Clin Infect Dis.* 1997;24:265–266.

183. Mitamura T, Kitaoka M, Watanabe M, et al. Study on Japanese encephalitis virus, the infectious agent which causes infectious encephalitis (summer encephalitis): Animal experiments and mosquito transmission experiments. *Kansai Iji.* 1936;260:3–4.

184. Huang CH, Liu SH. Acute epidemic encephalitis of Japanese type: Clinical report of six proven cases. *Chin Med J.* 1940;58:427–439.

185. Westaway EG, Brinton MA, Gaidamovich SY, et al. Flaviviridae. *Intervirology.* 1985;24(4):183–192.

186. Chambers TJ, Hahn CS, Galler R, Rice CM. Flavivirus genome organization, expression, and replication. *Annu Rev Microbiol.* 1990;44:649–688.

187. Sumiyoshi H, Mori C, Fuke I, et al. Complete nucleotide sequence of the Japanese encephalitis virus genome RNA. *Virology.* 1987;161:497–510.

188. Okuno T, Okada T, Kondo A, Suzuki M, Kobayashi M, Oya A. Immunotyping of different strains of Japanese encephalitis virus by antibody-absorption, haemagglutination-inhibition and complement-fixation tests. *Bull World Health Organ.* 1968;38:547–563.

189. Chen WR, Rico-Hesse R, Tesh RB. A new genotype of Japanese encephalitis virus from Indonesia. *Am J Trop Med Hyg.* 1992;47:61–69.

190. Scherer WF, Buescher EL, Flemings MB, Noguchi A, Scanlon J. Ecologic studies of Japanese encephalitis virus in Japan, III: Mosquito factors, zootropism, and vertical flight of *Culex tritaeniorhynchus* with observations on variations in collections from animal-baited traps in different habitats. *Am J Trop Med Hyg.* 1959;8:665–677.

191. Scherer WF, Kitaoka M, Okuno T, Ogata T. Ecologic studies of Japanese encephalitis virus in Japan, VII: Human infection. *Am J Trop Med Hyg.* 1959;8:707–715.

192. Goto H. Efficacy of Japanese encephalitis vaccine in horses. *Equine Vet J.* 1976;8(3):126–127.

193. Fujisaki Y, Sugimori T, Morimoto T, Miura Y, Kawakami Y, Nakano K. Immunization of pigs with the attenuated S-strain of Japanese encephalitis virus. *Natl Inst Anim Health Q (Tokyo).* 1975;15(2):55–60.

194. Vaughn DW, Hoke CH Jr. The epidemiology of Japanese encephalitis: Prospects for prevention. *Epidemiol Rev.* 1992;14:197–221.

195. Self LS, Shin HK, Kim KH, Lee KW, Chow CY, Hong HK. Ecological studies on *Culex tritaeniorhynchus* as a vector of Japanese encephalitis. *Bull World Health Organ.* 1973;49:41–47.

196. Mitchell CJ, Chen PS, Boreham PF. Host-feeding patterns and behaviour of 4 Culex species in an endemic area of Japanese encephalitis. *Bull World Health Organ.* 1973;49:293–299.

197. Hanna J, Ritchie S, Loewenthal M, et al. Probable Japanese encephalitis acquired in the Torres Strait. *Communicable Dis Intelligence.* 1995;19(9):206–207.

198. Tsai TF, Yu YX. Japanese encephalitis vaccines. Plotkin SA, Mortimer EA Jr, eds. *Vaccines.* 2nd ed. Philadelphia: W.B. Saunders; 1994: 671–713.

199. Igarashi A, Tanaka M, Morita K, et al. Detection of west Nile and Japanese encephalitis viral genome sequences in cerebrospinal fluid from acute encephalitis cases in Karachi, Pakistan. *Microbiol Immunol.* 1994;38:827–830.

200. Hoke CH Jr, Vaughn DW, Nisalak A, et al. Effect of high-dose dexamethasone on the outcome of acute encephalitis due to Japanese encephalitis virus. *J Infect Dis.* 1992;165:631–637.

201. Umenai T, Krzysko R, Bektimirov TA, Assaad FA. Japanese encephalitis: Current worldwide status. *Bull World Health Organ.* 1985;63:625–631.

202. Halstead SB, Grosz CR. Subclinical Japanese encephalitis, I: Infection of Americans with limited residence in Korea. *Am J Hyg.* 1962;75:190–201.

203. Benenson MW, Top FH Jr, Gresso W, Ames CW, Altstatt LB. The virulence to man of Japanese encephalitis virus in Thailand. *Am J Trop Med Hyg.* 1975;24:974–980.

204. Grossman RA, Edelman R, Willhight M, Pantuwatana S, Udomsakdi S. Study of Japanese encephalitis virus in Chiangmai Valley, Thailand, III: Human seroepidemiology and inapparent infections. *Am J Epidemiol.* 1973;98:133–149.

205. Chakraborty MS, Chakravarti SK, Mukherjee KK, Mitra AC. Inapparent infection by Japanese encephalitis (JE) virus in the West Bengal. *Indian J Public Health.* 1980;24(3):121–127.

206. Burke DS, Lorsomrudee W, Leake CJ, et al. Fatal outcome in Japanese encephalitis. *Am J Trop Med Hyg.* 1985;34:1203–1210.

207. Grossman RA, Edelman R, Chiewanich P, Voodhikul P, Siriwan C. Study of Japanese encephalitis virus in Chiangmai Valley, Thailand, II: Human clinical infections. *Am J Epidemiol.* 1973;98:121–132.

208. Matsumura R, Nakamuro T, Sugata T, Mano Y, Takayanagi T. A case of Japanese encephalitis demonstrating characteristic changes in MRI [in Japanese]. *Rinsho Shinkeigaku.* 1991;31:869–871.

209. Eguchi I, Miyao M, Yamagata T, Shimoizumi H, Yano S, Yanagisawa M. Computed cranial tomography, magnetic resonance imaging and brain echo imaging in Japanese B encephalitis [in Japanese]. *No To Hattatsu.* 1991;23:355–361.

210. Shoji H, Murakami T, Murai I, et al. A follow-up study by CT and MRI in 3 cases of Japanese encephalitis. *Neuroradiology.* 1990;32:215–219.

211. Shoji H, Hiraki Y, Kuwasaki N, Toyomasu T, Kaji M, Okudera T. Japanese encephalitis in the Kurume region of Japan: CT and MRI findings. *J Neurol.* 1989;236:255–259.

212. Schneider RJ, Firestone MH, Edelman R, Chieowanich P, Pornpibul R. Clinical sequelae after Japanese encephalitis: A one-year follow-up study in Thailand. *Southeast Asian J Trop Med Public Health.* 1974;5:560–568.

213. Simpson TW, Meiklejohn G. Sequelae of Japanese B encephalitis. *Am J Trop Med Hyg.* 1947;27:727–730.

214. Miyake M. The pathology of Japanese encephalitis: A review. *Bull World Health Organ.* 1964;30:153–160.

215. Johnson RT, Burke DS, Elwell M, et al. Japanese encephalitis: Immunocytochemical studies of viral antigen and inflammatory cells in fatal cases. *Ann Neurol.* 1985;18:567–573.

216. Burke DS, Nisalak A, Ussery MA, Laorakpongse T, Chantavibul S. Kinetics of IgM and IgG responses to Japanese encephalitis virus in human serum and cerebrospinal fluid. *J Infect Dis.* 1985;151:1093–1099.

217. Innis BL, Nisalak A, Nimmannitya S, et al. An enzyme-linked immunosorbent assay to characterize dengue infections where dengue and Japanese encephalitis co-circulate. *Am J Trop Med Hyg.* 1989;40:418–427.

218. Clarke DH, Casals J. Techniques for hemagglutination and hemagglutination inhibition with arthropod-borne viruses. *Am J Trop Med Hyg.* 1958;7:561–573.

219. Anderson R. Molecular considerations for the laboratory diagnosis of Japanese encephalitis virus. *Southeast Asian J Trop Med Public Health.* 1989;20:605–610.

220. Gadkari DA, Paranjape SG, Shah PS, Mourya DT. Detection of Japanese encephalitis virus infection in mosquitoes and cell culture by polymerase chain reaction (PCR). Bangkok: Second Asia-Pacific Congress of Medical Virology; November 1991. Abstract S11–71991.

221. Leake CJ, Burke DS, Nisalak A, Hoke CH Jr. Isolation of Japanese encephalitis virus from clinical specimens using a continuous mosquito cell line. *Am J Trop Med Hyg.* 1986;35:1045–1050.

222. Harinasuta C, Wasi C, Vithanomsat S. The effect of interferon on Japanese encephalitis virus in vitro. *Southeast Asian J Trop Med Public Health.* 1984;15:564–568.

223. Ghosh SN, Goverdhan MK, Sathe PS, et al. Protective effect of 6-MFA, a fungal interferon inducer against Japanese encephalitis virus in bonnet macaques. *Indian J Med Res.* 1990;91:408–413.

224. Wada Y. Control of Japanese encephalitis vectors. *Southeast Asian J Trop Med Public Health.* 1989;20:623–626.

225. Centers for Disease Control. Japanese encephalitis: Report of a World Health Organization working group. MMWR. 1984;33:119–125.

226. Chunsuttiwat S. Japanese encephalitis in Thailand. *Southeast Asian J Trop Med Public Health.* 1989;20:593–597.

227. Innis BL. Japanese encephalitis. Porterfield JS, ed. *Kass Handbook of Infectious Diseases: Exotic Viral Infections.* Vol 1. London: Chapman & Hall Medical; 1995.

228. Hoke CH Jr, Nisalak A, Sangawhipa N, et al. Protection against Japanese encephalitis by inactivated vaccines. *N Engl J Med.* 1988;319:608–614.

229. Poland JD, Cropp CB, Craven RB, Monath TP. Evaluation of the potency and safety of inactivated Japanese encephalitis vaccine in US inhabitants. *J Infect Dis.* 1990;161:878–882.

230. Sanchez JL, Hoke CH Jr, McCown J, et al. Further experience with Japanese encephalitis vaccine. *Lancet* 1990;335:972–973.

231. Gambel JM, DeFraites R, Hoke CH Jr, et al. Japanese encephalitis vaccine: Persistence of antibody up to 3 years after a three-dose primary series. *J Infect Dis.* 1995;171:1074.

232. Andersen MM, Ronne T. Side-effects with Japanese encephalitis vaccine. *Lancet.* 1991;337:1044.

233. Ruff TA, Eisen D, Fuller A, Kass R. Adverse reactions to Japanese encephalitis vaccine. *Lancet.* 1991;338:881–882.

234. Robinson HC, Russell ML, Csokonay WM. Japanese encephalitis vaccine and adverse effects among travellers. Can Dis Wkly Rep. 1991;17(32):173–174,177.

235. Mulhall BP, Wilde H, Sitprija V. Japanese B encephalitis vaccine: Time for a reappraisal? *Med J Aust.* 1994;160:795–797.

236. Nazareth B, Levin J, Johnson H, Begg N. Systemic allergic reactions to Japanese encephalitis vaccines. *Vaccine.* 1994;12:666.

237. Meyer KF, Haring CM, Howitt B. The etiology of epizootic encephalomyelitis of horses in the San Joaquin Valley, 1930. *Science.* 1931;74:227–228.

238. Giltner LT, Shahan MS. The 1933 outbreak of infectious equine encephalomyelitis in the eastern states. *North Am Vet.* 1933;14:25–27.

239. Ten Broeck C, Hurst EW, Traub E. Epidemiology of equine encephalitis in the eastern United States. *J Exp Med.* 1935;62:677–685

240. Kubes V, Rios FA. The causative agent of infectious equine encephalitis in Venezuela. *Science.* 1939;90:20–21.

241. Webster LT, Wright FH. Recovery of eastern equine encephalomyelitis virus from brain tissue of human cases of encephalitis in Massachusetts. *Science.* 1938;88:305–306.

242. Howitt BE. Recovery of the virus of equine encephalomyelitis from the brain of a child. *Science.* 1938;88:455–456.

243. Franck PT, Johnson KM. An outbreak of Venezuelan encephalitis in man in the Panama Canal zone. *Am J Trop Med Hyg.* 1970;19:860–865.

244. Sanchez JL, Takafuji ET, Lednar WM, et al. Venezuelan equine encephalomyelitis: Report of an outbreak associated with jungle exposure. *Mil Med.* 1984;149:618–621.

245. Chamberlain RW, Rubin H, Kissling RE, Eidson ME. Recovery of eastern equine encephalomyelitis from a mosquito, *Culiseta melanura* (Coquillett). *Proc Soc Exp Biol Med.* 1951;77:396–398.

246. Peters CJ, Dalrymple JM. Alphaviruses. In: Fields BN, ed. *Virology.* New York: Raven Press, Ltd.; 1990: 713–761.

247. Strauss JH, Strauss EG. The alphaviruses: Gene expression, replication, and evolution. Microbiol Rev. 1994;58: 491–562.

248. Anthony RP, Brown DT. Protein-protein interactions in an alphavirus membrane. *J Virol*. 1991;65:1187–1194.

249. Rice CM, Strauss JH. Association of sindbis virus glycoproteins and their precursors. *J Mol Biol*. 1982;154:325–348.

250. Paredes AM, Brown DT, Rothnagel R, et al. Three-dimensional structure of a membrane-containing virus. *Proc Natl Acad Sci USA*. 1993;90:9095–9099.

251. Roehrig JT, Hunt AR, Kinney RM, Mathews JH. In vitro mechanisms of monoclonal antibody neutralization of alphaviruses. *Virology*. 1988;165:66–73.

252. Davis NL, Grieder FB, Smith JF, et al. A molecular genetic approach to the study of Venezuelan equine encephalitis virus pathogenesis. *Arch Virol Suppl*. 1994;9:99–109.

253. Walton TE. Arboviral encephalomyelitides of livestock in the western hemisphere. *J Am Vet Med Assoc*. 1992;200:1385–1389.

254. Weaver SC, Salas R, Rico-Hesse R, et al. Re-emergence of epidemic Venezuelan equine encephalomyelitis in South America. *Lancet*. 1996;348:436–440.

255. Weaver SC, Rico-Hesse R, Scott TW. Genetic diversity and slow rates of evolution in New World alphaviruses. *Curr Topics Microbiol Immunol*. 1992;176:99–117.

256. Weaver SC, Bellew LA, Gousset L, Repik PM, Scott TW, Holland JJ. Diversity within natural populations of eastern equine encephalomyelitis virus. *Virology*. 1993;195:700–709.

257. Walton TE. Equine arboviral encephalomyelitides: A review. *J Equine Vet Sci*. 1988;8:49–53.

258. De Much-Macias J, Sanchez-Spindola I. Two human cases of laboratory infection with Mucambo virus. *Am J Trop Med Hyg*. 1965;14:475–478.

259. Dietz WH, Peralta PH, Johnson KM. Ten clinical cases of human infection with Venezuelan equine encephalomyelitis virus, subtype I-D. *Am J Trop Med Hyg*. 1979;28:329–334.

260. Galindo P. Endemic vectors of Venezuelan encephalitis. In: *Venezuelan Encephalitis: Proceedings of the Workshop–Symposium on Venezuelan Encephalitis Virus; 14-17 September 1971*. Washington, DC: Pan American Health Organization; 1972: 249–252. PAHO Science Publication 243.

261. Young NA, Johnson KM, Gauld LW. Viruses of the Venezuelan equine encephalomyelitis complex: Experimental infection of Panamanian rodents. *Am J Trop Med Hyg*. 1969;18:290–296.

262. Seymour C, Dickerman RW, Martin MS. Venezuelan encephalitis virus infection in neotropical bats, II: Experimental infections. *Am J Trop Med Hyg*. 1978;27:297–306.

263. Walton TE, Grayson MA. Venezuelan equine encephalomyelitis. In: Monath TP, ed. *The Arboviruses: Epidemiology and Ecology*. Vol 4. Boca Raton, Fla: CRC Press; 1988: 204–231.

264. Kinney RM, Tsuchiya KR, Sneider JM, Trent DW. Genetic evidence that epizootic Venezuelan equine encephalitis (VEE) viruses may have evolved from enzootic VEE subtype I–D virus. *Virology*. 1992;191:569–580.

265. Weaver SC, Bellew LA, Rico-Hesse R. Phylogenetic analysis of alphaviruses in the Venezuelan equine encephalitis complex and identification of the source of epizootic viruses. *Virology*. 1992;191:282–290.

266. Hardy JL. The ecology of western equine encephalomyelitis virus in the central valley of California, 1945–1985. *Am J Trop Med Hyg*. 1987;37(Suppl):18S-32S.

267. Smith CEG. Factors influencing the transmission of western equine encephalomyelitis virus between its vertebrate maintenance hosts and from them to humans. *Am J Trop Med Hyg.* 1987;37(Suppl):33S-39S.

268. Weaver SC, Scott TW, Lorenz LH. Patterns of eastern equine encephalomyelitis virus infection in *Culiseta melanura* (Diptera: Culicidae). *J Med Entomol.* 1990;27:878–891.

269. Scott TW, Weaver SC. Eastern equine encephalitis virus: Epidemiology and evolution of mosquito transmission. *Adv Virus Res.* 1989;37:277–328.

270. Johnson KM, Martin DH. Venezuelan equine encephalitis. *Adv Vet Sci Comp Med.* 1974;18:79–116.

271. Hess AD, Hayes RO. Seasonal dynamics of western encephalitis virus. *Am J Med Sci.* 1967;253:333–348.

272. Reisen WK, Hardy JL, Presser SB. Evaluation of domestic pigeons as sentinels for detecting arboviruses in southern California. *Am J Trop Med Hyg.* 1992;46:69–79.

273. Scherer WF, Dickerman RW, Diaz-Najera A, Ward BA, Miller MH, Schaffer PA. Ecologic studies of Venezuelan encephalitis virus in southeastern Mexico, III: Infection of mosquitoes. Am J Trop Med Hyg. 1971;20:969–979.

274. Cupp EW, Scherer WF, Ordonez JV. Transmission of Venezuelan encephalitis virus by naturally infected *Culex (Melanoconion) opisthopus. Am J Trop Med Hyg.* 1979;28:1060–1063.

275. Scherer WF, Dickerman RW, Cupp EW, Ordonez JV. Ecologic observations of Venezuelan encephalitis virus in vertebrates and isolations of Nepuyo and Patois viruses from sentinel hamsters at Pacific and Atlantic habitats in Guatemala, 1968–1980. *Am J Trop Med Hyg.* 1985;34:790–798.

276. Groot H. The health and economic impact of Venezuelan equine encephalitis (VEE). In: *Venezuelan Encephalitis: Proceedings of the Workshop–Symposium on Venezuelan Encephalitis Virus; 14-17 September 1971.* Washington, DC: Pan American Health Organization; 1972: 7–27 PAHO Science Publication 243.

277. Reta G. Equine disease: Mexico. In: *Venezuelan Encephalitis: Proceedings of the Workshop–Symposium on Venezuelan Encephalitis Virus; 14-17 September 1971.* Washington, DC: Pan American Health Organization; 1972: 209–214. PAHO Science Publication 243.

278. Sharman R. Equine disease. In: *Venezuelan Encephalitis: Proceedings of the Workshop–Symposium on Venezuelan Encephalitis Virus; 14-17 September 1971.* Washington, DC: Pan American Health Organization; 1972: 221–224. PAHO Science Publication 243.

279. Colombian Ministry of Health. Vigilance de salud pública de la EEV en La Guajira. *Informe Quincenal de Casos y Brotes de Enfermedades.* 1995;1(4):19–20.

280. Tsai T, Monath TP. Alphaviruses. In: Richmond DD, Whitley RJ, Heyden FG, eds. *Clinical Virology.* New York: Churchill and Livingstone; 1997: 1217–1256.

281. Bigler WJ, Lasting EB, Buff EE, Prather EC, Beck EC, Hoff GL. Endemic eastern equine encephalomyelitis in Florida: A twenty-year analysis, 1955–1974. *Am J Trop Med Hyg.* 1976;25:884–890.

282. de la Monte S, Castro F, Bonilla NJ, Gaskin de Urdaneta A, Hutchins GM. The systemic pathology of Venezuelan equine encephalitis virus infection in humans. *Am J Trop Med Hyg.* 1985;34:194–202.

283. Jackson AC, SenGupta SK, Smith, JF. Pathogenesis of Venezuelan equine encephalitis virus infection in mice and hamsters. *Vet Pathol.* 1991;28:410–418.

284. Gleiser, CA, Gochenour WS, Berge TO, Tigertt WD. The comparative pathology of experimental Venezuelan equine encephalomyelitis infection in different animal hosts. *J Infect Dis.* 1962;110:80–97.

285. Austin FJ, Scherer WF. Studies of viral virulence, I: Growth and histopathology of virulent and attenuated strains of Venezuelan encephalitis virus in hamsters. *Am J Pathol.* 1971;62:195–210.

286. Walker DH, Harrison A, Murphy K, Flemister M, Murphy FA. Lymphoreticular and myeloid pathogenesis of Venezuelan equine encephaltitis in hamsters. *Am J Pathol*. 1976;84:351–370.

287. Monath TP, Cropp CB, Short WF, et al. Recombinant vaccinia–Venezuelan equine encephalomyelitis (VEE) vaccine protects nonhuman primates against parental and intranasal challenge with virulent VEE virus. *Vac Res*. 1992;1:55–68.

288. Gochenour WS. The comparative pathology of Venezuelan encephalitis virus infection in selected animal hosts. In:*Venezuelan Encephalitis: Proceedings of the Workshop–Symposium on Venezuelan Encephalitis Virus; 14-17 September 1971*. Washington, DC: Pan American Health Organization; 1972: 113–119. PAHO Science Publication 243.

289. Sanmartin C, Mackenzie RB, Trapido H, et al. Encefalitis equina Venezolana en Colombia, 1967. *Bol Oficina Sanit Panam*. 1973;74:104–137.

290. Sanmartin C. Diseased hosts: man. In: *Venezuelan Encephalitis: Proceedings of the Workshop–Symposium on Venezuelan Encephalitis Virus; 14-17 September 1971*. Washington, DC: Pan American Health Organization; 1972: 186–188. PAHO Science Publication 243.

291. Garcia-Tamayo J, Esparza J, Martinez AJ. Placental and fetal alterations due to Venezuelan equine encephalitis virus in rats. *Infect Immun*. 1981;32:813–821.

292. Garcia-Tamayo J, de Garcia SE, Esparza, J. Alteraciones iniciales inducidas en los vasos placentarios de la rata por el virus de la Encefalitis equina Venezolana. *Invest Clin*. 1983;24:3–15.

293. McGowan JE Jr, Bryan JA, Gregg MB. Surveillance of arboviral encephalitis in the United States, 1955–1971. *Am J Epidemiol*. 1973;97:199–207.

294. Ayres JC, Feemster RF. The sequelae of eastern equine encephalomyelitis. *N Engl J Med*. 1949;240:960–962.

295. Finley, KG. Post encephalitis manifestations of viral encephalitides. In: Fields NS, Blattner RF, eds. *Viral Encephalitis*. Springfield, Ill: Charles Thomas; 1959: 69–91.

296. Sanmartin-Barberi C, Groot H, Osborno-Mesa E. Human epidemic in Colombia caused by the Venezuelan equine encephalomyelitis virus. *Am J Trop Med Hyg*. 1954;3:283–293.

297. Feemster RF. Equine encephalitis in Massachusetts. *N Engl J Med*. 1958;257:107–113.

298. Calisher CH, Monath TP. *Togaviridae* and *Flaviviridae*: The alphaviruses and flaviviruses. In: Lennette EH, Halonen P, Murphy FA, eds. *Laboratory Diagnosis of Infectious Diseases: Principles and Practice*. Vol 2. New York: Springer-Verlag; 1988: Chap 22.

299. Burke DS, Nisalak A, Ussery MA. Antibody capture immunoassay detection of Japanese encephalitis virus immunoglobulin M and G antibodies in cerebrospinal fluid. *J Clin Microbiol*. 1982;16:1034–1042.

300. Monath TP, Nystrom RR, Bailey RE, Calisher CH, Muth DJ. Immunoglobulin M antibody capture enzyme-linked immunosorbent assay for diagnosis of St. Louis encephalitis. *J Clin Microbiol*. 1984;20:784–790.

301. Calisher CH, el-Kafrawi AO, Al-Deen Mahmud MI, et al. Complex-specific immunoglobulin M antibody patterns in humans infected with alphaviruses. *J Clin Microbiol*. 1986;23:155–159.

302. Briceño Rossi AL. The frequency of VEE virus in the pharyngeal material of clinical cases of encephalitis. *Gac Med Caracas*. 1964;72:5–22.

303. Wenger F. Venezuelan equine encephalitis. *Teratol*. 1977;16:359–362.

304. Casamassima AC, Hess LW, Marty A. TC-83 Venezuelan equine encephalitis vaccine exposure during pregnancy. *Teratol*. 1987;36:287–289.

305. Rehle TM. Classification, distribution and importance of arboviruses. *Trop Med Parasit.* 1989;40:391–395.

306. McNeil JG, Lednar WM, Stansfield SK, et al. Central European tick-borne encephalitis: Assessment of risk for persons in the armed services and vacationers. *J Infect Dis Suppl.* 1985;152:650–651.

307. Gustafson R. Epidemiological studies of Lyme borreliosis and tick-borne encephalitis. *Scand J Infect Dis Suppl.* 1994;92:1–63.

308. Treib J. First case of tick-borne encephalitis (TBE) in the Saarland. *Infection.* 1994;22:368–369.

309. Westaway EG, Brinton MA, Gaidamovich SY, et al. Flaviviridae. *Intervirology.* 1985;24:183–192.

310. Chambers TJ, Hahn CS, Galler R, Rice CM. Flavivirus genome organization, expression, and replication. *Annu Rev Microbiol.* 1990;44:649–688.

311. Heinz FX, Berger R, Tuma W, et al. A topological and functional model of epitopes on the structural glycoprotein of tick-borne encephalitis virus defined by monoclonal antibodies. *Virology.* 1983;126:525–537.

312. Gresíková M, Calisher C. Tick-borne encephalitis. In: Monath TP, ed. *The Arboviruses: Epidemiology and Ecology.* Vol 4. Boca Raton, Fla: CRC Press; 1989: 177–198.

313. Mandl CW, Holzmann H, Kunz C, Heinz FX. Complete genomic sequence of Powassan virus: Evaluation of genetic elements in tick-borne versus mosquito-borne flaviviruses. *Virology.* 1993;194:173–184.

314. Gresíková M, Sekeyová M. Antigenic relationships among viruses of the tick-borne encephalitis complex as studied by monoclonal antibodies. *Acta Virol.* 1984;28:64–68.

315. Korenberg EI, Horáková M, Kovalevsky JV, Hubalek Z, Karavanos AS. Probability models of the rate of infection with tick-borne encephalitis virus in *Ixodes persulcatus* ticks. *Folia Parasitol.* 1992;39:85–92.

316. Gresíková M, Kozuch O, Sekeyov· M, Nosek J . Studies on the ecology of tick-borne encephalitis virus in the Carpathian and Pannonian type of natural foci. *Acta Virol.* 1986;30:325–331.

317. Kozuch O, Gresíková M, Nosek J, Lichard M, Sekeyová M. The role of small rodents and hedgehogs in a natural focus of tick-borne encephalitis. *Bull World Health Organ.* 1967;36(Suppl 1):61–66.

318. Nuttall PA, Jones LD, Labuda M, Kaufman WR. Adaptations of arboviruses to ticks. *J Med Entomol.* 1994;31:1–9.

319. Rehácek J. Transovarial transmission of tick-borne encephalitis virus by ticks. *Acta Virol.* 1962;6:220–226.

320. Chunikhin SP, Stefutkina LF, Korolev MB, et al. Sexual transmission of tick-borne encephalitis virus in Ixodids. *Parazitol.* 1983;17:214–217.

321. Labuda M, Jones LD, Williams T, Danielova V, Nuttall PA. Efficient transmission of tick-borne encephalitis virus between cofeeding ticks. *J Med Entomol.* 1993;30:295–299.

322. Gresíková M. Recovery of tick-borne encephalitis virus from the blood and milk of subcutaneously infected sheep. *Acta Virol.* 1958;2:113–119.

323. Ernek E, Kozuch O, Nosek J. Isolation of tick-borne encephalitis virus from blood and milk of goats grazing in the Tribec focus zone. *J Hyg Epidemiol Microbiol Immunol.* 1968;12:32–36.

324. Sixl W, Stünzner D, Withalm H, Kock M. Rare transmission mode of FSME (tick-borne encephalitis) by goat's milk. *Geographia Medica Suppl.* 1989;2:11–14.

325. Gresíková M, Sekeyová M, Stúpalová S, Necas S. Sheep milk-borne epidemic of tick-borne encephalitis in Slovakia. *Intervirology.* 1975;5(1-2):57–61.

326. Gresíková M. Excretion of the tick-borne encephalitis virus in the milk of subcutaneously infected cows. *Acta Virol.* 1958;2:188–192.

327. Blaskovic D, Nosek J. The ecological approach to the study of tick-borne encephalitis. *Prog Med Virol.* 1972;14: 275–320.

328. Blaskovic D, Pucekova G, Kubínyi S, Stúpalová S, Oravcova V. An epidemiological study of tick-borne encephalitis in the Tribec region: 1953–63. *Bull World Health Organ.* 1967;36(Suppl 1):89–94.

329. Molnár E, Kubászova T. Tick-borne encephalitis: A comparative serological survey in Hungary. *Acta Microbiol Acad Sci Hung.* 1966;13:289–294.

330. Ogawa M, Okubo H, Tsuji Y, Uasui N, Someda K. Chronic progressive encephalitis occurring 13 years after Russian spring-summer encephaltis. *J Neurol Sci.* 1973;19:363–373.

331. Grinschgl G. Virus meningo-encephalitis in Austria: Clinical features, pathology, and diagnosis. *Bull World Health Organ.* 1955;23:535–564.

332. McNair AN, Brown JL. Tick-borne encephalitis complicated by monoplegia and sensorineural deafness. *J Infect.* 1991;22:81–86.

333. Artsob H. Powassan encephalitis. In: Monath TP, ed. *The Arboviruses: Epidemiology and Ecology.* Vol 4. Boca Raton, Fla: CRC Press; 1989: 29–50.

334. Tsai TF. Arboviral diseases of North America. In: Feigin RD, Cherry JD, eds. *Textbook of Pediatric Infectious Diseases.* 3rd ed. Philadelphia: W.B. Saunders; 1992: 132–133.

335. Shiu SY, Ayres MD, Gould EA. Genomic sequence of the structural proteins of louping ill virus: Comparative analysis with tick-borne encephalitis virus. *Virology.* 1991;180:411–415.

336. Venugopal K, Gritsun T, Lashkevich VA, Gould EA. Analysis of the structural protein gene sequence shows Kyasanur Forest disease virus as a distinct member in the tick-borne encephalitis virus serocomplex. *J Gen Virol.* 1994;75:227–232.

337. Rao TR. Immunological surveys of arbovirus infections in South-East Asia, with special reference to dengue, chikungunya, and Kyasanur Forest disease. *Bull World Health Organ.* 1971;44:585–591.

338. Roggendorf M, Heinz F, Deinhardt F, Kunz C. Serological diagnosis of acute tick-borne encephalitis by demonstration of antibodies of the IgM class. *J Med Virol.* 1981;7:41–50.

339. Albrecht P, Kozuch O. Rapid identification of tick-borne encephalitis virus by the fluorescent antibody technique. *Bull World Health Organ.* 1967;36(Suppl 1):85–88.

340. Hofmann H, Frisch-Niggemeyer W, Heinz F. Rapid diagnosis of tick-borne encephalitis by means of enzyme linked immunosorbent assay. *J Gen Virol.* 1979;42:505–511.

341. Whitby JE, Ni H, Whitby HE, et al. Rapid detection of viruses of the tick-borne encephalitis virus complex by RT-PCR of viral RNA. *J Virol Methods.* 1993;45:103–114.

342. Barrett PN, Dorner F. Tick-borne encephalitis vaccine. In: Plotkin SA, Mortimer EA, eds. *Vaccines.* 2nd ed. Philadelphia: W.B. Saunders; 1994: 715–727.

343. Stephenson JR. Flavivirus vaccines. *Vaccine.* 1988;6:471–480.

344. Bock H, Klockmann U, Jungst C, Schindel-Kunzel F, Theobald K, Zerban R. A new vaccine against tick-borne encephalitis: Initial trial in man including a dose-response study. *Vaccine.* 1990;8:22–24.

345. Harabacz I, Bock H, Jungst C, Klockmann U, Praus M, Weber R. A randomized phase II study of a new tick-borne encephalitis vaccine using three different doses and two immunization regimens. *Vaccine.* 1992;10:145–150.

346. Stephenson JR, Lee JM, Easterbrook LM, Timofeev AV, Elbert LB. Rapid vaccination protocols for commercial vaccines against tick-borne encephalitis. *Vaccine*. 1995;13:743–746.

347. Kunz C, Heinz FX, Hofmann H. Immunogenicity and reactogenicity of a highly purified vaccine against tick-borne encephalitis. *J Med Virol*. 1980;6:103–109.

348. Klockmann U, Krivanec K, Stephenson JR, Helfenhaus S. Protection against European isolates of tick-borne encephalitis virus after vaccination with a new tick-borne encephalitis vaccine. *Vaccine*. 1991;9:210–212.

349. Harabacz I, Bock H, Jüngst C, Klockmann U, Praus M, Weber R. A randomized phase II study of a new tick-borne encephalitis vaccine using three different doses and two immunization regimens. *Vaccine*. 1992;10:145–150.

350. Klockmann U, Bock HL, Kwasny H, et al. Humoral immunity against tick-borne encephalitis virus following manifest disease and active immunization. *Vaccine*. 1991;9:42–46.

351. Zoulek G, Roggendorf M, Deinhardt F, Kunz C. Different immune responses after intradermal and intramuscular administration of vaccine against tick-borne encephalitis virus. *J Med Virol*. 1986;19:55–61.

352. Zoulek G, Roggendorf M, Deinhardt F. Immune response to single dose, multisite, intradermal and to intramuscular administration of vaccine against tick-borne encephalitis virus. *Lancet*. 1984;2:584.

353. Bohus M, Glocker FX, Jost S, Deuschl G, Lucking CH. Myelitis after immunization against tick-borne encephalitis. *Lancet*. 1993;342:239–240.

354. von Hendenstrom M, Heberle U, Theobald K. Vaccination against tick-borne encephalitis (TBE): Influence of simultaneous application of TBE immunoglobulin on seroconversion and rate of adverse events. *Vaccine*. 1995;13:759-762.

355. Girgsdies OE, Rosenkranz G. Tick-borne encephalitis: Development of a pediatric vaccine. A controlled, randomized, double-blind and multicenter study. *Vaccine*. 1996;14:1421–1428.

356. Weber W. Germany halts tick-borne encephalitis vaccine. *Lancet*. 2000;356:52.

357. Craig SC, Pittman PR, Lewis TE, et al. An accelerated schedule for tick-borne encephalitis vaccine: The American military experience in Bosnia. *Am J Trop Med Hyg*. 1999;61:874–878.

358. Sabin AB. Phlebotomus fever. In: TM Rivers, ed. *Viral and Rickettsial Infections of Man*. 2nd ed. Philadelphia: J.B. Lippincott Co; 1952.

359. Tesh RB, Saidi S, Gajdamovic SJ, Rodhain F, Vesenjak-Hirjan J. Serological studies on the epidemiology of sandfly fever in the Old World. *Bull World Health Organ*. 1976;54:663–74.

360. Gaidamovich SY, Khutoretskaya NV, Azyamov YV, Tsyupa VI, Mel'nikova EE. Virological study of cases of sandfly fever cases in Afghanistan. *Vopr Virusol*. 1990;35(1):45–47.

361. Robeson G, el Said LH, Brandt W, Dalrymple J, Bishop DH. Biochemical studies on the Phlebotomus fever group viruses (Bunyaviridae family). *J Virol*. 1979;30:339–350.

362. Birt C. Phlebotomus fever and dengue. *Trans R Soc Trop Med Hyg*. 1913;6:243–262.

363. Whittingham HE. The etiology of phlebotomus fever. *J State Med*. 1924;32:461–469.

364. Newstead R. The papataci flies (Phlebotomus) of the Maltese Islands. *Ann Trop Med Parasitol*. 1911;5:139–186.

365. Taussig S. Die Hundskrankheit, endemischer Magankatarrh in der Herzegowina. *Wien Klin Wchnschr*. 1905;18:129–136,163–169.

366. Doerr R, Franz K, Taussig S. *Das Papatacifieber*. Leipzig, Germany: Deuticke; 1909.

367. McClain DJ, Summers PL, Pratt WD, Davis K, Jennings GB. Experimental of nonhuman primates with Sandfly fever virus. *Am J Trop Med Hyg.* 1997;56:554–560.

368. Sabin AB, Philip CB, Paul JR. Phlebotomus (pappataci or sandfly) fever. *JAMA.* 1944;125:603–606.

369. Hertig M, Sabin AB. Sandfly fever (pappataci, phlebotomus, three-day fever). In: Coates JB Jr, Hoff EC, Hoff PM, eds. *Communicable Diseases: Arthropodborne Diseases Other than Malaria.* Vol 7. *Preventive Medicine in World War II.* Washington, DC: Office of the Surgeon General, US Department of the Army; 1964:.

370. Paul JR, Melnick JL, Sabin AB. Experimental attempts to transmit phlebotomus (sandfly, pappataci) and dengue fevers to chimpanzees. *Proc Soc Exp Biol Med.* 1948:68:193–198.

371. Sabin AB. Experimental studies on Phlebotomus (papataci, sandfly) fever during World War II. *Arch Gesamte Virus Forsch.* 1951;4:367–410.

372. Tesh RB, Papaevangelou G. Effect of insecticide spraying for malaria control on the incidence of sandfly fever in Athens, Greece. *Am J Trop Med Hyg.* 1977;26:163–166.

373. Tesh RB, Chaniotis BN, Peralta PH, Johnson KM. Ecology of viruses isolated from Panamanian phlebotomine sandflies. *Am J Trop Med Hyg.* 1974;23:258–269.

374. Tesh RB, Peters CJ, Meegan JM. Studies on the antigenic relationship among phleboviruses. *Am J Trop Med Hyg.* 1982;31:149–155.

375. Tesh RB, Peralta PH, Shope RE, Chaniotis BN, Johnson KM. Antigenic relationships among phlebotomus fever group arboviruses and their implication for the epidemiology of sandfly fever. *Am J Trop Med Hyg.* 1975;24:135–144.

376. Verani P, Nicoletti L, Ciufolini MG. Antigenic and biological characterization of Toscana virus, a new Phlebotomus fever group virus isolated in Italy. *Acta Virol.* 1984;28(1):39–47.

377. Ehrnst A, Peters CJ, Niklasson B, Svedmyr A, Holmgren B. Neurovirulent Toscana virus (a sandfly fever virus) in Swedish man after visit to Portugal. *Lancet.* 1985;1:1212–1213.

378. Schwarz TF, Jager G, Gilch S, Pauli C. Serosurvey and laboratory diagnosis of imported sandfly fever virus, serotype Toscana, infection in Germany. *Epidemiol Infect.* 1995;114:501–510.

379. Eitrem R, Niklasson B, Weiland O. Sandfly fever among Swedish tourists. *Scand J Infect Dis.* 1991;23:451–457.

380. Verani P, Lopes MC, Nicoletti L, Balducci M. Studies on *Phlebotomus*-transmitted viruses in Italy. I: Isolation and characterization of a sandfly fever Naples-like virus. In: Vesenjak-Hirjan J, ed. *Arboviruses in the Mediterranean Countries, Zbl Bakt.Suppl 9.* Stuttgart: Gustav Fischer Verlag; 1980: 195–201.

381. George JE. Isolation of Phlebotomus fever virus from *Phlebotomus papatasi* and determination of the host ranges of sandflies (*Diptera: Psychodidae*) in West Pakistan. *J Med Entomol.* 1970;7:670–676.

382. Le-Lay-Rogues G, Valle M, Chastel C, Beaucournu JC. Small wild mammals and arboviruses in Italy. *Bull Soc Pathol Exot Filiales.* 1983;76:333–345.

383. Mochkovski SD, Diomina NA, Nossina VD, Pavlova EA, Livshitz JL, Pels HJ, et al. Researches on sandfly fever, 8: transmission of sandfly fever virus by sandflies hatched from eggs laid by infected females. *Med Parazitol Parazitarn Bolezni.* 1937;6:922–937.

384. Ciufolini MG, Maroli M, Verani P. Growth of two phleboviruses after experimental infection of their suspected sand fly vector, *Phlebotomus perniciosus* (*Diptera: Psychodidae*). *Am J Trop Med Hyg.* 1985;34:174–179.

385. Endris RG, Tesh RB, Young DG. Transovarial transmission of Rio Grande virus (*Bunyaviridae: Phlebovirus*) by the sand fly, *Lutzomyia anthophora.* *Am J Trop Med Hyg.* 1983;32:862–864.

386. Ciufolini MG, Maroli M, Guandalini E, Marchi A, Verani P. Experimental studies on the maintenance of Toscana and Arbia viruses (*Bunyaviridae*: *Phlebovirus*). *Am J Trop Med Hyg*. 1989;40:669–675.

387. Cullinan ER, Whittaker SRF. Outbreak of sandfly fever in two general hospitals in the Middle East. *Brit Med J*. 1943;2:543–545.

388. Tesh RB, Modi GB. Studies on the biology of phleboviruses in sand flies (*Diptera: Psychodidae*). I: Experimental infection of the vector. *Am J Trop Med Hyg*. 1984;33:1007–1016.

389. Petrischeva PA, Alymov AY. On transovarial transmission of virus of pappataci fever by sandflies. *Arch Biol Sci (Moscow)*. 1938;53:138–144.

390. Saidi S, Tesh R, Javadian E, Sahabi Z, Nadim A. Studies on the epidemiology of sandfly fever in Iran, II: the prevalence of human and animal infection with five phlebotomus fever virus serotypes in Isfahan province. *Am J Trop Med Hyg*. 1977;26:288–293.

391. Travassos da Rosa AP, Tesh RB, Pinheiro FP, Travassos da Rosa JF, Peterson NE. Characterization of eight new phlebotomus fever serogroup arboviruses (Bunyaviridae: *Phlebovirus*) from the Amazon region of Brazil. *Am J Trop Med Hyg*. 1983;32:1164–1171.

392. Shope RE, Peters CJ, Walker JS. Serological relation between Rift Valley fever virus and viruses of phlebotomus fever serogroup. *Lancet*. 1980;1:886–887.

393. Shope RE, Meegan JM, Peters CJ, Tesh RB, Travassos da Rosa AP. Immunologic status of Rift Valley fever virus. *Contr Epidem Biostatist*. 1981;3:42–52.

394. McCloskey RV, Shelokov A. Further characterization and serological identification of Chagres virus, a new human isolate. *Am J Trop Med Hyg*. 1965;14:152–155.

395. Sather GE. Punta toro (PT) strain. *Am J Trop Med Hyg*. 1970;19:1103–1104.

396. Srihongse S, Johnson KM. Human infections with Chagres virus in Panama. *Am J Trop Med Hyg*. 1974;23:690–693.

397. Whittingham HE, Rook AF. The prevention of phlebotomus fever. *Trans R Soc Trop Med Hyg*. 1923;17:290–330.

398. Eitrem R, Vene S, Niklasson B. Incidence of sandfly fever among Swedish United Nations soldiers on Cyprus during 1985. *Am J Trop Med Hyg*. 1990;43:207–211.

399. Nikolayev VP, Perepelkin VS, Rayevskiy KK, Prusakova ZM. A natural focus of Sandfly-borne fevers in the Republic of Afghanistan [in Russian]. *Zh Mikrobiol Epid Immunogiol*. 1991;Mar:39–41.

400. Bartelloni PJ, Tesh RB. Clinical and serologic responses of volunteers infected with phlebotomus fever virus (Sicilian type). *Am J Trop Med Hyg*. 1976;25:456–462.

401. Bellanti JA, Krasner RI, Bartelloni PJ, Yang MC, Beisel WR. Sandfly fever: Sequential changes in neutrophil biochemical and bactericidal factors. *J Immunol*. 1972;108:142–151.

402. Nicoletti L, Verani P, Caciolli S, et al. Central nervous system involvement during infection by *Phlebovirus toscana* of residents in natural foci in central Italy (1977–1988). *Am J Trop Med Hyg*. 1991;45:429–434.

403. Schwarz TF, Gilch S, Jager G. Aseptic meningitis caused by sandfly fever virus, serotype Toscana. *Clin Infect Dis*. 1995;21:669–671.

404. Fleming J, Bignall JR, Blades AN. Sandfly fever: Review of 664 cases. *Lancet*. 1947;1:443–445.

405. Tesh RB, Chaniotis BN. Transovarial transmission of viruses by phlebotomine sandflies. *Ann N Y Acad Sci*. 1975;266:125–134.

406. Robert LL, Perich MJ. Phlebotomine sand fly (*Diptera*: *Psychodidae*) control using a residual pyrethroid insecticide. *J Am Mosq Control Assoc*. 1995;11:195–199.

407. Tesh RB. The genus *Phlebovirus* and its vectors. *Ann Rev Entomol*. 1988;33:169–181.

408. Basimike M, Mutinga MJ. Effects of permethrin-treated screens on phlebotomine sand flies, with reference to *Phlebotomus martini* (*Diptera*: *Psychodidae*). *J Med Entomol*. 1995;32:428–432.

409. Peters CJ, Jones D, Trotter R, et al. Experimental Rift Valley fever in rhesus macaques. *Arch Virol*. 1988;99:31–44.

410. Dattwyler RS, Luft BJ. *Borrelia burgdorferi*. In: Gorbach SL, Bartlett JG, Blacklow NR, eds. *Infectious Diseases*. 2nd ed. Philadelphia: W.B. Saunders; 1998: 1937–1946.

411. Barbour AG, Fish D. The biological and social phenomenon of Lyme disease. *Science*. 1993;260:1610–1616.

412. Centers for Disease Control and Prevention. Lyme Disease—United States, 1996. *MMWR*. 1997;46:531–535.

413. Bowen SG, Schulze TL, Hayne C, Parkin WE. A focus of Lyme disease in Monmouth County, New Jersey. *Am J Epidemiol*. 1984;120:387–394.

414. Anderson JF, Duray PH, Magnarelli LA. Prevalence of *Borrelia burgdorferi* in white-footed mice and *Ixodes dammini* at Fort McCoy, Wis. *J Clin Microbiol*. 1987;25:1495–1497.

415. Centers for Disease Control. Lyme Disease—U.S. Navy and U.S. Marine Corps, 1989. *Lyme Disease Surveillance Summary*. 1990;1(2).

416. Underwood PK, Armour VM. Cases of Lyme disease reported in a military community. *Mil Med*. 1993;158:116–119.

417. Welker RD, Narby GM, Legare EJ, Sweeney DM. Lyme disease acquired in Europe and presenting in CONUS. *Mil Med*. 1993;158:684–685.

418. Burgdorfer W, Barbour AG, Hayes SF, et al. Lyme disease—a tick-borne spirochetosis? *Science*. 1982;216: 1317–1319.

419. Falco RC, Daniels TJ, Fish D. Increase in abundance of immature *Ixodes scapularis* (*Acari*: *Ixodidae*) in an emergent Lyme disease endemic area. *J Med Entomol*. 1995;32:522–526.

420. Burgdorfer W, Lane RS, Barbour AG, Gresbrink RA, Anderson JR. The western black-legged tick, *Ixodes pacificus*: A vector of *Borrelia burgdorferi*. *Am J Trop Med Hyg*. 1985;34:925–930.

421. Asbrink E. Erythema chronicum migrans Afzelius and acrodermatitis chronica atrophicans: Early and late manifestations of *Ixodes ricinus*-borne *Borrelia* spirochetes. *Acta Derm Venereol Suppl (Stockh)*. 1985;118:1–63.

422. Kawabata M, Baba S, Iguchi K, Yamaguti N, Russell H. Lyme disease in Japan and its possible incriminated tick vector, *Ixodes persulcatus*. *J Infect Dis*. 1987;156:854.

423. Anderson JF, Magnarelli LA, Burgdorfer W, Barbour AG. Spirochetes in *Ixodes dammini* and mammals from Connecticut. *Am J Trop Med Hyg*. 1983;32:818–824.

424. Battaly GR, Fish D. Relative importance of bird species as hosts for immature *Ixodes dammini* (Acari: Ixodidae) in a suburban residential landscape of southern New York State. *J Med Entomol*. 1993;30:740–747.

425. Stafford KC 3rd, Bladen VC, Magnarelli LA. Ticks (Acari: Ixodidae) infesting wild birds (Aves) and white-footed mice in Lyme, CT. *J Med Entomol*. 1995;32:453–466.

426. Ginsberg HS. *Ecology and Management of Ticks and Lyme Disease at Fire Island National Seashore and Selected Eastern National Parks*. Denver, Colo: National Parks Service, Natural Resources Publication Office; 1992.

427. Mannelli A, Kitron U, Jones CJ, Slajchert, TL. Role of the eastern chipmunk as a host for immature *Ixodes dammini* (Acari: Ixodidae) in northwestern Illinois. *J Med Entomol*. 1993;30:87–93.

428. Luttrell MP, Nakagaki K, Howerth EW, Stallknecht DE, Lee KA. Experimental infection of *Borrelia burgdorferi* in white-tailed deer. *J Wildlife Dis*. 1994;30:146–154.

429. Oliver JH Jr, Stallknecht D, Chandler FW, James AM, McGuire BS, Howerth E. Detection of *Borrelia burgdorferi* in laboratory-reared *Ixodes dammini* (Acari: Ixodidae) fed on experimentally inoculated white-tailed deer. J *Med Entomol*. 1992;29:980–984.

430. Telford SR 3rd, Mather TN, Moore SI, Wilson ML, Spielman A. Incompetence of deer as reservoirs of the Lyme disease spirochete. *Am J Trop Med Hyg*. 1988;39:105–109.

431. Lane RS, Burgdorferi W. Spirochetes in mammals and ticks (Acari: Ixodidae) from a focus of Lyme borreliosis in California. *J Wildlife Dis*. 1988;24:1–9.

432. Lang JD. Ixodid ticks (Acari: Ixodidae) found in San Diego County, California. *J Vector Ecology*. 1999;24:61–69.

433. Wright SA, Thompson MA, Miller MJ, et al. Ecology of *Borrelia burgdorferi* in ticks (Acari: Ixodidae), rodents, and birds in the Sierra Nevada foothills, Placer County, California. *J Med Entomol*. 2000;37:909–918.

434. United States Army Environmental Hygiene Agency. White-tailed deer population trends. *Focus on Lyme Disease*. 1993;1(1):10–11.

435. Piesman J, Mather TN, Sinsky RJ, Spielman A. Duration of tick attachment and *Borrelia burgdorferi* transmission. *J Clin Microbiol*. 1987:25:557–558.

436. Santino I, Dastoli F, Sessa R, Del Piano M. Geographical incidence of infection with *Borrelia burgdorferi* in Europe. *Panminerva Med*. 1997;39:208–214.

437. Shih CM, Wang JC, Chao LL, Wu TN. Lyme disease in Taiwan: First human patient with characteristic erythema chronicum migrans skin lesion. *J Clin Microbiol*. 1998;36:807–808.

438. Strijdom SC, Berk M. Lyme disease in South Africa. *S Afr Med J*. 1996;86(6 Suppl):741–744.

439. Yoshinari NH, deBarros PJ, Bonoldi VL, et al. Outline of Lyme borreliosis in Brazil [in Portuguese]. *Rev Hosp Clin Fac Med Sao Paulo*. 1997:52:111–117.

440. Neira O, Cerda C, Alvarado MA, et al. Lyme disease in Chile: Prevalence study in selected groups [in Spanish]. *Rev Med Chile*. 1996;124:537–544.

441. Aoun K, Kechrid A, Lagha N, Zarrouk A, Bouzouaia N. Lyme disease in Tunisia, results of a clinical and serological study (1992-1996) [in French]. *Sante*. 1998;8:98–100.

442. United States Army Environmental Hygiene Agency. The role of the white-tailed deer. *Focus on Lyme Disease*. 1994;1(2):9.

443. Centers for Disease Control and Prevention. Established and reported distribution of the Lyme disease vectors *Ixodes scapularis* (*I. dammini*) and *Ixodes pacificus*, by county, United States, 1907–1996. CDC Lyme Disease web page. http://www.cdc.gov/ncidod/dvbid/tickmap.htm. Accessed on 16 Sept 1998.

444. Meek JI, Robert CL, Smith EV Jr., Cartter ML. Underreporting of Lyme disease by Connecticut physicians. *J Public Health Manage Practice*. 1996;2:61–65.

445. Steere AC, Taylor E, McHugh GL, Logigian EL. The overdiagnosis of Lyme disease. *JAMA*. 1993;269:1812–1816.

446. Logigian EL, Kaplan RF, Steere AC. Chronic neurologic manifestations of Lyme disease. *N Engl J Med*. 1990;323:1438–1444.

447. Gaudino EA, Coyle PK, Krupp LB. Post-Lyme syndrome and chronic fatigue syndrome: Neuropsychiatric similarities and differences. *Arch Neurol.* 1997;54:1372–1376.

448. Preac-Mursic V, Weber K, Pfister HW, et al. Survival of *Borrelia burgdorferi* in antibiotically treated patients with Lyme borreliosis. *Infection.* 1989;17:355–359.

449. Bayer ME, Zhang L, Bayer MH. *Borrelia burgdorferi* DNA in the urine of treated patients with chronic Lyme disease symptoms: A PCR study of 97 cases. *Infection.* 1996;24:347–353.

450. Centers for Disease Control and Prevention. CDC recommendations for the use of Lyme disease vaccine: Recommendation of the Advisory Committee on Immunization Practices (ACIP). *MMWR.* 1999;48(RR-7):1–17.

451. Dennis DT, Meltzer MI. Antibiotic prophylaxis after tick bites. *Lancet.* 1997;350:1191–1192.

452. Magid D, Schwartz B, Craft J, Schwartz JS. Prevention of Lyme disease after tick bites: A cost-effectiveness analysis. *N Engl J Med.* 1992;327:534–541.

453. Nadelman RB, Nowakowski J, Fish D, et al. Prophylaxis with single-dose doxycycline for the prevention of Lyme disease after an Ixodes scapularis tick bite. *N Engl J Med.* 2001;345:79–84.

454. Centers for Disease Control and Prevention. Lyme disease: Questions and Answers. http://www.cdc.gov/ncidod/dvbid/lyme_AQ.htm. Accessed 17 Apr 2001.

455. Wormser GP, Nadelman RB, Dattwyler RJ, et al. Practice guidelines for the treatment of Lyme disease. *Clin Infect Dis.* 2000;31(Suppl 1):1–14.

456. Nadelman RB, Horowitz HW, Hsieh TC, et al. Simultaneous human granulocytic ehrlichiosis and Lyme disease. *N Engl J Med.* 1997;337:27–30.

457. Centers for Disease Control and Prevention. Update: Self-induced malaria associated with malariotherapy for Lyme disease—Texas. *MMWR.* 1991;40:665–666.

458. Moore JA. Jarisch-Herxheimer reaction in Lyme disease. *Cutis.* 1987;39:397–398.

459. Falco RC, Fish D. Epidemiology of tick bites acquired in a Lyme disease endemic area of southern New York State. *Am J Epidemiol.* 1988;128:1146–1152.

460. Maupin GO, Fish D, Zultowsky J, Campos EG, Piesman J. Landscape ecology of Lyme disease in a residential area of Westchester County, New York. *Am J Epidemiol.* 1991;133:1105–1113.

461. Deblinger RD, Rimmer DW. Efficacy of a permethrin-based acaricide to reduce the abundance of *Ixodes dammini* (*Acari: Ixodidae*). *J Med Entomol.* 1991;28:708–711.

462. Stafford KC III. Third-year evaluation of host-targeted permethrin for the control of *Ixodes dammini* (*Acari: Ixodidae*) in southeastern Connecticut. *J Med Entomol.* 1992;29:717–720.

463. Schulze TL, Taylor GC, Vasvary LM, Simmons W, Jordon RA. Effectiveness of an aerial application of carbaryl in controlling *Ixodes dammini* (*Acari: Ixodidae*) adults in a high-use recreational area in New Jersey. *J Med Entomol.* 1992;29:544–547.

464. Schulze TL, Jordan RA. Potential influence of leaf litter depth on effectiveness of granular carbaryl against subadult *Ixodes scapularis* (*Acari: Ixodidae*). *J Med Entomol.* 1995;32:205–208.

465. Solberg VB, Keidhardt K, Sardelis MR, et al. Field evaluation of two formulations of cyfluthrin for control of *Ixodes dammini* and *Amblyomma americanum* (*Acari: Ixodidae*). *J Med Entomol.* 1992;29:634–638.

466. Pound JM, Miller JA, George JE, Lemeilleur CA. The "4-Poster" passive topical treatment device to apply an acaricide for controlling ticks (Acari: Ixodidae) feeding on white-tailed deer. *J Med Entomol.* 2000;37:588–594.

467. Sigal LH. A Symposium: National Clinical Conference on Lyme Disease. *Am J Med.* 1995;98(4A):1S-89S.

468. Felz MW, Durden LA. Attachment sites of four tick species (Acari: Ixodidae) parasitizing humans in Georgia and South Carolina. *J Med Entomol.* 1999;36:361–364.

469. Couch P, Johnson CE. Prevention of Lyme disease. *Am J Hosp Pharm.* 1992;49:1164–1171.

470. Schoen RT, Meurice F, Brunet CM, et al. Safety and immunogenicity of an outer surface protein A vaccine in subjects with previous Lyme disease. *J Infect Dis.* 1995;172:1324–1329.

471. Steere AC, Sikand VK, Meurice F, et al. Vaccination against Lyme disease with recombinant *Borrelia burgdorferi* outer-surface lipoprotein A with adjuvant. *N Engl J Med.* 1998;339:209–215.

472. Sigal LH, Zahradnik JM, Lavin P, et al. A vaccine consisting of recombinant *Borrelia burgdorferi* outer-surface protein A to prevent Lyme disease. *N Engl J Med.* 1998;339:216–222.

473. Nightingale SL. From the Food and Drug Administration: Lyme disease vaccine approved. *JAMA.* 1999;281:408.

474. Bakken JS, Dumler JS, Chen SM, Eckman MR, Van Etta LL, Walker DH. Human granulocytic ehrlichiosis in the upper midwest United States: A new species emerging? *JAMA.* 1994;272:212–218.

475. Petersen LR, Sawyer LA, Fishbein DB, et al. An outbreak of ehrlichiosis in members of an Army Reserve unit exposed to ticks. *J Infect Dis.* 1989;159:562–568.

476. Harkess JR, Ewing SA, Crutcher JM, Kudlac J, McKee G, Istre GR. Human ehrlichiosis in Oklahoma. *J Infect Dis.* 1989;159:576–579.

477. Eng TR, Harkess JR, Fishbein DB, et al. Epidemiologic, clinical, and laboratory findings of human ehrlichiosis in the United States, 1988. *JAMA.* 1990;264:2251–2258.

478. McDade JE. Ehrlichiosis—a disease of animals and humans. *J Infect Dis.* 1990;161:609–617.

479. Dumler JS, Chen SM, Asanovich K, Trigiani E, Popov VL, Walker DH. Isolation and characterization of a new strain of *Ehrlichia chaffeensis* from a patient with nearly fatal monocytic ehrlichiosis. *J Clin Microbiol.* 1995;33:1704–1711.

480. Chen SM, Dumler JS, Bakken JS, Walker DH. Identification of a granulocytotropic *Ehrlichia* species as the etiologic agent of human disease. *J Clin Microbiol.* 1994;32:589–595.

481. Yevich SJ, Sánchez JL, DeFraites RF, et al. Seroepidemiology of infections due to spotted fever group rickettsiae and *Ehrlichia* species in military personnel exposed in areas of the United States where such infections are endemic. *J Infect Dis.* 1995;171:1266–1273.

482. Walker DH, Dumler JS. Emergence of the ehrlichioses as human health problems. *Emerging Infec Dis.* 1996;2(1):18–29.

483. Chen SM, Popov VL, Feng HM, Walker DH. Analysis and ultrastructural localization of *Ehrlichia chaffeensis* proteins with monoclonal antibodies. *Am J Trop Med Hyg.* 1996;54:405–412.

484. Fishbein DB, Dawson JE, Robinson LE. Human ehrlichiosis in the United States, 1985 to 1990. *Ann Intern Med.* 1994;120:736–743.

485. Centers for Disease Control and Prevention. Human granulocytic ehrlichiosis—New York, 1995. *MMWR.* 1995;44:593–595.

486. Standaert SM, Dawson JE, Schaffner W, et al. Ehrlichiosis in a golf-oriented retirement community. *N Engl J Med.* 1995;333:420–425.

487. Dumler JS, Bakken JS. Human granulocytic ehrlichiosis in Wisconsin and Minnesota: A frequent infection with the potential for persistence. *J Infect Dis.* 1996;173:1027–1030.

488. Brouqui P, Raoult D. In vitro antibiotic susceptibility of the newly recognized agent of ehrlichiosis in humans, *Ehrlichia chaffeensis*. *Antimicrob Agents Chemother*. 1992;36:2799–2803.

489. Philip CB. Tsutsugamushi disease (scrub typhus) in World War II. *J Parasitol*. 1948;34:169–191.

490. Tamura A, Ohashi N, Urakami H, Miyamura S. Classification of *Rickettsia tsutsugamushi* in a new genus, *Orientia* gen. nov., as *Orientia tsutsugamushi* comb. nov. *Int J Syst Bacteriol*. 1995;45:589–591.

491. Traub R, Wisseman CL Jr. The ecology of chigger-borne rickettsioses (scrub typhus). *J Med Entomol*. 1974;11:237–303.

492. Watt G, Strickman D. Life-threatening scrub typhus in a traveler returning from Thailand. *Clin Infect Dis*. 1994;18:624–626.

493. Brown GW, Shirai A, Jegathesan M, et al. Febrile illness in Malaysia—an analysis of 1,629 hospitalized patients. *Am J Trop Med Hyg*. 1984;33:311–315.

494. Takada N, Khamboonruang C, Yamaguchi T, Thitasut P, Vajrasthira S. Scrub typhus and chiggers in northern Thailand. *Southeast Asian J Trop Med Public Health*. 1984;15:402–406.

495. Strickman D, Tanskul P, Eamsila C, Kelly DJ. Prevalence of antibodies to rickettsiae in the human population of suburban Bangkok. *Am J Trop Med Hyg*. 1994;51:149–153.

496. Olson JG, Bourgeois AL. Changing risk of scrub typhus in relation to socioeconomic development in the Pescadores Islands of Taiwan. *Am J Epidemiol*. 1979;109:236–243.

497. Taylor AC, Hii J, Kelly DJ, Davis DR, Lewis GE Jr. A serological survey of scrub, tick, and endemic typhus in Sabah, East Malaysia. *Southeast Asian J Trop Med Public Health*. 1986;17:613–619.

498. Eamsila C, Singsawat P, Duangvaraporn A, Strickman D. Antibodies to *Orientia tsutsugamushi* in Thai soldiers. *Am J Trop Med Hyg*. 1996;55:556–559.

499. Brown GW, Shirai A, Groves MG. Development of antibody to *Rickettsia tsutsugamushi* in soldiers in Malaysia. *Trans R Soc Trop Med Hyg*. 1983;77:225–227.

500. Olson JG, Irving GS, Bourgeois AL, Hodge FA, Van Peenen PF. Seroepidemiological evidence of infectious diseases in United States Marine Corps personnel, Okinawa, Japan, 1975-1976. *Mil Med*. 1979;144:175–176.

501. Berman SJ, Kundin WD. Scrub typhus in South Vietnam: A study of 87 cases. *Ann Intern Med*. 1973;79:26–30.

502. Watt G, Strickman D, Kantipong P, Jongsakul K, Paxton H. Performance of a dot blot immunoassay for the rapid diagnosis of scrub typhus in a longitudinal case series. *J Infect Dis*. 1998;177:800–802.

503. Strickman D. Serology of scrub typhus: New directions for an old disease. *Clin Immunol Newsletter*. 1994;14:62–65.

504. Smadel JE, Woodward TE, Ley HL, Philip CV, Traub R. Chloromycetin in the treatment of scrub typhus. *Science*. 1948;108:160–161.

505. Watt G, Chouriyagune C, Ruangweerayud R, et al. Scrub typhus infections poorly responsive to antibiotics in northern Thailand. *Lancet*. 1996;348:86–89.

506. Strickman D, Sheer T, Salata K, et al. In vitro effectiveness of azithromycin against doxycycline-resistant and -susceptible strains of *Rickettsia tsutsugamushi*, etiologic agent of scrub typhus. *Antimicrob Agents Chemother*. 1995;39:2406–2410.

507. Watt G, Kantipong P, Jongsakul K, Watcharapichat P, Phulsuksombati D. Azithromycin activities against *Orientia tsutsugamushi* strains isolated in cases of scrub typhus in Northern Thailand. *Antimicrob Agents Chemother*. 1999;43:2817–2818.

508. Armed Forces Pest Management Board. *Personal Protective Techniques Against Insects and Other Arthropods of Military Significance*. Washington, DC: AFPMB; 1996. Technical Information Memorandum No. 36.

509. Twartz JC, Shirai A, Selvaraju G, Saunders JP, Huxsoll DL, Groves MG. Doxycycline prophylaxis for human scrub typhus. *J Infect Dis*. 1982;146:811–818.

510. Moe JB, Pederson CE. The impact of rickettsial disease on military operations. *Mil Med*. 1980;145:780–785.

511. Raoult D, Dasch GA. Immunoblot cross-reactions among *Rickettsia*, *Proteus* spp. and *Legionella* spp. in patients with Mediterranean spotted fever. *FEMS Immunol Med Microbiol*. 1995;11:13–18.

512. Traub R, Wisseman CL. The ecology of murine typhus—a critical review. *Trop Dis Bull*. 1978;75:237–317.

513. Woodward TE, Philip CB, Loranger GL. Endemic typhus in Manila, Philippine Islands. *J Infect Dis*. 1946;78:167–172.

514. Plotz H, Woodward TE, Philip CB, Bennett BL. Endemic typhus in Jamaica, B.W.I. *Am J Public Health*. 1943;33: 812–814.

515. Taylor JP, Betz TG, Rawlings JA. Epidemiology of murine typhus in Texas, 1980 through 1984. *JAMA*. 1986;255:2173–2176.

516. Brown AE, Meek SR, Maneechai N, Lewis GE. Murine typhus among Khmers living at an evacuation site on the Thai-Kampuchean border. *Am J Trop Med Hyg*. 1988;38:168–171.

517. Duffy PE, LeGuillouzic H, Gass RF, Innis BL. Murine typhus identified as a major cause of febrile illness in a camp for displaced Khmers in Thailand. *Am J Trop Med Hyg*. 1990;43:520–526.

518. Dupont HT, Brouqui P, Faugere B, Raoult D. Prevalence of antibodies to *Coxiella burnetii*, *Rickettsia conorii*, and *Rickettsia typhi* in seven African countries. *Clin Infect Dis*. 1995;21:1126–1133.

519. Silpapojakul K, Woodtayagone J, Lekakula A, Vimuktalaba A, Krisanapan S. Murine typhus in southern Thailand. *J Med Assoc Thai*. 1987;70:55–62.

520. Richards AL, Soeatmadji DW, Widodo A, et al. Seroepidemiological evidence for murine and scrub typhus in Malang, Indonesia. *Am J Trop Med Hyg*. 1997;57:91–95.

521. Silpapojakul K, Pradutkanchana J, Pradutkanchana S, Kelly DJ. Rapid, simple serodiagnosis of murine typhus. *Trans R Soc Trop Med Hyg*. 1995;89:625–628.

522. Kelly DJ, Chan CT, Paxton H, Thompson K, Howard R, Dasch GA. Comparative evaluation of a commercial enzyme immunoassay for the detection of human antibody to *Rickettsia typhi*. *Clin Diagnostic Lab Immunol*. 1995;2:356–360.

523. Scoville AB Jr. Epidemic typhus fever in Japan and Korea. In: Soule MH, ed. *Rickettsial Diseases of Man*. Washington, DC: American Association for the Advancement of Science; Thomas, Adams & Davis, Inc; 1948: 28–35.

524. Raoult D, Ndihokubwayo JB, Tissot-Dupont H, et al. Outbreak of epidemic typhus associated with trench fever in Burundi. *Lancet*. 1998;352:353–358.

525. Woodward TE. Murine and epidemic typhus rickettsiae: How close is their relationship? *Yale J Biol Med*. 1982;55:335–341.

526. Goddard J, McHugh CP. Impact of a severe tick infestation at Little Rock AFB, Arkansas on Volant Scorpion military training. *Mil Med*. 1990;155:277–280.

527. Weiss E. Rickettsias. In: *Encyclopedia of Microbiology*. Vol 3. San Diego,Calif: Academic Press; 1992: 585–610.

528. Sanchez JL, Candler WH, Fishbein DB, et al. A cluster of tick-borne infections: Associations with military training and asymptomatic infections due to *Rickettsia rickettsii*. *Trans R Soc Trop Med Hyg*. 1992;86:321–325.

529. Smoak BL, McClain JB, Brundage JF, et al. An outbreak of spotted fever rickettsiosis in US Army troops deployed to Botswana. *Emerging Infect Dis*. 1996;2:217–221.

530. Williams WJ, Radulovic S, Dasch GA, et al. Identification of *Rickettsia conorii* infection by polymerase chain reaction in a soldier returning from Somalia. *Clin Infect Dis*. 1994;19:93–99.

531. Dalton MJ, Clarke MJ, Holman RC, et al. National surveillance for Rocky Mountain spotted fever, 1981–1992: Epidemiologic summary and evaluation of risk factors for fatal outcome. *Am J Trop Med Hyg*. 1995;52:405–413.

532. Sirisanthana T, Pinyopornpanit V, Sirisanthana V, Strickman D, Kelly DJ, Dasch GA. First cases of spotted fever group rickettsiosis in Thailand. *Am J Trop Med Hyg*. 1994;50:682–686.

533. Uchida T, Uchiyama T, Kumano K, Walker DH. *Rickettsia japonica* sp. nov., the etiologic agent of spotted fever group rickettsiosis in Japan. *Int J Syst Bacteriol*. 1992;42:303–305.

534. Centers for Disease Control and Prevention. Summary—cases of specified notifiable diseases, United States, cumulative, week ending December 16, 1995 (50th week). *MMWR*. 1996;45:12.

535. Sexton DJ, Muniz M, Corey GR, et al. Brazilian spotted fever in Espirito Santo, Brazil: Description of a focus of infection in a new endemic region. *Am J Trop Med Hyg*. 1993;49:222–226.

536. Raoult D, Weiller PJ, Chagnon A, Chaudet H, Gallias H, Casanova P. Mediterranean spotted fever: Clinical, laboratory and epidemiological features of 199 cases. *Am J Trop Med Hyg*. 1986:845–850.

537. Benenson AS. Immunization and military medicine. *Rev Infect Dis*. 1984;6:1–12.

538. Cavanaugh DC, Cadigan FC, Williams JE, Marshall JD. Plague. In: Ognibene AJ, Barrett O Jr, eds. *General Medicine and Infectious Diseases*. Vol 2. *Internal Medicine in Vietnam*. Washington, DC: Office of the Surgeon General and Center of Military History, US Army; 1982.

539. Cartwright FF, Biddiss MD. *Disease and History*. New York: Dorset Press; 1972: 29–53.

540. Walker DH, Barbour AG, Oliver JH, et al. Emerging bacterial zoonotic and vector-borne diseases: Ecological and epidemiological factors. *JAMA*. 1996;275:463–469.

541. Centers for Disease Control and Prevention. Update: human plague—India, 1994. *MMWR*. 1994;43:761–762.

542. Friese K, Mahurka U, Rattanani L, Kattyar A, Rai S. The plague peril: Are you at risk? *India Today*. 15 October 1994.

543. Campbell GL, Hughes JM. Plague in India: A new warning from an old nemesis. *Ann Intern Med*. 1995;122:151–153.

544. Pollitzer R. *Plague*. Geneva: World Health Organization; 1954. WHO Monograph Series No. 22.

545. Kohn GC, ed. *Encyclopedia of Plague and Pestilence*. New York: Facts on File, Inc; 1995: 25–26, 255–256.

546. Butler T. *Plague and Other Yersinia Infections*. New York: Plenum Medical Book Company; 1983.

547. Anderson RS, Hoff EC, Hoff PM, eds. *Special Fields*. Vol 9. *Preventive Medicine in World War II*. Washington, DC: Office of the Surgeon General, Department of the Army; 1969.

548. Cavanaugh DC, Elisberg BL, Llewellyn CH, et al. Plague immunization, V: Indirect evidence for the efficacy of plague vaccine. *J Infect Dis*. 1974;129(Suppl):S37–40.

549. US Army Medical Research Institute of Infectious Diseases. *Diagnosis and Treatment of Exotic Diseases of Tactical Importance to U.S.Centcom Forces—1991*. Fort Detrick, Md: USAMRIID; 1991.

550. Mobley JA. Biological warfare in the twentieth century: Lessons from the past, challenges for the future. *Mil Med*. 1995;160:547–553.

551. Rolicka M. New studies disputing allegations of bacteriological warfare during the Korean War. *Mil Med*. 1995;160:97–100.

552. US Army Center for Health Promotion and Preventive Medicine. *Prevention and Control of Plague*. Aurora, CO: USACHPPM Direct Support Activity–West, Fitzsimmons AMC ; 1995. Technical Guide TG-103.

553. Morris JT, McAllister CK. Bubonic plague. *Southern Med J*. 1992;85:326–327.

554. Craven RB, Barnes AM. Plague and tularemia. *Infect Dis Clin N Am*. 1991;5:165–175.

555. Legters LJ, Cottingham, AJ Jr, Hunter DH. Clinical and epidemiologic notes on a defined outbreak of plague in Vietnam. *Am J Trop Med Hyg*.1970;19:639–652.

556. Butler T. Yersinia infections: Centennial of the discovery of the plague bacillus. *Clin Infect Dis*. 1994;19:655–663.

557. Mann JM, Martone WJ, Boyce JM, Kaufmann AF, Barnes Am, Weber NS. Endemic human plague in New Mexico: Risk factors associated with infection. *J Infect Dis*. 1979;140:397–401.

558. Centers for Disease Control and Prevention. Human plague—United States, 1993–1994. *MMWR*. 1994;43:242–246.

559. World Health Organization. Human plague in 1992. *Wkly Epidemiol Rec*. 1994;69(2):8–10.

560. Butler T. *Yersinia* species, including plague. In: Mandell GL, Bennett JE, Dolin R. *Principles and Practice of Infectious Diseases*. Philadelphia: Churchill, Livingstone: 2000: 2406–2414.

561. Immunization Practices Advisory Committee (ACIP). Plague vaccine. *MMWR*. 1982;31:301–304.

562. Conrad FG, LeCocq FR, Krain R. A recent epidemic of plague in Vietnam. *Arch Intern Med*. 1968;122:193–198.

563. Migden D. Bubonic plague in a child presenting with fever and altered mental status. *Ann Emerg Med*. 1990;19:207–209.

564. McCrumb FR Jr, Mercier S, Robic J, et al. Chloramphenicol and terramycin in the treatment of pneumonic plague. *Am J Med*. 1953;14:284–293.

565. Crook LD, Tempest B. Plague: A clinical review of 27 cases. *Arch Intern Med*. 1992;152:1253–1256.

566. Butler T. Plague. In: Strickland GT, ed. *Hunter's Tropical Medicine*. 7th ed. Philadelphia: W.B. Saunders Company; 1991: Chap 47.

567. World Health Organization. *International Health Regulations*. Geneva: WHO; 1969, 3rd annotated edition 1983; updated and reprinted 1992.

568. Williamson ED, Eley SM, Stagg AJ, Green M, Russell P, Titball RW. A subunit vaccine elicits IgG in serum, spleen cell cultures and bronchial washings and protects immunized animals against pneumonic plague. *Vaccine*. 1997;15:1079–1084.

569. Heath DG, Anderson GW, Mauro JM, et al. Protection against experimental bubonic and pneumonic plague by a recombinant capsular F1-V antigen fusion protein vaccine. *Vaccine*. 1998;16:1131–1137.

570. Headquarters, Departments of the Army, the Navy, the Air Force, and Transportation. *Immunizations and Chemoprophylaxis*. Washington, DC: DA, DN, DAF, DT; 1 November 1995. Air Force Joint Instruction 48-110, Army Regulation 40-562, BUMEDINST 6230.15, CG COMDTINST M6230.4E.

571. Departments of the Army, the Navy, and the Air Force, and Commandant, Marine Corps. *Treatment of Biological Warfare Agent Casualties.* Washington, DC: DA, DN, DAF, CMC; 17 July 2000. Army FM 8-284, Navy NAVMED P-5042, Air Force AFMAN(I) 44-156, Marine Corps MCRP 4-11.1C.

572. Kortepeter MG, Christopher GW, Cieslak TJ, et al. *Medical Management of Biological Casualties Handbook.* 4th ed. Fort Detrick, Md: US Army Medical Research Institute of Infectious Diseases; 2001.

573. Kortepeter MG, Parker GW. Potential biological weapons threats. *Emerg Infect Dis.* 1999;5:523–527.

574. Henderson DA. The looming threat of bioterrorism. *Science.* 1999;283:1279–1282.

575. Khan AS, Ashford DA, Craven RB, et al. Biological and chemical terrorism: Strategic plan for preparedness and response. Recommendations of the CDC Strategic Planning Workgroup. *MMWR.* 2000;49(RR04):1–14.

576. Inglesby TV, Dennis DT, Henderson DA, et al. Plague as a biological weapon: Medical and public health management. *JAMA.* 2000;283:2281–2290.

577. Buck AB. Filarial infections. In Strickland GT, ed. *Hunter's Tropical Medicine.* 7th ed. Philadelphia: Saunders; 1991: 711–744.

578. Keeling JH. Tropical parasitic infections. In: James WD, ed. *Military Dermatology.* In: *Textbook of Military Medicine.* Washington, DC: Office of the Surgeon General, US Department of the Army, and Borden Institute; 1994: 274–279.

579. Gratz NG, Jany WC. What role for insecticides in vector control programs? *Am J Trop Med Hyg.* 1994;50(Suppl 6):11–20.

580. Sudomo M, Kasnodiharjo, Oemijati S. Social and behavioral aspects of filariasis transmission in Kumpeh, Jambi, Indonesia. *Southeast Asian J Trop Med Public Health.* 1993;24(Suppl 2):26–30.

581. Committee on Infectious Diseases. Filariasis. In: Peter G, ed. *1993 Pediatric Red Book: Report of the Committee on Infectious Diseases.* Elk Grove Village, Ill: American Academy of Pediatrics; 1994: 191–193.

582. Ottenson EA. The filariases and tropical eosinophilia. In: Warren KS, Mahmoud AAF, eds. *Tropical and Geographical Medicine.* 2nd ed. New York: McGraw-Hill; 1990: 407–429.

583. World Health Organization. http://www.filariasis.org/dis_diagnosis.shtml, accessed April 2001.

584. Andrade LD, Medeiros Z, Pires ML, et al. Comparative efficacy of three different diethylcarbamazine regimens in lymphatic filariasis. *Trans R Soc Trop Med Hyg.* 1995;89:319–321.

585. Drugs for parasitic infection. *Med Lett Drugs Ther.* 1993;35(911):111–122.

586. Gelband H. Diethylcarbamazine salt in the control of lymphatic filariasis. *Am J Trop Med Hyg.* 1994;50(Suppl 6):655–662.

587. Moulia-Pelat JP, Nguyen LN, Hascoet H, Luquiaud P, Nicolas L. Advantages of an annual single dose of ivermectin 400 micrograms/kg plus diethylcarbamazine for community treatment of bancroftian filariasis. *Trans R Soc Trop Med Hyg.* 1995;89:682–685.

588. Maxwell CA, Curtis CF, Haji H, Kisumku S, Thalib AI, Yahya SA. Control of Bancroftian filariasis by integrating therapy with vector control using polystyrene beads in wet pit latrines. *Trans R Soc Trop Med Hyg.* 1990;84:709–714.

589. ADAPCO, Inc. Larvicides. http://www.adapcoinc.com/larvicides.php, accessed April 2001.

590. Curtis CF, Morgan PR, Minjas JN, Maxwell CA. Insect-proofing of sanitation systems. In: Curtis CF, ed. *Appropriate Technology in Vector Control.* Boca Raton, Fla: CRC Press, 1990: Chap 10.

591. Ottesen EA. Filarial infections. *Infect Dis Clin North Am.* 1993;7:619–633.

592. Fischer P, Supali T, Wibowo H, Bonow I, Williams SA. Detection of DNA of nocturnally periodic *Brugia malayi* in night and day blood samples by a polymerase chain reaction–ELISA-based method using an internal control DNA. *Am J Trop Med Hyg.* 2000;62:291–296.

593. McMahon JE, Simonsen PE. Filariases. In: Cook GC, ed. *Manson's Tropical Diseases.* 20th ed. London: WB Saunders; 1996.

594. Greene BM. Onchocerciasis. In: Warren KS, Mahmoud AAF, eds. *Tropical and Geographical Medicine.* 2nd ed. New York: McGraw-Hill; 1990: 429–439.

595. Robert LL, Coleman RE, Lapointe DA., Martin DJ, Kelly R, Edman JD. Laboratory and field evaluation of five repellents against the black flies *Prosimulium mixtum* and *P. fuscum* (*Diptera: Simuliidae*). *J Med Entomol.* 1992;29(2:267–272.

596. Renz A, Enyong P. Trials of garments impregnated with "Deet" repellent as an individual protection against *Simulium damnosum* s.l., the vector of onchocerciasis in the savanna and forest regions of Cameroon. *Zeitschrift fur Angewandte Entomologie.* 1983;95(1):92–102.

597. Schmidt ML. Relative effectiveness of repellents against *Simulium damnosum* (Diptera: Simuliidae) and *Glossina morsitans* (Diptera: Glossinidae) in Ethiopia. *J Med Entomol.* 1977;14(3):276–278.

598. Mommers EC, Dekker HS, Richard P, Garcia A, Chippaux JP. Prevalence of *L. loa* and *M. perstans* filariasis in southern Cameroon. *Trop Geogr Med.* 1994;47(1):2–5.

599. Meyers WM, Connor DH, Neafle RC. Dipetalonemiasis. In: Binford CH, Connor DH, eds. *Pathology of Tropical and Extraordinary Diseases.* Vol 2. Washington, DC: Armed Forces Institute of Pathology; 1976: 384–389.

600. Hoegaerden MV, Invanoff B, Flocard F, Salle A, Chabaud B. The use of mebendazole in the treatment of filariases due to *Loa loa* and *Mansonella perstans. Ann Trop Med Parasitol.* 1987;81:275–282.

601. Cunningham D. On the presence of peculiar parasitic organisms in the tissue of a specimen of Delhi Boil. *Scient Mem Med Offrs Army India.* 1885;1:21–31. As cited in: Kean BH, Mott KE, Russell AJ, eds. *Tropical Medicine and Parasitology: Classic Investigations.* Vol 1. Ithaca, NY: Cornell University Press; 1978.

602. Borovsky PF. On Sart sore. *Voenno-Medicinskij Zurnal (Mil Med J).* 1898;Pt.CXCV(11):925–941. As cited in: Kean BH, Mott KE, Russell AJ, eds. *Tropical Medicine and Parasitology: Classic Investigations.* Vol 1. Ithaca, NY: Cornell University Press; 1978.

603. Hoare C. Early discoveries regarding the parasite of Oriental sore. *Trans R Soc Trop Med Hyg.* 1938;32:67–92.

604. Leishman W. On the possibility of the occurrence of trypanosomiasis in India. *BMJ.* 1903;1:1252–1254.

605. Donovan C. Aetiology of one of the heterogenous fevers of India. *BMJ.* 1903;2:1401.

606. Swaminath CS, Shortt HE, Anderson LAP. Transmission of Indian Kala-azar to man by the bites of *Phlebotomus argentipes. Indian J Med Res.* 1942;30:473–477.

607. Most H. Leishmaniasis. Anderson RS, Haven WP, eds. *Infectious Diseases and General Medicine.* Vol. 3. In: *Internal Medicine in World War II.* Washington, DC, Office of the Surgeon General, Dept of the Army; 1968: 1–48.

608. Most H, Lavietes PH. Kala-azar in American military personnel: Report of 30 cases. *Medicine.* 1947;26:221–284.

609. Angevine D, Hamiliton T, Wallace F, Hazard J. Lymph nodes in leishmaniasis. *Am J Med Sci.* 1945;210:33–38.

610. Cole A, Cosgrove P, Robinson G. A preliminary report of an outbreak of kala-azar in a battalion of King's African Rifles. *Trans R Soc Trop Med Hyg.* 1942;36:25–34.

611. Corkill NL. Activation of latent kala-azar and malaria by battle experience. *Ann Trop Med Parasitol*. 1948;42:224–229.

612. Broughton R. Ten cases of dermal leishmaniasis near Aden. *J R Navy Med Services*. 1964;50:176–178.

613. Michie I. Visceral leishmaniasis in the Aden Protectorate. *J R Army Med Corps*. 1966;112:27–35.

614. Bell D, Carmichael J, Williams R, Hohman R, Stewart P. Localized leishmaniasis of lymph nodes. *BMJ*. 1968;1:740.

615. Naggan L, Isler I, Michaeli D, Levin C. Cutaneous leishmaniasis in the Jericho Valley: An epidemiological and clinical survey. *Harefuah*. 1968;75:175–177.

616. Giladi M, Danon YL, Greenblatt C, Schinder E, Nili E. Keziot—a new endemic site of cutaneous leishmaniasis in Israel: An epidemiological and clinical study of a non-immune population entering an endemic area. *Trop Geogr Med*. 1985;37:298–303.

617. Dunn MA, Smerz RW. Medical support of the Sinai Multinational Force and Observers, 1982. *Mil Med*. 1983;10:773–778.

618. Mansour NS, Youssef FG, Mohareb EW, Dees WH, Karuru ER. Cutaneous leishmaniasis in north Sinai. *Trans R Soc Trop Med Hyg*. 1987;81:747.

619. Mansour NS, Youssef FG, Mohareb EW, Dees WH, Karuru ER. Cutaneous leishmaniasis in the peace keeping forces in East Sinai. *J Egypt Soc Parasitol*. 1989;19:725–732.

620. Norton SA, Frankenburg S, Klaus SN. Cutaneous leishmaniasis acquired during military service in the Middle East. *Arch Dermatol*. 1992;128:83–87.

621. Nadim A, Javadian E. Leishmanization in the Islamic Republic of Iran. In: Walton B, Wijeyaretne P, Modabber F, eds. *Research and Control for the Leishmaniases*. Ottawa: International Development Research Centre; 1988: 336–339.

622. Magill AJ, Grogl M, Gasser RA Jr, Sun W, Oster CN. Visceral infection caused by *Leishmania tropica* in veterans of Operation Desert Storm. *N Engl J Med*. 1993;328:1383–1387.

623. Magill AJ, Grogl M, Johnson SC, Gasser RA Jr. Visceral infection due to *Leishmania tropica* in a veteran of Operation Desert Storm who presented 2 years after leaving Saudi Arabia. *Clin Infect Dis*. 1994;19:805–806.

624. Hepburn NC, Tidman MJ, Hunter JA. Cutaneous leishmaniasis in British troops from Belize. *Br J Dermatol*. 1993;128:63–68.

625. Kean B. Cutaneous leishmaniasis on the isthmus of Panama. *Arch Dermatol Syphilology*. 1948;50:90–101.

626. Lansjoen P. Cutaneous leishmaniasis: A report of 10 cases. *Ann Intern Med*. 1956;45:623–639.

627. Walton BC, Person DA, Bernstein R. Leishmaniasis in the US military in the Canal Zone. *Am J Trop Med Hyg*. 1968;17:19–24.

628. Minkin W, Lynch PJ. Central American leishmaniasis. *Mil Med*. 1969;134:698–700.

629. Kern F, Pedersen JK. Leishmaniasis in the United States: A report of ten cases in military personnel. *JAMA*. 1973;226:872–874.

630. Takafuji ET, Hendricks LD, Daubek JL, McNeil KM, Scagliola HM, Diggs CL. Cutaneous leishmaniasis associated with jungle training. *Am J Trop Med Hyg*. 1980;29:516–520.

631. Sanchez JL, Diniega BM, Small JW, et al. Epidemiologic investigation of an outbreak of cutaneous leishmaniasis in a defined geographic focus of transmission. *Am J Trop Med Hyg*. 1992;47:47–54.

632. Chulay JD, Oster CN, McGreevy PB, Hendricks LD, Kreutzer RD. American cutaneous leishmaniasis: Presentation and problems of patient management. *Rev Soc Bras Med Trop*. 1988;21:165–172.

633. Aronson NE, Wortmann GW, Johnson SC, et al. Safety and efficacy of intravenous sodium stibogluconate in the treatment of leishmaniasis: Recent U.S. military experience. *Clin Infect Dis*. 1998;27:1457–1464.

634. Magill A. The epidemiology of the leishmaniases. In: Weinstock M, ed. *Dermatologic Clinics*. Vol. 13. Philadelphia: W.B. Saunders; 1995: 505–523.

635. Grimaldi G Jr, Tesh RB. Leishmaniases of the New World: Current concepts and implications for future research. *Clin Microbiol Rev*. 1993;6:230–250.

636. Ashford RW, Bettini S. Ecology and epidemiology: Old World. In: Peters W, Killick-Kendrick R, eds. *The Leishmaniases in Biology and Medicine*. Vol. 1. London: Academic Press Inc; 1987: 365–424.

637. Shaw J, Lainson R. Ecology and epidemiology: New World. In: Peters W, Kilick-Kendrick R, eds. *The Leishmaniases in Biology and Medicine*. Vol. 2. London: Academic Press, Inc.; 1987: 291–363.

638. Grimaldi G Jr, Tesh RB, McMahon-Pratt D. A review of the geographic distribution and epidemiology of leishmaniasis in the New World. *Am J Trop Med Hyg*. 1989;41:687–725.

639. World Health Organization. *Control of the Leishmaniases*. Geneva: WHO; 1990. Technical Report No 793.

640. Lane R. Phlebotamine sandflies. In: Cook G, ed. *Manson's Tropical Medicine*. 20th ed. London: W.B. Saunders; 1996: 1666–1674.

641. Christensen HA, Fairchild GB, Herrer A, Johnson CM, Young DG, de Vasquez AM. The ecology of cutaneous leishmaniasis in the Republic of Panama. *J Med Entomol*. 1983;20:463–484.

642. Herwaldt BL, Arana BA, Navin TR. The natural history of cutaneous leishmaniasis in Guatemala. *J Infect Dis*. 1992;165:518–527.

643. Marsden P. Mucosal leishmaniasis ("espundia" Escomel, 1911). *Trans R Soc Trop Med Hyg*. 1986;80:859–876.

644. Wortmann GW, Aronson NE, Miller RS, Blazes D, Oster CN. Cutaneous leishmaniasis following local trauma: A clinical pearl. *Clin Infect Dis*. 2000;31:199–201.

645. Walton B. American cutaneous and mucocutaneous leishmaniasis. In: Peters W, Killick-Kendrick R, eds. *The Leishmaniases in Biology and Medicine*. Vol. 2. London: Academic Press; 1987: 637–664.

646. Pampiglione S, La Placa M, Schlick G. Studies on Mediterranean leishmaniasis, 1: An outbreak of visceral leishmaniasis in northern Italy. *Trans R Soc Trop Med Hyg*. 1974;68:349–359.

647. Pampiglione S, Manson-Bahr PE, Giungi F, Giunti G, Parenti A, Canestri Trotti G. Studies on Mediterranean leishmaniasis, 2: Asymptomatic cases of visceral leishmaniasis. *Trans R Soc Trop Med Hyg*. 1974;68:447–453.

648. Badaro R, Jones TC, Carvalho EM, et al. New perspectives on a subclinical form of visceral leishmaniasis. *J Infect Dis*. 1986;154:1003–1011.

649. Navin TR, Arana FE, de Merida AM, Arana BA, Castillo AL, Silvers DN. Cutaneous leishmaniasis in Guatemala: Comparison of diagnostic methods. *Am J Trop Med Hyg*. 1990;42:36–42.

650. Burns JM Jr, Shreffler WG, Benson DR, Ghalib HW, Badaro R, Reed SG. Molecular characterization of a kinesin-related antigen of *Leishmania chagasi* that detects specific antibody in African and American visceral leishmaniasis. *Proc Natl Acad Sci USA*. 1993;90:775–779.

651. Qu JQ, Zhong L, Masoom-Yasinzai M, et al. Serodiagnosis of Asian leishmaniasis with a recombinant antigen from the repetitive domain of a *Leishmania* kinesin. *Trans R Soc Trop Med Hyg*. 1994;88:543–545.

652. Singh S, Gilman-Sachs A, Chang KP, Reed SG. Diagnostic and prognostic value of K39 recombinant antigen in Indian leishmaniasis. *J Parasitol.* 1995;81:1000–1003.

653. Badaro R, Benson D, Eulalio MC, et al. rK39: A cloned antigen of *Leishmania chagasi* that predicts active visceral leishmaniasis. *J Infect Dis.* 1996;173:758–761.

654. Herwaldt BL, Berman JD. Recommendations for treating leishmaniasis with sodium stibogluconate (Pentostam) and review of pertinent clinical studies. *Am J Trop Med Hyg.* 1992;46:296–306.

655. Ballou WR, McClain JB, Gordon DM, et al. Safety and efficacy of high-dose sodium stibogluconate therapy of American cutaneous leishmaniasis. *Lancet.* 1987;2:13–16.

656. Gasser RA Jr, Magill AJ, Oster CN, Franke ED, Grogl M, Berman JD. Pancreatitis induced by pentavalent antimonial agents during treatment of leishmaniasis. *Clin Infect Dis.* 1994;18:83–90.

657. Magill A. Leishmaniasis. In: Rakel R, ed. *Conn's Current Therapy.* Philadelphia: W. B. Saunders; 1995: 83–87.

658. Olliaro P, Bryceson A. Practical progress and new drugs for changing patterns of leishmaniasis. *Parasitol Today.* 1993;9:323–328.

659. Berman JD. Human leishmaniasis: clinical, diagnostic, and chemotherapeutic developments in the last 10 years. *Clin Infect Dis.* 1997;24:684–703.

660. Beaver PC, Jung RC, Cupp EW. *Clinical Parasitology.* 9th ed. Philadelphia: Lea & Febiger; 1984: Chap 10.

661. Kirchhoff LV. American trypanosomiasis (Chagas' disease). *Gastroenterol Clin North Am.* 1996;25:517–532.

662. Goddard J. *Physician's Guide to Arthropods of Medical Importance.* Boca Raton, Fla: CRC Press; 1993: Chap 12.

663. Cross JH, Uniformed Services University of the Health Sciences. Personal Communication, 1987.

664. Kirchhoff LV. Chagas' disease, American trypanosomiasis. *Infect Dis Clin North Am.* 1993;7:487–502.

665. Salazar-Schettino PM. Customs which predispose to Chagas' disease and cysticercosis in Mexico. *Am J Trop Med Hyg.* 1983;32:1170–1180.

666. Prata A. Chagas' disease. *Infect Dis Clin North Am.* 1994;8:61–76.

667. Espinosa R, Carrasco HA, Belandria F, et al. Life expectancy analysis in patients with Chagas' disease: Prognosis after one decade (1973–1983). *Int J Cardiol.* 1985;8:45–56.

668. Maguire JH, Hoff R. American trypanosomiasis. In: Hoeprich P, ed. *Infectious Diseases.* Philadelphia: J.B. Lippincott; 1994: 1258–1267.

669. Marr JJ, Docampo R. Chemotherapy for Chagas' disease: A perspective on current therapy and considerations for future research. *Rev Infect Dis.* 1986;8:884–903.

670. Kirchhoff LV. American trypanosomiasis (Chagas' disease)—a tropical disease now in the United States. *N Engl J Med.* 1993;329:639–644.

671. Gallerano RH, Marr JJ, Sosa RR. Therapeutic efficacy of allopurinol in patients with chronic Chagas' disease. *Am J Trop Med Hyg.* 1990;43:159–166. Published erratum: *Am J Trop Med Hyg,* 1991;44:580.

672. Bales JD, Harrison SM. African trypanosomiasis. In: Hoeprich P, ed. *Infectious Diseases.* Philadelphia: J.B. Lippincott; 1994: 1214–1218.

673. Panosian CB, Cohen L, Bruckner D, Berlin G, Hardy WD. Fever leukopenia, and a cutaneous lesion in a man who had recently traveled in Africa. *Rev Infect Dis.* 1991;13:1131–1138.

674. Bales JD. African trypanosomiasis. In: Strickland GT, ed. *Hunter's Tropical Medicine*. Philadelphia: W.B. Saunders; 1991: 617–628.

675. Goddard J. *Physician's Guide to Arthropods of Medical Importance*. Boca Raton, Fla: CRC Press; 1993: Chap 18.

676. Burke J. Apropos of congenital African trypanosomiasis [in French]. *Ann Soc Belg Med Trop*. 1973;53:63–64.

677. Kuzoe FA. Current situation of African trypanosomiasis. *Acta Trop*. 1993;54:153–162.

678. Pepin J, Milford F. The treatment of human African trypanosomiasis. *Adv Parasitol*. 1994;33:1–47.

Chapter 36

DISEASES TRANSMITTED PRIMARILY FROM ANIMALS TO HUMANS

PATRICK W. KELLEY, MD, DRPH
KENT E. KESTER, MD
CLIFTON A. HAWKES, MD
ARTHUR M. FRIEDLANDER, MD
JULIE PAVLIN, MD, MPH

KELLY T. MCKEE, JR., MD, MPH
WILLIAM R. BYRNE, MD
CHRISTIAN F. OCKENHOUSE MD, PhD
LISA A. PEARSE, MD, MPH
COLONEL DAVID HOOVER, MD

LEPTOSPIROSIS

HANTAVIRUSES

TOXOPLAMOSIS

Q FEVER

VIRAL HEMORRHAGIC FEVERS

RABIES

TULAREMIA

ANTHRAX

BRUCELLOSIS

P.W. Kelley; Colonel, Medical Corps, US Army (Retired); Director, Board on Global Health, Institute of Medicine, 500 Fifth Street, NW, Washington, DC 20001; Formerly, Director, Division of Preventive Medicine, Walter Reed Army Institute of Research, Director, DoD Global Emerging Infections System, Silver Spring, MD 20910-7500

K.T. McKee, Jr., Colonel, Medical Corps US Army (Retired); Director of Extramural Clinical Research, US Army Medical Research Institute of Infectious Diseases,1425 Porter Street, Fort Detrick, MD 21702; Formerly, Chief, Medical Operations Division, US Army Medical Research Institute of Infectious Diseases

K.E. Kester, MD, Lieutenant Colonel, Medical Corps, US Army; Chief, Department of Clinical Trials, Division of Communicable Diseases and Immunology, Walter Reed Army Institute of Research, Silver Spring, MD 20910-7500

W.R. Byrne, MD, Colonel, Medical Corps US Army; Infectious Disease Officer, Infectious Disease Service, Walter Reed Army Medical Center, Washington, DC 20307-5001; Formerly, Chief, Medical Division, United States Army Medical Research Institute of Infectious Diseases, Fort Detrick, MD 21702-5011

C.A. Hawkes, MD, Colonel, Medical Corps, US Army; Chief, Infectious Disease Service, Walter Reed Army Medical Center, Washington, DC 20307-5001

C.F. Ockenhouse MD, PhD, Colonel, Medical Corps, US Army; Infectious Disease Officer, Department of Immunology, Division of Communicable Diseases and Immunology, Walter Reed Army Institute of Research, Silver Spring, Maryland 20910-7500

A.M. Friedlander, MD, Colonel, Medical Corps, US Army (Retired); Senior Military Scientist, US Army Medical Research Institute of Infectious Diseases, Fort Detrick, MD 21702-5011; Adjunct Professor of Medicine, Uniformed Services University of the Health Sciences, 4301 Jones Bridge Road, Bethesda, Maryland 20814-4799

L.A. Pearse, MD, MPH, Major, Medical Corps, US Army; Chief, Mortality Surveillance Division, Armed Forces Institute of Pathology, 1413 Research Boulevard, Building 102, Rockville, MD 20850; Formerly, Chief, Preventive Medicine Service, William Beaumont Army Medical Center, El Paso, TX 79920-5001

J. Pavlin, MD, MPH, Lieutenant Colonel, Medical Corps, US Army; Chief, Department of Field Studies, Walter Reed Army Institute of Research, Silver Spring, MD 20910-7500

D. Hoover, MD, Colonel, Medical Corps, US Army; Infectious Disease Officer, Department of Bacterial Diseases, Division of Communicable Diseases and Immunology, Walter Reed Army Institute of Research, Silver Spring, MD 20910-7500

LEPTOSPIROSIS

Introduction and Military Relevance

Leptospirosis is a zoonotic infection in which humans are incidentally infected when they have direct or indirect skin or mucous membrane contact with the contaminated urine of infected wild and domestic animals. Leptospirosis has been well documented in military populations with a history of exposures to mud or various bodies of water in endemic locales.[1,2] It is caused by a spirochete, and transmission can occur in urban, suburban, and rural settings in both tropical and temperate areas. The clinical spectrum ranges from an asymptomatic or influenza-like infection (the most common presentation) through hemorrhagic manifestations, meningismus, jaundice, and renal failure. The more severe end of the spectrum is called Weil's syndrome. Although efforts at prevention can include immunization of domestic animals, the major means of prevention used in the military setting include education, rodent control, and, when appropriate, weekly doxycycline prophylaxis.

Description of the Pathogen

There are more than 200 antigenically distinct serovars or strains of leptospire classified into about 23 groups under the species *Leptospira interrogans*. The distribution of serovars varies around the world. The pathogenicity of serovars varies from animal to animal and even between "identical" serovars from different regions.[3] A newly recognized species, *L fainei*, may also affect humans. A nonpathogenic species, *L biflexa*, also exists. Advances in molecular genetics are leading to a variety of new classification schemes that do not relate to traditional serological groupings.

Leptospires are obligate aerobes. They are flexible, tightly coiled, helicoidal rods with one or both ends usually hooked. Due to its thinness and motility, darkfield microscopy is necessary for optimal visualization even with staining.

Epidemiology

Transmission

Leptospires can live free or in association with human and animal hosts. Animals that survive the acute infection may shed the organisms in their urine for years. In a 1982 survey of 139 small animals trapped at the Jungle Operations Training Center in Panama, 42% had leptospira in their urine (Takafuji ET. 1982. Unpublished data). Even dogs immunized to prevent clinical disease can develop renal shedding.[4] In the environment, *L interrogans* can survive under favorable conditions for as long as 6 months. Tropical, unpolluted, nonsaline, slightly alkaline waters provide an ideal environment.

Although leptospires usually enter the person through breaks in skin or mucous membranes, prolonged immersion in water may facilitate infection through otherwise intact skin. Service members seem to be at particular risk during operations in swamps, streams, ponds, and muddy areas. Leptospirosis has been particularly noteworthy among US forces operating in Panama and Vietnam.[1,2] Other professions that are notably at risk include agriculture and aquaculture, sewer and construction work, animal husbandry, veterinary and slaughterhouse work, mining, and laboratory work. Increasingly, recreational pursuits have been shown to be correlated with risk; this includes care of pets, hunting, fishing, swimming in ponds and other bodies of fresh water, rafting, and playing sports on muddy fields.[5–7] Other possible routes of infection implicated include contaminated drinking water and food preparation surfaces, and, rarely, animal bites. Extremely rare routes of transmission include human-to-human transmission through urine, breast milk, and sex.[8,9]

Geographic Distribution

Leptospirosis can be found in almost every country, though the distribution within a country reflects the variations in host-animal populations and the environment.[3] Cases have been recognized in virtually all states in the United States, though most reports are from Hawaii and the less-arid southern states.[5]

As was clearly evident with US troops training in Panama, risk may increase significantly in the rainy season. Rains or flooding can enhance the flushing of subsurface leptospires into surface waters and draw shedding rodents and other animals to swampy areas.[8] Urban flooding following hurricanes and other heavy rains is also associated with increased risk. The seasonality of reported cases may also reflect the cyclic nature of human agricultural or recreational activity. Though persons in arid areas tend to be at lesser risk of leptospirosis, significant transmission can occur under the right environmental conditions, carrier prevalence, and human behaviors. For example, the concentration of shedding animals and people around scarce water holes or oases may create opportunities for transmission.

Incidence

The incidence of leptospirosis is grossly underreported because the clinical presentation is often that of a nonspecific influenza-like illness. Most cases are not specifically diagnosed or are misdiagnosed as a more common febrile infection such as dengue. On occasion this can be a fatal mistake. Clinical awareness of the patient's epidemiologic history and a high index of suspicion are essential to making this diagnosis and instituting timely, effective therapy.

Leptospirosis occurs both sporadically and in common-source outbreaks. Probably the highest incidence documented has been in US forces training in Panama. Between 1977 and 1982, close surveillance was conducted on seven US Army units attending the 3-week course at the Jungle Operations Training Center during the fall rainy season. This surveillance yielded 91 confirmed and probable cases, for an annualized incidence estimate of 41,000 per 100,000 person years (Takafuji ET. 1984. Unpublished data) (Figure 36-1). Since these troops in training did not have daily exposure, the real risk was probably even higher. Clearly these attack rates indicate that an intense operational exposure to contaminated environments can have a major impact on not only individual health but also unit capability and mission accomplishment.

Pathogenesis and Clinical Findings

The underlying pathologic effect of acute leptospirosis resembles a vasculitis with damage to the endothelial lining of capillaries coupled with hepatitic and renal tubular dysfunction.[10] Historically most leptospirosis deaths have been due to renal failure, but dialysis has reduced the fatality of this factor. Cardiac effects, to include myocarditis and arrhythmias, are now the leading cause of death in leptospirosis. Hemorrhagic manifestations are also common in severe cases. Jaundice is a major feature of severe leptospirosis and appears to reflect hepatic cell dysfunction more than hemolysis. Survivors generally have no lasting liver or renal dysfunction. Repeated infections with other serovars can occur. Intrauterine infections can cause fetal loss, premature labor, and congenital infection.

The incubation period for leptospirosis is typically 7 to 12 days (range: 2 to 26 days). Very short incubations have been seen in laboratory exposures. Although about 90% of recognized cases present as a mild, self-limited febrile illness, in a prospective serosurvey of soldiers that identified 24 infected persons, only one denied any symptomatology.[2] It is quite possible that if all cases were ascertained, even more than 90% would be recognized as mild.

Mild, anicteric patients often present with the sudden onset of fever that peaks at 38°C to 40°C. Other complaints may include headache, chills, back and joint pain, neck stiffness, and intense myalgia. Even lightly touching the skin over the thighs, calves, and lumbosacral muscles may elicit notable pain. A commonly described finding dur-

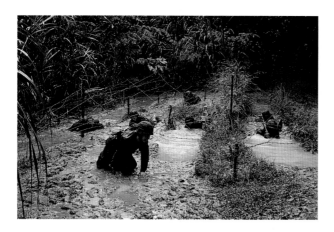

Fig. 36-1. A typical occupational exposure: soldiers in the mud at the Jungle Operations Training Center, Panama.
US Army photograph.

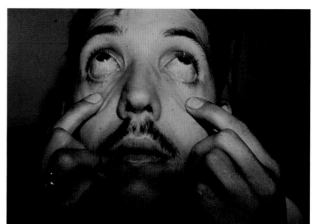

Fig. 36-2. Conjunctival suffusion in a soldier with leptospirosis Photograph: Courtesy of Colonel Ernest Takafuji, Medical Corps, US Army.

ing the first 3 days of illness is conjunctival suffusion, a dilation of the conjunctival vessels without associated signs of inflammation (Figure 36-2). Generalized abdominal pain is sometimes noted and may suggest a "surgical abdomen" or enteric fever. Nausea, vomiting, diarrhea, and constipation may also be reported. Skin manifestations of mild leptospirosis can include a variety of rashes, mainly but not exclusively on the trunk. Meningeal irritation, photophobia, and a variable degree of physiological dysfunction may also noted in mild disease.

Although often not noted by clinicians, classically leptospirosis is described as having an initial leptospiremic phase followed after a 1- to 5-day fairly asymptomatic period by a secondary leptospiuric phase. The leptospiremic phase typically lasts 4 to 7 days and ends about the time antibodies appear. During the leptospiruric phase, fever returns and may be associated with signs of aseptic meningitis[10] (Figure 36-3). The severity of the meningitis is variable. The second phase may last 4 to 30 days or longer. In a review of 150 cases in service members serving in Vietnam, however, only 48% of cases were noted to have this second phase, which usually lasted only 1 day.[1]

In that minority of cases with severe leptospirosis, the initial fever and generalized abnormalities can progress to manifest jaundice, azotemia, hemorrhage, anemia, shock, and altered mental status. As the disease progresses into the second week, hemorrhagic manifestations may be noted in the skin, conjunctiva, and sputum.[10] Deaths due to adrenal hemorrhage have been noted but are rare. Renal failure, acute respiratory distress syndrome, congestive heart failure, and arrhythmias are additional manifestations of severe leptospirosis. Hemorrhagic pneumonitis has been a significant manifestation in infections acquired in Korea, other Far Eastern locales, and Nicaragua. Mild proteinuria is a notable laboratory finding. Vitamin K can correct the prothrombin deficiency that is sometimes seen. Other common laboratory findings include elevated creatinine phosphokinase and amalyse levels, neutrophilia, and thrombocytopenia. During the secondary phase, the cerebrospinal fluid may show a pleocytosis. A variety of chest roentgenogram abnormalities are common and may include pulmonary opacities, pleural effusion, and evidence of myositis or pericardial effusion. Electrocardiographic abnormalities are also noted.

Published case fatality rates vary widely, probably reflecting geographic variation in serovars and in the low proportion of mild cases that are specifically diagnosed. Overall, the true case fatality is

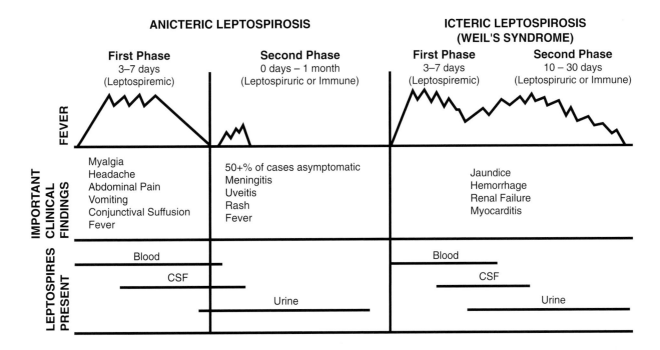

Fig. 36-3. The clinical course of leptospirosis
Reprinted with permission from: Feigin Rd, Anderson DC. Leptospirosis. In: Feigin RD, Cherry JD, eds. *Textbook of Pediatric Infectious Disease.* Vol 2. Philadelphia: W.B. Saunders; 1998: 1534.

probably less than 1.0%, but severe cases may have rates of well over 10%. In survivors, convalescence may extend to several months. In a small percentage of survivors, a variety of delayed ocular complications, including anterior uveal tract inflammation, may become manifest during convalescence or as long as a year later. These and headaches may persist for years.[11]

Diagnostic Approaches

Early diagnosis is important in leptospirosis for antibiotic therapy to be effective and to prevent future cases. Key to diagnosis is a good epidemiologic history, especially when patients present with a febrile illness associated with an abrupt onset, myalgias, and severe headache. The differential diagnosis includes heat injury, influenza, dengue, rickettsioses, typhoid fever, brucellosis, relapsing fever, toxoplasmosis, malaria, yellow fever, septicemia, toxic shock syndrome, Kawasaki syndrome, Hantaan virus infection, and Legionnaires' disease. In the Caribbean region, the relative frequency of dengue has contributed to the missed diagnosis of leptospirosis, sometimes with fatal consequences. In the Balkans, distinguishing between leptospirosis and hantavirus infection has also been difficult.

The specific diagnosis of leptospirosis usually requires paired sera to document a 4-fold rise in antibody titer and is thus often retrospective. Commercial enzyme immunosorbent assays or macroagglutination serologic screening tests are typically used. Polymerase chain reaction methods are also available in some laboratories and can help with early diagnosis. The definitive antibody assay is the microagglutination test, but this is found only in reference laboratories and requires that the battery of live leptospiral organisms used reflect the serovars prevalent in the location where the putative exposure occurred.[8] The importance of this is illustrated by the report that 70% of the leptospirosis acquired by US soldiers in Panama could be diagnosed serologically by the microagglutination test only when Panamanian isolates were used as antigen.[12] Presumptive diagnosis can be made when there are compatible clinical findings and either a positive macroagglutination slide test or a microagglutination titer of at least 1 in 100. Many other assays are under development, including rapid dipstick-type tests.

Cultures of blood and cerebrospinal fluid established during the first week or so on specific media are also valuable in confirming the diagnosis, but it may take 6 to 8 weeks for the leptospires to grow.[8]

After the first week, successful cultures of urine are possible. Specimens of blood, cerebrospinal fluid, and urine for culture must be innoculated into special culture media such as Tween 80-albumin (EMJH) media. To reduce the effect of inhibitory substances, three serial dilutions should be made to yield specimen to media concentrations of 1:10, 1:100, and 1:1000. The cultures should be incubated in the dark at 28°C to 30°C. If an appropriate leptospiral growth medium is not immediately available, leptospira can survive for a week or longer after collection in a tube of blood anticoagulated with heparin or sodium oxalate. In one study of US soldiers who trained in Panama in which blood and urine cultures were taken within 3 days of fever onset, more than 94% of patient cultures were positive.[2] Culture results are sometimes positive in the face of negative serologies.

Recommendations for Therapy and Control

Most experts feel that antibiotic therapy of leptospirosis is useful if given early in the illness. Doxycycline, 100 mg by mouth twice a day for 7 days, has been shown to be effective in soldiers who acquired leptospirosis in Panama if given within the first 4 days of illness.[13] Penicillin has also been used with success in some studies[14–16] but not in others. Erythromycin, some of the newer penicillins, and cephalosporins may also be effective.[17] Jarisch-Herxheimer reactions (ie, temperature rise, drop in blood pressure, and precipitation or exacerbation of other symptoms and signs) have been reported to occur after antibiotic therapy for leptospirosis. Concern over these reactions, however, does not justify avoiding antibiotics. Nonspecific therapy may be useful to manage pain, fever, mental status changes, vomiting, renal failure, hypotension, and hemorrhage.

Prevention in humans is based on exposure reduction and antibiotic prophylaxis. Exposure reduction requires an understanding of the epidemiology of the infection in a particular setting. Education of service members, commanders, operational planners, and health care personnel on the epidemiology of leptospirosis is important. Although military operational imperatives may require exposure to potentially contaminated soil and water, an awareness of leptopsirosis may strengthen consideration of tactical alternatives that can mitigate exposures. Knowledge of the epidemiology of leptospirosis can also help influence a commander to put some areas off limits for recreational use. Other methods (eg, rodent control in camps, use of protective clothing and surface disinfectants) have a place in some occupational exposure settings. Simply wearing shoes rather than going barefoot reduces the risk of leptospirosis for individuals walking around fields, farms, bivouac sites, lawns, or other areas where infected wild and domestic animals may urinate. Prevention programs in domesticated animals can

include immunization.

Chemoprophylaxis with weekly doxycycline (200 mg) has been extremely effective in preventing troops training in Panama during the high-risk rainy season from getting leptospirosis; such a regimen should only be used for short, high-risk exposures.[2,7]

[Patrick W. Kelley]

HANTAVIRUSES

Introduction and Military Relevance

Infectious febrile syndromes complicated by renal and hematological abnormalities have been described in northern Europe, the Balkans, and throughout the Far East for many decades. Since the 1930s, these geographically distinct but clinically and epidemiologically similar entities have frequently been cited in association with the military and its operations. During World War II, huge outbreaks of these diseases were documented among Japanese and Soviet soldiers encamped along the Amur River valley in the Far East, while more than 1,000 German and Finnish troops were stricken in Lapland.[18,19] Beginning in the 1950s, hemorrhagic nephroso-nephritis became increasingly recognized as a hazard to military camps in central Europe.[20] Despite their widespread recognition across the Eurasian landmass, however, these disorders were unknown to US military physicians until the Korean War, when more than 3,000 United Nations military personnel developed so-called epidemic (or Korean) hemorrhagic fever between 1951 and 1953.[21] Although these diseases were widely assumed to be infectious zoonoses, details of their epidemiology and pathogenesis remained undefined until Lee and colleagues recognized the causative agent of Korean hemorrhagic fever, Hantaan virus, in 1976.[22] Since that time, these disorders, now known collectively as hemorrhagic fever with renal syndrome (HFRS), have been linked to a variety of similar but serologically distinct agents called hantaviruses. As evidenced by repeated severe and occasionally lethal outbreaks among soldiers in Korea[23] and Europe,[24] hantaviruses continue to plague the field operations of US military forces in endemic areas.

Description of the Pathogens

Hantaviruses are negative-stranded RNA viruses sharing morphological and biochemical characteristics of the family *Bunyaviridae*. Taxonomically, they are classified as a separate genus within this large

virus family.[25] Each hantavirus has evolved in association with a predominant rodent host in which it establishes a chronic, inapparent infection.[26] As of 1997, more than 25 hantaviruses had been described belonging to four phylogenetic and antigenic groups. About half of the currently recognized hantaviruses have been linked to human disease.[27–29] Hantaviruses of particular interest to military populations include the Seoul, Hantaan, Puumala, Dobrava/Belgrave, and the so-called "American" viruses (eg, Sin Nombre, Andes).

Epidemiology

Transmission and Geographic Distribution

Chronically infected rodents shed large amounts of virus in urine, saliva, and, to a lesser extent, feces.[30] Humans most likely become infected either by contact with these contaminated excreta and secreta through inhalation of small particle aerosols or by percutaneous or mucous membrane contact with infectious materials. Individuals at highest risk include those living or working in rural areas, such as farmers and foresters. Military personnel in the field also represent a high-risk group. Person-to-person spread of hantaviruses associated with HFRS has never been documented.

Hantaviruses have been found on every continent except Antarctica. The epidemiology of each different virus is a function of the ecology, population dynamics, and geographic distribution of its predeominant rodent host. Hantavirus reservoirs tend to be among the most abundant rodents found in a given disease-endemic area. However, infection within rodent populations is not uniform—a characteristic reflected in the microfocal distribution of human disease.[31]

With the exception of Seoul virus, hantaviruses typically cause human disease in rural settings. Hantaan virus, the cause of classic severe ("Far Eastern") HFRS, circulates across China, northern Asia, and the Korean peninsula.[32] Its reservoir, *Apodemus agrarius*, is the ubiquitous striped field mouse. The etiologic agent of a generally milder disease variant known as nephropathia epidemica, Puumala virus, is associated primarily with the bank vole *Clethrionomys glareolus*. This rodent ranges throughout Scandinavia and the rest of northern Europe south into the Balkan states.[32,33] Dobrava/Belgrade virus is associated epidemiologically with severe HFRS. This agent is carried (perhaps along with Hantaan-like viruses) in central Europe and the Balkans by the yellow-necked field mouse, *Apodemus flavicollis*.[34–36] *Rattus* species serve as reservoirs for Seoul virus. Seoul virus is recognized worldwide and has been linked to comparatively mild human illness, most frequently in eastern Asia, but it can also cause severe HFRS.

Until relatively recently, hantaviruses were thought to be associated exclusively with HFRS and to cause disease largely in Europe and Asia. In late 1993, however, an outbreak of a rapidly progressive respiratory syndrome among inhabitants of the Four Corners region of the southwestern United States was shown to be caused by a novel hantavirus (ultimately called Sin Nombre) associated with deer mice (*Peromyscus maniculatus*).[37–39] As efforts intensified to define the geographical extent of what came to be known as hantavirus pulmonary syndrome (HPS), some cases were identified outside the known distribution of *P maniculatus*. It soon became evident that hantaviruses other than Sin Nombre were probably responsible for this disorder as well.[40,41] As of 1997, more than 150 domestic cases of HPS had been identified, and it became clear that several different hantaviruses could cause the syndrome. With expansion of surveillance to other parts of the Western hemisphere and application of newer molecular diagnostic technologies, numerous related but clearly distinct agents have been identified throughout North, Central, and South America.[28,29,41,42] Some viruses (eg, Sin Nombre, Andes, Laguna Negra, Black Creek Canal, Bayou, Monongahela, Juquitiba, New York-1) have been associated with acute, symptomatic human disease. Other viruses (eg, Prospect Hill, Muleshoe, Cano Delgatido, El Moro Canyon, Rio Segundo, Rio Mamore) have been found only in rodents. With increasing awareness, it is highly likely that additional hantaviruses indigenous to the Americas will be identified.

Incidence

Numerically, HFRS is the most important of the viral hemorrhagic fevers, with tens to hundreds of thousands of cases occurring annually across endemic areas. HFRS is recognized year-round, but the highest incidences coincide with periods of maximal rodent activity: late autumn and early winter (with a smaller peak in the spring) in Asia and central Europe; late summer and early fall in colder areas of western Europe (eg, Scandinavia); and spring in warmer parts of Europe (eg, France, Belgium).[33,43]

Pathogenesis and Clinical Findings

The basic pathological abnormality in human hantaviral infection is vascular endothelial damage, probably due to both direct (cytopathic) and indirect (immunopathologic) virus effects. While pathological changes are found in virtually all organ systems, a characteristic triad of lesions is associated with fatal, classic HFRS: hemorrhagic necrosis of the renal medulla, anterior pituitary gland, and cardiac right atrium.

Classic HFRS seen in the Far East is a complex, multiphasic disorder that poses significant challenges in clinical management[21] (Table 36-1). While HFRS may present as a fulminant, rapidly progressive and fatal hemorrhagic fever, most cases (70% to 80%) are more benign. Asymptomatic infections occur but are probably uncommon. After an incubation period of 2 to 3 weeks (range: 4 to 42 days), onset of illness is usually abrupt and nonspecific, with fever, myalgia, headache, and anorexia most frequently reported. Severe abdominal or lower back pain, facial flushing, periorbital edema, and injection of the conjunctivae, together with axillary and palatal petechiae, are typical early disease features. As the clinical course evolves, hypotension (which may be severe) and oliguria or anuria are seen. With recovery of renal function, massive diuresis occurs. Convalescence is prolonged. Complete recovery often takes months. Leukocytosis, thrombocytopenia, and massive proteinuria are characteristic laboratory features during the acute stages of disease, while anemia and hyposthenuria are generally seen during convalescence. Similar clinical features, though of lesser severity, are seen in most western European HFRS (nephropathia epidemica-like) patients. Mortality in Hantaan or Dobrava/Belgrade infections may approach 15% or more, while deaths due to Puumala virus are uncommon. Severe and occasionally fatal cases of HFRS among animal handlers and scientists have been caused by Seoul virus transmitted from colonized laboratory rats with inapparent infections,[44] and Seoul virus has been epidemiologically linked to chronic renal disease in some areas.[45]

TABLE 36-1

FAR EASTERN HEMORRHAGIC FEVER WITH RENAL SYNDROME: TYPICAL CLINICAL AND
LABORATORY CHARACTERISTICS

Stage	Duration	Prominent Clinical Features	Laboratory Findings
Febrile	3-7 d	Fever, malaise, headache, myalgia, back pain, abdominal pain, nausea, vomiting, facial flush, petechiae (face, neck, trunk), conjunctival hemorrhage	WBC: normal or elevated Platelets: decreasing Hematocrit: rising Urine: proteinuria 1+ to 3+
Hypotensive	2 h-3 d	Nausea, vomiting, tachycardia, hypotension, shock, visual blurring, hemorrhagic signs, ±oliguria (late)	WBC: increasing with left shift Platelets: markedly decreasing Bleeding time: increasing, prothrombin time may be prolonged Hematocrit: markedly increasing Urine: proteinuria 4+ hematuria 1+ hyposthenuria BUN and creatinine rising rapidly
Oliguric	3-7 d	Oliguria ± anuria, blood pressure may rise, nausea and vomiting may persist, 1/3 with severe hemorrhage (epistaxis, cutaneous, gastrointestinal, genitorurinary, central nervous system)	WBC: normalizes Platelets: normalize Hematocrit: normalizes then falls Urine: proteinuria 4+ hematuria 1+ to 4+ BUN and creatinine: markedly increasing Na^+, Ca^{++}: falling; K^+ rising
Diuretic	Days to weeks	Polyuria (up to 3-6 L/d)	BUN and creatinine: normalize electrolytes: may be abnormal (diuresis) Urine: normalizes
Convalescent	Weeks to months	Strength and function regained slowly	Anemia and hyposthenuria may persist for months

NOTE: All phases may not be present in a given patient; phases may "blend" in some individuals
WBC: white blood count, BUN: blood urea nitrogen
Reprinted with permission from Military Medicine, the official journal of the Association of Military Surgeons of the United States (AMSUS): McKee, KT Jr, MacDonald C, LeDuc JW, Peters CJ. Hemorrhagic fever with renal syndrome—a clinical perspective. *Mil Med*. 1985;150:640–647.

In contrast to disease caused by hantaviruses across Eurasia, the clinical features of American hantavirus infections center primarily on the cardiorespiratory systems[46] (Table 36-2). HPS is a serious disease with high mortality. After a 3- to 6-day prodromal period of fever, myalgia, and often gastrointestinal symptoms, dyspnea, cough, and hypotension appear and progress rapidly; patients may be in extremis within hours. Renal abnormalities tend to be relatively insignificant. Progressive hypoxemia and pulmonary edema, followed by cardiac arrhythmias and intractable hypotension, challenge survival. Fatality rates approach 50% of cases reported to date, with most deaths occurring within 24 hours of onset of pulmonary decline.[46,47] Among survivors, recovery from acute illness may be rapid, with normalization of most clinical and laboratory parameters. However, lassitude and weakness continue for weeks to months, and pulmonary function abnormalities may persist in some patients.[48] Leukocytosis and thrombocytopenia are common laboratory findings, as is mild proteinuria. Atypical lymphocytes frequently can be found on peripheral blood smears.

Diagnostic Approaches

A high index of suspicion is critical to diagnosing hantavirus infections. Any patient presenting in or returning from a hantavirus-endemic area with fever of abrupt onset, headache, gastrointestinal symptoms, respiratory distress, lower back or abdominal pain, or any combination of these symptoms should be evaluated for possible HFRS or HPS.

TABLE 36-2

HANTAVIRUS PULMONARY SYNDROME: TYPICAL CLINICAL AND LABORATORY FEATURES

Stage	Duration	Prominent Clinical Features	Laboratory Features
Prodrome	3-7 d	Fever, myalgia (especially back, lower extremities), nausea, vomiting, diarrhea, abdominal pain; occasional headache, dizziness	WBC: normal or rising Platelets: normal or falling Hematocrit: normal or rising
Cardiopulmonary	3-16 d	Fever, dyspnea, cough, tachypnea, tachycardia, rapidly progressive respiratory failure, hypotension; cardiogenic/hypotensive shock, cardiac arrhythmias	WBC: rising with left shift and atypical lymphocytes Platelets: falling Hematocrit: rising PTT: rising Mild proteinuria Metabolic acidosis
Convalescent	Weeks to months	Rapid normalization of cardio-respiratory function, diuresis; strength and function regained slowly	Normalization of most parameters, pulmonary function abnormalities may persist

WBC: white blood count, PTT: partial thromboplastin time

An elevated white blood cell count, low platelet count, or proteinuria in this setting should precipitate serological testing for hantavirus infection. The differential diagnosis of HFRS includes rickettsiosis, leptospirosis, meningococcemia, leukemia, hemolytic-uremic syndrome, other viral infections, and poststreptococcal syndromes. HPS can be confused with pneumonic plague; legionellosis; psittacosis; other pneumonic processes of viral, bacterial, or fungal origin; autoimmune disorders, such as thrombotic thrombocytopenic purpura; or pancreatitis accompanied by adult respiratory distress syndrome. Diagnosis is established either by demonstrating hantavirus-specific IgM antibodies in acute serum using enzyme immunoassay or by a 4-fold or greater rise in IgG antibodies using enzyme immunoassay or immunofluorescence.[49] Viral antigens or nucleic acid sequences can be detected in tissue samples by immunohistochemical or molecular amplification techniques.[50] Recovery of hantaviruses from clinical specimens is typically difficult and efforts to cultivate those agents from body fluids are generally unrewarding.

Recommendations for Therapy and Control

Bed rest and early hospitalization in an intensive care environment are critical to successful treatment of hantavirus-infected patients. With HFRS, evacuation from outlying areas should be as atraumatic as possible, to avoid damage to an already compromised microvascular bed. Where facilities exist, patients should be hospitalized locally (ie, "in-country"). Aeromedical evacuation, particularly over long distances and at altitude, should be avoided. Patient isolation is not required. Wide fluctuations in fluid status and the attendant biochemical disturbances are important considerations in patient care and require careful attention. Peritoneal dialysis or hemodialysis is often required in managing metabolic complications.

In HPS, adequate oxygenation and tissue perfusion are the goals of treatment; therefore, mechanical ventilation and use of pressor agents are important adjuncts to general supportive care. Respiratory management should be provided in an intensive care setting. Fluids must be meticulously managed to avoid overhydration and exacerbation of pulmonary edema. As with HFRS, transfer should be avoided if possible; if the patient must be moved, hypoxia and trauma to the fragile vascular beds should be minimized. Isolation of patients with HPS is generally considered unnecessary. In the United States, person-to-person transmission has not been seen, but a single report has suggested interpersonal spread during an outbreak in Argentina.[51] Hantaviruses are sensitive in vitro to the antiviral drug ribavirin. This drug has been shown to reduce morbidity and mortality in Chinese HFRS patients[52]; however, its utility has not been proven elsewhere. In the case of HPS, ribavirin appeared to be ineffective in reducing mortality in an open-label trial.[47] Experience to date is therefore insufficient to rec-

---

EXHIBIT 36-1

MEASURES TO MINIMIZE EXPOSURE TO RODENTS IN HANTAVIRUS-ENDEMIC AREAS

- Store human and animal food under rodent-proof conditions
- Burn or bury garbage or discard it in rodent-proof containers
- Inspect vacant cabins or other enclosed shelters (to include seasonal latrines) for evidence of rodent infestation before use; do not use such structures until appropriately cleaned and disinfected; regularly inspect occupied buildings for evidence of rodent activity
- Disinfect rodent-contaminated areas by spraying a disinfectant, such as dilute bleach, before cleaning
- Avoid inhalation of dust by wearing approved respirators when cleaning previously unoccupied areas*; mist these areas with water before sweeping or mopping
- Remove dead rodents promptly from the area; wear disposable gloves or plastic bags over the hands when handling dead rodents; place all dead rodents into a plastic bag (preferably a bag containing sufficient disinfectant to wet the carcass) before disposal
- Never attempt to feed, handle, or keep wild or stray animals as pets or mascots
- Do not pitch tents or place sleeping bags near potential rodent shelters (eg, burrows, garbage dumps, woodpiles)
- Sleep above the ground on cots if feasible
- Use bottled water or water from approved sources for drinking, cooking, washing dishes, and brushing teeth
- Launder or dry clean rodent-contaminated clothing and bedding, using rubber or plastic gloves when handling contaminated materials
- Be on the lookout for rodents and their burrows or nests and avoid contact; be aware that exposures may not seem significant in all cases

---

*If clear evidence of infestation is present, HEPA-filtered respirators, goggles, solvent-resistant gloves, coveralls, and boots should be worn while cleaning.
HEPA: high efficiency particulate air

---

ommend its unqualified use in HPS.

Elimination or significant reduction of reservoir rodent populations in the field setting is logistically impossible. Exposure to rodent-contaminated brush, dusts, or fomites constitutes a theoretical infection risk to humans, but these have not been documented as routes of hantavirus transmission. General avoidance of rodents, together with their burrows and nesting areas, is useful advice in all endemic areas. Additional measures to control exposure to rodents and their habitats should also be undertaken[53] (Exhibit 36-1).

Hantavirus vaccines produced outside the United States are in use in some endemic areas, but these products are of unproven utility. A candidate vaccinia-vectored recombinant immunogen developed by the US Army is under study.

[Kelly T McKee, Jr.]

TOXOPLASMOSIS

Introduction and Military Relevance

Owing to its widespread distribution, soil reservoir, and association with suboptimal food preparation and inadequate personal sanitation practices, toxoplasmosis has particular relevance for service members deployed in the field and the military physicians who support them. Reports have documented toxoplasmosis outbreaks among deployed US Army troops.[54] *Toxoplasma gondii*, the etiologic agent of toxoplasmosis, was first described in 1908 by Nicolle and Marceaux,[55] with the first case of human disease described 15 years later.[56] The organism is a ubiquitous parasite with a worldwide distribution. While infection of humans is common, most primary infections in immunocompetent individuals are relatively asymptomatic. Greater morbidity and mortality is instead associated with toxoplasmosis affecting immunocompromised patients, especially those with HIV infection, and congenitally infected neonates.[57p500–503] *T gondii* is associated with three major syndromes: lymphadenopathy (usually in immunocompetent hosts), opportunistic infections in immunocompromised hosts, and congenital disease associated with an acute maternal infection.[58] In addition, ocular toxoplasmosis may occur either as a result of an acute infection or a reactivation of a congenital infection.[59]

Description of the Pathogen

Initially discovered in 1908 in a northern African rodent, the gondi, *Toxoplasma gondii* has been subsequently found in an unusually wide array of animals.[60] It is a crescentic-appearing, obligate intracellular coccidian parasite that can multiply in virtually any cell of its vertebrate hosts.[61] Felines serve as the definitive host, and many other animals function as intermediate hosts.[62] While only one species has been identified, strain variation based on differences in virulence has been characterized.[63] Three distinct life forms have been described: oocyst, tachyzoite, and tissue cyst.

Oocysts

Oocysts are the infective form shed by infected cats in their feces. After release, the oocysts require a maturation step, known as sporulation, to become infective. The time to completion of sporulation may vary widely and depends on the ambient temperature (2 to 3 days at 24°C; 14 to 21 days at 11°C). Sporulation will not occur at temperatures less than 4°C or greater than 37°C. Oocysts may remain viable in moist soil for as long as 18 months, leading to an additional environmental reservoir that may prove difficult to eradicate.[64,65] Oocysts are generally shed for 1 to 3 weeks by primarily infected cats; prolonged shedding may be associated with feline immune system defects.[66,67] Oocyst shedding usually occurs only once in an infected cat's lifetime; however, it may occasionally recur with repeated *Toxoplasma* exposure or infection with the coccidian protozan *Isospora felis*.[61,68] At peak release, an infected cat may shed 20 million oocysts in its feces per day.[67]

Tachyzoites

Tachyzoites represent the rapidly dividing asexual invasive form found in an acute *Toxoplasma* infection. These rapidly dividing organisms, best seen with a Wright-Giemsa stain (Figure 36-4) can infect virtually all mammalian cells except nonnucleated erythrocytes.[69] Spread of tachyzoites into the bloodstream accounts for the disseminated nature of *Toxoplasma* infections. Tissue invasion leads to expanding focal lesions.[62] The tachyzoite form of *Toxoplasma* is susceptible to desiccation, freezing

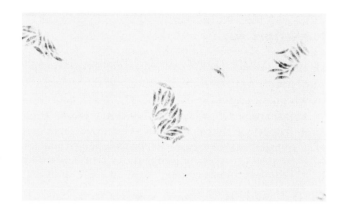

Fig. 36-4. Tachyzoites of *Toxoplasma gondii* from cerebrospinal fluid stained with Wright-Giemsa and photographed at x1,200.
Photograph: Courtesy of Lieutenant Colonel Kent Kester, Walter Reed Army Institute of Research.

followed by thawing, and gastric acid.[69] Unpasteurized milk from infected goats and cattle has been found to harbor viable tachyzoites.[57]

Tissue Cysts

Tissue cysts are the end result of all *T gondii* infections; these are collections of dormant organisms, termed bradyzoites, formed by tachyzoite dissemination (Figure 36-5). They serve as a tissue reservoir for recurrent infection.[60] Bradyzoites tend to reactivate in the context of immune impairment, cre-

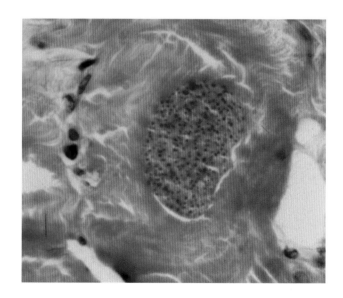

Fig. 36-5. A toxoplasmic cyst in skeletal muscle, stained with hematoxylin-eosin an photographed at x1,200.
Photograph: Courtesy of the Armed Forces Institute of Pathology. AFIP negative 73-7677.

ating a significant hazard in immunocompromised hosts. Cysts may form in any tissue, but they are commonly localized in the cardiac and skeletal muscle and the brain, possibly because of suboptimal immune surveillance in those sites.[61] Encysted organisms persist for the life of the host.[66,70]

The *Toxoplasma* life cycle splits into an exoenteric cycle and an enteric cycle. The exoenteric cycle occurs in most warm-blooded mammals. Tachyzoites invade macrophages and divide within vacuoles. Later, cellular rupture occurs, and the released organisms proceed to infect adjacent cells. Some of these successive infections may lead to the formation of tissue cysts. In the enteric cycle, which occurs only in felines, the liberated parasites enter the cells of the small intestine and develop; released merozoites subsequently infect adjacent cells. As the cycle is repeated, gametogenesis occurs. Fusion of two gametes leads to the formation of a zygote, which then becomes an oocyst.[61]

Epidemiology

Transmission

Infection occurs predominantly via the ingestion of either viable oocysts or tissue cysts. Consuming oocysts is related to contamination of the food or drink with feces from infected cats. Consuming viable tissue cysts is due to a lack of proper food preparation, often in raw or undercooked meat.[60]

While the seropositivity rate of domestic cats ranges between 30% and 80%, pet cats are probably not the direct source of human infection. They tend to be fastidious animals, rarely having fecal material present on their coats long enough for oocysts to sporulate.[67] Transmission from pet cats is more likely from careless handling of litter box contents by their owners. Other members of the family Felidae, such as ocelots and jaguarundis, have also been shown to pass viable *Toxoplasma* oocysts in their feces.[71] Thus, wild felines probably also play a role in transmission of toxoplasmosis.[54] Infected domestic and wild animals, including cattle, pigs, dogs, horses, and rodents, may serve as intermediate hosts and carry viable cysts in their tissues for long periods of time.[70]

Contamination of foodstuffs by cat feces may lead to the presence of infectious oocysts. Additionally, cat feces may contaminate other items, such as soil and drinking water. Ingestion of any of these items may lead to infection with *Toxoplasma*. It has been estimated that the simple act of handling soil contaminated with feces from infected cats may lead to the deposition of 10 to 100 oocysts under the fin-

gernails. Suboptimal personal hygiene may lead to the transfer of the oocysts into the mouth, leading to the development of a primary infection. Various coprophagic insects, including filth flies, cockroaches, and dung beetles, may also serve as transfer agents for infectious oocysts.[60]

Ingestion of viable tissue cysts may be the more common method of infection in the Western world. The large number of bradyzoites found within a tissue cyst makes the probability of infection following cyst ingestion quite high.[60] This mode of infection, which results from the consumption of raw or undercooked meat that contains tissue cysts, likely contributes to the very high *Toxoplasma* seropreva-lences in countries such as France, where less emphasis is placed on thorough cooking of meat. Conversely, the seroprevalence rate in Great Britain, where meat is more likely to be cooked thoroughly, is much lower.[66]

Infection can also be passed from an infected woman to her fetus. Congenital toxoplasmosis occurs as a direct consequence of acute maternal infection during pregnancy. Laboratory accidents have been reported as a cause of acute *Toxoplasma* transmission.[69] Occasionally, organ transplants from seropositive donors are compromised by *Toxoplasma* reactivation in the transplant recipient, often with devastating circumstances.[61,70] Rarely, blood transfusions may serve as a means of transmission, especially if circulating tachyzoites are present. Tachyzoites may survive up to 60 days in citrated blood.[69]

Geographic Distribution

Both animals and humans on five continents have serologic evidence of *Toxoplasma* infection.[72] Higher prevalence is present in areas with warm and humid climates, such as Haiti, Tahiti, or the lowlands of Guatemala, where nearly all people are seropositive.[72,73] This is presumably related to greater oocyst survival in the warm, moist soil characteristic of these areas.[64,65] In addition, areas with higher cat populations also have higher prevalence rates. Dryer and colder environments are associated with lower rates of seroprevalence because oocysts are less likely to survive.[72] Specific area variations are often due to changes in weather and animal populations.

Incidence

Approximately 500,000,000 persons worldwide are estimated to be seropositive for *Toxoplasma* antibodies.[66] Overall, serosurveys suggest that 30% to

40% of the US population is seropositive for *Toxoplasma* by age 50. The majority of these have no symptoms and never come to medical attention.[69] Regional differences in seropositivity have been described, with the highest levels found in the southeastern United States; seroprevalence rates are much lower in the western and northwestern portions of the country. Interestingly, an assessment of seroprevalence data of military recruits showed a significant decrease in overall seropositivity rates as compared with similar, older studies; this is possibly related to a decline in the presence of viable *T gondii* cysts in meat products.[74,75] *Toxoplasma* antibody prevalence rates vary as much in animals as in humans.[73,76]

The incidence of congenital toxoplasmosis varies in the United States, occurring in between 1/1,000 and 1/8,000 live births, leading to 500 to 4,100 congenitally infected infants born each year. Seroprevalence among US women ranges from 3.3% to 30%.[77]

Pathogenesis and Clinical Findings

There are two major patterns of toxoplasmosis in humans: postnatally acquired toxoplasmosis and congenital infection. While both are characterized by dissemination of *Toxoplasma* organisms throughout the body, the manifestations and complications of these two disease variants are quite distinct. Since most human infection with *T gondii* is asymptomatic, it is important to make a clear distinction between infection and disease. The clinical disease of toxoplasmosis may occur at any time during or after parasitemia.[58]

Infection of Postnatal Hosts

In contrast to the congenital form, toxoplasmosis acquired after birth is characterized by a much different course. Most cases remain asymptomatic. The most common clinical manifestation of acquired toxoplasmosis in children and young adults is lymphadenopathy involving single or multiple nodes[58,61] (Figure 36-6). Incubation periods are variable and are likely influenced by the number of viable organisms ingested. The affected nodes are usually in the 1- to 2-cm range and, while tender to the touch, are usually not intrinsically painful. Node suppuration is not a typical finding. Most patients with symptomatic acquired toxoplasmosis present with a syndrome, typified by malaise and fever, similar to that seen in infectious mononucleosis.[58] Other manifestations, such as encephalitis, myocarditis, pericarditis, hepatitis, pneumonitis, and

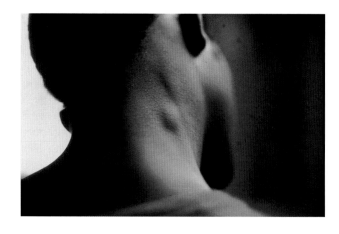

Fig. 36-6. This photograph shows a node in a US soldier who was deployed to the Jungle Operations Training Center in Panama from Fort Bragg, NC, in 1981.
Photograph: Courtesy of Colonel Ernest T. Takafuji, Medical Corps, US Army.

macular papular rash are much less common in immunocompetent individuals.[78] While clinical involvement of the heart, brain, lungs, and liver is rare during an acute acquired infection, *T gondii* can disseminate to these and other organs and may cause clinical disease.[79]

Patients may have localized lymphadenopathy and an elevated number of atypical lymphocytes in their peripheral blood smear; 10% to 20% may have peripheral eosinophilia.[78] A minority of patients have an elevated erythrocyte sedimentation rate.[79] Hepatomegaly and splenomegaly have been described.[78] Heterophile antibodies are negative and hepatic transaminases are usually normal, but severe hepatitis has been reported.[79] Occasionally, the lymphadenopathy may involve retroperitoneal, mesenteric, and mediastinal nodes.[78] During the course of the illness, symptoms and lymphadenopathy may fluctuate. Resolution occurs in most patients after a few months.[58] It has been estimated that as much as 15% of unexplained lymphadenopathy in normal hosts may be caused by toxoplasmosis.[80] Failure to consider toxoplasmosis as a cause of lymphadenopathy may lead to unnecessary lymph node biopsies. McCabe[77] assessed 107 cases of histologically confirmed toxoplasmosis with lymphadenopathy. The majority presented with a solitary node in the head or neck area without other symptoms, but nearly one third had significant malaise. The overall clinical course of these patients was typically benign. Some patients, however, did have serious extranodal disease, including myocarditis, pneumonitis, encephalitis, and fetal transmission. Both brief and prolonged illnesses were described.

Retinochoroiditis may also be seen in immunocompetent adolescents and adults and may be either a late sequela of congenital infection or a manifestation of acute infection.[58,59,76]

Reactivation of latent *Toxoplasma* in immunocompromised patients, including those infected with human immunodeficiency virus, is often associated with serious illness, typically encephalitis. *Toxoplasma* encephalitis in patients with acquired immunodeficiency syndrome remains a significant cause of morbidity and mortality in those infected with human immunodeficiency virus.[67]

Congenital Toxoplasmosis

Congenital toxoplasmosis results from an acute *Toxoplasma* infection of a pregnant woman. Nearly 50% of fetuses exposed become infected. Of these, between 10% and 20% have clinical symptoms of infection at birth and the remainder appear normal.[77] The classical triad of congenital toxoplasmosis consists of retinochoroiditis, hydrocephalus, and intracranial calcifications.[60,81] While the symptoms are often mild, severely affected infants may bear evidence of generalized or central nervous system infection. Other clinical findings of infected infants may include prematurity, intutero growth retardation, hepatosplenomegaly, jaundice, vasculitis, vascular thrombosis, seizures, and microcephaly.[60,77,81]

Diagnostic Approaches

While the definitive method for the diagnosis of an active *Toxoplasma* infection is mouse inoculation, it is normally only found in research laboratories. Serologic tests are the primary means of diagnosis for *Toxoplasma* infections elsewhere.[80] The gold standard serological test has been the Sabin-Feldman dye test (DT).[82] This assay, which measures specific IgG directed against *T gondii*, is not always readily available because it requires live parasites. The IgG immunofluorescent assay (IFA) is generally in agreement with the DT. Unfortunately, neither the DT or the IFA is very specific for acute infection. IgG is detectable approximately 2 weeks after the onset of infection and peaks within 1 to 2 months. High titers may persist for months in some patients.[80] IgM antibodies, as determined by IFA, usually appear during the first week of infection and peak within a month. IgM titers often return to undetectable levels within a few months of the initial infection. Sulzer[83] examined the immune responses of 32 individuals who became acutely infected with *Toxoplasma* during military jungle training in Panama. Rapid rises of both IgM and IgG antibod-

ies occurred within 2 weeks of infection. Interestingly, IgM did not precede IgG in any of the subjects. Many of the patients had persistently elevated IgM levels for 6 months to 1 year. A newer double sandwich IgM enzyme-linked immunosorbent assay (DS-IgM-ELISA) appears to be even more sensitive and specific for acute *Toxoplasma* infection and can be performed in about 2 hours.[84,85] All other available *Toxoplasma* antibody tests are associated with chronic infection and are not useful for the diagnosis of acute infection.[58] Newborns from mothers who are antibody positive have passively transferred maternal IgG. Demonstration of IgM antibodies in the neonate's circulation is thought to provide a more accurate indication of infection in the newborn because IgM does not cross the placenta.[81]

The diagnostic approach for a patient who may have acute toxoplasmosis with lymphadenopathy would include obtaining an IgM IFA or a DS-IgM-ELISA or both. A positive result on either test suggests an acute infection occurring within the past 3 to 4 months.[86] If negative, however, these tests do not rule out an acute infection, although a negative DS-IgM-ELISA greatly decreases the chance of an acute *Toxoplasma* infection being present.[87] A negative IgG IFA virtually excludes an acute infection.[79] High levels of specific IgG may block the IgM assays, giving a false-negative result. Removal of IgG from the sample may yield a more reliable IgM determination.[88] A 4-fold rise in IgG level by IFA over a 3-week period also provides supportive evidence of an acute infection.[83] Using the polymerase chain reaction, it may be possible to identify those patients with active toxoplasmosis who have equivocal or negative serologic tests.[87,88] While not yet standardized, polymerase chain reaction–based identification offers the possibility of very specific diagnosis based on the detection of circulating *Toxoplasma* DNA. Unfortunately, assays for *Toxoplasma* serology are not generally found in forward-deployed medical units. Thus, the issue of screening febrile military personnel for toxoplasmosis, especially in tropical areas, remains problematic.

Recommendations for Therapy and Control

Therapy

Therapy for toxoplasmosis varies with the type of infection present. Immunocompetent patients with acute acquired toxoplasmosis probably do not require any therapy unless their symptoms are particularly severe or persistent.[61] Immunodeficient patients with acute toxoplasmosis require longer courses of therapy, while acquired immunodeficiency syndrome patients with encephalitis require lifelong suppressive therapy. Immediate treatment of acute maternal infections in pregnant women may decrease the chance of fetal infection. Although treatment will not reverse tissue damage, congenitally infected infants probably benefit from therapy.[58] Active retinochoroiditis should be treated to prevent vision loss. Minimally symptomatic or asymptomatic patients do not require therapy.[69]

The most effective regimen for therapy of toxoplasmosis consists of the synergistic combination of pyrimethamine and sulfadiazine.[69] This combination exerts a growth-inhibiting effect rather than a parasiticidal effect on proliferating *Toxoplasma* tachyzoites.[61] Unfortunately, the cyst form of the organism is resistant to this therapy and persists in tissues. Substitution of the antibiotic clindamycin for sulfadiazine appears not to affect efficacy and toxicity, although the specific effect of clindamycin on *Toxoplasma* is unclear.[89,90] Both regimens appear to reduce symptoms in acute acquired disease. For immunocompetent patients with acute toxoplasmosis, pyrimethamine is first given as a loading dose of 200 mg in two divided doses. Follow-on therapy is given at a dose of 25 to 50 mg/day for 2 to 4 additional weeks.[69] Since pyrimethamine is a folic acid antagonist, hematologic toxicity is commonly seen as a dose-related myelosuppression. Twice weekly blood counts during therapy will help to identify those patients at risk of significant myelotoxicity. Addition of folinic acid (5 to 10 mg with pyrimethamine) will help to prevent or ameliorate the myelosuppression.[61] Sulfadiazine is given along with pyrimethamine, first as a loading dose of 75 mg/kg up to a dose of 4 g, then as 1 to 1.5 g every 6 hours.[69] Maintenance of good urine output is essential to prevent crystalluria and oliguria. Clindamycin is given at a dose of 600 mg every 6 hours, either orally or intravenously.[61]

Control

The most important goal in the prevention of toxoplasmosis is the protection of seronegative pregnant women and patients with immunodeficiencies.[69] These two groups, however, are not usually associated with military deployments. Thus, without an effective vaccine, toxoplasmosis prevention for the military revolves around the prevention of acute infection in immunocompetent individuals, most of whom will not become symptomatic even after infection. Prevention of infection will help them in the future should they ever become immunocompromised. To date, no immunization scheme directed against *Toxoplasma* has proved effective.[61]

The major goal in controlling the spread of toxoplasmosis is the reduction in the number of potentially infectious organisms present. Full cooking of all meat products will effectively prevent transmission from viable tissue cysts. While freezing meat can reduce the infectivity of tissue cysts, it does not completely eliminate the risk of infection.[57] Individuals should also avoid raw eggs and unpasteurized dairy products, especially goat's milk.[61] Bradyzoites within tissue cysts are killed by irradiation of at least 25 rads, temperatures higher than 61°C for at least 4 minutes, or freezing at -20°C for 24 hours followed by thawing.[69] Salting, pickling, and curing of meat also kills tissue cysts.[66]

Ideally, cats should be maintained only as indoor pets to prevent them from acquiring *Toxoplasma* from the environment. In addition, cats should not be fed raw meat, because they may acquire an acute infection from the ingestion of viable tissue cysts.[60] Cat feces should be disposed of daily to prevent sporulation of oocysts. Wastes may be buried, burned, or flushed into a waste collection system that has no communication with the drinking water system. Gloves should be worn whenever handling containers bearing cat wastes. Care should be taken to prevent aerosolization of cat wastes via shaking. Pregnant women should not clean cat litter containers, and they should wear gloves during any encounter with soil (eg, gardening). Strict handwashing before eating should be mandated. Similarly, hand washing is important for all who handle raw meats or soil. Stray cats should be removed from sand-containing structures to prevent their depositing oocyst-containing feces. Open sandboxes or sand piles should be covered when not in use so as not to attract cats. Since agricultural produce may be contaminated with oocysts, it is important that all such items be thoroughly washed with clean water.[57] Additionally, local drinking water supplies may also be contaminated with infectious oocysts.[87] Benenson and colleagues[54] reported an outbreak of acute toxoplasmosis in 39 US soldiers associated with the ingestion of oocyst-contaminated drinking water in the Panamanian jungle. Effective source protection and water purification schemes need to be in place to prevent this type of contamination. Vector control should focus on control of potential transfer vectors, such as flies and cockroaches.[61] Stray cats should be eliminated from encampment sites. There is no need for isolation of patients presenting with acute symptomatic toxoplasmosis, since person-to-person spread is not a part of the parasite's normal life cycle.[57]

Primitive sanitary conditions associated with a mass deployment increase the risk of acquiring toxoplasmosis. Proper personal hygiene, food preparation, and water supplies should effectively prevent most *Toxoplasma* infections from occurring.

Consideration of toxoplasmosis in the differential diagnosis of lymphadenopathy syndromes may obviate the need for immediate patient evacuation for lymph node biopsy.

[Kent E. Kester]

Q FEVER

Introduction and Military Relevance

Q Fever is a zoonotic disease caused by *Coxiella burnetii*, a rickettsia-like organism of low virulence but remarkable infectivity. There is a sporelike form of the organism that is extremely resistant to heat, pressure, and desiccation, allowing it to induce infection by airborne dissemination at sites miles distant from an infected source. The sporelike form may also persist in the environment for weeks or months under harsh conditions and subsequently cause infection after indirect exposure. The acute clinical disease associated with Q fever infection in humans is usually benign but temporarily incapacitating.

Since description of the disease in Australia in 1937, thousands of cases involving military personnel of many countries have been reported.[91] Many US soldiers in Italy during World War II were affected, with five confirmed outbreaks.[92–95] In one of these outbreaks, approximately 1,700 cases occurred at an airbase in southern Italy as a result of sheep and goats herded in pastures nearby.[94]

Hundreds of cases of atypical pneumonia consistent with Q fever were also observed during World War II in German soldiers in Serbia, southern Yugoslavia, Italy, Crimea, Greece, Ukraine, and Corsica,[91] usually in the apparent absence of disease in the indigenous population.

Q fever has been identified even in service members stationed or training in their home countries close to sheep or goats, particularly parturient animals[91]; outbreaks have been described among Swiss soldiers, Greek soldiers, and British airmen on the Isle of Man. Outbreaks have also been described in deployed British and Swedish troops stationed in Cyprus, US airmen in Libya, and French soldiers in Algeria.[91,96,97] Among US military personnel in the Persian Gulf War, one case of meningoencephalitis associated with acute Q fever was reported, with the onset of symptoms 2 weeks after the individual's return from the Persian Gulf.[98]

Because the infectivity of *C burnetii* is at least equivalent to that of anthrax and tularemia,[99] Q fever has been evaluated as a potential biological warfare agent by the United States, but stocks and munitions (except for strains necessary for vaccine research) were destroyed between May 1971 and May 1972, in accordance with the executive order signed by President Richard Nixon.[100]

Description of the Pathogen

C burnetii is classified in the family *Rickettsiaceae*, but it is not included in the genus *Rickettsia* and therefore is not a true rickettsia. It is not closely related to any other bacterial species when comparative 16s ribosomal RNA analysis is performed[101]; the genus *Coxiella* has only one species.

C burnetii must occupy an intracellular environment to grow or reproduce, similar to true rickettsia, but the sporelike form can survive extracellularly and transmit infection by itself.[102] The sporelike form may also be seen in human tissue.[103] *C burnetii* in the host occupies the phagolysosome of eukaryotic cells, which is usually a very destructive, acidic environment with numerous digestive enzymes.

Phase variation has been described with *C burnetii*.[104] Phase I, the virulent form associated with natural infection, has a smooth lipopolysaccharide (LPS) component of the outer membrane; phase II, an avirulent form resulting from serial laboratory passage of the organism in eggs or cell culture, has a rough, incomplete LPS.

Epidemiology

Transmission

Human infection with *C burnetii* is usually the result of inhaling infected aerosols, although tickborne disease does occur, as do cases resulting from ingesting unpasteurized milk from infected animals. *C burnetii* is extremely infectious; under experimental conditions, a single organism is capable of producing infection and disease in humans.[105]

The primary reservoirs for human infection are livestock animals, such as sheep, cattle, and goats, particularly parturient females. *C burnetii* also infects a large number of other species of wild and domesticated animals, including cats, dogs, pigs, camels, birds, and poultry. Numerous species of ticks harbor the infection, and transovarial transmission of the organism can maintain the infection in the wild.

During gestation in infected animals, the proliferation of *C burnetii* in the placenta facilitates aerosolization of large numbers of the pathogen during parturition. Unpasteurized eggs from infected poultry may also transmit the infection, as can unpasteurized milk. *C burnetii* is shed in the urine and feces of infected animals, in addition to being present in the blood and tissues. Humans who work with animal products or in animal husbandry, especially abattoir workers or animal handlers and veterinary personnel who assist during parturition (eg, calving, lambing), are thus at increased risk for acquiring Q fever.

Survival of the sporelike form of *C burnetii* as an aerosol or on inanimate surfaces, such as straw, hay, or clothing, allows for transmission to individuals who are not in direct contact with infected animals. Examples include service members sleeping in barns previously occupied by infected animals[93]; laundry workers handling infected clothing[106]; coworkers of an individual with an infected parturient cat at home[107]; and residents of an urban community living along a road used by farm vehicles.[108] Investigations of outbreaks of Q fever frequently report a significant proportion of patients who have no direct contact with animals and cases among people who live or work miles from an infected source. Human-to-human transmission has been reported, but it is a very rare event.[109]

Geographical Distribution

The distribution of *C burnetii* is worldwide,[110] and the host range is very diverse, including a large number of mammalian species and arthropods. Q fever has been identified in most countries where an attempt has been made to identify evidence of infection in humans or animals, except New Zealand. Outbreaks of fever are infrequently reported, however, and the disease may be endemic in areas where cases are rarely or never reported.

In the United States, the epidemiology of Q fever is variable. Isolated but regularly occurring cases have been observed in areas with endemic foci in cattle.[111] Clusters of cases have been described in areas with infected dairy herds.[112] A small outbreak in Maine associated with exposure to a parturient cat has been described,[113] similar to an outbreak in Nova Scotia, Canada.[114] Between 1981 and 1992, five outbreaks of Q fever in the United States were reported from five different states.[115–119] Four of these outbreaks occurred in research facilities using sheep.

Incidence

Although reported outbreaks of Q fever in the United States have been relatively uncommon in recent years,[120,121] underreporting undoubtedly occurs. For example, although the first two cases of Q fever were reported from two adjacent rural counties in Michigan in 1984, a study published 4 years later showed that 15% of the general population surveyed in those two counties and 43% of goat owners were seropositive.[122]

Pathogenesis and Clinical Findings

After an individual inhales an infected aerosol, ingests infected milk, or suffers a tick bite, *C burnetii* organisms are phagocytized, predominately by unstimulated macrophages. There is little host reaction at the portal of entry, either in the lung, skin, or alimentary tract. After phagocytosis, conditions within the phagolysosome trigger growth and multiplication of *C burnetii*, with little initial damage to the host cell. Eventually the phagolysosome and cytoplasm become engorged with *C burnetii* organisms, and the host cell lyses. Dissemination of the pathogen occurs as the organisms circulate freely in the plasma, are carried on the surface of cells, and are carried by circulating macrophages.

In animals, infection with *C burnetii* frequently lasts for the life of the animal in a dormant state. The acute infection is usually inapparent in animals, except for an increased rate of spontaneous abortion in some species.

In humans, after multiplication and dissemination of the organism, polyclonal antibody production represents the initial immune response to *C burnetii*, but control of the infection by the host eventually requires the development of specific cell-mediated immunity, with killing by activated macrophages and natural killer cells. This process may result in a granulomatous reaction without the scarring and tissue reaction observed with true granulomata.

The incubation period for Q fever in humans varies from 10 to 40 days, and the infection may be manifested by, in order of frequency, asymptomatic seroconversion, acute illness, or chronic disease. In epidemiologic surveys, most seropositive individuals do not recall having the illness. The tendency for *C burnetii* to produce asymptomatic seroconversion, particularly when the infecting inoculum is low, has been documented in several publications. In outbreaks, the incidence of asymptomatic seroconversion is usually about 50%.[105,107,123] These observations underscore the value of an epidemiologic investigation when even a single case of acute Q fever is recognized.

There is no characteristic illness for acute Q fever,[124,125] and manifestations may vary considerably among locations where the disease is acquired. The onset of Q fever may be abrupt or insidious, with fever, chills (including frank rigors), and headache being the most common symptoms (Table 36-3). The headache is usually described as severe, throbbing, and frontal or retro-orbital. Diaphoresis, malaise, fatigue, and anorexia are very common. Myalgias

TABLE 36-3

FREQUENCY OF SYMPTOMS IN ACUTE Q FEVER (%)

Symptoms	%
Fever	80-100
Chills, rigors	75-100
Headache, retro-orbital pain	50-100
Malaise	50-100
Diaphoresis	40-100
Myalgias	45-85
Weakness, fatigue	40-85
Weight loss (≥ 7kg)	50-80
Cough	50-60
Chest pain	25-50
Anorexia	35-45
Neurological	10-35
Sore throat	5-35
Nausea, vomiting	15-20
Arthralgias	10-20
Diarrhea	5-20
Neck stiffness	5-7

Data sources: Robbins FC, Ragan CA. Q fever in the Mediterranean area: Report of its occurrence in allied troops, I: Clinical features of the disease. *Am J Hyg.* 1946;44:6–22; Feinstein M, Yesner R, Marks JL. Epidemics of Q fever among troops returning from Italy in the spring of 1945, I: Clinical aspects of the epidemic at Camp Patrick Henry, Virginia. *Am J Hyg.* 1946;44:72–87; Langley JM, Marrie TJ, Covert A, Waag DM, Williams JC. Poker players' pneumonia: An urban outbreak of Q fever following exposure to a parturient cat. *N Engl J Med.* 1988;319:354–356; Raoult D, Marrie TJ. State-of-the-art clinical lecture: Q fever. *Clin Infect Dis.* 1995;20:489–496; Tissot Dupont H, Raoult D, Brouqui P. Epidemiologic features and clinical presentation of acute Q fever in hospitalized patients: 323 French cases. *Am J Med.* 1992;93:427–434; Smith DL, Ayres JG, Blair I, et al. A large Q fever outbreak in the West Midlands: Clinical aspects. *Respir Med.* 1993;87:509–516; and Derrick EH. The course of infection with *Coxiella burnetii. Med J Aust.* 1973;1:1051–1057.

are also a frequent complaint, while arthralgias are relatively unusual. Cough tends to appear later in the illness than some of the other more common symptoms and may not be a prominent complaint.[126] Chest pain occurs in a minority of patients and may be pleuritic or a vague substernal discomfort. A weight loss of more than 7 kg is relatively common, particularly when the initial illness is prolonged. Although nonspecific evanescent skin eruptions have been reported, there is no characteristic rash.

For unknown reasons, cigarette smokers are more likely than nonsmokers to develop symptomatic infection with Q fever.[126] The temperature tends to fluctuate, with peaks of 39.5°C to 40.5°C (103°F-105°F), and in approximately one fourth of the cases is biphasic; in two thirds of patients with acute disease, the febrile period lasts 13 days or less.[127] Neurological symptoms are not uncommon and have been observed in up to 23% of acute cases reported in a recent outbreak.[126]

Physical findings in acute Q fever are also relatively nonspecific. Rales are probably the most commonly observed physical finding; evidence of pleural effusion (including friction rub) and consolidation may also be noted but not in the majority of infections. Although hepatomegaly, splenomegaly, jaundice, pharyngeal injection, and hepatic and splenic tenderness have all been reported, they are relatively unusual in acute infection.

Reports of abnormalities on chest x-ray examination vary with locale but can probably be identified in 50% to 60% of patients. An abnormal chest radiograph may be seen in the absence of pulmonary symptoms, while a normal chest radiograph may be observed in a patient with pulmonary symptoms.[128]

Laboratory abnormalities associated with acute Q fever most commonly involve tests of liver function, and patients may present with a clinical and laboratory picture consistent with acute hepatitis. In 50% to 75% of patients, 2- to 3-fold elevations of the aspartate aminiotransferase or alanine aminotransferase (AST or ALT) or both are observed, while elevations of either the alkaline phosphatase or total bilirubin or both are observed in only 10% to 15%.[126] The white blood count is usually normal; the erythrocyte sedimentation rate is elevated in approximately one third of patients.[97] Mild anemia or thrombocytopenia may also be observed.

The case fatality rate of acute Q fever is low, even without treatment, and chronic disease, usually manifested by endocarditis, probably develops in less than 1% of acute infections. Q fever endocarditis usually occurs on heart valves with preexisting abnormalities. Those with prosthetic heart valves or other vascular prostheses are also at increased risk of infection.[124] Granulomatous hepatitis also occurs as a chronic complication of Q fever, more commonly after ingestion of unpasteurized infected milk.[125] A syndrome of protracted fatigue following acute Q fever has been described.[129–131]

Diagnostic Approaches

Diagnosis of Q fever is usually accomplished by serological testing. A number of methods have been used,[132] the most common being antibody detection by indirect fluorescent antibody or enzyme-linked immunosorbent assay (ELISA). Significant antibody titers are usually not identifiable until 2 to 3 weeks into the illness; convalescent antibody titers, 2 to 3 months after onset, almost always demonstrate a typical 4-fold rise. After infection, significant antibody titers may persist for years.

In general, antibodies to the phase II organism are identified earlier in the illness, during the first few months after infection, followed by a decline in antibody to the phase II organism and a rise in antibody to the phase I organism. Antibodies of the IgM type are usually observed within the first 6 to 12 months after infection, with persistence of IgG antibodies afterward. Of the methods currently used for the diagnosis of Q fever, the ELISA is the most sensitive and easiest to perform; the utility of the ELISA for epidemiologic screening and diagnosis of Q fever has been confirmed.[133,134] The sensitivity of this test in the convalescent phase of illness or in the first 1 to 2 years after infection approaches 100%.[134] Polymerase chain reaction may also be useful in the future for the diagnosis of Q fever[135–137] but remains to be validated in acute clinical cases.

Recommendations for Therapy and Control

Antibiotic treatment of acute Q fever shortens the course of the disease and is effective in preventing disease when administered during the incubation period.[105] Tetracyclines remain the mainstay of therapy for acute disease.[138] Macrolide antibiotics, such as erythromycin and azithromycin, are also effective.[139,140] Quinolones, chloramphenicol, and trimethoprim-sulfamethoxazole have also been used to treat Q fever,[138] but experience with these antibiotics is very limited.

Q fever in humans can be prevented by immunization with a formalin-killed whole cell vaccine. Although a very effective Q fever vaccine is licensed in Australia (Q-Vax, CSL, Victoria, Australia), all Q fever vaccines used in the United States are currently investigational. Existing vaccines are generally well tolerated after subcutaneous injection, although individuals already immune to Q fever may develop severe local reactions at the site of injection.[141,142] These reactions can be avoided by prior screening with an intradermal skin test to detect presensitized or immune individuals.[143]

Control of Q fever requires, most importantly, recognition of the disease (which may be difficult considering the nonspecific clinical findings) and awareness of the potential risk of infection in appropriate settings. Areas such as cow or sheep sheds that are or have been occupied by animals that may harbor the infection should be avoided. Considering the large number of mammalian species that may carry the infection, close contact with animals, both domestic and wild, outside of the United States should be avoided, especially if birthing is occurring. Disposal of animal products of conception should be accomplished as soon as possible. Unpasteurized or uncooked animal products should never be consumed. In spite of an innate resistance to heat, *C burnetii* organisms are inactivated by pasteurization at 62.7°C (145°F) for 30 minutes, 71.6°C (161°F) for 15 seconds, or boiling.[57p407–411] Dead animals and animal products should also be handled with care, because Q fever may be transmitted by contact with these materials.

If contamination with *C burnetii* has occurred, disinfection of areas or articles soiled by infected blood, tissue, or other animal products is recommended with 0.05% hypochlorite, 5% peroxide, or a 1:100 solution of Lysol.[57] Although complete inactivation even with these measures is not certain, both 70% ethanol and a 5% solution of N-alkyl dimethyl benzyl and ethylbenzal ammonium chlorides have been shown to completely inactivate the organism after 30 minutes of exposure.[144]

[William R. Byrne]

VIRAL HEMORRHAGIC FEVERS

Introduction and Military Relevance

The hemorrhagic fevers are serious, widely distributed human infections caused by viruses from several different taxonomic families (Table 36-4). As a group, these diseases share many clinical, pathophysiologic, and epidemiologic features. Most are zoonoses; human infections occur as a result of incursion into the cycles of transmission established between each virus and its host or reservoir in nature.

TABLE 36-4

VIRAL HEMORRHAGIC FEVERS OF HUMANS

Family/Virus	Disease	Geographic Distribution	Natural Transmission
Arenaviridae			
Lassa	Lassa Fever	Rural west Africa	Rodent to human[*]
Junin	Argentine HF	Rural Argentina	Rodent to human[*]
Machupo	Bolivian HF	Rural Bolivia	Rodent to human[*]
Guanarito	Venezuelan HF	Rural Venezuela	Rodent to human[*]
Sabiá		Rural(?) Brazil	Unknown[*]
Bunyaviridae			
Hantaan	HFRS	Rural Asia, Far East, central Europe/Balkans(?)	Rodent to human
Puumala	HFRS	Rural western Europe, central Europe/Balkans	Rodent to human
Dobrava/Belgrade	HFRS	Central Europe/Balkans	Rodent to human
Seoul	HFRS	Worldwide	Rodent to human
Sin Nombre[†]	HPS	Americas	Rodent to human
Crimean-Congo Hemorrhagic Fever	CCHF	Rural Africa, west Asia, central Europe	Tick bite; inhalation or contact with blood of infected mammals[*]
Rift Valley Fever	RVF	Sub-Saharan Africa, Egypt	Mosquito bite; inhalation or contact with blood of infected mammals[*]
Filoviridae			
Ebola-Sudan	Ebola HF	Sudan	Unknown[*]
Ebola-Zaire	Ebola HF	Zaire	Unknown[*]
Ebola-Ivory Coast	Ebola HF	Ivory Coast	Unknown[*]
Marburg	Marburg HF	Sub-Saharan Africa	Unknown[*]
Flaviviridae			
Yellow fever	Yellow fever	Africa, South America	Mosquito bite
Dengue	Dengue HF	Tropical/subtropical regions worldwide	Mosquito bite
Omsk	Omsk HF	Northern Asia	Tick bite; contact with infected muskrats[*]
KFD	KFD	Rural India	Tick bite[*]

[*]The threat of severe nosocomial or laboratory-acquired infection or both is particularly high
[†]Other hantaviruses endemic to the Americas and associated with hantavirus pulmonary syndrome have also been described and characterized but are not included in this table
HF: hemorrhagic fever, HFRS: hemorrhagic fever with renal syndrome, HPS: hantavirus pulmonary syndrome, RVF: Rift Valley fever, KFD: Kayasanur Forest disease

Viral hemorrhagic fever should be considered in the differential diagnosis of febrile illnesses among military personnel living or working in disease-endemic areas. Military personnel tend to be among those at highest risk for acquiring viral hemorrhagic fevers because field operations and warfare are often conducted under adverse environmental conditions in remote regions where exposure to vectors or reservoir hosts for the etiologic agents is likely. The impact of dramatic, highly lethal infections on the morale and welfare of forces cannot be overestimated. Therapeutic interventions are time-critical for infected individuals, and rapid implementation of surveillance and control strategies may be essential to avoiding either panic, epidemic catastrophe, or both. Clinical management of these diseases is demanding and resource-intensive. Explosive nosocomial outbreaks are a well-documented consequence of unwitting introduction of viral hemorrhagic fevers into routine clinical care settings. Personnel at both clinical and research laboratories are at particularly high risk of infection. No licensed vaccines are currently available for the viral hemorrhagic fevers discussed in this chapter, but safe and effective immunogens have been or are being developed for use in high-risk populations (Table 36-5).

Many viral hemorrhagic fevers are efficiently spread by aerosol transmission from infected reservoirs. This fact, coupled with the recognized high morbidity and mortality associated with naturally acquired human disease and the stability of the etiologic agents under adverse environmental conditions, has generated considerable interest in their potential for use as biological warfare agents. Resources are available for advice and specific guidance from the US Army Medical Research Institute of Infectious Diseases, Fort Detrick, Md, and the Special Pathogens Branch of the National Center for Infectious Diseases at the Centers for Disease Control and Prevention, Atlanta, Ga.

In this chapter, hemorrhagic fevers caused by arenaviruses and filoviruses, together with Crimean-Congo hemorrhagic fever, are considered; else-where in this volume are discussions of hemorrhagic fevers caused by mosquito-borne flaviviruses (dengue, yellow fever), tick-borne flaviviruses (Omsk hemorrhagic fever, Kayasanur Forest disease), and other members of the *Bunyaviridae* (hemorrhagic fever with renal syndrome, hantavirus pulmonary syndrome, Rift Valley fever).

Arenavirus Hemorrhagic Fevers

Description of the Pathogens

The family *Arenaviridae* contains segmented, single-stranded RNA viruses. Each human pathogenic arenavirus is associated with a specific rodent species in which it establishes a chronic, persistent infection. Infected rodents shed large quantities of virus in secretions and excreta; humans become infected through inhalation of virus-containing aerosols and via mucous membrane or percutaneous inoculation of virus through contact with contaminated surfaces. Arenaviruses have been classified into 2 groups: the Old World complex (eg, lymphocytic choriomeningitis virus, Lassa virus), and the New World (or Tacaribe virus) complex. Lassa is the only Old World complex virus that causes hemorrhagic fever. Within the New World complex, four viruses are recognized causes of hemorrhagic fever

TABLE 36-5

THERAPEUTIC AND PREVENTIVE MEASURES SPECIFIC FOR SELECTED VIRAL HEMORRHAGIC FEVERS

Disease	Therapy	Prevention
Arenaviruses		
Lassa fever	Supportive, ribavirin	Rodent control, avoidance of reservoir
Argentine HF	Supportive, immune plasma, ribavirin(?)	Candid #1 Junin vaccine (IND)
Bolivian HF	Supportive, ribavirin(?)	Rodent control, Candid #1 vaccine(?)
Venezuelan HF	Supportive	Avoidance of reservoir
Sabiá HF	Supportive, ribavirin(?)	Unknown
Filoviruses		
Ebola HF	Supportive	Unknown
Marburg HF	Supportive	Unknown
Bunyaviruses		
Crimean-Congo HF	Supportive, ribavirin	Tick control, avoidance of slaughtered animals

Note: (?) indicates anecdotal experience or strong theoretical justification for use based upon in vitro findings or experimental models or both
HF: hemorrhagic fever, IND: investigational new drug

in humans: Junin (which causes Argentine hemorrhagic fever), Machupo (Bolivian hemorrhagic fever), Guanarito (Venezuelan hemorrhagic fever), and Sabiá (no specific disease designation).

Lassa Fever

Transmission. The sole reservoir for Lassa virus is *Mastomys natalensis*, the multimammate rat. This peri-domestic rodent is an important source of protein for people in disease-endemic areas, and it regularly contaminates houses and living areas with infectious urine and respiratory secretions.[145,146] Most cases of Lassa fever apparently are acquired through contact with rodents or their excreta, but human-to-human spread also occurs. Clustering of cases and seropositives is frequently found, and transmission of disease through contact with febrile patients and via sexual intercourse during incubation and convalescence has been seen. Nosocomial outbreaks are uncommon but are well documented.[147,148]

Geographic Distribution and Incidence. Lassa fever occurs in the West African nations of Sierra Leone, Liberia, Nigeria, Guinea, and probably in Senegal, Ivory Coast, Upper Volta, and Mali. Infection with Lassa virus is common in all ages and both sexes; estimates range from thousands to hundreds of thousands of incident cases annually.[149] In Sierra Leone, as many as 16% of adult medical admissions to hospitals, 47% of adult febrile admissions, 20% of pediatric febrile admissions, and 30% of adult medical deaths may be due to this disease.[150,151] Mortality in pregnant women is particularly high, reaching 30% or more during the third trimester.[152]

Pathogenesis and Clinical Findings. Lassa fever is a disease of insidious onset. Fever, malaise, and headache appear gradually, usually 8 to 14 days after exposure to the virus. As illness progresses, sore throat, myalgias, arthralgias, epigastric or retrosternal pain, vomiting, and dry cough appear. Physical findings include conjunctivitis, abdominal and muscle tenderness, lymphadenopathy, hypotension, and relative bradycardia. About 40% of patients develop a painful, purulent pharyngitis that is sometimes associated with vesicles or ulcers. A progressively "toxic" appearance is typically accompanied by edema of the face and neck. There is no characteristic skin rash, and neither cutaneous hemorrhage nor jaundice is evident early in the disease. Severe hypotension and bleeding from the nose and mouth, gastrointestinal tract, or vagina are associated with a fatal outcome; these complications occur in the minority of patients, however (15% to

20%). Pericardial rubs occur in about 20% of cases. Acute encephalitis has been described in many hospitalized patients, manifesting as seizures, dystonia, and neuropsychiatric changes.[153] More severe evidence of central nervous system involvement (stupor, coma, focal neurological signs) signifies a poor prognosis. Recovery may take a month or more. Convalescence may be complicated by ataxia, orchitis, uveitis, pericarditis, pleural effusion, or ascites. Eighth nerve deafness occurs in 25% to 30% of survivors and may be permanent; Lassa fever is considered to be among the most important causes of deafness in West Africa.[154]

Clinical laboratory findings in Lassa fever are generally unremarkable. White blood cell counts may be depressed early, but as the disease progresses they frequently are normal or elevated. Platelet counts are normal or elevated but platelet function is abnormal.[155] Proteinuria is inconsistent. High serum viremia ($> 10^{3.6}$ $TCID_{50}$/mL) and aspartate aminotransferase (AST > 150 IU/L) are each associated with a poor prognosis (50% and 73% mortality, respectively). If both factors coexist, mortality is 80%.[156,157]

Diagnostic Approaches. Diagnosis of Lassa fever is made by demonstration of a 4-fold rise in virus-specific antibodies, virus isolation, antigen detection by enzyme immunoassay, or demonstration of virus-specific IgM or high-titered IgG in the setting of a compatible clinical illness. The differential diagnosis includes malaria, typhoid fever, and other febrile illnesses common to West Africa. A single case-control study from Sierra Leone suggested that triads of either pharyngitis, retrosternal pain, and proteinuria or pharyngitis, retrosternal pain, and vomiting were useful to discriminate Lassa fever from other conditions.[150]

Recommendations for Therapy and Control. The specific therapy for Lassa fever is the antiviral drug ribavirin. Administration of ribavirin by both parenteral and oral routes has been shown to be effective in reducing mortality, but the parenteral route is more effective.[157] Optimal benefit is derived within the first 6 days of illness. Although of unproven benefit, prophylactic administration of oral ribavirin represents a prudent approach to management of a significant exposure to Lassa virus (eg, a needlestick). There is no vaccine presently available for Lassa fever; prevention consists of control and avoidance of reservoir rodents. Control of nosocomial spread has been accomplished in endemic areas through use of barrier precautions and care to avoid cross-contamination of needles and other devices. Clinical and diagnostic laboratory samples are highly hazardous and should be manipulated only by trained personnel in controlled, high-level biocontainment facilities.

South American Hemorrhagic Fevers

Argentine hemorrhagic fever (AHF), Bolivian hemorrhagic fever (BHF), Venezuelan hemorrhagic fever (VHF), and hemorrhagic fever caused by Sabiá virus often are referred to collectively as the South American hemorrhagic fevers. The hemorrhagic fevers they cause are clinically similar, but each disease has its own specific transmission patterns and geographic distribution.

AHF occurs in a progressively expanding endemic zone that includes portions of Buenos Aires, Cordoba, Santa Fe, and La Pampa provinces of north-central Argentina.[158] AHF is a seasonal disease, with a prominent peak in autumn that coincides with the summer grain harvests and the period of maximum population density for the Junin virus reservoir, *Calomys musculinus*, the field mouse. Disease is associated with inhalation of contaminated aerosols generated by mechanical grain harvesters and with exposure to linear habitats frequented by *C musculinus*, such as fencerows and railroad beds. Disease incidence before the introduction of the Junin virus vaccine was 200 to 1,000 cases per year. Although all ages and both sexes are affected, most cases are seen in male agricultural workers who are 20 to 60 years old.

Like AHF, the preponderance of BHF occurs in conjunction with peaks of agricultural activity. Although most BHF is thought to occur after exposure to aerosolized rodent urine, clusters of cases in Cochabamba in 1971 and near Magdelena in 1994 provide strong suggestive evidence for person-to-person spread of Machupo virus.[159,160] BHF is found naturally only in the Beni Department of northern Bolivia, although the range of the reservoir for Machupo virus, *C callosus*, also includes parts of Argentina, Paraguay, and Brazil. *C callosus* differs in habit from that of its Argentine congener in that it also has peri-domestic affinities. Between 2,000 and 3,000 cases of BHF have been recorded since the disease was recognized in 1959; many of these were associated with a series of devastating epidemics that occurred between 1962 and 1964 in and around the village of San Joachin.[161] Effective rodent control and surveillance programs that arose from these outbreaks eliminated epidemic BHF, and only sporadic cases have occurred since. Currently, cases number in the low double digits annually. Most cases of BHF occur in men from rural areas, but community and family outbreaks have involved all ages and both sexes.

VHF was first recognized in 1989 following an outbreak of hemorrhagic fever in Guanarito, Portuguesa State, Venezuela.[162] The reservoir for Guanarito virus is thought to be the cane rat, *Zygodontomys brevicauda*. The cotton rat, *Sigmodon alstoni*, cocirculates in the area and carries a closely related virus (putatively named Pirital virus) whose disease potential remains undefined at this time.[163] As is the case with AHF and BHF, both children and adults are susceptible to infection with VHF virus, although the highest risk tends to be among adult male farm workers. A seasonal peak in disease has been noted from November to January. As of 1997, fewer than 150 cases of this disease had been documented from the endemic area, most of them between 1989 and 1991.

Sabiá virus has been recovered only once from a human; under natural conditions it was acquired near Sao Paulo, Brazil, in 1990.[164] Its reservoir and mode of transmission to humans are unknown. Two subsequent human infections with Sabiá virus occurred following laboratory accidents, emphasizing the importance of confining work with this and related human-pathogenic arenaviruses to biosafety level 3 or 4 facilities.

Pathogenesis and Clinical Findings. The South American hemorrhagic fevers are clinically similar. The incubation period is generally 1 to 2 weeks. Patients experience the gradual development of fever, malaise, myalgia, and anorexia. Headache, dizziness, backache, epigastric pain, vomiting, and diarrhea follow shortly afterward, accompanied by flushing of the face and chest, conjunctival injection, and orthostatic hypotension. Cutaneous petechiae are frequent, appearing most commonly in the axillae and palate. Congestion and bleeding of the gums is frequently seen, and the appearance of hemorrhage along the gingival margin at the point of tooth insertion is a characteristic finding. Neurological changes are virtually universal, with tremors (most commonly of the tongue and hands), lethargy, depressed deep tendon reflexes, and hyperaesthesia being most frequently noted. In most cases, improvement begins after 7 to 10 days, and patients go on to a prolonged recovery that may be accompanied by weakness, autonomic instability, and alopecia. About one third will progress to more severe illness, however, with evolution along one of three fairly distinctive patterns: a hemorrhagic diathesis with mucous membrane and puncture wound bleeding; a progressive neurological deterioration with convulsions, delirium, obtundation, and coma; or a mixed hemorrhagic-neurologic syndrome with shock. Untreated, mortality may exceed 25%.

Thrombocytopenia (platelets < 100,000/mm^3) and leukopenia (white blood cell count < 4,000/mm^3) are almost universal. Proteinuria with or without microscopic hematuria is freqently seen. In AHF, serum alpha interferon levels may be exceedingly high (1,000-16,000 IU/mL); higher levels correlate with poorer prognoses.

Diagnostic Approaches. Diagnosis of South American arenavirus infections can be accomplished by serology (eg, indirect immunofluorescence, enzyme immunoassay, neutralization tests), antigen detection (eg, antigen detection enzyme immunoassay), or virus isolation. Clinical samples should be considered infectious and handled under biosafety level 4 conditions until treated with radiation or chemicals to inactivate the virus. The differential diagnosis includes lymphocytic choriomeningitis, hantavirus diseases, typhoid fever, and a host of other viral and bacterial diseases endemic to rural South America.

Recommendations for Therapy and Control. Convalescent immune plasma has been shown to be effective in treating AHF when administered within 8 days of disease onset.[165] Effectiveness of plasma therapy correlates with quantity (titer) of neutralizing antibody delivered.[166] A neurological syndrome of uncertain etiology is associated with immune plasma therapy in about 10% of treated survivors. This condition typically begins 4 to 6 weeks after treatment and is characterized by fever, headache, ataxia, and intention tremor but is usually benign. Intravenous ribavirin has shown promise in preliminary studies for therapy of AHF, but controlled trials have not been conducted. The drug has been successful in limited numbers of patients with Machupo and Sabiá virus infections as well, but additional experience is needed to document efficacy.

Rodent avoidance and control constitute the principal nonmedical modalities for preventing South American hemorrhagic fevers. A live-attenuated Junin virus vaccine codeveloped by the US Army and the Argentine government was shown in controlled trials[167] to be 95% efficacious in preventing AHF. This vaccine, called Candid #1, has been administered to more than 160,000 persons in the AHF-endemic area; its use has been associated with a dramatic decrease in disease incidence. Candid #1 successfully protected experimental animals against BHF but not VHF; it has not yet been assessed in humans for these diseases.

Filovirus Hemorrhagic Fevers

The *Filoviridae* are morphologically unique RNA viruses for which neither the reservoirs nor the modes of natural infection to humans are known. Although biochemically similar, the filoviruses are serologically distinctive. They have been classified into the Marburg and the Ebola groups. The Ebola group has three subtypes: Ebola-Sudan, Ebola-Zaire, and Ebola-Reston. A probable fourth Ebola strain recovered from a human infected in the Ivory Coast is incompletely classified at present. All but Ebola-Reston have been documented as causing hemorrhagic fevers in humans.

Epidemiology

The epidemiology of filoviruses is marked by the occurrence of dramatic, explosive outbreaks, typically with high mortality. Despite repeated and extensive efforts, no natural reservoir for any filovirus has been identified. Person-to-person spread of filoviruses has been documented repeatedly in association with parenteral or mucous membrane exposure to contaminated body fluids; health care workers regularly contribute substantially to morbidity and mortality statistics during epidemics.[168] Aerosol transmission is unproved in human infection, but airborne transmission of both Marburg and Ebola has been demonstrated experimentally, and there are indications that droplets or aerosols played a role in the spread of Ebola-Reston among quarantine cynomolgus macaques.

Marburg virus was the cause of simultaneous clusters of viral hemorrhagic fever in 1967 among individuals in Marburg, West Germany, and Belgrade, Yugoslavia, who were connected directly or indirectly with African green monkeys shipped from Uganda.[169] Marburg virus has since been recognized usually in the context of individual infections, both with and without secondary transmission.

Ebola-Zaire and Ebola-Sudan, in contrast, have been associated with repeated large epidemics in sub-Saharan Africa; the former more frequently and recently (1995 and 1996-1997).[170] In each of these outbreaks, case-fatality rates have been high (50% to 90%). Ebola-Ivory Coast virus has been seen only sporadically and has infected both humans and chimpanzees. Ebola-Reston has caused widespread morbidity and mortality of greater than 75% among colonies of cynomolgus macaques exported from the Philippines.[171] Several humans have been infected with Ebola-Reston virus in association with primate epizootics, but, to date, none have become ill.

Pathogenesis and Clinical Findings

Human filovirus infections are severe, debilitating, and frequently fatal. The experience to date with Asian filoviruses (eg, Ebola-Reston) suggests avirulence for humans; but that is based on very limited information. The incubation period for African filoviruses is generally 3 to 8 days but may be longer in secondarily acquired infections. Disease onset is abrupt, with frontal headache, fever, chills, myalgias, anorexia, and extreme malaise. Nausea, vomiting, and diarrhea are common early in the disease course, and conjunctivitis, pharyngitis, and oral ulcerations may be seen. Patients typically are prostrate and apathetic. A maculopapular rash appears on the trunk and back around the fifth day of illness and desquamates in survivors. Petechiae and oozing from venipunctures are frequent, and bleeding from mucous membranes of the gastrointestinal and genitourinary tracts and of the nasopharynx is commonly observed. Death due to intractable shock occurs between 6 and 16 days following disease onset. Infections in pregnancy are particularly severe, and fetal wastage is universal. The catabolic toll of these infections is huge; patients are severely wasted, and convalescence for survivors is prolonged.

Diagnostic Approaches

Platelet and leukocyte counts are depressed early, and a left shift is common. As disease progresses, neutrophilia appears. Serum transaminases are increased (AST > ALT), but bilirubin is generally normal or only slightly elevated. Viremia is present from early in the disease course and may persist for weeks (especially in semen and the anterior chamber of the eye) in survivors. Diagnosis of human filovirus infection is made by serology (enzyme immunoassay), antigen detection (antigen-capture enzyme immunoassay in serum, immunohistochemistry in tissues), visualization of virus particles in tissues by electron microscopy, and virus isolation. Initially developed immunofluorescent antibody tests are not reliable for serological diagnosis. Body fluid and tissue samples are highly infectious, and specimens should be handled only by trained personnel at the highest possible levels of biocontainment. The differential diagnosis includes a wide variety of diseases that occur in sub-Saharan Africa, including malaria, typhoid fever, and rickettsial diseases, as well as other viral hemorrhagic fevers.

Recommendations for Therapy and Control

There is no specific treatment available for filovirus diseases. Supportive care (eg, fluids, pressors, management of shock and hemorrhage) is most important. Exclusion of other, treatable conditions must always be considered. In the absence of insight regarding natural hosts or vectors of filoviruses, control measures are limited to interruption of person-to-person spread through early case identification, quarantine, decontamination, and barrier nursing precautions. The risk of nosocomial infection is high. There is no vaccine currently available for any filovirus.

Crimean-Congo Hemorrhagic Fever

Description of the Pathogen

Crimean-Congo hemorrhagic fever (CCHF) virus is a member of the *Nairovirus* genus in the large *Bunyaviridae* family. This RNA virus is maintained in nature via complex relationships between its arthropod vectors (multiple species of ixodid [hard] ticks) and nonhuman vertebrate hosts. The virus was initially identified in 1947 as the cause of Crimean hemorrhagic fever, but it was not until 1969 that its identity with an agent recovered from a febrile patient in the Belgian Congo in 1956 was recognized and the name revised to reflect the linkage.[172]

Epidemiology

Ticks presumably serve as both vectors and reservoirs for CCHF. Both transstadial and transovarial transmission of virus have been documented in several ixodid species. These ticks feed on a wide variety of domestic and wild animals, including birds. The predominant vertebrate reservoirs for the virus include large herbivores and wild hares; it is likely that vertebrate amplification in these hosts contributes substantively to natural sustainment and spread of the virus. Human CCHF occurs following the bite of an infected tick; through exposure to blood, tissues, or excreta of infected vertebrate reservoirs; or nosocomially.

The CCHF-endemic area is widespread, covering portions of three continents; infections have been recognized in eastern and central Europe, the Middle East, northern Asia, and throughout Africa. Since most CCHF occurs in rural and often remote regions, accurate incidence and prevalence data is scanty. Illness-to-infection ratios approach 50% in some countries, but infected ticks or seropositive animals or both have been recovered from other areas where human infections are unreported. The reasons for such wide variability in disease expression are unknown. Shepherds, farmers, abbatoir workers, and others engaged in outdoor activities in rural areas (eg, hunters, boy scouts) constitute the majority of those infected through natural exposure. The risk of nosocomial infection is high; explosive outbreaks have been repeatedly documented among hospital staff engaged in the surgical or medical management of unsuspected CCHF cases.[173,174]

Pathogenesis and Clinical Findings

Onset of CCHF is abrupt. After a 2- to 7-day incubation period, patients suddenly develop high fever, chills, myalgias, severe headache, weakness, epigastric pain, nausea, and vomiting. Flushing of the face and chest, palatal petechiae, and conjunctival injection are frequently seen. Between 3 and 5 days later, a remission of several hours duration occurs in one half to two thirds of patients. Subsequently, a second phase of the illness, the "hemorrhagic" phase, ensues and is characterized by the appearance of petechiae, epistaxes, bradycardia, profound hypotension, and pulmonary edema. In severe cases, uncontrolled hemorrhage from puncture wounds and mucosal surfaces occurs. The second stage may last 3 to 10 days. For survivors, recovery is prolonged.

Thrombocytopenia, leukopenia, and elevated serum enzyme levels appear early in the disease course and carry prognostic significance. In South Africa, leukocytosis, platelets levels of less than 20,000/mm^3, marked transaminase elevations, or profound coagulation abnormalities each was more than 90% predictive of a fatal outcome if seen during the initial 5 days of illness.[175]

Diagnostic Approaches

Diagnosis of CCHF is made by serology (eg, indirect immunofluorescence, enzyme immunoassay), antigen detection, or virus isolation. Virus is readily recovered from body fluids and tissues during acute illness. These materials constitute a substantial hazard for health care workers and laboratory personnel, so patients should be managed in isolation and diagnostic samples handled only under biosafety level 4 containment levels. The differential diagnosis of CCHF includes typhoid fever, malaria, and other bacterial or rickettsial diseases. Other viral hemorrhagic fevers should also be considered, particularly those caused by hantaviruses (in eastern and central Europe and Asia) and filoviruses (in Africa).

Recommendations for Therapy and Control

CCHF virus is sensitive in vitro to ribavirin, and the drug has become an important adjunct to intensive supportive care for CCHF in South Africa and perhaps elsewhere.[176] Use of personal protective measures (eg, repellents containing DEET for the skin, permethrin treatment of clothing [see chapter 22, Personal Protection Measures Against Arthropods]) to discourage tick bites is the most effective means available to prevent natural infection. In endemic areas, awareness of the disease in ungulates and hares and avoidance of blood and fluids from these animals as they are slaughtered or marketed should be emphasized. Postexposure prophylaxis with ribavirin is probably indicated after high-risk exposures (eg, needlesticks, resuscitation), though its efficacy in this setting is unproven. A formalin-inactivated mouse brain CCHF vaccine has been produced and used in Bulgaria and the former Soviet Union, but its safety and efficacy are also unproved.

[Kelly T. McKee, Jr.]

RABIES

Introduction and Military Relevance

Rabies is an acute encephalomyelitis caused by a number of closely related rhabdoviruses. It is transmissible, primarily by direct contact, through the secretions of infected animals. The possibility of contact with such animals during the course of field training or deployment and the worldwide occurrence of rabies make it a disease of military importance. Recent deployments to Africa, the Car- ibbean region, and Latin America, where animal rabies is highly endemic, underscores the significant risk deployed military personnel may face. Military physicians must have a firm understanding of the principles of rabies prevention and management. Despite advances in preexposure and postexposure prophylaxis, rabies as an infectious disease remains almost always fatal.

Rabies ("rage" or "madness" in Latin) was first described in dogs by Democritus circa 500 BC.[177]

Since that time, it has become one of the most feared infectious diseases known. Treatment involved cauterization with a hot iron until 1885. In that year, Louis Pasteur introduced the first effective rabies vaccine, which was prepared from a virus strain isolated from the brain of a rabid cow in 1882 and subsequently passed through rabbits. Today rabies still represents a significant health threat. Although it usually can be prevented with timely immunization, once infection is established, recovery is extremely rare.

The threat of rabies has been a longstanding concern for the US military. Outbreaks of skunk-transmitted disease were reported by the US Army as a source of rabies among horses and soldiers in the western frontier in the 1870s.[178] After World War II, US service members were redeploying from many parts of the world. At the time, there was no reliable data on the distribution of rabies in the United States. The US Army Veterinary Corps, the only source of information, found that rabies was rampant in all the theaters of war except parts of the Pacific, but it was enzootic in the Philippines, Taiwan, and Japan.[179] The global rabies problem in the late 1940s received various degrees of attention, depending on where the US Army veterinarians were posted. In the Philippines, they attempted to control rabies with the Kelser chloroform-treated vaccine, with little success.[180] General MacArthur's staff gave a high priority to the control of rabies, first by educating the civilian population and then by animal control through reduction in numbers and vaccination.

The postwar rabies problem in the United States also caused great concern. This led to a national rabies program, which included animal control through education, elimination of stray animals, preexposure vaccination of pet dogs, and preexposure prophylaxis and postexposure treatment for humans. Since World War II, the Centers for Disease Control has been active in promoting rabies control. But until there are major advances in the primary prevention of rabies among animals and in the control of human disease, it will remain a significant challenge to the military medical community.

Description of the Pathogen

Rabies is caused by a number of different strains of highly neurotropic, single-stranded RNA viruses. Most of those that infect vertebrates and invertebrates are bullet-shaped and belong to the genus *Lyssavirus* and the genus *Vesiculovirus* in the family *Rhabdoviridae*. The lyssaviruses include the classic

rabies virus, which has been isolated from terrestrial mammals (eg, dogs, cats) and bats. There are, in addition, a number of rabies-related viruses that on rare occasions may cause human infection; examples include the Lagos bat virus (isolated from bats and cats), the Mokola virus (shrews and dogs), the European bat virus, and the Duvenhage virus prototype strains (bats). These viruses differ antigenically from the classic rabies viruses, engendering concern that current vaccines may not protect against them.

Despite its lethal effect on living tissue, the rabies virus survives very poorly in the environment. It is rapidly inactivated by desiccation, ultraviolet and x-ray irradiation, sunlight, trypsin, B-propiolactone, ether, and detergents.[181] It is, however, stable for many years when frozen at -70°C or freeze-dried and held at 0°C to 4°C.

Epidemiology

Transmission

Rabies viruses are transmitted largely by the bite of an infected animal; however, nonbite exposures have also been reported in which the victim was licked by an animal suspected of being rabid.[182,183] Airborne transmission has been confirmed in two settings: in caves inhabited by bats (from aerosolized bat urine) and in the laboratory.[184] Bats found in private homes may also pose a threat for rabies transmission. A fatal case of human rabies reported in 1995 involving a child illustrates this concern. A bat had been found in the child's bedroom approximately 3 weeks prior to symptoms, but there had been no evidence of a bite. The bat brain was later found to be positive for rabies by direct fluorescent antibody and nucleotide sequence analysis. This case suggests that even apparently limited contact with bats or other animals infected with rabies virus may be associated with transmission.[185] Rabies transmission has also been documented to occur via corneal transplants from infected donors.[186] The risk for transmission of rabies from a patient to family members or healthcare workers is extremely low; human-to-human transmission has been documented only in corneal transplant cases.

The rabies virus can be found in wild and domestic animals, primarily carnivores such as dogs, wolves, domestic cats, foxes, skunks, raccoons, ferrets, jackals, and mongooses. It is also found in bats but rarely in rabbits, rodents, or opossums. The relative importance of each animal species as a vector in the spread of this disease varies according to geographical location. In highly industrialized countries such as the United States, Canada, and many European countries, canine rabies has been effectively curtailed through canine vaccination. Dogs, therefore, account for less than 5% of the cases of animal rabies. The most common rabid domestic animal is now the cat. In the United States until 1989, the most commonly rabid animal was the skunk. A marked transition in animal rabies has occurred with the recent emergence of raccoons as the most common rabies reservoir and coyotes as the newest mammalian reservoir of a canine variant in Texas.[187] The ultimate reservoirs of variants indigenous to the United States are racoons, skunks, foxes, multiple species of insectivorous bats, and, most recently, coyotes, but in some developing countries (eg, parts of Asia, Africa, and Latin America) where canine rabies has not been adequately controlled, dogs still account for more than 90% of reported cases in animals, posing a substantially higher risk of transmission. Animals are usually infective (shedding virus) at least 3 to 5 days (and in some animals, such as Ethiopian dogs, up to 14 days) before clinical signs of rabies appear. As a general rule, suspected rabid animals should be observed for at least 10 days after the bite. Since the preshedding incubation period in dogs may extend for several months, rabies-free areas such as Hawaii require a period of animal quarantine before entry. Rabid animals continue to shed virus during the course of the disease.

Geographic Distribution

The worldwide incidence of human rabies is not known, but it has been reported from every continent except Australia (the two Australian cases reported in 1987 and 1990 were contracted in other countries)[188] and the Antarctic. The rabies-related viruses appear to be limited to Africa and Europe, but these are areas to which American military personnel are frequently deployed.

Incidence

The World Health Organization estimates that 35,000 rabies deaths occur each year.[189] More than 99% of the cases have occurred in those areas where canine rabies is still endemic, especially China and India. In contrast, only 1 of 9 rabies cases believed acquired in the United States between 1980 and 1993 was canine-associated, while 10 of 11 cases acquired outside the United States were canine-associated.

Six of the nine rabies cases acquired in the United States were attributable to bats.[190–194]

The incidence of human rabies in the United States has recently increased, with rabies variants associated with bats predominating among indigenously acquired cases. Between January 1990 and June 1997, there were 24 human cases of rabies diagnosed in the United States, compared to only 10 cases diagnosed during the preceding decade. Among these 24 cases, 19 were acquired in the United States, with 17 (89%) attributable to bats. Five of those cases were caused by canine variants characteristic of those occurring in Mexico, Haiti, India, and Nepal.

Pathogenesis and Clinical Findings

The pathogenesis of rabies virus infection is not entirely understood. While it is highly neurotropic and the infection is largely restricted to nervous tissue, the first site of attachment is believed to be the plasma membrane of muscle cells.[195]

The incubation period following bite exposure is usually between 20 and 90 days; however, a wide range of incubation periods has been reported, varying from as short as 4 days to as long as 19 years.[196] Most cases have incubation periods of less than 1 year. Bites on the head generally have shorter incubation periods (25 to 48 days) than those involving the extremities (46 to 78 days).[197]

The prodrome associated with rabies infection is very nonspecific; symptoms include malaise, fatigue, headache, anorexia, fever, cough, chills, sore throat, abdominal pain, nausea, vomiting, and diarrhea. Prodomal sensations at the bite site are sometimes reported. This may last for 2 to 10 days, followed by the acute onset of neurologic symptoms that herald central nervous system involvement. This stage of the disease usually presents in either one of two ways—a "furious" form or "paralytic" form—and lasts for 2 to 7 days.

Furious rabies is the more common presentation and is characterized by hyperactivity, disorientation, hallucinations, bizarre behavior, and autonomic instability with hyperthermia, hypertension, and hypersalivation. Over half of these patients will experience pharyngeal, laryngeal, and diaphragmatic spasms when attempting to drink liquids. This causes choking, gagging, and aspiration and results in hydrophobia. Similarly, aerophobia may be present since blowing air in the face may also precipitate these spasms. Numerous potential complications may develop and require specific treatment. Some of the more serious ones include hypoxia, cardiac arrhythmias, hypotension, and cerebral edema.

The paralytic form of rabies occurs in approximately 20% of patients and is characterized by either a generalized and symmetric paralysis or an ascending paralysis. In contrast to furious rabies, hyperactivity is absent, but mental status changes are common. They usually progress from agitation to confusion and disorientation and finally to coma.

Diagnostic Approaches

For the patient presenting with clinical signs and symptoms of hydrophobia and hyperactivity, especially with known exposure to a rabid animal, rabies should be the leading diagnosis. Aside from this clinical scenario, it is very difficult to distinguish rabies from other forms of viral encephalitis. It is important, however, to consider other causes, particularly treatable ones such as herpes simplex encephalitis. Post-vaccinal encephalomyelitis following immunization with Semple type (nerve tissue-derived) rabies vaccine should also be considered. Other central nervous system processes may also mimic rabies, including seizure disorders, cerebrovascular accidents, intracranial mass lesions, and atropine poisoning. Hysterical reactions to animal bites (pseudohydrophobia) are sometimes seen in patients who are extremely fearful of developing rabies. Paralytic rabies may be confused with poliomyelitis, Guillain-Barre syndrome, and transverse myelitis.

Human rabies is very difficult to diagnose early in the course of the illness because of the nonspecific prodrome. A good history, especially of exposure, and a high index of suspicion are very important. Alterations in the hematologic profile and blood chemistries are mild, nonspecific, and not helpful diagnostically. Cerebrospinal fluid (CSF) examination is likely to demonstrate a mononuclear pleocytosis (60% to 85%), but CSF glucose and protein are usually normal. Electroencephalography may show generalized slowing or paroxysmal bursts of spike potentials. Computerized tomography and magnetic resonance imaging may show diffuse enhancement, but such findings are not specific for rabies encephalitis. Furthermore, these imaging techniques may be normal even in patients with advanced rabies encephalitis.

Definitive laboratory diagnosis is by detection of the rabies antigen or antibody or isolation of the virus. The most reliable test early in the disease requires a nuchal skin biopsy with immunofluorescent staining for rabies antibody. Procedurally, a 6- to 8-mm full-thickness wedge or punch biopsy specimen is taken from the nape of the neck above the hairline. It should be placed in a vial with a piece of moist filter paper and stored at -70°C until shipped; it should not be placed in formalin. This test is more sensitive than corneal impression smears for viral antigen and has about 50% positivity during the first week of illness.[198] Corneal impression tests, however, should still be done on every suspected case of human rabies, because the test may be positive before the neutralizing antibodies appear in serum.[199] This test involves the immunofluorescent antibody staining of epithelial cells, which are obtained by pressing a clean glass microscope slide firmly against the cornea and rocking gently to increase the number of cells that stick to the slide.[200] The sensitivity of this test varies anywhere from 31%[201] to 41%[202] and is greatly affected by the number of corneal epithelial cells on a slide.

The role and timing of brain biopsy in the diagnosis of rabies encephalitis is not clearly defined. Brain biopsy in the past has offered the best prospect for identifying virus by fluorescent antibody tests (sensitivity 99%, specificity 100%) or the presence of the characteristic cytoplasmic inclusions called Negri bodies (sensitivity 90%, specificity greater than 99%),[203] but the regions of the brain (eg, hippocampus, horn of Ammon, cerebellum, brain stem) where the virus is most commonly found are not easily accessible for biopsy. Specimens obtained from other areas of the brain may be normal, so a negative biopsy does not rule out rabies.

The standard test for rabies-neutralizing antibody is the rapid fluorescent focus inhibition test, which is positive in 50% of patients by the 8th day of clinical illness and in almost all patients by the end of the second week (sensitivity 95% to 100%, specificity 100%).[204]

Viral isolation has been a disappointing tool for identifying rabies infection. Rabies virus has been isolated ante mortem from a variety of human body fluids and tissues, including saliva, urine, tracheal secretions, CSF, and brain tissue, but the yield is very low. Postmortem, rabies virus has been isolated from skin at the site of the bite and from tissue from the pericardium, adrenal gland, pancreas, liver, and bladder. Nested polymerase chain reaction is a two-step amplification method that has been successful in detecting the rabies virus. The sensitivity of this technique is reported to be 8 picograms of rabies virus–specific RNA, with no false-positive results.[205] In addition, decomposition of specimens has minimal effect on nested polymerase chain reaction detection of rabies viral RNA.

Unfortunately, these specific diagnostic tests will rarely be available in the field setting, so clinical awareness is essential.

Recommendations for Therapy and Control

Therapy

Wounds should be thoroughly and vigorously washed immediately with a 20% soap solution, followed by debridement when appropriate. This simple maneuver alone reduces the risk of rabies by up to 90%.[206,207] Sutures should be avoided whenever possible and occlusive dressings or topical ointments should not be used. If sutures are used, they should be placed after local infiltration with human rabies immunoglobulin (HRIG) and should fit snugly but not too tightly. Antimicrobial prophylaxis should be considered for a moderate-to-severe injury that has occurred within 8 hours, especially if there is possible bone or joint penetration and for wounds involving the hands. The antibiotic of choice is the combination of amoxicillin/clavulanic acid 250-500 mg given three times a day for 3 to 5 days. This will kill most bacteria associated with bite wounds, which include *Pasteurella multocida, Staphylococcus aureus,* and anaerobic organisms. For those allergic to penicillin, a combination of clindamycin and ciprofloxacin should provide comparable antimicrobial coverage. In addition, the patient's tetanus immunization status should be addressed.

Antiviral agents, such as adenosine arabinoside and isoprinosine, have been ineffective for treatment of clinical rabies. Treatment with human leukocyte interferon (peripherally and intrathecally) has been unsuccessful.[208] HRIG also has been shown to be ineffective, and there is concern that it may exacerbate the disease process.

Management is largely supportive, with intensive respiratory and cardiovascular monitoring and support. In the field, the air-evacuation process must be started as soon as this diagnosis is suspected. Steroids, which are often administered for cerebral edema (one of the possible complications of rabies), should be avoided because they have been shown to increase rabies mortality in experimentally infected animals and to decrease the immune response to vaccines.

Control

Infection Control. Infection control procedures for patients with known or suspected rabies infection should include standard, contact, and droplet precautions.[209] Standard precautions apply to blood, all body fluids, secretions, excretions (except for sweat), nonintact skin, and mucous membranes. Handwashing and the use of gloves, nonsterile gowns, masks, and eye protection or face shields are extremely important when patient-care activities are likely to generate splashes or sprays. And in accordance with contact precautions, the patient should be placed in a private room and movement of the patient from the room should be limited to essential purposes only. Droplet precautions require the use of a mask whenever working within 3 feet of the patient, even if splashes or sprays are not likely. Special air handling and ventilation are not necessary.

For contacts of patients with proven rabies, exposures for which prophylaxis may be recommended include: (*a*) bites, with penetration of skin by teeth, (*b*) exposure to the patient's saliva or other potentially infectious material in direct contact with mucous membranes or broken skin, and (*c*) scalpel nicks or needle sticks if the instrument was in contact with the patient's CSF, nervous tissue, ocular tissue, or internal organs.[210]

Prevention. Rabies prevention includes a variety of components: vaccination of animals, minimization of exposure to potentially infected animals, proper management of animals that bite humans, preexposure prophylaxis for selected high-risk persons, and postexposure prophylaxis that includes wound management, passive immunization, and active immunization when indicated.

Animal Measures. In the United States, local governments are responsible for initiating and maintaining effective programs to ensure vaccination of all dogs and cats and to remove strays and unwanted animals. This has resulted in a decline of laboratory-confirmed rabies cases in dogs from 6,949 in 1947 to 130 in 1993. Preexposure vaccination is very important in the control of rabies in these animals. There are at least 28 rabies vaccines (inactivated) for animals marketed in the United States and recommended by the National Association of State Public Health Veterinarians.[211]

Livestock, as a rule, are not vaccinated, but immunization should be considered for animals that might have frequent contact with humans in areas where rabies is epizootic in wild animals. Rabies control in wildlife through oral vaccination (via aerial drops of bait containing the vaccine) has been successful in controlling rabies in red foxes in Europe and Canada.[212,213] Similar programs in the United States have targeted raccoons, coyotes and foxes. Population reduction of wildlife rabies reservoirs is not a recommended or cost-effective method for rabies control.[214] This is especially true with bats, so human and domestic animal contact with bats should be minimized. Bats should be physically excluded from houses and surrounding structures by sealing potential entrances.[211] In addition, bats should never be handled unless appropriate safety precautions are taken, especially by untrained and unvaccinated persons. Bats should never be kept as pets.

Other measures to limit exposure include the removal of all stray dogs and cats from the community. This is especially important when military personnel are deployed to areas where rabies is epizootic. Personnel deployed to countries where rabies is enzootic should avoid unnecessary contact with wild or domesticated animals. It may be useful to establish an official "no-mascot" policy, strictly forbidding such contact.

A healthy dog or cat that bites a person should be confined and observed for at least 10 days. This recommendation is based on studies that observed that the virus was not isolated from the saliva of a rabid cat earlier than 1 day before the onset of clinical rabies and was not isolated from a rabid dog earlier than 3 days before onset.[215,216] There are a few reports of long periods of symptom-free virus excretion in dogs infected with rabies viruses from Ethiopia and India; this prompted some rabies-free areas to require a 6-month quarantine before entrance is allowed.[217] Following a long campaign for change by the US Army, Hawaii, a rabies-free state, recently reduced the quarantine time for dogs and cats from 4 months to 30 days if certain conditions are met.[218] Dogs and cats under quarantine should be evaluated by a veterinarian at the first sign of illness. If signs of rabies are present, the animal should be euthanized and the head carefully removed to prevent damage to the brain that would preclude proper pathologic examination. The head should then be packed in ice but not frozen and sent for histologic examination and culture for the rabies virus. Any stray or unwanted dog or cat that bites someone should be euthanized immediately and examined for rabies.

Data regarding viral shedding are limited in bats, raccoons, and skunks, and the risk of their harboring rabies is high; therefore, unlike pet dogs and cats, quarantine for these animals is not recommended. Prophylaxis should be started promptly after a documented exposure, whether the animal is caught or not. If the biting animal or its carcass is available, its tissue should be tested for the presence of rabies. If the results are negative, prophy-

laxis may be discontinued.

Preexposure Immunization Preexposure immunization with rabies vaccine usually results in protective antibody levels. Preexposure immunization is particularly important for individuals who are at high risk and for persons whose postexposure therapy might be delayed. It promotes a rapid anamnestic antibody response when booster doses of the vaccine are given to bite victims and eliminates the need for passive immunization with HRIG. It also reduces the number of vaccine doses needed if postexposure prophylaxis is necessary.

Preexposure immunization is recommended for anyone involved in wildlife management, veterinarians, animal handlers, laboratory workers handling rabies-infected specimens, military personnel whose assignments expose them to an unusual risk of rabies, Special Operations personnel because they may be delayed in getting postexposure prophylaxis, and others with frequent exposure to dogs, cats, foxes, raccoons, skunks, or bats.[219]

Of the number of rabies vaccines available, the most widely used preparation in the United States is the human diploid cell rabies vaccine (HDCV), which contains inactivated whole virus and is manufactured in France as a preexposure immunization. It is administered intramuscularly (only in the deltoid region) as a 1.0 mL dose on days 0, 7, and 28. Immunity is assumed after proper vaccination in a healthy individual. Additional primary doses are generally not necessary unless the vaccinee received an incomplete series, is immunocompromised, or has documented inadequate antibody titers. The World Health Organization considers a level of 0.5 IU or greater to be an adequate titer,[220] which is roughly equivalent to complete neutralization at the 1:25 level by the rapid fluorescent focus inhibition test that is recommended by the Centers for Disease Control and Prevention 2 to 4 weeks after primary vaccination. For those individuals at consistently high risk of exposure (eg, rabies researchers), titers should be checked every 6 months; for all others, titers should be checked every 2 years if a rabies risk persists.

The rabies vaccine adsorbed, produced in rhesus monkey diploid cell cultures by Bioport Corporation of Lansing, Mich, is also licensed and available in the United States. It is administered intramuscularly as a 1.0 mL dose and has been shown to be as effective as the HDCV for both preexposure and postexposure prophylaxis.[221] The purified chick embryo cell culture vaccine (RabAvert, Chiron Behring GmbH and Company) has been licensed by the Food and Drug Administration for both preexposure and postexposure prophylactic use in humans. It provides another option for vaccine candidates who develop a sensitivity to one of the other vaccines. Preexposure vaccination for persons not previously vaccinated consists of three 1.0 mL doses injected intramuscularly in the deltoid region for

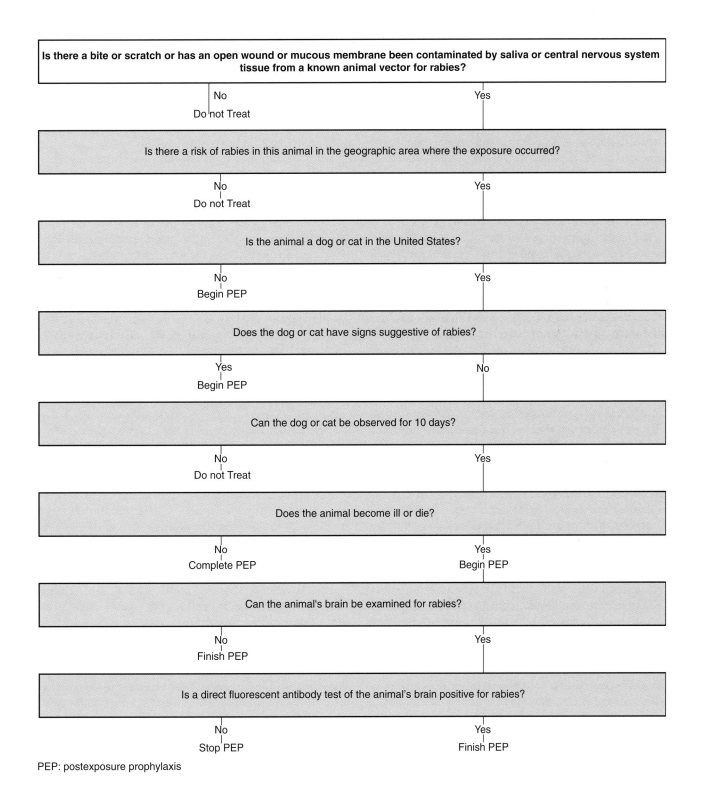

PEP: postexposure prophylaxis

Fig. 36-7. An algorithm for human rabies postexposure prophylaxis adults and in the anterolateral zone of the thigh for young children on days 0, 7, and either 21 or 28.[222]

Chloroquine phosphate, often given for malarial prophylaxis, may interfere with the antibody response to rabies vaccine.[186] Results of a randomized controlled study[223] indicated that chloroquine taken in the dose recommended for malaria prophylaxis can reduce the antibody response to primary immunization with HDCV; however, study participants were vaccinated by the reduced dose intradermal route, which is no longer recommended. It is believed that injecting rabies vaccine intramuscularly provides a reasonable margin of safety in this situation.

Postexposure Prophylaxis Very often the most difficult question facing the medical officer managing a possible rabies case is whether or not to initiate postexposure prophylaxis. A simplified approach to this management problem is illustrated in Figure 36-7. This process requires "yes" or "no" responses to several key questions designed to develop a rabies risk profile that addresses exposure and probability of the animal's being infected. For exposures to highly suspect animals, treatment should be started on the patient immediately and discontinued if fluorescent antibody testing of the animal brain is negative. In cases where the risk is low, treatment may be delayed for up to 48 hours pending the results of fluorescent antibody testing. Other factors often considered in deciding when to administer postexposure prophylaxis include suspicious animal behavior and whether the attack was provoked. Although such observations might suggest a higher likelihood of rabies, they are very subjective and are difficult to assess in wild animals.[224]

Expert guidance in making these decisions is provided at many military installations by a Rabies Advisory Board, which is composed of representatives from Preventive Medicine, Emergency Medicine, Pediatrics, Infectious Diseases (if available), and Veterinary Services. The chairman is usually the Preventive Medicine Officer, who is empowered to convene the board whenever there is suspicion of rabies exposure. Board members will have access to up-to-date information from local and state health departments on the occurrence of animal rabies in the area, which is critical in making decisions regarding postexposure prophylaxis. Local veterinary, animal control, and public health personnel may provide needed assistance in locating and quarantining animals suspected of having rabies.

The key elements of effective patient management following exposure to the rabies virus include local wound treatment, passive antibody administration, and vaccination (Table 36-6).

TABLE 36-6

RABIES POSTEXPOSURE PROPHYLAXIS RECOMMENDATIONS FOR ADULTS

Previously Vaccinated?	Treatment	Regimen
NO	Local wound care	Clean wound immediately with soap and water
	HRIG	20 IU/kg body weight: as much as possible infiltrated around wound site(s) and the remainder IM in buttocks
	Vaccine[*]	HDCV, RVA, or PCEC 1.0 mL IM (deltoid area) on days 0, 3, 7, 14, and 28
YES[†]	Local wound care	Clean wound immediately with soap and water
	Vaccine	HDCV, RVA, or PCEC 1.0 mL IM (deltoid), on days 0 and 3

[*]Do not inject using the same syringe as HRIG or into the same anatomic site
[†]Either (a) preexposure or postexposure vaccination with HDCV or RVA or (b) documentation of past antibody response to any other rabies vaccine
HRIG: human rabies immune globulin, HDCV: human diploid cell rabies vaccine, RVA: rabies vaccine adsorbed, PCEC: purified chick embryo cell culture

Passive immunization is achieved with the use of HRIG. This preparation has been well tolerated, with no reports of anaphylaxis or serum sickness and no reports of transmission of hepatitis or other viruses. A single dose of 20 IU/kg body weight is administered with as much of the total dose as is anatomically feasible infiltrated at the site of the wound. The remaining volume should be given intramuscularly in the upper outer quadrant of the buttocks or the anterolateral aspect of the thigh, but this should be an anatomical site distant from the site of vaccine administration. Local infiltration may, in some instances, be limited in wounds involving small anatomic areas such as fingertips. Any person with a previous history of preexposure or postexposure vaccination with HDCV or rabies vaccine adsorbed should not be given HRIG. The administration of HRIG is unnecessary and contraindicated because of the potential interference with an anamnestic response to booster vaccination.

During some overseas deployments, HRIG may be unavailable. In the past, the only available alternative had been heterologous antiserum of equine origin (ARS, anti-rabies serum), but this preparation was associated with serum sickness in 16% of recipients in one study.[225] Although not licensed in the United States, a purified antirabies sera of equine origin (ERIG, equine rabies immune globulin) is available. In developing countries, ERIG may be the only viable alternative. The incidence of adverse reactions with ERIG has been low (0.8% to 6.0%), and the reactions have largely been minor.[226]

If in an area where only ERIG (or even ARS) is available, the decision to prophylax should take into account individual sensitivity to horse serum and the severity and likelihood of rabies exposure. Predeployment planning should include consideration for preexposure prophylaxis when the area of operation is located in countries where HRIG is not likely to be available.

Active immunization in persons not previously vaccinated consists of five 1.0 mL intramuscular doses of HDCV, RVA, or RabAvert vaccine into the deltoid region in adults or the anterolateral zone of the thigh for children; the first dose is given as soon as possible after exposure (day 0) and repeated on days 3, 7, 14, and 28. If the patient has been previously immunized, only two 1.0 mL injections on days 0 and 3 are needed. Vaccine should not be injected by the same syringe used to inject HRIG or at the same.

Postexposure treatment failures are uncommon, but they do occur and are more likely when one or more of these measures is omitted. One of the most common errors is the omission of passive immunization.[227] In other cases, local wound cleansing was omitted or post-exposure treatment was delayed.[228]

[Clifton A. Hawkes]

TULAREMIA

Introduction and Military Relevance

Tularemia (rabbit fever, deer-fly fever, Ohara disease) is a zoonotic bacterial disease caused by *Francisella tularensis*. Clinical recognition of tularemia and the epidemiology, diagnosis, treatment, and prevention of this disease are important military medicine capabilities. Transmission of tularemia can occur by direct inoculation of contaminated animal tissue, by ingestion of contaminated meat or water, and by bites from infected ticks, deer flies, and mosquitoes. The variety of clinical presentations of tularemia and the confusion of it with other infectious diseases underscore the importance of rapid diagnosis and a detailed history of travel and animal and arthropod exposure. In addition, the virulence of the bacterium, its transmissibility, and its capacity to induce significant morbidity make *F tularensis* a potential biological warfare agent.

Description of the Pathogen

The causative agent of tularemia is *Francisella tularensis*. *F tularensis* is a small, gram-negative, oxidase-negative, aerobic, nonmotile coccobacillus that can cause disease with as few as 10 organisms.[229] There are two distinct subspecies: *F tularensis*, biovar *tularensis* (type A), which produces virulent infections, and *F tularensis*, biovar *palaearctica* (type B), which produces infections that are often milder and indolent. *Francisella* organisms can survive for extended periods of time in water, mud, and animal carcasses.

Epidemiology

Transmission

Reservoirs for this organism in nature include many species of birds and wild animals (eg, rabbits, muskrats, squirrels, skunks, coyotes, beavers, water rats) and domesticated cats.[230] Direct and indirect transmission to humans typically occurs through the bite of infected animals[231] or the handling of blood or tissue or both while skinning and dressing rabbits or other infected animals.[232,233] Tularemia can be acquired from the consumption or handling of insufficiently cooked meat contaminated with the organism, through drinking or skin contact with contaminated water, and through contact with contaminated animal skins (Figure 36-8). *F tularensis* is resistant to freezing; rabbit meat remains infectious after being frozen for more than 3 years. Inhalation of bacteria from the dust of contaminated soil and occupational exposure from farming have been reported.[234] Along with the respiratory route, other mucous membranes (eg, ocular, oropharyngeal) are potential points of entry for the organism. There is no person-to-person transmission. The potential for laboratory acquisition from aerosolized organisms is high, and cultures should not be obtained because of the danger to laboratory personnel.

Vectors that can transmit the disease to humans include mosquitoes, deer flies (*Chrysops discalis*), and ticks (eg, *Dermacentor andersoni*, *D variabilis*, *Amblyoma americanum*). Ticks may be infected

TULAREMIA

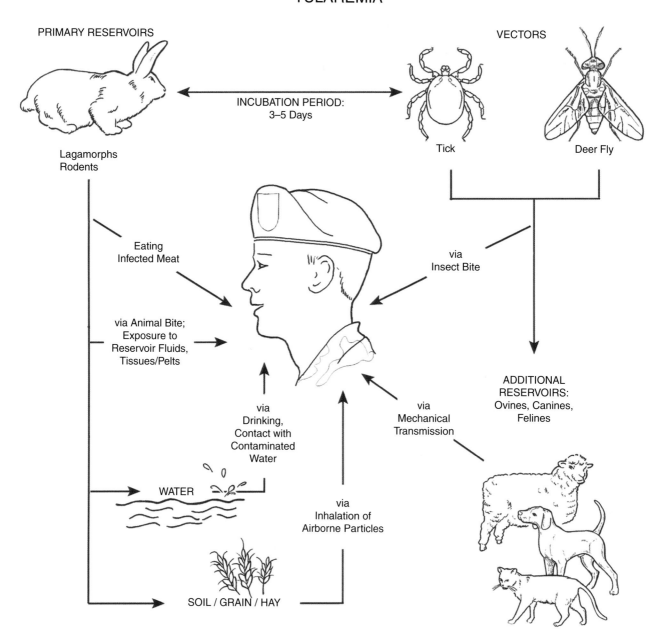

Fig. 36-8. The transmission cycle of *Francisella tularensis*. Art by Annabelle Wright, Walter Reed Army Institute of Research; research by Amelia Poisson.

throughout their lifetime and can transovarially pass the organisms to their progeny.

Geographic Distribution

Type A strains are limited to North America, particularly to the states of Arkansas, Oklahoma, South Dakota, and Missouri.[235] Type B strains are found in the northern hemisphere, including North America, Europe, Russia, China, and Japan. *F tularensis* has not been found in Africa or South America.

Incidence

Approximately 200 cases of tularemia are reported in the United States per year.[236] The highest incidence of tularemia occurs in the summer months, when tick-borne transmission occurs. A second peak occurs in the winter, presumably with the increase in hunting wild animals such as rabbits. Transmission of the organism is not stable and can vary from year to year.

Pathogenesis and Clinical Findings

F tularensis is highly infectious; as few as 10 to 50 organisms can establish an infection through intracutaneous inoculation or via inhalation of aerosolized bacteria. Factors that contribute to the pathogenesis of the disease include the virulence of the organism, route of entry, age and immune status of the patient, and systemic involvement. Type A organisms are typically more virulent than Type B organisms, and less virulent strains may cause infections that resolve without treatment. The molecular basis for virulence of the organisms is unknown. *F tularensis* is an intracellular organism primarily of cells of the reticuloendothelial system, including macrophages, edothelial cells, and hepatocytes. The organism multiplies within macrophages, resisting intracellular destruction by preventing lysosome-phagosome fusion. A cellular-mediated immune response by the host attempts to control the infection by activation of T lymphocytes with consequent production of interferon-gamma and tumor necrosis factor. These cytokines activate macrophages through the production of reactive oxygen and nitrogen products that kill the intracellular organism.

The route of inoculation of the bacteria often predicts the clinical presentation of the disease, and the severity of illness depends on the virulence of the organism.[237,238] The clinical presentation of this disease can be confused with other infections, such as plague, staphylococcal and streptococcal infections, cat-scratch fever, and sporotrichosis, so an accurate clinical description that leads to a rapid diagnosis and the expeditious institution of therapy is required. There are six clinical forms of tularemia: glandular, ulceroglandular, typhoidal, pulmonary, oculoglandular, and oropharyngeal.

The most common forms of infection are classified as glandular or ulceroglandular tularemia. A localized, nonhealing, punched-out circular ulcer with raised borders forms at the site of inoculation in the skin and leads to lymphadenopathy and lymphadenitis in 90% of ulceroglandular tulaeria. In many cases, an ulcer or erythematous papule may not be clinically evident in glandular tularemia, and the only manifestation of infection is a relatively nonspecific regional lymphadenitis and systemic illness. The incubation period for the disease is approximately 3 days (range of 2 to 10 days). Fever is the primary sign of infection, and flu-like symptoms appear before or concurrent with swelling and pain in regional lymph nodes. Fever may last for up to 3 weeks in approximately 20% of cases treated with appropriate antibiotics.

The other major classification of tularemia is a systemic illness called typhoidal tularemia. It is the most frequently fatal form of the disease and results from rapid dissemination of the organism into multiple organs by hematogenous spread. This form of the disease may occur in patients with underlying illness, poor nutritional state, alcohol abuse, or chronic renal failure. Splenomegaly may be observed in 15% to 20% of the patients, but hepatomegaly is less common. Typhoidal tularemia in a healthy service member suggests an aerosol exposure, as may occur in a laboratory or during a bioterrorist event.

A major complication of typhoidal tularemia is the appearance of tularemic pneumonia, which may occur regardless of the initial route of entry but is three times more common in typhoidal disease than other forms of tularemia. Pulmonary symptoms are characterized by a nonproductive cough, pleuritic chest pain, dyspnea on exertion, malaise, fever, and myalgias. Radiographic findings may be normal or may show pulmonary infiltrates that mimic fungal and other bacterial pneumonias, tuberculosis, or malignancy.[236] Hilar adenopathy can be seen in 36% of tularemia pneumonia.[234] Pleural effusions complicating tularemic pneumonia are rare, but pleural-based granulomatous inflammation secondary to *F tularensis* infection has been reported and can be confused with the more common *Mycobacterium tuberculosis* infection.[238] The mortality rate from tularemic pneumonia is high.[236]

Other less common forms of tularemia include oropharyngeal tularemia; this results from the ingestion of infectious organisms and may induce pharyngitis, diarrhea, abdominal pain, and emesis. Oculoglandular tularemia is extremely rare and is acquired by the direct inoculation of bacteria into the conjunctival sac. Dermatological manifestations of the disease may include erythema nodosum and erythema multiforme.[237]

Rarely, *Francisella* organisms can cause meningitis, with cerebral spinal fluid findings of an elevated protein level and a predominance of mononuclear cells.[239] A precise history of rabbit and cat exposure should be elicited and therapy immediately initiated if other more common causes of meningitis are excluded.

Diagnostic Approaches

The current methods for the diagnosis of infections caused by *F tularensis* are unsatisfactory. The diagnosis of tularemia by serology, either by serum agglutination or enzyme-linked immunosorbent assay, remains the method of choice.[240] Serum agglutination titers documenting a 4-fold increase in titer between acute and convalescent sera or an absolute titer of 1:160 or greater aid in the diagnosis of exposure to *F tularensis,* but cross-reactions with *Brucella* species, *Proteus* species, and heterophile antibodies are known to occur. Antibodies to the *Francisella* organism typically appear after the second week of infection, and it is not unusual to have negative serologic agglutination tests despite acute infection. Therefore in the absence of definitive diagnosis, a presumptive diagnosis based on clinical presentation and epidemiologic exposure mandates aggressive treatment. The organism may be identified directly by fluorescent antibody assays on specimens obtained from an ulcer exudate or a lymph node aspirate. If a biopsy is done, appropriate antibiotics may be given to avoid the potentially resultant bacteremia.

In some rare cases, *F tularensis* can be directly cultured from aspirates of ulcers, from pleural fluid, or from blood.[241] However, culture of this highly infectious bacterium should only be attempted in a biosafety level 3 laboratory. Special media containing cysteine or cystine for growth are required to isolate the organism. Modified Muellar-Hinton broth, chocolate blood agar, and modified charcoal yeast extract agar have been used to isolate the bacterium.[240] The bacteria grow as smooth, blue-gray colonies, and identification as *Francisella* can be made by slide agglutination using commercially available antisera. The polymerase chain reaction has been used to rapidly and accurately identify *Francisella* from clinical specimens but is currently a research tool not generally available in the clinical microbiology laboratory.[242,243]

Recommendations for Therapy and Control

Therapy

Factors to be considered in the treatment of tularemia include the natural resistance of *F tularensis* to all penicillins and other β-lactams, the intracellular environment of the organism, the organism's tendency to cause suppurative adenitis, and the need for both parenteral antibiotics in severe infection and oral antibiotics for localized ulceroglandular

disease. Another consideration when choosing an antibiotic regimen is whether the infection has been diagnosed with certainty or the diagnosis is based solely on the history or clinical examination. Since treatment with antibiotics that cannot penetrate cells fails to eliminate the bacteria and frequently results in clinical relapse, treatment should be directed toward the elimination of both extracellular and intracellular forms of the bacteria. Factors that increase the risk of clinical relapse include underlying immunosuppression, insufficient duration of therapy, and the use of bacteriostatic rather than bacteriocidal antibiotics.[236]

The antibiotic of choice in the treatment of tularemia is streptomycin (1 g intramuscularly four times a day for 10 to 14 days).[244,245] However, alternative antibiotics with comparable efficacy to streptomycin but with less potential for the adverse side effects of ototoxicity and nephrotoxicity have been sought. Gentamicin, another bactericidal aminoglycoside, is an adequate alternative to streptomycin and has been successfully used to treat the disease in both the adult[246] and pediatric population,[247] albeit with a greater relapse rate (6%).[248] Caution should be exercised when using gentamicin alone because of its variability in cell penetration, the higher frequency of relapses, and the need to maintain high blood levels of the antibiotic. Treatment with gentamicin (5 mg/kg) to maintain blood levels at approximately 5 µg/mL should continue for 10 to 14 days. Tetracycline is efficacious, but again, higher relapse rates occur, which may be a function of its bacteriostatic activity. Oral quinolones, such as ciprofloxacin (500-750 mg twice a day for 10 to 30 days), have been shown to be particularly efficacious, with resolution of fever within 2 days of beginning therapy and fewer documented relapses than tetracycline or the aminoglycosides.[248,249] Because of its excellent bactericidal activity, stability in an acidic environment, and levels of antibiotic achieved in soft tissues, ciprofloxacin is an excellent alternative in culture-proven *Francisella* infections and may become the antibiotic of choice for suspected but not proven infection.

In vitro antimicrobial susceptibility testing does not correlate with clinical response and should not be used to direct the choice of antibiotics. Cephalosporins, such as cefotaxime, ceftazidime, and ceftriaxone, have in vitro activity against *Francisella*[250] but no in†vivo efficacy.[251] For cases of suspected tularemic meningitis, chloramphenicol should be added to the streptomycin treatment regimen.[252] A single case report showed that imipenem (500 mg intravenously every 8 hours for 14 days) can achieve clinical cure with no relapse.[253] The best indicator of response to therapy is the resolution of fever, which usually falls within 3 days of instituting therapy.[247]

Control

Protective measures that minimize contact with and infection by *F tularensis* include avoiding potentially contaminated drinking water, refraining from bathing and swimming in untreated water, and wearing protective clothing and insect repellent to protect against transmission by mosquitoes, ticks, and flies. Wild rabbit and rodent meat must be carefully handled and thoroughly cooked. For laboratory workers who may come in contact with the bacteria, the importance of the use of gloves and masks is obvious. Although quarantine is not indicated, universal secretion precautions should be taken when working with patients who have open lesions.

There is no licensed vaccine against tularemia. However, a live attenuated vaccine for laboratory personnel exposed to *F tularensis* has been shown to be safe and partially efficacious.[254] This vaccine is held under an investigational new drug protocol by the US Army Medical Research Institute of Infectious Diseases, Fort Detrick, Md. Postexposure prophylaxis with doxycycline, as may occur after a biological warfare incident, may be beneficial.[255]

[Christian F. Ockenhouse]

ANTHRAX

Introduction

Anthrax, a zoonotic disease caused by *Bacillus anthracis*, occurs in domesticated and wild animals—primarily herbivores such as goats, sheep, cattle, horses, and swine. Humans usually become infected by contact with infected animals or contaminated animal products. Natural infection occurs most commonly via the cutaneous route and only very rarely via the respiratory or gastrointestinal routes. There are typical manifestations associated with each of these three routes.

The US military's primary concern with anthrax is with its potential use as a biological weapon, for which anthrax is suited because of the infectiousness of its spores by the respiratory route and the high mortality of inhalational anthrax. This concern was heightened after the revelation that the largest epidemic of inhalational anthrax in the 20th century occurred when anthrax spores were accidentally released from a military research facility in Sverdlovsk, USSR, in 1979. Cases were also reported in animals located more than 50 km from the site.[256,257] Another concern is that as the US military's mission expands to include more worldwide humanitarian efforts, service members are increasingly likely to encounter unvaccinated livestock that may have anthrax.

Description of the Pathogen

Bacillus anthracis is a large, gram-positive, spore-forming, nonmotile bacillus (1-1.5 μm by 3-10 μm) that forms a prominent capsule in tissue. The encapsulated bacterium occurs singly or in chains of two or three bacilli. The organism does not form spores in living tissue; sporulation occurs only after the infected body has been opened and exposed to oxygen. The spores are very stable and may survive in soil for decades under favorable conditions.

Epidemiology

Transmission

Anthrax in humans is nearly always associated with direct exposure to infected animals or to contaminated animal products. Animals, either domestic or wild, become infected when they ingest spores from the soil. Humans rarely, if ever, contract anthrax directly from the soil unless they are working with contaminated bone meal fertilizer. Exposure usually occurs through handling spore-laden carcasses, hides, wool, hair, or bones, often in an industrial setting. Cutaneous lesions, by far the most common form of anthrax, occur on exposed parts of the body (eg, arms, neck, face). Inhalation of a sufficient quantity of spores results in inhalational anthrax. This uncommon but lethal disease occurs most often in those processing contaminated wool or animal hair in an enclosed space. This is the form of anthrax that has potential as a biologic weapon. Finally, oropharyngeal or gastrointestinal anthrax can arise from eating poorly cooked, contaminated meat. This form of the disease is also quite rare.

There is no proven vector for transmission, although it has been suggested that anthrax in animals has been spread by biting flies carrying spores from one grazing area to another.[258] No evidence exists for a similar mechanism in humans. Human-to-human transmission does not occur in inhalational anthrax and has been reported in only two cases of cutaneious disease.[259–261]

Geographic Distribution

Anthrax occurs worldwide, existing as a spore. Human cases of anthrax continue to be reported from Africa, Asia, Europe, and the Americas.[262] The threat of anthrax is increased when there is a concurrent epizootic in the region, particularly in cattle. Environmental conditions such as drought, which may promote trauma to the oral cavity of grazing animals, are thought to increase the chances of an animal acquiring anthrax.[263]

Incidence

In the United States, the annual incidence of human anthrax has steadily declined from approximately 127 cases in the early years of the 20th century to about 1 per year in the 1990s. The vast majority of cases have been cutaneous. Under natural conditions, inhalational anthrax is exceedingly rare, with only 18 cases having been reported in the United States in the 20th century.[264] During times of economic hardship and disruption of veterinary and human public health practices, such as occurs during war, there have been large epidemics of anthrax. The largest reported epidemic of human anthrax occurred in Zimbabwe from 1978 through 1980, with an estimated 10,000 cases. Nearly all these were cutaneous.[258,265,266] Incidence increases during the spring and summer months.

Units located in rural areas, particularly those in which there has been recent socioeconomic disruption leading to poor animal husbandry, should be aware of the increased risk of human anthrax in the presence of animal anthrax. If the stay is prolonged, it may be worthwhile to assist the community in immunizing their herds against anthrax.

Pathogenesis and Clinical Findings

B anthracis possesses three known virulence factors, which are an antiphagocytic capsule and two protein exotoxins (called the lethal and the edema toxins). The anthrax toxins possess two components: (1) a shared cell-binding, or B, domain and (2) a distinct active, or A, domain that has the toxic activity. Both components are required for biologic activity.[267–269]

Infection begins when the spores are inoculated through the skin or mucosa. It is thought that spores are ingested at the local site by macrophages and germinate into the vegetative bacilli that produce a capsule and toxins. At these sites, the bacilli are released from the macrophage, proliferate, and produce the edema and lethal toxins that impair host leukocyte function and lead to the distinctive pathological findings of edema, hemorrhage, tissue necrosis, and a relative lack of leukocytes.

In inhalational anthrax, the spores are ingested by alveolar macrophages, which transport them to the regional tracheobronchial lymph nodes, where germination occurs.[270] Once in the tracheobronchial lymph nodes, the local production of toxins by extracellular bacilli gives rise to the characteristic pathological picture of massive hemorrhagic, edematous, and necrotizing lymphadenitis, and the mediastinitis that is almost pathognomonic of this disease.[271] The bacilli can then spread to the blood, leading to septicemia with seeding of other organs and frequently causing hemorrhagic meningitis. Death is the result of respiratory failure that is associated with pulmonary edema, overwhelming bacteremia, and, often, meningitis.

Cutaneous Anthrax

More than 95% of cases of anthrax are cutaneous (Figure 36-9). After inoculation, the incubation period is 1 to 5 days. The disease first appears as a small papule that progresses over one to two days to a vesicle containing serosanguinous fluid with

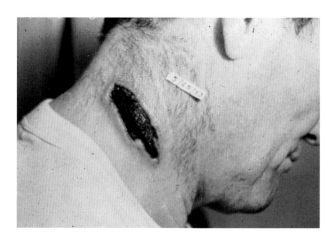

Fig. 36-9. A cutaneous lesion of anthrax with eschar on a patient's neck, occurring on approximately day 15 of disease. The patient had worked with air-dried goat skins from Africa.
Photograph: Courtesy of the Armed Forces Institute of Pathology, Washington, DC. AFIP Negative 75-4203-7.

many organisms and few leukocytes. The vesicle, which may be 1 to 2 cm in diameter, ruptures and leaves a necrotic ulcer. Satellite vesicles may also be present. The lesion is usually painless, and varying degrees of edema may surround it. The edema may occasionally be massive, encompassing the entire face or limb, and is called "malignant edema." Patients usually have fever, malaise, and headache, which may be severe in those with extensive edema. There may also be local lymphadenitis. The ulcer base develops a characteristic black eschar; after 2 to 3 weeks the eschar separates, usually leaving no scar. Septicemia is very rare, and with treatment mortality should be less than 1%. The case-fatality rate for untreated cutaneous anthrax is 5% to 20%.

Inhalational Anthrax

Inhalational anthrax begins after an incubation period of 1 to 6 days with nonspecific symptoms of malaise, fatigue, myalgia, and fever. There may be an associated nonproductive cough and mild chest discomfort. These symptoms usually persist for 2 or 3 days, and in some cases there may be a short period of improvement. This is followed by the sudden onset of increasing respiratory distress with dyspnea, stridor, cyanosis, increased chest pain, and diaphoresis. There may be associated edema of the chest and neck. Chest X-ray examination may show the characteristic widening of the mediastinum and

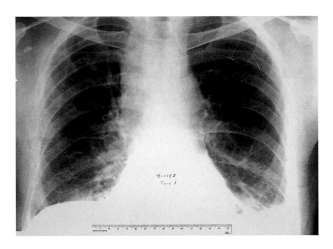

Fig. 36-10. This roentgenogram, taken on day 2 of illness, shows the lungs of a 51-year-old laborer with occupational exposure to airborne anthrax spores. Marked mediastinal widening is evident with small parenchymal infiltrate. Photograph: Courtesy of the Armed Forces Institute of Pathology, Washington, DC. AFIP Negative 71-12790-2.

pleural effusions (Figure 36-10). Bacterial pneumonia is an uncommon finding but can occur in some patients.[256] While cases of inhalational anthrax have been rare in the 20th century, several have occurred in patients with underlying pulmonary disease, suggesting increased susceptibility in these patients.[264] Meningitis is present in up to 50% of cases, and some patients may present with seizures. The onset of respiratory distress is followed by the rapid onset of shock and death within 24 to 36 hours. Mortality has been essentially 100% in reported cases, and there are no reliable human data on the effectiveness of current treatment regimens and supportive care.

Oropharyngeal and Gastrointestinal Anthrax

Oropharyngeal and gastrointestinal anthrax result from the ingestion of undercooked, infected meat. After an incubation period of 2 to 5 days, patients with oropharyngeal disease present with a severe sore throat or a local oral or tonsillar ulcer, usually associated with fever, toxicity, and swelling of the neck due to cervical or submandibular lymphadenitis and edema. Dysphagia and respiratory distress may also be present. Gastrointestinal anthrax begins with nonspecific symptoms of nausea, vomiting, and fever; these are followed in most cases by severe abdominal pain. The presenting sign may be an acute abdomen, which may be associated with hematemesis, massive ascites, and diarrhea. Mortality in each of these forms may be as high as 50% even with treatment.

Meningitis

Meningitis usually follows bacteremia as a complication of the disease. Meningitis may also occur, but very rarely, without a clinically apparent primary focus. It is very often hemorrhagic, which is important diagnostically, and is almost invariably fatal.

Diagnostic Approaches

The most critical aspect in making a diagnosis of anthrax is a high index of suspicion associated with a compatible history of exposure. Cutaneous anthrax should be considered following the development of a painless pruritic papule, vesicle, or ulcer that often is surrounded by edema and develops into a black eschar. With extensive or massive edema, such a lesion is almost pathognomonic. Gram's stain or culture of the lesion will usually confirm the diagnosis. The differential diagnosis should include tularemia, staphylococcal or streptococcal disease, and orf (a zoonotic viral disease of sheep and goats).

The diagnosis of inhalational anthrax is extraordinarily difficult, but the disease should be suspected in those with a history of exposure to a *B anthracis*–containing aerosol. The early symptoms are entirely nonspecific, but two situations suggest the diagnosis: (1) the development of respiratory distress in association with radiographic evidence of a widened mediastinum due to hemorrhagic mediastinitis and (2) the presence of hemorrhagic pleural effusion or hemorrhagic meningitis. Sputum examination is not helpful in making the diagnosis, since pneumonia is not usually a feature of inhalational anthrax.

Gastrointestinal and oropharyngeal anthrax are exceedingly difficult to diagnose because of the rarity of the diseases and their nonspecific symptoms. Only with an appropriate epidemiologic history in the setting of an outbreak are these diagnoses usually considered. Microbiological cultures are not helpful in confirming the diagnosis. Gram's stain or Giemsa stain of the peripheral blood may allow visualization of the organism, and standard blood culture may yield the organism but not until late in the course of the disease.

Meningitis due to anthrax can be clinically indistinguishable from meningitis due to other causes. An important distinguishing feature is that the cerebral spinal fluid is grossly hemorrhagic in as many as 50% of the cases. The diagnosis can be confirmed by identifying the organism in cerebral spinal fluid by microscopy or culture.

Serology is generally only of use in making a retrospective diagnosis. Antibody to protective antigen or the capsule develops in 68% to 93% of reported cases of cutaneous anthrax.[272–275] Bacterial identification is confirmed by demonstration of the protective antigen toxin component, lysis by a specific bacteriophage, detection of capsule by fluorescent antibody, or virulence for mice and guinea pigs. Additional confirmatory tests to identify the organism by the presence of toxin and capsule genes using the polymerase chain reaction have also been developed as research tools. An enzyme-linked immunosorbent assay for circulating toxins will be positive but not until late in the course when bacteremia is present. A hand-held form of this assay has been shown to be of value in the field for rapid diagnosis in animals and is available on a research basis for use in human disease.

Recommendations for Therapy and Control

Therapy

Penicillin is the drug of choice for anthrax. Cutaneous anthrax without toxicity or systemic symptoms may be treated with oral penicillin. If spreading infection or systemic symptoms are present, then intravenous therapy with high-dose penicillin (2 million units administered every 6 hours) may be initiated until a clinical response is obtained. Effective therapy will reduce edema and systemic symptoms but will not change the evolution of the skin lesion itself. Treatment should be continued for 7 to 10 days. Tetracycline, erythromycin, and chloramphenicol have also been used successfully. These drugs may be used for treatment of the rare case caused by naturally occurring penicillin-resistant organisms or in penicillin-allergic patients. Other drugs, including the fluoroquinolones, first-generation cephalosporins, and doxycycline, are effective in vitro but have not been used in human cases.

Inhalational, oropharyngeal, and gastrointestinal anthrax should be aggressively treated with large doses of intravenous penicillin (2 million units administered every 2 hours), and appropriate vasopressors, oxygen, and other supportive therapy should also be used.

Illness after a suspected or known attack with *B anthracis* spores should be treated based on antibiotic sensitivities because of the possibility of inducing antibiotic resistance in weaponized spores. In the absence of information regarding antibiotic sensitivities, treatment should be instituted at the earliest signs of disease with intravenous ciprofloxacin (400 mg every 8 to 12 hours) or intravenous doxycycline (200 mg initially, followed by 100 mg every 12 hours).

Control

Service members on deployment should avoid contact with animals, hides, or products made from hide. To avoid potential cases of gastrointestinal anthrax, they should also take care to avoid the consumption of meat from infected animals. This issue applies primarily when there is local acquisition of food supplies. Additionally, all meat should be thoroughly cooked.

When service members encounter sick or dead animals, samples should be taken for microbiological diagnosis. If anthrax is confirmed, the dead animals should be incinerated and the remaining bones buried deeply. Caution must be used when handling carcasses to avoid direct contact with skin, especially broken skin. If incineration is impossible, the animal should be buried to a depth of at least 6 feet and covered with lime.[259]

Prophylactic Treatment After Exposure

Experimental evidence from animals has demonstrated that postexposure antibiotic treatment, beginning 1 day after exposure to a lethal aerosol challenge with anthrax spores, can provide significant protection against death. All three drugs used in this study—ciprofloxacin, doxycycline, and penicillin—were effective.[276] In vitro sensitivity tests demonstrate very good activity against *B anthracis* with the quinolone antimicrobial agents.[277,278] Optimal protection is afforded by combining antibiotics with active immunization.[276] Oral antibiotics should be continued for at least 4 weeks, during which the unimmunized patient should be given 3 doses of vaccine 2 weeks apart. For those already immunized with at least 3 doses of the vaccine, the status of vaccination should be checked and any necessary boosters given. Regardless of immunization status, if the exposure has been confirmed and antibiotic supplies are sufficient, everyone exposed should be given 30 days of antibiotic treatment. Treatment for unimmunized personnel should be extended to 60 days if no vaccine is available, and the patient should be observed carefully for any signs and symptoms once antibiotic therapy has been discontinued.

Active Immunization

As of 1999, the only licensed human vaccine against anthrax is produced by BioPort Inc. (formerly the Michigan Biologic Products Institute). This vaccine was licensed in the early 1970s and has been given to thousands of people. This vaccine is made from sterile filtrates of microaerophilic cultures of an attenuated, unencapsulated, nonproteolytic, strain (V770-NP 1-R) of *B anthracis*. The recommended schedule for vaccination is 0.5 mL given subcutaneously at 0, 2, and 4 weeks, followed by doses at 6, 12, and 18 months. Annual boosters are recommended if the potential for exposure continues. When tested by an enzyme-linked immunosorbent assay, more than 95% of vaccinees seroconvert after the initial three doses.[279,280] Local side effects, consisting of erythema, tenderness, induration, and edema, may occur in up to 30% of recipients, but systemic side effects are rare.[281] Nontender subcutaneous nodules at the site of vaccination can occur and resolve without treatment. No long-term sequelae from the vaccine have been reported.[282]

The vaccine should be given to industrial workers exposed to potentially contaminated animal products imported from countries in which animal anthrax remains uncontrolled. People in direct contact with potentially infected animals and laboratory workers should also be immunized. Contraindications for use of the vaccine include a hypersensitivity reaction to the vaccine or one of its components. Reasons for temporary deferment of the vaccine include active febrile illness, corticosteroid or other immunosuppressive regimen, and pregnancy. Servicemembers who are scheduled to receive the vaccine and believe they may be pregnant should be referred for pregnancy testing, and vaccination should be suspended until the patient is no longer pregnant.

In 1998, the Department of Defense initiated the Anthrax Vaccination Immunization Program, a military-wide program to immunize all active duty and reserve forces against anthrax over several years. All immunizations given under the program are tracked centrally and documented in patient medical records. As of February 2001, more than 2 million doses have been given.

Anthrax Vaccination Immunization Program guidelines stipulate that if there is deviation from the vaccination schedule, the next dose should be given as soon as possible and then all remaining doses given based on the time of the last dose. The series should only be restarted if only one dose has been received and more than 2 years have elapsed since receiving that dose.

[Arthur M. Friedlander, Lisa A. Pearse, Julie Pavin]

BRUCELLOSIS

Introduction and Military Relevance

Brucellosis is a zoonotic infection of domesticated and wild animals caused by bacteria of the genus *Brucella*. Humans become infected by ingestion of animal food products, direct contact with infected animals, or inhalation of infectious aerosols. Onset is acute or insidious and is characterized by fever and a variety of systemic symptoms or by a local inflammatory process.

In 1751, Cleghorn, a British army surgeon stationed on the Mediterranean island of Minorca, described cases of a chronic, relapsing febrile illness and cited Hippocrates' description of a similar disease more than 2,000 years earlier.[283] David Bruce isolated the causative organism from the spleens of five fatal cases in 1897 but termed it a micrococcus.[284] In 1897, Hughes coined the name "undulant fever" and described 844 cases.[285] In that same year, Bang identified a "Bacillus of abortion" in placentas and fetuses of cattle suffering from contagious abortion.[286] Twenty years later, Evans recognized that Bang's organism was identical to the causative agent of human brucellosis described by Hughes.

The organism infects a borad range of mammals, causing abortion, fetal death, and genital infection.[287,288] Humans, who are usually infected incidentally by contact with infected animals or ingestion of dairy foods, may develop numerous symptoms in addition to the usual ones of fever, malaise, and muscle pain that might incapacitate military personnel in a theater of operations. Disease frequently becomes chronic and may relapse, even with treatment. The ease of transmission by aerosol suggests that *Brucella* organisms might be a candidate for use as a biological warfare agent.

Description of the Pathogen

Brucellae are small, nonmotile, nonsporulating, nontoxigenic, nonfermenting, aerobic, gram-negative coccobacilli that may, based on DNA homology, represent a single species.[289] Conventionally, however, they are classified into six species, each comprising several biovars. Each species has a characteristic but not absolute predilection to infect certain animals (Table 36-7). A novel species (proposed nomen *B maris*) has recently been isolated from marine mammals.[290] Only *Brucella melitensis, B suis, B abortus, B canis* and *B manis* cause disease in humans.

TABLE 36-7

TYPICAL HOST SPECIFICITY OF *BRUCELLA* SPECIES

Brucella Species	Animal Host	Human Pathogenicity
B suis	Swine	High
B melitensis	Sheep, goats	High
B abortus	Cattle, bison	Intermediate
B canis	Dogs	Intermediate
B ovis	Sheep	None
B neotomae	Rodents	None
B maris	Marine mammals	Not known

Epidemiology

Transmission

Natural transmission is through contact with infectious tissues or secretions, through ingestion of raw milk and dairy products, or by inhalation of aerosolized bacteria in animal enclosures, laboratories, or slaughterhouses. Brucellosis is rarely, if ever, transmitted from person to person. The incidence of human disease is thus closely tied to the prevalence of infection in sheep, goats, swine, camels, and cattle and to practices that allow exposure of humans to potentially infected animals or their products.[291–293] In the United States, where most states are free of infected animals and where dairy products are routinely pasteurized, illness has historically occurred primarily in individuals who have occupational exposure to infected animals (eg, veterinarians, shepherds, cattlemen, slaughterhouse workers). In many other countries, humans more commonly acquire infection by ingestion of unpasteurized dairy products, especially cheese. In the last 2 decades, food-borne acquisition has also become relatively more frequent in the United States because of importation of contaminated food from Mexico.[294]

Less obvious exposures can also lead to infection. In Kuwait, for example, disease with a relatively high proportion of respiratory complaints has occurred in individuals who camped in the desert during the spring lambing season.[295] In Australia, an outbreak of *B suis* infection was noted in hunters of feral pigs.[296] Brucellae are also highly infectious in laboratory settings.

Geographic Distribution and Incidence

Brucella organisms are distributed worldwide. Fewer than 200 total cases per year (0.04 cases per 100,000 population) are reported in the United States. The incidence is much higher in the Middle East, countries bordering the Mediterranean Sea, China, India, Mexico, and Peru. For example, the incidence rate in Jordan was 33 cases per 100,000 population (1987)[297] and in Kuwait was 88 cases per 100,000 (1985).[298]

Pathogenesis and Clinical Findings

Brucellae can enter mammalian hosts through skin abrasions or cuts, the conjunctiva, the respiratory tract, and the gastrointestinal tract.[299] In the gastrointestinal tract, the organisms are phagocytosed by lymphoepithelial cells of gut-associated lymphoid tissue, from which they gain access to the submucosa.[300] Organisms are rapidly ingested by polymorphonuclear leukocytes, which generally fail to kill them,[301,302] and are also phagocytosed by macrophages. Bacteria transported in macrophages may eventually localize in lymph nodes, liver, spleen, mammary glands, joints, kidneys, and bone marrow. This wide distribution of infected macrophages throughout the mononuclear phagocyte system and other organs explains the prominence of nonspecific constitutional symptoms and diverse localization of abnormalities in this disease.

If unchecked by macrophages, the bacteria destroy their host cells and infect additional cells. Brucellae can also replicate extracellularly. The host cellular response may range from abscess formation to lymphocytic infiltration to granuloma formation with caseous necrosis.

In ruminants, *Brucella* organisms target embryonic and trophoblastic tissue. When septic abortion occurs, the intense concentration of bacteria and aerosolization of infected tissue during parturition often result in infection of other animals and people.

Clinical manifestations of brucellosis are diverse.[303] Patients may present with an acute, systemic febrile illness, an insidious chronic infection, or a localized inflammatory process. Disease may be abrupt or insidious in onset, with an incubation period of 3 days to several weeks. Patients usually complain of nonspecific symptoms such as fever, sweats, fatigue, anorexia, and muscle or joint aches (Table 36-8). Neuropsychiatric symptoms, notably depression, headache, and irritability, occur frequently. In addition, focal infection of bone, joints,

TABLE 36-8

SYMPTOMS AND SIGNS OF BRUCELLOSIS

Symptom or Sign	Patients Affected (%)
Fever	90-95
Malaise	80-95
Sweats	40-90
Body Aches	40-70
Hepatomegaly	10-70
Arthralgia	20-40
Splenomegaly	10-30

Data sources: Mousa AR, Elhag KM, Khogaii M, Marafie AA. The nature of human brucellosis in Kuwait: Study of 379 cases. *Rev Infect Dis.* 1988;10:211–217; Buchanan TM, Faber LC, Feldman RA. Brucellosis in the United States, 1960-1972: An abattoir-associated disease, I: Clinical features and therapy. *Medicine (Baltimore).* 1974;53:403–413; and Gotuzzo E, Alarcon GS, Bocanegra TS, et al. Articular involvement in human brucellosis: A retrospective analysis of 304 cases. *Semin Arthritis Rheum.* 1982;12:245–255.

or genitourinary tract may cause local pain. Cough, pleuritic chest pain, and dyspepsia may also be noted. Chronically infected patients frequently lose weight. Symptoms often last for 3 to 6 months and occasionally for a year or more. Physical examination is usually normal, although hepatomegaly, splenomegaly, or lymphadenopathy may occur. Brucellosis does not usually cause leukocytosis, and some patients may be moderately neutropenic. Although disease manifestations cannot be strictly related to the infecting species, *B melitensis* tends to cause more severe, systemic illness than the other brucellae, and *B suis* is more likely to cause localized, suppurative disease.

Infection with *B melitensis* leads to bone or joint disease in about 30% of patients; sacroiliitis3 develops in 6% to 15%, particularly in young adults.[304,305] Arthritis of all large joints combined occurs with about the same frequency as sacroiliitis. Joint inflammation seen in patients with *B melitensis* is mild, and erythema of overlying skin is uncommon. Synovial fluid is exudative, but cell counts are in the low thousands with predominantly mononuclear cells. Spondylitis, another important osteoarticular manifestation of brucellosis, tends to affect middle-aged or elderly patients, causing back (usually lumbar) pain, local tenderness, and occasionally radicular symptoms.

Magnetic resonance imaging, computer assisted tomography, and bone scintigraphy are more sensitive than plain films for demonstration of bone and joint abnormalities.[306] In sacroiliitis and peripheral joint infections, destruction of bone is unusual. In spondylitis, erosion and sclerosis of the anterosuperior portion of the vertebrae, often accompanied by osteophyte formation, occur early. Magnetic resonance imaging shows an increased T2-weighted signal. Later, diffuse involvement of vertebrae may lead to further destruction of vertebral bodies and nuclear herniation into the softened vertebral bodies. Paravertebral abscess occurs rarely. In contrast with frequent infection of the axial skeleton, osteomyelitis of long bones is rare.[307]

Infection of the genitourinary tract may lead to signs and symptoms of disease in humans.[308] Pyelonephritis and cystitis and, in males, epididymoorchitis, may occur. Both diseases may mimic their tuberculous counterparts, with "sterile" pyuria on routine bacteriologic culture. With bladder and kidney infection, *Brucella* organisms can be cultured from the urine. Brucellosis in pregnancy can lead to placental and fetal infection.[309] Whether abortion is more common in brucellosis than in other severe bacterial infections, however, is unknown.

Lung infections have also been described, particularly before the advent of effective antibiotics. Although up to one quarter of patients with brucellosis may complain of respiratory symptoms (eg, cough, dyspnea, or pleuritic pain), chest X-ray examinations are usually normal.[310] Diffuse or focal infiltrates, pleural effusion, abscess, and granulomas may be noted.

Hepatitis and, rarely, liver abscess also occur. Mild elevations of serum lactate dehydrogenase and alkaline phosphatase are common. Biopsy may show well-formed granulomas or nonspecific hepatitis with collections of mononuclear cells.[303] Other sites of infection include the heart, central nervous system, and skin. Brucella endocarditis, a rare but most feared complication, accounts for 80% of deaths from brucellosis.[311] Central nervous system infection usually manifests itself as chronic meningoencephalitis, but subarachnoid hemorrhage and myelitis also occur.

Diagnostic Approaches

A thorough history that elicits details of possible exposure (eg, laboratories, animals, animal products, or environmental exposure to locations inhabited by potentially infected animals) is the most important diagnostic tool. Personnel with certain military occupations and symptoms compatible with brucellosis should be questioned particularly closely. Veterinary medicine officers assume responsibility for meat inspection and may visit slaughterhouses, especially during deployments. Special Forces personnel may subsist on the local economy during some actions and ingest unpasteurized dairy products. Brucellosis should also be strongly considered in the differential diagnosis of febrile illness if service members have been exposed to a presumed biological attack. Polymerase chain reaction and antibody-based antigen detection systems may demonstrate the presence of the organism in environmental samples collected from the attack area.

When the disease is considered, diagnosis is usually made by serology. The tube agglutination test remains the standard method.[312] Use of the tube agglutination test after treatment of serum with 2-mercaptoethanol or dithiothreitol to dissociate IgM into monomers detects IgG antibody. A titer of 1:160 or higher is considered diagnostic. Most patients already have high titers at the time of clinical presentation, so a 4-fold rise in titer may not occur. IgM rises early in disease and may persist at low levels (eg, 1:20) for months or years after successful treatment. Persistence or increase of 2-mercaptoethanol–

resistant titers has been associated with persistent disease or relapse. Serum testing should always include dilution to at least 1:320, since inhibition of agglutination at lower dilutions may occur. The tube agglutination test does not detect antibodies to *B canis*. Enzyme-linked immunosorbent assays have been developed but are not well standardized.

Diagnosis should be pursued by microbiologic culture of blood or body fluid samples. Cultures should be held for at least 2 months and subcultured weekly onto solid medium. Because it is extremely infectious for laboratory workers, the organism should be subcultured only in a biohazard hood. The reported frequency of isolation from blood varies widely, from less than 10% to 90%; *B melitensis* is said to be more readily cultured than *B abortus*. Culture of bone marrow may increase the yield.[313]

Recommendations for Therapy and Control

Brucellae are sensitive in vitro to a number of oral antibiotics and to aminoglycosides. Therapy with a single drug has resulted in a high relapse rate, so combined regimens should be used whenever possible.[314] A 6-week regimen of doxycycline 200 mg per day administered orally with streptomycin 1 g per day administered intramuscularly for the first 2 to 3 weeks is effective therapy for adults with most forms of brucellosis.[315] Gentamicin, 2 to 5 mg per kg per day, is now often substituted for streptomycin.[291] A 6-week oral regimen of both rifampin (900 mg/day) and doxycycline (200 mg/day) is also effective and should result in nearly 100% response and a relapse rate of lower than 10%. Treatment with a combination of streptomycin and doxycycline may result in less frequent relapse than treatment with the combination of rifampin and doxycycline.[315]

Spondylitis, endocarditis, and central nervous system infections generally require prolonged therapy. Spondylitis should be treated with a regimen that includes an aminoglycoside, as notable failures have occurred in patients treated with the combination of rifampin and doxycycline. Endocarditis may best be treated with rifampin, streptomycin, and doxycycline; infected valves should be replaced early in therapy.[316] Central nervous system disease responds to a combination of rifampin and trimethoprim/sulfamethoxazole. This antibiotic combination is also effective for children under 8 years of age.[315] The Joint Food and Agriculture Organization–World Health Organization Expert Committee recommends treatment of pregnant women with rifampin.[317] Trimethoprim/sulfamethoxazole is a reasonable alternative drug in pregnancy.[291]

Organisms used in a biological attack may be resistant to these first-line antimicrobial agents. Medical officers should make very effort to obtain tissue and environmental samples for bacteriological culture, so that the antibiotic susceptibility profile of the infecting brucellae may be determined and the therapy adjusted accordingly.

Effective livestock immunization programs will markedly reduce the incidence of human disease. Animal handlers should wear appropriate protective clothing when working with infected animals. Meat should be well-cooked, and milk should be pasteurized. Service members in endemic areas should be counseled to avoid eating uncooked foods, particularly dairy products, obtained from the local economy. Sheep, goats, cattle, swine, and camels in endemic areas should be considered infected. Locating camps close to these animals should be avoided, particularly during birthing seasons; animals should be segregated from military personnel. Laboratory workers should culture the organism only with appropriate biosafety level 2 (clinical samples) or 3 (research) containment.

In the event of a biological attack, the standard gas mask should adequately protect personnel from airborne brucellae, because the organisms are probably unable to penetrate intact skin. After personnel have been evacuated from the attack area, clothing, skin, and other surfaces can be decontaminated with standard disinfectants to minimize risk of infection by accidental ingestion or by conjunctival inoculation of viable organisms.

There is no commercially available vaccine for humans. In the event of known percutaneous or mucosal exposure to virulent or vaccinal strains of *Brucella*, prophylactic administration of rifampin and tetracycline for 3 to 6 weeks seems reasonable.[57p75–78,291]

[David Hoover]

REFERENCES

1. Berman SJ, Tsai C, Holmes K, Fresh JW, Watten RH. Sporadic anicteric leptospirosis in South Vietnam: A study in 150 patients. *Ann Intern Med*. 1973:79:167–173.

2. Takafuji ET, Kirkpatrick JW, Miller RN, et al. An efficacy trial of doxycycline chemoprophylaxis against leptospirosis. *N Engl J Med*. 1984;310:497–500.

3. Torten M. Leptospirosis. In: Steele JH, ed. *Handbook Series in Zoonoses*. Vol 1. Boca Raton, Fla: CRC Press; 1979: pp 363–421.

4. Feigin RD, Lobes LA, Anderson D, Pickering L. Human leptospirosis from immunized dogs. *Ann Intern Med*. 1973;79:777–785.

5. Kaufmann AF. Epidemiologic trends of leptospirosis in the United States, 1965-1974. In: Johnson RC, ed. *The Biology of Parasitic Spirochetes*. New York: Academic Press; 1976: pp 177-190.

6. Wilkins E, Cope A, Waitkins S. Rapids, rafts, and rats. *Lancet*. 1988;2:283–284.

7. Sanford JP. Leptospirosis—time for a booster. *N Engl J Med*. 1984;310:524–525.

8. Faine S, ed. *Guidelines for the Control of Leptospirosis*. Geneva: World Health Organization; 1982.

9. Bolin CA, Koellner P. Human-to-human transmission of *Leptospira interrogans* by milk. *J Infect Dis*. 1988;158:246–247.

10. Feigin RD, Anderson DC. Human leptospirosis. *CRC Crit Rev Clin Lab Sci*. 1975;5:413–467.

11. Shpilberg O, Shaked Y, Maier MK, Samra D, Samra J. Long-term follow-up after leptospirosis. *South Med J*. 1990;83:405–407.

12. Thiermann AB: Leptospirosis: Current developments and trends. *J Am Vet Med Assoc*. 1984;184;722–725.

13. McClain JB, Ballou WR, Harrison SM, Steinweg DL. Doxycycline therapy for leptospirosis. *Ann Intern Med*. 1984;100:696–698.

14. Kocen RS. Leptospirosis: A comparison of symptomatic and penicillin therapy. *Br Med J.* 1962;1:1181.

15. Watt G, Padre LP, Tuazon ML, Everard CO, Callender J. Placebo-controlled trial of intravenous penicillin for severe and late leptospirosis. *Lancet.* 1988;1:433–435.

16. Edwards CN, Nicholson GD, Hassell TA, et al. Penicillin therapy in icteric leptospirosis. *Am J Trop Med Hyg.* 1988;39:388–390.

17. Alexander AD, Rule PL. Penicillins, cephalosporins, and tetracyclines in treatment of hamsters with fatal leptospirosis. *Antimicrob Agents Chemother.* 1986;30:835–839.

18. Gajdusek DC. Virus hemorrhagic fevers with special reference to hemorrhagic fever with renal syndrome (epidemic hemorrhagic fever). *J Peds.* 1962;60:841–857.

19. Lahdevirta J. Nephropathia epidemica in Finland: A clinical, histological and epidemiological study. *Ann Clin Res (Helsinki).* 1971;3(suppl 8):1–154.

20. Trencseni T, Keleti B. *Clinical Aspects and Epidemiology of Haemorrhagic Fever with Renal Syndrome: Analysis of Clinical and Epidemiological Experiences in Hungary.* Budapest: Akademiai Kiado; 1971.

21. McKee KT Jr, LeDuc JW, Peters CJ. Hantaviruses. In: Belshe RB, ed. *Textbook of Human Virology.* 2nd ed. St. Louis: Mosby Year Book; 1991: 615–632.

22. Lee HW, Lee P-W, Johnson KM. Isolation of the etiological agent of Korean hemorrhagic fever. *J Infect Dis.* 1978;137:298–308.

23. Pon E, McKee KT Jr, Diniega BM, Merrel B, Corwin A, Ksiazek TG. Outbreak of hemorrhagic fever with renal syndrome among U.S. Marines in Korea. *Am J Trop Med Hyg.* 1990;42:612–619.

24. Underwood PK. Chief, Preventive Medicine Service, US Army Medical Department Activity, Neurnberg. Personal communication, 1992.

25. Schmaljohn CS, Hasty SE, Dalrymple JM, et al. Antigenic and genetic properties of viruses linked to hemorrhagic fever with renal syndrome. *Science.* 1985;227:1041–1044.

26. LeDuc JW. Epidemiology of Hantaan and related viruses. *Lab Anim Sci.* 1987;37:413–418.

27. Chapman LE, McKee KT Jr, Peters CJ. Hantaviruses. In: Feigin RD, Cherry JD, eds. *Textbook of Pediatric Infectious Diseases.* 4th ed. Philadelphia: W.B. Saunders; 1998: 2141–2150.

28. Schmaljohn C, Hjelle B. Hantaviruses: A global disease problem. *Emerg Infect Dis.* 1997;3:95–104.

29. Peters CJ. Hantavirus pulmonary syndrome—the Americas. Scheld WM, Craig WA, Hughes JM, eds. *Emerging Infections.* Washington, DC: ASM Press; 1998.

30. Lee HW, French GR, Lee PW, Baek LJ, Tsuchiya K, Foulke RS. Observations on natural and laboratory infection of rodents with the etiologic agent of Korean hemorrhagic fever. *Am J Trop Med Hyg.* 1981;30:477–482.

31. Yanagihara R. Hantavirus infection in the United States: Epizootology and epidemiology. *Rev Infect Dis.* 1990;12:449–457.

32. Lee HW, Lee PW, Baek LJ, Chu YK. Geographical distribution of hemorrhagic fever with renal syndrome and hantaviruses. *Arch Virol.* 1990;115 (Suppl 1):5–18.

33. Settergren B. Nephropathia epidemica (hemorrhagic fever with renal syndrome) in Scandinavia. *Rev Infect Dis.* 1991;13:736–744.

34. Avsic-Zupanc T, Likar M, Navakovic S, et al. Evidence of the presence of two hantaviruses in Slovenia. *Arch Virol*. 1990;115(Suppl 1):87–94.

35. Avsic-Zupanc T, Xiao SY, Stojanovic R, Gligic A, van der Groen G, LeDuc JW. Characterization of Dobrava virus: A hantavirus from Slovenia, Yugoslavia. *J Med Virol*. 1992;38:132–137.

36. Gligic A, Dimkovic N, Xiao SY, et al. Belgrade virus: A new hantavirus causing severe hemorrhagic fever with renal syndrome in Yugoslavia. *J Infect Dis*. 1992;166:113–120.

37. Nichol ST, Spiropoulou CF, Morzunov S, et al. Genetic identification of a hantavirus associated with an outbreak of acute respiratory illness. *Science*. 1993;262:914–917.

38. Elliott LH, Ksiazek TG, Rollin PE, et al. Isolation of the causative agent of hantavirus pulmonary syndrome. *Am J Trop Med Hyg*. 1994;51:102–108.

39. Ksiazek TG, Peters CJ, Rollin PE, et al. Identification of a new North American hantavirus that causes acute pulmonary insufficiency. *Am J Trop Med Hyg*. 1995;52:117–123.

40. Rollin PE, Ksiazek TG, Elliott LH, et al. Isolation of Black Creek Canal virus, a new hantavirus from *Sigmodon hispidus* in Florida. *J Med Virol*. 1995;46:35–39.

41. Morzunov SP, Feldmann H, Spiropoulou CF, et al. A newly recognized virus associated with a fatal case of hantavirus pulmonary syndrome in Louisiana. *J Virol*. 1995;69:1980–1983.

42. Khan AS, Ksiazek TG, Peters CJ. Hantavirus pulmonary syndrome. *Lancet*. 1996;347:739–741.

43. Lee HW. Epidemiology. In: Lee HW, Dalrymple JM, eds. *Manual of Hemorrhagic Fever with Renal Syndrome*. Seoul: World Health Organization Collaborating Center for Virus Reference and Research Institute for Viral Diseases and Korea University; 1989: 39–48.

44. Desmyter J, LeDuc JW, Johnson KM, Brasseur, Deckers C, van Ypersele de Strihou C. Laboratory rat associated outbreak of haemorrhagic fever with renal syndrome due to Hantaan-like virus in Belgium. *Lancet*. 1983;2:1445–1448.

45. Glass GE, Watson AJ, LeDuc JW, Kelem GD, Quinn TC, Childs JE. Infection with ratborne hantavirus in US residents is consistently associated with hypertensive renal disease. *J Infect Dis*. 1993;167:614–620.

46. Butler JC, Peters CJ. Hantaviruses and hantavirus pulmonary syndrome. *Clin Infect Dis*. 1994;19:387–394.

47. Chapman LE. Hantaviruses. *Sem Ped Infect Dis*. 1996;7:97–100.

48. Koster FT. Professor of Medicine, University of New Mexico Health Sciences Center, June 1997. Personal communication

49. Lee PW, Meegan JM, LeDuc JW, et al. Serologic techniques for detection of Hantaan virus infection, related antigens and antibodies. In: Lee HW, Dalrymple JM, eds. *Manual of Hemorrhagic Fever with Renal Syndrome*. Seoul: World Health Organization Collaborating Center for Virus Reference and Research Institute for Viral Diseases, and Korea University; 1989: 75–106.

50. Feldmann H, Sanchez A, Morzunov S, et al. Utilization of autopsy RNA for the synthesis of the nucleocapsid antigen of a newly recognized virus associated with hantavirus pulmonary syndrome. *Virus Res*. 1993;30:351–367.

51. Enria D, Padula P, Segura EL, et al. Hantavirus pulmonary syndrome in Argentina: Possibility of person to person transmission. *Medicina (B Aires)* 1996; 56: 709–711.

52. Huggins JW, Hsiang CM, Cosgriff TM, et al. Prospective, double-blind, concurrent, placebo-controlled clinical trial of intravenous ribavirin therapy of hemorrhagic fever with renal syndrome. *J Infect Dis*. 1991;164:1119–1127.

53. Armed Forces Pest Management Board. *Protection from Rodent-Borne Diseases, With Special Emphasis on Occupational Exposure to Hantavirus.* Washington, DC: Defense Pest Management and Information and Analysis Center and the Deputy Under Secretary of Defense for Environmental Security; 1999. Technical Information Memorandum 41.

54. Benenson MW, Takafuji ET, Lemon SM, Greenup RL, Sulzer AJ. Oocyst-transmitted toxoplasmosis associated with ingestion of contaminated water. *N Engl J Med.* 1982;307:666–669.

55. Nicolle C, Manceaux LH. Sur une infection á corps de Leishman (ou organismes voisins) du gondi. *Comptes Rendus Hebdomadaires des Séances de l'Académie des Sciences.* 1908;147:763–766.

56. Jank J. Pathogenesa a pathologická anatomie tak nazuného vrozeného kolobome zluté skvrny v oku normálne velikém a mikrophthalmickém s nálezem parazitu v sítnici. *Cas Lék Ces.* 1923;62:1021–1027,1054–1059,1081–1085,1111–1115,1138–1144.

57. Chin J, ed. *Control of Communicable Diseases Manual.* 17th ed. Washington, DC: American Public Health Association; 2000.

58. Krick JA,Remington JS. Toxoplasmosis in the adult—an overview. *N Engl J Med.* 1978;298:550–553.

59. Nussenblatt RB, Belfort R. Ocular toxoplasmosis: An old disease revisited. *JAMA.* 1994;271:304–307.

60. Jackson MH, Hutchison WM. The prevalence and source of *Toxoplasma* infection in the environment. *Adv Parasitol.* 1989;28:55–105.

61. Scott RJ. Toxoplasmosis. *Trop Dis Bull.* 1978;75:809–827.

62. Garcia LS, Sulzer AJ, Healy GR, Grady KK, Brukner DA. Blood and tissue protozoa. In: Murray PR, Baron EJ, Pfaller MA, Tenover FC, Yolken RH, eds. *Manual of Clinical Microbiology.* 6th ed. Washington, DC: ASM Press; 1995: 1171–1195.

63. Sibley LD, Boothroyd JC. Virulent strains of *Toxoplasma gondii* comprise a single clonal lineage. *Nature.* 1992;359:82–85.

64. Frenkel JK, Ruiz A, Chinchilla M. Soil survival of *Toxoplasma* oocysts in Kansas and Costa Rica. *Am J Trop Med Hyg.* 1975;24:439–443.

65. Yilmaz SM, Hopkins SH. Effects of different conditions on duration of infectivity of *Toxoplasma gondii* oocysts. *J Parasitol.* 1972;58:938–939.

66. Dubey JP, Beattie CP. Toxoplasmosis of animals and man. Boca Raton, Fla: CRC Press; 1988.

67. Glaser CA, Angulo FJ, Rooney JA. Animal-associated opportunistic infections among persons infected with the human immunodeficiency virus. *Clin Infect Dis.* 1994;18:14–24.

68. Dubey JP. Reshedding of *Toxoplasma* oocysts by chronically infected cats. *Nature.* 1976;262:213–214.

69. Beaman MH, McCabe RE, Wong SY, Remington JS. *Toxoplasma gondii.* In: Mandell GL, Bennett JE, Dolin R, eds. *Principles and Practice of Infectious Diseases.* 4th ed. New York: Churchill Livingstone; 1995: 2455–2475.

70. Feldman HA. Toxoplasmosis. *N Engl J Med.* 1968;279:1370–1375.

71. Jewell ML, Frenkel JK, Johnson KM, Reed V, Ruiz A. Development of *Toxoplasma* oocysts in neotropical *Felidae.* *Am J Trop Med Hyg.* 1972;21:512–517.

72. Frenkel JK. Toxoplasmosis. In: Binford CH, Connor DH, eds. *Pathology of Tropical and Extraordinary Diseases.* Vol 1. Washington, DC: Armed Forces Institute of Pathology; 1976: 284–300.

73. Feldman HA, Miller LT. Serological study of toxoplasmosis prevalence. *Am J Hyg*. 1956;64:320–335.

74. Smith KL, Wilson M, Hightower AW, et al. Prevalence of *Toxoplasma gondii* antibodies in US military recruits in 1989: Comparison with data published in 1965. *Clin Infect Dis*. 1996;23:1182–1183.

75. Feldman HA. A nationwide serum survey of United States military recruits, 1962, VI: *Toxoplasma* antibodies. *Am J Epidemiol*. 1965;81:385–391.

76. Feldman HA. Toxoplasmosis. *N Engl J Med*. 1968;279:1431–1437 (conclusion).

77. McCabe RE, Brooks RG, Dorfman RF, Remington JS. Clinical spectrum in 107 cases of toxoplasmic lymphaden-opathy. *Rev Infect Dis*. 1987;9:754–774.

78. Wong SY, Remington JS. Toxoplasmosis in pregnancy. *Clin Infect Dis*. 1994;18:853–862.

79. Remington JS. Toxoplasmosis in the adult. *Bull N Y Acad Med*. 1974;50:211–227.

80. Elliot DL, Tollf SW, Goldberg L, Miller JB. Pet-associated illness. *N Engl J Med*. 1985;313:985–995.

81. Remington JS, McLeod R, Desmonts G. Toxoplasmosis. In: Remington JS, Klein JO, eds. *Infectious Diseases of the Fetus and Newborn Infant*. 4th ed. Phildelphia: W.B. Saunders; 1995: 140–267.

82. Sabin AB, Feldman HA. Dyes as microchemical indicators of a new immunity phenomenon affecting a proto-zoon parasite (*Toxoplasma*). *Science*. 1948;108:660–663.

83. Sulzer AJ, Franco EL, Takafuji ET, Benenson MW, Walls KW, Greenup RL. An oocyst-transmitted outbreak of toxoplasmosis: Patterns of immunoglobulin G and M over one year. *Am J Trop Med Hyg*. 1986;35:290–296.

84. Brooks RG, McCabe RE, Remington JS. Role of serology in the diagnosis of toxoplasmic lymphadenopathy. *Rev Infect Dis*. 1987;9:1055–1062.

85. Tomasi JP, Schlit AF, Stadtsbaeder S. Rapid double-sandwich enzyme-linked immunosorbent assay for detec-tion of human immunoglobulin M anti-*Toxoplasma gondii* antibodies. *J Clin Microbiol*. 1986;24:849–850.

86. Desmonts G, Couvreur J. Congenital toxoplasmosis: A prospective study of 378 pregnancies. *N Engl J Med*. 1974;290:1110–1116.

87. Ho-Yen DO, Joss AWL, Balfour AH, Smyth ET, Baird D, Chatterton JM. Use of the polymerase chain reaction to detect *Toxoplasma gondii* in human blood samples. *J Clin Pathol*. 1992;45:910–913.

88. Depouy-Camet J, de Souza SL, Maslo C, et al. Detection of *Toxoplasma gondii* in venous blood from AIDS pa-tients by polymerase chain reaction. *J Clin Microbiol*. 1993;31:1866–1869.

89. Dannemann BR, Israelski DM, Remington JS. Treatment of toxoplasmic encephalitis with intravenous clindamycin. *Arch Intern Med*. 1988;148:2477–2482.

90. Dannemann B, McCutchan JA, Israelski D, et al. Treatment of toxoplasmic encephalitis in patients with AIDS: A randomized trial comparing pyrimethamine plus clindamycin to pyrimethamine plus sulfadizine. *Ann In-tern Med*. 1992;116:33–43.

91. Spicer AJ. Military significance of Q fever: A review. *J R Soc Med*. 1978;71:762–767.

92. Robbins FC, Ragan CA. Q fever in the Mediterranean area: Report of its occurrence in allied troops, I: Clinical features of the disease. Am J Hyg. 1946;44:6–22.

93. Robbins FC, Gauld RL, Warner FB. Q fever in the Mediterranean area: Report of its occurrence in allied troops, II: Epidemiology. Am J Hyg. 1946;44:23–50.

94. The Commission of Acute Respiratory Diseases. Epidemics of Q fever among troops returning from Italy in the spring of 1945, III: Etiological studies. Am J Hyg. 1946;44:88–102.

95. Feinstein M, Yesner R, Marks JL. Epidemics of Q fever among troops returning from Italy in the spring of 1945, I: Clinical aspects of the epidemic at Camp Patrick Henry, Virginia. *Am J Hyg.* 1946;44:72–87.

96. Spicer AJ, Crawther RW, Vella EE, Bengtsson E, Miles R, Ritzolis G. Q fever and animal abortion in Cyprus. Trans R Soc Trop Med Hyg. 1977;71:16–20.

97. Rombo L, Bengtsson E, Grandien M. Serum Q fever antibodies in Swedish UN soldiers in Cyprus: Reflecting a domestic or foreign disease? *Scand J Infect Dis.* 1978;10:157–158.

98. Ferrante MA, Dolan MJ. Q fever meningoencephalitis in a soldier returning from the Persian Gulf War. *Clin Infect Dis.* 1993;16:489–496.

99. World Health Organization. *Health Aspects of Chemical and Biological Weapons: Report of a WHO Group of Consultants.* Geneva: WHO; 1970: 72, 99.

100. Department of the Army. *US Army Activity on the US Biological Warfare Programs: 1942-1977: Annexes.* Vol 2. DA; 1977.

101. Weisburg WG, Dobson ME, Samuel JE, et al. Phylogenetic diversity of the rickettsias. *J Bacteriol.* 1989;171:4202–4206.

102. Williams JC. Infectivity, virulence, and pathogenicity of *Coxiella burnetii* for various hosts. In: Williams JC, Thompson HA, eds. *Q Fever: The Biology of* Coxiella burnetii. Boca Raton, Fla: CRC Press; 1991.

103. McCaul TF, Dare AJ, Gannon JP, Galbraith AJ. In vivo endogenous spore formation by *Coxiella burnetii* in Q fever endocarditis. *J Clin Pathol.* 1994;47:978–981.

104. Stoker MGP, Fiset P. Phase variation of the Nine Mile and other strains of *Rickettsia burnetii. Can J Microbiol.* 1956;2:310–321.

105. Tigertt WD, Benenson AS. Studies on Q fever in man. *Trans Assoc Am Phys.* 1956;69:98–104.

106. Oliphant JW, Gordon DA, Meis A, Parker RR. Q fever in laundry workers presumably transmitted from contaminated clothing. *Am J Hyg.* 1949;49:76–82.

107. Marrie TJ, Langille D, Papukna V, Yates L. Truckin' pneumonia—an outbreak of Q fever in a truck repair plant probably due to aerosols from clothing contaminated by contact with newborn kittens. *Epidemiol Infect.* 1989;102:119–127.

108. Salmon MM, Howells B, Glencross EJ, Evans AD, Palmer SR. Q fever in an urban area. *Lancet.* 1982;1:1002–1004.

109. Mann JS, Douglas JG, Inglis JM, Leitch AG. Q fever: Person to person transmission within a family. *Thorax.* 1986;41:974–975.

110. Kaplan MM, Bertagna P. The geographical distribution of Q fever. *Bull World Health Organ.* 1955;13:829–860.

111. Wisniewski HJ, Piraino FF. Review of virus respiratory infections in the Milwaukee area, 1955–1965. *Public Health Reports.* 1969;84:175–181.

112. Epidemiology of a Q fever outbreak in Los Angeles County, 1966. *HSMHA Health Reports.* 1972;87:71–74.

113. Pinsky RL, Fishbein DB, Greene CR, Gensheimer KF. An outbreak of cat-associated Q fever in the United States. J Infect Dis. 1991;164:202–204.

114. Langley JM, Marrie TJ, Covert A, Waag DM, Williams JC. Poker players' pneumonia: An urban outbreak of Q fever following exposure to a parturient cat. *N Engl J Med.* 1988;319:354–356.

115. Centers for Disease Control. Q fever among slaughterhouse workers—California. *MMWR.* 1986;35:223–226.

116. Meiklejohn G, Reimer LG, Graves PS, Helmick C. Cryptic epidemic of Q fever in a medical school. *J Infect Dis.* 1981;144:107–113.

117. Rauch AM, Tanner M, Pacer RE, Barrett MJ, Brokopp CD, Schonberger LB. Sheep-associated outbreak of Q fever, Idaho. *Arch Intern Med.* 1987;147:341–344.

118. Graham CJ, Yamauchi T, Rountree P. Q fever in animal laboratory workers: An outbreak and its investigation. *Am J Infect Control.* 1989;17:345–348.

119. Hamadeh GN, Turner BW, Trible W Jr, Hoffmann BJ, Anderson RM. Laboratory outbreak of Q fever. *J Fam Pract.* 1992;35:683–685.

120. D'Angelo LJ, Baker EF, Schlosser W. Q fever in the United States, 1948–1977. *J Infect Dis.* 1979;139:613–615.

121. Sawyer LA, Fishbein DB, McDade JE. Q fever in patients with hepatitis and pneumonia: Results of a laboratory-based surveillance in the United States. *J Infect Dis.* 1988;158:497–498.

122. Sienko DG, Bartlett PC, McGee HB, Wentworth BB, Herndon JL, Hall WN. Q fever: A call to heighten our index of suspicion. *Arch Intern Med.* 1988;148:609–612.

123. Dupuis G, Petite J, Peter O, Vouilloz M. An important outbreak of human Q fever in a Swiss Alpine valley. *Int J Epidemiol.* 1987;16:282–287.

124. Raoult D, Marrie TJ. State-of-the-art clinical lecture: Q fever. *Clin Infect Dis.* 1995;20:489–496.

125. Tissot Dupont H, Raoult D, Brouqui P. Epidemiologic features and clinical presentation of acute Q fever in hospitalized patients: 323 French cases. *Am J Med.* 1992;93:427–434.

126. Smith DL, Ayres JG, Blair I, et al. A large Q fever outbreak in the West Midlands: Clinical aspects. *Respir Med.* 1993;87:509–516.

127. Derrick EH. The course of infection with *Coxiella burnetii. Med J Aust.* 1973;1:1051–1057.

128. Smith DL, Wellings R, Walker C, Ayres JG, Burge PS. The chest x-ray in Q fever: A report on 69 cases from the 1989 West Midlands outbreak. *Br J Radiol.* 1991;64:1101–1108.

129. Marmion BP, Shannon M, Maddocks I, Storm P, Penttila I. Protracted fatigue and debility after Q fever. *Lancet.* 1996;347:977–978.

130. Ayres JG, Smith EG, Flint N. Protracted fatigue and debility after acute Q fever. *Lancet.* 2996;347:978–979.

131. Ayres JG, Flint N, Smith EG, et al. Post-infection fatigue syndrome following Q fever. *QJM.* 1998;91:105–123.

132. Peter O, Dupuis G, Peacock MG, Burgdorfer W. Comparison of enzyme-linked immunosorbent assay and complement fixation and indirect fluorescent-antibody tests for detection of *Coxiella burnetti* antibody. *J Clin Microbiol.* 1987;25:1063–1067.

133. Uhaa IJ, Fishbein DB, Olson JG, Rives CC, Waag DM, Williams JC. Evaluation of specificity of indirect enzyme-linked immunosorbent assay for diagnosis of human Q fever. *J Clin Microbiol.* 1994;32:1560–1565.

134. Waag D, Chulay J, Marrie T, England M, Williams J. Validation of an enzyme immunoassay for serodiagnosis of acute Q fever. *Eur J Clin Microbiol Infect Dis.* 1995;14:421–427.

135. Hoover TA, Vodkin MH, Williams JC. A *Coxiella burnetii* repeated DNA element resembling a bacterial insertion sequence. *J Bacteriol.* 1992;174:5540–5548.

136. Stein A, Raoult D. Detection of *Coxiella burnetii* by DNA amplification using polymerase chain reaction. *J Clin Microbiol.* 1992;30:2462–2466.

137. Willems H, Thiele D, Krauss H. Plasmid based differentiation and detection of *Coxiella burnetii* in clinical samples. *Eur J Epidemiol.* 1993;9:411–418.

138. Raoult D. Treatment of Q fever. *Antimicrob Agents Chemother.* 1993;37:1733–1736.

139. Tselentis Y, Gikas A, Kofteridis D. Q fever in the Greek island of Crete: Epidemiologic, clinical, and therapeutic data from 98 cases. *Clin Infect Dis.* 1995;20:1311–1316.

140. Sobradillo V, Zalacain R, Capelastegui A, Uresandi F, Corral J. Antibiotic treatment in pneumonia due to Q fever. *Thorax.* 1992;47:276–278.

141. Benenson AS. Q fever vaccine: Efficacy and present status. In: Smadel JE, ed. *Symposium on Q Fever by the Committee on Rickettsial Diseases.* Washington, DC: Armed Forces Epidemiology Board; 1959: 47–60.

142. Bell JF, Lackman DB, Meis A, Hadlow WJ. Recurrent reaction at site of Q fever vaccination in a sensitized person. *Mil Med.* 1964;124:591–595.

143. Lackman DB, Bell EJ, Bell JF, Pickens EG. Intradermal sensitivity testing in man with a purified vaccine for Q fever. *Am J Public Health.* 1962;52:87–93.

144. Scott GH, Williams JC. Susceptibility of *Coxiella burnetii* to chemical disinfectants.

145. Monath TP, Newhouse VF, Kemp GE, Setzer HW, Cacciapouti A. Lassa virus isolation from *Mastomys natalensis* rodents during an epidemic in Sierra Leone. *Science.* 1974;185:263–265.

146. Ter Meulen J, Lukashevich I, Sidibe K, et al. Hunting of peridomestic rodents and consumption of their meat as possible risk factors for rodent-to-human transmission of Lassa virus in the Republic of Guinea. *Am J Trop Med Hyg.* 1996;55:661–666.

147. Carey DC, Kemp GE, White HA, et al. Lassa fever—epidemiological aspects of the 1970 epidemic, Jos, Nigeria. *Trans R Soc Trop Med Hyg.* 1972;66:402–408.

148. Monath TP, Mertens PE, Patton R, et al. A hospital epidemic of Lassa fever in Zorzor, Liberia, March-April 1972. *Am J Trop Med Hyg.* 1973;22:773–779.

149. McCormick JB. Epidemiology and control of Lassa fever. *Curr Top Microbiol Immunol.* 1987;134:69–78.

150. McCormick JB, King IJ, Webb PA, et al. A case-control study of the clinical diagnosis and course of Lassa fever. *J Infect Dis.* 1987;155:445–455.

151. Webb PA, McCormick JB, King IJ, et al. Lassa fever in children in Sierra Leone, West Africa. *Trans R Soc Trop Med Hyg.* 1986;80:577–582.

152. Price ME, Fisher-Hoch SP, Craven RB, McCormick JB. A prospective study of maternal and fetal outcome in acute Lassa fever infection during pregnancy. *BMJ.* 1988;297:584–587.

153. Solbrig MV. Lassa virus and central nervous system diseases. In: Salvato MS, ed. *The Arenaviruses.* New York: Plenum Press; 1993: 325–330.

154. Cummins D, McCormick JB, Bennet D, et al. Acute sensorineural deafness in Lassa fever. *JAMA.* 1990;264: 2093–2096.

155. Fisher-Hoch S, McCormick JB, Sasso D, Craven RB. Hematologic dysfunction in Lassa fever. *J Med Virol.* 1988;26:127–135.

156. Johnson KM, McCormick JB, Webb PA, Smith EC, Elliott LH, King IJ. Clinical virology of Lassa fever in hospitalized patients. *J Infect Dis*. 1987;155:456–464.

157. McCormick JB, King IJ, Webb PA, et al. Lassa fever: Effective therapy with ribavirin. *N Eng J Med*. 1986;314:20–26.

158. Maiztegui JI, Feuillade M, Briggiler A. Progressive extension of the endemic area and changing incidence of Argentine hemorrhagic fever. *Med Microbiol Immunol*. 1986;175:149–152.

159. Peters CJ, Kuehne RW, Mercado RR, Le Bow RH, Spertzel RO, Webb PA. Hemorrhagic fever in Cochabamba, Bolivia, 1971. *Am J Epidimiol*. 1974;99:425–433.

160. Centers for Disease Control and Prevention. Bolivian hemorrhagic fever—El Beni Department, Bolivia, 1994. *MMWR*. 1994;43:943–946.

161. MacKenzie RB. Epidemiology of Machupo virus infection, I: Pattern of human infection, San Joachin, Bolivia, 1962–1964. *Am J Trop Med Hyg*. 1965;14:808–813.

162. Salas R, de Manzione N, Tesh RB, et al. Venezuelan haemorrhagic fever. *Lancet*. 1991;338:1033–1036.

163. Fulhorst CE, Bowen MD, Salas RA, et al. Isolation and characterization of Pirital virus, a newly discovered South American arenavirus. *Am J Trop Med Hyg*. 1997;56:548–553.

164. Lisieux T, Coimbra M, Nassar ES, et al. New arenavirus isolated in Brazil. *Lancet*. 1994;343:391–392.

165. Maiztegui JI, Fernandez NJ, de Damilano AJ. Efficacy of immune plasma in treatment of Argentine haemorrhagic fever and association between treatment and a late neurological syndrome. *Lancet*. 1979;2:1216–1217.

166. Enria DA, Briggiler AM, Fernandez NJ, Levis SC, Maiztegui JI. Importance of dose of neutralizing antibodies in treatment of Argentine haemorrhagic fever with immune plasma. *Lancet*. 1984;2:255–256.

167. Maiztegui JI, McKee, KT Jr, Barrera Oro JG, et al. Protective efficacy of a live attenuated vaccine against Argentine hemorrhagic fever. *J Infect Dis*. 1998;177:277–283.

168. World Health Organization. Ebola haemorrhagic fever. *Wkly Epidemiol Rec*. 1995;70:149–151.

169. Martini GA, Siegert R, eds. *Marburg Virus Disease*. New York: Springer-Verlag; 1971.

170. Peters CJ, Sanchez A, Rollin PE, Ksiazek TG, Murphy FA. *Filoviridae*: Marburg and Ebola viruses. In: Fields BN, Knipe DM, Channock RM, Melnick JL, Roizman B, Shope RE, eds. *Virology*. 3rd ed. New York: Raven Press; 1996: 1161–1176.

171. Jahrling PB, Geisbert TW, Dalgard DW, et al. Preliminary report: Isolation of Ebola virus from monkeys imported to USA. *Lancet*. 1990;335:502–505.

172. Casals J. Antigenic similarity between the virus causing Crimean hemorrhagic fever and Congo virus. *Proc Soc Exp Biol Med*. 1969;131:233–236.

173. Burney MI, Ghafoor A, Saleen M, Webb PA, Casals J. Nosocomial outbreak of viral hemorrhagic fever caused by Crimean hemorrhagic fever-Congo virus in Pakistan, January 1976. *Am J Trop Med Hyg*. 1980;29:941–947.

174. Watts DM, Ksiazek TG, Linthicum KJ, Hoogstraal H. Crimean-Congo hemorrhagic fever. In: Monath TP, ed. *The Arboviruses: Epidemiology and Ecology*. Vol 2. Boca Raton, Fla: CRC Press; 1986: 177–222.

175. Swanepoel R, Gill DE, Shepherd AJ, Leman PA, Mynhardt JH, Harvey S. The clinical pathology of Crimean-Congo hemorrhagic fever. *Rev Infect Dis*. 1989;11(Suppl 4):S794–S800.

176. Fisher-Hoch SP, Khan JA, Rehman S, Mirza S, Khurshid M, McCormick JB. Crimean Congo-haemorrhagic fever treated with oral ribavirin. *Lancet*. 1995;346:472–475.

177. Steele JH, Fernandez PJ. History of rabies and global aspects. In: Baer GM, ed. *The Natural History of Rabies*. 2nd ed. Boca Raton, Fla: CRC Press; 1991: 1–24.

178. Steele JH. Rabies in the Americas and remarks on global aspects. *Rev Infect Dis*. 1988;10(Suppl 4):S585–S597.

179. Miller EB, Caldwell GL, Coates JB, eds. *United States Army Veterinary Service in World War II*. Washington, DC: Office of the Surgeon General, Department of the Army; 1961.

180. Kelser RA. Chloroform-treated rabies vaccine: Preliminary report. *Veterinary Bull*. 1928;22:95–98.

181. Kaplan C, Turner GS, Warrell DA. *Rabies: The Facts*. 2nd ed. Oxford: Oxford University Press; 1986.

182. Centers for Disease Control. Human rabies death—Alabama. *MMWR*. 1963;12:300.

183. Constantine DG. Rabies transmission by the non-bite route. *Public Health Rep*. 1962;77:287–289.

184. Winkler WG, Fashinell TR, Leffingwell L, Howard P, Conomy P. Airborne rabies transmission in a laboratory worker. *JAMA*. 1973;226:1219–1221.

185. Centers for Disease Control and Prevention. Human rabies—Washington, 1995. *MMWR*. 1995;44:625–627.

186. Houff SA, Burton RC, Wilson RW, et al. Human-to-human transmission of rabies virus by corneal transplant. *N Engl J Med*. 1979;300:603–604.

187. Hanlon CA, Koprowski H. Rabies: Issues in transmission and infectivity. *Mediguide to Infectious Diseases*. 1997;17(4):1–7.

188. McColl KA, Gould AR, Selleck PW, Hooper PT, Westbury HA, Smith JS. Polymerase chain reaction and other laboratory techniques in the diagnosis of long incubation rabies in Australia. *Aust Vet J*. 1993;70:84–89.

189. World Health Organization. Global health situation, IV: Selected infectious and parasitic diseases due to identified organisms. *Wkly Epidemiol Rec*. 1993;68:43–44.

190. Centers for Disease Control. Human rabies—Michigan. *MMWR*. 1983;32:159–160.

191. Centers for Disease Control. Human rabies—Pennsylvania. *MMWR*. 1984;33:633–635.

192. Centers for Disease Control. Human rabies—Texas, 1991. *MMWR*. 1991;40:132–133.

193. Centers for Disease Control. Human rabies—Texas, Arkansas, and Georgia, 1991. *MMWR*. 1991;40:765–769.

194. Centers for Disease Control and Prevention. Human rabies—New York, 1993. *MMWR*. 1993;42:805–806.

195. Tsiang H. Pathophysiology of rabies virus infection of the nervous system. *Adv Virus Res*. 1993;42:375–412.

196. Fishbein DB, Bernard KW. Rabies virus. In: Mandel G, Dolin RG, Bennett J, eds. *Principles and Practice of Infectious Diseases*. 4th ed. New York: Churchill Livingstone; 1995: 1527–1543.

197. Warrell DA. The clinical picture of rabies in man. *Trans R Soc Trop Med Hyg*. 1976;70:188–195.

198. Blenden DC, Creech W, Torres-Anjel MJ. Use of immunofluorescence examination to detect rabies virus antigen in the skin of humans with clinical encephalitis. *J Infect Dis*. 1986;154:698–701.

199. Schneider LG. The cornea test; a new method for the intra-vitam diagnosis of rabies. *Zentralbl Veterinarmed (B)*. 1969;16:24–31.

200. Zaidman GW, Billingsley A. Corneal impression test for the diagnosis of acute rabies encephalitis. *Ophthalmology*. 1998;105:249–251.

201. Larghi OP, Gonzalez E, Held JR. Evaluation of the corneal test as a laboratory method for rabies diagnosis. *Appl Microbiol*. 1973;25:187–189.

202. Mathuranayagam D, Rao PV. Antemortem diagnosis of human rabies by corneal impression smears using immunofluorescent technique. *Indian J Med Res*. 1984;79:463–467.

203. Swoveland PT, Johnson KP. Identification of rabies antigen in human and animal tissues. *Ann N Y Acad Sci*. 1983;420:185–191.

204. Smith JS, Yager PA, Baer GM. A rapid reproducible test for determining rabies neutralizing antibody. *Bull World Health Organ*. 1973;48:535–541.

205. Kamolvarin N, Tirawatnpong T, Rattanasiwamoke R, Tirawatnpong S, Panpanich T, Hemachudha T. Diagnosis of rabies by polymerase chain reaction with nested primers. *J Infect Dis*. 1993;167:207–210.

206. Dean DJ, Baer GM, Thompson WR. Studies on the local treatment of rabies infected wounds. *Bull World Health Organ*. 1963;28:477–486.

207. Lin FT, Chen SB, Wang YZ, Sun CZ, Zeng FZ, Wang GF. Use of serum and vaccine in combination for prophylaxis following exposure to rabies. *Rev Infect Dis*. 1988;10(suppl 4):S766–S770.

208. Merigan TC, Baer GM, Winkler WG, et al. Human leukocyte interferon administration to patients with symptomatic and suspected rabies. *Ann Neurol*. 1984;16:82–87.

209. Bergen GA, Fitzmorris K. Viral encephalitis. In: *Infection Control and Applied Epidemiology: Principles and Practice*. St. Louis: Mosby; 1996.

210. Helmick CG, Tauxe RV, Vernon AA. Is there a risk to contacts of patients with rabies? *Rev Infect Dis*. 1987;9:511–518.

211. Centers for Disease Control and Prevention. Compendium of animal rabies control, 1997: National Association of State Public Health Veterinarians, Inc. *MMWR*. 1997;46(RR-4):1–9.

212. Brochier B, Kieny MP, Costy F, et al. Large-scale eradication of rabies using recombinant vaccinia-rabies vaccine. *Nature*. 1991;354:520–522.

213. Rosatte RC, Power MJ, MacInnes CD, Campbell JB. Trap-vaccinate-release and oral vaccination for rabies control in urban skunks, raccoons and foxes. *J Wildl Dis*. 1992;28:562–571.

214. National Association of State Public Health Veterinarians. Compendium of animal rabies control, 1994. *J Am Vet Assoc*. 1994;204:173–176.

215. Vaughn JB, Gerhardt P, Newell KW. Excretion of street rabies virus in the saliva of dogs. *JAMA*. 1965:193:363–368.

216. Vaughn JB Gerhardt P, Paterson J. Excretion of rabies virus in saliva of cats. *JAMA*. 1963;184:705.

217. Fekadu M, Shaddock JH, Baer GM. Intermittent excretion of rabies virus in the saliva of a dog two and six months after it had recovered from experimental rabies. *Am J Trop Med Hyg*. 1981;30:1113–1115.

218. Lopez T. Quarantine changes take effect in Hawaii. *J Am Vet Med Assoc*. 1997;211:817,819.

219. Roumiantzeff M, Ajjan N, Vincent-Falquet JC. Experience with preexposure rabies vaccination. *Rev Infect Dis*. 1988;10(suppl 4):S751–S757.

220. Centers for Disease Control. Rabies prevention—United States, 1991: Recommendations of the Immunization Practices Advisory Committee. *MMWR*. 1991;40:1–19.

221. Trimarchi CV, Safford M Jr. Poor response to rabies vaccination by the intradermal route. *JAMA*. 1992;268:874.

222. Centers for Disease Control and Prevention. Availability of new rabies vaccine for human use. *MMWR*. 1998;47:12,19.

223. Pappaioanou M, Fishbein DB, Dreesen DW, et al. Antibody response to preexposure human diploid-cell rabies vaccines given concurrently with chloroquine. *N Engl J Med*. 1986;314:280–284.

224. Siwasontiwat D, Lumlertdacha B, Polsuwan C, Hemachudha T, Chutvongse S, Wilde H. Rabies: Is provocation of the biting dog relevant for risk assessment? *Trans R Soc Trop Med Hyg*. 1992;86:443.

225. Karliner JS, Belaval GS. Incidence of adverse reactions following administration of antirabies serum: A study of 562 cases. *JAMA*. 1965:193:359.

226. Wilde H, Chomchey P, Punyaratabandhu P, Phanupak P, Chutivongse S. Purified equine rabies immune globulin: A safe and affordable alternative to human rabies immune globulin. *Bull World Health Organ*. 1989;67:731–736.

227. Centers for Disease Control. Human rabies despite treatment with rabies immune globulin and human diploid cell rabies vaccine—Thailand. *MMWR*. 1987;36:759–760,765.

228. Hatz CF, Bidaux JM, Eichenberger K, Mikulics U, Junghanss T. Circumstances and management of 72 animal bites among long-term residents in the tropics. *Vaccine*. 1995;13:811–815.

229. Schriker RL, Eigelsbach HT, Mitten JQ, Hall WC. Pathogenesis of tularemia in monkeys aerogenically exposed to *Francisella tularensis* 425. *Infect Immun*. 1972;5:734–744.

230. Sanford JP. Landmark perspective: Tularemia. *JAMA*. 1983;250:3225–3226.

231. Capellan J, Fong IW. Tularemia from a cat bite: Case report and review of feline-associated tularemia. *Clin Infect Dis*. 1993;16:472–475.

232. Francis E. Tularemia. *JAMA*. 1925;84:1243–1250.

233. Boyce JM. Recent trends in the epidemiology of tularemia in the United States. *J Infect Dis*. 1975;131:197–199.

234. Syrjala H, Kujala P, Myllyla V, Salminen A. Airborne transmission of tularemia in farmers. *Scand J Infect Dis*. 1985;17:371–375.

235. Centers for Disease Control and Prevention. Cases of selected notifiable diseases: United States, weeks ending December 11, 1993, and December 5, 1992. *MMWR*. 1993;42:955–958.

236. Gill V, Cunha BA. Tularemia pneumonia. *Semin Respir Infect*. 1997;12:61–67.

237. Evans ME, Gregory DW, Schaffner W, McGee ZA. Tularemia: A 30-year experience with 88 cases. *Medicine (Baltimore)*. 1985;64:251–269.

238. Schmid GP, Catino D, Suffin SC, Martone WJ, Kaufmann AF. Granulomatous pleuritis caused by *Francisella tularensis*: Possible confusion with tuberculous pleuritis. *Am Rev Respir Dis*. 1983;128:314–316.

239. Lovell VM, Cho CT, Lindsey NJ, Nelson PL. *Francisella tularensis* meningitis: A rare clinical entity. *J Infect Dis*. 1986;154:916–918.

240. Stewart SJ. *Francisella*. In: Murray PR, Baron EJ, Pfaller MA, Tenover FC, Yolken RH, eds. *Manual of Clinical Microbiology*. Washington, DC: ASM Press; 1995: 545–548.

241. Provenza JM, Klotz SA, Penn RL. Isolation of *Francisella tularensis* from blood. *J Clin Microbiol*. 1986;24:453–455.

242. Fulop M, Leslie D, Titball R. A rapid, highly sensitive method for the detection of *Francisella tularensis* in clinical samples using the polymerase chain reaction. *Am J Trop Med Hyg*. 1996;54:364–366.

243. Sjostedt A, Eriksson U, Berglund L, Tarnvik A. Detecton of *Francisella tularensis* in ulcers of patients with tularemia by PCR. *J Clin Microbiol.* 1997;35:1045–1048.

244. Enderlin G, Morales L, Jacobs RF, Cross JT. Streptomycin and alternative agents for the treatment of tularemia: Review of the literature. *Clin Infect Dis.* 1994;19:42–47.

245. Penn RL. *Francisella tularensis* (tularemia). In: Mandell GL, Bennett JE, Dolin R, eds. *Principles and Practice of Infectious Diseases.* 4th ed. New York: Churchill Livingstone; 1995: 2060–2068.

246. Mason WL, Eigelsbach HT, Little SF, Bates JH. Treatment of tularemia, including pulmonary tularemia, with gentamicin. *Am Rev Respir Dis.* 1980;121:39–45.

247. Cross JT, Schutze GE, Jacobs RF. Treatment of tularemia with gentamicin in pediatric patients. *Pediatr Infect Dis J.* 1995;14:151–152.

248. Risi GF, Pombo DJ. Relapse of tularemia after aminoglycoside therapy: Case report and discussion of therapeutic options. *Clin Infect Dis.* 1995;20:174–175.

249. Syrjala H, Schildt R, Raisainen S. In vitro susceptibility of *Francisella tularensis* to fluoroquinolones and treatment of tularemia with norfloxacin and ciprofloxacin. *Eur J Clin Microbiol Infect Dis.* 1991;10:68–70.

250. Baker CN, Hollis DG, Thornsberry C. Antimicrobial susceptibility testing of *Francisella tularensis* with a modified Mueller-Hinton broth. *J Clin Microbiol.* 1985;22:212–215.

251. Cross JT, Jacobs RF. Tularemia: Treatment failures with outpatient use of ceftriaxone. *Clin Infect Dis.* 1993; 17:976–980.

252. Hill B, Sandstrom G, Schroder S, Franzen C, Tarnvik A. A case of tularemia meningitis in Sweden. *Scand J Infect Dis.* 1990;22:95–99.

253. Lee HC, Horowitz E, Linder W. Treatment of tularemia with imipenem/cilastatin sodium. *South Med J.* 1991;84:1277–1278.

254. Saslow S, Eigelsbach HT, Prior JA, Wilson HE, Carhrt S. Tularemia vaccine study. *Arch Intern Med.* 1961;107:134–146.

255. Franz DR, Jahrling PB, Friedlander AM, et al. Clinical recognition and management of patients exposed to biological warfare agents. *JAMA.* 1997;278:399–411.

256. Abramova FA, Grinberg LM, Yampolskaya OV, Walker DH. Pathology of inhalational anthrax in 42 cases from the Sverdlovsk outbreak of 1979. *Proc Natl Acad Sci USA.* 1993;90:2291–2294.

257. Walker DH, Yampolska O, Grinberg LM. Death at Sverdlovsk: What have we learned? *Am J Pathol.* 1994;144: 1135-1141.

258. Davies JC. A major epidemic of anthrax in Zimbabwe, part II: Distribution of cutaneous lesions. *Cent Afr J Med.* 1983;29:8–12.

259. Brachman PS. Anthrax. In: Evans AS, Brachman PS, eds. *Bacterial Infections of Humans: Epidemiology and Control.* 2nd ed. New York: Plenum Medical Book Co; 1991: 75–86.

260. Christie AB. *Infectious Diseases: Epidemiology and Clinical Practice.* 2 Vols. New York: Churchill Livingston; 1987: 992.

261. Nunanusont D, Limpakarnjanarat K, Foy HM. Outbreak of anthrax in Thailand. *Ann Trop Med Parasitol.* 1990;84: 507–512.

262. Fujikura T. Current occurrence of anthrax in man and animals. *Salisbury Med Bull Suppl.* 1990;68:1.

263. Wilson GS, Miles AA. *Topley and Wilson's Principles of Bacteriology and Immunity.* Vol 2. Baltimore: Williams & Wilkins; 1955: 1940.

264. Brachman PS. Inhalation anthrax. *Ann N Y Acad Sci.* 1980:353:83–93.

265. Davies JC. A major epidemic of anthrax in Zimbabwe. *Cent Afr J Med.* 1982;28:291–298.

266. Davies JC. A major epidemic of anthrax in Zimbabwe: The experience at the Beatrice Road Infectious Diseases Hospital, Harare. *Cent Afr J Med.* 1985;31:176-180.

267. Ivins BE, Ezzell JW Jr, Jemski J, Hedlund KW, Ristroph JD, Leppla SH. Immunization studies with attenuated strains of *Bacillus anthracis. Infect Immun.* 1986;52:454-458.

268. Mikesell P, Ivins BE, Ristroph JD, Dreier TM. Evidence for plasmid-mediated toxin production in *Bacillus anthracis. Infect Immun.* 1983;39:371–376.

269. Cataldi A, Labruyere E, Mock M. Construction and characterization of a protective antigen-deficient *Bacillus anthracis* strain. *Mol Microbiol.* 1990;4:1111-1117.

270. Ross JM. The pathogenesis of anthrax following the administration of spores by the respiratory route. *J Pathol Bacteriol.* 1957;73:485–494.

271. Dutz W, Kohout E. Anthrax. *Pathol Annu.* 1971;6:209–248.

272. Turnbull PC, Leppla SH, Broster MG, Quinn CP, Melling J. Antibodies to anthrax toxin in humans and guinea pigs and their relevance to protective immunity. *Med Microbiol Immunol (Berl).* 1988;177:293–303.

273. Buchanan TM, Feeley JC, Hayes PS, Brachman PS. Anthrax indirect microhemagglutination test. *J Immunol.* 1971;107:1631–1636.

274. Sirisanthana T, Nelson KE, Ezell J, Abshire TG. Serological studies of patients with cutaneous and oral-oropharyngeal anthrax from northern Thailand. *Am J Trop Med Hyg.* 1988;39:575–581.

275. Harrison LH, Ezzell JW Jr, Abshire TG, Kidd S, Kaufmann AF. Evaluation of serologic tests for diagnosis of anthrax after an outbreak of cutaneous anthrax in Paraguay. *J Infect Dis.* 1989;160:706–710.

276. Friedlander AM, Welkos SL, Pitt ML, et al. Postexposure prophylaxis against experimental inhalation anthrax. *J Infect Dis.* 1993;167:1239–1243.

277. Doganay M, Aydin N. Antimicrobial susceptibility of *Bacillus anthracis. Scand J Infect Dis.* 1991;23:333–335.

278. Lightfoot NF, Scott RJ, Turnbull PC. Antimicrobial susceptibility of *Bacillus anthracis. Salisbury Med Bull Suppl.* 1990;68:95.

279. Turnbull PC, Broster MG, Carman JA, Manchee RJ, Melling J. Development of antibodies to protective antigen and lethal factor components of anthrax toxin in humans and guinea pigs and their relevance to protective immunity. *Infect Immun.* 1986;52:356–363.

280. Pittman PR. Lieutenant Colonel, Medical Corps, US Army. Chief, Clinical Investigation, Medical Division, US Army Medical Research Institute of Infectious Diseases, Fort Detrick, Frederick, Md. Personal communication, January 1994.

281. Anthrax vaccine adsorbed. Lansing, Mich: Michigan Dept of Public Health; 1987. Package insert.

282. Brachman PS, Gold H, Plotkin SA, Fekety FR, Werrin M, Ingraham NR. Field evaluation of a human anthrax vaccine. *Am J Public Health.* 1962;52:632–645.

283. Cleghorn G. *Observations of the Epidemical Diseases of Minorca (From the Years 1744 to 1749).* London, England; 1751. As cited in: Evans AC. Comments on the early history of human brucellosis. Larson CH, Soule MH, eds. *Brucellosis.* Baltimore, Md: Waverly Press; 1950: 1–8.

284. Bruce D. Note on the discovery of a micro-organism in Malta fever. *Practitioner (London).* 1887;39:161–170. As cited in: Evans AC. Comments on the early history of human brucellosis. Larson CH, Soule MH, eds. *Brucellosis.* Baltimore, Md: Waverly Press; 1950: 1–8.

285. Hughes ML. *Mediterranean, Malta or Undulant Fever.* London, England: Macmillan and Co; 1897. As cited in: Evans AC. Comments on the early history of human brucellosis. Larson CH, Soule MH, eds. *Brucellosis.* Baltimore, Md: Waverly Press; 1950: 1–8.

286. Bang B. Die Aetiologie des seuchenhaften ("infectiösen") Verwerfens. *Z Thiermed (Jena).* 1897;1:241–278. As cited in: Evans AC. Comments on the early history of human brucellosis. Larson CH, Soule MH, eds. *Brucellosis.* Baltimore, Md: Waverly Press; 1950: 1–8.

287. Meador VP, Hagemoser WA, Deyoe BL. Histopathologic findings in *Brucella abortus*–infected, pregnant goats. *Am J Vet Res.* 1988;49(2):274–280.

288. Nicoletti P. The epidemiology of bovine brucellosis. *Adv Vet Sci Comp Med.* 1980;24:69–98.

289. Grimont F, Verger JM, Cornelis P, et al. Molecular typing of *Brucella* with cloned DNA probes. *Res Microbiol.* 1992;143:55–65.

290. Jahans KL, Foster G, Broughton ES. The characterisation of Brucella strains isolated from marine mammals. *Vet Microbiol.* 1997;57:373–382.

291. Young EJ. Brucellosis: Current epidemiology, diagnosis, and management. *Curr Clin Top Infect Dis.* 1995;15:115–128.

292. Radwan AI, Bekairi SI, Prasad PV. Serological and bacteriological study of brucellosis in camels in central Saudi Arabia. *Rev Sci Tech.* 1992;11:837–844.

293. Yagoub IA, Mohamed AA, Salim MO. Serological survey of *Brucella abortus* antibody prevalence in the one-humped camel (*Camelus dromedarius*) from eastern Sudan. *Rev Elev Med Vet Pays Trop.* 1990;43:167–171.

294. Chomel BB, DeBess EE, Mangiamele DM, et al. Changing trends in the epidemiology of human brucellosis in California from 1973 to 1992: A shift toward foodborne transmission. *J Infect Dis.* 1994;170:1216–1223.

295. Mousa AR, Elhag KM, Khogali M, Marafie AA. The nature of human brucellosis in Kuwait: Study of 379 cases. *Rev Infect Dis.* 1988;10:211–217.

296. Robson JM, Harrison MW, Wood RN, Tilse MH, McKay AB, Brodribb TR. Brucellosis: Re-emergence and changing epidemiology in Queensland. *Med J Aust.* 1993;159:153–158.

297. Dajani YF, Masoud AA, Barakat HF. Epidemiology and diagnosis of human brucellosis in Jordan. *J Trop Med Hyg.* 1989;92:209–214.

298. Mousa AM, Elhag KM, Khogali M, Sugathan TN. Brucellosis in Kuwait: A clinico-epidemiological study. *Trans R Soc Trop Med Hyg.* 1987;81:1020–1021.

299. Buchanan TM, Hendricks SL, Patton CM, Feldman RA. Brucellosis in the United States, 1960–1972: An abattoir-associated disease, III: Epidemiology and evidence for acquired immunity. *Medicine (Baltimore).* 1974;53:427–439.

300. Ackermann MR, Cheville NF, Deyoe BL. Bovine ileal dome lymphoepithelial cells: Endocytosis and transport of *Brucella abortus* strain 19. *Vet Pathol.* 1988;25:28–35.

301. Elsbach P. Degradation of microorganisms by phagocytic cells. *Rev Infect Dis.* 1980;2:106–128.

302. Braude AI. Studies in the pathology and pathogenesis of experimental brucellosis, II: The formation of the hepatic granulomas and its evolution. *J Infect Dis*. 1951;89:87–94.

303. Young EJ. An overview of human brucellosis. *Clin Infect Dis*. 1995;21:283–289.

304. Gotuzzo E, Alarcon GS, Bocanegra TS, et al. Articular involvement in human brucellosis: A retrospective analysis of 304 cases. *Semin Arthritis Rheum*. 1982;12:245–255.

305. Mousa AR, Muhtaseb SA, Almudallal DS, Khodeir SM, Marafie AA. Osteoarticular complications of brucellosis: A study of 169 cases. *Rev Infect Dis*. 1987;9:531–543.

306. al Shahed MS, Sharif HS, Haddad MC, Aabed MY, Sammak BM, Mutairi MA. Imaging features of musculoskeletal brucellosis. *Radiographics*. 1994;14:333–348.

307. Rotes-Querol J. Osteo-articular sites of brucellosis. *Ann Rheum Dis*. 1957;16:63–68.

308. Ibrahim AI, Awad R, Shetty SD, Saad M, Bilal NE. Genito-urinary complications of brucellosis. Br J Urol. 1988;61:294–298.

309. Lubani MM, Dudin KI, Sharda DC, et al. Neonatal brucellosis. *Eur J Pediatr*. 1988;147:520–522.

310. Buchanan TM, Faber LC, Feldman RA. Brucellosis in the United States, 1960–1972: An abattoir-associated disease, I: Clinical features and therapy. *Medicine (Baltimore)*. 1974;53:403–413.

311. Peery TM, Belter LF. Brucellosis and heart disease, II: Fatal brucellosis. *Am J Pathol*. 1960;36:673–697.

312. Young EJ. Serologic diagnosis of human brucellosis: Analysis of 214 cases by agglutination tests and review of the literature. *Rev Infect Dis*. 1991;13:359–372.

313. Gotuzzo E, Carrillo C, Guerra J, Llosa L. An evaluation of diagnostic methods for brucellosis—the value of bone marrow culture. *J Infect Dis*. 1986:153:122–125.

314. Hall WH. Modern chemotherapy for brucellosis in humans. *Rev Infect Dis*. 1990;12:1060–1099.

315. Luzzi GA, Brindle R, Sockett PN, Solera J, Klenerman P, Warrell DA. Brucellosis: Imported and laboratory-acquired cases, and an overview of treatment trials. *Trans R Soc Trop Med Hyg*. 1993;87:138–141.

316. Chan R, Hardiman RP. Endocarditis caused by *Brucella melitensis*. *Med J Aust*. 1993;158:631–632.

317. *Joint FAO/WHO Expert Committee on Brucellosis, Sixth Report*. Geneva: FAO/WHO; 1986. WHO Technical Report Series 740.

Chapter 37

DISEASES TRANSMITTED BY FOOD, WATER, AND SOIL

DAVID N. TAYLOR, MD
SHARON L. LUDWIG, MD, MPH
LEONARD N. BINN, PhD
JAMES FLECKENSTEIN, MD
JOSE L. SANCHEZ, MD, MPH
WILLIAM A. PETRI, JR., MD, PhD
JOANNA M. SCHAENMAN, PhD

CHARLES W. HOGE, MD
JOHN H. CROSS, PhD
W. PATRICK CARNEY, MPH, PhD
NAOMI E. ARONSON, MD
DUANE R. HOSPENTHAL, MD, PhD
MAY-ANN LEE, PhD
ERIC P. H. YAP, MBBS, DPhil

D.N. Taylor, MD, Colonel, Medical Corps, US Army (Retired); Department of International Health, Johns Hopkins University Bloomberg School of Public Health, 624 North Broadway, Baltimore, MD 21205; Formerly, Research Coordinator for Prevention of Diarrheal Disease, Division of Communicable Diseases and Immunology, Walter Reed Army Institute of Research, Silver Spring, Maryland

S.L. Ludwig, MD, MPH, Commander, US Public Health Service, Operational Preventive Medicine/Epidemiology Staff Officer, US Coast Guard Commandant (G-WKH-1), 2100 Second Street SW, Washington DC 20593

L.N. Binn, PhD; Supervisory Research Microbiologist, Department of Virus Diseases, Division of Communicable Diseases and Immunology, Walter Reed Army Institute of Research, Silver Spring, MD 20910-7500

J. Fleckenstein, MD; Assistant Professor of Medicine, Departments of Medicine and Molecular Sciences, Infectious Disease Division, University of Tennessee Health Science Center and Veterans Affairs, 1030 Jefferson Avenue, Memphis, TN 38104; Formerly: Lieutenant Colonel, Medical Corps, US Army; Infectious Disease Service, Walter Reed Army Medical Center, Washington, DC 20307

J.L. Sanchez, MD, MPH, Colonel, Medical Corps, US Army; Medical Epidemiologist and Military Chief, Global Epidemiology and Threat Assessment, HIV Research Program, Walter Reed Army Institute of Research, 13 Taft Court, Rockville, MD 20850

W.A. Petri, Jr., MD, PhD; Professor of Medicine, Microbiology, and Pathology, Division of Infectious Diseases, Room 2115, MR4 Building, University of Virginia Health Sciences Center, Charlottesville VA 22908

J.M. Schaenman, PhD; Chief Resident, Department of Internal Medicine, Stanford University School of Medicine, 300 Pasteur Drive, Stanford, CA 94305

C.W. Hoge, MD, Colonel, Medical Corps, US Army; Chief, Department of Psychiatry and Behavioral Sciences, Division of Neuropsychiatry, Walter Reed Army Institute of Research, Silver Spring, MD 20910-7500; Formerly, Principal Investigator, Department of Enteric Infections, Division of Communicable Diseases and Immunology, Walter Reed Army Institute of Research

J.H. Cross, PhD; Professor of Tropical Public Health, Uniformed Services University of the Health Sciences, 4301 Jones Bridge Road, Bethesda MD 20814-4799

W.P. Carney, MPH, PhD, Captain, MSC, US Navy (Ret.); Professor, Department of Preventive Medicine and Biometrics, Uniformed Services University of the Health Sciences, 4301 Jones Bridge Road, Bethesda, MD 20814-4799

N.E. Aronson, MD, Colonel, Medical Corps, US Army; Director, Infectious Diseases Division, Room A3058, Uniformed Services University of the Health Sciences, 4301 Jones Bridge Road, Bethesda, MD 20814

D.R. Hospenthal, MD, PhD, Lieutenant Colonel, Medical Corps, US Army; Chief, Infectious Disease Service, Brooke Army Medical Center, 3851 Roger Brooke Drive, Fort Sam Houston, TX 78234-6200

M-A. Lee, PhD; Programme Head, Defence Medical and Environmental Research Institute, @DSO National Laboratories, 27 Medical Drive, Singapore 119597

E.P.H. Yap, MBBS, DPhil; Programme Head, Defence Medical and Environmental Research Institute, @DSO National Laboratories, 27 Medical Drive, Singapore 119597

DIARRHEA CAUSED BY *ESCHERICHIA COLI*

Escherichia coli is a gram-negative, facultatively anaerobic, rod-shaped bacterium that is generally a normal, nonpathogenic inhabitant of the intestine of mammals. It is a member of the large family of bacteria known as the Enterobacteriaceae, which also includes salmonellae and shigellae. *E coli* that compose the normal intestinal flora may become pathogenic when seeded outside the intestine, as a cause of sepsis, focal infections, or wound infections. *E coli* may acquire virulence factors that render them pathogenic to humans in the gut. These virulence factors are usually stabile genetic characteristics that are passed on from generation to generation resulting in a stable clone or strain.

Four general categories of *E coli* have been recognized as enteric pathogens:[1] Enterotoxigenic *E coli* (ETEC), enterohemorrhagic *E coli* (EHEC), enteroinvasive *E coli* (EIEC), and enteropathogenic *E coli* (EPEC). EPEC organisms are part of a larger group generally referred to as enteroadherent *E coli*.

Enterotoxigenic *Escherichia coli*

Introduction and Military Relevance

ETEC is one of the most common causes of diarrheal diseases among children in developing countries[2,3] and is the most common cause of traveler's diarrhea acquired in those countries.[4,5] Diarrheal

disease has accompanied military campaigns for centuries,[6] but traveler's diarrhea was only described as a clinical syndrome after World War II when travel to exotic locations by air became more feasible.[7] It was not until the early 1970s that ETEC was recognized as an enteric pathogen in both humans and animals.[8] One of the first known ETEC outbreaks occurred in British troops stationed in Aden in the Persian Gulf region in the 1960s.[9] Rowe identified a single *E coli* serotype (O148:H28) as the cause of illnesses that occurred in the first few weeks of the deployment. These strains of *E coli*, as well as others (O6:H16) from US military forces serving in Vietnam, were shown to be pathogenic in volunteers and were subsequently found to produce enterotoxins.[10] Ever since, ETEC has been found to be an important cause of diarrhea during many deployments in the developing world, most notably the Middle East and Africa (Table 37-1). Diarrheal disease was a major problem during the Persian Gulf War,[11] and ETEC and *Shigella* organisms caused the majority of these illnesses (Table 37-2).

Description of the Pathogen

ETEC produces either a heat-labile toxin (LT), a heat-stable toxin (ST), or both toxins (LT/ST). The isolation rates of ETEC producing these toxins from persons with diarrhea varies from survey to sur-

TABLE 37-1

ISOLATION RATES OF ENTEROTOXIGENIC *ESCHERICHIA COLI* AMONG PERSONNEL ON MILITARY DEPLOYMENTS (1987–1993)

Exercise (Country)	Year	Number cultured	Percentage ETEC	Reference
Operation Restore Hope (Somalia)	1992-1993	113	16	1
Operation Desert Shield (Saudi Arabia)	1990	432	29	2
Operation Bright Star (Egypt)	1989	104	57	3
USS Kennedy (Alexandria, Egypt*)	1988	118	34	4
Operation Bright Star (Egypt)	1987	183	33	5

*port visit

References: (1) Sharp TW, Thornton SA, Wallace MR, et al. Diarrheal disease among military personnel during Operation Restore Hope, Somalia, 1992-1993. *Am J Trop Med Hyg*. 1995;52:188–193. (2) Hyams KC, Bourgeois AL, Merrell BR, et al. Diarrheal disease during Operation Desert Shield. *N Engl J Med*. 1991;325:1423–1428. (3) Taylor DN, Sanchez JL, Candler W, Thornton S, McQueen C, Echeverria P. Treatment of travelers' diarrhea: Ciprofloxacin plus loperamide compared with ciprofloxacin alone; a placebo-controlled, randomized trial. *Ann Intern Med*. 1991;114:731–734. (4) Scott DA, Haberberger RL, Thornton SA, Hyams KC. Norfloxacin for the prophylaxis of travelers' diarrhea in U.S. military personnel. *Am J Trop Med Hyg*. 1990;42:160–164. (5) Haberberger RL Jr, Mikhail IA, Burans JP, et al. Traveler's diarrhea during joint American–Egyptian armed forces exercises in Cairo, Egypt. *Mil Med*. 1991;156:27–30.

TABLE 37-2

BACTERIAL ENTEROPATHOGENS IDENTIFIED IN STOOL SAMPLES FROM 432 US MILITARY PERSONNEL WITH ACUTE GASTROENTERITIS DURING OPERATION DESERT SHIELD

Enteropathogen	Isolation Rate	
	Number	Percent
ETEC*		
Heat-labile toxin	15	3.5
Heat-stable toxin	44	10.2
Heat-labile and heat-stable toxin	64	14.8
Mixed ETEC infection	2	0.5
Total of ETEC	125	28.9
Shigella organisms		
S dysenteriae	4	0.9
S flexneri	12	2.8
S boydii	8	1.9
S sonnei	89	20.6
Total of *Shigella* organisms	113	26.2
EIEC†	3	0.7
Salmonella	7	1.6
Campylobacter	2	0.5

*Enterotoxigenic *E coli*
†Enteroinvasive *E coli*
Reprinted from: Hyams KC, Bourgeois AL, Merrell BR, et al. Diarrheal disease during Operation Desert Shield. *N Engl J Med.* 1991;325:1423–1425. Copyright © 1991 Massachusetts Medical Society. All rights reserved.

vey, but in most studies the isolation rates of each toxin type are approximately equal.[12] Strains producing ST or LT/ST are more pathogenic than strains producing only LT and belong to a small number of O:H serotypes; most have recognized intestinal cell adherence or colonization factors.[1] Strains producing only heat-labile toxin belong to a much larger number of O:H serotypes and often do not possess known colonization factors.[12]

Epidemiology

Transmission. Most epidemiologic studies have implicated contaminated foods as the main source of ETEC. The human reservoir is large, and fecal spread to food via hands is probably the main method of contamination.[13,14] ETEC can also be isolated from domestic animals, and contamination of meats with intestinal contents may be another important source in food. Vegetables can be contami-

nated with human feces used as fertilizer or with untreated sewage. During the Persian Gulf War, vegetables acquired from local markets were an important source of contamination. Decontamination of salad vegetables in chlorinated water was unsuccessful because the volume of food required was too great to allow for the proper contact time.[15]

Geographic Distribution. In tropical climates, disease caused by ETEC occurs year-round; in more temperate climates, disease is more common in the warmer summer months. In the developed world, ETEC is a rare cause of diarrhea, and almost all of the epidemiologic data that are available is from foodborne or waterborne outbreaks.[16–18]

Incidence. Diarrhea caused by ETEC is a major health problem for infants and children in the developing world and is the major cause of traveler's diarrhea in those traveling to the developing world. Studies in areas of the developing world where hygiene is poor suggest that exposure to ETEC is nearly constant. Under these circumstances, the level of immunity is the key factor in determining susceptibility to disease. Infants and newly arriving travelers have the least immunity and more frequently develop severe diarrhea when infected. After repeated exposure, illnesses become less severe or less symptomatic. Because ETEC is endemic in developing countries, outbreaks are rare except in new arrivals, such as travelers. During the build-up stages of the Persian Gulf War (August to October 1990), diarrhea affected as many as 5% of the service member strength per week (Figure 37-1).

Pathogenesis and Clinical Findings

ETEC can cause a severe watery diarrhea similar to cholera. ETEC must adhere to the small intestinal mucosa to cause disease. ETEC adherence is mediated by fimbriae on the surface of the organism. These fimbriae, called colonization factor antigens, are encoded by plasmids that usually encode heat stable toxin and often heat labile toxin.[1] The pathophysiology of diarrhea caused by ETEC is primarily determined by the production of these enterotoxins. Similar to cholera toxin, heat labile toxin is composed of one A subunit and 5 B subunits that bind to ganglioside GM1 on eucaryotic cell surfaces. The A subunit undergoes proteolytic cleavage that produces two fragments designated A1 and A2. The A1 fragment activates adenylcyclase and increases cyclic adenosine monophosphate through adenosine diphosphate ribosylation of the cell membrane, which causes fluid secretion by inhibiting sodium and chloride absorption and chloride secretion.

ETEC causes a secretory diarrhea with fluid and electrolyte loss without evidence of inflammation. The amount of diarrhea may be mild or massive, cholera-like purging. Generally, an inoculum of about 10^8 organisms is required to infect 50% of persons exposed.[10] Disease severity increases with inoculum size and may also be associated with the quantity of toxin produced by the organism. In travelers, disease occurs most commonly in the first weeks of travel. The incubation period ranges from 12 to 48 hours and shortens with higher inoculum size. Symptoms that accompany ETEC diarrhea are malaise, anorexia, abdominal cramping, nausea, vomiting in 25%, and low-grade fever in 30%. Untreated the illness lasts 1 to 5 days but can last as long as 2 weeks. Stool frequency is usually around

10 episodes per day for 1 or 2 days.[7,19] Complications are usually associated with dehydration. These include lethargy, muscle cramping, loss of consciousness, renal failure, and death. Infants and children may have a decreased absorptive capacity of the small bowel for several weeks after the illness, which can lead to malnutrition.

Diagnostic Approaches

E coli is a gram-negative rod that grows readily on routine culture media under aerobic conditions. *E coli* is identified on MacConkey agar as a lactose-fermenter. *E coli* can be isolated after several days from fecal specimens preserved in Cary-Blair transport media. There is no biochemical or serological

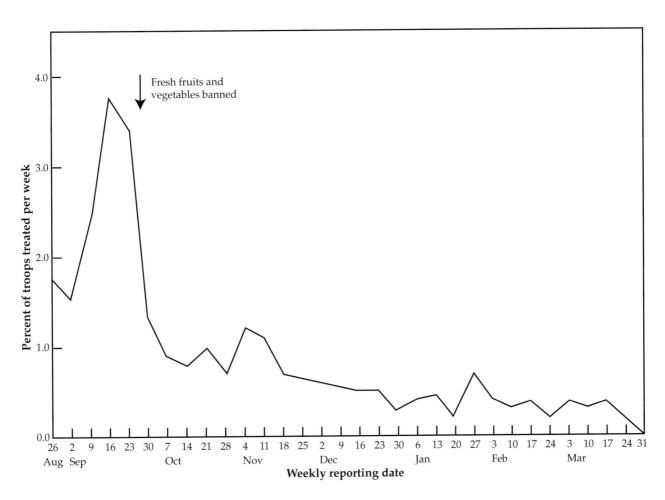

Fig. 37-1. This graph shows the weekly rates of gastroenteritis among 40,000 Marine Corps ground troops stationed in northeast Saudi Arabia in 1990 and 1991. The arrow indicates when fresh produce was removed from their diet, which was followed by a sharp decrease in the diarrheal disease incidence.
Reprinted with permission from: Hyams KC, Hanson K, Wignall FS, Escamilla J, Oldfield EC III. The impact of infectious diseases on the health of US troops deployed to the Persian Gulf during Operations Desert Shield and Desert Storm. *Clin Infect Dis.* 1995;20:1497–1504.

test that can be used to identify all ETEC serotypes, therefore methods to detect the heat-labile and heat-stable toxins must be used. The traditional methods have been Y1 or CHO cell culture assays to identify heat-labile toxin and the suckling mouse assay for heat-stable toxin.[19] These assays are difficult to maintain in most laboratories and are being replaced with DNA hybridization assays.[20] The hybridization can be detected using radioisotopes or by an enzyme-linked system. No commercial assays are available to detect ETEC.

Recommendations for Therapy and Control

In developing countries, diarrhea caused by ETEC is a disease of children younger than 5 years old. The mainstay of treatment is replenishing fluid and restoring electrolyte balance.[21] This can be accomplished with oral rehydration solution or, if that fails, with intravenous fluid. Breast feeding and the use of rice-based oral rehydration solution may provide some protection against malabsorption.[22] In addition, the use of vitamin A and zinc may prevent or shorten the illness.[23]

For travelers, other prophylactic and treatment modalities are useful. Treatment of traveler's diarrhea is aimed at decreasing the total amount of diarrhea and the number of days of illness. Many of the agents that can be used for prophylaxis can also be effectively used as treatment. Fluoroquinolones (eg, ciprofloxacin, norfloxacin) taken twice daily for 3 days are currently regarded the drugs of choice because of increased resistance among ETEC strains to trimethoprim-sulfamethoxazole (TMP/SMX) and the tetracyclines.[24]

Antimotility drugs also have a role in treatment. US military personnel in Thailand responded more rapidly to ciprofloxacin plus loperamide than to ciprofloxacin alone.[25] Loperamide acts more rapidly than antibiotics, so loperamide given in combination with ciprofloxacin provides the most rapid improvement. This regimen is generally recognized as the treatment of choice for adults.[24]

Good personal hygiene, in particular hand washing, is important in preventing all enteric infections. The warning to travelers to "cook it, boil it, peel it, or don't eat it" is good advice and reminds the individual that food left out at room temperature can easily become contaminated. To ensure that bacteria have been killed, foods should be served hot to the touch. Local water may not be adequately chlorinated and therefore should be avoided unless reboiled or chlorinated. Bottled water and boiled water are usually safe. Careful food inspection and food handling procedures are particularly important for military units working in the tropics. If food is bought from local sources, it must be assumed to be contaminated. Meats need to be prepared away from salad vegetables to prevent cross-contamination. Local produce should be decontaminated with chlorinated water.

Prophylaxis with antimicrobial agents (eg, doxycycline, TMP/SMX) is generally well tolerated but is only effective in areas where enteric pathogens are still susceptible to these antibiotics. Ciprofloxacin and norfloxacin once daily are currently the most effective prophylactic agents,[26] but because these agents are also used for treatment, they are not recommended for most travelers and all long-term residents abroad.[27] Bismuth subsalicylate in fairly large doses appears to decrease the incidence of diarrhea,[24] but this regimen is expensive, time consuming, and only partially effective.

The heterogeneity of the serotypes, adherence factors, and toxins have made vaccine development a difficult task. An oral, whole *E coli* cell plus CT B subunit vaccine is being developed.[28]

Enterohemorrhagic *Escherichia coli*

Introduction and Military Relevance

E coli serotype O157:H7, the most famous EHEC serotype, was first recognized as a pathogen in 1982 when two geographically separated outbreaks of hemorrhagic colitis associated with eating undercooked beef from a fast food restaurant occurred.[29] Since 1982, many well-described outbreaks and numerous sporadic cases have been reported, including a large outbreak of more than 600 cases again associated with undercooked hamburgers from a fast food restaurant in the northwestern United States.[30] Initial reports identified most cases from the northern United States (most frequently the Pacific Northwest) and Canada, but increasing awareness has identified cases throughout the United States. Outbreaks of EHEC have occurred in the United Kingdom, Germany, Argentina, and Japan.[31] Foodborne transmission has been associated with undercooked ground or roast beef, unpasteurized milk, improperly processed water and cider, contaminated mayonnaise, and vegetables fertilized with manure or irrigated with tainted water.[30] Service members consume as much, if not more, of these foodstuffs as their civilian neighbors and so are at risk of EHEC infection.

Description of the Pathogen

The prototype EHEC isolate is serotype O157:H7. A number of other serotypes of *E coli* causing an identical disease spectrum have been reported, including O26:H11, O111:H8, and O111:NM. EHEC is not invasive, nor does it produce enterotoxins. However, EHEC, like other enteric pathogens, must adhere to the intestinal epithelium to cause disease. The elaboration of cytotoxins distinguishes EHEC from other *E coli* pathogens.[32] The cytotoxins produced by EHEC are known as Shiga-like toxin 1 and 2 (for their similarities to Shiga toxin isolated from *Shigella dysenteriae* 1 [Shiga's bacillus]) or verotoxin 1 and 2 (for their effects on Vero tissue culture cells). EHEC strains can produce either of the Shiga-like toxins or both of them.

Epidemiology

Transmission and Geographic Distribution. Most outbreaks are foodborne, and ground beef is the most frequently implicated source. A cluster of cases in Connecticut were associated with a particular retail supermarket.[33] This study emphasizes the importance of meat-handling practices and the need for frequent decontamination. Widespread testing for *E coli* O157:H7 led to one of the largest recalls of frozen ground beef in 1997.[34] Several outbreaks have been associated with unpasteurized apple juice and sprouts.[35,36] Another outbreak was associated with swimming in a contaminated lake in Oregon.[37] *S sonnei* was also implicated in this outbreak. The findings demonstrated that transmission of these two organisms can be very similar. Although food, especially ground beef, seems to be the most important vehicle for acquisition of infection, person-to-person transmission has also been described.[38] Cattle appear to be the most important reservoir for EHEC. Three percent of dairy calves in the United States are estimated to be infected.[30]

Incidence. With the development of simple microbiologic screening tests has come the awareness that, at least in North America, *E coli* O157:H7 is a common cause of infectious bloody diarrhea. In a prospective, population-based study in Washington state,[39] *E coli* O157:H7 was identified in 25 (0.4%) of 6,485 stool specimens, and isolation of this serotype was associated with illness in all patients. In this study, and in two other studies conducted in Canada,[30] the isolation rates of *E coli* O157:H7 were similar to those for other well-recognized enteropathogens, such as shigella, salmonella, and campylobacter, and ranged

from 0.4% to 1.9%. Disease caused by EHEC occurs at all ages; however, the very young and very old are more likely to have severe disease or to develop complications such as hemolytic-uremic syndrome. The incidence of nonbloody diarrhea or asymptomatic infection caused by EHEC is not known.

Pathogenesis and Clinical Findings

EHEC, most commonly *E coli* O157:H7, is an important cause of nonbloody diarrhea, hemorrhagic colitis, and hemolytic-uremic syndrome.[40–42] EHEC produces two types of Shiga-like toxins, which mediate both hemorrhagic colitis and hemolytic uremic syndrome. There is a 5- to 9-day interval between the onset of diarrhea and the onset of hemolytic uremic syndrome. Reports from outbreaks and sporadic cases indicate that bloody diarrhea is the most common symptom of illness caused by EHEC. Some patients may have mild disease with nonbloody diarrhea. The frequency with which mild disease occurs is not known, although approximately 25% of cases in outbreaks may have nonbloody diarrhea.[30] The disease is typically ushered in by severe abdominal cramping and watery diarrhea, which is soon followed by grossly bloody stools. The amount of blood in the stool may range from streaking to frank blood. Indeed, many of the initial cases of hemorrhagic colitis were confused with gastrointestinal bleeding. The duration of bloody diarrhea is generally 2 to 4 days.[40] Vomiting occurs in approximately one third to one half of persons with bloody diarrhea. Fever occurs in the minority of patients and is usually low-grade (< 39°C [102°F]). Fecal leukocytes may be present but are not a common feature. The severity of abdominal cramping and the frequent absence of fever can lead clinicians to consider other diagnoses, such as acute abdomen, inflammatory bowel disease, ischemic bowel, and intussusception. Failure to consider EHEC may lead to unnecessary diagnostic and surgical procedures.

Hemolytic-uremic syndrome, consisting of hemolytic anemia and acute renal failure, is the most serious complication of disease caused by EHEC. Most outbreaks report hemolytic-uremic syndrome in less than 10% of ill persons[43] and almost always in young children and the elderly. *E coli* O157:H7 has also caused illness in elderly patients that is recognized by clinicians as thrombotic thrombocytopenic purpura. Hemolytic-uremic syndrome or thrombotic thrombocytopenic purpura in association with EHEC in the elderly carries a high risk of mortality.[42]

Diagnostic Approaches

On routine culture media, EHEC cannot be visually differentiated from nonpathogenic *E coli* flora. However, because *E coli* O157:H7 ferments sorbitol slowly and since only 6% to 7% of all *E coli* is sorbitol-negative, the use of MacConkey or similar media containing 1% sorbitol provides a simple screening method. Sorbitol-negative colonies can be picked and agglutinated with commercially available O157 antisera for presumptive identification. Definitive identification requires serotyping and assays for toxin production.

Recommendations for Therapy and Control

Although *E coli* O157:H7 is sensitive to most antibiotics in vitro, antibiotics have not been shown to limit the duration of the illness or ameliorate the symptoms.[41] The illness is self limited, but the time to resolution can vary from a few days to several weeks. Treatment is supportive. Immune globulin preparations have been reported to be beneficial in a few cases of hemolytic-uremic syndrome,[42] and the finding that commercially available preparations contain anticytotoxin-neutralizing antibodies supports further investigation of this therapeutic modality. Oral ingestion of a synthetic receptor for Shiga-like toxin may be useful in binding unbound toxin and may prevent hemolytic-uremic syndrome.[44]

The catastrophic nature of EHEC illness in elderly patients emphasizes the importance of impeccable technique in food preparation and early recognition and intervention in outbreaks. All *E coli*, including EHEC, are frequent contaminants of ground beef and may remain viable in undercooked food. In response to an increase in cases in 1993, the Food and Drug Administration issued an advisory that all ground meat be uniformly heated to at least 71°C (160°F) for at least 8 seconds to kill all contaminating *E coli*.[45,46] Cooking procedures should be monitored to assure that the time and temperature parameters are met. Milk and cider should be pasteurized, and drinking water should be adequately disinfected.

Enteroinvasive *Escherichia coli*

Introduction and Military Relevance

Certain strains of *E coli* are capable of penetrating cells of the intestinal epithelium, producing a disease spectrum virtually identical to that caused by *Shigella* organisms. The incidence of disease caused by EIEC is not well studied, primarily be-

cause of difficulties in identification of the organism. It appears to be a relatively infrequent cause of sporadic diarrhea and has been found less often than *Shigella* organisms in studies in which both pathogens have been looked for.[43] Military personnel are at risk under field conditions similar to their risk of shigellosis. Outbreaks have occurred in military settings in Israel.[45]

Description of the Pathogen

Strains recognized as EIEC belong to a number of *E coli* serotypes, including O28ac, O29, O112ac, O124, O136, O143, O144, O147, O152, O164, and O167.[1] The EIEC serotypes are distinct from those of ETEC, EPEC, and EHEC. There exists no simple method to reliably identify EIEC. EIEC shares many microbiologic features with *Shigella* organisms. Although many EIEC serotypes do not ferment lactose and most are lysine decarboxylase–negative and nonmotile, no biochemical test is absolutely specific in identifying these organisms. There are also cross-reactions between EIEC and *Shigella* O antigens, which may result in misidentification of some lactose-negative EIEC serotypes that agglutinate in *Shigella* antisera. The lactose-positive strains cannot be visually differentiated from nonpathogenic *E coli* flora.

Epidemiology

Outbreaks of illness due to EIEC from contaminated food have been described[47,48] but are infrequent. Person-to-person transmission has been described[49] and may be important for sporadic cases, but most cases have been associated with outbreaks that have been foodborne. EIEC is a recognized enteric pathogen in pediatric populations of some developing countries[47] and has been detected in travelers with diarrhea.[50]

Pathogenesis and Clinical Findings

The pathogenetic mechanisms of EIEC are similar to those of *Shigella* organisms. As with shigellae, EIEC possesses a large virulence plasmid, which confers the capacity for epithelial cell invasion and is necessary for full pathogenicity. The large virulence plasmids of EIEC and *Shigella* organisms are functionally identical and exhibit considerable DNA homology.[51] Like *Shigella* organisms, EIEC does not produce enterotoxins. One notable difference between EIEC and *Shigella* organisms is that a much larger inoculum of the former is required to cause disease (10^8 versus about 10^2 organisms, respectively);

however, this has only been definitively shown for one EIEC strain.[10]

Although the illness caused by EIEC cannot be differentiated from shigellosis, the overall severity of illness is probably less with EIEC.[43] Diarrhea, fever, nausea, and abdominal cramping are the most common symptoms.[10,47,48] Bloody diarrhea and severe illness requiring hospitalization are uncommon, and the disease is self-limited.

Diagnostic Approaches

When conventional methods do not identify pathogens associated with invasive disease, random lactose-positive *E coli* colonies can be picked and saved for further identification by a reference laboratory. The individual colonies can then be tested for invasiveness in the definitive biological test of guinea pig keratoconjunctivitis (Sereny test). An enzyme-linked immunosorbent assay that detects the presence of outer membrane proteins associated with the virulence plasmid has been shown to be a useful screening tool and correlates closely with a positive keratoconjunctivitis test.[43] DNA probes based on the virulence plasmid[43,52] have been shown to be sensitive epidemiologic tools for rapidly screening large numbers of *E coli* samples to identify EIEC.

Recommendations for Therapy and Control

Little is known about the antibiotic-resistance patterns of EIEC or about the usefulness of antibiotic treatment for EIEC-related illness. Keeping in mind the other similarities of EIEC-related illness to shigellosis, though, significant symptomatic illness with fever and dysentery should probably be treated with antibiotics such as TMP/SMX, ampicillin, or one of the quinolones.

Enteropathogenic *Escherichia coli* and Other Types of Enteroadherent *Escherichia coli*

Introduction and Military Relevance

EPEC strains are a common cause of diarrhea, particularly among children living in developing countries and may be a cause of traveler's diarrhea as well. It is significant for the military in that it is one of the many undiagnosed causes of diarrheal disease in the developing world. The first association with *E coli* and enteric infection was made in the 1940s when certain serotypes of *E coli* were incriminated by epidemiologic methods as important causes of infantile summer diarrhea and epidemic diarrhea in nurseries.[53] The most frequently incriminated serogroups (ie, O55, O86, O111, O114, O119, O125, O126, O127, O128, O142) were termed "enteropathogenic *E coli*" or EPEC.[54]

Description of the Pathogen

EPEC organisms do not produce enterotoxins or cytotoxins and do not invade and destroy intestinal epithelial cells. EPEC is now defined as a class of *E coli* capable of causing diarrhea in humans that attaches to and effaces the microvilli of enterocytes but does not produce high levels of Shiga-like toxins.[55] The in vitro adherence pattern of EPEC on HEp-2 cells is described as localized adherence.[56] *E coli* not belonging to the EPEC serotypes can adhere in patterns described as diffuse or enteroaggregative, and the role of these pathogens in causing diarrheal disease for adults in the developing world is unclear. One such strain was isolated from a traveler to Mexico.[57,58] The best documented association was a foodborne outbreak in 1991 in Minnesota that was associated with *E coli* O39 that produced the enteroaggregative heat-stabile toxin (EAST).[46] This class of *E coli* may be one of the undocumented causes of diarrhea in the developing world.

Epidemiology

EPEC and other adherent *E coli* possess a virulence factor known as enteroadherent factor (EAF). In a case-control study of endemic diarrheal disease, EAF-positive *E coli* was isolated from 7% of 272 Thai children under 6 months of age with diarrhea and 3% of controls.[3] There was no association with diarrhea in children older than 6 months of age. The two most commonly isolated EAF-positive *E coli* were classic EPEC serotypes O119:H6 and O127:H6. Overall, of the 64 EAF-positive *E coli* samples, 35 belonged to EPEC serogroups (21 were EPEC O:H serotypes) and 29 did not belong to EPEC serogroups. It is not clear if EPEC organisms of nonclassic serotypes are as pathogenic to humans as EPEC organisms of classic serotypes. Diffuse *E coli* was not associated with diarrhea. In Brazil, localized-adherence *E coli* was isolated from 23% of infants younger than 1 year old with diarrhea and 2% of controls, a significant difference.[59]

Pathogenesis and Clinical Findings

EPEC strains appear to cause disease by tightly adhering to the intestinal mucosa of animals and humans. Biopsies of the small bowel reveal that EPEC has the ability to adhere to the intestinal epithelium in discrete microcolonies, causing a destruction of the cell below. The histopathologic lesion is caused by

EPEC's adherence to the enterocyte surface.[60] In electron microscopic studies of EPEC, Knutton and colleagues[61] have found that EPEC causes effacement at the apical enterocyte membrane and localized destruction of brush border microvilli of the intestinal epithelial cell. The enterocyte membrane forms a pedestal or platform on which the bacteria adhere. Effacement appears to be a crucial step in the pathogenesis of EPEC diarrhea and requires the 80-kilobase EAF plasmid. Strains lacking the EAF plasmid no longer adhere to epithelial cells and are less virulent.[62] EPEC strains express bundle-forming pili that form a meshwork to stabilize the bacterial colony on the epithelium.[63] The gene coding for bundle-forming pili filament is encoded on the EAF plasmid.

In outbreaks occurring in infants in nurseries and daycare centers, infections can be severe and similar to rotavirus infection. In the developing world, EPEC may be a cause of acute and chronic diarrhea.[64] In adult volunteers, EPEC causes watery diarrhea 7 to 16 hours after ingestion of a large inoculum.[62] Three to four liters of diarrheal stool may be lost during the 2-day illness. Abdominal cramps, nausea, vomiting, malaise, and fever can also commonly occur.

Diagnostic Approaches

DNA probes for genes associated with virulence are now available for use in large epidemiologic investigations.[65,66] At present DNA probes are the most practical method for screening (followed by tissue culture assays) for further differentiating enteroadherent strains. *E coli* serotyping is also useful but can only be performed in a few reference laboratories.

Recommendations for Therapy and Control

The treatment guidelines for ETEC infection can be used for EPEC infection.

Very little is known about animal reservoirs for enteroadherent *E coli*. During EPEC outbreaks, standard public-health and infection-control procedures are important for interrupting transmission. Isolation of cases, cohorting by area and nursing personnel, institution of strict handwashing procedures, and prevention of common exposure to equipment, bedding, or solutions are all indicated.

[David N. Taylor]

CAMPYLOBACTER ENTERITIS

Introduction and Military Relevance

Campylobacter organisms are one of the most common causes of acute bacterial diarrhea in the world. They affect children in developing countries and military personnel and travelers to developing countries. They are also one of the most common bacterial causes of diarrhea among all ages in developed countries and have an epidemiology and food-borne transmission similar to *Salmonella* organisms. *Campylobacter jejuni* and *C coli* have their natural reservoirs in the intestinal tracts of wild and domestic animals, predominantly chickens and cattle. Transmission of the infection to humans occurs through ingestion of contaminated chicken, other meats, or milk or by direct contact with infectious animal feces. The disease is characterized by acute watery diarrhea or dysentery, fever, and abdominal pain that is usually self-limited over a few days. Military units have been affected through eating improperly cooked chicken, and a large waterborne outbreak occurred on a military post when a water tower became contaminated from nesting birds.[67]

Description of the Pathogen

Campylobacter species are gram-negative, curved, rod-shaped bacteria with a polar flagellum. *C jejuni* is the species most commonly associated with diarrhea. Other species associated with diarrhea include *C coli, C laridis, C hyointestinalis,* and *C upsaliensis.*[68] These species can be distinguished biochemically from *C jejuni* by their inability to hydrolyze hippurate. These hippurate-negative or atypical hippurate-positive *Campylobacter* strains may account for 5% to 15% of the total *Campylobacter* isolated from patients with diarrhea.[69,70]

Campylobacter organisms are microaerophilic: they grow best in reduced oxygen concentrations of about 5%. They will not grow in atmospheres with ambient oxygen or under anaerobic conditions. The importance of *Campylobacter* species as human pathogens was overlooked until the 1970s because they do not grow on routine bacteriological media for stool pathogens.[71] Selective growth conditions are used in identifying *Campylobacter* organisms to take advantage of their microaerophilic and thermophilic (42°C) characteristics. *C jejuni* and *C coli* are naturally resistant to vancomycin, polymyxin, and the cephalosporins. These antibiotics can be incorporated into the media to further select these *Campylobacter* species from other enteric flora. Two different serotyping schemes are used to distinguish among strains of *C jejuni and C coli.*[72] Over 100 Lior serotypes based on the heat-labile flagellar proteins have been described, and a scheme based on heat-stable, or Penner, serotypes has identified 60 different serotypes.

Epidemiology

Transmission and Geographic Distribution

Transmission of infection to humans occurs by ingestion of the organism, usually in contaminated food. Outbreaks affecting both children and adults may be traced to contaminated sources of drinking water, poultry, eggs, unpasteurized milk, and raw hamburger meat.[73] Chicken bought in retail stores can be contaminated with *Campylobacter* organisms, and improper cooking can lead to infection. Direct contact with animal feces is probably important in areas of poor sanitation or close contact with domestic animals. Waterborne outbreaks have been associated with surface water contamination and contamination in water towers from bird droppings. Food handlers who are asymptomatic excretors of *C jejuni* are not a significant source of infection.

Campylobacter infection has a cosmopolitan distribution. It has been reported as a cause of infection on all continents. These bacteria have a zoonotic reservoir.[74] They inhabit the intestinal tracts of a variety of birds, including chickens, turkeys, and water fowl; farm animals, including pigs, cows, sheep, goats, and horses; domestic dogs and cats; and wild rodents and monkeys. Frequently, these animals are infected but do not usually show signs of illness.

Incidence

Campylobacter organisms are one of the most common bacterial causes of diarrhea in developed countries.[68,75,76] The isolation from fecal samples is almost always associated with diarrheal disease or other enteric symptoms. It affects all age groups and has the highest incidence in children under 5 years old. There is also a marked increase in incidence in young adults that makes *Campylobacter* a particularly important cause of diarrhea in this age group.

Campylobacter organisms are a common cause of diarrhea in travelers[77] and military personnel from developed countries going to the tropics.[78] In developing countries *Campylobacter* enteritis ranks with rotavirus infection, enterotoxigenic *Escherichia coli* infection, and shigellosis as a leading cause of acute diarrhea in children.[79] Surveys of childhood diarrhea in the tropics showed that *Campylobacter* organisms were isolated from the stool cultures of 4% to 35% of cases, with the highest rate of infection reported in infants with diarrhea. Older children and adults are infected less frequently because of immunity acquired in early childhood.[80] Healthy children in developing countries frequently show asymptomatic infection. Infections caused by *C coli* are more likely to be asymptomatic than ones caused by *C jejuni*. The ratio of cases of diarrhea to all persons infected with *Campylobacter* organisms is highest in infancy and declines with increasing age. Second infections may be due to different serotypes of *Campylobacter*. Immunity, which can be total or partial, serves to prevent illness or decrease the severity of illness.

In developed countries, there is an increased incidence of infection during summer months. In tropical developing countries, infection occurs during all seasons. In more temperate developing countries, such as in north Africa, there is a higher prevalence of infection during the wet, winter months.

Pathogenesis and Clinical Findings

The infective dose is estimated to vary from 800 to 10^6 bacteria.[81] *C jejuni* is killed by normal gastric acidity (pH 2.3), indicating that gastric acid is an effective barrier against infection and that ingestion of organisms with milk or other food that neutralizes acid may enhance infection by reducing the required inoculum. The incubation period varies from 1 to 7 days and is usually 2 to 4 days. During the incubation period, illness, and convalescence, *C jejuni* multiplies in the intestine and is excreted in feces in quantities of 10^6 to 10^9 organisms per gram of stool. The duration of fecal excretion varies from about 8 days in children 1 to 5 years old, to 14 days in infants, to up to 3 months in adults not treated with antibiotics.[68,73]

Pathogenesis

C jejuni invades epithelial cells, which leads to ulcerated mucosa and bloody diarrhea.[82] The regions of the intestine most affected are the jejunum, terminal ileum, and colon. Biopsies of infected intestines show inflammatory infiltrates in the lamina propria, crypt abscesses, and mucosal ulceration. Bacteria gain access to the bloodstream, but bacteremia is uncommon because most strains of *C jejuni* are susceptible to the bacteriolytic action of serum complement.[83] There is evidence for the presence of cytotoxins, enterotoxins, invasiveness, and adherence properties in some isolates, but as yet there is no well-defined association between specific clinical syndromes and any putative virulence characteristic.[82]

Clinical Findings

The characteristic clinical features of *Campylobacter* enteritis are fever, diarrhea, and abdominal pain.[84]

The diarrhea may be either watery or dysenteric, with the presence of blood or mucus in liquid stool. In developing countries, most children present with watery diarrhea rather than dysentery, whereas a larger portion of patients in developed countries report dysenteric disease. Fever, nausea, vomiting, and malaise may precede the onset of diarrhea by a day or more, and such nonspecific constitutional symptoms may be more severe than the diarrhea itself. The disease is usually self-limited and lasts 1 to 7 days. Severity of disease varies widely: stool frequency may vary from one to more than eight times a day. Most cases are mild, but about 20% of cases will have prolonged, severe disease with high fever, grossly bloody stools, and relapses. The abdominal pain may be severe, and, because it is sometimes localized to the right lower quadrant, patients with this infection have been subjected to laparotomy for suspected appendicitis. Cases of toxic megacolon, pseudomembranous colitis, and massive rectal bleeding have been reported.[85] Usually examination of stool reveals fecal leukocytes and sometimes red blood cells. Often, a Gram's stain of stool shows bacterial forms, including spiral or "seagull" shapes, suggestive of *Campylobacter* morphology.

Fatalities from this illness are rare in the developed world, but children in developing countries with severe diarrheal syndromes commonly die. In Bangladesh, *Campylobacter* organisms were the fourth most common cause of diarrhea in children who died, and most of those children showed severe colitis and the complicating conditions of pneumonia, septicemias with other organisms, and malnutrition.[86] Less common complications reported in patients with *Campylobacter* enteritis include hypoglycemia, pancreatitis, peritonitis, and cholecystitis. A reactive arthritis may develop in patients who have the HLA-B27 haplotype.[87]

C jejuni infection has been identified as one of the triggers of Guillain–Barré syndrome (GBS), and acute motor axonal neuropathy.[87,88] Between 20% and 40% of GBS cases have serological or microbiologic evidence of a *C jejuni* infection, usually within a month of the onset of neurological symptoms. GBS cases with *C jejuni* infection were significantly associated with a slower recovery and a poorer outcome than GBS cases not associated with a *Campylobacter* infection.[88]

Diagnostic Approaches

The diagnosis of *Campylobacter* enteritis requires isolation of the bacterium from stool cultures. This requires selective media, such as Skirrow's or Campy-

BAP, incubation at 42°C, and a microaerophilic environment, such as a Gas-pak (BBL Microbiology Systems, Cockeysville, Md.) or, less optimally, a candle jar.[71,73] Identification follows standard bacteriological techniques. Fresh stool should be examined for the presence of leukocytes and to exclude the possible presence of trophozoites of *Entamoeba histolytica*. In the tropics, patients are frequently coinfected with more than one enteric pathogen. Endoscopy is not routinely advised; however, when inflammatory bowel disease is considered in the differential diagnosis, colonoscopy with biopsy may be useful. The colonic mucosa will show erythema, superficial ulcerations, and friability, and the biopsy will reveal characteristically acute inflammation and crypt abscesses.

Recommendations for Therapy and Control

Therapy

As in other diarrheal diseases, the most important therapeutic approach is rehydration, which can be carried out with either isotonic intravenous fluids or oral rehydration solutions. Severe dehydration due to this disease is infrequent. Use of antibiotics in *Campylobacter* infection is not routinely indicated, but they may be used to shorten illness when patients have bloody diarrhea.[73] In patients with bloody diarrhea, treatment with erythromycin should be considered. Most strains of *C jejuni* are susceptible to erythromycin, tetracyclines, aminoglycosides, clindamycin, chloramphenicol, and quinolones (eg, nalidixic acid, norfloxacin, ciprofloxacin, ofloxacin). Resistance to the fluoro-quinolone antibiotics can be a problem in treatment, particularly in the developing world. Azithromycin was evaluated as an alternative to ciprofloxacin for the treatment of ciprofloxacin-resistant *Campylobacter* acquired in Thailand by US military personnel.[78] In this study, nearly half of the *Campylobacter* infections were caused by ciprofloxacin-resistant organisms. Azithromycin was significantly more efficacious than ciprofloxacin in reducing the time of illness and the duration of shedding of the organism.

Control

Prevention of infection requires the provision of safe food and water. All meats, but especially poultry, should be handled with the assumption that they could be contaminated with *Campylobacter* organisms and other bacterial pathogens such as *Salmonella* organisms. Transmission of *Campylobacter* infection can be reduced by cooking meats thoroughly and avoiding contamination of other foods by the juices of uncooked meats. Travelers to developing countries should take the usual precautions to avoid most uncooked foods and to ensure that their cooked food is served fresh, thoroughly cooked, and still hot. Handwashing before meals is a good preventive measure against most enteric infections. As discussed with enterotoxigenic *Escherichia coli* infections (see earlier in this chapter), prophylactic antibiotics are not usually recommended. The presence of immunity after natural infection suggests that a vaccine

strategy might work. An oral, inactivated whole cell vaccine for *Campylobacter* is under development.

Reducing the hyperendemic transmission of *Campylobacter* infection in developing countries requires improvements in basic hygiene and living conditions of the people. Because children acquire infection in infancy and early childhood by ingesting contaminated food and by direct contact with animals, household methods of food preparation must be improved and animals, especially chickens, must be kept away from people's homes.

[David N. Taylor]

VIRAL GASTROENTERITIS

Introduction and Military Relevance

Diarrheal illness is one of the major causes of morbidity and mortality worldwide, especially in the developing world and among infants and young children everywhere. It is historically perhaps the most common cause of hospitalization and lost duty time for deployed military persons because of the difficulty in maintaining good hygienic standards in foreign and field environments. Diarrhea and accompanying gastrointestinal symptoms, such as bloating, cramping, and nausea, will be referred to here as gastroenteritis.

The first bacterial cause of gastroenteritis was discovered in 1883 when Koch isolated the cholera vibrio. Although many other bacterial sources have since been identified, the etiology of the majority of these illnesses has been elusive. Viruses were suspected but could not be etiologically confirmed, even during virology's golden age (the 1950s and 1960s) when tissue culture techniques lead to the discovery of hundreds of viruses.

The development of electron microscopic techniques permitted a quantum leap in understanding the etiology of diarrhea. In the single year from November 1972 to 1973, two of the most important diarrhea-causing viruses worldwide were discovered.[89] Immune electron microscopy—the direct visualization of antigen-antibody complexes—was used to detect the Norwalk virus, a primary cause of adult gastroenteritis. The following year, a thin section electron micrograph of duodenal mucosa revealed rotavirus, the single most important cause of severe diarrheal illness in infants and young children.

Further advances in electron microscopy and genomic sequencing have allowed the identification of other gastroenteritis-causing viruses that could not be detected with standard laboratory equipment and training. Special, well-resourced surveillance

programs, including advanced laboratory capabilities, are necessary for definitive diagnosis of viral gastroenteritis. In the military, only some tertiary care centers, research facilities, and contracted laboratories currently have this capability.

These viruses' wide geographic distribution and high infectivity in typical military living environments make them a high military medical priority. For example, in 1998 US Army recruits at Fort Bliss, Texas, experienced an outbreak of viral gastroenteritis apparently associated with a particular dining facility. Twelve percent of the soldiers in one unit (99 soldiers) were hospitalized. The causative agent was a Norwalk-like virus.[90]

In a survey of more than 2,000 servicemembers deployed to the Persian Gulf War in 1990 and 1991, 20% admitted to being kept from their duties at some time by diarrheal disease.[11] Using a variety of methods to identify causal pathogens, epidemiologists found Norwalk-like viruses to be the primary agent in servicemembers with vomiting and diarrhea. They may also have been a widespread cause of gastroenteritis during the colder months before surveillance started.

In the spring of 1992, a large outbreak of acute gastroenteritis on a US Navy aircraft carrier was caused by a Norwalk-like virus. The outbreak lasted 35 days, and during that time 8% of the crew of 4,500 sailors reported to sick-bay. A questionnaire survey of two thirds of the crew identified 13% of respondents with symptoms. (The remainder of the crew had work conflicts on the days the survey was distributed.) The outbreak all but disappeared when most of the sailors went on shore leave but reappeared when they returned. This outbreak virtually exhausted some of the carrier's critical medical supplies even though only 58% of sailors with symptoms sought medical care.[91]

A group of Air Force and Army Special Forces

personnel deployed for 1 month (February 1993) to northern Thailand experienced a gastroenteritis outbreak with an attack rate of 28%.[92] Stool specimens were obtained from 24 of 95 patients. Among the pathogens recovered was rotavirus, the most common cause of infantile diarrhea but a less-common cause in adults. These findings indicate that military populations may be at risk of infection from viruses that typically affect young children.

Viral diarrhea has a worldwide sinister reputation for its morbidity and mortality among infants and young children, but it is often considered a relatively minor nuisance for adults. In military populations, however, which experience travel, crowded and austere living conditions, and large dining facilities as a way of life, epidemics of viral diarrhea are more potent risks. The dangers are amplified by the importance of having each member of a unit functional.

Description of the Pathogens

Viruses that cause gastroenteritis generally fall into three categories: small and round with surface structures, small and round but featureless, and larger, less uniformly shaped viruses. The first group (small, round, surface-structured) consists of those that are the principal causes of viral diarrhea in adults. Classification has matured recently as genomic sequencing and other new techniques have added to observations of external structure as bases for categorization (Table 37-3).

Small Round Viruses with Surface Features

This group, whose prototype is the Norwalk virus, comprises two families. *Caliciviridae* includes Norwalk, Norwalk-like, and classic caliciviruses, and *Astroviridae* includes the astroviruses. They are approximately 30 nm in diameter and contain a single strand of positive-sense RNA. The surface features seen in this group consist of either indentations (small round structured viruses or SRSVs), cup-like hollows with six-pointed stars (classic calicivirus), or five- or six-pointed stars with a central stain (astrovirus).[93]

The subgroup of SRSVs are also known as Norwalk and Norwalk-like viruses. Each virus in the subgroup is named for the place of the outbreak from which it was first isolated; for example, the prototype virus was first isolated from an outbreak in Norwalk, Ohio. Antigenic studies by immune

TABLE 37-3

SIGNIFICANT VIRUSES ASSOCIATED WITH HUMAN GASTROENTERITIS

Morphology	Family	Virus	Remarks
Small Round			
With surface features	Caliciviridae	SRSV (Norwalk, Norwalk-like)	≥ four serotypes (Norwalk, Hawaii, Snow Mtn, Taunton)
		classic calicivirus	
	Astroviridae	astrovirus	seven serotypes
Without surface features	Picornaviridae	enterovirus (Hepatitis A, polio, echo, coxsackie)	diarrhea is a minor symptom
	Parvoviridae	parvovirus	
Larger, less uniform			
	Reoviridae	rotavirus	groups, subgroups, serotypes
	Adenoviridae	adenovirus (serotypes 40, 41)	

SRSV small round structured virus

Sources: (1) Hyams KC, Bourgeois AL, Merrell BR, et al. Diarrheal disease during Operation Desert Shield. *N Engl J Med.* 1991,325:1423–1428 (2) Sharp TW, Hyams KC, Watts D, et al. Epidemiology of Norwalk virus during an outbreak of acute gastroenteritis aboard a US aircraft carrier. *J Med Virol.* 1995;45:61–67 (3) Belliot G, Laveran H, Monroe SS. Outbreak of gastroenteritis in military recruits associated with serotype 3 astrovirus infection. *J Med Virol.* 1997;51:101–106 (4) Matsui SM, Greenberg HB. Astroviruses. In: Fields BN, Knipe DM, Howley PM, et al, eds. *Fields Virology.* 3rd ed. Philadelphia: Lippincott-Raven; 1996: 979–1016.

electron microscopy have resulted in the identification of at least four serotypes (ie, Norwalk, Hawaii, Snow Mountain, and Taunton). Three genotypes have also been distinguished,[94] but they do not directly correlate with the serotypes, which suggests the need for further study and refinement of the classification.

The astroviruses and classic caliciviruses are relatively minor causes of adult gastroenteritis.[1] Astrovirus serotype 3 was found in an outbreak of gastroenteritis in French military recruits.[95] No serotypes have been identified for classic caliciviruses.[96]

Small Round Featureless Viruses

Unstructured, or featureless, small viruses associated with gastroenteritis are parvoviruses and enteroviruses. Infection with the latter (including hepatitis A, polio, coxsackie, and echo viruses) is not mainly manifested by gastroenteritis, although these viruses may cause an incidental, mild diarrhea.[97,98] Hepatitis viruses are discussed in Chapter 38.

Larger, Variously Shaped Viruses

This group contains, most notably, rotaviruses and adenoviruses.

The rotaviruses are members of the Reoviridae family and are distinguished by their wheel-like (rota means "wheel" in Latin) appearance in an electron micrograph.[99] Members of the rotavirus genus infect humans and many domestic and laboratory animals. The rotaviruses contain group, subgroup, and serotype antigens. The rotaviruses have been divided into seven groups, designated A thru G, of which groups A, B, and C have been recovered from humans. The VP6 protein, making up 50% of the virion, contains the group-specific antigen. The group A rotaviruses have been antigenically classified into 14 serotypes.

Adenoviruses are icosahedral particles 70 to 100 nm in diameter[100] with fiber projections. The human adenoviruses are classified into at least 47 serotypes, which fall into 6 subgroups. They cause a variety of illnesses in humans, including respiratory, ocular, and diarrheal diseases. The subgroup F adenoviruses, serotypes 40 and 41, are responsible for diarrheal disease in humans and have been referred to as the fastidious adenoviruses because of the difficulty of propagating them in cell cultures.

Torovirus, coronavirus, pestivirus, and picobirnavirus have all been associated with diarrhea in humans but require further evaluation before they are widely accepted as causes of the illness.[89,97,98]

Epidemiology

Transmission

All diarrhea-causing viruses are transmitted mainly through the fecal-oral route.

Of the small round structured viruses, the Norwalk and Norwalk-like viruses, or SRSVs, are the most important cause of epidemic, nonbacterial gastroenteritis in the world. They may be the most common cause (including bacterial) of gastroenteritis in the developed countries. They are the only gastroenteritis-causing viruses that predominantly affect adults. The SRSV group has been shown to cause outbreaks in such diverse environments as family settings, health care institutions, travel situations, nursing homes, and schools.

Transmission of SRSVs, as well as being between persons by the fecal-oral route, can also be through common-source outbreaks associated with contaminated food or water. Virus particles occur in vomit and feces and are infective in very low doses (10 to 100 virus particles). Spread of infection therefore can occur via aerosol droplets, although this is not true respiratory transmission because the droplets are aerosolized by vomiting, rather than by coughing, sneezing, or other respiratory acts. Movement of contaminated laundry can also aerosolize viral particles. Not surprisingly, the spread of disease is rapid, and the secondary attack rate is high: over 50%.[101] Some shellfish-associated outbreaks have attack rates of 90%.[102]

Many other viruses causing gastroenteritis are also transmitted via common sources. Major sources of foodborne viral gastroenteritis are bivalve mollusks (eg, oysters, clams, cockles, mussels) and other shellfish contaminated from raw sewage. Fruits and vegetables can be contaminated with polluted irrigation water or with untreated sewage sludge used as fertilizer. So far, however, outbreaks attributed to salad items have been thought to be caused by contamination during preparation from infected food handlers.[102]

Among the small featureless viruses, Parvovirus-like particles have been associated with shellfish-related outbreaks. They are also found in well persons,[98] though, so their transmission by contaminated food is less certain.

One of the larger viruses, rotavirus (group A), is the major cause of pediatric morbidity and mortality from diarrhea throughout the world. A high inoculum (eg, from close contact with an infected infant, from drinking heavily contaminated water) or lowered immunity can produce minor illness in older children and adults. Waning immunity with age may also contribute to adult disease. Group B rotavirus has caused very large epidemics in adults in China but not elsewhere.[97]

Adenoviruses are not believed to be transmitted via food or water. Person-to-person transmission is probably the mechanism for spread of infection.

Geographic Distribution

All diarrhea-causing viruses are found worldwide, but there are differences in relative incidences among age groups and environmental settings. The SRSVs and enteric adenoviruses occur year-round, with peaks in the winter.[101] Rotavirus outbreaks occur during the cooler months in northern Europe and North America, where a yearly wave starts in the southwest in November and ends in New England in March.[97] The disease is year-round in areas within 10 degrees latitude of the equator.

Incidence

Figure 37-2 shows prevalences of the most common causes of viral gastroenteritis in school-aged children and adults in a developed country. In the United States, about 50% of adults have antibodies to Norwalk or Norwalk-like viruses by age 50.[102] In developing countries, however, SRSV antibody acquisition occurs in a similar fashion to that of rotavirus: neonates and very young children are more commonly affected.

SRSVs commonly circulate in communities and

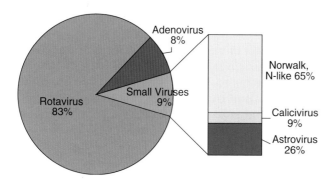

Fig. 37-2. The cumulative percentages of enteric viruses in the United Kingdom, 1990-1995.
Adapted from: Caul EO. Viral gastroenteritis: Small round structured viruses, caliciviruses and astroviruses, Part II: The epidemiological perspective. *J Clin Pathol.* 1996;49:960, with permission from the BMJ Publishing Group.

are believed to cause approximately 10% to 40% of gastrointestinal outbreaks in recreational camps, cruise ships, families, elementary schools and colleges, nursing homes, hospitals, cafeterias, and sports teams.[89,97,102] Although illness is relatively minor and short, the high attack rate causes a substantial loss of productivity at school and work.[93] For example, an SRSV outbreak associated with one infected bakery worker affected 3,000 persons and led to temporary closure of hospitals and schools in Minneapolis-St. Paul in 1982.[103] The similarities between the above settings and those found in military barracks, camps, and ships, along with the significance of lost productivity, suggests that the impact of SRSVs in the military may be substantial, but surprisingly little is known about viral gastroenteritis in these settings.

The other small structured viruses, calicivirus and astrovirus, are primarily found in the pediatric population. Calicivirus causes more pediatric diarrhea than any bacterial cause, but it is still less common than rotavirus. Calciviruses are rarely found in adults, except occasionally in nursing homes residents, where waning immunity may be a factor.[97,98,101] Enteric adenoviruses are considered the second-most important group of viruses associated with severe pediatric diarrhea.[89]

Pathogenesis and Clinical Findings

Gastroenteritis caused by SRSVs is usually a comparatively mild, self-limiting illness lasting approximately 12 to 60 hours. After an incubation period of about 24 to 48 hours, there is acute onset of nausea and vomiting (often explosive and projectile), abdominal cramping, and nonbloody diarrhea. Patients may have either vomiting or diarrhea or both, although vomiting is somewhat more prominent among children and diarrhea among adults. Symptoms, acuteness of onset, and a high secondary attack rate are characteristic enough to permit presumptive clinical diagnosis of SRSV.[89,104]

The SRSV seems to infect mature enterocytes of the proximal small intestine, causing malabsorption of D-xylose, lactose, and fat for up to 2 weeks after onset of illness. Gastric secretion of hydrochloric acid, pepsin, and intrinsic factor remain normal, but gastric emptying is slowed substantially. The latter finding probably accounts for the prominence of nausea and vomiting in this illness. Infection with SRSV induces both local gut and serum antibodies. The presence of serum antibodies, however, does not seem to protect against re-infection.

Classic calicivirus has an incubation period of 1

to 3 days, and illness lasts about 4 days. As in Norwalk-like illness, both vomiting and diarrhea may be present. Upper respiratory symptoms and fever occur less commonly. Unlike the case with SRSVs, antibodies to calicivirus may be protective.

In children, astrovirus disease is similar to but less severe than rotavirus.[105] Incubation is 24 to 36 hours, and illness lasts 1 to 4 days. Antibodies are probably protective.

Rotavirus has a 2-day incubation period. Watery diarrhea lasts 3 to 8 days and vomiting 3 days. Illness is often accompanied by fever and abdominal pain. Illness may be followed by temporary lactose intolerance. Infection confers long-term immunity to serious illness, but that immunity may wane with age.

The enteric adenovirus incubation period is 3 to 10 days, and illness lasts at least a week. Diarrhea is more prominent than vomiting or fever, and respiratory symptoms are often present. The long-term immunity conferred by infection may wane with age.

Viral gastroenteritis may be caused by multiple agents concurrently. This scenario is likely when shellfish or grossly contaminated water supplies are implicated. In outbreaks with mixed infections, differing incubation periods may create the impression that there is more than one outbreak.

Diagnostic Approaches

Except in instances where advanced laboratory capabilities (such as those found in the Theater Army Medical Laboratory or the Navy Joint Forward Laboratory) are deployed, field diagnosis usually depends on the clinical presentation of patients and the epidemiologic characteristics of outbreaks. Diagnoses based on these grounds are sufficient to initiate treatment and control measures.

Where laboratory confirmation of the diagnosis is available, it is valuable because it provides a better epidemiologic picture of the causes and illness patterns that are so disruptive to operations and training. Appropriate specimen collection, handling, and storage are crucial to establishing the etiology of gastroenteritis outbreaks. Particular care is necessary to prevent transmission of any agent to the personnel collecting or handling the specimens.

Since gastroenteritis-causing viruses are difficult to culture, other diagnostic tests are used. The tests include antigen and antibody detection by immunoassays, electron microscopy, and polymerase chain reaction. Electron microscopy is the classic procedure to detect viruses, and it is still the gold standard. These procedures are labor intensive, however, and few electron microscopes and experienced operators are available.

Fortunately for public health, the application of molecular biological procedures in the 1980s and 1990s resulted in determination of genome sequences and their product capsid proteins[106] that made many of the viral antigens available for rapid diagnostic tests. For example, commercial kits are available for the diagnosis of rotaviruses[107] and adenoviruses types 40 and 41.[108] The problem with these tests lies in their wide range of sensitivities (70% to 100%) and specificities (50% to 100%).[98]

Most individuals with viral gastroenteritis infection will have a rise in antibodies to that virus, but because these agents are so common, paired sera are necessary to demonstrate recent infection. At this time, though, antibody detection methods are available for Norwalk-like viruses only. Molecular studies are also permitting the application of reverse transcriptase polymerase chain reaction to SRSV diagnosis, although these procedures are not yet widespread.

Stool or serum specimens should be collected for diagnoses of suspected outbreaks of viral gastroenteritis, depending upon the tests to be used. The Centers for Disease Control and Prevention (CDC) recommends that stool specimens be collected within 48 hours of onset of symptoms (Exhibit 37-1). For outbreaks, electron microscopic examination or direct testing (antigen or reverse transcriptase polymerase chain reaction) requires that large volumes of stool be collected from at least 10 individuals who have unformed stool. Diagnostic yield is low if there are fewer specimens. These specimens should be refrigerated. If long-term storage is required, the stools should be stored at –70°C or colder. Stool samples to be sent to the CDC must be identified with a waterproof label and sealed in a plastic bag.

For antibody detection, serum is needed. Paired serum specimens should be collected during the first week and between the third and sixth weeks of illness.[98]

For the greatest yield, specimen collection should be accompanied by good clinical and epidemiologic information. Detailed directions for specimen collection and shipping are included in Exhibit 37-1.

Recommendations for Therapy and Control

The medical status of diarrhea patients should be assessed. Adults at risk for more severe illness[109] are those over 60 years of age, those who have a variety of chronic or immunosuppressive diseases or conditions, and those taking therapy that decreases gastric acidity (eg, hypochlorhydria, proton

---

EXHIBIT 37-1

CENTERS FOR DISEASE CONTROL AND PREVENTION GUIDELINES FOR COLLECTING SPECIMENS FOR VIRAL DIAGNOSIS

Stool

- **Collection in the first 48 hours.** Presently, viral diagnosis of a stool sample can be made only when the level of excretion is approximately 1 million particles/mL. For many viruses, this level of excretion is present only during the first 2 days of illness, and occasionally during the third. If specimens are not collected during the first 2 to 3 days of illness, an agent is unlikely to be detected. Thus, appropriate specimens should be collected as soon as an outbreak occurs. **Specimen collection should not await the results of epidemiologic and other investigations, since delay will almost certainly preclude a viral diagnosis.** If information gathered subsequently indicates that a viral etiology is unlikely, the specimens can be discarded before the cost of testing is incurred.

- **Ten diarrheal bulk specimens.** Bulk samples (enough to fill a large stool cup) are preferred, and only those specimens loose enough to assume the shape of their containers are likely to yield positive results. Serial specimens from persons with acute, frequent, high-volume diarrhea are particularly useful. The smaller the specimen and the more formed the stool, the lower the diagnostic yield. Rectal swabs are of little or no value. Specimens from at least 10 ill persons should be collected to maximize the chance that a diagnosis can be made. (The diagnostic yield is low when specimens from fewer than 10 persons are submitted.)

- **Storage at +4°C.** Because freezing may destroy the characteristic viral morphology that permits a diagnosis by electron microscopy, specimens should be kept at +4°C.

Paired Serum Specimens (essential for diagnosis)

- **Timing**   Acute: during the first week of symptoms
  Convalescent: 3rd to 6th week

- **Number**   10 pairs from ill persons (the same persons submitting stool specimens)
  10 pairs from well persons

- **Quantity**   Adults: 10 mL
  Children: 3 mL

- **Storage**   Tubes containing no anticoagulant (tubes with red tops) should be used for collection. Sera should be spun off and frozen. If a centrifuge is not available, a clot should be allowed to form, and the serum should be decanted and frozen. If this step cannot be taken, the whole blood should be refrigerated, not frozen.

Other Specimens

Viruses causing gastroenteritis cannot normally be detected in vomitus, water, food, or environmental samples. Although British researchers report electron microscope detection of virus in shellfish, no successful effort has yet been reported in the United States.

Source: Centers for Disease Control. Viral agents of gastroenteritis: Public health importance and outbreak management. *MMWR.* 1990;39(RR-5):19.

---

pump or histamine type 2 inhibitors, antacids). Angiotensin-converting enzyme inhibitors and diuretics may also predispose those taking them to more serious gastrointestinal infections.

At the same time, severity of illness (as measured by fever, shock, hematochezia, concomitant illness, and number of stools per 24 hours) and hydration status, including urine output, should be assessed and monitored. Treatment, which is mainly supportive, involves hydration and maintenance of fluids and electrolytes.

Fluid replacement is best accomplished with an oral rehydration solution (ORS). These solutions were developed to be a simple, non-invasive, and inexpensive therapy for victims of severe cholera.[110] It was known that sodium absorption was linked with other ions (eg, glucose, amino acids, dipeptides, tripeptides) at the intestinal brush border. However, early solutions contained higher levels of sodium than was optimal or even safe for less severe gastrointestinal infections and were associated with an increase in hypernatremia.

The need for a single ORS that could be administered to diarrhea patients regardless of age, etiologic agent, and initial serum sodium value resulted in a solution that contained the following (in mmol/L): sodium, 90; potassium, 20; chloride, 80; base, 30; and glucose, 111 (2%). This solution was approved by the World Health Organization and the United Nations International Children's Emergency Fund in 1975.[110] Oral rehydration solutions are available commercially and are encouraged for home use.

Patients with mild-to-moderate dehydration quickly improve clinically with simple rehydration. In these patients, the first 24 hours of illness should be managed with ORS as the only fluid intake (at least 2 L). Subsequently, 200 mL of ORS per loose stool should be given, along with unrestricted dietary and fluid intake.

Glucose-based ORS does not reduce the duration of illness or the volume of stool, but early feeding can reduce the severity and duration of illness.[110] It appears that glucose, in addition to providing the ORS sodium cotransport ion, also creates excessive osmotic load and therefore exacerbates diarrhea. More complex molecules, such as complex carbohydrates and larger proteins, are slowly digested by intestinal enzymes and then absorbed (as glucose or smaller peptides and amino acids, respectively) along with sodium. Therefore, a diet that emphasizes starches, cereals, yogurt, fruits, and vegetables is recommended after the first 24 hours. Foods high in simple sugars create too high an osmotic load and should be avoided.[110]

Symptoms of severe dehydration include profound apathy, weakness, confusion, or coma. Signs are tachycardia, rapid breathing, systolic blood pressure below 90 mm Hg, peripheral vasoconstriction (eg, cyanosis, cold extremities), uremia, and oliguria or anuria. If the patient is severely dehydrated or if ORS is not tolerated due to persistent vomiting, intravenous isotonic saline with potassium should be administered to replace fluid and electrolyte losses. In the event of acidosis due to severe dehydration, the replacement fluids should include 20% sodium bicarbonate (isotonic 1.26).

Antidiarrheal agents may be considered for treatment of symptoms. Bismuth subsalicylate may decrease abdominal cramping, but the reports are mixed on its effect on the duration of diarrhea.[98,105]

Antimotility drugs, including opiates, loperamide, and diphenoxylate, may reduce symptoms but should be avoided in anyone with dysenteric symptoms, since they are harmful in patients with shigella (bacterial) infection.

Unfortunately, viruses that infect via the gastrointestinal tract are relatively resistant to inactivation. Since they are acid-stable, they survive food processing and preservation methods that use a low-pH environment to inhibit bacterial and fungal organisms. Temperatures required to inactivate viruses are not well established but are higher than those that kill bacteria. Viruses can remain infectious after freezing.[102]

These difficulties in eliminating viruses from contaminated food make prevention of contamination and outbreak control all the more important. The highest-risk foods are shellfish. Methods for optimal depuration (the self-cleansing actions of live shellfish after they have been moved to clean waters) are recommended, but they are less effective for viruses than for bacteria (and testing for contamination typically focuses on *Escherichia coli*, a bacterium). No satisfactory system has yet been devised for removal of viruses.[102]

All foods for US servicemembers should be approved according to military regulations. In areas where raw sewage is discharged into waters that contain shellfish, shellfish should be avoided altogether. The same is true for fruits and vegetables grown where raw sewage sludge is used as a fertilizer.

In outbreak situations in military settings, aggressive intervention is necessary. First the common source, such as water, ice, or shellfish, must be identified and eliminated. If water is contaminated with SRSVs, shock chlorine concentration of at least 10 mg/L for at least 30 minutes may help.[98]

Next, interpersonal transmission must be prevented, but implementing preventive measures in the field setting is challenging. Workers at risk for transmission are health care providers, daycare center staff, and food handlers. It has been suggested that for at least 2 days after the resolution of their illness, infected workers be excluded from contact with susceptible persons. Handwashing must be emphasized. Safeguards must be employed with soiled laundry (eg, transported in an enclosed container and in a sanitary manner, washed promptly in a machine at maximum cycle length, machine dried). Soiled surfaces should be promptly cleaned and disinfected with a germicidal product. Persons performing these tasks should wear protective barriers, including face masks. Nosocomial spread is minimized by these outbreak control measures.

Finally, contact between well and ill persons should be minimized, and in environments such as cruise ships and camps, renewal of a susceptible population should be interrupted. Population dispersal has been suggested as an effective control measure,[91] but in the very setting where it is likely to be of greatest benefit—crowded military barracks or ships—it is of greatest impracticality. In some circumstances, it could also spread the outbreak.

Only one vaccine now exists for the prevention of viral gastroenteritis (other than hepatitis A), and it is not currently available. Rotavirus vaccine was licensed in the United States for prevention of infantile gastroenteritis. After an excess of intestinal intussusception in vaccinated babies, however, the CDC withdrew the recommendation to vaccinate.[111] The vaccine was subsequently withdrawn from the market.

[Sharon L. Ludwig; Leonard N. Binn]

TYPHOID FEVER

Introduction and Military Relevance

Typhoid fever has historically had a major impact on military campaigns. In the Spanish-American War, one in five soldiers contracted typhoid fever, and more than 1,500 men died during the typhoid epidemic of 1898.[112] This prompted formation of a typhoid fever commission, composed of Walter Reed, Victor Vaughn, and Edward Shakespeare. Their study[113] resulted in an improved understanding of the mechanisms of transmission, including an appreciation for the role of asymptomatic carriers. Early British and American efforts to develop an effective typhoid vaccine were largely driven by the need to protect soldiers.

Despite advances in field sanitation and the development of effective vaccines, typhoid fever continues to pose a significant threat to service members, who are frequently deployed to areas where the disease remains endemic.[114–118] Changes in the global epidemiology of typhoid fever, including the emergence of multidrug-resistant strains, have intensified the threat to service members.

Description of the Pathogen

Typhoid fever is caused by the gram-negative bacterium *Salmonella enterica* serovar Typhi, hereafter referred to as *S* Typhi. More than 100 phage types have been identified.

Epidemiology

Transmission and Geographic Distribution

Humans are the only known reservoir for *S* Typhi, and typhoid fever is perpetuated in regions where fecal-oral dissemination of the organism continues unabated because of the lack of clean water or appropriate sanitation. Epidemiologic data from developing countries suggests that the incidence of typhoid fever is highest in regions where contaminated water supplies serve large populations. Foodborne illness in these countries is associated with high attack rates, resulting from large inocula of organisms, and may vary seasonally as contaminated water is used to irrigate or "freshen" vegetables.[119–121] Susceptible personnel deployed to regions of high endemicity may become infected through consumption of locally obtained, contaminated food or water, or when typhoid carriers are employed to prepare food for service members.[122,123] Infections in recent immigrants and international travelers represent most reported *S* Typhi infections the United States.[124–128]

Incidence

Although there is no precise estimate of the global incidence of typhoid fever, the World Health Organization estimates that worldwide the number of typhoid fever cases exceeds 16 million annually,[129,130] which results in more than 600,000 deaths.[130] In many developing countries, rapid increases in population density, especially in urban areas, combined with inadequate sanitation have led to an increased incidence of typhoid fever.[129]

Pathogenesis and Clinical Findings

The incubation period of typhoid fever ranges from 3 to 60 days or more, but is most commonly 7 to 14 days. The incubation period is in part dependent on the inoculum size, as well as the host's susceptibility and the strain involved.[131] Generally a larger infectious dose is associated with a shorter incubation period and a more severe illness. On average, an inoculum of at least 10^5 organisms is necessary to produce disease in healthy adults, but some may become ill with lesser exposures.[132] As with other gastrointestinal pathogens, the number of organisms required may be significantly lower in those suffering from achlorhydria or in individuals taking H2 blockers.

S Typhi produces a spectrum of illnesses that vary widely with respect to severity, clinical signs, and symptomatology.[133–135] Classic typhoid fever often begins insidiously with nonspecific flu-like symptoms such as malaise, toxemia, fever, headache, anorexia, abdominal pain, and occasionally myalgias. One third to one half of patients present with diarrhea that varies in frequency from several to many stools per day.[136] Diarrhea appears to be more common in young children, while constipation occurs more commonly in adults.[136–139] Other symptoms that are less common and that may confound attempts at diagnosis are sore throat,[140] cough, dysuria, and bloody diarrhea.[141] Protracted diarrhea with few other symptoms may occur in young, malnourished children.[142] Many infections are mild and do not fit the classic description.

Physical signs ascribed to typhoid fever include a toxic appearance, dehydration, relative bradycardia, hepatosplenomegaly, abdominal tenderness, segmental ileus, rose spots (2- to 4-mm blanching, erythematous macules, frequently on the abdomen and chest), meningismus, and neuropsychiatric manifestations. Patients presenting early in the course of their illness may have relatively few signs or symptoms other than fever.[141,143] In travelers, typhoid fever is usually characterized by a persistent low-grade fever with headache.

In the preantibiotic era, many of the complications classically described in typhoid fever were appreciated after days of illness. These complications have taken on new importance with the emergence of multidrug-resistant strains, as patients fail to respond to antibiotics traditionally used to treat typhoid fever[144] and so have a greater tendency toward the complications that develop later in the course of the infection. Complications include intestinal perforation, gastrointestinal bleeding, pneumonia, pleural effusion, myocarditis, meningitis, sepsis, acute respiratory disease syndromes,[145] seizures, and coma.[146]

Intestinal perforation results from the proliferation of organisms in Peyer's patches of the small intestine and is one of the most feared complications of typhoid fever because of the high associated mortality rate. It occurs in approximately 3% of cases, particularly later in untreated cases.[147] With modern surgical techniques and antimicrobial therapy, the mortality rate has declined from nearly 100% in the preantibiotic era[148,149] to under 10% in a more recent study.[150]

Typical typhoid case fatality without treatment is 10%; with prompt treatment this can be reduced to less than 1%. Relapse rates as high as 20% may occur after therapy with appropriate antibiotics. Relapses occur in about 5% to 10% of untreated cases.

Immunity following natural infection with *S*

Typhi is incomplete and may be overcome by a high inoculum of organisms or infection with different phage types. Although reinfection does occur, it is felt to be rare.[151]

Diagnosis

Isolation of *S* Typhi from either blood or bone marrow is required for a definitive diagnosis of typhoid fever. In the absence of antimicrobial therapy, the majority of patients will be bacteremic in the first week of the illness. Isolation of the organism from stool supports but does not confirm the diagnosis. Occasionally, the organism can be isolated from urine or cultures of skin obtained from rose spots. A significant rise in typhoid O-type agglutinins or Vi antibody is helpful in confirming the diagnosis.

Recommendations for Therapy and Control

Typhoid fever presents the clinician with some unique therapeutic challenges. First, *S* Typhi can invade the intestinal epithelial cell and penetrate the lamina propria. From there, the organism enters the bloodstream, where it may multiply within mononuclear phagocytes, which protect it from some antimicrobial agents. Therefore, in vitro resistance may predict clinical failure, but sensitivity of the organism does not always translate to clinical success.[152] Because of the poor correlation between in vitro sensitivity testing and clinical outcome and because there is currently no valid, reliable animal model for typhoid fever; therapies should be based on the results of well-controlled clinical studies. Previous studies have demonstrated that early treatment with effective antimicrobial therapy may not prevent relapse,[153] so close scrutiny during convalescence is necessary. Emerging resistance to several of the agents used as standard therapy in many areas, including the Arabian Gulf, Africa, India, and Egypt,[154] has prompted the use of antibiotics that are more costly and less readily available in developing countries.

A number of different classes of antibiotics have been shown to be effective in the treatment of typhoid fever. Chloramphenicol has been a mainstay in the treatment of typhoid fever since it was first employed by Woodward and colleagues[155] in 1948. It remains useful in cases caused by chloramphenicol-sensitive *S* Typhi. However, the rare association of chloramphenicol with drug-induced aplastic anemia and the emergence of resistance to chloramphenicol in the 1970s[156] led to the investigation of alternative agents for treatment. Ampicilllin[157] and trimethoprim-sulfamethoxazole[158,159] were later shown to be effective therapies for typhoid fever. However, strains resistant to all of these traditional first-line therapies for typhoid fever have now emerged in many parts of the world,[154,160–166] leading to the introduction of different, newer antibiotics for treatment.

Fluoroquinolones are well suited for the treatment of typhoid fever and should be regarded as the agents of choice for adults in regions where multidrug-resistant strains of *S* Typhi are prevalent. These agents are highly active against salmonellae,[161,167] and they are concentrated in both macrophages and polymorphonuclear leukocytes, with intracellular levels as much as 10-fold higher than serum values.[168]

The third generation cephalosporins (eg, cefotaxime, cefoperazone, ceftriaxone, the orally administered cefixime) demonstrate excellent in vitro activity against many *Salmonella* species, including *S* Typhi.[169,170] Ceftriaxone and cefotaxime are effective against some ampicillin-resistant strains of *Salmonella*.[171] The minimal inhibitory concentrations for ceftriaxone are in the range of 0.05 µg/mL against most *Salmonella* species, and cellular penetration of ceftriaxone [172] indicates that it may be active against intracellular organisms. Its prolonged serum half-life and biliary excretion permit daily dosing.[173] Daily ceftriaxone for 3 [174], 5 [175], or 7 days [176] has compared favorably to standard 14-day courses of chloramphenicol in several randomized clinical trials. In a randomized clinical trial comparing ciprofloxacin to ceftriaxone, ciprofloxacin produced more rapid resolution of fever and had a higher success rate than ceftriaxone.[177] Although fluoroquinolones have been used successfully to treat typhoid fever in children, [178] there are persisting concerns about potential bone and cartilage toxicity of fluoroquinolones in young children.[179,180] The third generation cephalosporins are now considered the treatment of choice for children in regions where multidrug resistance is a problem.[181]

Patients presenting with severe toxemia from typhoid fever may benefit from the administration of corticosteroids. In a highly selected group of patients at high risk of death from typhoid fever in Jakarta, Indonesia, Hoffman and colleagues[182] demonstrated a significant reduction in mortality in patients treated with dexamethasone (3 mg/kg followed by 1 mg/kg every 6 hours) compared to placebo-treated controls. Others have suggested that patients receiving adjuvant steroids may have higher relapse rates.[183] Therefore, the use of corticosteroids in typhoid fever should be reserved for those cases complicated by profound mental status changes, severe toxemia, or impending shock.

Treatment of Typhoid Carriers

Between 1% and 5% of patients with typhoid fever become chronic carriers of *S* Typhi. The chronic carrier state is more common in women. The likelihood of becoming a carrier after having typhoid fever increases with age, paralleling an increased incidence of cholelithiasis. Infections with *Schistosoma haematobium* may result in chronic urinary carriage of *S* Typhi organisms,[184] which may reside in the gut of the worm or attached to the surface of the worm.[185] Antimicrobial treatment for acute disease does not prevent the development of the carriage state, and relapses have been reported as long as 24 months after initial therapy. Because humans are the only known reservoir for this organism, identification and treatment of carriers is of potential importance in interrupting the transmission of the organism to others.

Cure of typhoid carriers may be achieved with either antibiotics alone or through a combination of antimicrobial therapy and cholecystectomy. Most studies have demonstrated significantly lower cure rates for individuals with cholelithiasis, as calculi may serve as residual foci of infection. The finding of *S* Typhi in the bile of patients months after cholecystectomy supports the view that this organism may persist even after surgical intervention. Both intravenous ampicillin and oral amoxicillin, which is given with and without probenecid, have been employed successfully to eradicate the carriage state. Treatment with amoxicillin requires high doses (6 g daily) for 4 to 6 weeks and is frequently accompanied by intolerable gastrointestinal side effects.[186–188] Treatment with intravenous ampicillin has also been used, but prolonged intravenous therapy may be impractical. Oral trimethoprimsulfamethoxazole has been used with variable success.[189,190] Long-term followup examination is necessary to confirm successful clearance of the organism.

Fluoroquinolones have been used successfully to treat chronic carriers. Ciprofloxacin (750 mg orally twice a day for 28 days) eradicated the organism in 11 of 12 patients (92 %) with chronic *S* Typhi carriage.[191] Norfloxacin (400 mg twice a day for 28 days) was 86% effective in eradicating *S* Typhi from individuals without gallstones and 75% effective in those with cholelithiasis.[192]

Vaccines

The first successful US typhoid vaccine was developed by Colonel Frederick Fuller Russell and contributed significantly to the United States' dramatically lower incidence of typhoid fever in World War I than in the Spanish-American War. Later, volunteer trials of typhoid vaccines were initiated at the University of Maryland Hospital in collaboration with Joseph Smadel and others of the Walter Reed Army Institute of Research, Washington, DC.

Three vaccines for the prevention of typhoid fever are currently licensed for use in the United States[193] (Table 37-4). These include the live attenuated Ty21a oral typhoid vaccine and two parenteral vaccines: a heat-phenol inactivated vaccine and the recently licensed Vi capsular polysaccharide vaccine. A fourth vaccine, available only to the military, is the acetone-inactivated parenteral vaccine. The vaccines vary in their side effects, the time required for primary vaccination, and the need for booster immunizations.[194] Although each vaccine has been demonstrated to be effective in separate clinical trials, they have never been compared in prospective randomized studies. In clinical trials, the efficacy of the individual vaccines varies with the population studied and the intensity of exposure.

Parenteral killed whole cell typhoid vaccines, prepared by either heat-phenol or acetone inactivation methods, have been available for many years. In clinical trials, their efficacy varied from 50% to 88%.[194] Vaccination is often accompanied by side effects; nearly 25% of vaccinees develop fever, and 40% to 50% develop local side effects. The significant reactogenicity of these vaccines and the need

to administer two doses more than 1 month apart for the primary immunization limit their utility, especially in comparison to other available vaccines.

Another parenteral vaccine, prepared from purified Vi capsular polysaccharide,[195] an essential virulence determinant of *S* Typhi, was licensed for use in the United States in the mid 1990s. In one clinical trial, more than 90% of healthy US adult males seroconverted following a single 25 µg injection of purified Vi antigen.[196] In the same study, antibody levels remained significantly elevated for up to 34 months following primary immunization. Following a single dose of vaccine, the number of cases of typhoid fever was reduced by 55% to 74% when the vaccine was tested in endemic areas.[197,198]

The Ty21a oral typhoid vaccine is a live vaccine composed of a strain of *S* Typhi that has been attenuated by chemical mutagenesis[199] and has an efficacy rate similar to parenteral vaccines.[200] Because this vaccine is administered every other day for four doses, compliance needs to be reinforced.[201,202] Mefloquine and antibiotics may inhibit the growth of Ty21a,[203,204] so vaccination should be delayed 24 hours after consuming these drugs. The vaccine should not be administered to immunosuppressed individuals.

Typhoid vaccination should be directed at those individuals anticipating prolonged exposure in endemic areas. By US military regulation,[205] typhoid immunization is to be given to all alert forces. This

TABLE 37-4

DOSAGE AND SCHEDULES FOR ADULT TYPHOID FEVER VACCINATION

Vaccine	Dose	Number of doses	Dosing interval	Boosting interval
Ty21a				
primary series	1 capsule*	4	2 days	—
booster	1 capsule*	4	2 days	every 5 years
Vi capsular polysaccharide				
primary series	0.5 mL†	1	—	—
booster	0.5 mL†	1	—	every 2 years
Heat-phenol-inactivated				
primary series	0.5 mL‡	2	4 weeks	—
booster	0.5 mL‡	1	—	every 3 years

*oral
†intramuscularly
‡subcutaneously
Adapted from: Centers for Disease Control and Prevention. Typhoid immunization—recommendations of the Advisory Committee on Immunization Practices (ACIP). *MMWR*. 1994;43;RR-14:1–7.

generally includes Army personnel required to be ready for foreign deployment in 30 days or less, all foreign-deployed (except Canada) Navy and Marine Corps personnel, others subject to foreign deployment on short notice, and all Air Force rapid deployment personnel. It is also indicated for others deploying or traveling to high-risk areas. Vaccinees need to be reminded that typhoid vaccination does not obviate the need for caution in selecting food and drink in endemic areas because the vaccine is not 100% effective, immunity can be overcome by large inocula of organisms,[130] and the vaccine also offers no protection against other enteric pathogens.

Other Prevention Measures

In addition to vaccination, preventing cases of typhoid fever requires strict enforcement of measures designed to interrupt fecal–oral transmission of the organism. These include chlorination of water supplies, appropriate disposal of human waste, control of flies, strict attention to handwashing, and scrupulous management of food preparation. In endemic areas, local workers employed as food handlers should be closely screened using successive stool cultures to ensure that they are not typhoid carriers. Outbreaks of typhoid fever have often occurred after disasters, when disruption of water supplies and sanitation facilitate the transmission of S Typhi from infected carriers to a population of susceptible hosts. Mass vaccination of individuals at risk in this setting is of secondary importance to other efforts to halt transmission, such as restoration of clean water supplies and institution of appropriate levels of sanitation.

[James Fleckenstein]

NONTYPHOIDAL SALMONELLOSIS

Introduction and Military Relevance

Salmonellosis is an acute bacterial infection that can disrupt combat performance and readiness, most typically by causing cases of acute enterocolitis associated with fever, headache, abdominal pain, diarrhea, nausea, and sometimes vomiting. Salmonellosis has considerable impact in civilian and military arenas. It accounts for substantial health care expenditures, decreased productivity, and lost wages in Europe[206,207] and the United States. Annual health care costs in the United States resulting from these infections are estimated to exceed $50 million.[208] In the context of this chapter, salmonellosis will not include typhoid and paratyphoid fevers.

Salmonella organisms as a cause of enteric illness on deployments has been well documented[209–211] (Table 37-5). When good field sanitation is maintained, salmonella infections cease to be a major operational threat. When sanitation is compromised, though, the abrupt onset of salmonella infections and their tendency to present as epidemic case clusters can hinder readiness and performance. As was illustrated by an outbreak in US military personnel deployed to Croatia, personnel are at risk for salmonella infections when common dining facilities are used and hygienic practices are suboptimal.[212]

Description of the Pathogen

The salmonellae are nonspore-forming, gram-negative bacteria. Unlike *Salmonella typhi* and *S paratyphi*, for which humans constitute the only known reservoir, the nontyphoidal species of the genus are less host-adapted and may cause infections in multiple animal hosts. This large reservoir in lower animals constitutes a major source for infections in humans and in part accounts for the ubiquity of these infections. There are approximately 2,000 serotypes that can be distinguished by specific surface antigens. Their prevalence varies by region, with only a frac-

TABLE 37-5

INCIDENCE OF TYPHOID FEVER AND SALMONELLOSIS IN US ARMY TROOPS IN VIETNAM, 1965-1970

Year	Typhoid fever		Salmonellosis	
	No. of cases	Rate/1,000	No. of cases	Rate/1,000
1965	0	—	10	0.2
1966	1	0.01	17	0.01
1967	11	0.04	201	0.7
1968	8	0.02	70	0.2
1969	19	0.05	70	0.2
1970	23	0.08	30	0.1
Total	62	—	398	—

Reprinted from: Hedlund KW, Ognibene AJ. Typhoid fever and other salmonelloses. Ognibene AJ, Barrett O, eds. *General Medicine and Infectious Diseases*. Vol 2. In: *Internal Medicine in Vietnam*. Washington, DC: Office of the Surgeon General and Center of Military History, US Army; 1982: 365.

tion present at any time. These serotypes are grouped into four serogroups (A through D). Although serotype does not have significant implications for individual patient care, it has important public health significance with respect to surveillance and outbreak detection. This is particularly evident when an outbreak stems from widely distributed foods.

Epidemiology

Transmission

Transmission of *Salmonella* organisms may be direct or indirect. Nontyphoidal salmonellosis most commonly occurs after the consumption of contaminated food or water. *Salmonella* may be passed to humans because of a failure to cook food products thoroughly or by cross-contamination of salad or other uncooked foods. Sauces and custards that contain eggs are other potential sources. Cooked foods can be inoculated with salmonella when they are cooled (eg, by a food handler excreting organisms), and if the food is held improperly, multiplication of the organism may occur.

In the United States and other industrialized countries, the routine large-scale commercial preparation of food with national or international product distribution has served to disseminate *Salmonella* organisms and has resulted in massive outbreaks of nontyphoidal salmonellosis.[213,214] Outbreaks related to commercial food production are most frequently associated with consumption of dairy products,[214] eggs,[215] or meat[216]; however, the growing list of implicated food vehicles indicates that anything that can be contaminated and sustain growth of the organism can serve as a vehicle for transmission. International distribution of some foods has resulted in importation of novel strains of *Salmonella* and multinational epidemics on several occasions.[217,218]

In healthy volunteers, the median infective dose for salmonella infection is 10^7 organisms. This may be altered significantly by a number of important host factors that may increase the risk for the acquisition of salmonella infection, including reduced stomach acidity,[219] age, and depressed cell-mediated immunity. Exposure to antimicrobial agents increases the risk of infection by lowering natural colonization resistance through alteration of native colonic microflora.[220] Infection rates also appear to be dependent on the strain of *Salmonella,* and some infecting strains appear to cause more severe clinical manifestations.[221,222] Foods that buffer the effect of stomach acids, particularly fatty foods, may facilitate survival of the organism.[218,223]

Geographic Distribution

While *Salmonella* organisms are ubiquitous, certain serotypes may predominate in specific geographic or environmental niches, and these serotypes may evolve over time. In the United States, *S enteritidis* infections have spread from an initial focus in the Northeast to become a predominate serotype.[224] As in other countries, infections with *S enteritidis* largely can be traced to the distribution of infected eggs. Some strains may have an enhanced potential for spread, as has been evidenced by the rapid increase in *S enteritidis* phage type 4 in England and Wales[225] and the emergence of these strains in the United States.[226,227] Nontyphoidal salmonellosis is common in the developing world.

Incidence

Nontyphoidal *Salmonella* organisms cause numerous infections worldwide. While the incidence of typhoid fever in the United States has declined, the incidence of human nontyphoidal salmonellosis has steadily increased. In the United States alone, more than 40,000 cases are reported through passive surveillance to the Centers for Disease Control and Prevention annually.[228] It is estimated, however, that this represents only 1% to 5 % of the actual number of infections.

Pathogenesis and Clinical Findings

The incubation period for nontyphoidal salmonellosis is usually 12 to 36 hours. Approximately two thirds of all those with salmonella infections present with gastroenteritis and fever. These infections are often self-limited, require no therapy, and resolve over several days. Infected individuals may continue to excrete organisms for several weeks or months after the acute illness, but fewer than 1% of patients demonstrate carriage beyond 1 year.[229]

Bacteremia occurs in 3% to 10 % of all nontyphoidal salmonella infections,[230,231] and it has been reported to occur with most of the reported serotypes of *Salmonella*.[232] Some serotypes (eg, *S enterica* serovar Cholerasuis) may be more invasive than others, as is evidenced by their relatively frequent isolation from blood as compared with the number of stool isolates.[233]

At present, acquired immunodeficiency syndrome is the most common underlying condition associated with nontyphoidal salmonella bacteremia, followed by diabetes mellitus, malignancy, cirrhosis, chronic granulomatous disease, sickle cell disease, and collagen vascular diseases.[231,233] However, nearly half of the bacteremias arise in patients without a recognizable underlying disease.[234] In otherwise healthy patients, salmonella bacteremia is often associated with a clearly defined episode of gastroenteritis. Conversely, the possibility of underlying immunosuppression should be considered in individuals presenting with primary nontyphoidal salmonella bacteremia without gastrointestinal symptoms.[235] Malaria appears to predispose patients to concurrent septicemia with gram-negative organisms, particularly *Salmonella*.[236] The possibility of dual infection should be entertained in febrile service members who have been deployed to endemic areas.

Nontyphoidal salmonellosis is an infrequent cause of endocarditis. It occurs more frequently in individuals over the age of 50 with underlying heart disease.[237–239] Salmonella infections of the aorta, particularly the abdominal aorta,[240] occur more frequently and usually in patients with preexisting atherosclerotic disease.[241]

Numerous extraintestinal foci of salmonella infection have been reported, a reflection of the organism's predilection for invasion of the bloodstream.[237] Intraabdominal infections caused by *Salmonella* organisms usually involve the liver, spleen, or biliary tract, commonly in patients with underlying structural abnormalities. Mesenteric lymphadenitis causing an appendicitis-like syndrome has been reported.[242] Salmonella osteomyelitis, originally described by Sir James Paget in 1876,[243] most frequently affects the long bones and vertebrae,[244] although virtually any bone may be infected.[245] Sickle cell disease remains an important predisposing factor for salmonella osteomyelitis and septic arthritis, particularly in early childhood. Multiple, often symmetrical, sites may be involved. Central nervous system infections with *Salmonella* species are rare. Brain abscess, subdural and epidural empyema, and meningitis have all been reported.[246] Urinary tract infections due to nontyphoidal *Salmonella* species occur rarely and are often associated with underlying immunosuppression or structural abnormalities.[247] Chronic urinary carriage of salmonella occurs commonly in the Middle East in those with bladder malformations and concomitant infection with *Schistosoma hematobium*. Pneumonia may result from hematogenous spread of nontyphoidal *Salmonella* organisms.[248]

Diagnostic Approaches

A diagnosis is usually made by isolating salmonellae from feces or blood through use of enteric media. Serologic tests are not useful. To screen for enteric infections in asymptomatic persons, mul-tiple specimens of fecal material (3-10 g inoculated into enrichment media) should be obtained over several days because excretion may be intermittent. Investigation of close case contacts, especially those who may pose a significant ongoing risk to others, is indicated.

Recommendations for Therapy and Control

Therapy

The majority of nontyphoidal salmonella infections in immunocompetent hosts are cases of self-limited gastroenteritis and do not require treatment with antibiotics.[249,250] In most patients, antimicrobial therapy will serve to shorten the duration of symptoms by only 1 to 2 days and may extend the time of fecal excretion. Rehydration with oral electrolyte solutions is usually sufficient therapy.

In patients with particularly severe or protracted symptoms or in situations where performance is critical, antibiotic therapy is reasonable to speed recovery and return to duty. Because there is a higher risk of endothelial infection in older adults with bacteremia caused by *Salmonella*, some have suggested that patients older than 50 years receive antibiotic therapy for gastroenteritis.[251] In addition, immunosuppressed patients, particularly those with the human immunodeficiency virus,[252,253] may benefit from treatment of gastrointestinal infections to avoid subsequent bacteremia, which can be difficult to eradicate in this population. Infants younger than 2 months of age may also be candidates for antibiotic therapy.

For patients requiring therapy, initial treatment should ideally be based on some knowledge of local resistance patterns because of the emergence of strains resistant to multiple antimicrobial agents. Ampicillin, chloramphenicol, and trimethoprim-sulfamethoxazole have all been used successfully to treat nontyphoidal salmonellosis, but many strains are now resistant to these drugs. Alternatives are provided by newer agents, such as the fluoroquinolones and the third-generation cephalosporins, which demonstrate significantly more activity against *Salmonella* organisms in vitro.

Fluoroquinolones, in addition to being highly active against many salmonellae, possess favorable phamacokinetic parameters, including large volumes of distribution, long half lives, and good oral bioavailabilty.[254] High concentrations of fluoroquinolones are present in stool after oral dosing,[255] and fluoroquinolones also achieve high intracellular concentrations.[256] In double-blind trials of adults with diarrheal illness, ciprofloxacin shortened the duration of diarrhea by 1.5 to 2 days.[257–259] These agents have been used successfully to treat salmonella infections caused by strains resistant to multiple other classes of antibiotics.[260]

In vitro studies have shown that many *Salmonella* species are sensitive to third-generation cephalosporins (eg, cefotaxime, ceftriaxone, cefoperazone, ceftazidime), and these drugs have been used successfully to eradicate nontyphoidal salmonellae.[261] Because fluoroquinolones are not approved for use in children, third-generation cephalosporins are often employed in treating younger patients.

Many investigators have cautioned that the use of antimicrobial agents in animal husbandry for growth promotion has led to the emergence of drug-resistant infections in humans.[208,262,263] While the use of antibiotics in animal feeds has been discouraged, the practice remains widespread, and new multidrug-resistant infections continue to emerge throughout the world.[221,222,264,265] Occasionally, resistance may emerge during the course of therapy, particularly in the treatment of chronic deep-seated infections such as osteomyelitis.[266]

Prevention

Given the many modes of transmission of salmonella infections, it is unlikely that all infections will be prevented even with strict adherence to measures designed to prevent transmission of these organisms. However, most infections can be prevented through careful attention to food handling, sanitation, and education of those in charge of food preparation and procurement. Irradiation of processed foods, particularly those of animal origin, should be encouraged. Fresh fruits and vegetables obtained from local sources are often used to supplement the diet of service members during extended deployments; such foods should be viewed as potentially contaminated with multiple enteric pathogens, including *Salmonella*.[11] Veterinary inspection of locally procured foods on deployments is essential to reduce the risk of nontyphoidal salmonellosis. The proper chlorination of water supplies is also an important preventive measure and can prevent large-scale outbreaks of salmonellosis. Handwashing should be emphasized for food handlers, those caring for patients, patients with enteric illness, and those caring for infants and incontinent adults.

Ill individuals should not participate in food handling or the care of immunocompromised or hospitalized patients, the elderly, or young children. Known carriers of *Salmonella* should be prohibited from handling food until they no longer shed the organisms. Carriers should have at least two negative stool cultures documented before being permitted to prepare food. Care should be taken especially when employing foreign workers in military mess facilities, as asymptomatic foodhandlers have been implicated as sources of infection despite screening.[267,268]

[James Fleckenstein]

SHIGELLOSIS

Introduction and Military Relevance

Shigellosis, often referred to as bacillary dysentery, is a febrile diarrheal syndrome manifested by the passage of frequent, scant stools that are bloody, mucoid, or both bloody and mucoid. Symptoms of abdominal cramps and tenesmus are present due to direct invasion of the colonic mucosa by members of the *Shigella* species.[269] Descriptions of this syndrome can be found in the Old Testament and a like disease played a major role in many military campaigns as far back as the year 480 BC. Shigellosis is endemic throughout the world and is hyperendemic in many developing countries. Infection with *Shigella* species is the most common cause of dysentery in children less than 5 years of age, especially in developing countries, where affected children experience a higher rate of stunting and mortality.[270]

Shigellosis has had a significant impact on military forces throughout history. According to the Greek historian, Herodotus, epidemics of dysentery plagued Xerxes' Persian army (500,000 men strong) during their unsuccessful invasion of Greece around 480 BC, especially during the battle for Salamis, the most important victory in Greek history.[271] In the 18th century, Prussian forces fighting under Frederick William II in France suffered 12,000 cases among a unit of 42,000, forcing his withdrawal from combat and retreat across the Rhine.[272] The British during the Crimean War (1854–1856) suffered ten times more casualties from dysentery than from all the Russian weapons.[273]

Acute diarrheal diseases, to include shigellosis, have continued to be an important medical problem for US military personnel operating in areas where sanitation has been inadequate. In the US Civil War, acute diarrheal diseases accounted for more than 25% of the deaths in the Union Army.[274] During World War II in the Middle East theater of operations, attack rates as high as 50% per month and noneffective rates as high as 3.5% per week were documented.[275] In North Africa, the British

Army was also reported to have sustained a significant number of casualties due to dysentery.[276] Shigellosis also proved to be the most common enteric infection identified among US military personnel in Vietnam, with an annual hospitalization rate as high as 8% documented in 1965.[277]

US troops deployed to Lebanon in 1958 to help in the evacuation of the Palestinian Liberation Organization were severely stricken with dysentery. Approximately 30% to 50% of a 10,000-man Marine landing force was affected; a total of 527 hospitalizations were recorded.[278] During Operation Bright Star in Egypt in July 1983, approximately 30% of the 82nd Airborne Division troops developed dysentery in a 1-week period.[116] From 1981 to 1990, diarrheal diseases have affected 15% to 20% of US troops participating in short-term military exercises in Egypt and Thailand; up to 5% of troops have lost duty time because of their illnesses.[25,279–281] Among US military personnel deployed to South America and western Africa, *Shigella* species have been isolated in up to 5% of diarrhea cases.[282]

In a sample of 2,000 US military personnel deployed to Saudi Arabia during the Persian Gulf War, 57% reported a significant diarrheal illness during the first 3 months of deployment (September–November 1990); 20% reported that they were not able to perform their duties while affected. Multidrug-resistant *Shigella* species (principally *S sonnei*) infections accounted for 26% of the cases of diarrhea evaluated, second only to enterotoxigenic *Escherichia coli*, which was found in 29% of cases. There were at least 3 outbreaks of shigellosis in the first 3 months of the operation.[11] Outbreaks were associated mainly with consumption of fresh fruits and vegetables and, to a lesser extent, with contamination of communal latrines, lack of handwashing facilities, and a high number of desert filth flies.[15] During Operation Restore Hope in Somalia (1992-1993), one outbreak of shigellosis involving 10 cases and additional sporadic cases were well documented.[283]

Shigellosis has also been well documented in foreign military contingents, most notably in Israel among kibbutz dwellers and recruits of the Israeli Defence Force.[284] Historically, military outbreaks of shigellosis have been associated with consumption of contaminated food items prepared by infected foodhandlers, as well as facilitation of transmission by common houseflies (*Musca domestica*) in this setting.[285] Uncontrolled epidemics of shigellosis, especially due to *S dysenteriae* type 1, are potential "war stopper" illnesses, which cause significant incapacitation and decrement in unit effectiveness.

Description of the Pathogen

Shigellae are slender, gram-negative, nonmotile rod bacteria belonging to the family Enterobacteriaceae. They are closely related genetically to *E coli*, and their origin from a common ancestor has been postulated. There are four clinically important species of *Shigella*: *S dysenteriae*, *S flexneri*, *S boydii*, and *S sonnei*, which are also known as subgroups A, B, C, and D, respectively. Strains of *Shigella* can be serologically characterized by the O (somatic) antigens, which are made up of cell wall lipopolysaccharide antigens. Numerous serotypes exist among *S dysenteriae* (12 serotypes), *S flexneri* (6 serotypes and 13 subserotypes), and *S boydii* (18 serotypes) species and are determined by agglutination with *Shigella*-specific antisera.

S dysenteriae type 1, also known as the Shiga bacillus, is a pathogen of developing countries. It exhibits several unique features compared to other members of the genus *Shigella*, including the production of Shiga toxin and the propensity for epidemic spread. It has been associated with major dysentery epidemics among refugees; a significant proportion of the deaths during the most recent Rwandan civil war were due to *S dysenteriae* type 1 (as well as and *Vibrio cholerae* O1) infections.[286]

The shigellae are highly host-adapted; their only natural hosts are humans and a few nonhuman primates.[260] There are no known environmental reservoirs of infection. Only small numbers of inocula are necessary. Experimental studies in volunteers have shown that disease can result from ingestion of as few as 10 viable *S dysenteriae* type 1 organisms or a few hundred *S flexneri* 2a or *S sonnei* organisms.[287,288]

Epidemiology

Transmission

Direct, person-to-person contact is the most important mode of *Shigella* transmission. In regions with inadequate excreta disposal facilities, flies may also be an important vector.[285,289] The small inocula required to cause shigellosis facilitates transmission of the disease and explains the frequent failure of routine sanitary and hygienic measures to prevent shigellosis. Strict attention to handwashing after defecation[290] and measures to control houseflies[285] have been shown to reduce the incidence of shigellosis in military field studies.

Water and food also appear to be important vehicles of transmission of *Shigella* in developing countries.[291] Epidemics of waterborne shigellosis caused by fecally contaminated wells, lakes, ponds, pools, and other sources of surface water have been documented. In the United States during the 2-year period of 1993 to 1994, for example, 3 outbreaks of *S sonnei* associated with swimming in lakes (a total of 437 cases) and 4 outbreaks involving untreated water from wells dug and maintained by individuals and an individual cistern (a total of 279 cases) were documented.[292] Foodborne transmission, on the other hand, is not as common but, when it occurs, is associated with large outbreaks.[293] Shigellae are known to grow very well in food items such as rice, lentil soup, milk, cooked beef, cooked fish, mashed potato, raw cucumbers, and vegetables.[294,295]

Secondary cases during outbreaks of shigellosis are common, especially in households of index patients. The attack rate is higher if (*a*) the index case is a young, non–toilet-trained child, (*b*) the contacts are younger (rates of 40% to 60% in those 1 to 4 years of age but less than 20% in adults), (*c*) the houses have privies, and (*d*) improper handwashing practices are noted.[293,296] Other risk factors associated with secondary transmission are contact with a person with dysentery, sharing of latrines with other households, storing of water at home and hand-dipping with a hand-held cup, and consumption of food from street vendors.[297]

In industrialized countries, *Shigella* organisms are readily transmitted in certain populations at high risk where abnormal behavior or poor hygienic practices facilitate fecal-oral contamination.[298,299] High-risk groups include Native American populations,[298] children in childcare centers,[300,301] those in institutions for the mentally retarded,[302] those aboard ships,[303] those in penal institutions,[304] military units training under field conditions,[286] and those who practice anal-oral sex.[305]

Geographic Distribution

Shigellosis has a global distribution, but the prevalence of the various species and types varies geographically. In industrialized countries, such as the United States, endemic shigellosis is primarily a pediatric disease caused by *S sonnei*.[298] In developing countries, *S flexneri* is the most common species, with *S flexneri* 2a being a prominent serotype; *S boydii* is common in the Indian subcontinent.[306]

Incidence

It is estimated that 3 to 5 billion diarrhea cases occur worldwide every year; average rates range from 5 to 12 illnesses per child per year, with rates as high as 19 illnesses per child per year in the poorest areas. Approximately 5% to 10% of these diarrhea cases may be caused by *Shigella* organisms.[306] Diarrheal disease, including dysentery, also constitutes one of the leading causes of mortality, accounting for an estimated 5 to 10 million deaths per year. Most of these deaths (estimated at 12,600 deaths per day) occur in children less than 5 years of age in Asia, Africa, and Latin America.[307,308] The annual worldwide incidence of shigellosis is estimated at 200 million cases, with an annual death toll estimated at 650,000.[309]

Epidemics of Shiga dysentery, due to multidrug-resistant *S dysenteriae* type 1, caused an estimated 500,000 cases and 20,000 deaths between 1969 and 1973 in Central America.[310,311] Likewise, during major epidemics in Africa and the Indian subcontinent, a significant proportion of the population (up to 10%) were affected, with mortality rates as high as 10%.[297,312–314]

Pathogenesis and Clinical Findings

Shigellae cause disease by direct mucosal invasion of the distal small bowel and colon with concomitant inflammatory reaction. Enterotoxin production facilitates invasion and destruction of epithelial cells, which explains the findings of white blood cells and blood in stools. The incubation period for shigellosis is usually 12 to 96 hours, although *S dysenteriae* type 1 infections can take up to 1 week to manifest clinically.[315p451–455] Onset of fever, abdominal cramping, and malaise is followed by a variable amount of watery diarrhea before dysentery begins. In severe cases, it is not uncommon for an infected person to have 20 or 30 bowel movements per day, consisting of scant volumes of mucus or blood or both mucus and blood, often accompanied by severe abdominal cramping, tenesmus, and urgency. Depending on the infecting strain, a large proportion of patients may have only watery diarrhea, and some patients may have fever without intestinal symptoms. In general, *S sonnei* causes the mildest disease and *S dysenteriae* the most severe.

Most cases of shigellosis in well-nourished and healthy people are self-limited and resolve without sequelae. This is frequently not the case, however, in severe infections caused by *S dysenteriae* type 1 or by other serotypes in malnourished populations. In malnourished children, *Shigella* infection, particularly with *S dysenteriae* type 1, may result in a chronic type of relapsing diarrhea and a protein-losing enteropathy. Other complications in children can include convulsions, meningismus, and secondary spread with vaginitis. Intestinal complications of shigellosis include toxic megacolon, which carries a high fatality rate, and rectal prolapse, which requires early manual reduction. Intestinal perforation is rare.[316]

There are a number of unusual but important extraintestinal complications of *Shigella* infections. Peripheral leukocyte counts in excess of 50,000 have been seen in approximately 4% of patients during outbreaks caused by *S dysenteriae* type 1.[317] Having a leukemoid reaction carries a poor prognosis.[318] Hemolytic-uremic syndrome, consisting of the triad of microangiopathic hemolytic anemia, thrombocytopenia, and renal failure, occurs in a small percentage of cases of shigellosis, mostly those with *S dysenteriae* type 1 infections and mainly in children. Although the pathogenesis of hemolytic-uremic syndrome is not completely understood, there is an association between circulating endotoxin and the development of the syndrome.[314] Early dialysis to eliminate this toxin may be lifesaving.

Shigella bacteremia is generally considered an unusual occurrence.[319] Nevertheless, it has been documented to occur in as many as 4% of cases of *S dysenteriae* type 1 infections in a Bangladeshi population and was found to be associated with a high incidence of other complications and death.[320] In this study, young age and malnutrition were risk factors. Reiter's syndrome or reactive arthritis follows shigellosis in 1% to 2% percent of cases, usually 2 to 4 weeks after the acute illness. Persons with the HLA-B27 histocompatibility antigen are at much higher risk of this complication.[321]

A great majority of *Shigella*-infected patients will clear their infections within 2 weeks, more than 90% will clear within 1 to 4 weeks without antibiotic therapy. Even though long-term *Shigella* carriage has been well documented in less than 5% of cases, it may be important in the perpetuation of infection in the household and in the spread of infection to close contacts and by infected foodhandlers.[322] Carriage is reduced significantly (to less than 1 week) by antibiotic therapy.

A large body of evidence indicates that there is effective acquired immunity to *Shigella* infections. Introduction of a new strain in a previously nonimmune population, for example, is often followed by high attack rates greater than 5% to 10% in all age groups. Prospective studies among children in endemic areas, such as Guatemala[323] and Chile,[324] have shown that a prior bout of shigellosis

elicits about 75% protection against reinfection with a homologous serotype. Likewise, serological studies among Israeli military recruits have shown that preexisting anti-lipopolysaccharide (somatic antigen) antibodies protect individuals from subsequent *Shigella* infection.[325] Volunteer challenge studies done in the 1970s have also demonstrated that a previous bout of shigellosis confers 64% to 78% protection against dysentery caused by *S flexneri* type 2a and *S sonnei*.[326,327] Clearly, there is significant but by no means complete protection from clinical shigellosis caused by the same serotype. Unfortunately, such immunity can often be overcome with a large dose of *Shigella* organisms.[328]

Diagnostic Approaches

The definitive diagnosis of shigellosis depends on the isolation or identification of the organism from a stool specimen. In the near future, techniques such as rapid immunoassays for antigen detection, mononuclear antibody-based dipstick assays, DNA probes, and polymerase chain reaction kits may be used routinely for rapid diagnosis. *Shigella* rapidly loses viability in an acid environment and thus may be difficult to recover from stool specimens that are not processed within 2 to 4 hours. When direct plating from a stool sample is not possible, microbiologic recovery can be improved by the use of proper transport media; buffered glycerol saline has been reported to be the best.[329] Cary-Blair medium can also be used for transport but is not as good as buffered glycerol saline.[330] Although mucus or blood-flecked portions of stool samples are the preferred specimens for culture,[331] a properly obtained rectal swab, which samples the material in contact with the mucosal epithelium, can also be used for culture provided it is gathered from at least 2 cm past the anal sphincter. The specimens of choice are, in order of decreasing productivity, stool, rectal swab specimens, and anal swab specimens.[332]

A combination of nonselective media (eg, MacConkey's agar) and selective media (eg, Hektoen enteric agar, *Salmonella-Shigella* agar) are suggested for isolation.[329,331] Additionally, xylose-lysine-deoxycholate medium has been found to be especially good for isolating *Shigella* species.[333] Identity can be confirmed by agglutination tests using group-specific anti-lipopolysaccharide antibodies[334] against the four major serogroups: A (*S dysenteriae*), B (*S flexneri*), C (*S boydii*), and D (*S sonnei*).

In patients with febrile diarrhea or in those with mucoid, bloody stools but without fever, examination for fecal leucocytes by methylene blue staining of a fresh stool sample is indicated. The finding of fecal leukocytes in the stool strongly suggests, but is not diagnostic of, *Shigella* infection and should prompt stool culture for specific diagnosis.[335] The stool should also be examined for motile amoebic trophozoites containing ingested erythrocytes to rule out infection with *Entamoeba histolytica*.

Recommendations for Therapy and Control

Therapy

As in other diarrheal diseases, restoration of fluid deficit and maintenance of hydration status and serum electrolyte balance is indicated. Antimicrobial therapy has been shown to shorten the duration of symptoms in shigellosis,[336,337] and its use is justified in cases of moderate or severe disease. Throughout most of the world, *Shigella* organisms are resistant to multiple antibiotics that were previously useful in treatment. This makes effective therapy difficult, especially in countries where shigellosis is endemic and where the high cost of newer antibiotics prohibits their use.[338] In addition, major dysentery outbreaks since 1969 have increasingly involved multidrug-resistant strains of *S dysenteriae* type 1,[297,310–312,339–345] creating therapeutic difficulties. Interestingly, the first significant evidence of multidrug resistance occurred in 1967 and 1968 in Vietnam where widespread resistance to tetracycline, chloramphenicol, and ampicillin was found.[277,346] This rapid emergence of antibiotic resistance has been mediated by a drug-resistance (R) plasmid.[269]

The choice of an antimicrobial agent depends on the resistance patterns of *Shigella* in a particular geographic area.[269,293] Five-day regimens with ampicillin (100 mg/kg per day for children; 500 mg every 6 hours for adults) or trimethoprim-sulfamethoxazole (TMP-SMX, TMP: 10 mg/kg per day and SMX: 50 mg/kg per day in two divided doses) are good choices only in areas with sensitive strains. Tetracycline as a single oral adult dose of 2.5 g has been used successfully and may be effective even against antibiotic-resistant strains.[347] Short-course therapy with a quinolone (eg, norfloxacin 400 mg twice a day, ciprofloxacin 500 mg twice a day) or with TMP-SMX (TMP 160 mg and SMX 800 mg, 2 times a day) for 3 days is an alternative that has been useful in several military settings.[283,348] Single-dose therapeutic regimens with quinolones (eg, norfloxacin 800 mg, ciprofloxacin 1 g) have also been found to be effective in treating shigellosis in adults in developing countries.[349–351] Tetracycline and quinolones are not recommended for use in children younger than 8

years old. In such cases, nalidixic acid (55 mg/kg per day in 4 equally divided doses), TMP-SMX (TMP 10 mg/kg per day and SMX 50 mg/kg per day in 2 equally divided doses), or cefixime (8 mg/kg per day) for 5 days is indicated.[293,352] Antiperistaltic agents, such as diphenoxylate hydrochloride (Lomotil), may prolong clinical illness and could play a role in the development of toxic dilatation of the colon and, therefore, should not be used.[353] In contrast, a study done in Thailand among hospitalized patients with dysentery found that the addition of loperamide (Imodium) to a 3-day course of therapy with ciprofloxacin (500 mg twice a day) shortened the duration and frequency of diarrhea by more than 50%.[354]

Control

During acute illness, enteric precautions should be followed. Because of the low infecting dose, patients with *Shigella* infections should not be employed to handle food or to care for children until at least 2 successive fecal sample or rectal swab cultures are negative. The samples should be taken more than 24 hours apart and more than 48 hours after antimicrobial therapy ends. Patients and medical staff should be advised to always wash their hands with soap after defecation, before eating, and after patient contact. Fecally contaminated articles, such as clothing and linen, should be disinfected. Feces and vomitus should be disinfected with calcium hypochlorite or carbolic acid.[315] Active detection of other personnel infected with *Shigella* and treatment of close contacts of cases is not routinely indicated except in the case of foodhandlers, employees of child-care centers, hospital staff, and military personnel known to be exposed to a common source of infection during an epidemic. There is an urgent need to report all suspected outbreaks of shigellosis; early treatment of suspected cases with antibiotics is essential to limit transmissibility in the field setting.

Transmission of shigellosis can be decreased significantly in military populations by following some simple control measures (Exhibit 37-2).

Much effort has gone toward developing vaccines to prevent shigellosis in the past 30 years by many military and civilian investigators. Despite all this effort and despite the fact that *Shigella* was discovered almost a century ago, there are yet no licensed vaccines for the prevention of shigellosis.[355] Development of these vaccines has been hindered because there are no valid animal models for these pathogens and because there is no consensus about what constitute

---

EXHIBIT 37-2

SIMPLE AND EFFECTIVE MEASURES TO CONTROL TRANSMISSION OF SHIGELLOSIS IN MILITARY POPULATIONS

- Frequent effective handwashing with soap and water, especially after defecation and immediately before eating or preparing food

- Sanitary control and disposal of feces

- Provision of a safe water supply and protection from contamination, to include effective chlorination at the distribution point in military camps

- Avoidance of swimming in potentially contaminated bodies of fresh water (swimming in seawater is considered to be acceptable)

- Control of the vector (fly) populations in and around excreta disposal and dining facilities by use of insecticides, yeast-baited fly traps, garbage collection, and proper disposal of wastewater and sewage

- Proper cooking and subsequent refrigeration of potentially infected food items; leafy vegetables should be washed or chemically treated if they are to be eaten uncooked; all leftover food should be discarded, reheated to more than 60°C, or refrigerated or frozen immediately

- Avoidance of high-risk food items, such as food and drinks from street vendors

- Removal of persons with diarrhea from jobs as foodhandlers

- Early detection and treatment of cases to limit secondary transmission to other unit members

- Selective antibiotic prophylaxis of close contacts or potentially exposed personnel; doxycycline (100 mg/day for 14 days) has been found to protect contacts from clinical shigellosis;* in areas where *Shigella* organisms are antibiotic-resistant, ciprofloxacin (500 mg/day) or norfloxacin (400 mg/day) may be used as an alternative

---

*Ben-Yehuda O, Cohen D, Alkan M, Greenbaum A, Jelin N, Steinherz R. Doxycycline prophylaxis for shigellosis. *Arch Intern Med*. 1990;150:209–212.

---

the host protective immune factors.[356] Some scientists feel that protective immunity to shigellosis is mediated by mucosal factors, especially secretory immunoglobulin A (sIgA), and that only live, attenuated strains of bacteria are capable of eliciting an effective intestinal sIgA response. Under the hypothesis that antibodies secreted in the gut have an important role in protection against shigellosis, oral, enteroinvasive *Shigella* vaccines were developed in the 1980s and 1990s.[357]

Other investigators, though, feel that protection can be achieved by serum IgG and mucosal sIgA antibody response conferred by conjugate vaccines that elicit high levels of antibodies to the O-specific lipopolysaccharides of *Shigella* species.[358] Phase I and II studies among United States Army and Is-rael Defence Force soldiers has indicated that these injectable conjugate vaccines are safe and induce protective immunity that is equivalent to that present after shigellosis.[359,360] Moreover, a phase III study of a single-dose *S sonnei* conjugate vaccine conducted in Israel among male military recruits demonstrated a significant level (74%) of protective efficacy against culture-proven shigellosis caused by *S sonnei*.[361] Testing of other candidate oral, enteroinvasive, *Shigella* vaccines and subunit vaccines (part of the bacteria, administered parenterally, intranasally, or orally) is ongoing. A candidate oral, live, attenuated *S flexneri* 2a vaccine is presently undergoing trials in military personnel in the United States and among civilians in Bangladesh.[362]

[Jose L. Sanchez]

CHOLERA

Introduction and Military Relevance

The disease known as cholera has probably been endemic for over 2,000 years in the Indian subcontinent,[363] and the term "cholera" is first seen in the works of the great Greek physician Hippocrates.[364] The first well-documented clinical descriptions of cholera date back to 1503 in Gaspar Correa's book, *Lendas da India*.[365] The first recognized pandemic of the disease originated around 1817 in India. Since then, there have been an additional six pandemics. Nonimmune military forces, especially from Europe and India, have been repeatedly plagued by this dreaded disease. Infected military personnel have played a major role in the spread of what is now called classical cholera during the first six pandemics, in the 19th and early 20th centuries. Bengal troops traveling to Oman from Bombay in 1821 were principally responsible for the spread of classical cholera outside of the Indian subcontinent during the first pandemic. Death rates among British troops in India reached 21 per 1,000 in 1822.[366] During the second pandemic, Polish and French troops spread the disease in their homelands and in Austria in the spring of 1831.[367] In the largest recorded military outbreak, 350,000 cases occurred in Europe in 1866 among Austrian, Italian, and German forces. In the United States, Union troop movements during the Civil War were a key factor in spreading the disease to major Midwestern cities. During World War I, an epidemic affected 66,000 Russian prisoners in camps in Hungary, Austria, and Germany.[363]

Cholera caused by the El Tor biotype was first described at the El Tor quarantine station on the Sinai Peninsula in 1905 among pilgrims returning from Mecca. This same strain 55 years later gave rise to the seventh pandemic in 1960 and 1961 in Sulawesi, Indonesia.[363,368] Since then, the El Tor biotype has quickly replaced the classical as the predominant biotype worldwide.

Four important events in the 1990s have placed cholera high on the list of emerging infections. First among them was the reintroduction of cholera into Latin America in January 1991 after nearly 100 years of absence. This outbreak spread from Peru to Mexico within 2 years and in 5 years caused more than 1 million cases and 10,000 deaths.[367]

Second, during late 1992 a new serogroup, *Vibrio cholerae* O139 synonym Bengal, appeared in India and Bangladesh. This Bengal strain (initially detected in the countries bordering the Bay of Bengal) produced major epidemics of cholera-like illness (up to 200,000 cases from 1992 to 1996) in India, Bangladesh, and five other countries in Southeast Asia.[369–371] Travel-associated (ie, imported) cases have also been reported in the United States, the United Kingdom, Denmark, Germany, Japan, Hong Kong, and Singapore.[371–374]

Third, the massive outbreak of El Tor cholera in Rwandan refugees in Goma, Zaire, resulting in 70,000 cases and 12,000 deaths in July 1994, showed that during times of crisis cholera can be catastrophic.[375,376] The very high death rates caused by cholera (approximately 15 per 1,000), with case fatality ratios as high as 48% recorded at one camp,

were principally due to the rapid waterborne spread of cholera (as well as shigellosis), which quickly overwhelmed the existing medical support capabilities and the capacity for oral rehydration therapy at diarrhea treatment centers.[376] The Rwandan refugee experience contrasts sharply with the Peruvian experience during the peak of the Latin American epidemic (1991-1993). In Peru, case fatality ratios were kept consistently at or below 1% in comparison to significantly higher case fatality ratios for Africa (approximately 9%) and Asia (approximately 3%).[377]

Fourth, the resurgence of cholera has had an impact on nonimmune military personnel, expatriates, and travelers to endemic areas. During the Peruvian epidemic, for example, attack rates as high as 2% to 10% occurred among Peruvian military recruits (Sanchez JL, unpublished data). An increased incidence of cholera was also noted among Americans at the United States Embassy in Lima.[378] In the United States at the same time, a 10-fold increase in cholera cases was noted by Centers for Disease Control and Prevention investigators caused by the proximity of the Latin American outbreak and increased awareness.[379]

Description of the Pathogen

Cholera is caused by *Vibrio cholerae*, a motile, curved, gram-negative bacillus, first described in 1854 in Italy by Filippo Pacini. Subsequently, Robert Koch demonstrated in 1883 that cholera is caused by this organism, which he called *Kommabazillen*.[368] It is a well-defined species on the basis of biochemical tests and DNA homology studies.[380] The species can be subdivided into 139 different serogroups, based on the composition of the major surface antigen of the cell wall (the O somatic antigen). Only two of these 139 serogroups, O1 and O139, have been associated with epidemics of cholera; these two serogroups have been the only ones consistently found to produce cholera toxin (CT), the toxin responsible for fluid secretion into the bowel lumen.[381] Non-O1, non-O139 serogroups have been associated with only sporadic cases and small clusters of noncholera diarrheal illness.[382] Serogroup O1 can be further subdivided into 3 antigenic forms (or serotypes) named Ogawa, Inaba, and Hikojima based on quantitative differences of factors A, B, and C of the O antigen.[383] *V cholerae* O1 strains are also subdivided into 2 biotypes: classical and El Tor.

V cholerae O139 strains appear to be genetically related to the *V cholerae* O1 strains that caused the seventh pandemic. This non-O1 strain, identified in late 1992, is most likely an O antigen mutant with an array of virulence determinants typical of *V cholerae* O1, biotype El Tor.[384] The high attack rates of severe cholera from O139 seen among adults in areas long endemic for *V cholerae* O1 would seem to indicate that there is no cross-protection from previous infection by O1 serogroup strains. In contrast to O1 strains, these O139 strains have the capacity to produce a polysaccharide capsule and demonstrate an increased capacity for cholera toxin production, as well as for spread and proliferation within the environment.[385] These strains are also known to survive well in environmental water (eg, ponds, lakes, rivers, canals) unlike O1 and other non-O1 strains.[371,386]

V cholerae has, since the early 1980s, been identified as an integral part of the normal, free-living (autochtonous) bacterial flora in estuarine areas. The persistence of *V cholerae* within the environment (for months and probably years) is facilitated by its ability to enter a viable, nonculturable "dormant" state where the organism's requirements for nutrients and oxygen are markedly decreased.[387] It is also able to bind to chitin, a component of crustacean shells, and is able to colonize the surfaces of algae, phytoplankton, and copepods (zooplankton), in addition to the roots of aquatic plants such as water hyacinths. Environmental factors—such as increased water temperature, decreased salinity, increased pH, and an increase in the seawater's nutrients, among others—may trigger conversion of the organism from the viable, nonculturable phase to the culturable, and therefore infectious, phase. These environmental factors, in turn, may also lead to in-creases in the crustacean populations, with associated increases in the population of free-living *V cholerae*. The periodic introduction of such infectious environmental isolates into the human population, through ingestion of undercooked shellfish and seafood, is probably responsible for isolated foci of endemic disease on the US Gulf Coast and in Australia, as well as for the initial case clusters that gave rise to the Latin American epidemic.[378,388]

In addition, *V cholerae* O1 strains have been recently found to shift to a "rugose" form associated with the production of an exopolysaccharide that promotes cell aggregation. This form has been found to be resistant to disinfectants such as chlorine.[389] Chlorination of the water supply has been a key, effective intervention in controlling cholera outbreaks in the past.[390] If these rugose strains become prevalent in the potable water supply, they may serve as an important factor contributing to the waterborne transmission of cholera.

Epidemiology

The epidemiology of cholera can be roughly divided into two phases or patterns: the epidemic and the endemic[391,392] (Table 37-6).

Transmission

Cholera is caused by the ingestion of cholera bacilli in food or water that has been previously contaminated by feces or vomitus of infected persons.[315p100–110]

TABLE 37-6

EPIDEMIOLOGIC FEATURES OF CHOLERA

Feature	Epidemic phase	Endemic phase
Level of immunity	None, all susceptible	High, increasing with age until adulthood
Ages at greatest risk	All ages	Children 2–15 y, mothers of children < 2 y
Attack rates	Higher (1%-10%)	Lower (< 1%)
Primary transmission	Single food/water sources	Exposure to contaminated water, shellfish, seafood
Secondary transmission	Variable, intra-familial spread	Multiple food items, contaminated water sources, intra-familial spread (family clusters)
Asymptomatic infections	Less common	Very common
Principal reservoirs	Ill individuals and close contacts	Aquatic and environmental* asymptomatic shedders
Seasonality	Variable	Summer and monsoon months, times of algae blooms in coastal areas

*Viable, nonculturable (VNC) vibrios found in algae, phyto/zooplankton, estuarine waters, and roots of aquatic plants.
Sources: Colwell RR, Huq A. Vibrios in the environment: Viable but nonculturable *Vibrio cholerae*. In: Wachsmuth IK, Blake PA, Olsvik O, eds. *Vibrio cholerae and Cholera: Molecular to Global Perspectives*. Washington, DC: American Society for Microbiology; 1994: 117–133; Glass RI, Black RE. The epidemiology of cholera. In: Barua D, Greenough III WB, eds. *Cholera*. New York: Plenum Medical Book Co; 1992: 129–154; Shears P. Cholera. *Ann Trop Med Parasitol*. 1994;88:109–122.

Epidemics have followed the introduction of *V cholerae* into nonendemic areas and have been characterized by explosive outbreaks. Asymptomatically infected individuals have not played an important role in transmission in epidemic cholera, except for close household contacts (such as infected children or mothers), unit contacts, or foodhandlers. Control of transmission during the initial epidemic phase can be achieved more effectively than later, when the endemic phase is established.

The transition from the initial epidemic phase to a more protracted, chronic endemic phase is attained by the establishment of natural human reservoirs of infection in the population and in the aquatic environment. Once this occurs, cholera tends to settle into a clear seasonal pattern, with peaks of transmission during or at the end of the summer months or after the monsoon (rainy) season.

Contamination of food, whether at home, at common gatherings, in markets, or by street vendors, is common in areas that are endemic for cholera. *V cholerae* O1 can survive for 2 to 14 days in foods and can persist for many weeks in shellfish and mollusks.[388] Widespread contamination of surface water sources, such as lakes, rivers, streams, canals, springs, and wells, also contributes to the transmission of cholera.

The transmission patterns of O139 strains are similar to those of O1 strains.[371] The secondary infection rates among family members approximate 25% within 10 days of the index case. Household water (eg, from tubewells) has often been found to be the principal source of infection in Bangladesh. It appears, thus, that the predominant mode of transmission of *V cholerae* O139 is waterborne.

Geographic Distribution

Cholera is present worldwide and is particularly endemic in India and Bangladesh (surrounding the Bay of Bengal), as well as in South America.

Incidence

Attack rates of epidemic cholera occurring in nonimmune populations can be as high as 10%, affecting all age groups similarly. Considerable morbidity and mortality occur at the time of these outbreaks. For example, the introduction of cholera into West Africa in 1970 resulted in more than 150,000 cases and more than 20,000 deaths reported within 1 year.[393] Likewise, the introduction of cholera in Peru in 1991 resulted in more than 420,000 cases and more than 3,300 deaths reported within the first 15 months of that epidemic.[394]

Once cholera becomes endemic in an area, immunity is acquired early in life; higher attack rates occur in children 2 to 15 years of age and in women of childbearing age who are exposed to large inoculums of *V cholerae* organisms while caring for the very young.[395] Because of this relatively higher level of immunity, lower overall attack rates take place in the adult population (< 1% per year). Secondary transmission of cholera occurs principally by intra-familial spread, with usual rates of infection among family contacts in the range of 4% to 22% and sometimes as high as 50%.[395–397]

Diagnostic Approaches

Cholera is principally a clinical diagnosis. Any patient with watery diarrhea, especially if severely dehydrated, who is in or has traveled within the previous 5 days to an endemic area for cholera should be suspected of having cholera and treated accordingly. Definitive means of diagnosis is by isolation of the organism from culture of stool or rectal swab specimens. If processing is going to be delayed beyond 4 to 6 hours, the sample should be placed in Cary-Blair transport medium; *V cholerae* can be recovered from it for up to 4 weeks after sampling.[398] It is important not to refrigerate or freeze such samples because vibrios are more vulnerable to refrigeration or freezing than other enteric bacilli. Cultures in TCBS agar are detected as large, yellow, smooth colonies. Confirmation is done by slide agglutination in the presence of polyvalent O1 antisera in a microbiology laboratory.

Field Antigen Detection Tests

Rapid, reliable field identification methods are available. The most commonly used is darkfield microscopy, which relies on the identification of motile vibrios and their immobilization with specific O1 antisera. This method can identify cholera infections in 2 to 5 minutes in about 50% of cases.[399] Rapid diagnosis of both *V cholerae* O1 and O139 infections in the field has been made possible since 1992 by simple, rapid, field-expedient, immunological methods.[400–402] Direct detection of bacterial antigen in stool samples is done with coagglutination tests using monoclonal antibodies against the O1 and O139 antigens (CholeraScreen and BengalScreen, New Horizons Diagnostics Corp, Columbia, Md) or with colloidal-based colorimetric immunoassay kits (CholeraSMART and BengalSMART, New Horizons Diagnostics Corp, Columbia, Md). The cholera toxin can also be detected in stool samples by coagglutination tests using anti-cholera toxin (anti-

CT) antibodies.[403] DNA probes and polymerase chain reaction methods have been used in the 1990s in research laboratories for the detection of cholera toxin genes and to detect toxigenic *V cholerae* O1 in food and environmental samples.[380]

Serologic Antibody Detection Assays

Serologic assays can be useful in three settings: (1) in making a retrospective diagnosis of cholera, (2) in conducting epidemiologic investigations, or (3) in identifying infected contacts, (ie, cases where stool samples are unavailable or where many infections may be mild or asymptomatic). Antibacterial (or vibriocidal) and anti-CT antibody tests are described in detail in references 404 and 405. They tend to be used mostly in research settings. Serum vibriocidal antibodies have been associated with protection against disease in studies in endemic areas, as well as in volunteer studies.[380] This protection is related to the inhibition of vibrio colonization by secretory immunoglobulin A in the gut rather than as a result of a direct protective effect of serum (mainly IgG) antibodies. Vibriocidal antibody levels are seen to increase in only 50% to 60% of infected patients and remain elevated for 3 to 6 months after infection. By comparison, anti-CT antibodies are detected in more than 90% of patients and remain elevated for up to 2 years after initial infection. Therefore, anti-CT antibodies are more sensitive and useful in the serologic diagnosis of acute cases and for epidemiologic investigations in previously nonimmune populations, such as soldiers and travelers from developed countries. Serologic diagnosis is assisted by collection of acute phase (within 3 to 5 days of onset of illness) and convalescent phase (3 to 4 weeks thereafter) paired serum specimens. A 4-fold or greater rise in titers is considered diagnostic of recent infection with *V cholerae*.[405]

Pathogenesis and Clinical Findings

The toxin produced by *V cholerae* causes fluid secretion in the bowel lumen. The incubation period of cholera ranges from several hours to up to 5 days.[315] This is greatly determined by the inoculum size[391,406] and whether food serves as the vehicle of transmission because food protects vibrios from the action of stomach acid. As few as 100 to 1,000 organisms in food or in a bicarbonate buffering agent (as in volunteer studies) can cause disease.[406,407] Other host factors that increase the risk of cholera are the use of antacids or medications that reduce gastric acid secretion, the use of cannabis, and a history of gastric surgery.[408] It has also been found that individuals in the O blood group, while not at increased risk of infection, are at increased risk of developing severe cholera illness.[409,410] Breast-feeding appears to protect infants from developing cholera because of the protective effect of immunoglobulin A antibodies in breast milk.[411]

Only a minority of patients infected with *V cholerae* O1 develop severe cholera (cholera gravis). In Bangladesh, for example, it has been estimated that only 11% of classical infections and 2% of El Tor infections result in severe cholera.[412] Studies conducted among Peruvian military units (Sanchez J, unpublished data) and civilian populations [413] have documented that only 5% to 10% of diarrhea cases associated with *V cholerae* O1 infection resulted in severe disease or hospitalization.

The most marked features of severe cholera are the voluminous output of watery stool and the dehydration that results (Table 37-7). The rate of diarrhea can reach 500 to 1,000 mL per hour, leading rapidly to hypotension, tachycardia, and vascular collapse. The patient becomes lethargic or stuporous with sunken eyes and cheeks and dry mucous membranes. Decreased skin turgor (measured by the skin-pinch sign) is found in all such cases. Urine flow is decreased or absent, and serum specific gravity is consistently elevated. Clinical illness that goes untreated resolves in 4 to 6 days in most cases, unless circulatory collapse occurs. More than 90% of *V cholerae* O1-infected persons will be vibrio-free within 8 to 10 days, and rarely does excretion extend beyond 2 weeks.[396,397] Long-term carriers are exceedingly uncommon and do not play a significant role in disease transmission.

Detailed information regarding the clinical aspects of *V cholerae* O139 infections is limited.[371,414,415] Dhar and colleagues[416] have found in Bangladesh that the illnesses caused by O1 and O139 serogroups seem to be similar and that important clinical features, such as the duration of diarrhea and the degree of dehydration before hospital admission, were no different. In addition, they also found that patients with O139-serogroup infections responded to standard O1 serogroup cholera therapy.

Recommendations for Therapy and Control

Rehydration Therapy

The key to the treatment of cholera is the rapid rehydration of the patient, either with oral rehydration therapy (ORT) for mildly dehydrated patients or with a combination of ORT and intravenous re-

TABLE 37-7

GUIDELINES FOR CLINICAL EVALUATION OF DEHYDRATION AND RECOMMENDATIONS FOR REHYDRATION AND MAINTENANCE FLUID THERAPY

Parameter	Degree of Dehydration		
	Mild or none	Moderate	Severe
Mental status	Alert	Restless or lethargic	Lethargic, stuporous, or comatose
Thirst	Present	Present	Marked
Radial pulse	Normal	Rapid	Rapid and feeble or impalpable
Respirations	Normal	Tachypneic	Tachypneic, deep, labored
Skin-pinch sign	Skin retracts immediately	Skin retracts slowly (1 to 2 s)	Skin retracts very slowly (> 2 s)
Eyes	Normal	Sunken	Dramatically sunken
Urine flow	Normal	Scant and dark	Scant or absent
Serum specific gravity	≤ 1.027	1.028-1.034	> 1.034
Fluid deficit[*]	20 to 50	51 to 90	91 to 120
Preferred method of rehydration	ORT in 4-6 hrs	ORT or IVRT or both, depends on presence of vomiting and stool losses	IVRT, 2L in 30-60 m, remainder in 3-4 h
Preferred type of rehydration	WHO ORT (all ages) Rehydralyte (adults) Pedialyte (children) Infalyte (infants)	WHO ORT or IVRT or both, Normal saline[†‡]	Lactated Ringer's[†]
Maintenance	ORT for as long as diarrhea persists	NA	NA

ORT: Oral rehydration therapy, IVRT: Intravenous rehydration therapy, WHO: World Health Organization, NA: Not applicable.
[*]mL/kg of body weight
[†]Dextrose-containing solutions (2%–5%) are preferred because of the risk of hypoglycemia in cholera patients.
[‡]Addition of potassium chloride (10 mEq/L) is recommended to reduce risk of hypokalemia.
Reprinted with permission from: Sanchez JL, Taylor KN. Cholera. *Lancet*. 1997;349:1825–1830. (c) by The Lancet Ltd. 1997.

hydration therapy for moderate or severely dehydrated patients. The development of a practical, simple, and safe mode of oral rehydration in the 1960s has been lauded as one of the most important medical discoveries of this century.[417] Fluid therapy is divided into the rehydration phase and the maintenance phase.[418] Table 37-7 presents guidelines to follow for both phases of therapy.

Severely dehydrated patients have a major fluid deficit to make up in the first 4 hours (91 to 120 mL/kg of body weight). Intravenous rehydration therapy with a dextrose-containing solution of Ringer's Lactate (RL) or normal saline (NS) is indicated. In their absence, plain Ringer's Lactate or normal saline supplemented with potassium is indicated. Once the patient is alert and can tolerate oral fluids, ORT should be started. Stool losses, fluid intake, and serum-specific gravity should continue to be monitored closely at the patient's bedside on at least an hourly basis for the first 4 to 6 hours. Serum-specific gravity is the best objective parameter to evaluate success of rehydration; it can be measured using a simple and inexpensive hand-held refractometer. Once ORT is begun, the patient should be encouraged to drink freely to at least equal one and a half times the volume of stool losses. ORT should be continued for as long as the patient has diarrhea. Management of diarrhea can be easily done at the first or second echelon of care (eg, unit aid station, field clinic, hospital). Several ORT formulations are available in the United States and include: (*a*) World Health Organization (WHO) ORT (Janis Brothers Packaging Co., Kansas City, Mo.), (*b*) Rehydralyte (Ross Products Division, Abbott Laboratories, Columbus, Ohio), (*c*) Pedialyte (Ross Products Division, Abbott Laboratories, Columbus, Ohio), and (*d*) Infalyte (Mead Johnson Nutritionals, Bristol-Myers Squibb Co., Evansville, Ind.). Sports drinks (eg, Gatorade) and other high-sugar solutions (such as soft drinks) are not appropriate.[379]

Antimicrobial Therapy

Antimicrobial therapy is an important adjunctive therapy in cholera, whether caused by O1 or O139 strains[371,418] (Table 37-8). Duration of illness and stool volume losses can be cut in half with oral (not parenteral) antibiotics. In addition, the duration of excretion of *V cholerae* is also shortened to an average of 48 to 72 hours with antibiotics.[418] Tetracycline or doxycycline are the recommended first-line drugs. For children less than 8 years of age and pregnant women, erythromycin, furazolidone, or trimethoprim-sulfamethoxazole (TMP-SMX) are indicated. In areas where there has been significant resistance reported, quinolones such as norfloxacin or ciprofloxacin can be used.[416,419–422] Quinolones have great advantages in that they are effective as single-dose therapy and the rate of clearance of *V cholerae* from stools is faster than with tetracycline or furazolidone treatment.[419,420] This rapid clearance of the stools may help to reduce secondary transmission of cholera, especially in hospi-tals, treatment centers, and refugee settings where increased transmission is a serious problem.[419] Use of bismuth subsalicylate, albeit beneficial for traveler's diarrhea, has not been adequately evaluated in patients with cholera. Antiperistaltic agents, such as loperamide (Imodium) and diphenoxylate hydrochloride (Lomotil), should be avoided. Antiemetic agents, likewise, are of doubtful benefit and should be avoided because they may cause severe dystonic reactions in dehydrated patients.[418]

Control

Some strategies for the prevention and control of cholera follow. They are discussed in more detail in references 315, 378, 423, 424, and 425.

Early detection of incipient epidemics by establishing a continuous surveillance system for diarrheal diseases and investigating severe cases and clusters is crucial. All cases of watery diarrhea, especially if associated with severe dehydration or

TABLE 37-8

ANTIMICROBIAL THERAPY AND RESISTANCE PROFILE OF CHOLERA

Drug	Adult Dosage	Pediatric Dosage	Areas with Resistance
Tetracycline	500 mg four times daily for 3 days or 1 g single dose	50 mg/kg body weight divided in 4 daily doses for 3 days	Bangladesh, India, Thailand, Ecuador, eastern Africa, Zaire
Doxycycline	300 mg as a single dose	4–6 mg/kg as a single dose	Same as for tetracycline
Erythromycin	250 mg four times daily for 3 days	30 mg/kg body weight divided in 3 daily doses for 3 days	Bangladesh, India, Thailand, eastern Africa
Furazolidone	100 mg four times daily for 3 days	5 mg/kg body weight divided in 4 daily doses for 3 days or 7 mg/kg as a single dose	Bangladesh, India, Thailand, eastern Africa
TMP-SMX	320 mg TMP and 1.6 g SMX twice daily for 3 days	8 mg TMP and 40 mg SMX per kg body weight divided in 2 daily doses for 3 days	Bangladesh, India, Thailand, Ecuador, eastern Africa
Quinolones	Norfloxacin 400 mg twice daily for 3 days, or ciprofloxacin 250-500 mg, 1-2 times a day for 3 days or 1 g single dose	Not recommended	Not reported

TMP-SMX: Trimethoprim-sulfamethoxazole
Sources: Bennish ML. Cholera: pathophysiology, clinical features, and treatment. In: Wachsmuth IK, Blake PA, Olsvik O, eds. Vibrio cholerae *and Cholera: Molecular to Global Perspectives*. Washington, DC: American Society for Microbiology; 1994: 229–255; Swerdlow DL, Isaacson M. The epidemiology of cholera in Africa. In: Wachsmuth IK, Blake PA, Olsvik O, eds. Vibrio cholerae *and Cholera: Molecular to Global Perspectives*. Washington, DC: American Society for Microbiology; 1994: 297–307; Khan WA, Bennish ML, Seas C, et al. Randomised controlled comparison of single-dose ciprofloxacin and doxycycline for cholera caused by *Vibrio cholerae* O1 or O139. *Lancet*. 1996;348:296–300; Gotuzzo E, Seas C, Echevarria J, Carrillo C, Mostorino R, Ruiz R. Ciprofloxacin for the treatment of cholera: A randomized, double-blind, controlled clinical trial of a single daily dose in Peruvian adults. *Clin Infect Dis*. 1995;20:1485–1490; Yamamoto T, Nair GB, Albert MJ, Parodi CC, Takeda Y. Survey of *in vitro* susceptibilities of *Vibrio cholerae* O1 and O139 to antimicrobial agents. *Antimicrob Agents Chemother*. 1995;39:241–244; Mitra R, Basu A, Dutta D, Nair GB, Takeda Y. Resurgence of *Vibrio cholerae* O139 Bengal with altered antibiogram in Calcutta, India. *Lancet*. 1996;348:1181.

hospitalization, should be investigated. A simple clinical case definition—for example, watery diarrhea of sudden onset in a person of any age—is appropriate and can reliably predict *V cholerae* O1 or O139 infections in approximately 90% of cases.[424] Clustering in time or place or both (ie, spot mapping of cases) may suggest common modes of transmission amenable to control.

Good personal hygiene will limit spread within the unit or household. Proper handwashing with soap after defecation and before eating or preparing food is key, along with avoiding consumption of high-risk items prepared by the local population, such as food or drinks from street vendors, seafood or shellfish products (especially if raw), vegetables, uncarbonated drinks, and ice. Bathing in potentially contaminated bodies of water should also be prohibited.

Construction and proper maintenance of excreta disposal facilities will reduce the risk of spread of cholera in bivouacked units and refugee camp settings. Defecation on the ground and in or near drinking water sources should be avoided.

Provision of safe and plentiful water, as well as its protection and appropriate storage in the home, unit, or food serving areas, is important. Appropriate care in the preparation and handling of food items and consumption of cooked food while still hot are important. Foodborne spread of *V cholerae* is facilitated by bacterial multiplication in food kept at ambient temperatures after cooking.[388] Although the role of flies in cholera transmission is controversial, it is conceivable that they could represent a risk by inoculating food with *V cholerae*.[426] Therefore, fly-proofing of food service and fecal disposal facilities, as well as fly control by bait-traps or use of insecticides, is indicated.

Chemoprophylaxis

The use of tetracycline (500 mg twice a day for at least 2 days, half dose for children aged 8 to 13 years) or doxycycline (300 mg single dose, half dose for children aged 8 to 13 years) chemoprophylaxis reduces the rate of secondary transmission for household or unit contacts of cases.[423] For children younger than 8 years of age, pregnant women, and persons with kidney disease, tetracycline should be avoided; erythromycin or TMP-SMX may be used in the same dosages as for treatment (see Table 37-8). The use of single-dose ciprofloxacin (250 mg), on the other hand, has not been found to be effective in preventing *V cholerae* O1 infections among household contacts of cases.[427] It should be noted that mass chemoprophylaxis of a community or unit

is usually contraindicated, due to the risk of drug resistance and the appearance of potentially serious side effects.[381,423,428] It is indicated only when an outbreak of cholera has occurred in a closed group that has had a common exposure, and it is effective only if given within the first 5 days after exposure. Surveillance for cases among exposed personnel should be conducted for 5 days from the last exposure. No special isolation precautions are needed for cholera patients. Effective measures to limit nosocomial and intra-unit spread include handwashing with soap after each patient is seen, use of gloves for specimen handling, laundering of soiled clothing or bed linen, and disinfection of feces and vomitus with calcium hypochlorite or carbolic acid.[315]

Vaccines

Parenteral, whole-cell cholera vaccines have been in use since the late 19th century. Controlled trials in the 1960s in cholera-endemic areas demonstrated that parenteral vaccines were only 60% efficacious for the first 3 months, declining to 30% 4 to 6 months after vaccination.[429] Parenteral, phenol-inactivated vaccine (Wyeth Laboratories, Marietta, Penn), the only cholera vaccine licensed in the United States, has to be given in 2 doses at 1- to 4-week intervals and is associated with significant local reactions in up to 30% of vaccinees. A booster dose is recommended every 6 months. In addition, this vaccine does not reduce asymptomatic carriage of *V cholerae* O1, and its protective efficacy is very low (< 30%) in children.[430] Simultaneous administration with yellow fever vaccine can decrease subsequent antibody response to both vaccines. The cholera vaccine's usefulness for military forces or travelers to endemic areas is very limited.

The resurgence of cholera has renewed interest in vaccine development. In the past 15 years, inactivated oral cholera vaccine candidates have been developed and found to be protective in challenge studies. An oral vaccine, consisting of the B subunit of cholera toxin (1 mg) and 10^{11} cholera whole cells (WC/BS, Cholerix, SBL Vaccin AB, Stockholm, Sweden), was found to protect against diarrheal illness caused by *V cholerae* O1 and enterotoxigenic *Escherichia coli* in Bangladesh.[431] This vaccine provided 85% efficacy against cholera in the first 6 months and a cumulative efficacy of 50% over 3 years when 2 or 3 doses were given 6 weeks apart.[432] Protection, however, was evident only for the first 3 years of follow-up and was found to be better against classical than El Tor cholera, especially among children younger than 5 years of age.[432,433] A less expensive, recombinantly produced formulation of this vaccine (WC/rBS; Dukoral/oral cholera vaccine, SBL Vaccin AB, Stockholm, Sweden) was developed in the late 1980s and was subsequently found to be safe and immunogenic.[434] Immunity is conferred within 7 to 10 days of the second dose. This WC/rBS oral vaccine, given in 2 doses 1 to 2 weeks apart, provided 86% efficacy for 3 months against cholera among Peruvian military personnel immediately preceding an epidemic of El Tor cholera with attack rates of 2% to 3% in the summer of 1994.[435] Its efficacy in endemic areas where El Tor Ogawa is prevalent (eg, in Peru), however, has been limited. No efficacy was noted after two doses and 61% efficacy noted after a booster dose given a year later.[436] A similar inactivated oral cholera vaccine manufactured in Vietnam has shown a protective efficacy of 66% against El Tor cholera.[437] Protection in this study was found to be similar for young children (1 to 5 years old, 68%) as for older people (older than 5 years, 66%). It remains to be resolved whether this vaccine will be useful for travelers or military personnel without naturally acquired immunity.[438]

The oral, inactivated vaccines recently developed represent an unquestionable advance over the currently licensed parenteral vaccines. However, the need for two doses 1 to 2 weeks apart may make them a difficult option for rapid immunization of military forces or travelers and may limit their usefulness in the control of incipient or ongoing epidemics of cholera. Single-dose, live, attenuated, oral cholera vaccines would be ideal for these needs. The most well-studied of these vaccines is CVD 103–HgR (Mutacol Berna, Berna, Swiss Serum and Vaccine Institute, Bern, Switzerland). This vaccine confers an immune response (and protection in challenged volunteers) within 8 days of administration.[439] Volunteers attain 90% to 100% protection against subsequent challenge with El Tor and classical strains.[440] Unfortunately, this vaccine was not shown to protect against cholera in a recently completed, randomized, placebo-controlled, double-blind field trial in Indonesia.[441] This vaccine is licensed for use in Europe, Canada, and certain countries of Latin America. A booster dose is recommended after 6 months and chloroquine or antibiotics should be administered no sooner than 1 week after administration of this vaccine.

The rapid spread of *V cholerae* O139 among all ages in areas where *V cholerae* O1 is endemic indicates that immunity to O1-serogroup cholera is not protective against O139-serogroup infections.[369,381] Epidemiologic and laboratory studies suggest that natural immunity to *V cholerae* O1 is not protective against *V cholerae* O139.[433] This has been confirmed in recent studies in rabbits and in human volunteers.[371,442] The high rates of severe illness seen with this new strain and its potential impact in causing large epidemics among nonimmune adults predicate an urgent need to develop live, attenuated *V cholerae* O139-serogroup vaccines.

As of 2000, several O139-serogroup vaccine candidates have been developed and are in various stages of analysis.[443–446] Improved preparations of oral killed vaccines are also being developed, including combination *V cholerae* O1 and O139 vaccines and new parenteral cholera vaccines consisting of O antigens conjugated to a variety of proteins, including cholera toxin.[447]

The hope is that in the future, oral cholera vaccines, killed and live, will become readily available for use in vaccination programs in developing countries,[448] as well as for travelers, expatriates, and military personnel at risk. Another possibly important, although somewhat controversial, scenario is the use of these vaccines during acute emergencies (eg, famines, typhoons, floods) and among refugees in both primitive and well-established camps where the risk of impending cholera outbreaks is considered to be very high.[449] Such mass vaccination with the two-dose WC/rBS vaccine has been accomplished,[450] and cost-effectiveness evaluation performed by Naficy and colleagues found that this vaccine could be used for mass vaccination in refugee settings if the price per dose was low (< $0.22 per dose).[451]

[Jose L. Sanchez]

AMEBIASIS

Introduction and Military Relevance

Throughout history, soldiers involved in military campaigns have suffered from diarrheal illnesses, from Napoleon's troops invading Russia to Civil War soldiers along the banks of the Chickahominy River in Virginia. *Entamoeba histolytica* was first recognized as a diarrheal pathogen among US troops during the Philippine Insurrection in 1899, and since then it has been documented in every major war fought in the developing world. In World War II, for example, admission rates for amebic dysentery in the China-Burma-India theater were 22.39 per 1,000 per year.[452] Amebic dysentery, or amebic colitis, is the most common manifestation of *E histolytica* infection, but the protozoa can also gain access to the liver, presumably via the portal vein, where it causes liver abscesses. Less common target organs include the lung, brain, and skin, but wherever it invades, it demonstrates the lytic destruction of tissue befitting its species name. In the mid 1990s, *E histolytica* was separated from the nonpathogenic species *E dispar*. This reclassification has important ramifications for diagnosis and treatment because the two protozoa have identical morphology under the microscope but only *E histolytica* infection requires antiprotozoal therapy.

Description of the Pathogen

E histolytica is a pseudopod-forming protozoan parasite in the Sarcodina subphylum. *E histolytica* is the most invasive *Entamoeba,* a group that includes such other species that infect humans as *E hartmanni, E polecki, E coli, E gingivalis,* and *E dispar.* Only *E histolytica* causes dysentery and liver abscess. Its motile trophozoite form invades and causes disease, but the cyst form transmits disease from host to host (Figure 37-3). The quadrinucleate cyst averages from 10 to 15 mm in diameter, is excreted in the feces of an infected host, and is stable for weeks to months in an appropriately moist environment. In the small intestine, the cyst excysts to form eight trophozoites, mononucleate ameboid cells measuring from 10 to 60 mm in diameter. These trophozoites may then colonize the intestine as harmless commensals or invade into the colonic epithelium, causing inflammation and destruction of the bowel wall.

While *E histolytica* trophozoites may either colonize or invade host intestine, *E dispar* can only colonize and has never been documented to invade host tissue. As early as 1925, Brumpt suggested that the pathogenic and nonpathogenic types should be classified into two separate species.[453] However, the inability to distinguish morphologically between these two proposed species caused this proposal to languish until 1978, when differences in patterns of isoenzymes between "pathogenic" and "nonpathogenic zymodemes" of *E histolytica* suggested that two different species did in fact exist.[454] Since that initial observation, evidence has accumulated for the reclassification of *E histolytica* into pathogenic *(E histolytica)* and nonpathogenic *(E dispar)* species based on differences in monoclonal antibody epitopes,[455] Southern blot patterns of genomic DNA,[456] and ribosomal RNA sequences.[457] This reclassification is especially satisfying in that it helps to explain what was long a central conundrum in the study of amebiasis: of all the people who could be demonstrated by microscopic examination of stool samples to be carriers of "*E histolytica*" in the days before the two species were separated, only 10% manifested symptoms of amebiasis. Since *E dispar* is the more common organism and the two species are identical morphologically, it seems likely that most of the asymptomatic infections with "*E histolytica*" detected were actually caused by *E dispar.*

Epidemiology

Transmission

E histolytica cysts are transmitted by ingestion of fecally contaminated water and food or through direct fecal-oral contact; the trophozoite is not infectious because it is too fragile to resist the harsh pH and enzymatic conditions in the stomach. The

a 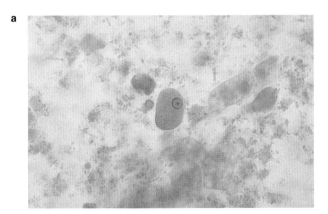 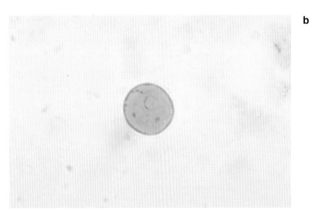 b

Fig. 37-3. *Entamoeba histolytica* or *E dispar* trophozoites (**a**: in a blue stain) and cyst (**b**: in an orange stain). Note that it is not possible to distinguish *E histolytica* form *E dispar* morphologically.
Photographs: Courtesy of the Centers for Disease Control and Prevention.

cyst, however, passes unscathed through the stomach to the small intestine. Intestinal trophozoites may also encyst and be excreted in the feces of the host, so that the cycle of infection is continued. The disease is considered communicable for as long as cysts are being passed, a situation that can last for years.[315p11-15] The incubation period for the development of amebic dysentery is variable but most commonly lasts from 2 to 4 weeks.

Geographic Distribution

Although *E histolytica* can be found throughout the world, it is endemic in the developing world where sanitary conditions allow infection to spread; examples include Central and South America, Africa, and the Indian subcontinent, where it is the third leading parasitic cause of death.[458]

Incidence

More than 10% of the world's population is thought to be infected by *E dispar* and *E histolytica*, with the approximately 50 million cases of invasive disease in the world each year resulting in as many as 100,000 deaths a year.[459] A 1988 survey in Mexico demonstrated that 8.4% of the population was seropositive for *E histolytica* as measured by the indirect hemagglutination assay, with a peak incidence occurring in the 5- to 9-year-old age group.[460] That year, there were an estimated 1 million cases of amebiasis and 1,216 deaths caused by *E histolytica* infection in Mexico.[461] In Bangladesh, studies using the stool antigen detection test showed that city-dwelling children with diarrhea had a 4.2% prevalence rate of infection with *E histolytica*.[462]

In developed countries, such as the United States, amebiasis is predominately a disease of recent immigrants and travelers returned from the tropics. One study in Germany documented that 0.3% of travelers abroad acquired invasive amebiasis, with the risk of infection increasing with the length of the trip.[463] One dramatic example was 160 Italian travelers who went on a 5-day trip to Thailand where 72% were infected; consumption of certain foods (ie, ice, ice cream, raw fruit) was significantly linked to *E histolytica* infection.[464]

Pathogenesis and Clinical Findings

E histolytica is thought to invade the colonic epithelium directly, adhering to host cells via the Gal/GalNAc lectin.[465] In vitro studies have demonstrated that lectin-mediated adherence is necessary for cytolysis, but the exact mechanism of cell killing is not known.[466] Tissue destruction begins as small foci of necrosis that progress to ulcers. The characteristic amebic lesion is a flask-shaped ulcer extending through the mucosa and muscularis mucosa into the submucosa. Factors that might influence the invasiveness of infection experienced by the host may include the particular strain of *E histolytica* present, the presence of anti-ameba antibodies, and the host's bacterial flora in the intestine, genetic predisposition, and nutritional state.

The most common clinical manifestation of intestinal amebiasis is amebic colitis, characterized by liquid stools (up to 25 a day) containing bloody mucus and accompanied by abdominal pain and tenderness (Table 37-9). The onset is usually gradual, building over the course of 1 to 3 weeks; when the diarrhea is severe, signs of dehydration and electrolyte imbalance may also be present. Essentially all patients have heme-positive stools, but fecal leukocytes may not be present, presumably due to the cytotoxic effect of amebic trophozoites on human neutrophils.

Acute necrotizing colitis, or fulminant colitis, is a more unusual and more severe manifestation of intestinal amebiasis, with a predisposition for occurring in debilitated hosts. These patients are severely ill with fever, leukocytosis, profuse bloody mucoid diarrhea, and abdominal pain and distention; the mortality rate is greater than 40%. Surgical intervention is often necessary to perform a partial or total colectomy.[467] Other uncommon results of intestinal invasion include ameboma, a carcinoma-like annular lesion of the colon, toxic megacolon, peritonitis, and cutaneous amebiasis.

TABLE 37-9

HISTORY, SYMPTOMS, AND SIGNS OF AMEBIC COLITIS

Male/female	1/1
Immigrant from or traveler to endemic area	Most
Gradual onset	Most
Length of symptoms > 1 wk	Most
Heme (+) stools	100%
Diarrhea	94-100%
Dysentery	94-100%
Abdominal pain	12-80%
Weight loss	44%
Fever > 38°C	10%

TABLE 37-10

HISTORY, SYMPTOMS, AND SIGNS OF AMEBIC LIVER ABSCESS

Male/female	9/1
Immigrant from or traveler to endemic area	Most
Length of symptoms > 4 weeks	21-51%
Fever	85-90%
Abdominal tenderness	84-90%
Weight loss	33-50%
Hepatomegaly	30-50%
Diarrhea	20-33%
Cough	10-30%
Jaundice	6-10%

From the intestine, invasion of submucosal venules can allow trophozoites to disseminate through the portal vein to the liver, where they can cause amebic liver abscess. Presenting symptoms of amebic liver abscess are usually fever and abdominal pain, often in the right upper quadrant (Table 37-10). On physical exam, there is often point tenderness over the liver, with or without hepatomegaly. Laboratory findings may include leukocytosis, mild anemia, and elevated alkaline phosphatase levels; hepatic imaging studies, such as ultrasound or computerized tomography, reveal an oval-shaped defect. Most patients do not experience concurrent diarrhea, although a history of dysentery within the past year is common.

Complications of liver abscess occur when the abscess expands to involve adjacent structures, such as the peritoneum, pericardium, diaphragm, pleural cavity, or lungs. Clinical manifestations of pleuropulmonary amebiasis are cough, pleuritic pain, and dyspnea. Less frequently, amebae spread to the brain by a hematogenous route, forming large necrotic lesions that rapidly prove fatal.

Diagnostic Approaches

Because *E histolytica* is endemic in the developing world, heme-positive diarrhea, especially in the absence of fever, in persons living in or returning from these areas should immediately raise the suspicion of amebic infection. Other invasive pathogens that should be included in the differential diagnosis are *Shigella* species, *Salmonella enteritidis, Campylobacter jejuni, Yersinia enterocolitica,* and the invasive species of *Escherichia coli.* Additionally, since amebiasis can

mimic inflammatory bowel disease, care must be taken to distinguish between these two diagnoses because steroid administration can cause amebic dysentery to develop into fulminant colitis.

The standard method for diagnosing intestinal amebiasis is to identify *E histolytica* trophozoites or cysts in the stool. This method, however, is flawed for two reasons. The first is that microscopic examination of a single stool specimen has a sensitivity of no more than 33% to 50% and, according to one study, a specificity of 79%. The second major problem is that this method fails to distinguish between the pathogen *E histolytica* and the morphologically identical *E dispar,* an organism that has never been documented to cause colitis or liver abscess. While it is true that hematophagous trophozoites are more likely to be *E histolytica,* they can also be *E dispar.*[468]

Taking advantage of the fact that *E histolytica* and *E dispar* possess divergent surface proteins, a stool antigen detection test that is specific for *E histolytica* has become available for clinical use from TechLab, Inc (Blacksburg, Va.). This test uses monoclonal antibodies specific for the *E histolytica* lectin in an enzyme-linked immunosorbent assay. Sensitivity and specificity are very high for this kit, at 93% and 98% respectively.[468] Another diagnostic test is the indirect hemagglutination test for anti-amebic antibody. This test is approximately 80% to 90% sensitive for amebic colitis and liver abscess but is problematic because it can be negative early in the course of infection and remain positive for years after an episode of amebiasis.[469] In endemic areas where a substantial number of residents have anti-amebic antibodies as detected by this test, a positive serologic test may reflect current or prior invasive amebiasis.[470]

If liver abscess is suspected, hepatic imaging can quickly establish the presence of a cavitary defect in the liver. However, because comparative studies using ultrasound, computerized tomography, and magnetic resonance imaging have shown that it is not possible to differentiate amebic from pyogenic abscess based on imaging alone,[471–473] information from epidemiologic risk factors must be used to suggest a diagnosis. Patients with amebic liver abscess tend to be younger in age (less than 45 years), predominantly male, and recent travelers or immigrants. Pyogenic liver abscess patients, on the other hand, often present with concurrent biliary tract disease. Serum anti-amebic antibodies can also be useful for establishing a diagnosis, and, if necessary, ultrasound-guided fine needle aspiration can be used to investigate the lesion. The stool antigen detection test is less effective for liver abscess, with a sensitivity of only 67%.[474]

Recommendations for Therapy and Control

Asymptomatic colonization with *E histolytica* can be treated with diloxanide furoate (500 mg three times a day for 10 days in adults) or with paromomycin (30 mg/kg in three divided doses for 7 days). Another luminal agent, diiodohydroxyquin, can cause optic atrophy and vision loss in children receiving chronic treatment and is not commercially available in the United States. All three of these agents are generally well tolerated.

Both amebic colitis and liver abscess can be treated with metronidazole (500-750 mg three times a day for 10 days) plus one of the luminal agents. Although metronidazole has some unpleasant side effects, such as headache, nausea, metallic taste, and a disulfuram-like reaction to alcohol, reaction is rarely severe, and treatment efficacy is greater than 90%. Uncommon neurologic side effects, such as vertigo, encephalitis, or neutropenia, may require discontinuation of treatment. Tinidazole, a nitroimidazole not available in the United States, is also an effective treatment. If patients with liver abscess fail to respond after 3 days, chloroquine or dehydroemetine may be added to the regimen. Needle aspiration of liver abscess is usually not required and has not been shown to speed recovery.

Control of amebic infection can be achieved by eradicating fecal contamination of food and water. Human feces must be disposed of in a sanitary manner, and persons working in endemic areas must be educated in personal hygiene and safe handling of locally obtained food and water supplies. Since cysts are resistant to low doses of chlorine or iodine, water can be boiled to make it safe to drink, and raw vegetables should be washed with soap and then soaked in vinegar for 15 minutes to ensure eradication of the cysts. Public water supplies can be protected from contamination by sand filtration, which removes most cysts.[315]

Although diarrheal pathogens such as *E histolytica* have long been a scourge of army encampments, recent military operations, such the Persian Gulf War, where the percentage of personnel treated for gastroenteritis per week dropped to below 1% after the first month, demonstrates that with proper precautions diarrheal disease does not have to be a major player in future military campaigns.

[William A. Petri, Jr.; Joanna M. Schaenman]

GIARDIASIS

Introduction and Military Relevance

Since the time of the Israelites fighting the Hittites, prevention of diarrheal disease has been a key factor in the successful mobilization of troops. A passage in Deuteronomy (23:9) exhorts the Israelites: "As part of your equipment have something to dig with, and when you relieve yourself dig a hole and cover up your excrement."

Giardiasis is an important parasitic cause of diarrheal disease. It is the most common parasite identified in stool samples of individuals in the United States, present in about 4% of stool specimens submitted to clinical laboratories.[475] The disease is quite common in developing countries, especially in urban slums where a substantial number of children are infected. Waterborne and foodborne transmission are the most frequent mechanisms of spread, with person-to-person spread important in daycare settings and among sexually active homosexual males.

In the military, giardiasis will most often be encountered in personnel during or after return from deployment to developing countries. In addition, it may be seen by those caring for native populations, refugees, and peacekeeping forces from developing nations. An example of the increased risk for giardiasis in developing countries is the experience with diarrheal illness in expatriate residents and tourists to Nepal, where 9% to 16% had *Giardia lamblia* identified in their stools.[77] In Operation Restore Hope in Somalia from 1992 to 1993, 0.8% of personnel sought care for diarrheal illness each week and less than 3% of all personnel reported a diarrheal illness per week. *G lamblia* was isolated from 4% of personnel with diarrhea, making it the third most common eneteropathogen identified (*Shigella* species were isolated from 33% and enterotoxigenic *Escherichia coli* from 16%). The relatively low overall attack rate of diarrhea (compared to previous deployments in developing countries) likely was due to the lack of consumption of local food products because of the economic devastation and security threats within Somalia. As in previous deployments, personnel drank bottled water from approved vendors and preprepared food from the United States.[283] A survey of 422 Marines returned from Operation Desert Storm similarly revealed a 2% prevalence of *G lamblia* cysts.[476] The risk of contracting giardiasis is not restricted to developing countries, however. In a Utah Army National Guard field training exercise in the Rocky Mountains of the United States, 15% of all personnel reported symptoms consistent with giardiasis, and symptoms were reported in 62% of personnel who supplemented their water supply with raw water from lakes, streams, and a cattle watering trough.[477]

Description of the Pathogen

Giardia lamblia has also been called *G intestinalis* and *G duodenalis.* The infective form of the parasite is the cyst, which is 7 to 10 μm wide and 8 to 12 μm long, with a refractile cell wall and 2 to 4 nuclei. Trophozoites are the motile form of the parasite, which emerge from the cyst in the small bowel lumen. They contain 2 nuclei and 4 flagella and are 12 to 15 μm long by 5 to 10 μm wide. The nuclei have a characteristic central karyosome, which gives the trophozoite its face-like appearance in stained specimens. The dorsal surface of the trophozoite is round and smooth, while the ventral surface has a concave anterior disc that is thought to help the trophozoite adhere to the intestinal epithelium.

Epidemiology

Transmission

Giardiasis is highly infectious—ingestion of as few as 10 to 25 cysts produces disease in human volunteers. Waterborne transmission is an important route of acquisition of giardiasis. Consumption of improperly treated surface water (as opposed to well water) is the most important risk factor. Military personnel, hikers, and campers who consume untreated stream or other surface water are at risk for infection with giardia. Surface water may be contaminated not only with giardia from human sources, but also with giardia from beavers, muskrats, and possibly other animals that have the potential to transmit giardia to humans.[478]

Foodborne transmission occurs. In one instance, 32 employees of a public school system developed symptomatic giardiasis after eating home-canned salmon. The salmon had been prepared by a grandmother who had just diapered her grandson, and the grandson was subsequently shown to have giardia infection.[479] Outbreak investigations need to consider the possibility of foodborne transmission, although waterborne transmission is more common.

Person-to-person spread of giardia infection is documented in children and employees in daycare centers, in sexually active male homosexuals, and in residents of institutions for the mentally handicapped.

Geographic Distribution

Giardiasis occurs in all parts of the world and is a common cause of waterborne outbreaks of diarrhea in the United States. Waterborne outbreaks have occurred in the Rocky Mountain areas of the United States and Canada and in the northwestern and northeastern United States. Even seemingly pristine mountain streams in North America can be contaminated with giardia; the infectious giardia cysts are extremely stable in cool water. In some urban slums in developing countries, rates of giardia infection approach 100%.[480]

Incidence

Surveys of children under the age of 3 years in daycare centers have measured giardia infection rates as high as 25% to 50%.[481] Most of these infections are asymptomatic: studies demonstrated that children with giardia infection had normal nutritional status and were not more likely to have enteric symptoms. Parents of children in day care and daycare workers have a higher rate of giardia infection than the overall population. Homosexual men seen in sexually transmitted disease clinics have rates of giardia infection as high as 10%.[482]

Pathogenesis and Clinical Findings

Pathogenesis

Infection is initiated by the ingestion of *G lamblia* cysts. Excystation follows ingestion, with the trophozoites multiplying in the small bowel. The infection remains luminal in almost all cases, with rare exceptions of mucosal invasion by the trophozoites. The parasite may adhere to the intestinal epithelium via its ventral disk or via a parasite carbohydrate-binding adhesin protein. Trophozoites encyst in the bowel lumen, with an encystation-specific secretory vesicle system implicated in synthesis of the cyst wall.[483]

The pathogenesis of diarrhea is not clear. No enterotoxin has been characterized, and the organism is normally not invasive. Damage to intestinal epithelial cells and atrophy of microvilli have been shown in biopsies of some patients with giardiasis. Malabsorption of protein, D-xylose, and fat soluble vitamins, as well as disaccharidase deficiency, occurs in some patients with giardiasis.

Different strains of the parasite differ in their ability to cause infection and diarrhea, as has been shown in human challenge studies. Parasite surface antigen variation has been documented in vitro and in experimental human infections, and the antibody response has been shown to be isolate-specific, suggesting that antigenic variation may be a mechanism of immune evasion.[484]

Evidence for acquired immunity to giardiasis includes the lower incidence of infection in adults than in children and the observation from epidemiological and human experimental challenge studies that symptomatic infections with giardia are more common with the first episode of infection than with later infections.[480,484]

Clinical Findings

Infection can be manifest after return from an endemic or high-risk area, as the average incubation period from infection to onset of diarrhea is 7 days and can be as long as 28 days. The typical patient with symptomatic giardiasis will have an illness lasting 7 days or more with some combination of symptoms including diarrhea, flatulence, foul-smelling stools, nausea, abdominal cramps, and excessive tiredness (Table 37-11). The most notable feature of the illness is the prolonged nature of the diarrhea and the malabsorption that may be present.[485] Lactase deficiency and malabsorption of D-xylose, protein, fat, and fat-soluble vitamins may all occur to varying degrees. Stool specimens are semiformed or loose, lack occult blood, and may contain mucus or fecal leukocytes or both. Especially in endemic settings, such as daycare centers in the developed world and urban slums in developing countries, most giardia infection is asymptomatic. Protection against symptomatic infection in children under 18 months of age has been associated with breast feeding.

Diagnostic Approaches

The diagnosis of giardiasis should be considered in outbreaks or individual cases of diarrheal illnesses lasting 5 to 7 days or more. Travel to a developing country, exposure to children in day care or to institutionalized individuals, and sex between male homosexuals should all increase the suspicion of giardiasis. Common source outbreaks can be either waterborne or foodborne.

Historically, giardiasis has been diagnosed by identification of the trophozoite or cyst in stool specimens. The motile trophozoite can sometimes be identified in a saline wet mount of fresh stool. Cysts can be stained with iodine; stools preserved in polyvinyl alcohol need trichrome or iron hematoxylin stains. Antigen detection assays are now available from at least six companies in immunofluorescent and enzyme immunoassay formats. These tests have comparable, and in many cases improved, sensitivity and specificity compared to microscopy. Sampling of duodenal contents for giardia by aspiration, biopsy, or string test is almost never necessary if careful examination of stool with antigen detection tests or stool microscopy is performed.

TABLE 37-11

PERCENTAGE OF PATIENTS WITH GIARDIASIS WHO HAVE SPECIFIC SYMPTOMS AND SIGNS OF GIARDIASIS

Prolonged diarrhea	100%
Fatigue	97%
Abdominal cramps	83%
Bloating	79%
Malodorous stool	79%
Flatulence	76%
Weight loss	59%
Fever	21%
Vomiting	17%

Reprinted with permission from Oxford University Press: Hopkins RS, Juranek DD. Acute giardiasis: an improved clinical case definition for epidemiologic studies. *Am J Epidemiol.* 1991;133:402–407.

Recommendations for Therapy and Control

Metronidazole is the drug of first choice for treatment of giardiasis, although it does not have a Food and Drug Administration indication for this use; tinidazole is also effective but is unavailable in the United States. Metronidazole (250 mg three times a day for adults or 15 mg/kg a day in three divided doses for 5 days for children) is 80% to 95% effective. Side effects of treatment include a disulfiram-like reaction when taken with alcohol, nausea, dry mouth, and headache. Dizziness, vertigo, paresthesias, and, rarely, encephalopathy or convulsions can be neurologic side effects and warrant disconting the drug. Neutropenia has been associated with metronidazole but is reversible after discontinuing the drug. There is no evidence of carcinogenicity or mutagenicity of metronidazole in humans, although use during the first trimester is not indicated. Alternative drugs include furazolidone, which can cause hemolysis in individuals with glucose-6-phosphate dehydrogenase deficiency; quinacrine, which is poorly tolerated because of nausea, vomiting, and cramping and is unavailable in the United States; and paromomycin, for which clinical experience in the treatment of giardiasis is limited.[486] In patients with a history of exposure and clinical findings consistent with giardiasis but with negative stool diagnostic studies for *G lamblia* and other enteropathogens, many authorities recommend empiric treatment with metronidazole because of the historic difficulties with sensitivity of the diagnostic tests.

Prevention of waterborne outbreaks requires proper flocculation, sedimentation, filtration, and chlorination of water supplies. Filtration is the single most important step of water purification for removal of the chlorine-resistant giardia cysts from community water supplies, as the cysts of giardia are not completely inactivated by the other steps. Good personal hygiene is required to prevent transmission by food handlers and in daycare centers. For military personnel in the field, all surface water should be considered to be contaminated with giardia. Approaches to field water purification include bringing the water to a boil for 1 minute, filtration through a 2 µm filter (but a 1 µm filter is best to also eliminate other cyst organisms), or treatment for 30 minutes with halazone (5 tablets per liter for 30 minutes), Globaline (tetraglycine hydroperiodide, 1 tablet per quart), or saturated crystalline iodine (12.5 mL/L for 30 minutes). Halazone or iodine treatment of water is less effective at 3°C than at 20°C.[487]

[William A. Petri, Jr.]

ENTERIC COCCIDIA INFECTIONS

Cryptosporidium

Introduction and Military Relevance

Cryptosporidium parvum, an intracellular coccidian protozoan, is an important emerging enteric pathogen associated with large waterborne outbreaks and cases related to person-to-person and zoonotic transmission. The control of this organism is challenging because of its high resistance to chlorine and other chemical disinfectants, small size (making filtration of the organism from potable water sources difficult), low infectious inoculum, and ubiquitous presence in various animal hosts and surface-water sources worldwide.[488]

Cryptosporidium was described in 1907 but first became recognized as an important human pathogen during the 1980s among immunocompromised persons, especially those infected with human immunodeficiency virus (HIV). Since then, the organism has increasingly been recognized as a common cause of diarrhea among immunocompetent persons in both developed and developing countries. *Cryptosporidium* is a well-recognized cause of traveler's diarrhea[489,490] and should be specifically considered in any water purification strategy used during a military deployment.

Description of the Pathogen

At least 20 species of *Cryptosporidium* have been reported, with *C parvum* the species associated with clinical illness in humans.[488] *C parvum* is found in a variety of mammals, including livestock and pets. It has a complex life cycle, which includes sexual and asexual stages and the ability to auto-infect and complete its development within a single host. The infectious inoculum has been proven to be as low as 30 organisms and theoretically may be as low as one organism.[491,492] Infectious oocysts, excreted by persons or animals, can exist in the environment for prolonged periods.

Epidemiology

Transmission. Fecal-oral transmission of oocysts can occur through person-to-person contact, animal-to-person contact, and ingestion of water or food that has been contaminated by human or animal feces.[493] Because of the widespread prevalence of the organism in animals, *Cryptosporidium* is ubiquitous in a variety of environmental water sources. Municipal drinking water outbreaks in the United States and other countries have occurred when *Cryptosporidium* has passed from surface-water sources (eg, lakes, rivers, and streams) through municipal treatment systems that met regulatory standards for filtration and chlorination.[493–495] The largest known *Cryptosporidium* diarrheal outbreak linked to public water occurred in 1993 and affected more than 400,000 residents of the Milwaukee, Wis., area.[495] In addition to common-source outbreaks linked to drinking water, outbreaks linked to public swimming facilities have also been well documented.[493,496]

Recent studies suggest that *Cryptosporidium* oocysts are present in 65% to 97% of surface water in the United States and that small numbers of oocysts regularly breach filtration systems; oocysts have been found in tap water in 27% to 54% of communities evaluated.[493]

Because of the low infectious inoculum, *Cryptosporidium* organisms are easily passed from person to person in a variety of settings, such as within families, at childcare and health care centers, at other institutional settings, and between sexual partners.[488,493,497] Animal-to-human transmission has been documented, especially from calves but also from other livestock, laboratory animals, and, occasionally, household pets.[488,493] There has been at least one case of cryptosporidiosis thought to be related to aerosol transmission.[498]

Geographic Distribution. *Cryptosporidium* has a world-wide distribution. However, the widespread nature of *Cryptosporidium* is often not well appreciated because of the lack of routine testing for this organism in clinical microbiology laboratories and research laboratories that specialize in enteric diseases.

Incidence. The organism has been estimated to cause 5% to 10% of diarrheal cases in developing countries and 1% to 3% of diarrheal cases in the United States and Europe,[488] but reported rates vary widely.[499] The high seroprevalence of *Cryptosporidium* that has been documented even in developed countries, where 17% to 58% of adults have detectable antibodies,[494,499,500] attests to the widespread exposure to the organism.

Pathogenesis and Clinical Findings

Sporozoites released from ingested oocysts invade and replicate in intestinal epithelial cells in both the small and large intestine. The exact mechanism of how the organism causes diarrhea is unknown. The average incubation period is 7 days, with a relatively wide range (1 to 28 days).[488,501,502]

In normal as well as immunocompromised hosts, infection can range from asymptomatic to severe, cholera-like diarrhea. Acute, watery diarrhea is the most common symptom and may be accompanied by loss of appetite, abdominal cramps, fatigue, malaise, nausea, vomiting, fever, and other symptoms.[488,495] Clues that may suggest a *Cryptosporidium* infection include prolonged diarrhea and diarrhea that is unresponsive to standard antibiotic treatment. In the Milwaukee outbreak, the mean duration of illness was 9 to 12 days for persons with laboratory-confirmed infection.[495,501] In normal hosts, the illness is self-limited, whereas immununocompromised hosts are predisposed to chronic *Cryptosporidium* infections.

Cryptosporidium can be excreted well after the resolution of symptoms. Although oocyst shedding for up to 2 months has been documented, the mean duration of shedding after resolution of symptoms is 7 days.[502] In the Milwaukee outbreak, 39% of patients developed recurrent episodes of watery diarrhea after 2 to 14 days of being free of symptoms.[501] The explanation for these recurrences, which lasted an average of 2 days (range 1 to 14 days), is uncertain but may relate to persons reinfecting themselves with oocysts that they are shedding.

Diagnostic Approaches

Cryptosporidium infection should be considered in the differential diagnosis of diarrheal episodes among US service members stationed in developing and developed countries. It is important for clinicians to determine whether routine ova and parasite examinations performed at their laboratory facilities include evaluation for *Cryptosporidium*. The diagnosis in a field setting is the same as in garrison. The diagnosis can be made in a field setting if there are capabilities for performing routine microscopy by a concentration procedure such as Sheather's sugar flotation or modified acid-fast staining.[488] Stool specimens may be examined fresh or after formalin fixative under routine light microscopy. Using the Sheather's sugar flotation method, *Cryptosporidium* species display a pink-tinged spherical shape under high-power light microscopy. Oocysts stain red or pink using the modified acid-fast procedure. Because other coccidia have similar microscopic and staining characteristics, it is important to measure the size of organisms detected. *Cryptosporidium* species are typically 4 to 6 μm in size, compared with 8 to 10 μm for *Cyclospora* and 20 to 30 μm for *Isospora*.[503] Newer assays using monoclonal antibodies, immunofluorescence, and enyzme-linked immunosorbent assay methods have been developed that may offer increased sensitivity in detecting *Cryptosporidium* in fecal specimens.[488,504]

Recommendations for Therapy and Control

Numerous drugs have been tried against *Cryptosporidium* with poor or limited success, although data from one study suggest that paromomycin, a poorly absorbed aminoglycoside, is effective in reducing oocyst excretion and improving clinical condition of patients with acquired immunodeficiency syndrome and cryptosporidiosis.[505] No treatment has been proven to shorten the course of infection in normal hosts.

Although data are limited on the risk of *Cryptosporidium* in military populations, based on data from civilian communities and travelers, *Cryptosporidium* may pose a significant threat of causing outbreaks related to the waterborne and person-to-person modes of transmission. The Centers for Disease Control and Prevention's (CDC's) strategy for prevention of infection [506] combines optimal potable water treatment with improved diagnostic and surveillance methods. The risk associated with low levels of oocysts, such as are commonly found in publicly treated water, is unknown but is generally not considered to be a serious hazard for immunocompetent persons unless other data suggest that water quality is not acceptable. Such data include epidemiologic evidence of an increase in the number of cases, water turbidity measurements, fecal coliform counts, and particle counts or turbidity measurements on filters. When evidence suggests that water quality may not be adequate, the CDC recommends boiling drinking water as the most reliable method of killing oocysts.[506] Bringing water to a boil for any length of time is adequate.[507] If a filtration system is used, only a filter capable of removing particles less than or equal to 1 µm should be used.[506] Filters in this category include those that produce water by reverse osmosis, those labeled as "Absolute" 1 µm filters, and those meeting American National Standards Institute (ANSI) (formally the National Sanitation Foundation) International Standard #53 "Cyst Removal." Systems that only employ ultraviolet light, activated carbon, or pentiodide-impregnated resins are not effective against *Cryptosporidium*. Bottled water does not guarantee that the water is free of oocysts unless it was distilled or filtered by methods that meet the criteria indicated above. Bottled-water labels have not been standardized regarding water source and whether treatment methods are adequate to remove oocysts. Generally, groundwater sources (eg, springs and wells) are much less likely to contain *Cryptosporidium* oocysts than surface-water sources, but the exclusive source of water is often not specified. Use of the terms "microfiltration" or "Nominal" 1 µm filters may not ensure that the filters used were effective against *Cryptosporidium*. Ozonation can kill oocysts, but the appropriate concentration and contact time relative to the allowable level of ozone has not been established for bottled water. Carbonated canned or bottled beverages are considered safe.

In addition to assuring adequate water treatment, secondary transmission through person-to-person spread needs to be carefully controlled because of the low infectious inoculum. Patients with *Cryptosporidium* infections should be instructed to wash their hands frequently (especially after using the toilet and before eating), avoid preparing food, avoid contact with hospitalized or institutionalized persons, and refrain from swimming in public bathing areas (such as swimming pools) while they have diarrhea. They should follow these precautions for 2 weeks after symptoms have resolved because of the likelihood that they will continue to shed viable organisms.[506]

Cyclospora Species

Introduction and Military Relevance

Cyclospora species (previously referred to as cyanobacterium-like bodies) has been associated with prolonged diarrhea among travelers[508–513] and indigenous persons living in developing counties.[514–517] Like *Cryptosporidium*, *Cyclospora* is also a cause of chronic diarrhea in HIV-infected persons.[511,512,518] Although the organism was first described in 1979,[519] it was not recognized as an important pathogen until the late 1980s and early 1990s.[508–514] Traveler's diarrhea cases caused by *Cyclospora* have been reported from all over the world, and a particularly high incidence of the infection has been documented among tourists and expatriate residents in Nepal.[508,509]

Description of the Pathogen

Initial reports in the 1980s and early 1990s described the organism either as resembling a cyanobacterium (blue-green algae), based primarily on the morphology in formalin-preserved specimens, or a coccidia, based on staining characteristics that were similar to *Cryptosporidium parvum*.[508,510–513,520] The organism, collected in potassium dichromate, was conclusively shown in 1993 to be a coccidia. Based on its sporulation characteristics, it was identified as a *Cyclospora*, a coccidia found in certain animals, and the name *Cyclospora cayetanensis* was proposed.[514,521] A *Cyclospora* oocyst, when induced to sporulate, develops four sporozoites within two sporocysts.

Epidemiology

Transmission. Studies provide compelling evidence that *Cyclospora* is a waterborne disease. In a case-control study of expatriates and travelers in Nepal, consumption of untreated water was significantly associated with disease.[509] *Cyclospora* infections in Nepal and other locations are highly seasonal, with virtually all cases occurring during the warm, rainy months.[508,509] This suggests that environmental factors are important in the life cycle of this organism. In 1990, an outbreak of diarrhea caused by *Cyclospora* occurred among 21 house-staff physicians and other staff working at a hospital in Chicago.[522] An epidemiologic investigation identified tap water in the physicians' dormitory as the most likely source, and an environmental investigation suggested that stagnant water in a rooftop storage tank may have contaminated the water supply after a pump failure. A 1995 outbreak of *Cyclospora*-induced diarrhea at a country club in New York was also traced to contaminated drinking water.[523]

Like *Cryptosporidium*, *Cyclospora* is difficult to

identify in water sources; the concentration of oocysts in water is likely to be low. However, there are at least three reports of the organism being identified in epidemiologically implicated water sources.[509,524,525] *Cyclospora* may be similar to *Cryptosporidium* in being resistant to chlorine. In 1994, an outbreak of diarrhea caused by *Cyclospora* occurred among British soldiers stationed at a Gurka military training camp in Pokhara, Nepal.[524] The organism was found in camp drinking water despite adequate chlorine levels.

In addition to the waterborne route of transmission, there is increasing evidence that *Cyclospora* is transmitted by food sources.[526–529] In the case-control study from Nepal, consumption of untreated water accounted for only 28% of cases studied,[509] suggesting that additional modes of transmission, such as by food or person-to-person contact, were likely. In one report from Nepal, *Cyclospora* was identified on a head of lettuce from which a patient had eaten 2 days before the onset of symptoms.[526]

In 1996 and 1997, large outbreaks of *Cyclospora* infection were detected in the United States and Canada.[529,530] Evidence implicated consumption of fresh raspberries from Guatemala and led to widespread recognition of the importance of this pathogen.

Geographic Distribution. A growing number of reports suggest that *Cyclospora* has a worldwide distribution. These include case reports of diarrhea among travelers and indigenous persons in numerous developing countries,[508–519] as well as reports of *Cyclospora* outbreaks and sporadic cases occurring in developed countries.[522,523,528–531]

Incidence. Although there have been many case reports throughout the world, there have been very few systematic studies of prevalence or incidence of *Cyclospora* in defined populations. Among expatriates and tourists in Nepal, the organism is identified in more than 10% of diarrhea cases occurring during the rainy season, and an annual incidence of 7% was documented among US Embassy personnel and dependents there in 1992.[509] In a subsequent year-long active-surveillance study of expatriate residents, an annual incidence of 32% (16 cases per 50 person-years) was detected.[532] Among Nepalese children younger than 5 years of age presenting to a clinic for treatment of diarrhea, 5% had *Cyclospora* identified in their stool.[515] There was a pronounced age variation, with a 12% prevalence among those children who were 18 months of age or older.

In a prospective study in Peru, 6% to 18 % of children younger than 2 years of age were found to have *Cyclospora* organisms at some time during a 2-year

period when stools were examined on a weekly basis.[514] Because the vast majority of stools were collected during times when children were well, only 22% of detected infections were associated with symptoms.

Cyclospora is likely to be a cause of low-level endemic disease in the United States, based on reports from the CDC and a prevalence study from Lahey Clinic in Massachusetts.[531] Of 1,042 consecutive stool samples examined at the Lahey Clinic's microbiology laboratory, 3 (0.3%) were positive for the organism. These three patients had no history of recent travel and presented with relapsing watery diarrhea that lasted from 12 days to 8 weeks.

Pathogenesis and Clinical Findings

Cyclospora causes a syndrome characterized by prolonged diarrhea and high morbidity if untreated. The largest case series that characterized the natural history of infection and small intestinal pathology was among adult travelers in Nepal.[508,509,533] Case-control data comparing patients with diarrhea to well controls provide strong evidence that *Cyclospora* is pathogenic.[509]

In the first few days of *Cyclospora* infection, symptoms can be indistinguishable from those caused by bacterial enteric pathogens, including the abrupt onset of watery diarrhea, fever, nausea, vomiting, and abdominal cramps. A protracted course of intermittent diarrhea, fatigue, upper intestinal symptoms (eg, loss of appetite, nausea, increased gas), and weight loss follows.[508,509] Among adult travelers in Nepal, the diarrheal illness associated with *Cyclospora* lasted a median of 7 weeks, compared with 9 days for persons with other causes of diarrhea.[509] Patients with *Cyclospora* averaged six diarrheal stools per day, which was similar to the number of stools seen in patients with bacterial diarrhea. Malabsorption of D-xylose is characteristic.[508] Without treatment, the disease is eventually self limited, and the disappearance of the organism from stool specimens is highly correlated with the resolution of symptoms.[508,509]

The incubation period is not well characterized but is likely to be as short as 1 or 2 days, based on data from studies in Nepal and the Chicago outbreak. Travelers in Nepal have acquired the infection within 2 days of arriving in country.[508] In the Chicago hospital outbreak, most cases occurred 1 to 8 days (with a peak at 2 days) after a water pump failure that was thought to be related to contamination of the water storage tank implicated in the outbreak.[522]

Little is known about the life cycle of *Cyclospora* or the pathogenic mechanisms responsible for symptoms. It is likely, however, that sporozoites released from ingested oocysts invade and replicate in upper intestinal enterocytes in a similar manner as other coccidia. Small intestinal biopsies from patients with the disease have shown inflammatory changes, villous atrophy, and crypt hyperplasia.[533,534] The organism has also been identified within jejunal enterocytes using electron microscopy.[534]

Diagnostic Approaches

Unsporulated *Cyclospora* oocysts are easily recognized in a fresh stool preparation using regular light microscopy.[514] However, up to 50% of infections will not be detected unless a concentration procedure, such as with formalin ethyl acetate, is used (Rajah R, Shlim DR, unpublished data, 2000). Like *Cryptosporidium*, the organism floats in Sheather's sucrose solution and can be detected using a modified acid-fast staining procedure.[514,520] Staining does not increase the rate of detection compared with a regular, concentrated, wet preparation (Rajah R, Shlim DR, unpublished data, 2000). Although most organisms appear red or pink on a modified acid-fast stain, some organisms resist the stain and appear white on the blue background.[520] It is important to measure the size of *Cyclospora* oocysts to make sure that they are in the 8- to 10-μm range, because they are morphologically similar but approximately twice the size of *Cryptosporidium* oocysts. *Cyclospora* organisms remain viable in potassium dichromate preservative for several months and will undergo sporulation within 5 days in vitro when incubated at 25°C to 32°C.[514] Formalin preservation tends to distort the internal structure of the unsporulated oocyst,[520] which is seen as round on examination of fresh stool (Figure 37-4).

Recommendations for Therapy and Control

Cyclospora infections in immunocompetent persons respond rapidly to a standard dose of trimethoprim-sulfamethoxazole (TMP-SMX)[535,536] and in this manner resemble *Isospora* infections. Immunocompromised persons with *Cyclospora* infections also respond to TMP-SMX treatment, but the dose used in patients with HIV infection is twice the dose used in healthy travelers in Nepal. In addition, chronic suppressive therapy is necessary to prevent relapse in HIV-infected persons.[518] There is evidence that cipro-

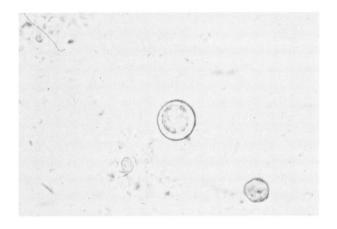

Fig. 37-4. This is a *Cyclospora* oocyst detected from a fresh stool preparation. Cell walls measuring 8 to 10 μm in diameter surround a single round unsporulated morula. Photograph: Courtesy of Lieutenant Colonel Charles W. Hoge, Medical Corps, US Army.

floxacin is an effective alternative, but its efficacy is less than that of TMP-SMX.[537]

Further studies are needed to determine optimal water purification strategies for *Cyclospora*, as well as the optimal methods to decontaminate suspect food. The outbreak in Nepal involving British soldiers suggested that *Cyclospora* is similar to *Cryptosporidium* in being resistant to chlorine.[524] Until additional data are available, the same strategies used to prevent *Cryptosporidium* oocyst transmission should be used to prevent transmission of *Cyclospora* oocysts.

Isospora belli

Isospora belli is mentioned in this chapter for completeness but is not considered an important military infectious disease. In contrast to *Cryptosporidium, Isospora* is strictly a human parasite. This characteristic, combined with its large, easily filterable size, limits or precludes chances of acquiring this organism from environmental or zoonotic sources. *Isospora* is a very rare cause of traveler's diarrhea,[538] but it is an important cause of chronic diarrhea in immunosuppressed (especially HIV-infected) persons living in developing countries.[503,539] The clinical features of illness and methods of diagnosis are similar to the two other intestinal coccidia. Like *Cyclospora, Isospora* infections respond to treatment with TMP-SMX.[539,540]

[Charles W. Hoge]

HELMINTHS

Introduction and Military Relevance

The world abounds in parasites and the majority are helminths. In 1947, Stoll [541] estimated the human population to be 2.16 billion and the number of helminthic infections in humans to be 2.25 billion. The human population in 2000 will be about 6 billion, and, based on current data, helminthic infections are keeping pace; at the end of the 20th century humanity's worm burden was 6 billion infections or more.

Military personnel are often assigned or deployed to areas of the world that are endemic for helminthic infections, have poor sanitation, or are scenes of unrest and devastation where public health facilities have been destroyed and good public health practices are absent. Soil and water may be contaminated with human and animal excrement, and safe water supplies may be cut off. In the past, military personnel have acquired helminthic infections directly from fecally contaminated soil, from food by eating raw or poorly cooked meat and vegetables, and from water by ingesting helminth eggs, larvae, or intermediate hosts harboring larval stages of the parasites. Some helminths relevant to military personnel and transmitted by food, water, and soil are presented here and helminths transmitted by snail and arthropod vectors, such as those that cause schistosomiasis and filariasis, are covered elsewhere.

Infections caused by *Strongyloides* worms, hookworm, and a number of other soil-transmitted helminths have been reported in US military personnel. Hookworm infection caused by *Ancylostoma duodenale* was documented in personnel deployed to Assam and Burma during World War II. Specific studies were also done on 50 selected hookworm-infected soldiers admitted to a hospital in Burma during World War II, and 80% of them had significant symptoms.[542] This parasite was also reported in personnel returning from the Pacific theater during World War II;[543] fortunately, little hookworm disease was seen in these cases. Ground troops were exposed to infection sleeping in foxholes, crawling through the jungle, and occupying native villages surrounded by soil previously contaminated with human excreta. A number of soldiers developed what was termed "trench cough" while in the foxholes. This was caused by the migration of hookworm larvae through the lungs. Coughing in the foxholes was a hazard since it could give the soldiers' position away. There were 22,238 cases of hookworm treated during the years 1942 to 1945.[544]

In an earlier publication covering the same years, Swartzwelder [545] reviewed the numbers of nematode and cestode infections and reported 1,242 admissions for strongyloidiasis, more than 5,000 cases of ascariasis, 285 hospital and quarters admissions for trichuriasis (most had been acquired in the United States), and approximately 2,000 cestode infections caused by *Taenia solium, T saginata,* and *Hymenolepsis nana.* In another review,[546] a number of infections with *Ascaris lumbricoides* were reported, especially in American troops in the vicinity of Manila. *Strongyloides stercoralis* was reported in 7.4% of 633 stools from troops in the Pacific theater. Trichuriasis, trichinosis, and even taeniasis were reported. Many Australian, British, and American ex–prisoners of war who worked on the Thai-Burma railway acquired strongyloidiasis, which was only detected years later in Veterans Administration hospitals.[547] Hookworm, *S stercoralis*, and *A lumbricoides* infections were also seen in US troops in Vietnam,[548] and these parasites, along with *Trichuris trichuria*, were diagnosed in patients with diarrhea seen at the Naval Support Activity Hospital in Danang, Vietnam.[549] Although many other helminthic infections were endemic in the Vietnamese, such as paragonimiasis, clonorchiasis, and fasciolopsiasis, none of these was seen in US service members.[550]

Helminthic infections among military personnel deployed to areas outside of Southeast Asia have also been reported. Dutch troops who had been in New Guinea became infected with *Ancylostoma ceylanicum* (erroneously reported as *A braziliensis*).[551] US military personnel stationed in Panama and troops going through jungle training there experienced eosinophilia, which was attributed to soil-transmitted helminths.[552] Hookworm infection was also associated with US military operations in Grenada in 1983.[553] More recently, hookworm and *S stercoralis* have been associated with gastrointestinal illness in troops returning from jungle training in Panama.[554] The eating of uncooked foods can also lead to infections during training exercises. During survival training on Okinawa, three US Marines acquired angiostrongyliasis by eating wild snails raw; others in the group ate only cooked snails and did not become ill.[555]

Description of the Pathogens

The worms that parasitize humans belong to three main groups: nematodes (or roundworms) and two within the flatworms: cestodes (or tapeworms) and trematodes (or flukes) (Table 37-12).

TABLE 37-12

HELMINTHS TRANSMITTED BY FOOD, WATER, AND SOIL

Parasite	Reservoir	Means of Transmission	Presenting Clinical Manifestations
Nematodes			
Ascaris lumbricoides	Humans	Eggs in soil	Vague intestinal symptoms, cough, pneumonitis, intestinal obstruction
Trichuris trichuria (whipworm)	Humans	Eggs in soil	Mucous diarrhea, abdominal discomfort, prolapsed rectum
Necator americanus (New World hookworm)	Humans	Larvae in soil	Dermatitis, eosinophilia, cough, abdominal pain, weakness, anemia
Ancylostoma duodenale (Old World hookworm)	Humans	Larvae in soil	Dermatitis, eosinophilia, cough, abdominal pain, weakness, anemia
Ancylostoma braziliense (hookworm)	Dogs	Larvae in soil	Cutaenous larva migrans, serpingineous tracts, dermatitis, pruritis
Ancylostoma ceylanicum (hookworm)	Dogs, cats	Larvae in soil	Anemia
Strongyloides stercoralis	Humans, dogs	Larvae in soil	Cough, eosinophilia, abdominal discomfort, larva currens
Trichinella spiralis	Pigs	Larvae in meat	Periorbital edema, muscle pain, eosinophilia, fever
Gnathostoma spinigerum	Dogs	Larvae in fish, frogs, tadpoles	Epigastric pain, vomiting, fever, edema, erythema, pruritis, rash, pain
Capillaria philippinensis	Birds	Larvae in fish	Diarrhea, abdominal pain, borborygmus
Anisakis simplex	Marine mammals	Larvae in marine fish, squid	Abdominal pain, eosinophilic granuloma, diarrhea, vomiting
Angiostrongylus cantonensis	Rats	Larvae in snails, slugs	Headache, eosinophilic meningitis, paresthesia
Angiostrongylus costaricensis	Cotton rats	Larvae in slugs	Abdominal pain, eosinophilia, palpable abdominal mass
Dracunculus medinensis	Humans	Larvae in copepods	Pruritis, blisters, ulcers, eosinophilia
Cestodes			
Diphyllobothrium latum	Fish-eating mammals	Fish	Anemia, vitamin B_{12} loss
Spirometra spp.	Dogs, cats	Frogs, tadpoles, snakes	Larval migrans, pain, periorbital edema, eosinophilia
Taenia saginata	Humans	Cysticercus larvae in beef	Vague gasterointestinal symptoms, anorexia
Taenia solium	Humans	Cysticercus larvae in pork	Vague gastrointestinal symptoms, anorexia
Taenia solium (Cysticercosis)	Humans	Eggs in soil	Epileptic seizures, nodules, muscle pain, visual disturbances
Hymenolepis nana	Rodents, beetles, fleas	Cysticercoid larvae in insects or eggs	Diarrhea, abdominal pain, anorexia, enteritis
Hymenolepis diminuta	Rats, beetles	Cysticercoid larvae in beetles	Diarrhea, abdominal pain, anorexia, enteritis
Trematodes: Liver			
Clonorchis sinensis	Humans, fish-eating mammals	Larvae in fish	Diarrhea, jaundice, hepatomegaly, eosinophilia, cirrhoses

(Table 37-12 *continues)*

Table 37-12 *continued*

Opisthorchis viverrini	Humans, fish-eating mammals	Larvae in fish	Diarrhea, jaundice, hepatomegaly, eosinophilia, cirrhoses
Opisthorchis felineus	Humans, fish-eating mammals	Larvae in fish	Diarrhea, jaundice, hepatomegaly, eosinophilia, cirrhoses
Fasciola hepatica	Sheep, goats, humans	Water plants, watercress	Abdominal pain, cirrhoses, jaundice, eosinophilia
Trematodes: Lung			
Paragonimus westermani	Crab-eating mammals	Larvae in crabs and crayfish	Cough, fever, hemoptysis, eosinophilia
Trematodes: Intestinal			
Fasciolopsis buski	Pigs, humans	Water plants	Abdominal pain, edema, diarrhea, eosinophilia, ascites
Metagonimus yokogawai	Fish-eating mammals	Fish	Vague abdominal pain, diarrhea, nausea
Heterophyes spp.	Fish-eating mammals	Fish	Vague abdominal pain, diarrhea, nausea
Echinostoma spp.	Rats, birds	Snails, tadpoles, fish	Abdominal pain, diarrhea, inflammation, ulcers

Nematodes

The nematodes are cylindrical and tapered at both ends. Their outer covering or skin consists of many layers of proteinaceous material that forms a cuticle. The size of these worms varies from a few millimeters to more than 50 cm. The mouth, at the anterior end, leads to a digestive tract and an anus at the posterior end. The sexes are separate: males have copulatory spicules and testes; some also have bursae, which are used to hold females during copulation. The females have one or two ovaries, a uterus, a vagina, and a vulva. The females produce eggs, larvae, or, rarely, both eggs and larvae.

Cestodes

The adult cestodes are flat and ribbon-like, consisting of chains of individual segments or proglottids collectively known as a strobila. The anterior end has a holdfast organ or scolex, with suckers and sometimes hooklets, followed by a neck. The neck is the area of growth or strobilization. Behind the neck region, the proglottids are of various sizes and stages of maturation: immature proglottids are followed by mature proglottids, with gravid proglottids filled with eggs at the extreme posterior. Tapeworms do not have a digestive tract and absorb nutrients through the integument or skin. Each proglottid possesses male and female sex organs. Tapeworms vary in length from millimeters to meters. Their width also varies depending on the location on the stroblia and may range from a few millimeters to a centimeter. Eggs may pass individually or within detached gravid proglottids.

Trematodes

Trematodes are flat or leaf-like and vary in size from a few millimeters to several centimeters; their width is variable. They possess two suckers or ascetabula, the anterior or oral sucker and the imperforate ventral sucker located along the median ventral line. The mouth is in the oral sucker and leads to a pharynx and two ceca (blind digestive tracts). Except for the schistosomes, all trematodes possess both male and female reproductive organs. They produce eggs of various sizes and shapes. Eggs may be embryonated when discharged from the human body or they may require a period of embryonation after they are deposited in water.

Epidemiology

Transmission

Helminthic infections in humans number in the billions. Animal and plant life, particularly when eaten raw or partially cooked, serve as major sources for human helminthic infections. Nearly one half of helminthic infections are acquired from the ingestion of fecally contaminated soil, water, or vegetation or by contact with the soil. Others are acquired by the ingestion of animal intermediate hosts containing infective stages of the parasites or by drinking water containing intermediate hosts. The life cycle and means of transmission of human helminthiasis is variable, depending on the species.

Nematodes. *Ascaris lumbricoides*, the giant intestinal roundworm, 20 to 35 cm long, resides in the small intestine, and the eggs pass with the feces. The eggs reach the soil, embryonate in a few weeks, and become infective. The hardy egg shell offers good protection, and the embryonated egg can withstand drying and other hazardous conditions for very long periods depending on conditions. When soil or vegetation contaminated with the eggs is ingested, the eggs hatch in the intestines and the liberated larvae penetrate the mucosa and migrate to the liver, heart, and lungs. After a period in the lungs, the young worms migrate up the pulmonary tree, are swallowed, and grow into adults in the small intestine. The prepatent period is 60 to 75 days.

Trichuris trichura or the whipworm, 30 to 55 mm long, lives in the large intestine, and eggs laid by females pass in the feces. The egg embryonates in the soil and is ingested with soil or contaminated vegetables or water. The eggs hatch in the intestine, and the larvae migrate down the bowel and develop directly into the adult stage in the large intestine. The prepatent period is 3 months.

There are several hookworm species that may infect humans, but the most important are *Ancylostoma duodenale*, the Old World hookworm, and *Necator americanus*, the New World hookworm. Adults of both species are about 8 to 13 mm in length and inhabit the small intestine. Eggs produced by the female worms pass in the feces into the environment. In the soil, rhabditiform larvae develop inside the eggs. The larvae hatch out of the eggs and, after a few days, develop into infective filariform larvae that are able to penetrate human skin. *A duodenale* larvae may also penetrate buccal mucosa with the drinking of contaminated water. In the soil, the filariform larvae will climb to the highest elevation on the grass and soil and congregate, a process called thigmotrophism, waiting to infect a victim through exposed feet or skin elsewhere on the body that contacts the contaminated area. *A duodenale* may also have a dormant stage in humans, called hypobiosis or arrested development, whereby the parasite remains in the larval stage somewhere in the body until it is ready to complete development. The larvae in the host migrate through the body to the lungs. After a period of further development in the lungs, the worms move up the respiratory pas-

sages to the throat, are swallowed, and mature in the small intestine. The prepatent period is 4 to 5 weeks.

Strongyloides stercoralis, only found as females in the definitive host, produces thin-shelled eggs containing larvae. The rhabditiform larvae hatch quickly from the eggs, pass in the feces, and develop into infective-stage filariform larvae. The larvae, like those of the hookworm, penetrate the skin and migrate through the body to the lungs and, eventually, to the small intestine. The prepatent period is 1 month. The larvae usually penetrate skin in contact with contaminated soil, but, like *A duodenale*, the larvae may also enter the body in drinking water and penetrate the buccal mucosa. Strains of *S stercoralis* may have a free-living cycle in the soil in which both male and female worms develop and reproduce. Furthermore, autoinfection can occur with certain strains of this parasite. Larvae may become infective while in the host, penetrate the gut, and migrate throughout the body, particularly in the immunosuppressed. This can lead to massive, disseminated infections decades after the initial infection.

Trichinella spiralis causes a widespread zoonotic parasitosis acquired by eating larva-laden muscle from infected pigs, wild game animals, or other carnivores. The meat is digested in the stomach and intestine; this releases the larvae, which enter the intestinal mucosa to mature. Adult worms reenter the gut and females release larvae, which enter the intestine wall, are picked up by the lymphatics or mesenteric venules, and are carried throughout the body to become encysted in striated muscle cells. The larvae remain in the musculature until eaten. Several other species of *Trichinella* have been described,[556] but *Trichinella spiralis* is considered the most important and the species that usually causes human infection. The other species are rarely reported in humans and are geographically limited. There are a plethora of carnivorous animal species scattered worldwide that serve as sources of infection.

Other exotic worms are acquired by humans who eat raw or poorly cooked animal life. *Gnathostoma spinigerum* is a parasite that is associated with eating raw freshwater fish and other aquatic animal life, especially in Southeast Asia. Adult worms are parasites of dogs, cats, and other carnivores; in the worm's life cycle, copepods are first-intermediate hosts and aquatic vertebrates are second-intermediate hosts. Larvae in the tissues of the second-intermediate host animals are released when the host's flesh is digested, and the larvae then migrate from the intestine to various parts of the body. Adult worms usually locate in the stomach wall and form tumors in the gastric mucosa of dogs and other carnivores. Humans are abnormal hosts in which the parasites do not mature. The larvae become migratory, wandering throughout the body, and cause disease. Raw or poorly cooked freshwater fish are the most common source of infection in humans.

Freshwater fish are also a source of a recently recognized parasite of humans, *Capillaria philippinensis*, reported primarily from the Philippines, Thailand, and a few other countries mostly in Asia. When humans eat small fish containing infective-stage larvae, the larvae are released after digestion of the fish and develop into adults in the intestine. Fish-eating birds are considered the natural host. If not treated early enough in humans, the parasitosis can cause death. Eggs passed in the feces embryonate in soil or water; eggs are eaten by the tiny fish and hatch in the fish intestine. The larvae become infective in about 3 weeks. In bird and human intestines, the larvae become adults, and females produce eggs or larvae. The larvae can also reach maturity in the host's gut, leading to autoinfection and hyperinfection.

Anisakiasis is another helminthiasis acquired from fish. *Anisakis simplex* is an intestinal parasite of marine mammals, with small marine crustaceans serving as the first-intermediate host and a variety of marine fish serving as the second-intermediate host. The infective larvae are usually in the mesenteries of the fish but migrate to the muscle when the fish dies. Humans acquire the infection by eating the fish raw in such dishes as ceviche, sashimi, or sushi. Larvae released from the fish muscle after digestion penetrate the intestinal mucosa of humans, provoking eosinophilic granulomas. Most cases of anisakiasis are reported from Japan.

Mollusks serve as intermediate hosts for rodent parasites of the genus *Angiostrongylus*. The rat lungworm, *Angiostrongylus cantonensis*, is found in the pulmonary vessels of *Rattus* species. Larvae produced by female worms leave the lungs, reach the intestine, and pass with the feces. These larvae enter land snails and develop into the infective stage. When the snails are eaten by rats, the larvae migrate to the brain, mature, and migrate to the pulmonary vessels. When humans eat infected snails, the larvae reach the brain, die, and cause an eosinophilic meningitis. The giant African snail, *Achatina fulica*, and *Pila* species are major sources of infection in Southeast Asia (mostly in Taiwan and Thailand). *Angiostrongylus costaricensis* is found in mesenteric arteries of cotton rats (*Sigmodon* species), and the slug *Vaginulus plebeius* serves as the inter-

mediate host. Humans eat this tiny slug accidentally with vegetation, and the parasite, after being digested out of the slug's tissues, penetrates the gut and causes eosinophilic granulomas in the cecum. Most infections are reported from Costa Rica.

Dracunculus medinensis, the longest nematode to parasitize humans, is acquired by ingesting infected copepods in drinking water. The larvae released from the arthropod as it is digested migrate through the tissue and usually settle in subcutaneous tissue in areas of the body that have contact with water. Female worms cause blisters to form in the skin through which they release larvae. The larvae are then taken up by the copepods. Dracunculiasis is endemic in African and some Middle Eastern and Southwest Asian countries.

Cestodes. Tapeworms are a common source of foodborne helminthic infections occurring worldwide. Infections are acquired in most cases by the ingestion of larvae in fish, meat, or arthropods. The large fish tapeworm *Diphyllobothrium latum* is acquired from fish, usually salmonoids, containing the pleurocercoid or sparganum stage of the worm. When the fish is eaten, the larva emerges from the fish tissue and attaches to the intestinal mucosa by a sucking groove or bothria at the head of the worm. Growth occurs at the neck region and segments form continuously. Eggs produced pass in the feces, which are deposited into water. A ciliated coracidium develops in the egg, hatches, swims around in the water, enters a copepod, and forms into a procercoid larva. The copepod is eaten by the fish, and the procercoid larva moves into the fish tissue and develops into a pleurocercoid larva. Pleurocercoid larvae or spargana of *Spirometra* species, which are parasites of canines and felines, may infect humans. The infections become visceral larva migrans or sparganosis. The life cycle and means of transmission of these parasites are similar to the fish tapeworms, with copepods and a variety of aquatic vertebrates serving as intermediate hosts or sources of infection. Sparganosis results from ingesting infected copepods or other aquatic animal life containing spargana or by using animal poultices infected with the parasite. The larvae emerge from the poultice and enter the body through the eye or wound upon which the poultice is placed.

Taenia saginata and *T solium* are tapeworms acquired by eating beef or pork containing cysticercus larvae. The larvae are released from the meat during digestion and attach to the intestinal mucosa with suckers and hooklets. Growth occurs in the neck region, with the developing proglottids or segments reaching sexual maturity as they move posteriorly. Eggs containing hexacanth embryos pass in the feces. The eggs are ingested by cattle and pigs and hatch in the intestine; the hexacanth then migrates to the tissues, usually muscle tissue. If eggs of *T solium* enter the intestinal tract of humans, the hexacanth embryos may enter tissue and develop into cysticercus larvae, causing the disease cysticercosis.

Other tapeworms that infect humans are the rodent cestodes *Hymenolepsis nana* and *H diminuta*. Both species are transmitted by the accidental ingestion of arthropods (eg, beetles, fleas) infected with cysticeroid larvae. *H nana* infections may also be acquired by ingesting eggs, and immunity to infection may develop in the definitive host. Infections caused by eating infected arthropods, however, do not confer immunity, and eggs produced by the adult worms hatch in the intestines and lead to autoinfection and hyperinfection.

Trematodes. There are myriad trematodes that infect humans. Most are foodborne and invade the liver, lungs, and intestines. These parasites are acquired by eating raw or partially cooked animal or plant life. Liver flukes, such as *Clonorchis sinensis* (Chinese liver flukes) in China and Korea and *Opisth orchis viverrini* in Thailand, are acquired by eating freshwater fish. The metacercaria is digested from the fish muscle and migrates into the bile passages. Eggs pass in human feces into water and are eaten by snails. The larvae in the snails multiply and release cercariae, which leave the snail, enter fish, and encyst in the fish musculature. In Eastern Europe and Russia, the cat liver fluke, *O felineus*, which also infects humans, has a similar life cycle.

The sheep liver fluke, *Fasciola hepatica*, found in sheep- and cattle-raising countries worldwide, will also invade the liver of humans. The adult flukes live in the bile ducts, the eggs pass with feces into a body of water, and a ciliated miracidum is released that enters snails. Cercariae emerge from the snail and encyst on aquatic vegetation as metacercariae. When humans eat the vegetation uncooked, the metacercariae migrate through the gut wall, enter the peritoneal cavity, penetrate the liver capsule, and migrate to the bile ducts. Human infections are frequent in European, African, and Latin American countries where people eat water plants (eg, watercress, water lettuce) uncooked.

There are approximately 40 species of *Paragonimus* worldwide, but the most important is the lung fluke *P westermani*, which is commonly found in China, Japan, Korea, Taiwan, and the Philippines. Other species are also found in Asia, North and South America, and Africa, but the prevalences are low. The worms, usually in pairs, are present in cystic cavities in lung parenchyma. Eggs are passed with sputum, but when they are swallowed, they pass in feces. A miracidium hatches from the egg in fresh water and penetrates a certain species of snail. The parasite multiplies in the snail, and the released cercariae encyst as metacercariae in crabs and crayfish. When humans eat these second-intermediate hosts raw or improperly cooked, the larvae migrate through the gut wall, into the peritoneal cavity, through the diaphragm, and into the lung tissue.

There are also a number of intestinal flukes of humans, such as *Fasciolopsis buski*, the giant intestinal fluke. It is only known to occur in certain parts of Asia, where pigs are the usual reservoir hosts. This large worm resides in the intestine and produces eggs that pass in the feces into water. The miracidia from the eggs enter snails, and the released cercariae encyst as metacercariae on a variety of water plants (eg, water caltrop, water chestnuts, water bamboo, water lettuce). The water plants are eaten, and the metacercariae encyst and grow into adults in the intestine.

Other intestinal flukes, such as *Metagoninus yokogawai* and *Heterophyes heterophyes*, are acquired from eating fish; *Echinostoma* species are acquired from eating fish, clams, snails, tadpoles, and other aquatic animal life. Most of these parasitoses are endemic in Asia, with sporadic reports from elsewhere in the world.

Geographic Distribution and Incidence

Human helminthic infections are found worldwide, with the highest prevalences in tropical countries where sanitation is poor or nonexistent and the population eats food that is raw or insufficiently cooked. Countries in Africa, Asia, the Middle East, and South and Central America are considered the most highly endemic. Warm climates foster helminthic infections. Intestinal roundworms infections are most common in Southeast Asia and Latin America, while trichinosis is more common in areas with a temperate climate and in the northern rather than in the southern hemisphere. Cestode infections are highly prevalent in Latin America, except for *H nana*, which is the most common tapeworm in North America. *Diphylloboth rium latum* infections are more common in temperate climates and are seen in populations living around the Great Lakes in North America and in Scandinavian countries. Other diphyllobothrid species are reported from Japan and South America. Trematode infections abound in Asian countries; they are associated with the habit of eating a variety of foods raw. Some trematode infections are common in Eastern Europe and in sheep-raising countries. Exotic parasitoses such as capillariasis, angiostrongyliasis, anisakiasis, and gnathostomiasis are also associated with eating raw freshwater and marine fish, snails, tadpoles, aquatic vegetation, and other aquatic life in Southeast Asia.

Pathogenesis and Clinical Findings

Helminths have intricate life cycles, and pathology is associated with their migratory pathways and final habitat in the host. Most humans have few worms and are free of disease, but there are occasions when there are massive infections and severe illness develops. It is usually the zoonotic parasites that cause serious disease. Most worms are commensals, but they can cause disease by (*a*) competing for essential nutrients, (*b*) obstructing, blocking, or perforating the intestinal tract or biliary tree, (*c*) sucking blood, (*d*) inducing inflammation and malabsorptive changes in the gut, and (*e*) inducing hypersensitivity reactions, usually caused by migrating larvae that secrete and excrete antigens that induce antibodies and cellular immune responses. In reinfection, host antibodies and memory cells respond and may affect the development of new infections.[557] Eosinophilia and pneumonitis are common, especially in helminthic infections with migrating larvae. Symptoms include abdominal pain and diarrhea, as well as malabsorption, iron deficiency anemia, and protein-losing enteropathy.

Nematodes

Intestinal infections involving *Ascaris lumbricoides* may cause allergic manifestations, gut obstruction, intussusception, blockage of bile ducts and cholangitis, perforation of the gut, and erratic ascariasis (worms passing out the nose, mouth, anus, or umbilicus).

Trichinella trichuria worms, especially in heavy infections, may affect intestinal integrity by burying their anterior ends in the mucosa, causing the bowel to appear villose. Sufficient edema develops to cause obstruction, and straining at defecation causes rectal prolapse. Whipworms are also known to suck blood, but the amount of blood loss is small.

Adult hookworms bite into the mucosa of the small intestine and suck blood. Large numbers of worms feeding at the same time may lead to iron deficiency anemia. Hookworm disease potentiates the effects of other intestinal parasitoses and contributes to malnutrition. There may be minor gut lesions with hemorrhage. The blood loss, depending on the species, is estimated to be 0.03 to 0.3 µL per day per worm. Larvae migrating through the lungs may cause pneumonitis. Larvae penetrating the skin may permit secondary bacterial infection, and hookworm larvae that are parasites of other animals, such as dog hookworms, may cause cutaneous larva migrans in humans (Figure 37-5).

Adult female *S stercoralis* worms buried in the mucosa of the small intestine damage the absorptive surface, causing chronic enteritis and sprue-like enteropathy, malabsorption, weight loss, and diarrhea. Hypersensitivity develops in some persons, and larvae may cause urticarial eruptions, larva currens, pneumonitis, and eosinophilia. Autoinfection in immunocompromised persons often leads to hyperinfections, disseminated strongyloidiasis, and death. In these individuals, the parasites may be present in undetectable levels for years, but when the host becomes immunosuppressed, the parasite multiplies rapidly. In many cases the sputum may contain rhabditiform larvae, indicating adult females in the lungs. The larvae spread to the liver, heart, adrenals, kidneys, and central nervous system (CNS). Persons with human t-cell lymphotrophic virus type I (HTLV-I) are highly susceptible to strongyloidiasis.

When muscle from an animal infected with *Trichinella spiralis* is eaten, the larvae enter the intestinal mucosa and cause a transitory enteritis and

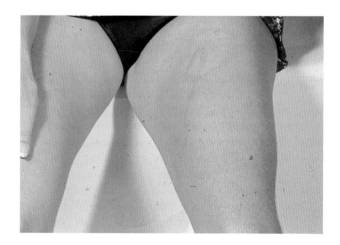

Fig. 37-5. This is an example of creeping eruption. Note the tract made by a migrating larva of dog hookworm on the thigh of family member of an American service member. She was sun bathing on a beach in Taiwan.
Photograph: Courtesy of Dr. John H Cross, Uniformed Services University of the Health Sciences.

malabsorption. Adults in the intestine reproduce, and the larvae migrate throughout the body to striated muscle. Once in the muscle, the larvae enter a cell, eventually die, and become calcified. Typhoidal-like symptoms occur early in the infections, and when the larvae are migrating, eosinophilia, muscle soreness and pain, and periorbital edema result. Cell destruction may cause acute inflammatory changes and an interstitial myocarditis. Trapped larvae in the lungs are known to precipitate edema, focal hemorrhage, and eosinophilia.

Gnathostoma larvae migrate to various parts of the human body. Larvae in subcutaneous tissues may cause transient, warm, erythematous swelling or migrate through the tissues, producing serpingenous tracts. The wandering larvae may also enter the eye and CNS, causing death. Eosinophilic neuritis, meningitis, and encephalitis may develop. In the eye, the infection may result in uveitis, hemorrhage, retinal detachment, and blindness.

Abdominal pain, diarrhea, and borborygmy are characteristic of infections with *Capillaria philippinensis*. Intestinal capillariasis as a result of autoinfection and hyperinfection causes malabsorption, protein-losing enteropathy, electrolyte imbalance, weight loss, wasting, and death. Thousands of *C philippinensis* organisms in all stages are present in the small intestine.[558] The parasite does not become disseminated but remains in the small intestine. The electrolyte imbalance and other physiological changes are responsible for pathological damage in other organs.

Anisakid nematode larvae, upon entering the human gastrointestinal tract, attempt to penetrate the mucosa and cause an eosinophilic granuloma. In addition, protease secretions from the worms can cause tunnels in the gastric mucosa. The larval worms are also known to enter the peritoneal cavity and other organs. Symptoms of an acute abdomen are produced by anisakid infections. In some species, the larvae remain in the throat and cause a condition termed "tickle throat."

Angiostrongylus cantonensis larvae in humans reach the CNS and cause an eosinophilic meningitis or eosinophilic meningoencephalitis. Dead worms rather than living ones are thought to cause disease. Eosinophilic pleocytosis is common. The larvae may also enter eyes and cause blindness. *Angiostrongylus costaricensis* larvae are responsible for abdominal angiostrongyliasis. The larvae enter the mesenteric blood vessels, causing a granulomatous inflammation in the intestinal wall and obstruction.

Dracunculus larvae migrate throughout the tissue, and in approximately 1 year adult females provoke the formation of a vesicle in the skin. Allergic manifestations result from toxic secretions from the worm and a painful, burning sensation occurs. When an infected area is immersed in water, the vesicle breaks and larvae emerge from the uterus of the female worm and escape into the water. Secondary bacterial infections can also occur.

Cestodes

Cestodes that inhabit the intestinal tract usually cause little pathology. Taenid scolices may cause some inflammation at sites of attachment in the mucosa, but the parasites have little other effect except competing with the host for food. *Diphyllobothrium latum*, on the other hand, competes with the host for vitamin B_{12}, which may result in megaloblastic anemia. Spargana of diphyllobothrids that infect a variety of mammals, especially of dogs and cats (*Spirometra* species), may invade tissues of humans who ingest copepods, eat infected intermediate hosts, or use animal poultices. The spargana migrate, causing larval migrans and disease to the invaded organs. Spargana have been found in transient erythematous swellings in many parts of the body and in eyes of Asians who used incised frog abdomens as a poultice. Infections caused by *Taenia saginata*, *H nana*, or *H diminuta* usually cause little pathology.

Cysticercosis occurs in humans who ingested eggs of *T solium*. The egg hatches in the intestine and the hexacanth embryo migrates to tissues and develops into a cysticercus. Brain, heart, muscle, and skin are preferred locations. Palpable nodules can be found in the skin, and in such cases there is usually CNS involvement. Cysticercosis involving the CNS will provoke symptoms of epilepsy. The cysticercus may degenerate, causing granulomas, calcification, and neurologic symptoms in the CNS.

Trematodes

Trematode infections are acquired with the ingestion of plant or animal life harboring the infective stage (metacercaria) of the parasite. There is usually little pathology associated with infections, except when a large number of worms are involved.

Opisthochid species, such as *O viverrini*, *O felineus*, and *Clonorchis sinensis*, are acquired by eating raw freshwater fish. After being released from the fish muscle following digestion, the larvae migrate up the bile duct and may cause jaundice, epigastric pain, diarrhea, and eosinophilia. Long-term infection causes chronic cholanigitis, liver damage, and gallstones. In endemic areas, the parasitosis is considered carcinogenic and is responsible for a high frequency of cholangiocarcinoma. Increased endogenous production of *N*-nitrosodimethylamine and *N*-nitrosodiisopropanolamine or hepatic activation of dietary carcinogens, plus chronic hyperplasia of the bile duct epithelium, may enhance susceptibility to cancer.[559]

There are several trematodes that inhabit the hepatobiliary system. The sheep liver fluke (*Fasciola hepatica*) damages the liver parenchyma while migrating through liver tissue to the bile ducts and causing hepatomegaly, necrosis, and hemorrhage along the migratory tracts. Adult worms in the bile ducts cause dilatation, inflammation, thickening of the walls, and obstruction. Extensive fibrotic changes in the bile ducts seem to be mostly caused by the large amount of proline produced by the adult worms.[560]

The normal habitat of the Asian lung fluke, *Paragonimus westermani,* is the lung, where cystic and inflammatory lesions develop. Lung infections are often misdiagnosed as tuberculosis because of hemoptysis and other pulmonary symptoms (eg, cough, bronchiectasis). Other organs, such as the brain and abdominal cavity, are occasionally invaded by the parasite. *Paragonimus* infections may cause symptoms of fever, cough, dyspnea, chest pain, and hemoptysis. Cerebral paragonimiasis simulates brain tumors, Jacksonian-like seizures, epilepsy, or meningitis.

Intestinal flukes such as *Fasciolopsis buski* are large and may cause intestinal obstruction and toxemia resulting in fascial paralysis and periorbital edema. Death is rare but does occur. Heterophyids, such as *Metagonimus* species and *Heterophyes* species, are small flukes that are also relatively short-lived. They live attached to the wall of the small intestine and cause disease by releasing tiny eggs that are picked up by the lymphatics and are carried to ectopic locations such as the brain, spinal cord, and heart. Large numbers of adults may cause diarrhea, nausea, and vague abdominal complaints. There are many other species of tiny flukes that inhabit the intestines of those who eat raw or undercooked vegetables, fish, and meat, particularly in Asia; these usually cause little disease, however. Echinostome infections are common throughout Asia, but they are short lasting and cause little disease.

Diagnostic Approaches

Most intestinal parasitic helminthiasis can be diagnosed under field conditions provided that standard field laboratory conditions, equipment, and supplies (eg, microscope, slides, cover glasses,

laboratory reagents) are available. Tissue helminthic infections diagnosed by biopsy or serologic methods require more sophisticated conditions, however. Direct and concentration methods can also be used if the equipment and supplies are available. Rapid dipstick enzyme-linked immunosorbent assay tests are under development that will have field applicability.

Intestinal parasitic infection may be diagnosed by examining the feces for eggs, larvae, or adult stages of the parasites. New techniques for detecting antigens and DNA by polymerase chain reaction may be used in the future. The definitive diagnosis, however, is by detecting the parasite or its products. Manuals on the laboratory diagnosis of parasitic diseases are available.[561,562] The parasitologic diagnosis is made by gross examination of the fecal specimen for large worms or the microscopic examination for eggs, larvae, and adults. Since some parasites produce eggs cyclically, eggs may not be present all the time. Therefore, multiple stools (seven stools over 10 days) should be examined if parasites are suspected. A small sample of stool may be placed onto a slide, a drop of saline or iodine solution added, and the mixture covered with a cover-glass and examined under a microscope. Stools can also be examined after concentration by sedimentation, formalin-ethyl-acetate, or zinc sulfate flotations. Microscopic examination is satisfactory for ascariasis, hookworm infections, trichuriasis, strongyloidiasis, intestinal capillariasis, and cestode and trematode infections. Culture methods such as the Harada-Mori filter paper-tube technique may be used to recover larvae of hookworm and *S stercoralis*. Placing stool into agar and observing larval tracts may also be used to isolate larvae of *S stercoralis*. Biopsied tissue can be examined histologically or pressed between two microscope slides and examined microscopically for evidence of trichinosis, cysticercosis, or sparganosis. Diagnosis of other tissue parasitoses can be presumptive, based on symptoms, or by serologic methods for angio-strongyliasis, gnathostomiasis, trichinosis, cysticercosis, sparganosis, disseminated strongyloidiasis, paragonimiasis, and liver fluke infections.

Recommendations for Therapy and Control

Therapy

Helminthic infections are commonly asymptomatic and simply require specific anthelmintic treatments. Some infections require antidiarrheal drugs and fluid replacement (eg, intestinal capillariasis), and some specific infections require symptomatic treatment with immunosuppressants (eg, steroids for trichinosis). Hookworm diseases may require blood transfusions and ferrous sulfate followed by an anthelmintic. Antipyretics are recommended where fever is encountered (eg, paragonimiasis) and analgesics when pain is involved (eg, dracunculiasis). Vitamin B$_{12}$ and folic acid may be given after the expulsion of *Diphyllobothrium latum.*

A number of anthelmintics are available to treat intestinal nematode infections.[563] Mebendazole (100 mg twice a day for 3 days or 500 mg once) or albendazole (400 mg once) are effective against ascariasis, trichuriasis, and hookworm; pyrantel pamoate (11 mg/kg once) is effective against ascariasis and hookworm. Thiabendazole (50 mg/kg per day in divided doses for 2 days), ivermectin (an investigational drug in the United States, 200 µg/kg per day for 1 to 2 days) or albendazole (200 mg twice a day for 3 days) are effective against strongyloidiasis. Gnathostome infections can be treated surgically or by the use of albendazole (400 mg once or twice daily for 21 days).[564] Mebendazole (200 mg twice a day for 20 days) or albendazole (200 mg twice a day for 10 days) is recommended for intestinal capillariasis. Anisakid nematodes are removed surgically or by endoscopy. Angiostrongyliasis has been treated in children with mebendazole (100 mg twice a day for 5 days) or thiabendazole (75 mg/kg per day in 3 doses for 3 days). Some authorities, however, do not recommend using anthelmintics for angiostrongyliasis because the disease is self-limiting and killing massive numbers of worms at one time may cause more pathology than if worms die off gradually. Dracunculiasis may be treated with metronidazole (250 mg three times a day for 10 days).

Most cases of trematodiasis respond to praziquantel (60-75 mg/kg per day in 3 doses for 1 to 2 days). The only drug presently available that is effective against fascioliasis, however, is triclabendazole (10 mg once).[560] Bithionol, once used for the treatment of fascioliasis, is no longer available. Praziquantel (5-10 mg/kg once) may be used to treat intestinal pork and beef tapeworms, as well as the fish tapeworm (ie, *Diphyllobothrium latum*). Cysticercosis has been known to respond to praziquantel (50 mg/kg per day in 3 doses for 15 days) or albendazole (400 mg twice a day for 8 to 30 days). Sparganosis is usually treated surgically or with praziquantel (60-75 mg/kg for 2 days).

Control

Helminthic infection prevalences are highest in areas where indiscriminate defecation and poor sanitation practices persist. When populations dispose of feces under sanitary conditions, most intestinal parasitic infections decrease and eventually disappear. South Korea, once highly endemic for intestinal helminthiasis, has nearly eradicated the worms through mass treatments, sanitary disposal of feces, and education.[565] Investigations into environmental sources of infection should be conducted. Military personnel under field conditions in endemic countries should avoid areas where human and animal feces have contaminated the soil. Sanitary latrines should be constructed for the military and even civilians where toilet facilities are absent. Fresh vegetables and fruits should be avoided if they have been fertilized with human feces (night soil) unless the produce has been cooked thoroughly and the fruits have been washed with safe water and peeled. Fecally contaminated water may contain helminth eggs and should not be consumed unless boiled or filtered; chemical purification has little effect on helminth eggs. Some species of hookworm larvae may be acquired in water, and copepods in water may be infected with *Dracunculus* or tapeworm larvae. Those living next to bodies of water should not use the water as latrines. Fresh sewage should not be dumped into the water unless treated first to destroy parasites and other pathogens. Parasites and vectors can be eliminated from water by boiling or passing water through fine-mesh filters, especially to remove copepods. Wearing shoes will protect the feet from skin-penetrating hookworm and *S stercoralis* larvae.

An abundance of helminthic infections are acquired from food. These diseases can be controlled by thoroughly cooking all meats. Pork should always be cooked well to prevent trichinosis; pork, beef, and fish should be cooked completely to prevent tapeworm infections. Dry cereals often contain beetles that serve as intermediate hosts for hymenolepid tapeworm infections; the cereal should not be eaten uncooked, if at all. There are many exotic parasitoses acquired from wild animals, which should never be eaten raw, especially fish, snails, other aquatic animal life, and carnivores. Domestic and wild animal pets should be examined and periodically treated for helminthic infections. Pet feces, especially from dogs, cats, and even raccoons and skunks, should be buried or burned and not permitted to lie on the ground. Eggs from *Toxocara* species (from dogs and cats) and *Baylisascaris procyonis* (from raccoons), when eaten by humans, can cause visceral larva migrans. Aquatic plants and nuts should also be eaten well cooked. Irradiation has been shown to be an excellent tool that sterilizes infected foods, but obtaining public support for the use of this potential disease prevention technique has been a problem.[566] At present this technology is not applicable to the field.

Indigenous populations and deployed military personnel should be educated to the dangers of helminthic parasites endemic to the area. Paragonimiasis and fasciolopsiasis have been nearly eradicated from Taiwan because children were taught in school not to eat crabs and water plants raw.[567] When children are educated about parasitic diseases in school, they often return home and tell their parents, who in turn become aware of the problems. Using television, radio, and other public relations avenues is a valuable means to educate populations.

[John H. Cross]

SCHISTOSOMIASIS

Introduction and Military Relevance

Schistosomiasis (also known as bilharziasis, snail fever, and Katayama fever) is a parasitic disease in tropical and semitropical regions. It requires amphibious or freshwater snails as intermediate hosts for development of the larval forms that can infect humans. It is a disease complex, with multiple ecological agents, that has mission-aborting potential. A basic understanding of its epidemiology, pathogenesis, clinical presentation, diagnosis, treatment, prevention, and control is crucial to military medicine.

Schistosomiasis has been implicated as a factor in military operations since biblical times.[568] In World War II, the US Army hospitalized 2,088 patients with schistosomiasis. The average number of days lost per admission was 159, resulting in 124,192 days lost to commanders.[569] During the reinvasion of Leyte alone, 1,500 cases were reported in US troops.[570]

In late 1949, a massive outbreak of acute schistosomiasis in soldiers from the People's Republic of China, who were training for an amphibious invasion of Taiwan in early 1950, resulted in an estimated 30,000 to 50,000 medical casualties. The impact of those casualties delayed the planned invasion of Taiwan for 6 critical months,[571] long enough for the US 7th Fleet to establish a Taiwan Defense Command and provide routine naval patrols through the Strait of Formosa.

The impact of schistosomiasis on a military operation comes from its acute syndrome, which can occur as early as 2 to 4 weeks after exposure. If left untreated, infected service members can be noneffective for weeks to months, depending on the species of schistosome involved and the intensity of the infection.

Description of the Pathogen

Microbiology

Schistosomes are parasitic flatworms found in the blood vessels of vertebrates. They are unique among the trematodes for having separate sexes. More than 15 species have been reported in humans; however, the major agents of human infections are *Schistosoma mansoni*, *S haematobium*, and *S japonicum*.[572] Three other species (*S intercalatum*, *S mekongi*, and *S malayensis*) are responsible for human disease in geographically limited areas of Africa and Asia.[573] Other schistosomes

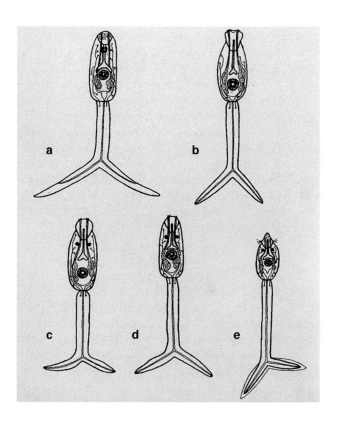

Fig. 37-6. Some fork-tailed (furcocercous) cercariae found in freshwater and amphibious mollusks: (**a**) strigeid cercaria, (**b**) human-infecting schistosome cercaria, (**c**) cercaria of *Schistosomatium douthitti*, (**d**) cercaria of a bird schistosome, and (**e**) cercaria of spirorchid trematode from turtles.

Reprinted with permission from: World Health Organization. *Snail Control in the Prevention of Bilharziasis.* Geneva: WHO; 1965: 193.

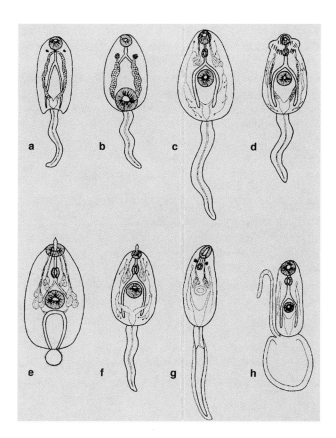

Fig. 37-7. Common types of cercariae found in freshwater and amphibious mollusks that should be distinguished from fucocercous cercariae: (**a**) gymnophallid, (**b**) monstome, (**c**) amphistome, (**d**) echinostome, (**e**) pleurolophocercous, (**f**) xiphidiocercaria, (**g**) microcercous, and (**h**) gasterotome.
Reprinted with permission from: World Health Organization. *Snail Control in the Prevention of Bilharziasis.* Geneva: WHO; 1965: 193.

found in humans are zoophilic, and humans are incidental hosts. *Human Schistosomiasis,*[574] published in 1993, is the most recent comprehensive source of information on this disease complex.

The cercariae, or larval forms, of the schistosomes that infect humans have a fork-tail, a characteristic that distinguishes them from most cercariae (Figure 37-6). In addition, schistosome cercariae lack other common surface features of many other types of cercariae (Figure 37-7), such as a stylet (see Figure 37-7e,f) or rings of spines (see Figure 37-7d) in the oral sucker region. Schistosome cercariae can be distinguished from other fork-tail cercariae by two characteristics: a lack of eye spots in the anterior half of the body and a ratio of the length of the forks of the tail to the total tail length of approximately 1:2.[575]

Life Cycle

Schistosomiasis is acquired from free-swimming cercariae, which are released from snails (Figure 37-8). The cercariae seek out and penetrate human skin, metamorphose to the schistosomula stage, and penetrate into veins; they are then carried passively to the lungs. In the lungs, they elongate into slender organisms that can negotiate the capillaries leading to the systemic circulatory system. Larval schistosomes must enter the mesenteric arteries, their capillaries, and then the hepatic portal veins to reach the liver, where they mature into adults and mate. The male then transports the female to a branch of the superior mesenteric veins of the intestine or to the veins associated with the urinary bladder, where egg laying commences. Pairs of schistosomes produce hundreds to thousands of eggs per day, depending on the species. Adults of *S mansoni, S japonicum, S mekongi,* and *S intercalatum* usually migrate to the superior mesenteric veins. *S haematobium* adults usually migrate into the vascu-

SCHISTOSOMIASIS

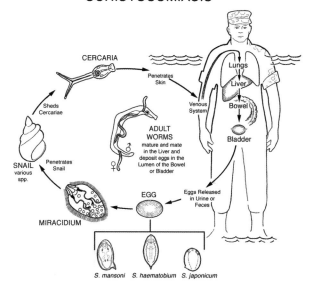

Fig. 37-8. Adult worms mature and mate in the liver. Males carry females to veins and capillaries of the bowel or bladder where eggs are deposited. Less than 50% of eggs deposited in capillaries reach the lumen of the intestine or bladder and are viable when passed in feces. Most are encapsulated by the host reactions, die, and contribute to pathology associated with chronic disease in either liver and intestine or urinary systems.
Drawing by Annabelle Wright, Walter Reed Army Institute of Research; research by Amelia Pousson.

lature surrounding the urinary bladder. In either location, eggs are released in small venules. Some eggs escape into the lumen of the intestine or urinary bladder and are voided in feces or urine. Those that do not escape (usually more than 50%) are trapped in tissues and become the focus of the host's immunological responses; this accounts for much of the pathology associated with chronic schistosomiasis.

The first free-living stage, the miracidium, hatches from the egg in a freshwater environment, then seeks out and penetrates a snail. In the snail, it undergoes a series of asexual (sporocyst) generations. Each miracidium that establishes a patent infection in a snail produces thousands of cercariae. The cercariae are the second free-living stage; more importantly, they are the infective stage for humans.

Epidemiology

Transmission

Transmission requires three factors: freshwater, infected snails, and susceptible mammalian hosts. The most limiting of these factors is the distribution of the snail that serves as the intermediate host. *S haematobium* is principally transmitted through aquatic *Bulinus* species (Figure 37-9), *S mansoni* through aquatic *Biomphalaria* species (Figure 37-10), and *S japonicum* through amphibious *Oncomelania* species (Figure 37-11). *Neotricula aperta* is the intermediate host of *S mekongi*, *S malayensis* is transmitted through *Robertsiella* species,[576] and *S intercalatum* is transmitted through *Bulinus* species.[573] In Asia, where schistosomiasis is a true zoonosis, infections in other mammalian hosts and the vector snails maintain significant transmission potential even in the absence of human populations. Sources of malacological expertise are identified in *Snail Hosts of Schistosomiasis and Other Snail-transmitted Diseases in Tropical America: A Manual*[577] and *Medical and Economic Malacology*.[575]

All military personnel who enter freshwater habitats in an endemic area are at risk of contracting schistosomiasis. The transmission potential of an area is directly related to the density of the molluscan host population and the infection rate in that population. In endemic areas, a 2% infection rate in the molluscan host population can maintain a more than 50% infection rate in the indigenous human population. The transmission potential of an area can be assessed by sampling suspected molluscan hosts and examining them for the cercarial stage using either photo-stimulation or crushing techniques.[575,577] When handling snails, forceps and rubber or latex gloves should be used, and 70% alcohol should be available

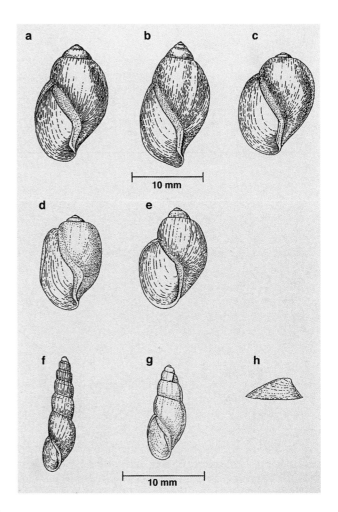

Fig. 37-9. Illustrations of shells of the intermediate hosts of *Schistosoma*: (***a***) *Bulinus (Physopsis) africanus* from Kenya, (***b***) *B (Phys) nasutus* from Tanganyika, (***c***) *B (Phys) globosus* from Angola, (***d***) *B (Phys) abyssinicus* from Somalia, (***e***) *B (Bulinus) truncatus* from Egypt, (***f***) *B (B) forskalii* from Sudan, (***g***) *B (B) senegalensis* from Gambia, and (***h***) *Ferrissia tenuis* from India.
Reprinted with permission from: World Health Organization. *Snail Control in the Prevention of Bilharziasis.* Geneva: WHO; 1965: 19.

to immediately disinfect any accidentally exposed skin.

Outbreaks of "swimmer's itch" or "clam digger's itch" are due to avian or mammalian schistosomes that are transmitted through local freshwater, amphibious, or estuarine snails. These zoophilic schistosomes are able to penetrate human skin but are unable to develop to maturity. Transmission is usually seasonal along the shores of freshwater lakes and estuarine waterways in temperate climates with peaks in the spring or early summer, but in tropical regions transmission can occur throughout the year. Sources of expertise identified in references 8 and

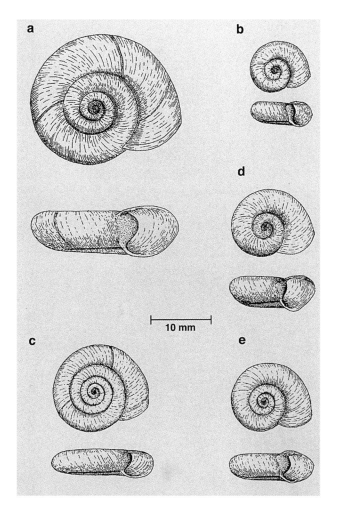

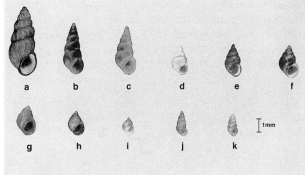

Fig. 37-11. Shells of snail hosts of oriental schistosomes: (**a**) *Oncomelania hupensis* from China, (**b**) *O nosophora* from Japan, (**c**) *O fortrwsana* from Taiwan, (**d***) *O hupensis chiui* from Taiwan, (**e**) *O quadrasi* from the Philippines, (**f**) *O lindoensis* from Indonesia, (**g**) *Neotricula aperta* alpha race from Thailand, (**h**) *N aperta* beta race from Thailand, (**i**) *N aperta* gamma race from Thailand, (**j**) *Tricula bollingi* from Thailand, and (**k**) *Robertsiella kaporensis* from Malaysia.

Reprinted with permission from: Sobhon P, Upatham ES. *Snail Hosts, Life Cycle, and Tegumental Structure of Oriental Schistosomes.* Geneva: United Nations Development Programme/World Bank/World Health Organization, Special Programme for Research and Training in Tropical Diseases; 1990: 20.

Fig. 37-10. Illustrations of shells of the intermediate hosts of *Schistosoma mansoni*: (**a**) *Biomphalaria glabratus* from Brazil, (**b**) *B straminea* from Brazil, (**c**) *B sudanica* from Uganda, (**d**) *B pfeifferi* from Rhodesia (now Zimbabwe), and (**e**) *B alexandria* from Egypt.

Reprinted with permission from: World Health Organization. *Snail Control in the Prevention of Bilharziasis.* Geneva: WHO; 1965: 18.

10 will be helpful in determining the identity of both animal schistosomes and their molluscan hosts.

Geographic Distribution

Schistosomiasis is endemic in 74 countries and territories[573] (Figures 37-12 and 37-13). *S haematobium* is found in 54 countries in Africa, the islands off the west coast of Africa, and the eastern Mediterranean region; *S mansoni* occurs in 52 countries and territories in South America, the Caribbean islands, Africa, Madagascar, and the eastern Mediterranean region; *S intercalatum* is present in at least five coun-

tries in western and central Africa (Cameroon, Equatorial Guinea, Gabon, Sao Tome and Principe, and Zaire); and *S japonicum* has been reported from Japan, Taiwan, China, the Philippines, Indonesia, and Thailand. (However, *S japonicum* is no longer considered endemic in Japan, the strain of *S japonicum* in Taiwan is zoophilic,[578] and the strain originally reported from peninsular Thailand[579] is now considered to be *S mekongi*.[576]) *S mekongi* has been reported from the Mekong River delta in Cambodia, Laos, and Thailand, and the distribution of *S malayensis* is limited to peninsular Malaysia.[573]

Prevalence

The most comprehensive summary of distribution and prevalence of schistosomiasis, based on data collected in the mid-1980s, is found in the *Atlas of the Global Distribution of Schistosomiasis*.[572] The World Health Organization[573] estimates that 600 million persons are exposed and 200 million persons are infected with schistosomiasis, but rates of infection vary considerably in any endemic area. Most cases have few symptoms, while a small, heavily infected cohort demonstrates severe disease. Where programs emphasizing morbidity control have been

Fig. 37-12. Global distribution of schistsosomiasis caused by *Schistosoma haematobium, S japonicum*, and *S mekongi*. Reprinted with permission from: World Health Organization Expert Committee. *The Control of Schistosomiasis.* Geneva: WHO; 1993: 16. WHO Technical Report Series 830.

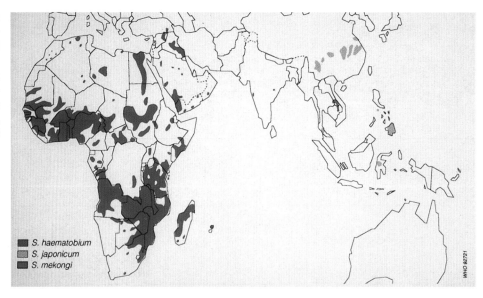

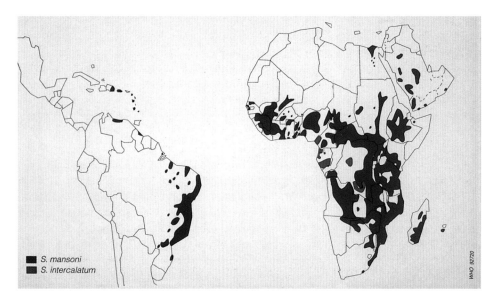

Fig. 37-13. Global distribution of schistosomiasis caused by *Schistosoma mansoni* and *S intercalatum*. Reprinted with permission from: World Health Organization Expert Committee. *The Control of Schistosomiasis*: Geneva: WHO; 1993: 17. WHO Technical Report Series 830.

initiated and sustained, prevalence rates and, more importantly, the morbidity associated with worm burdens have been greatly reduced.

Pathogenesis and Clinical Findings

Cercarial Dermatitis

The initial exposure to cercariae of a schistosome that infects humans produces a transient dermatitis, particularly in nonindigenous populations, that is difficult to distinguish from other forms of dermatitis. However, a recent history of water contact, itching between 12 and 24 hours after exposure, and distribution of papular or blistering lesions only on parts of the body that were immersed in water should suggest schistosome dermatitis in an endemic region.[580,581] Dermatitis (Figure 37-14) is more commonly seen after exposure to *S haematobium* and *S mansoni* than after exposure to *S japonicum*.[582]

The dermal reactions to zoophilic species of schistosomes are similar to those of the anthropophilic species but are usually more severe and are especially severe in individuals sensitized by previous exposures. Itching at the site of entry is common and is followed by a short-lived macular rash. Within 24 hours, pruritic, urticarial, or papular eruptions appear that can last a week or longer.[583,584]

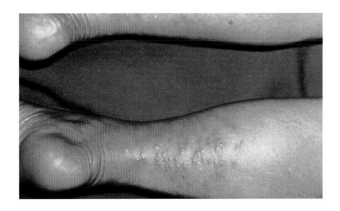

Fig. 37-14. Cercarial dermatitis. Note the typical distribution of lesions around the ankle, which was exposed to schistosome cercariae.
Photograph: Courtesy of Colonel Llewellyn J. Legters, Medical Corps, US Army (ret).

Acute Disease

Acute schistosomiasis is the result initially of immune responses to antigens of developing worms and subsequently of the formation of immune complexes to eggs released by sexually mature females.[581,585] The syndrome is usually reported after an initial heavy infection with any of the major anthropophilic species.[582] Although symptoms are similar regardless of the species of schistosome infecting humans, the intensity of the syndrome varies in proportion to the number of pairs of worms present and to the number of eggs produced. Females of *S japonicum* produce one egg per minute, of *S mansoni* one egg every 5 minutes, and of *S haematobium* one egg every 10 minutes.[586] Thus, it is not surprising that the acute syndrome is most severe in cases of *S japonicum* infection and least severe in cases of *S haematobium* infection.

Central nervous system manifestations are frequently reported in acute cases caused by *S japonicum*; they also occur, however, in acute cases caused by *S haematobium* and *S mansoni*. Most cases of acute cerebral schistosomiasis are caused by *S japonicum*, and most cases of schistosomal transverse myelitis are caused by *S mansoni*.[578,587,588] There were two case reports in 1992 of acute schistosomiasis caused by *S haematobium* involving the central nervous system in two Peace Corps volunteers: a 30-year-old exposed while swimming in Lake Malawi approximately 3 months before evaluation at a US medical center was diagnosed with acute cerebral schistosomiasis and a 26-year-old who had snorkeled in Lake Malawi a month before onset of symptoms was diagnosed with acute (transverse) myelitis.[589]

Acute schistosomiasis resembles serum sickness or an allergic syndrome, which is initially mediated by immediate and delayed-type hypersenstivity to cercarial and larval antigens. There is an abrupt onset of fever (usually late in the evening or at night), chills, abdominal pain followed by coughing, sweating, diarrhea, vomiting, headache, urticaria, hepatosplenomegaly, lymphadenopathy, and often marked elevations of IgE and IgG levels and eosinophil counts.[578,582,590,591] The more severe manifestations occur when egg production starts and large numbers of schistosome eggs are released.[581] This usually occurs 4 to 6 weeks after exposure in *S haematobium* infections,[590] 2 to 12 weeks after exposure in *S japonicum* infections,[578] and 3 to 9 weeks after exposure in *S mansoni* infections.[586] Gastrointestinal disturbances and recurrent diarrhea with mucoid and bloody stools are common features in the late stage of acute disease in its intestinal forms,[578,591] while hematuria is a common feature in the late stage of acute urinary schistosomiasis.[582,590]

In Chinese hospitals, before praziquantel (the current treatment of choice) was available, the mortality related to acute schistosomiasis varied from 2% to 20%. In the Orient, acute schistosomiasis (Katayama fever) has been observed in chronically infected persons and persons with documented cures after they have been exposed to many cercariae in a brief period.[578] In Egypt, acute schistosomiasis caused by *S haematobium* or *S mansoni* is not commonly diagnosed in rural populations of endemic areas, but it is frequently diagnosed in urban children visiting relatives in rural areas for the first time.[590,591] In contrast, acute oriental schistosomiasis is frequently observed in rural inhabitants after their first exposure, as well as in urban residents visiting relatives in rural areas.[578]

Chronic Disease

Chronic schistosomiasis develops gradually as a result of immunological responses to schistosome eggs deposited in tissues. The degree of disease is directly related to the number of eggs deposited in host tissue and the host reaction to them. In turn, egg deposition is a function of the number of worm pairs and duration of an infection.[581,583] Symptoms in heavily infected individuals, such as bleeding, ulceration, or polyposis, are due to the initial granulomatous response. In intestinal schistosomiasis (caused by *S japonicum* and *S mansoni*), ulceration and polyp formation occur in the bowel; in urinary schistosomiasis (*S haematobium*), those symptoms occur in the mucosa of the ureter and bladder.[581] In endemic regions, bleeding, ulceration, and polyposis are more common in teenagers than adults. The classical symptoms of intestinal schistosomiasis (ie, liver "pipestem" fibrosis and portal hypertension) and urinary schistosomiasis (ie, hydronephrosis, hydroureter, and bladder calcification) develop in adults who have been repeatedly infected over a long time. Pulmonary symptoms occur in all forms but are most common in cases caused by *S haematobium*. Central nervous system involvement is most common in *S japonicum* infections and least common in *S haematobium* infections.[592–594] Since eggs of *S japonicum* are relatively small and round and have a minute spine (Figure 37-15c), their size and shape may be responsible for their more frequent deposition in ectopic locations such as the central nervous system. Chronic disease sequelae can be prevented by prompt treatment of suspected and confirmed cases.

Diagnostic Approaches

Signs and symptoms of cercarial dermatitis and acute schistosomiasis must be considered in a differential diagnosis under field conditions, as it takes weeks for a patent infection to be diagnosed by stool, urine, or serological methods. History of freshwater contact, dermatitis on regions of the body that were submersed, and itching within the past few days should suggest schistosomiasis. In the following weeks, malaise, fever, urticaria, and vague intestinal complaints associated with transient toxic and allergic manifestations are common in light-to-moderate exposures. If an individual is initially exposed to many cercariae, there is an abrupt onset of fever with chills, abdominal pain, diarrhea, nausea, vomiting, cough, headache, urticaria, hepatosplenomegaly, frequently high eosinophilia counts (> 50), and elevated IgG and IgE levels. These acute symptoms, which can last for several days or weeks, are most common upon exposure to *S japonicum* cercariae and least common upon exposure to *S haematobium* cercariae.[593]

Definitive diagnosis has depended on the demonstration of eggs either in stool or urine specimens or in intestinal or bladder biopsy specimens from suspected cases.[595] Stool and urine examinations can be made with minimum laboratory support. Eggs of schistosomes are relatively large, are distinct in shape, and contain a fully developed embryo (miracidum) (Figure 37-15). Eggs of *S haematobium* and *S intercalatum* possess a distinct terminal spine

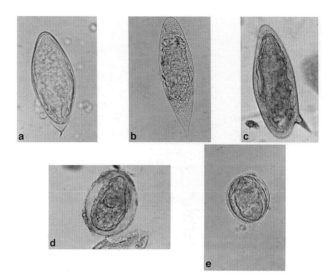

Fig. 37-15. Eggs of schistosomes commonly infecting humans are relatively large and nonoperculate with a transparent shell and either a lateral or terminal spine. (**a**) *S haematobium* (110-70 x 40-70 µ) and (**b**) *S intercalatum* (140-240 x 40-70 µ) eggs possess a distinct terminal spine. Eggs of *S intercalatum* are usually found in feces whereas eggs of *S haematobium* are usually found in urine. (**c**) *Schistosoma mansoni* eggs (115-175 x 45-70 µ) possess a distinct lateral spine and are usually recovered from feces. (**d**) Eggs of *S japonicum* (70-10 x 55-65 µ) and (**e**) *S mekongi* (51-78 x 39-66 µ) are round with a short, dull spines. Note that a short, dull spine is clearly visible on the *S mekongi* egg shell, whereas a short, dull spine on the shell of the *S japonicum* egg could easily be obscured by debris or orientation.
Photomicrographs: Courtesy of Dr. Lawrence R. Ash, Department of Epidemiology, School of Public Health, University of California, Los Angeles.

(Figure 37-15a,b). The latter eggs are usually found in feces, are larger, and frequently have an equatorial bulge. *S mansoni* eggs possess a distinctive lateral spine (Figure 37-15c), whereas those of *S japonicum* and *S mekongi* are round with a short, dull spine (Figure 37-15d,e). Concentration methods and multiple stool or urine examinations are recommended.[595,596] Clinical dipsticks for hematuria are efficient and effective screens for patent infections with *S haematobium* because hematuria is usually indicative of urinary schistosomiasis in areas where individuals are continually exposed.[596] However, hematuria is not a common sign of urinary schistosomiasis in light infections.

Even though current serological assays are unable to distinguish past infection from current ones, they are valuable in establishing a diagnosis of schistosomiasis in US military personnel, because most US forces have not been exposed to anthropophilic schistosomes or even to related helminths. The Centers for Disease Control and Prevention's Division of Parasitic Diseases has developed very sensitive and specific antibody assays for both *S haematobium* and *S mansoni*.[597] Serological assays are particularly useful for the diagnosis of acute schistosomiasis cases, as most cases are symptomatic before eggs can be detected in fecal or urine specimens.[581] Antigen detection assays for *S mansoni* and *S haematobium*, which can be used with either urine or serum samples, are as reliable as the Kato-Katz stool and urine filtration examinations, and antigen levels correlate well with egg counts for quantification of parasitemia.[598] Reagents for circulating cathodic antigen and circulating anodic antigen detection in urine and sera are available through the Laboratory of Parasitology, Medical Faculty, University of Leiden, Netherlands. If a suspected infection cannot be determined by stool or urine examination, sera should be tested for schistosome antigen or antibodies to schistosome antigens or both. If a suspected case demonstrates neurological symptoms in the absence of eggs in fecal or urine specimens, antibody or antigen assays may be the only means of establishing a diagnosis.

Recommendations for Therapy and Control

Therapy

Currently three anhelminthic drugs are used to treat schistosomiasis: praziquantel, oxamniquine, and metrifonate. Praziquantel is the drug of choice for treatment of all acute and patent cases of schistosomiasis.[573,563] Oxamniquine is an alternative treatment for both acute and patent cases of *S mansoni* infection, and metrifonate is an alternative treatment for cases of *S haematobium* infection.[573] All cases of schistosomiasis, whether or not they are symptomatic, and all suspected cases chould be treated to prevent potential pathological sequelae.

Praziquantel is exceptionally well tolerated. Side effects, such as abdominal discomfort, bloody diarrhea, nausea, vomiting, headache, dizziness, and drowsiness, are usually associated with heavy worm burdens. Praziquantel is better tolerated if given with meals, and side effects are fewer if it is given in divided doses. The World Health Organization[573] recommends 40 mk/kg of praziquantel as a single dose for infections with all species of schistosomes. *The Medical Letter*[563] recommends 60 mg/kg of praziquantel, divided in three equal doses over 1 day for *S japonicum* and *S mekongi* infections, and 40 mg/kg in three equal doses over 1 day for *S*

haematobium and *S mansoni* infections. Praziquantel is the only drug now recommended to treat infections with *S japonicum*, *S intercalatum*, and *S mekongi* because these parasites are unresponsive to oxamniquine. All patent cases, whether or not they are symptomatic, and all suspected cases should be treated to prevent potential pathological sequelae of chronic infections.

Effective doses of oxamniquine for *S mansoni* infections range between 15 and 60 mg/kg and should be given over 2 or 3 days.[573] *The Medical Letter*'s generic recommendations for treatment of *S mansoni* infections with oxamniquine are 15 mg/kg once for adults and 20 mg/kg divided into two doses for children; however, in East Africa they recommend that the dose be increased to 30 mg/kg, and in Egypt and South Africa to 30 mg/kg per day for 2 days.[563] Shekhar[599] recommends 40-60 mg/kg of oxamniquine over 2 to 3 days to treat *S mansoni* infections throughout Africa. In north Senegal, where *S mansoni* responds poorly to standard praziquantel therapy (36% cure rate), oxaminquine is highly recommended.[600]

Cercarial Dermatitis. If the dermatitis needs treatment, palliative topical agents such as corticosteroid creams should be used. In more severe cases, oral or parenteral antihistamines can be administered.[582] Usually, however, species of schistosomes that readily infect humans are well adapted to humans, and the dermatitis elicited is mild in comparison to that elicited by cercariae of zoophilic schistosomes.

Acute Disease. The combined use of steroids and praziquantel to treatment of acute schistosomiasis syndrome is based on clinical and experimental evidence that steroids act synergistically with schistosomicides. This combination augments cure and speeds recovery, even though there is an occasional worsening of clinical status and praziquantel is less effective against immature worms.[573,581,583,591,601] Prompt treatment with praziquantel and concurrent use of nonsteroid anti-inflammatory agents is recommended for persons with mild symptoms; corticosteroids should be used only for persons who appear extremely toxic or whose symptoms fail to respond to or worsen with treatment.[583] Farid[591] recommends 75 mg/kg of praziquantel, divided into 3 equal doses over 1 day, for treatment of acute *S mansoni* infections in Egypt.

Exposed Personnel. There are no clinical reports of the efficacy of any Food and Drug Administration–approved schistosomicidal drug against the schistosomal stage or immature schistosomes, but derivatives of artemisinin have been reported to suppress development of immature schistosomes.[602]

Two studies[603,604] in regions of rural China where *S japonicum* is endemic have demonstrated the efficacy of artemether in the reduction of acute schistosomiasis, both in the infection and reinfection rates and in the intensity of infections. In the two field trials, no cases of acute schistosomiasis were seen in groups treated with artemether, whereas in 4% and 9% of the control groups, acute schistosomiasis was diagnosed. While subsequent infection rates in the control groups were 13.6% and 15%, they were 5.5% and 4.2%, respectively, in the artemether groups. Similarly, the intensity of infection, as measured by eggs per gram using the Kato-Katz method, was reduced more than 5-fold in one field trial and 1.5-fold in the other. In neither field trial were adverse side effects observed. These results are encouraging and suggest that artemether, and probably other artemisinin derivatives, may provide a means of safely reducing the number of acute schistosomiasis cases and the rate and intensity of patent infections in persons who cannot avoid exposure.

An experimental study[605] in mice suggested that the efficacy curve of praziquantel is bimodal. Worm reduction rates ranged from 80% to 50% in the first 2 weeks, varied between 0% and 20% in the third and fourth week, and climbed back to 95% to 100% by the sixth week after exposure. Since praziquantel is well tolerated and its known side effects are related to worm burden,[573] its preemptive use should be seriously considered in personnel who have been exposed in order to prevent or lessen the impact of the acute state of this disease.

Prevention and Control

From a military perspective, control is prevention. Cases are a direct consequence of contact with or use of snail-infested freshwater contaminated with feces or urine containing schistosome eggs. The basic preventive options fall into four categories: limiting water contact, treating water, controlling snails, and educating personnel.

Limiting Water Contact

Since the intensity of the acute disease is directly related to the number of egg-depositing female schistosomes present, any protective barrier is better than none at all. Thus, clothing; gloves of rubber, latex, or vinyl; rubber boots; or anything that prevents a cercaria from contacting skin will reduce the chance of transmission.[606] For example, uniform trousers will provide some protection for legs if they are tucked into the top of combat boots with enough slack to form a cuff over the boot top, but the protective effect diminishes as the exposure lengthens.[607] If feasible, skin that contacts suspect water should be vigorously toweled dry as soon as possible, and 70% alcohol should be applied to the skin immediately.

No topical repellent is presently available that provides long-term protection against cercarial penetration. Field trials of 1% niclosamide as a topical antipenetrant demonstrate approximately 20% reduction in reinfections from *S mansoni*[608] but no significant reduction in reinfection rates from *S haematobium*[609] among Egyptian farmers. Pellegrino[606] summarizes numerous studies, conducted in the 1940s and 1950s, demonstrating that many compounds could provide relatively effective protection for limited periods of time. Repellents containing dibutylphthalate and benzylbenoate as principal agents in a turpentine base have been used with success in China.[610] Most oily substances that are hydrophobic offer some degree of protection for short periods, and a limited degree of protection is offered by topical insect repellents.[568,606]

A recent report[611] suggests that DEET, probably one of the most widely used insect repellents in the world, at concentrations of 7.5% or higher was 100% effective in immobilizing and killing cercariae of *S mansoni* in vitro, and cutaneous application of DEET in an isopropanol vehicle or as a commercial insect repellent preparation (Off with 7.5% DEET) was more than 99% effective in preventing entry of *S mansoni* cercariae into mouse tail skin. DEET may not only be a safe prophylactic agent in the control of human schistosomiasis, but it may also be potentially useful in the control of cercarial dermatitis associated with exposure to schistosomes of birds and mammals. A follow-up study[612] reported that DEET incorporated into liposomes (LIPODEET) appears to prolong the activity of DEET for more than 48 hours after a single application. In addition, LIPODEET was found to be minimally absorbed through the skin and loss from washing off was limited, suggesting that LIPODEET may be a safe, long-acting formulation of DEET that is effective in preventing successful penetration of schistosome cercariae.

The time of day can be a factor. Cercarial emergence from the snail is circadian, but the periodicity varies depending on the species involved. Cercariae of *S mansoni*, *S haematobium*, and *S japonicum* are usually shed in the mid to late morning. However, snails infected with *S mansoni* in the Caribbean region or with *S japonicum* in the Philippines and Indonesia usually shed cercariae in the late afternoon or early evening when rodents that are important reservoir hosts of schistosomiasis are active.[613,614] Risk can be minimized by restricting water contact during and for a few hours after this peak transmission period.

Treating Water

Before surface water is used for drinking, bathing, and washing clothes, it must be treated to remove or inactivate cercariae. If available, subsurface water should be used for these purposes. Surface water can be held in tanks that do not contain any infected snails for 24 hours before use,[615] boiled, or heated to either 50°C for 5 minutes or 80°C for 30 seconds to inactivate cercariae.[568] Drinking water treated with iodine is safe. Cercariae are killed within 30 minutes by 1 ppm chlorine residual in a pH range of 7.5 to 8.9, by 0.3 ppm at pH 5, and by 5 ppm at pH 10.[615] Sand grains smaller than 0.35 mm and diatomaceous earth filters remove cercariae.[616] US Army mobile water purification units employing either diatomite filters or a reverse-osmosis system are effective in removing cercariae.[568]

Controlling Snails

Niclosamide (Bayluscide [Bayer AG], Mollutox in the Middle East and North Africa) is the only highly effective synthetic molluscicide. In addition, nicolsamide is toxic to cercariae and will have a rapid and focal impact on transmission when applied.[615] A classic reference for snail control, *Snail Control in the Prevention of Bilharziasis*,[617] has chapters on both chemical and environmental methods of control. A more recent text, *Molluscicides in Schistoso-miasis Control*,[618] is an excellent review of the use of chemicals to control molluscan hosts of schistosomes.

There are a number of environmental and biological measures that can be used to control snail populations. One example comes from Asia: habitats of amphibious oncomelanid snails can simply be buried or flooded to drastically reduce snail populations. In regions where aquatic snails are involved, a well-designed irrigation system allows snail habitats to be dried out, and ditches drained and cleaned on a regular schedule. Although these measures may not be practical in a traditional military operation, they may be very useful in nontraditional military operations, such as humanitarian assistance and peacekeeping missions, in endemic areas.

Educating Personnel

Personnel must be alerted to hazards of freshwater contact (eg, swimming, bathing, washing clothes) before deployment to an endemic area. Any activity or intervention that reduces the frequency or duration of exposure to snail-infested waters will reduce the chance of infections. Military personnel should be taught that the first symptom of an exposure is a dermatitis affecting areas exposed to surface water within 6 to 48 hours of exposure. If exposed, they should seek medical attention.

[W. Patrick Carney]

COCCIDIOIDOMYCOSIS

Introduction and Military Relevance

Coccidioidomycosis was first recognized in 1892 in an Argentinean soldier who died of a disseminated case of this fungal infection. Pivotal to understanding the epidemiology and clinical course of this mycosis is surveillance work using the coccidioidin skin test and serologies done in the US Army air bases of the San Joaquin Valley in California during World War II. Smith[619,620] found that this inhalationally acquired infection from soil caused high morbidity among the military in endemic areas, although the majority of those infected had mild symptoms. Many soldiers were symptomatic, requiring 4 to 6 weeks of hospitalization for respiratory illness. A small percentage of those infected had serious, often fatal, infection, and persons of color were predisposed to having this severe course. Those who had reactive skin tests seemed immune to reinfection. It was also found that there were seasonal differences in infection rates and that dust control could significantly decrease the incidence of primary infection.

In the military, outbreaks have been associated with maneuvers of nonimmune units. For example, in 1992 a Tennessee-based US Marine Corps Reserve unit experienced an outbreak after training in San Luis Obispo County, Calif.[621] Other reports include an outbreak associated with moving earth to provide foundations for a housing project at Edwards Air Force Base, Calif.,[622] coccidioidomycosis as a sequela of a dust storm at Lemoore Naval Air Station, Calif.,[623] infection among German air defense artillery trainees in El Paso, Tex.,[624] and cases in those deployed to the Desert Training Center in Fort Irwin, Calif.[625]

Description of the Pathogen

Coccidioides immitis is a dimorphic fungus found in soil. In nature and in laboratory culture, it exists as a mycelial-arthrospore form. Animal studies suggest inhalation of as few as 7 to 12 arthroconidia suffice to cause infection.[626] In the host, the arthroconidia develop into spherules—spheres 20 to 60 μm in diameter—with small endospores inside.

Coccidioides is a hardy organism and has remained viable in dry soil and beach sand for more than 10 years.[627] It can be sterilized by soaking in hypochlorite, phenols, iodophors, or formaldehyde for at least 15 minutes.

Epidemiology

Transmission

Coccidioidomycosis is transmitted by inhalation of arthrospores from dust or soil in endemic areas. Reactivation can occur, principally in immunosuppressed hosts, such as organ transplantees and those with chemotherapy-induced lymphopenia and human immunodeficiency virus (HIV) infection. Infection has been reported to have been caused by fomites such as cotton, dirt moved from an endemic area, packing material around archaeological artifacts, fruit, and dust on cars driven through an endemic region. Infections in laboratory workers have usually been inhalationally acquired, but some have been primary inoculations leading to skin lesions. Inoculation from barbed wire and splinters has also been reported.[628] Person-to-person transmission has occurred—in a cast covering a draining sinus, the spherule form had converted to the mycelial phase. The organism aerosolized when the cast was opened, exposing many health care workers.[629]

Transmission seems to be most intense from August to November, especially if there is prolonged drought followed by heavy spring rains.[620] California had a marked increased incidence of primary *Coccidioides* infection due to this pattern in 1991 and 1992; incidence also increased later because of the disruption and construction related to the 1994 earthquake.[630] Large dust storms facilitate the transmission of coccidioidomycosis.

Geographic Distribution

The endemic zone for *Coccidioides* is restricted to the Western hemisphere between 40° north (California) and 40° south (Argentina) latitude (Figure 37-16). *Coccidioides* is usually found in arid climates of low rainfall, hot summers, few winter freezes, and alkaline soil. In the United States, this includes the deserts of Arizona, west Texas, and the central valleys of California; some areas of southern New

Mexico; Las Vegas, Nev.; and southwest Utah. Outside the United States, endemic areas are found in Mexico, Guatemala, El Salvador, Honduras, Colombia, Argentina, Brazil, Venezuela, and Paraguay.[631] It should be emphasized that areas of endemicity are focal within this distribution.

Incidence

Estimates suggest that 100,000 persons in the United States are infected each year.[632] In endemic areas of the Southwest, 30% to 50% of long-term residents are *Coccidioides* skin-test positive. Studies in Tucson, Ariz., suggest an annual infection risk of 2% to 4% per year.[633] There are several factors associated with a higher risk of dissemination once coccidioidomycosis is acquired. These include race and

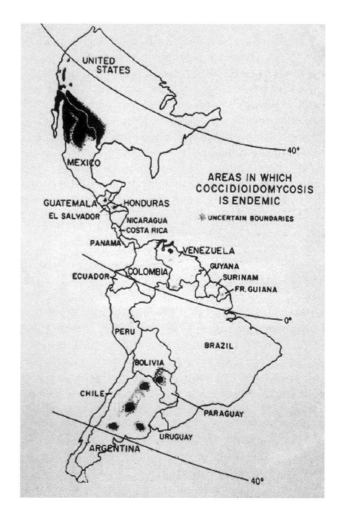

Fig. 37-16. Areas in which coccidiomycosis is endemic. Reprinted with permission from: Pappagianis D. *Coccidioidomycosis: A Text*. New York: Plenum Publishing; 1980.

ethnic origin (especially black and Filipino), HIV infection with CD4 counts of less than 250, having received an organ transplant, having Hodgkins disease or uremia, taking steroids for collagen vascular disease, and being in the second or third trimester of pregnancy.

The US military's experience in World War II suggests that immunity develops to exogenous reinfection.[619] In the San Joaquin Army air fields, active infection occurred only in those patients who had negative skin tests or were untested.

Occupational risk groups for the acquisition of coccidioidomycosis include agricultural laborers; archaeologists; geologists; paleontologists; construction, highway, pipeline, and oil-well drilling workers; laboratory technicians; and military personnel. Coccidioidomycosis is recognized as an occupational illness under the California worker's compensation law.

Pathogenesis and Clinical Findings

The arthroconidia are inhaled and establish infection in the small bronchi. The initial host response is neutrophilic, but the spherules are not killed by polymorphonuclear leukocytes. Cell-mediated immunity is essential to kill the fungus. Dissemination has been related to hematogenous spread of the fungus from suppurating lymph nodes in the hilae and mediastinum.

The majority (60%) of cases are asymptomatic or have symptoms similar to an upper respiratory tract infection.[619] Forty percent are symptomatic, mainly with an acute febrile illness lasting 7 to 28 days that often includes cough (usually nonproductive), malaise, pleuritic chest pain, night sweats, fatigue, occasional dyspnea, headache, pharyngitis, arthralgia, and, infrequently, hemoptysis. About 10% of symptomatic patients (especially females) may have a syndrome known as desert rheumatism or valley fever, which includes erythema nodosum (painful erythematous nodules often over the pretibial area, Figure 37-17) with or without symmetrical nonmigratory arthralgias and occasionally arthritis. Another skin manifestation of an early immune response to *C immitis* is toxic erythema, which can be scarlatiniform, morbilliform, or urticarial. Erythema multiforme can also occur, usually in the upper half of the body, and is sometimes accompanied by palmar desquamation. Valley fever is self limited, is associated with very large reactions to spherulin skin testing, and generally has a good prognosis. In these acute cases, spherulin skin test reagent should be diluted to 1:1,000 or 1:10,000 to avoid large local reactions.

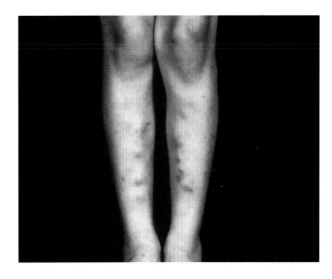

Fig. 37-17. Erythema nodosum is associated with acute coccidioidal infection. An immunologic phenomenon, it portends a benign course of infection.
Photograph: Courtesy of William Beaumont Army Medical Center, El Paso, Tex.

Disseminated extrapulmonary coccidioidomycosis occurs in 1% of symptomatic white persons and 10% of symptomatic black persons.[619] This is often a severe, relapsing, potentially life-threatening complication. Disseminated infection usually develops within a year of initial infection. The most common sites are skin, bone, joint, and meninges; other sites include the genitourinary tract, peritoneum, thyroid, lymph nodes, and spleen. It often manifests in a miliary pattern. The skin is frequently involved in disseminated coccidioidomycosis and may be the manifestation that a deployed military health care provider is most likely to see. Most commonly, the lesion is verrucous; it can also be a chronic ulcer (Figure 37-18), draining sinus tract, plaque, nodule, subcutaneous abscess, or sporotrichoid lesion with regional lymphadenitis.

Findings on chest radiograph include infiltrates (which can be single or multiple), hilar adenopathy, and occasionally ipsilateral pleural effusion or cavitary lesions. Five percent have chronic radiograph findings, which include nodules and thin-walled cystic lesions. Diffuse reticulonodular infiltrates suggest disseminated disease and are more frequently seen in immunocompromised hosts.

Laboratory clues are an elevated erythrocyte sedimentation rate and a fairly normal total white blood cell count. More than 25% will have an eosinophilia count of greater than 5%.

a
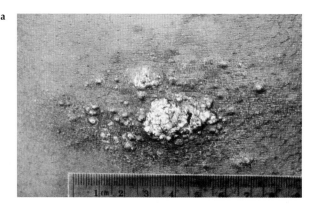
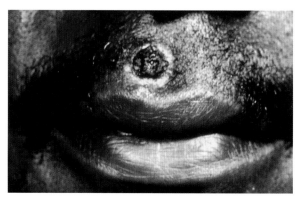
b

Fig. 37-18. Photograph (**a**) shows Verrucous cutaneous coccidioidomycosis. Photograph (**b**) shows the ulcerative form of cutaneous coccidioidomycosis above the lip. This lesion represents disseminated infection. Photographs: Courtesy of William Beaumont Army Medical Center, El Paso, Tex.

Diagnostic Approaches

In the field, coccidioidomycosis should be considered in cases of respiratory illness occurring approximately 1 to 3 weeks after exposure in endemic areas. Spherulin skin testing (1:100) designates those who have been infected; however, like the tuberculin skin test, it is better to have baseline data so as to detect conversion. A significant reaction is an induration of greater than or equal to 5 mm at either 24 or 48 hours. For febrile patients, a chest radiograph is recommended, as those at highest risk for dissemination may have an anergic result on the spherulin skin test. A positive coccidioidin skin test can be seen 2 to 21 days after exposure in 99% of those infected.[634] Causes of false-positive tests include the merthiolate preservative used in the skin test, histoplasmosis, paracoccidioidomycosis, and, possibly, recurrent recent (within 2 months) skin testing.[635] Causes described for false-negative skin tests include dissemination, placement too early, and methodologic problems with skin test placement such as subdermal injection or inaccurate measurement of the induration.

In garrison, several additional diagnostic aids may be employed. Coccidioidal serology can be very helpful. IgM antibodies can be seen in 7 to 10 days and measured by several assays (eg, tube precipitins, latex particle agglutination, immunodiffusion). Serum IgG antibodies occur later (50% by 4 weeks) and persist for a long time. Complement fixation IgG titers of greater than 1:16 to 1:32 are of concern because they are associated with a higher risk of dissemination, particularly if the test is standardized to the antigen of Smith.[636]

The spherules are rarely seen in sputum, pus, si-

nus tract drainage, or other body fluids. In tissue sections, the spherules may be seen with hematoxylin, hematoxylineosin, and Gomori's methenamine silver stain. *Coccidioides* can also autofluoresce.

The organism grows well on artificial media in 3 to 5 days. The mycelial form that is generated is highly infectious, so the laboratory should be warned that *C immitis* is suspected so safety measures will be carefully maintained.

Recommendations for Therapy and Control

Those with severe primary infection and those at risk for disseminated illness should be treated. This includes persons who are immunocompromised and those who have had a large inoculum exposure, have had symptoms for longer than 6 weeks, have an anergic reaction to the spherulin skin test, have an increased complement fixation titer, or are in the second or third trimester of pregnancy. All patients with extrapulmonary coccidioidomycosis should receive therapy. For patients who do not receive specific therapy, a repeat encounter at 1 to 2 years to document resolution or identify complications is suggested.

The current guidelines for treatment are in flux, with the availability since the early 1990s of the oral triazoles.[637] For severe illness, intravenous amphotericin B (1.5 to 3 g total dose, 0.5-0.7 mg/kg per day) is given; intrathecal amphotericin B (0.01-1.5 mg) must be given as well for meningeal coccidioidomycosis. During pregnancy, amphotericin B is the treatment of choice. For mild-to-moderate nonmeningeal coccidioidomycosis, itraconazole 200 mg orally twice a day or fluconazole 400 to 800 mg per day may be used; the regimen must be continued for at least 6 months after the disease becomes inactive. For meningeal coccidioidomycosis, fluconazole 600 to 800 mg per day is considered first-line therapy; in limited experience it is effective and less toxic than intrathecal amphotericin.[638] Some would initiate therapy for meningitis with amphotericin B intrathecally as well, trying for a more rapid treatment response. Therapy should be continued lifelong.

Overall, response rates of less than 75% are the norm in the treatment of coccidioidomycosis, and all patients with disseminated infection should be considered at risk for relapse.[639]

Data gathered at the San Joaquin Valley Army air bases support the utility of dust control in decreasing the incidence of infection in susceptible persons.[620] Lawns and trees should be aggressively planted, roads and airfields paved, and athletic fields oiled (optimal dosage is 1 qt of highly refined oil per square yard of dry field[619]). Temporary benefit has been observed with soil fumigation using 1-chloro-2-nitropropene.[640] Local authorities should be consulted about the legality of this measure. For optimal control, ground maneuvers in focal areas known to be highly endemic, especially in the late summer and fall, should be curtailed or limited to those persons known to have positive spherulin skin tests (although heavy reexposure may overwhelm this immunity). For those involved with earth-moving equipment, use of vehicles with air conditioned cabs is recommended. Buildings in endemic areas should have filtered air or air conditioning. Vehicles covered with dust from endemic areas should be thoroughly cleaned before departure. The use of personal respirators or masks for potentially heavy but limited exposure may be in theory useful but in practice very uncomfortable, given the hot, dry environment where *Coccidioides* is endemic.

In the clinical setting, dressings or casts over active coccidioidomycosis infections (eg, draining skin lesions) should be completely wetted before removal and the dressing treated with phenol or sodium hypochlorite solution to decrease any subsequent transmission.

Laboratory personnel should maintain *Coccidioides* isolates in sealed containers and handle culture samples with appropriate biosafety equipment for a class 3 biologic agent. For the first 3 to 5 days of growth, though, the sample is not particularly infectious.

There is as yet no successful vaccine for the prevention of coccidioidomycosis. While azole prophylaxis in high-risk patients (eg, those with HIV or transplanted organs) has been considered, it has not yet been adequately studied. Of note, in three reported cases in immunosuppressed hosts, disseminated coccidioidomycosis developed while the patients were receiving ketoconazole.[641]

Control in military units from a nonendemic region training in or deployed to endemic, nonimproved areas of the US Southwest should include a surveillance and education program. Optimally, this would include spherulin skin testing before training and 1 to 2 months after training, surveillance for clustering of febrile respiratory illness within a month of potential exposure, and observation for cases of erythema nodosum. Military personnel should be educated about the significance of symptoms consistent with disseminated infection. Dissemination will often occur once service members have redeployed to a nonendemic region where health care providers may not readily consider coccidioidomycosis in the differential diagnosis.

Coccidioidomycosis is a reportable medical condition in the US military and several southwestern states.

[Naomi E. Aronson]

HISTOPLASMOSIS

Introduction and Military Relevance

Histoplasmosis, caused by the fungal pathogen *Histoplasma capsulatum* var. *capsulatum*, is an infection of worldwide distribution. Usually an asymptomatic infection, histoplasmosis can be a severe and sometimes fatal disease. Outbreaks of acute histoplasmosis have been associated with military operations in the past. These epidemics have most frequently been associated with cleaning and clearing contaminated debris from structures such as infrequently used bunkers. Some of the earliest epidemics were reported in soldiers in Camp Gruber, Okla, and Camp Crowder, Mo, in the 1940s.[642] More recent outbreaks include those described in 1977 and 1982 associated with troop activity in Panama.[643,644] Histoplasmosis has the potential to affect the readiness and effectiveness of service members in situations where contaminated structures are cleaned or cleared for use.

First described by Samuel Darling in 1906, histoplasmosis was initially thought to be a parasitic infection.[645] Describing an autopsy performed while working in the Panama Canal Zone, Darling reported finding organisms in histiocytes that resembled plasmodia and appeared to have a capsule. Because of these observations, he recommended naming the new parasite *Histoplasma capsulata*. De Monbreun established that the causative agent, *H capsulatum*, was a dimorphic fungus.[646] He described the cultural characteristics of both the yeast and mycelial phases and fulfilled Koch's postulates by producing disease in animals with the isolate.

From its discovery and up until the late 1940s, histoplasmosis was considered to be widespread in distribution but rare and fatal. That a nonfatal infection could also occur was not elucidated until the introduction of histoplasmin skin testing. In the early 1940s, it was noted that military recruits from Kentucky and many south-central states had a higher than usual rate of calcifications on chest roentgenogram, changes suspicious of healed tuberculosis. Many people in those areas with abnormal chest roentgenograms had negative tuberculin skin tests. In the mid-1940s, studies by Palmer[647,648] and Christie[649] showed that reaction to the new skin test for histoplasmosis was widespread in the midwestern United States and correlated with asymptomatic pulmonary calcification in subjects with negative tuberculin tests. These studies, along with other epidemiologic work, firmly established histoplasmosis as a predominantly self-limiting infection of humans and animals.

Description of the Pathogen

H capsulatum var. *capsulatum* is a temperature-dependent, dimorphic, fungal pathogen.[650,651] In its natural habitat (soil) and in culture at room temperature, *H capsulatum* forms a mycelium of septate hyphae, which can produce both microconidia (2-5 µm) and tuberculate macroconidia (8-16 µm). It is this form of the fungus (and especially aerosolized microconidia) that is the infectious inoculum. In its pathogenic form or in culture at 37°C, *H capsulatum* var. *capsulatum* is a small yeast (2-5 µm). Conversion of the mycellial form, grown from clinical isolates, to a yeast at 37°C can be used in the identification of this organism. The mycelial form of *H capsulatum* grows well in soils with high nitrogen content and is found in soil contaminated by guano and debris of birds and bats. The most common niche of the fungus is in soil contaminated with the droppings of starlings, bats, or chickens. In addition to causing infection in humans, histoplasmosis is common in both wild and domesticated mammals. *H capsulatum* consists of three varieties: *capsulatum*, *duboisii*, and *farciminosum*. Most cases of histoplasmosis are caused by *H capsulatum* var. *capsulatum*. *H capsulatum* var. *duboisii* (*H duboisii*, African histoplasmosis) is a second variety of the fungus, which is found principally in Africa and causes disease usually limited to bone and skin. *H capsulatum* var. *farciminosum* is a pathogen that has thus far been limited to horses and mules.

Epidemiology

Transmission and Geographic Distribution

Inhalation of aerosolized conidia is the route of transmission. Histoplasmosis has been reported throughout the world, with greatest prevalence from 45° north latitude to 30° south latitude.[652] The distribution of this disease is concentrated in and around the Mississippi and Ohio River valleys in the United States.

Incidence

Clinically apparent disease is more common in males (4:1 ratio), although skin testing does not support a difference in exposure or infection between the sexes.[653] In the less-commonly seen forms of histoplasmosis, including disseminated disease, immunocompromised patients (eg, those who have a hematologic malignancy, have acquired immunodeficiency syndrome [AIDS], or have taken steroid or immunosuppressive therapies) and the very young are at higher risk.

The world's highest concentration of skin-test–positive individuals exists in the Mississippi and Ohio River valleys, with 80% to 90% of residents there testing positive. In the more highly endemic areas of this region, 80% to 90% of the population is skin-test–positive by age 20.[654] Large-scale skin testing of Navy recruits has enhanced the understanding of the epidemiology of histoplasmosis in the United States (Figure 37-19).[655] The annual incidence of histoplasmosis is thought to be approximately 250,000 in the United States.[656] In addition to endemic disease, about 200 small epidemics of histoplasmosis have also been described. Epidemics of histoplasmosis usually present with acute pulmonary disease in subjects exposed to large inoculum loads, although at least one outbreak presented as undifferentiated febrile syndrome without pulmonary signs or symptoms.[644] The source and causation of these epidemics is usually the disruption of debris, soil, or guano through cleaning or removing structures that are heavily contaminated by starlings, bats, or chickens. Examples include outbreaks associated

Fig. 37-19. Prevalence of histoplasmin skin test reactivity in the continental United States.
Reprinted with permission from: Edwards LB, Acquaviva FA, Livesay VT, Cross FW, Palmer CE. An atlas of sensitivity to tuberculin, PPD-B, and histoplasmin in the United States. *Am Rev Respir Dis.* 1969;99(Suppl):1–132.

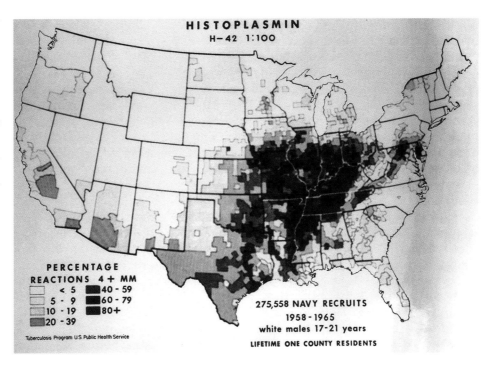

with cleaning buildings, bunkers, caves, silos, and areas of bird roosts; excavation of soil; and removal of dead trees. Attack rates of 90% to 100% have been reported in such outbreaks.[642] Disease caused by such high-inoculum exposure is often severe and incapacitating, requiring intensive care acutely and long periods of convalescence.

Pathogenesis and Clinical Findings

Histoplasmosis in humans can be manifested in many forms, from acute to chronic and localized or disseminated.[657,658] *H capsulatum* is not present in humans as normal flora or colonies and is not spread person-to-person. Infection most commonly occurs after inhalation of conidia of the fungus from the sources previously mentioned. Infection of normal, healthy adults usually results in mild, self-limiting pulmonary disease. The pathogenesis of these infections is complex and not completely understood. It is estimated by skin testing and chest roentgenogram findings that approximately 95% of infections are asymptomatic.[650,651] Symptomatic illness most commonly presents 10 days after a heavy exposure as an influenza-like illness with pulmonary infiltrates and development of mediastinal lymphadenopathy. Although the lungs are the most commonly affected site in acute symptomatic disease, nonspecific febrile illness without pulmonary signs or symptoms has been reported in at least one US Army outbreak.[644] The prevalence of this atypical form of histoplasmosis is not known.

Acute pulmonary histoplasmosis is the most common form of histoplasmosis, presenting as an acute respiratory illness. Most of these infections do not come to medical attention and resolve spontaneously. Symptoms develop 3 to 21 days following exposure, often occurring sooner in patents exposed to large amounts of inoculum or developing infection following reexposure. Symptoms and disease severity are believed to be correlated with host immunity and inoculum size. In symptomatic cases, signs and symptoms most commonly seen can be difficult to distinguish from influenza or "atypical" community-acquired pneumonias. These include fever, chest pain, cough, headache, malaise, chills, abdominal pain, and myalgias. Chest roentgenogram findings include hilar or mediastinal lymphadenopathy with or without patchy, often bilateral infiltrates. Hilar and splenic calcifications are common radiographic findings in patients who have previously had acute pulmonary disease. Mild anemia and transient increases in alkaline phosphatase can be noted. Rheumatologic signs and symptoms may be present in up to 5% of patients. More commonly presenting in white females, these include arthralgias, arthritis, erythema multiforme, and erythema nodosum. In severe cases, adult respiratory distress syndrome with diffuse reticulonodular infiltrates can occur.

Isolated mediastinitis or pericarditis may occur in persons with clinically inapparent infection. Mediastinitis due to histoplasmosis can present with a wide spectrum of disease. It can range from acute pulmonary disease presenting as only mediastinal adenopathy and pain that quickly resolves to a progressively destructive fibrosis that obstructs or destroys the mediastinal structures. Mediastinal granulomatosis is a description given to histoplasmosis that causes the coalescence and enlargement of mediastinal and hilar lymph nodes. Depending on the severity of this disease, patients may develop symptoms of esophageal or superior vena caval compression. Appearing as a central mass lesion on radiologic studies, this process may resolve spontaneously. Mediastinal fibrosis is a localized, progressive scarring reaction secondary to previous histoplasmosis. This process may cause obstruction and compression as described previously for granuloma formation and may ultimately lead to obliteration of mediastinal structures. Symptoms can include cough, dyspnea, hemoptysis, chest pain, and wheezing, plus those of superior vena cava syndrome. With mediastinal fibrosis, chest roentgenograms may reveal only mild mediastinal widening.

Chronic pulmonary histoplasmosis is a disease that most often affects middle-aged, white, male smokers with underlying emphysema. This form of histoplasmosis occurs in patients with underlying lung disease; it presents and progresses in a fashion similar to tuberculosis. Chronic pulmonary histoplasmosis usually causes upper lobe disease, often with progression to cavitation and fibrosis. Patients usually present with persistent or worsening cough, weight loss, malaise, and low-grade fever. Because of this, it is difficult to distinguish this disorder from exacerbation of chronic bronchitis, tuberculosis, and malignancy. Chest roentgenogram may show bullae, calcified granulomas or mediastinal nodes, pleural thickening with upper lobe infiltrates, or cavitation. Hilar adenopathy is rare. Disease may spontaneously resolve with linear scarring with or without cavity formation. Patients who develop thick-walled cavities usually do not have spontaneous resolution.

Acute, progressive, disseminated histoplasmosis is usually a primary infection, which can occur in normal, healthy adults but is much more common in immunocompromised persons and those at the extremes of age. It is very common in endemic areas in persons with AIDS, with attack rates possibly as high as 27%.[659] Patients with Hodgkin's lymphoma and lymphocytic leukemia are also at high risk. In acute disease, *H capsulatum* is found throughout the reticuloendothelial system, including bone marrow, blood, liver, spleen, and lymph nodes. Untreated, acute disseminated histoplasmosis is usually a fatal disease. In small children and infants, fever, malaise, weight loss, hepatosplenomegaly, and cervical adenopathy is common. Chest roentgenograms may show a miliary infiltrate or hilar adenopathy. Laboratory changes, including anemia, leukopenia, thrombocytopenia, and elevated alanine transaminase and alkaline phosphatase levels, are frequently noted. In adults with AIDS, acute disease usually results in fever, weight loss, malaise, cough, and dyspnea. Subacute and chronic forms of disseminated histoplasmosis can also occur, particularly in the elderly. These have common features, which include weight loss, malaise, fatiguability, and low-grade fever. Ulcers of the gums, tongue, tonsillar areas, and larynx can occur in up to one third of those affected with the chronic form. Chronic disease is often localized to specific organs, producing clinical disease associated with that particular site. The adrenal glands, gastrointestinal tract, central nervous system, and heart valves are the more frequently involved sites.

Diagnostic Approaches

As the majority of cases of histoplasmosis are asymptomatic, diagnosis is often retrospective and epidemiologic in nature, using histoplasmin skin testing or observation of calcified granuloma on chest roentgenogram. Diagnosis of symptomatic histoplasmosis may be difficult. Histoplasmosis should be included in the differential diagnosis of clusters of acute febrile disease, especially respiratory disease, in groups of personnel who have been performing duties that expose them to organic debris contaminated with bird or bat guano. Direct visualization on biopsy or smears and growth of the organism in culture are the most accurate means of diagnosis. Serological tests are of limited value. Detection of *H capsulatum* antigen in urine or blood is a newer method that has been shown to be most useful in acute, progressive, disseminated disease.[660]

Histopathological diagnosis is possible when infected tissue is available. Finding small budding yeasts in a granulomatous infection strongly suggests the diagnosis. These yeasts are difficult to see on routine staining but become readily apparent on Gomori methenamine silver staining. *H capsulatum* occasionally may be seen in peripheral blood smears of patients with acute disseminated disease. Calcofluor white preparations are useful in detecting *H capsulatum* in bronchoalveolar lavage.

Culture of sputum, blood, and bone marrow for *H capsulatum* is usually done on brain-heart infusion agar or diphasic medium at room temperature. Growth usually takes 4 to 6 weeks. Use of lysis centrifugation with blood samples may increase the recovery and decrease the time to grow the organism. Identification of *H capsulatum* from culture is made by either DNA probe, conversion of the mycelial phase to the yeast phase at 37°C, or, less commonly, by exoantigen testing.

Two available serologic tests for histoplasmosis are complement fixation (CF) and immunodiffusion (ID). These tests may be used in the retrospective confirmation of infections: CF by documentation of a 2-fold rise in titer, ID by the appearance of M or H identity bands. CF develops faster than ID but is less sensitive. Because of this, ID is often considered the confirmatory test. CF antibodies can be detected in most presentations of histoplasmosis but may take 4 to 6 weeks to develop.

Diagnosis by radioimmunoassay testing for antigen in blood and urine has become commercially available. Although this test has been shown to be very sensitive in patients who develop disseminated disease (especially in those who have AIDS[661]), less than 20% of patients with acute, self-limited, pulmonary infection have been shown to have a positive test.[660] The sensitivity of this test is highest when used with urine samples. It is currently only available at one site in the United States and the its full usefulness is not known.

The role of skin testing in histoplasmosis is limited and may be counterproductive. Skin-test positivity from endemic exposure is common, especially in the midwestern United States. Up to two thirds of those with active disease may have negative skin tests. Exposure to skin testing has also been shown to cause seroconversion in uninfected subjects, leading to false-positive complement fixation and immunodiffusion testing.

Recommendations for Therapy and Control

Asymptomatic and mild symptomatic cases of histoplasmosis do not require specific antifungal therapy. In general, antifungal therapy consists of intravenous amphotericin B (AMB) in life-threatening infections and oral itraconazole in less severe disease.[653,658] Moderate-to-severe acute pulmonary disease may be treated with itraconazole (400 mg/day for 3 to 6 weeks), ketoconazole (400 mg/day for 3 to 6 weeks), or AMB (0.5 mg/kg per day intravenously for 2 to 3 weeks). Overwhelming disease,

including that with adult respiratory distress syndrome, should always be treated with AMB. Chronic pulmonary disease may be treated with itraconazole (400 mg/day for 6 to 12 months). Acute disseminated histoplasmosis is usually treated with AMB, given as 0.5 mg/kg per day to a total dose of 35 mg/kg or 2.5 g. Itraconazole (200 mg orally three times a day for 3 days, then 200 mg orally two times a day for 6 to 12 months) has been shown to be effective therapy in milder cases.[662] Patients with subacute or chronic disseminated histoplasmosis may be treated with AMB as in acute disease or with long courses of azole (6 to 12 months of ketoconazole or itraconazole). Treatment of the other forms of histoplasmosis is generally based on clinical disease activity.

As exposure to soil and guano with high concentrations of the organism is the major source of infections, avoidance of areas that are most likely to be contaminated is the key to prevention and control measures (Figure 37-20). These areas include chicken houses, bird roosts, caves with bats, and

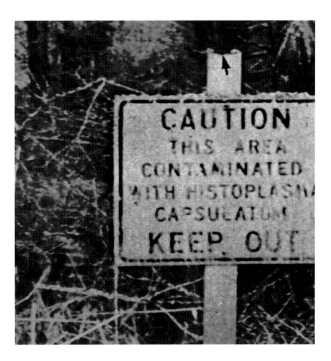

Fig. 37-20. An area in the vicinity of Fort Campbell, Ky, posted to warn potential visitors of the risk of histoplasmosis. The area had a heavy accumulation of starling guano contaminated with *Histoplasma capsulatum*.
Reprinted with permission from: Rippon JW. Histoplasmosis (*Histoplasmosis capsulati*). In: *Medical Mycology: The Pathogenic Fungi and the Pathogenic Actinomycetes*. 3rd ed. Philadelphia, Penn: WB Saunders; 1988: 386.

any structure with deposits of bird droppings. Presence of *H capsulatum* in these droppings or debris is most prevalent where deposits of guano are deep or longstanding. Disturbing these areas in any manner that leads to the production of dusts and aerosols is more likely to lead to infections. It makes sense to avoid placing helicopter landing zones in the vicinity of these areas and to use care in the clean up or destruction of structures contaminated by bird or bat guano. When these areas or structures need to be entered, use of water or oil spraying to decrease dust and aerosols during clean up should lower the risk of infection. Sweeping or shoveling of dry material should be avoided. Material removed should not be left uncovered and can be buried without posing a health risk. Use of personal protective (nuclear-biological-chemical) masks or HEPA (high efficiency particulate air) filter masks should adequately protect individuals. The United States Army Center for Health Promotion and Preventive Medicine (USACHPPM, formerly the United States Army Environmental Hygiene Agency) suggests avoidance in preference to decontamination for histoplasmosis-contaminated sites.[663] USACHPPM recommends use of full-face respirators with HEPA filters or supplied air. They also recommend wearing disposable garments, hats, boots, and gloves (using duct tape to seal at wrists and ankles), using low velocity water mist spraying, double bagging of removed droppings (in 3 mil or thicker plastic bags), disposing of wastes in landfills, removing and disposing of contaminated clothing properly (ie, as infectious waste), and showering before putting on clean clothing. Masks and nondisposable items should be decontaminated in a bag. Three percent formalin has been used in the past to decontaminate sites. However, such a strategy should be limited or avoided and only employed after consultation with appropriate local and federal authorities because of the possible detrimental impact of this action on individuals and the environment.

[Duane R. Hospenthal]

MELIOIDOSIS

Introduction and Military Relevance

Melioidosis is a tropical disease found in regions that within 20° north and south of the equator, which includes Southeast Asia and northern Australia. Melioidosis can occur in humans and a wide variety of animals such as goats, pigs, monkeys, dogs, birds, and reptiles. The disease may be contracted through soil contamination of skin abrasions, by inhalation of soil particles, or by aspiration of contaminated water. The disease is caused by a gram-negative bacterium, *Burkholderia pseudomallei* (previously known as *Pseudomonas pseudomallei*). The range of clinical presentations include inapparent infections, asymptomatic pulmonary infiltration to acute pulmonary infection, acute septicemic infections or chronic suppurative infections, and localized abscesses in those who acquired the infection through skin abrasions. Fatality rates in severe infections may approach 40%.[644,645]

Melioidosis was diagnosed among French soldiers involved in armed conflicts in Indochina from 1948 to 1954.[646] In the 1970s, cases were reported in US service members fighting in Vietnam.[547,648] Cases continued to manifest in US military personnel many years after their exposure to the bacteria during the war. Meliodosis has been referred to as the "time-bomb disease."[649]

Description of the Pathogen

This organism, previously placed in the genus *Pseudomonas*, has been placed in the genus *Burkholderia* based on phylogenetic analysis of 16S rRNA sequences.[650] *B pseudomallei*, a motile, gram-negative, rod-shaped organism, appears as wrinkled colonies with a yeasty odor when cultured on agar (Figure 37-21). A closely related species, *B mallei*, is a nonmotile organism that causes glanders in horses. Although genetically indistinguishable, it is recognized as a separate species because of zoonotic and epidemiologic considerations. Both *B pseudomallei* and *B mallei* are known to cause disease in many animal species, but the only direct evidence of zoonotic disease transferable to humans is glanders. *B pseudomallei* is thought to be a ubiquitous environmental contaminant and only an accidental or opportunistic pathogen. A closely related avirulent environmental strain of *B pseudomallei* has been isolated in Thailand, and the name *B thailandensis* has been proposed for it.[651,652]

The bacteria survive optimally between 24°C and 32°C in vitro [653] and can usually be found at a soil depth of between 25 cm and 45 cm.[654] The bacteria survive best under laboratory conditions when the pH is kept between 5.0 and 8.0. *B pseudomallei* is more easily killed by ultraviolet light than other soil bacteria.[653]

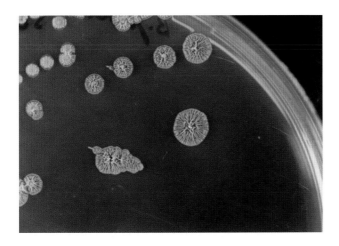

Fig. 37-21. Wrinkled colonies of *B pseudomallei* on modified Ashdown's medium agar.
Photograph: Courtesy of J.T.W. Thong and E.H. Yap, Department of Microbiology, National University of Singapore.

Epidemiology

Transmission

Humans are usually infected by inhalation or ingestion of contaminated soil and water or through the contamination of wounds. Most of the infections of US military personnel during the Vietnam War were attributed to inhalation of the organisms in dust raised by helicopter rotors.[655]

Geographic Distribution

B pseudomallei is widely distributed in soil and water in the tropics but is mainly found between the 20° north and 20° south (Figure 37-22). *B pseudomallei* has been frequently isolated from wet rice fields and cleared cultivated areas; the organisms have even been isolated from sport fields in the more urban environment of Singapore.[656] Human cases of melioidosis have been reported in the Caribbean islands of Guadeloupe and Puerto Rico.[657,658]

Incidence

Because of the failure to diagnose this infection in many topical countries besides northern Australia and Southeast Asian countries such as Thailand, Malaysia, and Singapore, little is known of the epidemiology of the disease. In Thailand, 2,000 to 3,000 cases of clinical melioidosis occur each year. The incidence rate in highly endemic areas is 3.5 to 5.5 cases per 100,000 population and is seasonal, with more cases occurring during the rainy season.[659] In Malaysia, antibodies to *B pseudomallei* have been detected in 6% of diabetics, 5% of pyrexics, 8% of pregnant women, and 3% of farmers.[660] Among 420 military personnel recruited by Malaysian Military serving in Sabah and Sarawak, 65.7% were found to have antibodies to the whole cell antigens of *B pseudomallei*.[661] Antibodies to *B pseudomallei* were also found in 18 of 905 British Commonwealth soldiers serving in West Malaysia.[662]

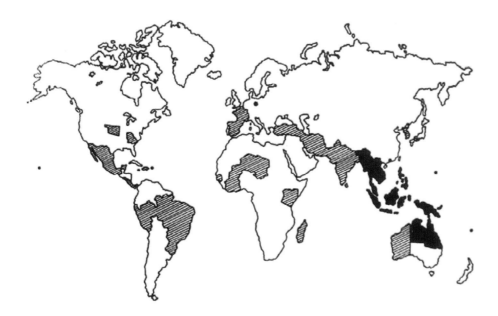

Fig. 37-22. World Distribution of *B pseudomallei* and *B pseudomallei*-like organisms from clinical and environmental isolates. The shaded areas show the main endemic areas; the hatched areas and asterisks show areas from which sporadic isolates have been gathered.
Reprinted with permission from: Dance DAB, Melioidosis: The Tip of the Iceberg? *Clin Microbiol Rev.* 1991, 4:52-60.

In Singapore between 1987 and 1994, 23 cases of melioidosis were diagnosed in persons serving in the Singapore Armed Forces.[663] During the period of 1989 to 1996, 372 cases of melioidosis with 147 deaths were reported in Singapore, giving a mean annual incidence rate of 1.7 per 100,000 population.[664]

Eight cases of melioidosis were diagnosed on Hainan Island in China from October 1995 to October 1996.[665] From 1989 to 1998, 206 cases of melioidosis were confirmed in the northern part of the Northern Territory of Australia, giving an incidence of 16.5 per 100,000 population.[666]

During the 1950s, cases of melioidosis were reported in French troops returning from Indochina after their military operations in the region. The US Army faced similar cases in troops returning from Vietnam.[667] A serological survey of US military personnel who served on active duty in Vietnam for at least two months showed that 20.7% had positive titers, as opposed to 5.7% in the control group.[655]

Pathogenesis and Clinical Findings

The incubation period for the infection can be as short as 2 days, or the infection can remain latent for more than 25 years. The clinical spectrum of melioidosis is protean, including acute fulminant septicemia, subacute illness, chronic infections, and subclinical disease. When latently infected patients manifest the disease after many years, usually it is in association with an immunocompromising illness such as diabetes mellitus, renal failure, systemic lupus, cirrhosis, alcoholism, or severe traumatic injury such as burns.[668] The infection can mimic various acute or chronic infections (eg, typhoid fever, malaria, tuberculosis, coccidiodomycosis, histoplasmosis). Correct clinical diagnosis at initial presentation is usually very difficult. Obtaining a compatible travel history should lead to inclusion of melioidosis in the differential diagnosis of any patient who is febrile and has an underlying disease or injury that could compromise host defenses.

The clinical presentation of septicemic melioidosis varies from an ill-defined febrile illness to fulminant septicemia. A history or clinical evidence of diabetes or uremia might suggest the diagnosis. In northern Thailand, melioidosis usually presents as acute septicemia, often resulting in metastatic abscesses in lungs, liver, and spleen and a rapid deterioration to shock and death.[669]

Subacute melioidosis can result from a primary infection that remains subacute or a reactivation of a previous infection. Most cases of melioidosis seen in nonendemic areas belong to this group. Patients may be asymptomatic or have symptoms indistinguishable from the common presentation of pulmonary tuberculosis. Recrudescent disease often involves the lungs, resembling reactivation tuberculosis with cavity formation in upper lobes.[668]

Chronic melioidosis may take the form of suppurative abscesses involving numerous anatomic sites. Patients can have infections lasting for years without symptoms. Chest radiographs usually show apical cavitary disease resembling tuberculosis; occasionally, patients may present with fever of unknown origin.

Subclinical melioidosis results in a chronic carrier state. The immune system probably suppresses the infection so no clinical disease develops. Once the host is immunocompromised, however, clinical disease can occur.

Diagnostic Approaches

Prompt diagnosis of melioidosis is important for initiation of treatment with the right combination of antibiotics. Definitive diagnosis of melioidosis is by culturing *B pseudomallei* from blood, sputum, pus, or urine during acute or subacute infections from any affected body fluid or source. The bacterium has been cultured from every body fluid except stool. It can be cultured on most routine laboratory media, and this is the main method of identification. The colonies appear rough and wrinkled, with a characteristic yeasty odor after 3 to 4 days' incubation. The use of selective media, such as the Ashdown's selective-differential agar medium, significantly increases the recovery of *B pseudomallei* from specimens with extensive normal flora (eg, sputum, specimens from the throat, rectum, and wounds).[669,670]

Serological methods such as the enzyme-linked immunosorbent assay, latex agglutination, and indirect hemagglutination assay can also be used to diagnose melioidosis. Indirect hemagglutination is commonly used for diagnosis; it detects antibodies that can agglutinate the *B pseudomallei* crude antigens coated onto the surface of erythrocytes. Use of the assay as a diagnostic tool in endemic regions is limited because of the background antibodies in a large portion of the healthy population living in endemic regions. In nonendemic regions, the assay is more sensitive and the cut-off titer of the assay is lower.[671]

Polymerase chain method has been developed for the detection of bacterial DNA in clinical samples. The method is rapid and sensitive, and it eliminates the need to propagate the pathogen.[672,673] Rapid immunoassays that work in 10 minutes have been developed for the detection of melioidosis. The assays have a sensitivity of 100% for the IgG tests and 93% for the IgM tests, while specificity is 95% for both.[674]

Recommendations for Therapy and Control

B pseudomallei has been shown to be susceptible in vitro to ceftazidime, tetracyclines, sulfonamides, chlorophenicol, kanamycin, and novobiocin.[668] Combinations of two or more antibiotics are usually used for treatment of melioidosis.[675] The use of high-dose intravenous ceftazidime, with or without trimethoprim-sulfamethoxazole (TMP-SMX), is the choice of treatment for severe melioidosis. Other suitable antibiotic regimens include imipenem with amoxycillin/clavulanate and cefoperazone/sulbactam with TMP-SMX. Potentially contaminated wounds should be well cleaned as soon as possible.

Exposure to *B pseudomallei* in the environment can be minimized by taking precautions when in contact with soil and water. This includes wearing boots and gloves, especially for those at high risk because of traumatic wounds or a debilitating illness. Person-to-person and zoonotic spread is virtually nonexistent, and quarantine of patients is unnecessary. Laboratory-acquired acute melioidosis, probably from the inhalation of an infectious aerosol, has been reported.[676] This underscores the need to take standard biosafety precautions when handling respiratory and sinus drainage and the wastes and body fluids of infected persons and animals.

[May-Ann Lee; Eric P. H. Yap]

REFERENCES

1. Levine MM. *Escherichia coli* that cause diarrhea: Enterotoxigenic, enteropathogenic, enteroinvasive, enterohemorrhagic, and enteroadherent. *J Infect Dis.* 1987;155:377–389.

2. Black RE, Brown KH, Becker S, Alim AR, Huq I. Longitudinal studies of infectious diseases and physical growth of children in rural Bangladesh, II: Incidence of diarrhea and association with known pathogens. *Am J Epidemiol.* 1982;115:315–324.

3. Echeverria P, Taylor DN, Lexsomboon U, Bhaibulaya M, Blacklow NR, Tamura K, Sakazaki R. Case-control study of endemic diarrheal disease in Thai children. *J Infect Dis.* 1989;159:543–548. Published erratum: *J Infect Dis.* 1989;160:1827.

4. Black RE. Pathogens that cause travelers' diarrhea in Latin America and Africa. *Rev Infect Dis.* 1986;8(Suppl 2):S131–135.

5. Taylor DN, Echeverria P. Etiology and epidemiology of travelers' diarrhea in Asia. *Rev Infect Dis.* 1986;8 (supp 2):S136–S141.

6. Tramont EC, Gangarosa EJ. Cholera, dysentery, and diarrhea. In: Blaser MJ, Smith PD, Ravdin JI, Greenberg HB, Guerrant RL, eds. *Infections of the Gastrointestinal Tract.* New York: Raven Press; 1995.

7. Kean BH. The diarrhea of travelers to Mexico: Summary of five-year study. *Ann Intern Med.* 1963;59:605–614.

8. Sack RB, Gorbach SL, Banwell JG, Jacobs B, Chatterjee BD, Mitra RC. Enterotoxigenic *Escherichia coli* isolated from patients with severe cholera-like disease. *J Infect Dis.* 1971;123:378–385.

9. Rowe B, Taylor J, Bettelheim KA. An investigation of travellers' diarrhoea. *Lancet.* 1970;1:1–5.

10. DuPont HL, Formal SB, Hornick RB, et al. Pathogenesis of *Escherichia coli* diarrhea. *N Engl J Med.* 1971;285:1–9.

11. Hyams KC, Bourgeois AL, Merrell BR, et al. Diarrheal disease during Operation Desert Shield. *N Engl J Med.* 1991;325:1423–1428.

12. Wolf MK, Taylor DN, Boedeker EC, et al. Characterization of enterotoxigenic *Escherichia coli* isolated from U.S. troops deployed to the Middle East. *J Clin Microbiol.* 1993:31;851–856.

13. Tjoa W, DuPont HL, Sullivan P, et al. Location of food consumption and traveler's diarrhea. *Am J Epidemiol.* 1977;106:61–66.

14. Rasrinaul L, Suthienkul O, Echeverria P, et al. Foods as a source of enteropathogens causing childhood diarrhea in Thailand. *Am J Trop Med Hyg.* 1988;39:97–102.

15. Hyams KC, Hanson K, Wignall FS, Escamilla, Oldfield EC III. The impact of infectious diseases on the health of US troops deployed to the Persian Gulf during Operations Desert Shield and Desert Storm. *Clin Infect Dis.* 1995;20:1497–1504.

16. Rosenberg ML, Koplan JR, Wachsmuth IK, et al. Epidemic diarrhea at Crater Lake from enterotoxigenic *Escherichia coli*: A large waterborne outbreak. *Ann Intern Med.* 1977;86:714–718.

17. Taylor WR, Schell WL, Wells JG, et al. A foodborne outbreak of enterotoxigenic *Escherichia coli* diarrhea. *N Engl J Med.* 1982;306:1093–1095.

18. MacDonald KL, Eidson M, Strohmeyer C, et al. A multistate outbreak of gastrointestinal illness caused by enterotoxigenic *Escherichia coli* in imported semisoft cheese. *J Infect Dis.* 1985;151:716–720.

19. Merson MH, Morris GK, Sack DA, et al. Travelers' diarrhea in Mexico: A prospective study of physicians and family members attending a congress. *N Engl J Med.* 1976;294:1299–1305.

20. Moseley SL, Echeverria P, Seriwatana J, et al. Identification of enterotoxigenic *Escherichia coli* by colony hybridization using three enterotoxin gene probes. *J Infect Dis.* 1982;145:863–869.

21. Avery ME, Snyder JD. Oral therapy for acute diarrhea: The underused simple solution. *N Engl J Med.* 1990;323;891–894.

22. International Study Group on Reduced-Osmolality ORS Solutions. Multicentre evaluation of reduced-osmolarity oral rehydration salts solution. *Lancet.* 1995;345:282–285.

23. Sazawal S, Black RE, Bhan MK, Bhandari N, Sinha A, Jalla S. Zinc supplementation in young children with acute diarrhea in India. *N Engl J Med.* 1995;333:839–844.

24. DuPont HL, Ericsson CD. Prevention and treatment of traveller's diarrhea. *N Engl J Med.* 1993;328:1821–1827.

25. Taylor DN, Sanchez JL, Candler W, Thornton S, McQueen C, Echeverria P. Treatment of travelers' diarrhea: Ciprofloxacin plus loperamide compared with ciprofloxacin alone; a placebo-controlled, randomized trial. *Ann Intern Med.* 1991;114:731–734.

26. Scott DA, Haberberger RL, Thornton SA, Hyams KC. Norfloxacin for the prophylaxis of travelers' diarrhea in U.S. military personnel.*Am J Trop Med Hyg.* 1990;42:160–164.

27. Taylor DN. Quinolones as chemoprophylactic agents for travelers' diarrhea. *J Travel Med.* 1994;1:119–121.

28. Svennerholm AM, Holmgren J, Sack DA. Development of oral vaccines against enterotoxigenic *Escherichia coli* diarrhoea. *Vaccine.* 1989;7:196–198.

29. Riley LW, Remis RS, Helgerson SD, et al. Hemorrhagic colitis associated with a rare *Escherichia coli* serotype. *N Engl J Med.* 1983;308:681–685.

30. Griffin PM, Tauxe RV. The epidemiology of infections caused by *Escherichia coli* O157:H7, other enterohemorrhagic *E. coli*, and the associated hemolytic uremic syndrome. *Epidemiol Rev.* 1991;13:60–98.

31. Watanabe H, Wada A, Inagaki Y, Itoh KI, Tamura K. Outbreaks of enterohaemorrhagic *Escherichia coli* O157:H7 infection by two different genotype strains in Japan,1996. *Lancet.* 1996;348:831–832.

32. O'Brien AD, Holmes RK. Shiga and Shiga-like toxins. *Microbiol Rev.* 1987;51:206–220.

33. Banatvala N, Magnano AR, Cartter ML, et al. Meat grinders and molecular epidemiology: Two supermarket outbreaks of *Escherichia coli* O157:H7 infection. *J Infect Dis.* 1996;173:480–483.

34. Centers for Disease Control and Prevention. *Escherichia coli* O157:H7 infections associated with eating a nationally distributed commercial brand of frozen ground beef patties and burgers—Colorado, 1997. *MMWR.* 1997;278:891.

35. McCarthy M. E coli O157:H7 outbreak in USA traced to apple juice. *Lancet.* 1996;348:1299.

36. Centers for Disease Control and Prevention. Outbreaks of *Escherichia coli* O175:H7 infection associated with eating alfalfa sprouts—Michigan and Virginia, June–July 1997. *MMWR.* 1997;46:741–744.

37. Keene WE, McAnulty JM, Hoesly FC, et al. A swimming-associated outbreak of hemorrhagic colitis caused by *Escherichia coli* O157:H7 and *Shigella sonnei. N Engl J Med.* 1994;331:579–584.

38. Spika JS, Parsons JE, Nordenberg D, Wells JG, Gunn RA, Blake PA. Hemolytic uremic syndrome and diarrhea associated with *Escherichia coli* O157:H7 in a day care center. *J Pediatr.* 1986;109:287–291.

39. MacDonald KL, O'Leary MJ, Cohen ML, et al. *Escherichia coli* O157:H7, an emerging gastrointestinal pathogen: Results of a one-year, prospective, population-based study. *JAMA.* 1988;259:3567–3570.

40. Griffin PM, Ostroff SM, Tauxe RV, et al. Illnesses associated with *Escherichia coli* O157:H7 infections: A broad clinical spectrum. *Ann Intern Med.* 1988;109:705–712.

41. Su C, Brandt LJ. *Escherichia coli* O157:H7 infection in humans. *Ann Intern Med.* 1995;123:698–714.

42. Boyce TG, Swerdlow DL, Griffin PM. *Escherichia coli* O157:H7 and the hemolytic-uremic syndrome. *N Engl J Med.* 1995;333:364–368.

43. Taylor DN, Echeverria P, Sethabutr O, et al. Clinical and microbiologic features of *Shigella* and enteroinvasive *Escherichia coli* infections detected by DNA hybridization. *J Clin Microbiol.* 1988;26:1362–1366.

44. Armstrong GD, Rowe PC, Goodyer P, et al. A phase I study of chemically synthesized verotoxin (Shiga-like toxin) Pk-trisaccharide receptors attached to chromosorb for preventing hemolytic-uremic syndrome. *J Infect Dis.* 1995;171:1042–1045.

45. Ephros M, Cohen D, Yavzori M, Rotman N, Novics B, Ashkenazi S. Encephalopathy associated with enteroinvasive *Escherichia coli* O144:NM infection. *J Clin Microbiol.* 1996;34:2432–2434.

46. Hedberg CW, Savarino SJ, Besser JM, et al. An outbreak of foodborne illness caused by *Escherichia coli* O39:NM, an agent not fitting into the existing scheme for classifying diarrheogenic *E coli. J Infect Dis.* 1997;176:1625–1628.

47. Marier R, Wells JC, Swanson RC, Callahan W, Mehlman IJ. An outbreak of enteropathogenic *Escherichia coli* foodborne disease traced to imported French cheese. *Lancet.* 1973;2:1376–1378.

48. Snyder JD, Wells JG, Yashuk J, Puhr N, Blake PA. Outbreak of invasive *Escherichia coli* gastroenteritis on a cruise ship. *Am J Trop Med Hyg.* 1984;33:281–284.

49. Harris JR, Mariano J, Wells JG, Payne BJ, Donnell HD, Cohen ML. Person-to-person transmission in an outbreak of enteroinvasive *Escherichia coli. Am J Epidemiol.* 1985;122:245–252.

50. Wanger AR, Murray BE, Echeverria P, Mathewson JJ, DuPont HL. Enteroinvasive *Escherichia coli* in travelers with diarrhea. *J Infect Dis.* 1988;158:640–642.

51. Hale TL, Sansonetti PJ, Schad PA, Austin S, Formal SB. Characterization of virulence plasmids and plasmid-associated outer membrane proteins in *Shigella flexneri, Shigella sonnei,* and *Escherichia coli. Infect Immun.* 1983;40:340–350.

52. Venkatesan M, Buysse JM, Vandendries E, Kopecko DJ. Development and testing of invasion-associated DNA probes for detection of *Shigella* spp. and enteroinvasive *Escherichia coli. J Clin Microbiol.* 1988;26:261–266.

53. Robins-Browne RM. Traditional enteropathogenic *Escherichia coli* of infantile diarrhea. *Rev Infect* Dis. 1987;9:28–53.

54. Ewing WH. *Edwards' and Ewing's Identification of Enterobacteriaceae.* 4th ed. New York: Elsevier Science Publishing; 1986.

55. Donnenberg MS. Enteropathogenic *Escherichia coli.* In: Blaser MJ, Smith PD, Ravdin JI, Greenberg HB, Guerrant RL, eds. *Infections of the Gastrointestinal Tract.* New York: Raven Press; 1995.

56. Scaletsky IC, Silva MLM, Trabulsi LR. Distinctive patterns of adherence of enteropathogenic *Escherichia coli* to HeLa cells. *Infect Immun.* 1984;45:534–536.

57. Mathewson JJ, Johnson PC, DuPont HL, et al. A newly recognized cause of travelers diarrhea: Enteroadherent *Escherichia coli. J Infect Dis.* 1985;151:471–475.

58. Mathewson JJ, Johnson PC, DuPont HL, Satterwhite TK, Winsor DK. Pathogenicity of enteroadherent *Escherichia coli* in adult volunteers. *J Infect Dis.* 1986;154:524–527.

59. Gomes TAT, Blake PA, Trabulsi LR. Prevalence of *Escherichia coli* strains with localized, diffuse, and aggregative adherence to HeLa cells in infants with diarrhea and matched controls. *J Clin Microbiol.* 1989;27:266–269.

60. Cravioto A, Gross RJ, Scotland SM, Rowe B. An adhesive factor found in strains of *Escherichia coli* belonging to the traditional enteropathogenic serotypes. *Curr Microbiol.* 1979;3:95–99.

61. Knutton S, Lloyd DR, McNeish AS. Adhesion of enteropathogenic *Escherichia coli* to human intestinal enterocytes and cultured human intestinal mucosa. *Infect Immun.* 1987;55:69–77.

62. Levine MM, Nataro JP, Karch H, et al. The diarrheal response of humans to some classic serotypes of enteropathogenic *Escherichia coli* is dependent on a plasmid encoding an enteroadhesiveness factor. *J Infect Dis.* 1985;152:550–559.

63. Giron JA, Ho ASY, Schoolnik GK. An inducible bundle-forming pilus of enteropathogenic *Escherichia coli. Science.* 1991;254:710–713.

64. Bhan MK, Raj P, Levine MM, et al. Enteroaggregative *Escherichia coli* associated with persistent diarrhea in a cohort of rural children in India. *J Infect Dis.* 1989;159:1061–1064.

65. Levine MM, Prado V, Robins-Browne R, et al. Use of DNA probes and Hep-2 cell adherence assay to detect diarrheagenic *Escherichia coli. J Infect Dis.* 1988;158:224–228.

66. Nataro JP, Baldini MM, Kaper JB, Black RE, Bravo N, Levine MM. Detection of an adherence factor of enteropathogenic *Escherichia coli* with a DNA probe. *J Infect Dis.* 1985;152:560–565.

67. DeFraites RF, Kadlec RP. *Waterborne Campylobacter Enteritis Outbreak at Fort Knox, KY.* Washington, DC: Walter Reed Army Institute of Research; 1991. Epidemiologic Consultant Service Final Report.

68. Taylor DN, Blaser MJ. *Campylobacter* infections. In: Evans AS, Brachman PS, eds. *Bacterial Infections of Humans: Epidemiology and Control.* 2nd ed. New York: Plenum Publishing; 1990: 151–172.

69. Totten PA, Patton CM, Tenover FC, et al. Prevalence and characterization of hippurate-negative *Campylobacter jejuni* in King County, Washington. *J Clin Microbiol.* 1987;25:1747–1752.

70. Taylor DN, Kiehlbauch JA, Tee W, Pitarangsi C, Echeverria P. Isolation of Group 2 aerotolerant *Campylobacter* species from Thai children with diarrhea. *J Infect Dis.* 1991;163:1062–1067.

71. Skirrow MB. *Campylobacter* enteritis: A "new" disease. *Br Med J.* 1977;2:9–11.

72. Patton CM, Barrett TJ, Morris GK. Comparison of the Penner and Lior methods for serotyping *Campylobacter* spp. *J Clin Microbiol.* 1985;22:558–565.

73. Blaser MJ, Reller LB. *Campylobacter* enteritis. *New Engl J Med*. 1981;1444–1452.

74. Blaser MJ, Taylor DN, Feldman RA. Epidemiology of *Campylobacter* infections. In: Campylobacter *Infections in Man and Animals*. CRC Press: Boca Raton, Fla; 1983: 144–161.

75. Blaser MJ, Wells JG, Feldman RA, Pollard RA, Allen JR, Collaborative Diarrheal Disease Study Group. *Campylobacter* enteritis in the United States: A multicenter study. *Ann Intern Med*. 1983;98:360–365.

76. Skirrow MB. A demographic survey of *Campylobacter*, *Salmonella*, and *Shigella* infections in England: A public health laboratory service survey. *Epidem Infect*. 1987;99:647–657.

77. Hoge CW, Shlim DR, Echeverria P, Rajah R, Herrmann JE, Cross JH. Epidemiology of diarrhea among expatriate residents living in a highly endemic environment. *JAMA*. 1996;275:533–538.

78. Kuschner R, Trofa AF, Thomas RJ, et al. Use of azithromycin for the treatment of *Campylobacter* enteritis in travelers to Thailand, an area where ciprofloxacin resistance is prevalent. *Clin Infect Dis*. 1995;21:536–541.

79. Taylor DN. *Campylobacter* infections in developing countries. In: Nachamkin I, Blaser MJ, Tompkins LS, eds. Campylobacter jejuni: *Current Status and Future Trends*. Washington, DC: American Society of Microbiology; 1992: 20–30.

80. Taylor DN, Echeverria P, Pitarangsi C, et al. Influence of strain characteristics and immunity on the epidemiology of *Campylobacter* infections in Thailand. *J Clin Microbiol*. 1988;26:863–868.

81. Black RE, Levine MM, Clements ML, Hughes TP, Blaser MJ. Experimental *Campylobacter jejuni* infection in humans. *J Infect Dis*. 1988;157:472–479.

82. Walker RI, Caldwell MB, Lee EC, Guerry P, Trust TJ, Ruiz-Palacios GM. Pathophysiology of *Campylobacter* enteritis. *Microbiol Rev*. 1986;50:81–94.

83. Blaser MJ, Perez GP, Smith PF, et al. Extraintestinal *Campylobacter jejuni* and *Campylobacter coli* infections: Host factors and strain characteristics. *J Infect Dis*. 1986;153:552–559.

84. Blaser MJ, Berkowitz ID, LaForce FM, Cravens FM, Reller LB, Wang WLL. *Campylobacter* enteritis: Clinical and epidemiologic features. *Ann Intern Med*. 1979;91:179–185.

85. Skirrow MD, Blaser MJ. Campylobacter jejuni. In: Blaser MJ, Smith PD, Ravid JI, Greenberg HB, Guerrant RL, eds. *Infections of the Gastrointestinal Tract*. New York: Raven Press; 1995.

86. Butler T, Islam M, Azad AK, Islam MR, Speelman P. Causes of death in diarrhoeal diseases after rehydration therapy: An autopsy study of 140 patients in Bangladesh. *Bull World HealthOrgan*. 1987;65:317–323.

87. Allos BM, Blaser MJ: *Campylobacter jejuni* and the expanding spectrum of related infections. *Clin Infect Dis*. 1995;20:1092–1099.

88. Rees JH, Soudain SE, Gregson NA, Hughes RA. *Campylobacter jejuni* infection and Guillain-Barre syndrome. *N Engl J Med*. 1995;333:1374–1379.

89. Kapikian AZ. Overview of viral gastroenteritis. *Arch Virol Suppl*. 1996;12:7–19.

90. Centers for Disease Control and Prevention. Norwalk-like viral gastroenteritis in U.S. Army trainees—Texas, 1998. *MMWR*. 1999;48;225–227.

91. Sharp TW, Hyams KC, Watts D, et al. Epidemiology of Norwalk virus during an outbreak of acute gastroenteritis aboard a US aircraft carrier. *J Med Virol*. 1995;45:61–67.

92. Echeverria P, Jackson LR, Hoge CW, Arness MK, Dunnavant GR, Larsen RR. Diarrhea in US troops deployed to Thailand. *J Clin Microbiol*. 1993,31:3351–3352.

93. Kapikian AZ, Estes MK, Chanock RM. Norwalk group of viruses. In: Fields BN, Knipe DM, Howley PM, et al., eds. *Fields Virology*. 3rd ed. Philadelphia: Lippincott- Raven; 1996: 783–810.

94. Jiang X, Matson DO, Cubitt WD, Estes MK. Genetic and antigenic diversity of human caliciviruses (HuCVs) using RT-PCR and new EIAs. *Arch Virol Suppl*. 1996;12:251–262.

95. Belliot G, Laveran H, Monroe SS. Outbreak of gastroenteritis in military recruits associated with serotype 3 astrovirus infection. *J Med Virol*. 1997;51:101–106.

96. Chiba S. Immunological aspects of viral gastroenteritis. In: Paradise LJ, Bendinelli M, Friedman H, eds. *Enteric Infections and Immunity*. New York: Plenum Press; 1996.

97. Blacklow NR, Greenberg HB. Viral gastroenteritis. *N Engl J Med*. 1991;325:252–264.

98. Centers for Disease Control. Viral agents of gastroenteritis: Public health importance and outbreak management. *MMWR*. 1990;39(RR-5):1–24.

99. Kapikian AZ, Chanock RM. Rotaviruses. In: Fields BN, Knipe DM, Howley PM, et al., eds. *Fields Virology*. 3rd ed. Philadelphia: Lippincott-Raven; 1996: 1657–1708.

100. Shenk T. Adenoviridae: The viruses and their replication. In: Fields BN, Knipe DM, Howley PM, et al., eds. *Fundamental Virology*, 3rd ed. Philadelphia: Lippincott-Raven; 1996: 979–1016.

101. Caul EO. Viral gastroenteritis: Small round structured viruses, caliciviruses, and astroviruses, Part II: The epidemiological perspective. *J Clin Pathol*. 1996;49:959–964.

102. Appleton H. Norwalk viruses and the small round viruses causing foodborne gastroenteritis. In: Hui YH, Gorham JR, Murrell KD, Cliver DO, eds. *Diseases Caused by Viruses, Parasites, and Fungi*. Vol 2. In: *Foodborne Disease Handbook*. New York: Marcel Dekker; 1994.

103. Kuritsky JN, Osterholm MT, Greenberg HB, et al. Norwalk gastroenteritis: A community outbreak associated with bakery product consumption. *Ann Infect Dis*. 1984;100:519–521.

104. Caul EO. Viral gastroenteritis: Small round structured viruses, caliciviruses, and astroviruses, Part I: The clinical and diagnostic perspective. *J Clin Pathol*. 1996;49:874–880.

105. Matsui SM, Greenberg HB. Medical management of foodborne viral gastroenteritis and hepatitis. In: Hui YH, Gorham JR, Murrell KD, Cliver DO, eds. *Diseases Caused by Viruses, Parasites, and Fungi*. Vol 2. In: *Foodborne Disease Handbook*. New York: Marcel Dekker; 1994.

106. Cubitt D, Bradley DW, Carter MJ, et al. Caliciviridae. *Arch Virol*. 1995;Suppl 10:359–363.

107. Christensen ML. Rotaviruses. In: Murray PR, Barron EJ, Pfaller MA, Tenover FC, Yolken RH, eds. *Manual of Clinical Microbiology*. 6th ed. Washington, DC: ASM Press; 1996: 1012–1016.

108. Petric M. Caliciviruses, astroviruses, and other diarrhea viruses. In: Murray PR, Barron EJ, Pfaller MA, Tenover FC, Yolken RH, eds. *Manual of Clinical Microbiology*. 6th ed. Washington, DC: ASM Press; 1996: 1017–1024.

109. Farthing M, Feldman R, Finch R, et al. Management of infective gastroenteritis in adults: A consensus statement by an expert panel convened by the British Society for the Study of Infection. *J Infect*. 1996;33:143–152.

110. Centers for Disease Control and Prevention. Management of acute diarrhea in children: Oral rehydration, maintenance, and nutritional therapy. *MMWR*. 1992;41(RR-16).

111. Centers for Disease Control and Prevention. Withdrawal of rotavirus vaccine recommendation. *MMWR*. 1999;48:1007.

112. Benenson AS. Immunization and military medicine. *Rev Infect Dis*. 1984;6:1–12.

113. Bayne-Jones S. *The Evolution of Preventive Medicine in the United States Army, 1607–1939*. Office of the Surgeon General, Department of the Army: Washington, DC; 1968.

114. Daoud AS, Zaki M, Pugh RN, al-Mutairi G, Beseiso R, Nasrallah AY. Clinical presentation of enteric fever: Its changing pattern in Kuwait. *J Trop Med Hyg*. 1991;94:341–347.

115. Heppner DG Jr, Magill AJ, Gasser RA Jr, Oster CN. The threat of infectious diseases in Somalia. *N Engl J Med*. 1993;328:1061–1068.

116. Oldfield EC, Wallace MR, Hyams KC, Yousif AA, Lewis DE, Bourgeois AL. Endemic infectious diseases of the Middle East. *Rev Infect Dis*. 1991;13(Suppl 3):S197–S217.

117. Oldfield EC 3d, Rodier GR, Gray GC. The endemic infectious diseases of Somalia. *Clin Infect Dis*. 1993;16(Suppl 3):S132–S157.

118. Ollé-Goig JE, Ruiz L. Typhoid fever in rural Haiti. *Bull Pan Am Health Org*. 1993;27:382–388.

119. Hornick RB. Selective primary health care: Strategies for control of disease in the developing world, XX: Typhoid fever. *Rev Infect Dis*. 1985;7:536–546.

120. Sears SD, Ferreccio C, Levine MM, et al. The use of Moore swabs for isolation of *Salmonella typhi* from irrigation water in Santiago, Chile. *J Infect Dis*. 1984;149:640–642.

121. Morris J, Ferreccio C, Garcia J, et al. Typhoid fever in Santiago, Chile: A study of household contacts of pediatric patients. *Am J Trop Med Hyg*. 1984;33:1198–1202.

122. Birkhead GS, Morse DL, Levine WC, et al. Typhoid fever at a resort hotel in New York: A large outbreak with an unusual vehicle. *J Infect Dis*. 1993;167:1228–1232.

123. Convery HT, Frank L. Management issues in a major typhoid fever outbreak. *Am J Public Health*. 1993;83:595–596.

124. Feldman RE, Baine WB, Nitzkin JL, Saslaw MS, Pollard RA. Epidemiology of *Salmonella typhi* infection in a migrant labor camp in Dade County, Florida. *J Infect Dis*. 1974;130:334–342.

125. Mathieu JJ, Henning KJ, Bell E, Frieden TR. Typhoid fever in New York City, 1980 through 1990. *Arch Intern Med*. 1994;154:1713–1718.

126. Rice PL, Baine WB, Gangarosa EJ. *Salmonella typhi* infections in the United States, 1967–1972: Increasing importance of international travelers. *Am J Epidemiol*. 1977;106:160–166.

127. Ryan CA, Hargrett-Bean NT, Blake PA. *Salmonella typhi* infections in the United States, 1975–1985: Increasing role of foreign travel. *Rev Infect Dis*. 1989;11:1–8.

128. Taylor DN, Pollard RA, Blake PA. Typhoid fever in the United States and risk to international travelers. *J Infect Dis*. 1983;148:599–602.

129. Edelman R, Levine MM. Summary of an international workshop on typhoid fever. *Rev Infect Dis*. 1986;8:329–349.

130. Ivanoff B, Levine MM, Lambert PH. Vaccination against typhoid fever: Present status. *Bull World Health Org*. 1994;72:957–971.

131. Naylor G. Incubation period and other features of food-borne and water-borne outbreaks of typhoid fever in relation to pathogenesis and genetics of resistance. *Lancet*. 1983;1:864.

132. Hornick RB, Greisman SE, Woodward TE, DuPont HL, Dawkins AT, Snyder MJ. Typhoid fever: Pathogenesis and immunologic control (first of two parts). *N Engl J Med*. 1970;283:686-691.

133. Boomsma LJ. Clinical aspects of typhoid fever in two rural Nigerian hospitals: A prospective study. *Trop Geogr Med*. 1988;40:97–102.

134. Thisyakorn U, Mansuwan P, Taylor DN. Typhoid and paratyphoid fever in 192 hospitalized children in Thailand. *Am J Dis Childhood*. 1987;141:862–865.

135. Yew FS, Chew SK, Goh, KT Monteiro EH, Lim YS. Typhoid fever in Singapore: A review of 370 cases. *J Trop Med Hyg*. 1991;94:352–357.

136. Roy S, Speelman P, Butler T, Nath S, Rahman H, Stoll BJ. Diarrhea associated with typhoid fever. *J Infect Dis*. 1985;151:1138–1143.

137. Kuri-Bulos N. Enteric fevers in children: The importance of age in the varying clinical picture. *Clin Pediatr*. 1981;20:448–452.

138. Sen S, Mahakur A. Enteric fever—a comparative study of adult and paediatric cases. *Indian J Pediatr*. 1972;39:354–360.

139. Stoll BJ, Glass RI, Banu H, Alam M. Enteric fever in patients admitted to a diarrhoeal disease hospital in Bangladesh. *Trans R Soc Trop Med Hyg*. 1983;77:548–551.

140. Stuart BM, Pullen RL. Typhoid: Clinical analysis of three hundred and sixty cases. *Arch Intern Med*. 1946;78:629–661.

141. Wicks AC, Holmes GS, Davidson L. Endemic typhoid fever: A diagnostic pitfall. *Q J Med*. 1971;40:341–354.

142. Mishra S, Srinivasan G, Chaturvedi P. Persistent diarrhoea: An unusual presentation of typhoid fever. *J Trop Pediatr*. 1994;40:314–315.

143. Klotz SA, Jorgensen JH, Buckwold FJ, Craven PC. An epidemic with remarkably few clinical signs and symptoms. *Arch Intern Med*. 1984;144:533–537.

144. Butta Z, Naqvi S, Razzaq R, Farooqui B. Multidrug-resistant typhoid in children: Presentation and clinical features. *Rev Infect Dis*. 1991;13:832–836.

145. Buczko GB, McLean J. Typhoid fever associated with adult respiratory distress syndrome. *Chest*. 1994;105:1873–1874.

146. Woodward TE, Smadel JE. Management of typhoid fever and its complications. *Ann Intern Med*. 1964;60:144–157.

147. van Basten JP, Stockenbrügger R. Typhoid perforation: A review of the literature since 1960. *Trop Geogr Med*. 1994;46:336–339.

148. Bitar R, Tarpley J. Intestinal perforation in typhoid fever: A historical and state-of-the-art review. *Rev Infect Dis*. 1985;7:257–271.

149. Butler T, Knight J, Nath SK, Speelman P, Roy SK, Azad MA. Typhoid fever complicated by intestinal perforation: A persisting fatal disease requiring surgical management. *Rev Infect Dis*. 1985;7:244–256.

150. Mock CN, Amaral J, Visser LE. Improvement in survival from typhoid ileal perforation: results of 221 operative cases. *Ann Surg*. 1992;215:244–249.

151. Hornick RB, Greisman SE, Woodward TE, DuPont HL, Dawkins AT, Snyder MJ. Typhoid fever: Pathogenesis and immunologic control (second of two parts). *N Engl J Med*. 1970;283:739–746.

152. Keusch GT. Antimicrobial therapy for enteric infections and typhoid fever: State of the art. *Rev Infect Dis*. 1988;10:S199–S205.

153. Hornick R. Typhoid fever. In: Evans A, Feldman H, ed. *Bacterial Infections in Humans: Epidemiology and Control*. New York: Plenum; 1982:659–676.

154. Mourad AS, Metwally M, Nour el Deen A, et al. Multiple-drug resistant *Salmonella typhi*. *Clin Infect Dis*. 1993;17:135.

155. Woodward T, Smadel J, Ley H, Green R, Mankikar D. Preliminary report on the beneficial effect of chloromycetin in the treatment of typhoid fever. *Ann Intern Med*. 1948;29:131–134.

156. Paniker C, Vimala K. Transferable chloramphenicol resistance in *Salmonella typhi*. *Nature*. 1972;239:109–110.

157. Sanders WL. Treatment of typhoid fever: A comparative trial of ampicillin and chloramphenicol. *Br Med J*. 1965;2:1226–1227.

158. Snyder MJ, Gonzolez O, Palomino C, et al. Comparative efficacy of chloramphenicol, ampicillin, and co-trimoxazole in the treatment of typhoid fever. *Lancet*. 1976;1155–1157.

159. Kamat S. Evaluation of therapeutic efficacy of trimethoprim-sulfamethoxazole and chloramphenicol in enteric fever. *B Med J*. 1970;3:320–322.

160. Olarte J, Galinda E. *Salmonella typhi* resistant to chloramphenicol, ampicillin, and other antimicrobial agents: Strains isolated during an extensive typhoid fever epidemic in Mexico. *Antimicrob Agents Chemother*. 1973;4:597–601.

161. Goldstein FW, Chumpitaz JC, Guevara JM, Papadopoulou B, Acar JF, Vieu JF. Plasmid-mediated resistance to multiple antibiotics in *Salmonella typhi*. *J Infect Dis*. 1986;153:261–266.

162. Threlfall EJ, Ward LR, Rowe B, et al. Widespread occurence of multiple drug-resistant *Salmonella typhi* in India. *Eur J Clin Microbiol Infect Dis*. 1992;11:990–993.

163. Gupta A. Multidrug-resistant typhoid fever in children: Epidemiology and therapeutic approach. *Pediatr Infect Dis J*. 1994;13:134–140.

164. Rowe B, Ward L, Threlfall E. Treatment of multidrug resistant typhoid fever. *Lancet*. 1991;337:1422.

165. Rowe B, Ward L, Threlfall E. Spread of multiresistant *Salmonella typhi*. *Lancet*. 1990;336:1065.

166. Rao PS, Rajashekar V, Varghese GK, Shivananda PG. Emergence of multidrug-resistant *Salmonella typhi* in rural southern India. *Am J Trop Med Hyg*. 1993;48:108–111.

167. Dupont HL. Quinolones in *Salmonella typhi* infection. *Drugs*. 1993;45:119–124.

168. Pocidalo J. Use of fluoroquinolones for intracellular pathogens. *Rev Infect Dis*. 1989;11:S979–S984.

169. Soe GB, Overturf GD. Treatment of typhoid fever and other systemic salmonelloses with cefotaxime, ceftriaxone, cefoperazone, and other newer cephalosporins. *Rev Infect Dis*. 1987;9:719–736.

170. Brittain D, Scully B, Hirose T, Neu H. The pharmacokinetic and bacterial characteristics of oral cefixime. *Clin Pharmacol Ther*. 1985;38:590–594.

171. Cherubin C, Eng R, Smith S, Goldstein E. Cephalosporin therapy for salmonellosis: questions of efficacy and cross resistance with ampicillin. *Arch Intern Med*. 1986;146:2149–2152.

172. Kuhn H, Angehrn P, Havas L. Autoradiographic evidence for penetration of 3H-ceftriaxone (Rocephin) into cells of spleen, liver, and kidney of mice. *Chemotherapy*. 1986;32:102–112.

173. Acharya G, Crevoisier C, Butler T, et al. Pharmacokinetics of ceftriaxone in patients with typhoid fever. *Antimicrob Agents Chemother*. 1994;38:2415–2418.

174. Acharya G, Butler T, Ho M, et al. Treatment of typhoid fever: Randomized trial of a three-day course of ceftriaxone versus a fourteen-day course of chloramphenicol. *Am J Trop Med Hyg*. 1995;52:162–165.

175. Islam A, Butler T, Kabir I, Alam NH. Treatment of typhoid fever with ceftriaxone for 5 days or chloramphenicol for 14 days: A randomized clinical trial. *Antimicrob Agents Chemother.* 1993;37:1572–1575.

176. Islam A, Butler T, Nath SK, et al. Randomized treatment of patients with typhoid fever by using ceftriazone or chloramphenicol. *J Infect Dis.* 1988;158:742–747.

177. Wallace MR, Yousif AA, Mahroos GA, et al. Ciprofloxacin versus ceftriaxone in the treatment of multiresistant typhoid fever. *Eur J Clin Microbiol Infect Dis.* 1993;12:907–910.

178. Dutta P, Rasaily R, Saha MR, et al. Ciprofloxacin for treatment of severe typhoid fever in children. *Antimicrob Agents Chemother.* 1993;37:1197–1199.

179. Lumbiganon, P, Pengsaa K, Sookpranee T. Ciprofloxacin in neonates and its possible adverse effect on the teeth. *Pediatr Infect Dis.* 1991;10:619–620.

180. Douidar S, Snodgrass W. Potential role of fluoroquinolones in pediatric infections. *Rev Infect Dis.* 1989;11:878–889.

181. Mandal BK. Modern treatment of typhoid fever. *J Infect.* 1991;22:1–4.

182. Hoffman SL, Punjabi NH, Kumala S, et al. Reduction of mortality in chloramphenicol-treated severe typhoid fever by high-dose dexamethosone. *N Engl J Med.* 1984;310:82–88.

183. Cooles P. Adjuvant steroids and relapse of typhoid fever. *Am J Trop Med Hyg.* 1986;89:229–231.

184. Hathout S, El-Ghaffar Y, Awny A, Hassan K. Relation between urinary schistosomiasis and chronic enteric urinary carrier state among Egyptians. *Am J Trop Med.* 1966;15:156–161.

185. Melhem R, LoVerde P. Mechanism of interaction of *Salmonella* and *Schistosoma* species. *Infect Immun.* 1984;44:274–281.

186. M͵nnich D, Békési S. Curing of typhoid carriers by cholecystectomy combined with amoxycillin plus probenecid treatment. *Chemotherapy.* 1979;25:362–366.

187. Münnich D, Békési S, Lakatos M, Bardovics E. Treatment of typhoid carriers with amoxicillin and in combination with probenicid. *Chemotherapy.* 1974;20:29–38.

188. Nolan CM, White PC. Treatment of typhoid carriers with amoxicillin: Correlates of successful therapy. *JAMA.* 1978;239:2352–2354.

189. Brodie J, MacQueen I, Livingstone D. Effect of trimethoprim-sulfamethoxazole on typhoid and *Salmonella* carriers. *Br Med J.* 1970;3:318–319.

190. Iwarson S. Long-term cotrimoxazole treatment of chronic *Salmonella* carriers. *Scand J Infect Dis.* 1977;9:297–299.

191. Ferreccio C, Morris J, Valdivieso C, et al. Efficacy of ciprofloxacin in the treatment of chronic typhoid carriers. *J Infect Dis.* 1988;157:1235–1239.

192. Gotuzzo E, Guerra JG, Benavente L, et al. Use of norfloxacin to treat chronic typhoid carriers. *J Infect Dis.* 1988;157:1221–1225.

193. Typhoid vaccines—which one to choose? *Drug Ther Bull.* 1993;31:9–10.

194. Centers for Disease Control and Prevention. Typhoid immunization—recommendations of the Advisory Committee on Immunization Practices (ACIP). *MMWR.* 1994;43(RR-14):1–7.

195. Robbins J, Robbins J. Reexamination of the protective role of the capsular polysaccharide (Vi antigen) of *Salmonella typhi. J Infect Dis.* 1984;150:436–449.

196. Keitel W, Bond M, Zahradnik J, Cramton T, Robbins J. Clinical and serological responses following primary and booster immunization with *Salmonella typhi* Vi capsular polysaccharide vaccines. *Vaccine*. 1994;12:195–199.

197. Acharya IL, Lowe CU, Thapa R, et al. Prevention of typhoid fever in Nepal with the Vi capsular polysaccharide of *Salmonella typhi*: A preliminary report. *N Engl J Med*. 1987;317:1101–1104.

198. Klugman K, Gilbertson I, Koornhof H, et al. Protective activity of Vi capsular polysaccharide vaccine against typhoid fever. *Lancet*. 1987;2:1165–1169.

199. Germanier R, Fürer E. Isolation and characterization of Gal E Mutant Ty21a of *Salmonella typhi*: A candidate strain for a live, oral typhoid vaccine. *J Infect Dis*. 1975;131:553–558.

200. Cryz SJ Jr, Que JU, Levine MM, Wiedermann G, Kollaritsch H. Safety and immunogenicity of a live oral bivalent typhoid fever (*Salmonella typhi* Ty21a)-cholera (*Vibrio cholerae* CVD 103-HgR) vaccine in healthy adults. *Infect Immun*. 1995;63:1336–1339.

201. Rahman S, Barr W, Hilton E. Use of oral typhoid vaccine strain Ty21a in a New York state travel immunization facility. *Am J Trop Med Hyg*. 1993;48:823–826.

202. Kaplan DT, Hill DR. Compliance with live, oral Ty21a typhoid vaccine. *JAMA*. 1992;267:1074.

203. Kozarsky PE. Effects of antimalarial chemotherapeutic agents on the viability of the Ty21a typhoid vaccine strain. *Clin Infect Dis*. 1992;15:1057–1058.

204. Cryz SJ. Post-marketing experience with live oral Ty21a vaccine. *Lancet*. 1993;341:49–50.

205. Departments of the Air Force, Army, Navy, and Transportation. *Immunizations and Chemoprophylaxis*. Washington, DC: DoD; 1995. Air Force Joint Instruction 48-110, Army Regulation 40-562, BUMEDINST 6230.15, CG COMDTINST M6230.4E.

206. Barnass S, O'Mahony M, Sockett PN, Garner J, Franklin J, Tabaqchali S. The tangible cost implications of a hospital outbreak of multiply-resistant *Salmonella*. *Epidemiol Infect*. 1989;103:227–234.

207. Sockett PN, Roberts JA. The social and economic impact of salmonellosis: A report of a national survey in England and Wales of laboratory-confirmed Salmonella infections. *Epidemiol Infect*. 1991;107:335–347.

208. Cohen ML, Tauxe RV. Drug-resistant *Salmonella* in the United States: An epidemiologic perspective. *Science*. 1986;234:964–969.

209. Hedlund KW, Ognibene AJ. Typhoid fever and other salmonelloses. Ognibene AJ, Barrett O, eds. *General Medicine and Infectious Diseases*. Vol 2. In: *Internal Medicine in Vietnam*. Washington, DC: Office of the Surgeon General and Center of Military History, US Army; 1982: 360–377.

210. Echeverria P, Jackson LR, Hoge CW, et al. Diarrhea in U.S. troops deployed to Thailand. *J Clin Microbiol*. 1993;31:3351–3352.

211. Petruccelli BP, Murphy GS, Sanchez JL, et al. Treatment of traveler's diarrhea with ciprofloxacin and loperamide. *J Infect Dis*. 1992;165:557–560.

212. Intrepido A. Diarrhea outbreak—Croatia. *Med Surveil Monthly Rep*. 1996;08:7,10.

213. Centers for Disease Control and Prevention. Outbreak of *Salmonella enteritidis* associated with nationally distributed ice cream products—Minnesota, South Dakota, and Wisconsin, 1994. *MMWR*. 1994;43:740–741.

214. Ryan CA, Nickels MK, Hargrett-Bean NT, et al. Massive outbreak of antimicrobial-resistant salmonellosis traced to pasteurized milk. *JAMA*. 1987;258:3269–3274.

215. St. Louis ME, Morse DL, Potter ME, et al. The emergence of grade A eggs as a major source of *Salmonella enteritidis* infections: New implications for the control of salmonellosis. *JAMA.* 1988;259:2103–2107.

216. Spika JS, Waterman SH, Hoo GW, et al. Chloramphenicol-resistant *Salmonella newport* traced through hamburger to dairy farms: A major persisting source of human salmonellosis in California. *N Engl J Med.* 1987;316:565–570.

217. Pönkä A, Andersson Y, Siitonen A, et al. Salmonella in alfalfa sprouts. *Lancet.* 1995;345:462–463.

218. Craven PC, Mackel DC, Baine WB, Barker WH, Gangarosa EJ. International outbreak of *Salmonella eastbourne* infection traced to contaminated chocolate. *Lancet.* 1975;1:788–792.

219. Giannella RA, Broitman SA, Zamcheck N. Influence of gastric acidity on bacterial and parasitic enteric infections: A perspective. *Ann Intern Med.* 1973;78:271–276.

220. Pavia AT, Shipman LD, Wells JG, et al. Epidemiologic evidence that prior antimicrobial exposure decreases resistance to infection by antimicrobial-sensitive *Salmonella. J Infect Dis.* 1990;161:255–260.

221. Centers for Disease Control and Prevention. Multidrug-resistant *Salmonella* serotype Typhimurium—United States, 1996. *MMWR.* 1997;46:308–310.

222. Wall PG, Morgan D, Lamden K, et al. A case control study of infection with an epidemic strain of multiresistant *Salmonella typhimurium* DT104 in England and Wales. *Commun Dis Rep CDR Rev.* 1994;4:R130–R135.

223. Blaser MJ, Newman LS. A review of human salmonellosis, I: Infective dose. *Rev Infect Dis.* 1982;4:1096–1105.

224. Mishu B, Koehler J, Lee LA, et al. Outbreaks of *Salmonella enteritidis* infections in the United States, 1985–1991. *J Infect Dis.* 1994;169:547–552.

225. Salmonella in humans, England and Wales: Quarterly report. *Commun Dis Rep CDR Wkly.* 1995;5:133–134.

226. Boyce TG, Koo D, Swerdlow DL, et al. Recurrent outbreaks of *Salmonella enteritidis* infections in a Texas restaurant: Phage type 4 arrives in the United States. *Epidemiol Infect.* 1996;117:29–34.

227. *Salmonella enteritidis* phage type 4: Chicken and egg. *Lancet.* 1988:720–722. Editorial.

228. Chalker RB, Blaser MJ. A review of human salmonellosis, III: Magnitude of *Salmonella* infection in the United States. *Rev Infect Dis.* 1988;10:111–124.

229. Buchwald DS, Blaser MJ. A review of human salmonellosis, II: Duration of excretion following infection with nontyphi *Salmonella. Rev Infect Dis.* 1984;6:345–356.

230. Mandal B, Lyons M. Bacteremia in salmonellosis: A 15-year retrospective study from a regional infectious diseases unit. *Br Med J.* 1988;297:242–243.

231. Cherubin CE, Neu HC, Imperato PJ, Harvey RP, Bellen N. Septicemia with non-typhoid salmonella. *Medicine (Baltimore).* 1974;53:365–376.

232. Blaser MJ, Feldman RA. Salmonella bacteremia: Reports to the Centers for Disease Control, 1968–1979. *J Infect Dis.* 1981;143:743–746.

233. Lee SC, Yang PH, Shieh WB, Lasserre R. Bacteremia due to non-typhi *Salmonella*: Analysis of 64 cases and review. *Clin Infect Dis.* 1994;19:693–696.

234. Bassa A, Parras F, Reina J, Villar E, Gil J, Alomar P. Non-typhi *Salmonella* bacteraemia. *Infection.* 1989;17:290–293.

235. Ramos JM, Garcia-Corbeira P, Aguado JM, Arjona R, Ales JM, Soriano F. Clinical significance of primary vs. secondary bacteremia due to nontyphoid *Salmonella* in patients without AIDS. *Clin Infect Dis.* 1994;19:777–780.

236. Gopinath R, Keystone JS, Kain KC. Concurrent falciparum malaria and *Salmonella* bacteremia in travelers: Report of two cases. *Clin Infect Dis.* 1995;20:706–708.

237. Cohen JI, Bartlett JA, Corey GR. Extra-intestinal manifestations of salmonella infections. *Medicine (Baltimore).* 1987;66:349–388.

238. Fernández Guerrero ML, Torres Perea R, Gomez Rodrigo J, Nunez García A, Jusdado JJ, Ramon Rincón JM. Infectious endocarditis due to non-typhi *Salmonella* in patients infected with human immunodeficiency virus: Report of two cases and review. *Clin Infect Dis.* 1996;22:853–855.

239. Moss PJ, McKendrick MW, Channer KS, Read RC. Persisting fever after gastroenteritis. *Lancet.* 1996;347:1662.

240. Parsons R, Gregory J, Palmer DL. Salmonella infections of the abdominal aorta. *Rev Infect Dis.* 1983;5:227–231.

241. Oskoui R, Davis WA, Gomes MN. Salmonella aortitis: A report of a successfully treated case with a comprehensive review of the literature. *Arch Intern Med.* 1993;153:517–525.

242. García-Corbeira P, Ramos JM, Aguado JM, Soriano F. Six cases in which mesenteric lymphadenitis due to non-typhi *Salmonella* caused an appendicitis-like syndrome. *Clin Infect Dis.* 1995;21:231–232.

243. Paget J. On some of the sequels of typhoid fever. *St. Bartholomew's Hosp Rep.* 1876;12:1–4.

244. Ortiz-Neu C, Marr JS, Cherubin CE, Neu HC. Bone and joint infections due to *Salmonella. J Infect Dis.* 1978;138:820–828.

245. Kamarulzaman A, Briggs RJ, Fabinyi G, Richards MJ. Skull osteomyelitis due to *Salmonella* species: Two case reports and review. *Clin Infect Dis.* 1996;22:638–641.

246. Rodriguez RE, Valero V, Watanakunakorn C. *Salmonella* focal intracranial infections: Review of the world literature (1884–1984) and report of an unusual case. *Rev Infect Dis.* 1986;8:31–41.

247. Ramos JM, Aguado JM, Garcia-Corbeira P, Alés JM, Soriano F. Clinical spectrum of urinary tract infections due to nontyphoidal *Salmonella* species. *Clin Infect Dis.* 1996;23:388–390.

248. Aguado JM, Obeso G, Cabanillas JJ, Fernandez-Guerrero M, Ales J. Pleuropulmonary infections due to nontyphoid strains of *Salmonella. Arch Intern Med.* 1990;150:54–56.

249. Reid T. The treatment of non-typhi salmonellosis. *J Antimicrob Chemother.* 1992;29:4–8.

250. Kazemi M, Gumpert T, Marks M. A controlled trial comparing sulfamethoxazole-trimethoprim, ampicillin, and no therapy in the treatment of salmonella gastroenteritis in children. *J Pediatr.* 1973;83:646–650.

251. Cohen PS, O'Brien TF, Schoenbaum SC, Medeiros AA. The risk of endothelial infection in adults with salmonella bacteremia. *Ann Intern Med.* 1978;89:931–932.

252. Levine WC, Buehler JW, Bean NH, Tauxe RV. Epidemiology of nontyphoidal *Salmonella* bacteremia during the human immunodeficiency virus epidemic. *J Infect Dis.* 1991;164:81–87.

253. Nelson MR, Shanson DC, Hawkins DA, Gazzard BG. *Salmonella, Campylobacter* and *Shigella* in HIV-seropositive patients. *AIDS.* 1992;6:1495–1498.

254. DuPont H, Ericsson C, Robinson A, Johnson P. Current problems in antimicrobial therapy for bacterial enteric infection. *Am J Med.* 1987;82:324–328.

255. Cofsky R, DuBouchet L, Landesman S. Recovery of norfloxacin in feces after administration of a single oral dose to human volunteers. *Antimicrob Agents Chemother.* 1984;26:110–116.

256. Easmon CS, Crane JP, Blowers A. Effect of ciprofloxacin on intracellular organisms: In-vitro and in-vivo studies. *J Antimicrob Chemother*. 1986;18(suppl D):43–48.

257. Pichler HE, Diridl G, Stickler K, Wolf D. Clinical efficacy of ciprofloxacin compared with placebo in bacterial diarrhea. *Am J Med*. 1987;82:329–332.

258. Pichler HE, Diridl G, Wolf D. Ciprofloxacin in the treatment of acute bacterial diarrhea: A double blind study. *Eur J Clin Microbiol*. 1986;5:241–243.

259. Dryden MS, Gabb RJ, Wright SK. Empirical treatment of severe acute community-acquired gastroenteritis with ciprofloxacin. *Clin Infect Dis*. 1996;22:1019–1025.

260. Barnass S, Franklin J, Tabaqchali S. The successful treatment of multiresistant nonenteric salmonellosis with seven day oral ciprofloxacin. *J Antimicrob Chemother*. 1990;25:299–300.

261. Soe G, Overturf G. Treatment of typhoid fever and other systemic salmonelloses with cefotaxime, ceftriaxone, cefoperazone, and other newer cephalosporins. *Rev Infect Dis*. 1987;9:719–736.

262. Holmberg SD, Osterholm MT, Senger KA, Cohen ML. Drug-resistant *Salmonella* from animals fed antimicrobials. *N Engl J Med*. 1984;311:617–622.

263. O'Brien TF, Hopkins JD, Gilleece ES, et al. Molecular epidemiology of antibiotic resistance in *Salmonella* from animals and human beings in the United States. *N Engl J Med*. 1982;307:1–6.

264. Lee LA, Puhr ND, Maloney EK, Bean NA, Tauxe RV. Increase in antimicrobial-resistant *Salmonella* infections in the United States, 1989–1990. *J Infect Dis*. 1994;170:128–134.

265. Threlfall EJ, Frost JA, Ward LR, Rowe B. Increasing spectrum of resistance in multiresistant *Salmonella typhimurium*. *Lancet*. 1996;347:1053–1054.

266. Workman MR, Philpott-Howard J, Bragman S, Britio-Babapulle F, Bellingham AJ. Emergence of ciprofloxacin resistance during treatment of Salmonella osteomyelitis in three patients with sickle cell disease. *J Infect*. 1996;32:27–32.

267. Khuri-Bulos NA, Abu Khalaf M, Shehabi A, Shami K. Foodhandler-associated *Salmonella* outbreak in a university hospital despite routine surveillance cultures of kitchen employees. *Infect Control Hosp Epidemiol*. 1994;15:311–314.

268. Dryden MS, Keyworth N, Gabb R, Stein K. Asymptomatic foodhandlers as the source of nosocomial salmonellosis. *J Hosp Infect*. 1994;28:195–208.

269. Keusch GT, Bennish ML. Shigellosis. In: Evans AS, Brachman PS, eds. *Bacterial Infections of Humans: Epidemiology and Control*. New York: Plenum Medical Book Co; 1991: 593–620.

270. Henry FJ, Alam N, Aziz KM, Rahaman MM. Dysentery, not watery diarrhoea, is associated with stunting in Bangladeshi children. *Hum Nutr Clin Nutr*. 1987;41:243–249.

271. Durant W. *The Life of Greece*. New York: Simon and Schuster; 1939: 239–242.

272. Hare R. Pomp and pestilence. In: *Infectious Disease, Its Origins, and Conquest*. New York: The Philosophical Library; 1955: 103–108.

273. McNeill WH. *Plagues and Peoples*. New York: Anchor Books, Doubleday; 1976: 251.

274. Philbrook FR, Gordon JE. Diarrhea and dysentery. In: Hoff EC, ed. *Communicable Disease Transmitted Chiefly Through Respiratory and Alimentary Tracts*. Vol 4. *Preventive Medicine in World War II*. Washington, DC: Office of the Surgeon General, US Department of the Army; 1958: 319–376.

275. Quin NE. The impact of diseases on military operations in the Persian Gulf. *Mil Med*. 1982;147:728–734.

276. Gear HS. Hygiene aspects of the El Alamein victory, 1942. *BMJ*. 1944;1:382–387.

277. Gentry LO, Hedlund KW, Wells RF, Ognibene AJ. Bacterial diarrheal diseases. In: Wells RF, ed. *General Medicine and Infectious Diseases*. Vol 2. *Internal Medicine in Vietnam*. Washington, DC: Office of the Surgeon General, US Department of the Army; 1977: 355–395.

278. Daniell FD, Crafton LD, Walz SE, Bolton HT. Field preventive medicine and epidemiologic surveillance: The Beirut, Lebanon experience, 1982. *Mil Med*. 1985;150:171–176.

279. Haberberger RL, Mikhail IA, Burans JP, et al. Travelers' diarrhea among United States military personnel during joint American–Egyptian armed forces exercises in Cairo, Egypt. *Mil Med*. 1991;156:27–30.

280. Sanchez JF. Gelnett J, Petruccelli, BP, DeFraites RF, Taylor DN. Diarrheal disease incidence and morbidity among United States military personnel during short-term missions overseas. *Am J Trop Med Hyg*. 1998;58:299–304.

281. Beecham III HJ, Lebron CI, Echeverria P. Short report: Impact of traveler's diarrhea on United States troops deployed to Thailand. *Am J Trop Med Hyg*. 1997;57:699–701.

282. Bourgeois AL, Gardiner CH, Thornton SA, et al. Etiology of acute diarrhea among United States military personnel deployed to South America and West Africa. *Am J Trop Med Hyg*. 1993;48:243–248.

283. Sharp TW, Thornton SA, Wallace MR, et al. Diarrheal disease among military personnel during Operation Restore Hope, Somalia, 1992–1993. *Am J Trop Med Hyg*. 1995;52:188–193.

284. Green MS, Block C, Cohen D, Slater PE. Four decades of shigellosis in Israel: Epidemiology of a growing public health problem. *Rev Infect Dis*. 1991;13:248–253.

285. Cohen D, Green M, Block C, et al. Reduction of transmission of shigellosis by control of houseflies (*Musca domestica*). *Lancet*. 1991;337:993–997.

286. Goma Epidemiology Working Group. Public health impact of the Rwandan refugee crisis: What happened in Goma, Zaire, in July 1994? *Lancet*. 1995;345:339–344.

287. DuPont HL, Levine MM, Hornick RB, Formal SB. Inoculum size in shigellosis and implications for expected mode of transmission. *J Infect Dis*. 1989;159;1126–1128.

288. Levine MM, DuPont HL, Formal SB, et al. Pathogenesis of *Shigella dysenteriae* (Shiga) dysentery. *J Infect Dis*. 1973;127:261–270.

289. Levine OS, Levine MM. Houseflies (*Musca domestica*) as mechanical vectors of shigellosis. *Rev Infect Dis*. 1991;13:688–696.

290. Khan MU. Interruption of shigellosis by hand washing. *Trans R Soc Trop Med Hyg*. 1982;76:164–168.

291. Boyce JM, Hughes JM, Alim AR, et al. Patterns of *Shigella* infection in families in rural Bangladesh. *Am J Trop Med Hyg*. 1982;31:1015–1020.

292. Centers for Disease Control and Prevention. Surveillance for waterborne-disease outbreaks—United States, 1993–1994. *MMWR*. 1996;45(SS-1):1–33.

293. DuPont HL. *Shigella* species (bacillary dysentery). In: Mandell GL, Douglas RG, Bennett JE, eds. *Principles and Practice of Infectious Diseases*. Vol. 2. New York: Churchill Livingstone; 1990: 1716–1722.

294. Islam MS, Hasan MK, Khan SI. Growth and survival of *Shigella flexneri* in common Bangladeshi foods under various conditions of time and temperature. *Appl Environ Microbiol*. 1993;59:652–654.

295. Hedberg CW, Levine WC, White KE, et al. An international foodborne outbreak of shigellosis associated with a commercial airline. *JAMA*. 1992;268:3208–3212.

296. Hardy A, Watt J. Studies of the acute diarrheal diseases, XVIII: Epidemiology. *Public Health Rep.* 1948;63:363.

297. Tuttle J, Ries AA, Chimba RM, Perera CU, Bean NH, Griffin PM. Antimicrobial-resistant epidemic *Shigella dysenteriae* type 1 in Zambia: Modes of transmission. *J Infect Dis.* 1995;171:371–375.

298. Blaser MJ, Pollard RA, Feldman RA. *Shigella* infections in the United States, 1974–1980. *J Infect Dis.* 1983;147:771–775.

299. Black RE, Craun GF, Blake PA. Epidemiology of common-source outbreaks of shigellosis in the United States, 1961–1975. *Am J Epidemiol.* 1978;108:47–52.

300. Pickering LK, Evans DG, DuPont HL, Vollet JJ, Evans Jr DJ. Diarrhea caused by *Shigella*, rotavirus, and *Giardia* in day-care centers: Prospective study. *J Pediatr.* 1981;99:51–56.

301. Pickering LK, Bartlett AV, Woodward WE. Acute infectious diarrhea among children in day care: Epidemiology and control. *Rev Infect Dis.* 1986;8:539–547.

302. Eyre JWH. Asylum dysentery in relation to *S. dysenteriae*. *BMJ.* 1904;1:1002–1004.

303. Merson MH, Tenney JH, Meyers JD, et al. Shigellosis at sea: An outbreak aboard a passenger cruise ship. *Am J Epidemiol.* 1975;101:165–175.

304. DuPont HL, Gangarosa EJ, Reller LB, et al. Shigellosis in custodial institutions. *Am J Epidemiol.* 1970;92:172–179.

305. Mildvan D, Gelb AM, William D. Venereal transmission of enteric pathogens in male homosexuals: Two case reports. *JAMA.* 1977;238:1387–1389.

306. Guerrant RL, Hughes JM, Lima NL, Crane J. Diarrhea in developed and developing countries: Magnitude, special settings, and etiologies. *Rev Infect Dis.* 1990;12:S41–S50.

307. Walsh JA, Warren KS. Selective primary health care: An interim strategy for disease control in developing countries. *N Engl J Med.* 1979;301:967–974.

308. Snyder JD, Merson MH. The magnitude of the global problem of acute diarrhoeal disease: A review of active surveillance data. *Bull World Health Organ.* 1982;60:605–613.

309. Institute of Medicine. The prospects for immunizing against *Shigella* spp. In: *New Vaccine Development: Establishing Priorities, Diseases of Importance in Developing Countries.* Vol 2. Washington, DC: National Academy Press; 1986: 329–337.

310. Mata LJ, Gangarosa EJ, Caceres A, Perera DR, Mejicanos ML. Epidemic Shiga bacillus dysentery in Central America, I: Etiologic investigations in Guatemala, 1969. *J Infect Dis.* 1970;122:170–180.

311. Gangarosa EJ, Perera DR, Mata LJ, Mendizabal-Morris C, Guzman G, Reller LB. Epidemic Shiga bacillus dysentery in Central America, II: Epidemiologic studies in 1969. *J Infect Dis.* 1970;122:181–190.

312. Ries AA, Wells JG, Olivola D, et al. Epidemic *Shigella dysenteriae* type 1 in Burundi: Panresistance and implications for prevention. *J Infect Dis.* 1994;169:1035–1041.

313. Rahaman MM, Khan MM, Aziz KM, Islam MS, Kibriya AK. An outbreak of dysentery caused by *Shigella dysenteriae* type 1 on a coral island in the Bay of Bengal. *J Infect Dis.* 1975;132:15–19.

314. Khan MU, Roy NC, Islam R, Huq I, Stoll B. Fourteen years of shigellosis in Dhaka: An epidemiological analysis. *Int J Epidemiol.* 1985;14:607–613.

315. Chin J, ed. *Control of Communicable Diseases Manual.* 17th ed. Washington, DC: American Public Health Association; 2000.

316. Azad MA, Islam M, Butler T. Colonic perforation in *Shigella dysenteriae* 1 infection. *Ped Infect Dis*. 1986;5:103–104.

317. Koster F, Levin J, Walker L, et al. Hemolytic-uremic syndrome after shigellosis: Relation to endotoxemia and circulating immune complexes. *N Engl J Med*. 1978;298:927–933.

318. Butler T, Islam MR, Bardhan PK. The leukemoid reaction in shigellosis. *Am J Dis Child*. 1984;138:162–165.

319. Barrett-Connor E, Conner JD. Extraintestinal manifestations of shigellosis. *Am J Gastroenterol*. 1970;53:234–245.

320. Struelens MJ, Patte D, Kabir I, Salam A, Nath SK, Butler T. *Shigella* septicemia: Prevalence, presentation, risk factors, and outcome. *J Infect Dis*. 1985;152:784–790.

321. Calin A, Fries JF. An experimental epidemic of Reiter's syndrome revisited: Follow-up evidence on genetic and environmental factors. *Ann Intern Med*. 1976;84:564–566.

322. Levine M, DuPont H, Khodabandelou M, Hornick RB. Long-term shigella-carrier state. *N Engl J Med*. 1973;288:1169–1171.

323. Mata LJ. *The Children of Santa Maria Cauque: A Prospective Field Study of Health and Growth*. Cambridge, Mass: MIT Press; 1978.

324. Ferreccio C, Prado V, Ojeda A, et al. Epidemiologic patterns of acute diarrhea and endemic *Shigella* infections in children in a poor periurban setting in Santiago, Chile. *Am J Epidemiol*. 1991;134:614–627.

325. Cohen D, Green MS, Block C, Slepon R, Ofek I. A prospective study on the association between serum antibodies to lipopolysaccharide and attack rate of shigellosis. *J Clin Microbiol*. 1991;29:386–389.

326. DuPont HL, Hornick RB, Snyder MJ, Libonati JP, Formal SB, Gangarosa EJ. Immunity in shigellosis, II: Protection induced by oral live vaccine or primary infection. *J Infect Dis*. 1972;125:12–16.

327. Herrington DA, Van de Verg L, Formal SB, et al. Studies in volunteers to evaluate candidate *Shigella* vaccines: Further experience with a bivalent *Salmonella typhi-Shigella sonnei* vaccine and protection conferred by previous *Shigella sonnei* disease. *Vaccine*. 1990;8:353–357.

328. Levine MM, Gangarosa EJ, Werner M, Morris GK. Shigellosis in custodial institutions, 3: Prospective clinical and bacteriologic surveillance of children vaccinated with oral attenuated *Shigella* vaccines. *J Pediatr*. 1974;84:803–806.

329. Morris GK, Koehler JA, Gangarosa EJ, Sharrar RG. Comparison of media for direct isolation and transport of shigellae from fecal specimens. *Appl Microbiol*. 1970;19:434–437.

330. Wells JG, Morris GK. Evaluation of transport methods for isolating *Shigella*. *J Clin Microbiol*. 1981;13:789–790.

331. Rahaman MM, Huq I, Dey CR. Superiority of MacConkey's agar over salmonella-shigella agar for isolation of *Shigella dysenteriae* type 1. *J Infect Dis*. 1975;131:700–703.

332. Echeverria P, Sethabutr O, Pitarangsi C. Microbiology and diagnosis of infections with *Shigella* and enteroinvasive *Escherichia coli*. *Rev Infect Dis*. 1991;13(Suppl 4):S220–S225.

333. Hunt AL, Goldsmid JM. An investigation of culture media for the isolation of shigellae. *Med Lab Sci*. 1990;47:151–157.

334. Gray LD. *Escherichia, Salmonella, Shigella,* and *Yersinia*. In: Murray Pr, Bayou EF, Pfaller MA, Tenover FC, Yollcen RH, eds. *Manual of Clinical Microbiology*. Washington, DC: American Society of Microbiology Press; 1995: 450–456.

335. Korzeniowski DM, Barada FA, Rouse JD, Guerrant RL. Value of examination for fecal leukocytes in the early diagnosis of shigellosis. *Am J Trop Med Hyg*. 1979;28:1031–1035.

336. Haltalin KC, Nelson JD, Ring 3rd R, Sladoje M, Hinton LV. Double-blind treatment study of shigellosis comparing ampicillin, sulfadiazine, and placebo. *J Pediatr*. 1967;70:970–981.

337. Tong MJ, Martin DG, Cunningham JJ, Gunning JJ. Clinical and bacteriological evaluation of antibiotic treatment in shigellosis. *JAMA*. 1970;214:1841–1844.

338. Murray BE. Resistance of *Shigella, Salmonella*, and other selected enteric pathogens to antimicrobial agents. *Rev Infect Dis*. 1986;8(Suppl 2):S172–S181.

339. Shahid NS, Rahaman MM, Haider K, Banu H, Rahman N. Changing pattern of resistant Shiga bacillus (*Shigella dysenteriae* type 1) and *Shigella flexneri* in Bangladesh. *J Infect Dis*. 1985;152:1114–1119.

340. Paniker CK, Vimala KN, Bhat P, Stephen S. Drug-resistant shigellosis in South India. Indian *J Med Res*. 1978;68:413–417.

341. Frost JA, Rowe B, Vandepitte J, Threlfall EJ. Plasmid characterization in the investigation of an epidemic caused by multiply resistant *Shigella dysenteriae* type 1 in Central Africa. *Lancet*. 1981;2:1074–1076.

342. Bennish M, Eusof A, Kay B, Wierzba T. Multiresistant *Shigella* infections in Bangladesh. *Lancet*. 1985;2:441.

343. Macaden R, Bhat P. The changing pattern of resistance to ampicillin and co-trimoxazole in *Shigella* serotypes in Bangalore, southern India. *J Infect Dis*. 1985;152:1348.

344. Munshi MH, Sack DA, Haider K, Ahmed ZU, Rahaman MM, Morshed MG. Plasmid-mediated resistance to nalidixic acid in *Shigella dysenteriae* type 1. *Lancet*. 1987;2:419–421.

345. Taylor DN, Bodhidatta L, Brown JE, et al. Introduction and spread of multi-resistant *Shigella dysenteriae* I in Thailand. *Am J Trop Med Hyg*. 1989;40:77–85.

346. Martin DG, Tong MJ, Ewald PE, Kelly HV. Antibiotic sensitivities of *Shigella* isolates in Vietnam, 1968–1969. *Mil Med*. 1970;135:560–562.

347. Pickering LK, DuPont HL, Olarte J. Single-dose tetracycline therapy for shigellosis in adults. *JAMA*. 1978;239:853–854.

348. Bassily S, Hyams KC, El-Masry NA, et al. Short-course norfloxacin and trimethoprim-sulfamethoxazole treatment of shigellosis and salmonellosis in Egypt. *Am J Trop Med Hyg*. 1994;51:219–223.

349. Rogerie F, Ott D, Vandepitte J, Verbist L, Lemmens P, Habiyaremye I. Comparison of norfloxacin and nalidixic acid for treatment of dysentery caused by *Shigella dysenteriae* type 1 in adults. *Antimicrob Agents Chemother*. 1986;29:883–886.

350. Bennish ML, Salam MA, Khan WA, Khan AM. Treatment of shigellosis, III: Comparison of one- or two-dose ciprofloxacin with standard 5-day therapy, a randomized, blinded trial. *Ann Intern Med*. 1992;117:727–734.

351. Gotuzzo E, Oberhelman RA, Maguina C, et al. Comparison of single-dose treatment with norfloxacin and standard 5-day treatment with trimethoprim-sulfamethoxazole for acute shigellosis in adults. *Antimicrob Agents Chemother*. 1989;33:1101–1104.

352. Ashkenazi S, Amir J, Waisman Y, et al. A randomized, double-blind study comparing cefixime and trimethoprim-sulfamethoxazole in the treatment of childhood shigellosis. *J Pediatr*. 1993;123:817–821.

353. DuPont HL, Hornick R. Adverse effects of Lomotil therapy in shigellosis. *JAMA*. 1973;226:1525–1528.

354. Murphy GS, Bodhidatta L, Echeverria P, et al. Ciprofloxacin and loperamide in the treatment of bacillary dysentery. *Ann Intern Med*. 1993;118:582–586.

355. World Health Organization. Research priorities for diarrhoeal disease vaccines: Memorandum from a WHO meeting. *Bull World Health Organ*. 1991;69:667–676.

356. World Health Organization. Development of vaccines against shigellosis: Memorandum from a WHO meeting. *Bull World Health Organ*. 1987;65:17–25.

357. Hale TL. Shigella Vaccines. In: Ala' Aldeen DAA, Hormaeche CE, eds. *Molecular and Clinical Aspects of Bacterial Vaccine Development.* John Wiley & Sons; 1995: 179–204.

358. Robbins JB, Chu C-Y, Schneerson R. Hypothesis for vaccine development: Protective immunity to enteric diseases caused by nontyphoidal *Salmonellae* and *Shigellae* may be conferred by serum IgG antibodies to the O-specific polysaccharide of their lipopolysaccharides. *Clin Infect Dis.* 1992;15:346–361.

359. Taylor DN, Trofa AC, Sadoff J, et al. Synthesis, characterization, and clinical evaluation of conjugate vaccines composed of the O-specific polysaccharides of *Shigella dysenteriae* type 1, *Shigella flexneri* type 2, *Shigella sonnei* (*Plesiomonas shigelloides*) bound to bacterial toxoids. *Infect Immun.* 1993;61:3678–3687.

360. Cohen D, Ashkenazi S, Green MS, et al. Safety and immunogenicity of investigational *Shigella* conjugate vaccines in Israeli volunteers. *Infect Immun.* 1996;64:4074–4077.

361. Cohen D, Ashkenazi S, Green MS, et al. Double-blind vaccine-controlled randomized efficacy trial of an investigational *Shigella sonnei* conjugate vaccine in young adults. *Lancet.* 1997;349:155–159.

362. Taylor DN, Research Coordinator for Prevention of Diarrheal Disease, Walter Reed Army Institute of Research. Oral communication, 2000.

363. Barua D. History of cholera. In: Barua D, Greenough III WB, eds. *Cholera.* New York: Plenum Medical Book Co: 1992: 1–24.

364. MacPherson J. *Annals of Cholera from the Earliest Periods to the Year 1817.* London: HK Lewis; 1884.

365. Gaskoin G. On the literature on cholera. *Medico-Chirurgical Rev.* 1867;40:217–232 (English translation of work of Gaspar Correa).

366. MacNamara C. *A History of Asiatic Cholera.* London: MacMillan and Co; 1876.

367. Lacey SW. Cholera: Calamitous past, ominous future. *Clin Infect Dis.* 1995;20:1409–1419.

368. Pollitzer R. Cholera. In: Monograph No. 43. Geneva, Switzerland: World Health Organization; 1959.

369. Albert MJ, Siddique AK, Islam MS, et al. A large outbreak of clinical cholera due to *Vibrio cholerae* non-O1 in Bangladesh. *Lancet.* 1993;341:704.

370. Nair GB, Ramamurthy T, Bhattacharya SK, et al. Spread of *Vibrio cholerae* O139 Bengal in India. *J Infect Dis.* 1994;169:1029–1034.

371. Sack RB, Albert MJ, Siddique AK. Emergence of *Vibrio cholerae* O139. *Curr Clin Topics Infect Dis.* 1996;16:172–193.

372. Popovic T, Fields PI, Olsvik O, et al. Molecular subtyping of toxigenic *Vibrio cholerae* O139 causing epidemic cholera in India and Bangladesh, 1992–1993. *J Infect Dis.* 1995;171:122–127.

373. Echeverria P, Hoge CW, Bodhidatta L, et al. Molecular characterization of *Vibrio cholerae* O139 isolates from Asia. *Am J Trop Med Hyg.* 1995;52:124–127.

374. Dalsgaard A, Nielsen GL, Echeverria P, Larsen JL, Schonheyder HC. *Vibrio cholerae* O139 in Denmark. *Lancet.* 1995;345:1637–1638.

375. Centers for Disease Control and Prevention. Morbidity and mortality surveillance in Rwandan refugees—Burundi and Zaire, 1994. *MMWR.* 1996;45:104–107.

376. Siddique AK, Salam A, Islam MS, et al. Why treatment centres failed to prevent cholera deaths among Rwandan refugees in Goma, Zaire. *Lancet.* 1995;345:359–361.

377. Tauxe R, Seminario L, Tapia R, Libel M. The Latin American epidemic. In: Wachsmuth IK, Blake PA, Olsvik O, eds. Vibrio cholerae *and Cholera: Molecular to Global Perspectives*. Washington, DC: American Society for Microbiology; 1994: 321–344.

378. Sanchez JL, Taylor KN. Cholera. *Lancet*. 1997;349:1825–1830.

379. Besser RE, Feikin DR, Eberhart-Phillips JE, Mascola L, Griffin PM. Diagnosis and treatment of cholera in the United States: Are we prepared? *JAMA*. 1994;272:1203–1205.

380. Kaper JB, Morris JG Jr, Levine MM. Cholera. *Clin Microbiol Rev*. 1995;8:48–86. Published erratum: *Clin Microbiol Rev*. 1995;8:316.

381. Waldor MK, Mekalanos JJ. ToxR regulates virulence gene expression in non-O1 strains of *Vibrio cholerae* that cause epidemic cholera. *Infect Immun*. 1994;62:72–78.

382. Swerdlow DL, Ries AA. *Vibrio cholerae* non-O1—the eighth pandemic? *Lancet*. 1993;342:382–383.

383. Sakazaki R, Tamuru K. Somatic antigen variation in *Vibrio cholerae*. *Japan J Med Sci Biol*. 1971;24:93–100.

384. Hall RH, Khambaty FM, Kothary M, Keasler SP. Non-O1 *Vibrio cholerae*. *Lancet*. 1993;342:430.

385. Morris JG, the Cholera Laboratory Task Force. *Vibrio cholerae* O139 Bengal. In: Wachsmuth IK, Blake PA, Olsvik O, eds. Vibrio cholerae *and Cholera: Molecular to Global Perspectives*. Washington, DC: American Society for Microbiology; 1994: 95–115.

386. Islam MS, Hasan MK, Miah MA, et al. Isolation of *Vibrio cholerae* O139 Bengal from water in Bangladesh. *Lancet*. 1993;342:430.

387. Colwell RR, Huq A. Vibrios in the environment: Viable but nonculturable *Vibrio cholerae*. In: Wachsmuth IK, Blake PA, Olsvik O, eds. Vibrio cholerae *and Cholera: Molecular to Global Perspectives*. Washington, DC: American Society for Microbiology; 1994: 117–133.

388. Kolvin JL, Roberts D. Studies on the growth of *Vibrio cholerae* biotype El Tor and biotype classical in foods. *J Hyg (Lond)*. 1982;89:243–252.

389. Morris JG Jr, Sztein MB, Rice EW, et al. *Vibrio cholerae* O1 can assume a chlorine-resistant rugose survival form that is virulent for humans. *J Infect Dis*. 1996;174:1364–1368.

390. Deb BC, Sircar BK, Sengupta PG, et al. Studies on interventions to prevent El Tor cholera transmission in urban slums. *Bull World Health Organ*. 1986;64:127–131.

391. Glass RI, Black RE. The epidemiology of cholera. In: Barua D, Greenough III WB, eds. *Cholera*. New York: Plenum Medical Book Co; 1992: 129–154.

392. Shears P. Cholera. *Ann Trop Med Parasitol*. 1994;88:109–122.

393. Goodgame RW, Greenough WB. Cholera in Africa: A message for the West. *Ann Intern Med*. 1975;82:101–106.

394. Swerdlow DL, Mintz ED, Rodriguez M, et al. Waterborne transmission of epidemic cholera in Trujillo, Peru: Lessons for a continent at risk. *Lancet*. 1992;340:28–32.

395. Glass RI, Becker S, Huq MI, et al. Endemic cholera in rural Bangladesh, 1966–1980. *Am J Epidemiol*. 1982;116:959–970.

396. Dizon JJ, Fukumi H, Barua D, et al. Studies on cholera carriers. *Bull World Health Organ*. 1967;37:737–743.

397. Feachem RG. Environmental aspects of cholera epidemiology, III: Transmission and control. *Trop Dis Bull*. 1982;79:1–47.

398. Kelly MT, Hickman-Brenner FW, Farmer III JJ. Vibrio. In: Balows A, Hausler WJ, Herrmann KO, Isenberg HD, Shadomy HJ, eds. *Manual of Clinical Microbiology*. Washington, DC: American Society for Microbiology; 1991: 384–395.

399. Benenson AS, Islam MR, Grenough III WB. Rapid identification of *Vibrio cholerae* by darkfield microscopy. *Bull World Health Organ*. 1964;30:827–831.

400. Colwell RR, Hasan JA, Huq A, et al. Development and evaluation of a rapid, simple, sensitive, monoclonal antibody-based co-agglutination test for direct detection of *Vibrio cholerae* O1. *FEMS Microbiol Lett*. 1992;96:215–219.

401. Hasan JA, Huq A, Tamplin ML, Siebeling RJ, Colwell RR. A novel kit for rapid detection of *Vibrio cholerae* O1. *J Clin Microbiol*. 1994;32:249–252.

402. Hasan JA, Huq A, Nair GB, et al. Development and testing of monoclonal antibody-based rapid immunodiagnostic test kits for direct detection of *Vibrio cholerae* O139 synonym Bengal. *J Clin Microbiol*. 1995;33:2935–2939.

403. Ramamurthy T, Bhattacharya SK, Uesaka Y, et al. Evaluation of the bead enzyme-linked immunosorbent assay for detection of cholera toxin directly from stool specimens. *J Clin Microbiol*. 1992;30:1783–1786.

404. Sack RB, Sack DA. Immunologic methods for the diagnosis of infections by Enterobacteriaceae and Vibrionaceae. In: Rose NR, Conway de Macario E, Fahey JL, Friedman H, Penn GM, eds. *Manual of Clinical Laboratory Immunology*. Washington, DC: American Society for Microbiology; 1992: 482–488.

405. Barrett TJ, Feeley JC. Serologic diagnosis of *Vibrio cholerae* O1 infections. In: Wachsmuth IK, Blake PA, Olsvik O, eds. Vibrio cholerae *and Cholera: Molecular to Global Perspectives*. Washington, DC: American Society for Microbiology; 1994: 135–141.

406. Levine MM, Black RE, Clements ML, Nalin DR, Cisneros L, Finkelstein RA. Volunteer studies in development of vaccines against cholera and enterotoxigenic *Escherichia coli*: A review. In: Holme T, Holmgren J, Merson MH, Mollby R, eds. *Acute Enteric Infections in Children: New Prospects for Treatment and Prevention*. Amsterdam: Elsevier/North-Holland Biomedical Press; 1981: 443–459.

407. Cash RA, Music SI, Libonati JP, Snyder MJJ, Wenzel RP, Hornick RB. Response of man to infection with *Vibrio cholerae*, I: Clinical, serologic, and bacteriologic responses to known inoculum. *J Infect Dis*. 1974;129:45–52.

408. van Loon FP, Clemens JD, Shahrier M, et al. Low gastric acid as a risk factor for cholera transmission: Application of a new, non-invasive gastric acid field test. *J Clin Epidemiol*. 1990;43:1361–1367.

409. Glass RI, Holmgren J, Haley CE, et al. Predisposition for cholera of individuals with O blood group: Possible evolutionary significance. *Am J Epidemiol*. 1985;121:791–796.

410. Clemens JD, Sack DA, Harris JR, et al. ABO blood groups and cholera: New observations on specificity of risk and modification of vaccine efficacy. *J Infect Dis*. 1989;159:770–773.

411. Glass RI, Svennerholm AM, Stoll BJ, et al. Protection against cholera in breast-fed children by antibodies in breast milk. *N Engl J Med*. 1983;308:1389–1392.

412. Gangarosa EJ, Mosley WH. Epidemiology and surveillance of cholera. In: Barua D, Burrows W, eds. *Cholera*. Philadelphia: WB Saunders; 1974: 381–403.

413. Begue RE, Castellares G, Hayashi KE, et al. Diarrheal disease in Peru after the introduction of cholera. *Am J Trop Med Hyg*. 1994;51:585–589.

414. Battacharya SK, Battacharya MK, Nair GB, et al. Clinical profile of acute diarrhoea cases infected with the new epidemic strain of *Vibrio cholerae* O139: Designation of the disease as cholera. *J Infect*. 1993;27:11–15.

415. Mahalanabis D, Faruque AS, Albert MJ, Salam MA, Hoque SS. An epidemic of cholera due to *Vibrio cholerae* O139 in Dhaka, Bangladesh: Clinical and epidemiological features. *Epidemiol Infect*. 1994;112:463–471.

416. Dhar U, Bennish ML, Khan WA, et al. Clinical features, antimicrobial susceptibility, and toxin production in *Vibrio cholerae* O139 infection: Comparison with *V. cholerae* O1 infection. *Trans Roy Soc Trop Med Hyg.* 1996;90:402–405.

417. Water with sugar and salt. *Lancet.* 1978;2:300–301. Editorial.

418. Bennish ML. Cholera: Pathophysiology, clinical features, and treatment. In: Wachsmuth IK, Blake PA, Olsvik O, eds. Vibrio cholerae *and Cholera: Molecular to Global Perspectives.* Washington, DC: American Society for Microbiology; 1994: 229–255.

419. Khan WA, Bennish ML, Seas C, et al. Randomized controlled comparison of single-dose ciprofloxacin and doxycycline for cholera caused by *Vibrio cholerae* O1 or O139. *Lancet.* 1996;348:296–300.

420. Gotuzzo E, Seas C, Echevarria J, Carrillo C, Mostorino R, Ruiz R. Ciprofloxacin for the treatment of cholera: A randomized, double-blind, controlled clinical trial of a single daily dose in Peruvian adults. *Clin Infect Dis.* 1995;20:1485–1490.

421. Yamamoto T, Nair GB, Albert MJ, Parodi CC, Takeda Y. Survey of in vitro susceptibilities of *Vibrio cholerae* O1 and O139 to antimicrobial agents. *Antimicrob Agents Chemother.* 1995;39:241–244.

422. Mitra R, Basu A, Dutta D, Nair GB, Takeda Y. Resurgence of *Vibrio cholerae* O139 Bengal with altered antibiogram in Calcutta, India. *Lancet.* 1996;348:1181.

423. Barua D, Merson MH. Prevention and control of cholera. In: Barua D, Greenough III WB, eds. *Cholera.* New York: Plenum Medical Book Co; 1992: 329–349.

424. Vugia DJ, Rodriguez M, Vargas R, et al. Epidemic cholera in Trujillo, Peru 1992: Utility of a clinical case definition and shift in *Vibrio cholerae* O1 serotype. *Am J Trop Med Hyg.* 1994;50:566–569.

425. Clark RN. The purification of water on a small scale. *Bull World Health Organ.* 1956;14:820–826.

426. Deb BC, Sircar BK, Sengupta PG, et al. Intra-familial transmission of *Vibrio cholerae* biotype El Tor in Calcutta slums. *Indian J Med Res.* 1982;76:814–819.

427. Echevarria J, Seas C, Carrillo C, Mostorino R, Ruiz R, Gotuzzo E. Efficacy and tolerability of ciprofloxacin prophylaxis in adult household contacts of patients with cholera. *Clin Infect Dis.* 1995;20:1480–1484.

428. Mhalu FS, Mmari PW, Ijumba J. Rapid emergence of El Tor *Vibrio cholerae* resistant to antimicrobial agents during the first six months of the fourth cholera epidemic in Tanzania. *Lancet.* 1979;1:345–347.

429. Feeley JC, Gangarosa EJ. Field trials of cholera vaccine. In: *Cholera and Related Diarrheas: 43rd Nobel Symposium, Stockholm, Sweden, 1978.* Basel, Switzerland: S. Karger; 1980: 204–210.

430. Joo I. Cholera vaccines. In: Barua D, Burrows W, eds. *Cholera.* Philadelphia: WB Saunders; 1974: 333–335.

431. Holmgren J, Osek J, Svennerholm AM. Protective oral cholera vaccine based on a combination of cholera toxin B subunit and inactivated cholera vibrios. In: Wachsmuth IK, Blake PA, Olsvik O, eds. Vibrio cholerae *and Cholera: Molecular to Global Perspectives.* Washington, DC: American Society for Microbiology; 1994: 415–424.

432. Clemens JD, Sack DA, Harris JR, et al. Field trial of oral cholera vaccines in Bangladesh: Results from three-year follow-up. *Lancet.* 1990;335:270–273.

433. van Loon FP, Clemens JD, Chakraborty J, et al. Field trial of inactivated oral cholera vaccines in Bangladesh: Results from 5 years of follow-up. *Vaccine.* 1996;14:162–166.

434. Sanchez JL, Trofa AF, Taylor DN, et al. Safety and immunogenicity of the oral, whole cell/recombinant B subunit cholera vaccine in North American volunteers. *J Infect Dis.* 1993;167:1446–1449.

435. Sanchez JL, Vasquez B, Begue RE, et al. Protective efficacy of oral whole-cell/recombinant-B-subunit cholera vaccine in Peruvian military recruits. *Lancet*. 1994;344:1273–1276.

436. Taylor DN, Cardenas V, Sanchez JL, et al. Two-year study of the protective efficacy of the oral whole cell plus recombinant B subunit cholera vaccine in Peru. *J Infect Dis*. 2000;181:1667–1673.

437. Trach DD, Clemens JD, Ke NT, et al. Field trial of a locally produced, killed, oral cholera vaccine in Vietnam. *Lancet*. 1997;349:231–235.

438. Taylor DN, Sanchez JL, Cardenas V, Gilman RE, Sadoff J. Jury still out on dosage regimen for oral inactivated WC/rCTB cholera vaccine. *J Infect Dis*. In press.

439. Tacket CO, Losonsky G, Nataro JP, et al. Onset and duration of protective immunity in challenged volunteers after vaccination with live oral cholera vaccine CVD 103–HgR. *J Infect Dis*. 1992;166:837–841.

440. Levine MM, Tacket CO. Recombinant live cholera vaccines. In: Wachsmuth IK, Blake PA, Olsvik O, eds. Vibrio cholerae *and Cholera: Molecular to Global Perspectives*. Washington, DC: American Society for Microbiology; 1994:395–413.

441. Richie EE, Punjabi NH, Disharta YY, et al. Efficacy trial of single-dose live oral cholera vaccine CVD 103-HgR in north Jakarta, Indonesia, a cholera-endemic area. *Vaccine*. 2000;18:2399–2410.

442. Morris JG Jr, Losonsky GE, Johnson JA, et al. Clinical and immunologic characteristics of *Vibrio cholerae* O139 Bengal infection in North American volunteers. *J Infect Dis*. 1995;171:903–908.

443. Taylor DN, Killeen KP, Hack DC, et al. Development of a live, oral, attenuated vaccine against El Tor cholera. *J Infect Dis*. 1994;170:1518–1523.

444. Tacket CO, Morris JG, Losonsky GA, et al. Volunteer studies investigating the pathogenicity of *Vibrio cholerae* O139 and the protective efficacy conferred by both primary infection and by vaccine strain CVD 112. In: *Proceedings of the 30th Joint Conference on Cholera and Related Diarrheal Diseases*. Fukuoka, Japan: US–Japan Cooperative Medical Science Program; 1994: 142–147.

445. Waldor MK, Coster TS, Killeen KP, et al. Vibrio cholerae O139: Genetic analysis, immunobiology, and volunteer studies of live attenuated vaccines. In: *Proceedings of the 30th Joint Conference on Cholera and Related Diarrheal Diseases*. Fukuoka, Japan: US–Japan Cooperative Medical Science Program; 1994: 148–152.

446. Coster TS, Killeen KP, Waldor MK, et al. Safety, immunogenicity, and efficacy of live attenuated *Vibrio cholerae* O139 vaccine prototype. *Lancet*. 1995;345:949–952.

447. Ryan ET, Calderwood SB. Cholera vaccines. *J Infect Dis*. 2000;31:561–565.

448. Levine MM. Oral vaccines against cholera: Lessons from Vietnam and elsewhere. *Lancet*. 1997;349:220–221.

449. World Health Organization. The potential role of new cholera vaccines in the prevention and control of cholera outbreaks during acute emergencies: Report of a meeting. 13–14 February 1995. Geneva, Switzerland. Document No. CDR/GPV/95.1.

450. Legros D, Paquet C, Perea W, et al. Mass vaccination with a two-dose oral cholera vaccine in a refugee camp. *Bull World Health Organ*. 1999;77:837–842.

451. Naficy A, Rao MR, Paquet C, Antona D, Sorkin A, Clemens JD. Treatment and vaccination strategies to control cholera in sub-Saharan refugee settings. *JAMA*. 1998;279:521–525.

452. Ognibene A, Wells R. Amebiasis and other parasistic diseases. In: Ognibene A, Barrett O, eds. *General Medicine and Infectious Diseases*. Vol. 2. *Internal Medicine in Vietnam*. Washington, DC: Office of the Surgeon General and Center for Military History, US Army, 1982; 397–412.

453. Brumpt E. Étude sommaire de l' *"Entamoeba dispar"* n. sp. Amibe á kystes quadrinuclées, parasite de l'homme. *Bull Acad Med (Paris).* 1925;94:943–952.

454. Sargeaunt PG, Williams JE, Grene JD. The differentiation of invasive and non-invasive *Entamoeba histolytica* by isoenzyme electrophoresis. *Trans R Soc Trop Med Hyg.* 1978;72:519–521.

455. Petri WA Jr, Jackson TF, Gathiram V, et al. Pathogenic and nonpathogenic strains of *Entamoeba histolytica* can be differentiated by monoclonal antibodies to the galactose-specific adherence lectin. *Infect Immun.* 1990;58:1802–1806.

456. Tannich E, Horstmann RD, Knobloch J, Arnold HH. Genomic DNA differences between pathogenic and non-pathogenic *Entamoeba histolytica. Proc Natl Acad Sci USA.* 1989;86:5118–5122.

457. Clark CG, Diamond LS. The Laredo strain and other *"Entamoeba histolytica*-like" amoebae are *Entamoeba moshkovskii. Mol Blochem Parasitol.* 1991;46(l):11–18.

458. Walsh JA. Prevalence of *Entamoeba histolytica* infection. In: Ravdin JI, ed. *Amebiasis: Human Infection by* Entamoeba histolytica. New York: John Wiley and Sons; 1988: 93–105.

459. World Health Organization. *The World Health Report 1995: Bridging the Gaps; Report of the Director-General.* Geneva: WHO; 1996.

460. Caballero-Salcedo A, Viveros-Rogel M, Salvatierra B, et al. Seroepidemiology of amebiasis in Mexico. *Am J Trop Med Hyg.* 1994;50:412–419.

461. Petri WA Jr, Clark GC, Mann BJ, Braga LL. International seminar on amoebiasis. *Parasitol Today.* 1993;9:73.

462. Haque R, Faruque AS, Hahn P, Lyerly DM, Petri WA Jr. *Entamoeba histolytica* and *Entamoeba dispar* infection in children in Bangladesh. *J Infect Dis.* 1997;175:734–736.

463. Weinke T, Friedrich-Janicke B, Hopp P, Janitschke K. Prevalence and clinical importance of *Entamoeba histolytica* in two high-risk groups: Travelers returning from the tropics and male homosexuals. *J Infect Dis.* 1990;161:1029–1031.

464. de Lalla F, Rinaldi E, Santoro D, Nicolin R, Tramarin A. Outbreak of *Entamoeba histolytica* and *Giardia lamblia* in travellers returning from the tropics. *Infection.* 1992;20(2):78–82.

465. Ravdin JI, Guerrant RL. Role of adherence in cytopathogenic mechanisms of *Entamoeba histolytica*: Study with mammalian tissue culture cells and human erythrocytes. *J Clin Invest.* 1981;68:1305–1313.

466. Ravdin JI, John JE, Johnston LI, Innes DJ, Guerrant RL. Adherence of *Entamoeba histolytica* trophozoites to rat and human colonic mucosa. *Infect Immun.* 1985;48:292–297.

467. Aristizabal H, Acevedo J, Botero M. Fulminant amebic colitis. *World J Surg.* 1991;15:216–221.

468. Haque R, Neville LM, Hahn P, Petri WA Jr. Rapid diagnosis of *Entamoeba* infection by using *Entamoeba* and *Entamoeba histolytica* stool antigen detection kits. *J Clin Microbiology.* 1995;33(10):2558–2561.

469. Kagan IG. Serologic diagnosis of parasitic diseases. *N Engl J Med.* 1970;282:685–686.

470. Ximenez C, Leyva, O, Moran P, et al. *Entamoeba histolytica*: Antibody response to recent and past invasive events. *Ann Trop Med Parasitol.* 1993;87:31–39.

471. Ralls PW, Barnes PF, Radin DR, Colletti P, Halls J. Sonographic features of amebic and pyogenic liver abscesses: A blinded comparison. *Am J Roentgenol.* 1987;149:499–501.

472. Radin DR, Ralls PW, Colletti PM, Halls JM. CT of amebic liver abscess. *Am J Roentgenol.* 1987;150:1297–1301.

473. Elizondo G, Weissleder R, Stark DD, et al. Amebic liver abscess: Diagnosis and treatment evaluation with MR imaging. *Radiology.* 1987;165:795–800.

474. Abd-Alla MD, Jackson TF, Gathiram V, el-Hawey AM, Ravdin JI. Differentiation of pathogenic *Entamoeba histolytica* infections from nonpathogenic infections by detection of galactose-inhibitable adherence protein antigen in sera and feces. *J Clin Microbiol*. 1993;31:2845–2850.

475. Hill DR. *Giardia lamblia*. In: Mandell GL, Bennett JE, Dolin R, eds. *Principles and Practice of Infectious Diseases*. 4th ed. New York: Churchill Livingstone; 1995: 2487–2492.

476. Malone JD, Paparello S, Thornton S, Mapes T, Haberberger R, Hyams KC. Parasitic Infection in troops returning from Operation Desert Storm. *N Engl J Med*. 1991;325:1448–1449.

477. Laxer MA. Potential exposure of Utah Army National Guard personnel to giardiasis during field training exercises: A preliminary survey. *Mil Med*. 1985;150:23–26.

478. Erlandsen SL, Sherlock LA, Januschka M, et al. Cross-species transmission of *Giardia* spp.: Inoculation of beavers and muskrats with cysts of human, beaver, mouse, and muskrat origin. *Appl Environ Microbiol*. 1988;54:2777–2785.

479. Osterholm MT, Forfang JC, Ristinen TL, et al. An outbreak of foodborne giardiasis. *N Engl J Med*. 1981;304:24–28.

480. Oyerinde JP, Ogunbi O, Alonge AA. Age and sex distribution of infections with *Entamoeba histolytica* and *Giardia intestinalis* in the Lagos population. *Int J Epidemiol*. 1977;6:231–234.

481. Pickering LK, Woodward WE, DuPont HL, Sullivan P. Occurrence of *Giardia lamblia* in children in day care centers. *J Pediatr*. 1984;104:522–526.

482. Quinn TC, Stamm WE, Goodell SE, et al. The polymicrobial origin of intestinal infections in homosexual men. *N Engl J Med*. 1983;309:576–582.

483. Reiner DS, McCaffery M, Gillin FD. Sorting of cyst wall proteins to a regulated secretory pathway during differentiation of the primitive eukaryote, *Giardia lamblia*. *Eur J Cell Biol*. 1990;53:142–153.

484. Nash TE, Herrington DA, Levine MM, Conrad JT, Merritt JW Jr. Antigenic variation of *Giardia lamblia* in experimental human infections. *J Immunol*. 1990;144:4362–4369.

485. Hopkins RS, Juranek DD. Acute giardiasis: An improved clinical case definition for epidemiologic studies. *Am J Epidemiol*. 1991;133:402–407.

486. Tracy JW, Webster LT. Drugs used in the chemotherapy of protozoal infections: Trypanosomiasis, leishmaniasis, amebiasis, giardiasis, trichomoniasis, and other protozoal infections. In: Hardman JG, Limbird LE, eds. *Goodman & Gilman's The Pharmacological Basis of Therapeutics*. 9th ed. New York: McGraw Hill; 1996: 987–1008.

487. Kahn FH, Visscher BR. Water disinfection in the wilderness: A simple, effective method of iodination. *West J Med*. 1975;122:450–453.

488. Ungar BLP. *Cryptosporidium*. In: Mandel GL, Bennett JE, Dolin R, eds. *Principles and Practice of Infectious Diseases*. 4th ed. New York: Churchill Livingstone; 1995: 2500–2510.

489. Ma P, Kaufman DL, Helmick CG, D'Souza AJ, Navin TR. Cryptosporidiosis in tourists returning from the Caribbean. *N Engl J Med*. 1985;312:647–648.

490. Taylor DN, Houston R, Shlim DR, Bhaibulaya M, Ungar BL, Echeverria P. Etiology of diarrhea among travelers and foreign residents in Nepal. *JAMA*. 1988;260:1245–1248.

491. DuPont HL, Chappell CL, Sterling CR, Okhuysen PC, Rose JB, Jakubowski W. Infectivity of *Cryptosporidium parvum* in healthy volunteers. *N Engl J Med*. 1995;332:855–859.

492. Haas CN, Rose JB. Reconciliation of microbial risk models and outbreak epidemiology: The case of the Milwaukee outbreak. In: *Proceedings of the American Water Works Association 1994 Annual Conference: Water Quality*. Denver: American Water Works Association; 1994: 517–523.

493. Juranek DD. Cryptosporidiosis: Sources of infection and guidelines for prevention. *Clin Infect Dis*. 1995;21(Suppl 1):S57–S61.

494. Hayes EB, Matte TD, O'Brien TR, et al. Large community outbreak of cryptosporidiosis due to contamination of a filtered public water supply. *N Engl J Med*. 1989;320:1372–1376.

495. MacKenzie WR, Hoxie NJ, Proctor ME, et al. A massive outbreak in Milwaukee of *Cryptosporidium* infection transmitted through the public water supply. *N Engl J Med*. 1994;331:161–167.

496. McAnuity JM, Fleming DW, Gonzalez AH. A community-wide outbreak of cryptosporidiosis associated with swimming at a wave pool. *JAMA*. 1994;272:1597–1600.

497. Cordell RL, Addiss DG. Cryptosporidiosis in child care settings: A review of the literature and recommendations for prevention and control. *Pediatr Infect Dis J*. 1994;13:310–317.

498. Hojlyng N, Holten-Andersen W, Jepsen S. Cryptosporidiosis: A case of airborne transmission. *Lancet*. 1987;2:271–272.

499. Kuhls TL, Mosier DA, Crawford DL, Griffis J. Seroprevalence of cryptosporidial antibodies during infancy, childhood, and adolescence. *Clin Infect Dis*. 1994;18:731–735.

500. Ungar BL, Mulligan M, Nutman TB. Serologic evidence of *Cryptosporidium* infection in US volunteers before and during Peace Corps service in Africa. *Arch Intern Med*. 1989;149:894–897.

501. MacKenzie WR, Schell WL, Blair KA, et al. Massive outbreak of waterborne *Cryptosporidium* infection in Milwaukee, Wisconsin: Recurrence of illness and risk of secondary transmission. *Clin Infect Dis*. 1995;21:57–62.

502. Jokipii L, Jokipii AM. Timing of symptoms and oocyst excretion in human cryptosporidiosis. *N Engl J Med*. 1986;315:1643–1647.

503. Goodgame RW. Understanding intestinal spore-forming protozoa: *Cryptosporidia, Microsporidia, Isospora*, and *Cyclospora*. *Ann Intern Med*. 1996;124:429–441.

504. Alles AJ, Waldron MA, Sierra LS, Mattia AR. Prospective comparison of direct immunofluorescence and conventional staining methods for detection of *Giardia* and *Cryptosporidium* spp. in human fecal specimens. *J Clin Microbiol*. 1995;33:1632–1634.

505. White AC Jr, Chappell CL, Hayat CS, Kimball KT, Flanigan TP, Goodgame RW. Paromomycin for cryptosporidiosis in AIDS: A prospective, double-blind trial. *J Infect Dis*. 1994;170:419–424.

506. Centers for Disease Control and Prevention. Assessing the public health threat associated with waterborne cryptosporidiosis: Report of a workshop. *MMWR*. 1995;44(RR-6):1–19.

507. Fayer R. Effect of high temperature on infectivity of *Cryptosporidium parvum* oocysts in water. *Appl Environ Microbiol*. 1994;60:2732–2735.

508. Shlim DR, Cohen MT, Eaton M, Rajah R, Long EG, Ungar BL. An alga-like organism associated with an outbreak of prolonged diarrhea among foreigners in Nepal. *Am J Trop Med Hyg*. 1991;45:383–389.

509. Hoge CW, Shlim DR, Rajah R, et al. Epidemiology of diarrhoeal illness associated with coccidian-like organism among travellers and foreign residents in Nepal. *Lancet*. 1993;341:1175–1179.

510. Pollok RC, Bendall RP, Moody A, Chiodini PL, Churchill DR. Traveller's diarrhoea associated with cyanobacterium-like bodies. *Lancet*. 1992;340:556–557.

511. Wurtz RM, Kocka FE, Peters CS, Weldon-Linne CM, Kuritza A, Yungbluth P. Clinical characteristics of seven cases of diarrhea associated with a novel acid fast organism in the stool. *Clin Infect Dis*. 1993;16:136–138.

512. Long EG, Ebrahimzadeh A, White EH, Swisher B, Callaway CS. Alga associated with diarrhea in patients with acquired immunodeficiency syndrome and in travelers. *J Clin Microbiol*. 1990;28:1101–1104.

513. Soave R, Dubey JP, Ramos LJ, Tummings M. A new intestinal pathogen? *Clin Res*. 1986;34:533A. Abstract.

514. Ortega YR, Sterling CR, Gilman RH, Cama VA, Diaz F. *Cyclospora* species: A new protozoan pathogen of humans. *N Engl J Med*. 1993;328:1308–1312.

515. Hoge CW, Echeverria P, Rajah R, et al. Prevalence of *Cyclospora* species and other enteric pathogens among children less than 5 years of age in Nepal. *J Clin Microbiol*. 1995;33:3058–3060.

516. Albert MJ, Kabir I, Azim T, Hossain A, Ansaruzzaman M, Unicomb L. Diarrhea associated with *Cyclospora* species in Bangladesh. *Diagn Microbiol Infect Dis*. 1994;19:47–49.

517. Sifuentes-Osornio J, Porras-Cortes G, Bendall RP, Morales-Villarreal F, Reyes-Teran G, Ruiz-Palacios GM. *Cyclospora cayetanensis* infection in patients with and without AIDS: Biliary disease as another clinical manifestation. *Clin Infect Dis*. 1995;21:1092–1097.

518. Pape JW, Verdier RI, Boncy M, Boncy J, Johnson WD. *Cyclospora* infection in adults infected with HIV: Clinical manifestations, treatment, and prophylaxis. *Ann Intern Med*. 1994;121:654–657.

519. Ashford RW. Occurrence of an undescribed coccidian in man in Papua New Guinea. *Ann Trop Med Parasitol*. 1979;73:497–500.

520. Long EG, White EH, Carmichael WW, et al. Morphologic and staining characteristics of a cyanobacterium-like organism associated with diarrhea. *J Infect Dis*. 1991;164:199–202.

521. Ortega YR, Gilman RH, Sterling CR. A new coccidian parasite (Apicomplexa: Eimeriidae) from humans. *J Parasitol*. 1994;80:625–629.

522. Huang P, Weber JT, Sosin DM, et al. The first reported outbreak of diarrheal illness associated with *Cyclospora* in the United States. *Ann Intern Med*. 1995;123:409–414.

523. Carter RJ, Guido F, Jacquette G, Rapoport M. Outbreak of cyclosporiasis at a country club—New York, 1995. In: *45th Annual Epidemic Intelligence Service (EIS) Conference*. Atlanta, Ga: US Department of Health and Human Services, Public Health Service; April 1996: 58. Abstract.

524. Rabold JG, Hoge CW, Shlim DR, Kefford C, Rajah R, Echeverria P. *Cyclospora* outbreak associated with chlorinated drinking water. *Lancet*. 1994;344:1360–1361.

525. Hale D, Aldeen W, Carroll K. Diarrhea associated with Cyanobacterialike bodies in an immunocompetent host: An unusual epidemiological source. *JAMA*. 1994;271:144–145.

526. Centers for Disease Control. Outbreaks of diarrheal illness associated with cyanobacteria (blue-green algae - like bodies—Chicago and Nepal, 1989 and 1990. *MMWR*. 1991;40:325–327.

527. Connor BA, Shlim DR. Foodborne transmission of *Cyclospora*. *Lancet*. 1995;346:1634.

528. Koumans EH, Katz D, Malecki J, et al. Novel parasite and modes of transmission: *Cyclospora* infection—Florida. In: *45th Annual Epidemic Intelligence Service (EIS) Conference*. Atlanta, Ga: US Department of Health and Human Services, Public Health Service; April 1996: 60. Abstract.

529. Herwaldt BL, Ackers ML, the Cyclospora Working Group. An outbreak in 1996 of cyclosporiasis associated with imported raspberries. *N Engl J Med*. 1997;336:1548–1556.

530. Herwaldt BL, Beach MJ, the Cyclospora Working Group. The return of cyclospora in 1997: Another outbreak of cyclosporiasis in North American associated with imported raspberries. *Ann Intern Med*. 1999;130:210–220.

531. Ooi WW, Zimmerman SK, Needham CA. *Cyclospora* species as a gastrointestinal pathogen in immunocompetent hosts. *J Clin Microbiol.* 1995;33:1267–1269.

532. Shlim DR, Hoge CW, Rajah R, Scott RMcN, Pandy P, Echeverria P. Persistent high risk of diarrhea among foreigners in Nepal during the first two years of residence. *Clin Infect Dis.* 1999;29:613–616.

533. Connor BA, Shlim DR, Scholes JV, Raybum JL, Reedy J, Rajah R. Pathologic changes in the small bowel in nine patients with diarrhea associated with a coccidia-like body. *Ann Intern Med.* 1993;119:377–382.

534. Bendall RP, Lucas S, Moody A, Tovey G, Chiodini PL. Diarrhoea associated with cyanobacterium-like bodies: A new coccidian enteritis in man. *Lancet.* 1993;341:590–592.

535. Madico G, Gilman RH, Miranda E, Cabrera L, Sterling CR. Treatment of *Cyclospora* infections with co-trimoxazole. *Lancet.* 1993;342:122–123.

536. Hoge CW, Shlim DR, Ghimire M, et al. Placebo-controlled trial of co-trimoxazole for *Cyclospora* infections among travelers and foreign residents in Nepal. *Lancet.* 1995;345:691–693.

537. Verdier RI, Fitzgerald DW, Johnson WD, Pape JW. Trimethoprim-sulfamethoxazole compared with ciprofloxacin for treatment and prophylaxis of *Isospora belli* and *Cyclospora cayatenensis* infection in HIV-infected patients: A randomized controlled trial. *Ann Intern Med.* 2000;132:885–888.

538. Godiwala T, Yaeger R. Isospora and travelers' diarrhea. *Ann Intern Med.* 1987;106:908–909.

539. Dehovitz JA, Pape JW, Boncy M, Johnson WD Jr. Clinical manifestations and therapy of *Isospora belli* infection in patients with the acquired immunodeficiency syndrome. *N Engl J Med.* 1986;315:87–90.

540. Drugs for parasitic infections. *Med Lett Drugs Ther.* 1993;35(911):111–122.

541. Stoll NR. This wormy world. *J Parasit.* 1947;33:1–18.

542. Rogers AM, Dammin GJ. Hookworm infection in American troops in Assam and Burma. *Am J Med Sci.* 1946;211:531–538.

543. Most H, Hayman JM, Wilson TB. Hookworm infections in troops returning from the Pacific. *Am J Med Sci.* 1946;212:347–350.

544. Swartzwelder C. Nematode and cestode infections. In: *Communicable Diseases Transmitted Chiefly through Respiratory and Alimentary Tracts.* Vol 4. *Preventive Medicine in World War II.* Washington, DC: Office of the Surgeon General, Department of the US Army; 1958: 503–517.

545. Swartzwelder C. Hookworm. In: *Communicable Diseases Transmitted through Contact or By Unknown Means.* Vol 5. *Preventive Medicine in World War II.* Washington, DC: Office of the Surgeon General, Department of the US Army; 1960: 15–24.

546. Most H. Helminthiasis. In: *Infectious Diseases and General Medicine.* Vol 3. *Internal Medicine in World War II.* Washington, DC: Office of the Surgeon General, Department of the US Army; 1968: 145–156.

547. Pawlowski K. Epidemiology prevention and control. In: Grove DA, ed. *Strongyloidiasis: A Major Roundworm Infection of Man.* London: Taylor and Francis; 1989: 235–249.

548. Sheeby TW. Digestive disease as a national problem, VI: Enteric disease among United States troops in Vietnam. *Gastroenterology.* 1968;55:105–112.

549. Forman DW, Tong NJ, Murrell KD, Cross JH. Etiologic study of diarrheal disease in Vietnam. *Am J Trop Med Hyg.* 1971;20:598–601.

550. Barrett O. Other parasitic diseases. In: *General Medicine and Infectious Diseases*. Vol 2. *Internal Medicine in Vietnam*. Washington, DC: Office of the Surgeon General, Department of the US Army; 1982: 412–417.

551. Beaver PC, Jung RC, Cuff EW. *Clinical Parasitology*. Philadelphia: Lea and Febiger; 1984: 825.

552. Takafuji ET, Kelley PW, Wiener HA, et al. Eosinophilia and soil transmitted helminthiasis related to jungle training in Panama. Washington, DC: Walter Reed Army Institute of Research; 1984. Epidemiology Consultant Service (EPICON) Report.

553. Kelley PW, Takafuji ET, Wiener H , et al. An outbreak of hookworm infection associated with military operations in Granada. *Mil Med*. 1989;154:55–59.

554. Stoute JA, Brundage J, Petruccelli B, Bell C, Keep L. Outbreak of eosinophilia and gastrointestinal illness in soldiers returning from jungle training in Panama. Washington, DC: Walter Reed Army Institute of Research; 1994. Epidemiology Consultant Service (EPICON) Report.

555. Cross JH. Clinical manifestation and laboratory diagnoses of eosinophilic meningitis syndrome associated with angiostrongyliasis. *Southeast Asian J Trop Med Public Health*. 1978;9:161–170.

556. Pozio E, LaRosa G, Murrell KD, Lichtenfels JR. Taxonomic revision of the genus *Trichinella*. *J Parasitol*. 1992;78:654–659.

557. Von Lichtenberg F. Infectious diseases. In: Cotran R, Kumar V, Robbins S, eds. *Robins Pathologic Basis of Disease*. 4th ed. Philadelphia: WB Saunders: 307–434.

558. Cross JH. Intestinal capillariasis. *Clin Microbiol Rev*. 1992 5:120–129.

559. Srivatanakul P, Ohshima H, Khlat M, et al. Opisthorchis viverrini infestation and endogenous nitrosamines as risk factors for cholangiocarcinoma in Thailand. *Int J Cancer*. 1991;48:821–825.

560. World Health Organization. *Control of Foodborne Trematode Infections*. Geneva: WHO; 1995: 849. WHO Technical Report.

561. Ash LR, Orhiel TC. *Parasites: A Guide to Laboratory Procedures and Identification*. Chicago: ASCP Press; 1987.

562. Garcia LS, Bruckner DA. *Diagnostic Medical Parasitology*. 3rd ed. Washington, DC: ASM Press; 1997.

563. Drugs for parasitic infections. *Med Lett Drugs Ther*. 1998;40:1–12.

564. Kraivichian P, Kulkumthorn M, Yingyourd P, Akarabovorn P, Paireepai CC. Albendazole for treatment of human gnathostomiasis. *Trans R Soc Trop Med Hyg*. 1992;86:418–421.

565. Chin Thack Soh. Professor, Yonsei University Medical School. Personal Communication, 1984.

566. Laoharanu P, Murrell D. A role for irradiation in the control of foodborne parasites. *Trends Food Sci Tech*. 1994;5:190–195.

567. Cross JH. Changing patterns of some trematode infections in Asia. *Arzneimittelforschung*. 1984;34:1224–1226.

568. Michelson EH. A *Concise Guide for the Detection, Prevention, and Control of Schistosomiasis in the Uniformed Services*. Washington, DC: Armed Forces Pest Management Board, Forest Glen Section; 1987. Technical Information Memorandum No. 23.

569. Reister SA, ed. *Medical Statistics in World War II*. Washington, DC: Office of the Surgeon General, Department of the Army; 1975: 410–411.

570. Wright WH. Bilharzia as a public health problem in the Pacific. *Bull World Health Organ*. 1950;2:581–595.

571. Kiernan FA Jr. The blood fluke that saved Formosa. *Harpers Magazine.* 1959;April:45–47.

572. Doumenge JP, Mott KE, Cheung C, et al. *Atlas of the Global Distribution of Schistosomiasis.* Bordeaux, France: Centre d'Etudes de Geographie Tropicale/World Health Organization, Presses Universitaires de Bordeaux; 1987.

573. World Health Organization. *Control of Schistosomiasis.* Geneva: WHO; 1993. Technical Report Series 830.

574. Jordan P, Webbe G, Sturrock RF, eds. *Human Schistosomiasis.* Wallingford, UK: CAB International; 1993.

575. Malek EA, Cheng TC. *Medical and Economic Malacology.* New York: Academic Press; 1974.

576. Sobhon P, Upatham ES. *Snail Hosts, Life Cycle, and Tegumental Structure of Oriental Schistosomes.* Geneva: United Nations Development Programme/World Bank/World Health Organization, Special Programme for Research and Training in Tropical Diseases; 1990: 1–36.

577. Malek EA. *Snail Hosts of Schistosomiasis and other Snail-transmitted Diseases in Tropical America: A Manual.* Washington, DC: Pan American Health Organization; 1985. Scientific Publication No. 478.

578. Chen MG. *Schistosoma japonicum* and *S. japonicum*-like infections: Epidemiology, clinical and pathological aspects. In: Jordan P, Webbe G, Sturrock RF, eds. *Human Schistosomiasis.* Wallingford,UK: CAB International; 1993: 237–270.

579. Lee HF, Wykoff DE, Beaver PC. Two cases of human schistosomiasis in new localities in Thailand. *Am J Trop Med Hyg.* 1966;15:303–306.

580. Appleton CC. Schistosome dermatids: An unrecognized problem in South Africa. *S Afr Med J.* 1984;65:467–469.

581. King CH. Acute and chronic schistosomiasis. *Hosp Pract (Off Ed).* 1991;263:117–130.

582. Strickland GT, Abdel-Wahab MF. Schistosomiasis. In: Strickland GT, ed. *Hunter's Tropical Medicine.* Philadelphia: W.B. Saunders; 1991.

583. Lucey DR, Maguire JH. Schistosomiasis. *Infect Dis Clin North Am.* 1993;7:635–653.

584. Centers for Disease Control. Cercarial dermatitis outbreak at a state park—Delaware, 1991. *MMWR.* 1992;41:225–228.

585. Mansour MM, Ali PO, Farid Z, Simpson AJ, Woody JW. Serological differentiation of acute and chronic schistosomiasis mansoni by antibody responses to keyhole limpet hemocyanin. *Am J Trop Med Hyg.* 1989:41:338–344.

586. Basch PF. *Schistosomes: Development, Reproduction, and Host Relations.* New York: Oxford University Press; 1991.

587. Scrimgeour EM, Gajdusek DC. Involvement of the central nervous system in *Schistosoma mansoni* and *S. haematobium* infection. *Brain.* 1985;108:1023–1038.

588. Marcial-Rojas RA, Fiol RE. Neurologic complications of schistosomiasis: Review of the literature and report of two cases of transverse myelitis due to *Schistosoma mansoni. Ann Intern Med.* 1963;59:2115–2130.

589. Centers for Disease Control and Prevention. Schistosomiasis in U.S. Peace Corps volunteers—Malawi, 1992. *MMWR.* 1995;42:565–570.

590. Farid Z. Schistosomes with terminal-spined eggs: Pathology and clinical aspects. In: Jordan P, Webbe G, Sturrock RF, eds. *Human Schistosomiasis.* Wallingford, UK: CAB International; 1993: 159–193.

591. Farid Z, Woody J, Kamal M. Praziquantel and acute urban schistosomiasis. *Trop Geogr Med.* 1989;412:172.

592. Chen MG, Mott KE. Progress in assessment of morbidity due to *Schistosoma haematobium* infection: A review of the literature. *Trop Dis Bull.* 1989;86:(4) R1-R36.

593. Chen MG, Mott KE, Progress in assessment of morbidity due to *Schistosoma japonicum* infection: a review of the literature. *Trop Dis Bull.* 1988;85:6 R1-R45.

594. Chen MG, Mott KE, Progress in assessment of morbidity due to *Schistosoma mansoni* infection: a review of the literature. *Trop Dis Bull.* 1988;85:10R1-R56.

595. Peters PA, Kasura JW. Update on diagnostic methods for schistosomiasis. *Baillieres Clin Trop Med Commun Dis.* 1987;2:419–433.

596. Ash LR, Orihel TC. *Parasites: a Guide to Laboratory Procedures and Identification.* Chicago: ASCP Press; 1987.

597. Tsang VCW, Wilkins PP. Immunodiagnosis of schistosomiasis: Screen with FAST-ELISA and confirm with immunoblot. *Clin Lab Med.* 1991;11:1029–1039.

598. Ndhlovu P, Cadman H, Gundersen S, et al. Circulating anodic antigen (CAA) levels in different age groups in a Zimbabwean rural community endemic for *Schistosoma haematobium* determined using the magnetic beads antigen-capture enzyme-linked immunoassay. *Am J Trop Med Hyg.* 1996;54:537–542.

599. Shekhar KC. Schistosomiasis drug therapy and treatment considerations. *Drugs.* 1991;42:379–405.

600. Stelma FF, Sall S, Daff B, Sow S, Niang M, Gryseels B. Oxamniquine cures *Schistosoma mansoni* infection in a focus in which cure rates with praziquantel are unusually low. *J Infect Dis.* 1997;176:304–307.

601. Lambenucci JR. *Schistosoma mansoni:* Pathological and clinical aspects. In: Jordan P, Webbe G, Sturrock RF, eds. *Human Schistosomiasis.* Wallingford, UK: CAB International; 1993.

602. Xiao SH, You JQ, Yang YQ, Wang CZ. Experimental studies on early treatment of schistosomal infection with artemether. *Southeast Asian J Trop Med Public Health* . 1995;26:306–318.

603. Xiao S, Shi Z, Zhuo S, et al. Field studies on the preventive effect of oral artemether against schistosomal infection. *Chin Med J (Engl).* 1996;109(4):272–275.

604. Xiao SH, Booth M, Tanner M. The prophylactic effects of artemether against *Schistosoma japonicum* infections. *Parasitol Today.* 2000;16:122–126.

605. Sabah AA, Fletcher C, Webbe G, Doenhoff MJ. *Schistosoma mansoni:* Chemotherapy of infections of different ages. *Exp Parasitol.* 1986;61:294–303.

606. Pellegrino J. Protection against human schistosome cercariae. *Exp Parasitol.* 1967;21(1):112–131.

607. Chen KY, Kuo JS. Protection experiments against the cercariae of *Schistosoma japonicum. Chin Med J (Engl).* 1958;77:580.

608. Abu-Elyazeed RR, Podgore JK, Mansour NS, Kilpatrick, ME. Field trial of 1% niclosamide as a topical antipenetrant to *Schistosoma mansoni* cercariae. *Am J Trop Med Hyg.* 1993;49:403–409.

609. Podgore JK, Abu-Elyazeed RR, Mansour NS, Youssef FG, Hibbs RG, Gere JA. Evaluation of a twice-a-week application of 1% niclosamide lotion in preventing *Schistosoma haematobium* reinfection. *Am J Trop Med Hyg.* 1994;51:875–879.

610. Hsu HF, Hsu SYL. Schistosomiasis in the Shanghai area. In: Quinn JR, ed. *China Medicine as We Saw It.* Bethesda, Md: Department of Health, Education, and Welfare/Public Health Service/National Institutes of Health; 1974. DHEW (NIH) Publication 75–684.

611. Salafsky B, Ramaswany R, He YX, Anderson GL, Nowicki DK, Dhibuya T. Evaluation of N,N-diethyl-m-tolumide (DEET) as a topical agent for preventing skin penetration by cercariae of *Schistosoma mansoni. Am J Trop Med Hyg.* 1998;58:828–834.

612. Salafsky B, Ramaswamy K, He YX, Li J, Shibuya T. Development and evaluation of LIPODEET, a new long-acting formulation of N,N-diethyl-m-tolumide (DEET) for the prevention of schistosomiasis. *Am J Trop Med Hyg.* 1999;58:828–834.

613. Sturrock RF. The intermediate hosts and host-parasite relationships. In: *Human Schistosomiasis.* Jordan P, Webbe G, Sturrock RF, eds. Wallingford, UK: CAB International; 1993.

614. Carney WP, Sudomo M. Schistosomiasis in Indonesia. *Proceedings Symposium Parasitic Dis Problems.* 1980: 58–63.

615. Webbe G, Jordan P. Control. In: *Human Schistosomiasis.* Jordan P, Webbe G, Sturrock RF, eds. Wallingford, UK: CAB International; 1993.

616. Bemade MA, Johnson B. Schistosome cercariae removal in the control of schistosomiasis. *J Am Water Works Ass.* 1971;63:449–453.

617. World Health Organization. *Snail Control in the Prevention of Bilharziasis.* Geneva: WHO; 1965.

618. Cheng TC, ed. *Molluscicides in Schistosomiasis Control.* New York: Academic Press; 1974.

619. Smith CE. Coccidioidomycosis. In: Anderson RS, ed. *Communicable Diseases Transmitted Chiefly Through Respiratory and Alimentary Tracts.* Vol 4. *Preventive Medicine in World War II.* Washington, DC: Office of the Surgeon General; 1958.

620. Smith CE, Beard RR, Rosenberger HG, Whiting EG. Effect of season and dust control on coccidioidomycosis. *JAMA.* 1946;132:833–838.

621. Standaert SM, Schaffner W, Galgiani JN, et al. Coccidicidomycosis among visitors to a *Coccidioides immitis*-endemic area: An outbreak in a military reserve unit. *J Infect Dis.* 1995;171:1672–1675.

622. Joffe B. An epidemic of coccidioidomycosis probably related to soil. *N Engl J Med.* 1960:262:720–722.

623. Williams PL, Sable DL, Mendez P, Smyth LT. Symptomatic coccidioidomycosis following a severe natural dust storm: An outbreak at the Naval Air Station, Lemoore, Calif. *Chest.* 1979;76:566–570.

624. Sturde HC. Skin test reactivity and residua of coccidioidal pulmonary infections in German airmen. In: Einstein HE, Catanzaro A, eds. *Coccidioidomycosis.* Washington, DC: National Foundation for Infectious Diseases; 1985: 43–45.

625. Miller RN, Gertz C. *Assessment of Risk of Coccidioidomycosis at Fort Irwin During Exercise, Mohave Chief, 3rd Brigade, 4th Infantry Division (MECH), Fort Carson, Colorado.* Washington, DC: Walter Reed Army Institute of Research; 1979. Final Epidemiology Consultant Service (EPICON) Report.

626. Kong YCM, Levine HB, Madin SH, Smith CE. Fungal multiplication and histopathologic changes in vaccinated mice infected with *Coccidioides immitis. J Immunol.* 1964;92:779–790.

627. Swatek FE, Omieczynski DT, Plunkett OA. *Coccidioides immitis* in California. In: Ajello L, ed. *Coccidioidomycosis.* Tucson: University of Arizona Press; 1967: 255–264.

628. Winn WA. Primary cutaneous coccidioidomycosis. *Arch Dermatol.* 1965;92:221–228.

629. Eckmann BN, Schaefer GL, Huppert M. Bedside interhuman transmission of coccidioidomycosis via growth on fomites. *Am Rev Respir Dis.* 1964;89:175–185.

630. Pappagianis D. Marked increase in cases of coccidioidomycosis in California: 1991, 1992, and 1993. *Clin Infect Dis.* 1994;19(suppl 1):S14–S18.

631. Pappagianis D. Epidemiology of coccidioidomycosis. *Curr Top Med Mycol.* 1988;2:199–238.

632. Galgiani JN. Coccidioidomycosis. *West J Med.* 1993;1592:153–171.

633. Dodge RR, Lebowitz MD, Barbee RA, Burrows B. Estimates of *C. immitis* infection by skin test reactivity in an endemic community. *Am J Public Health.* 1985;75:863–865.

634. Smith CE, Whiting EG, Baker EE, Rosenberger HG, Beard RR, Saito MT. The use of coccidioidin. *Am Rev Tuberc.* 1948;57:330–360.

635. Galgiani JN, Valley Fever Vaccine Study Group. Development of dermal hypersensitivity to coccidioidal antigens associated with repeated skin testing. *Am Rev Respir Dis.* 1986;134:1045–1047.

636. Smith CE, Saito MT, Beard RR, Kepp RM, Clark RW, Eddie BU. Serological tests in the diagnosis and prognosis of coccidioidomycosis. *Am J Hyg.* 1950;52:1–21.

637. Galgiani JN, Ampel NM, Catanzaro A, Johnson R, Stevens DA, Williams PL. Practice guidelines for the treatment of coccidioidomycosis. *Clin Infect Dis.* 2000;30:658–661.

638. Tucker RM, Galgiani JN, Denning DW, et al. Treatment of coccidioidal meningitis with fluconazole. *Rev Infect Dis.* 1990;12(suppl 3):S380–S389.

639. Graybill JR. Treatment of coccidioidomycosis. *Curr Top Med Mycol.* 1993;5:151–179.

640. Elconin AF, Egeberg MC, Bald JG, et al. A fungicide effective against *Coccidioides immitis* in soil. In: L. Ajello, ed. *Coccidioidomycosis.* Tucson, Ariz: University of Arizona Press; 1967: 319–321.

641. Fish DG, Ampel NM, Galgiani JN, et al. Coccidioidomycosis during human immunodeficiency virus infection: A review of 77 patients. *Medicine (Baltimore).* 1990;69:384–391.

642. Grayston JT, Furcolow ML. The occurrence of histoplasmosis in epidemics—Epidemiological studies. *Am J Public Health.* 1953;43:665–676.

643. Larrabee WF, Ajello L, Kaufman L. An epidemic of histoplasmosis on the isthmus of Panama. *Am J Trop Med Hyg.* 1978;27:281–285.

644. Burke DS, Gaydos JC, Churchill FE, Kaufman L. Epidemic histoplasmosis in patients with undifferentiated fever. *Mil Med.* 1982;147:466–467.

645. Darling ST. A protozoon general infection producing pseudotubercules in the lungs and focal necroses in the liver, spleen and lymph nodes. *JAMA.* 1906;46:1283–1285.

646. De Monbreun WA. The cultivation and cultural characteristics of Darling's *Histoplasma capsulatum. Am J Trop Med.* 1934;14:93–135.

647. Palmer CE. Geographic differences in sensitivities to histoplasmin among student nurses. *Public Health Rep.* 1946;61:475–487.

648. Palmer CE. Nontuberculous pulmonary calcification and sensitivity to histoplasmin. *Public Health Rep.* 1945;60:513–520.

649. Christie A, Peterson JC. Pulmonary calcification in negative reactors to tuberculin. *Am J Public Health.* 1945;35:1131–1147.

650. Kwon-Chung KJ, Bennett JE. Histoplasmosis. In: *Medical Mycology.* Philadelphia, Penn: Lea & Febiger; 1992: 464–513.

651. Rippon JW. Histoplasmosis (*Histoplasmosis capsulati*). In: *Medical Mycology: The Pathogenic Fungi and the Pathogenic Actinomycetes.* 3rd ed. Philadelphia, Penn: WB Saunders; 1988: 381–423.

652. Furcolow ML. Epidemiology of histoplasmosis. In: Sweany HC, ed. *Histoplamosis*. Springfield, Ill: Charles C Thomas; 1960: 113–148.

653. Bullock WE. *Histoplasma capsulatum*. In: Mandell GL, Bennett JE, Dolin R, eds. *Mandell, Douglas, and Bennett's Principles and Practice of Infectious Diseases*. 4th ed. New York: Churchill Livingstone; 1995: 2340–2353.

654. Furcolow ML. Recent studies on the epidemiology of histoplasmosis. *Ann N Y Acad Sci*. 1953;72:127–164.

655. Edwards LB, Acquaviva FA, Livesay VT, Cross FW, Palmer CE. An atlas of sensitivity to tuberculin, PPD-B, and histoplasmin in the United States. *Am Rev Respir Dis*. 1969;99(Suppl):1–132.

656. Ajello L. Distribution of *Histoplasma capsulatum* in the United States. In: Ajello L, Chick W, Furcolow MF, eds. *Histoplamosis: Proceedings of the 2nd National Conference*. Springfield, Ill: Charles C Thomas; 1971: 103–122.

657. Goodwin RA, DesPrez RM. Histoplasmosis: State of the art. *Am Rev Respir Dis*. 1978;117:929–956.

658. Wheat J. Histoplasmosis: Recognition and treatment. *Clin Infect Dis*. 1994;19(Suppl 1):S19–S27.

659. Wheat LJ, Connolly-Stringfield PA, Baker RL, et al. Disseminated histoplasmosis in the acquired immune deficiency syndrome: Clinical findings, diagnosis and treatment, and review of the literature. *Medicine*. 1990;69:361–374.

660. Wheat LJ, Kohler RB, Tewari RP. Diagnosis of disseminated histoplasmosis by detection of *Histoplasma capsulatum* antigen in serum and urine specimens. *N Engl J Med*. 1986;314:83–88.

661. Wheat LJ, Connolly-Stringfield P, Kohler RB, Frame PT, Gupta MR. *Histoplasma capsulatum* polysaccharide antigen detection in diagnosis and management of disseminated histoplasmosis in patients with acquired immunodeficiency syndrome. *Am J Med*. 1989;87:396–400.

662. Wheat LJ, Hafner R, Korzun AH, et al. Itraconazole treatment of disseminated histoplasmosis in patients with the acquired immunodeficiency syndrome. *Am J Med*. 1995;98:336–342.

663. United States Army Environmental Hygiene Agency. *Managing Health Hazards Associated with Bird and Bat Droppings*. Aberdeen Proving Ground, Md: USAEHA; December 1992. Technical Guide 142.

664. While NJ, Dance DA, Chaowagul W, Wattanagoon Y, Wuthiekanun V, Pitakwatchara N. Halving of mortality of severe melioidosis by ceftazidime. *Lancet*. 1989;2:1040.

665. Chaowagul W, White NJ, Dance DA, et al. Melioidosis: A major cause of community-acquired septicemia in northeastern Thailand. *J Infect Dis*. 1989;159:890–899.

666. Rubin HL, Alexander AD, Yager RH. Melioidosis—a military medical problem? *Mil Med*. 1963;128:538–542.

667. Sanford JP. *Pseudomonas* species (including melioidosis and glanders). In: Mandell GL, Douglas RG, Bennett, eds. *Principles and Practice of Infectious Diseases*. 2nd ed. New York: John Wiley & Sons; 1250–1254.

668. Dance DA. Melioidosis: The tip of the iceberg? *Clin Microbiol Rev*. 1991;4:52–60.

669. Howe C, Sampath A, Spotnitz M. The *pseudomallei* group: A review. *J Infect Dis*. 1971;124:598–606.

670. Yabuuchi E, Kosako Y, Oyaizu H, et al. Proposal of *Burkholderia* gen. nov. and transfer of seven species of the genus *Pseudomonas* homology group II to the new genus, with the type species *Burkholderia cepacia* (Palleroni and Holmes 1981) comb. nov. *Microbiol Immunol*. 1992;36:1251–1275.

671. Smith MD, Angus BJ, Wuthiekanun V, White NJ. Arabinose assimilation defines a nonvirulent biotype of *Burkholderia pseudomallei*. *Infect Immunol*. 1997;65:4319–4321.

672. Brett PJ, DeShazer D, Woods DE. *Burkholderia thailandensis* sp. nov., a *Burkholderia pseudomallei*-like species. *Int J Syst Bacteriol*. 1998;48:317–320.

673. Tong S, Yang S, Lu S, He W. Laboratory investigation of ecological factors influencing the environmental presence of *Burkholderia pseudomallei*. *Microbiol Immunol*. 1996;40:451–453.

674. Thomas AD, Forbes-Faulker JC. Persistence of *Pseudomonas pseudomallei* in soil. *Aust Vet J*. 1981;57:535–536.

675. Clayton AJ, Lisella RS, Martin DG. Melioidosis: A serological survey in military personnel. *Mil Med*. 1973;138:24–26.

676. Dance DA. Ecology of *Burkholderia pseudomallei* and the interactions between environmental *Burkholderia* spp. and human-animal hosts. *Acta Trop*. 2000;74:159–168.

677. Dorman SE, Gill VJ, Gallin JI, Holland SM. *Burkholderia pseudomallei* infection in a Puerto Rican patient with chronic granulomatous disease: Case report and review of occurrences in the Americas. *Clin Infect Dis*. 1998;26:889–894.

678. Perez JM, Petiot A, Adjide C, Gerry F, Goursaud R, Juminer B. First case report of melioidosis in Guadeloupe, a French West Indies archipelago. *Clin Infect Dis*. 1997;25:164–165.

679. Suputtamongkol Y, Hall AJ, Dance DA, et al. The epidemiology of melioidosis in Ubon Ratchatani, northeast Thailand. *Int J Epidemiol*. 1994;23:1082–1090.

680. Vadivelu J, Puthucheary SD, Gendeh GS, Parasakthi N. Serodiagnosis of melioidosis in Malaysia. *Singapore Med J*. 1995;36:299–302.

681. Embi N, Suhaimi A, Mohamed R, Ismail G. Prevalence of antibodies to *Pseudomonas pseudomallei* exotoxin and whole cell antigens in military personnel in Sabah and Sarawak, Malaysia. *Micro Immunol*. 1992;36:899–904.

682. Thin RN. Melioidosis antibodies in Commonwealth soldiers. *Lancet*. 1976;1:31–33.

683. Lim MK, Tan EH, Soh CS, Chang TL. *Burkholderia pseudomallei* infection in the Singapore Armed Forces from 1987 to 1994—an epidemiological review. *Ann Acad Med Singapore*. 1997;26:13–17.

684. Heng BH, Goh KT, Yap EH, Loh H, Yeo M. Epidemiological surveillance of melioidosis in Singapore. *Ann Acad Med Singapore*. 1998;27:478–484.

685. Yang S, Tong S, Mo C, et al. Prevalence of human melioidosis on Hainan Island in China. *Microbiol Immunol*. 1998;42:651–654.

686. Currie BJ, Fisher DA, Howard DM, et al. The epidemiology of melioidosis in Australia and Papua New Guinea. *Acta Trop*. 2000;74:121–127.

687. Brundage WG, Thuss CJ, Walden DC. Four fatal cases of melioidosis in US soldiers in Vietnam: Bacteriologic and pathologic characteristics. *Am J Trop Med Hyg*. 1968;17:183–191.

688. Ip M, Osterberg LD, Chua PY, Raffin TA. Pulmonary melioidosis. *Chest*. 1995;108:1420–1424.

689. Chaowagul W, White NJ, Dance DA, et al. Melioidosis: A major cause of community-acquired septicemia in northeastern Thailand. *J Infect Dis*. 1989;159:890–899.

690. Ashdown LR. An improved screening technique for isolation of *Pseudomonas pseudomallei* from clinical specimens. *Pathology*. 1979;11:293–297.

691. Dharakul T, Songsivilai S. Recent developments in the laboratory diagnosis of melioidosis. *J Infect Dis Antimicrob Agents*. 1996;13:77–80.

692. Rattanathongkom A, Sermswan RW, Wongratanacheewin S. Detection of *Burkholderia pseudomallei* in blood samples using polymerase chain reaction. *Mol Cell Probes*. 1997;11:25–31.

693. Sura T, Smith MD, Cowan GM, Walsh AL, White NJ, Krishna S. Polymerase chain reaction for the detection of *Burkholderia pseudomallei. Diagn Microbiol Infect Dis.* 1997;29:121–127.

694. Cuzzubbo AJ, Chenthamarakshan V, Vadivelu J, Puthucheary SD, Rowland D, Devine PL. Evaluation of a new commercially available immunoglobulin M and immunoglobulin G immunochromatographic test for diagnosis of melioidosis infection. *J Clin Microbiol.* 2000;38:1670–1671.

695. Chaowagul W. Recent advances in the treatment of severe melioidosis. *Acta Trop.* 2000;74:133–137.

696. Green RN, Tuffnell PG. Laboratory acquired melioidosis. *Am J Med.* 1968;44:599–605.

Chapter 38

DISEASES SPREAD BY CLOSE PERSONAL CONTACT

GREGORY C. GRAY, MD, MPH; BRIAN FEIGHNER, MD, MPH; DAVID H. TRUMP, MD, MPH;
S. WILLIAM BERG, MD, MPH; MARGAN J. ZAJDOWICZ, MD; AND THADDEUS R. ZAJDOWICZ, MD

RESPIRATORY PATHOGENS

MENINGOCOCCAL DISEASE

TUBERCULOSIS

SEXUALLY TRANSMITTED DISEASES AND HUMAN
   IMMUNODEFICIENCY VIRUS INFECTION

VIRAL HEPATITIS

G.C. Gray, MD, MPH Captain, Medical Corps, US Navy, (Retired); Professor, Department of Epidemiology, University of Iowa College of Public Health, 200 Hawkins Drive, Iowa City, IA 52242; Formerly, Director, DoD Center for Deployment Health Research, Naval Health Research Center, San Diego, CA 92186-5122

B. Feighner, MD, MPH, Colonel, Medical Corps, US Army; Interim Chair, Department of Military and Emergency Medicine, Uniformed Services University of the Health Sciences, 4301 Jones Bridge Road, Bethesda, MD 20814-4799

D.H. Trump, MD, MPH, Captain, Medical Corps, US Navy; Associate Professor and Director, Medical Student Education Programs,, Department of Preventive Medicine and Biometrics, Uniformed Services University of the Health Sciences, 4301 Jones Bridge Road, Bethesda, MD 20814-4799

S.W. Berg, MD, MPH, Captain, Medical Corps, US Navy (Retired); Director, Hampton Health District, 3130 Victoria Boulevard, Hampton, VA 23661-1588; Formerly, Director for Organizational Development, Navy Environmental Health Center, Norfolk, Virginia

M.J. Zajdowicz, MD, Captain, Medical Corps, US Navy; Directorate for Medical Affairs, Naval Medical Center, Portsmouth, VA 23708

T.R. Zajdowicz, MD, Captain, Medical Corps, US Navy; Command Surgeon, Joint Task Force Civil Support, US Joint Forces Command, Fort Monroe, VA 23551

RESPIRATORY PATHOGENS

Introduction and Military Relevance

Respiratory pathogens have plagued military populations throughout US history. Records from the War of 1812, the Spanish American War, and World War I document the devastation respiratory pathogens have caused and the inability of public health officials to control them.[1–3] Especially well documented are the epidemics that occurred during the mobilization for World War I. In 1918, a 30-day epidemic of *Streptococcus pneumoniae* infections occurred at a military camp in Illinois, causing 2,349 hospital admissions for pneumonia and a 50% mortality rate.[4] During 1918, a 2-month military epidemic of influenza in Little Rock, Arkansas, affected 12,393 men and led to 1,499 cases of pneumonia, 31% of whom died during treatment.[5] Other reports record that hemolytic streptococci (*Streptococcus pyogenes*) were a continual cause of military epidemics of bronchopneumonia, empyema, and pharyngitis. In total, it was estimated that more than 1.4 million US Army personnel suffered from respiratory disease during World War I, accounting for more than 41% of all forms of disease and causing more than 77% (45,000) of Army disease deaths.[2]

Before antimicrobials were widely available, strategies to prevent military epidemics of respiratory disease were not very successful. Generally, military public health officers could do little more than attempt to isolate and treat the afflicted with various therapies against streptococci, which included digitalis, whiskey, strychnine, and various horse sera.[6–8] Following the success of researchers in South Africa, US military officials attempted to control *S pneumoniae* epidemics at select US Army camps during World War I with a crude vaccine,[9,10] but their efforts were unsuccessful.[3,11] Commenting on the trade-off between isolating the ill and compromising the mission, one military physician of 1917 wrote that "Exposure to infection and hardships which will result in deaths from pneumonia may be just as necessary as going into action with resulting deaths from gunshot wounds."[7]

Despite the limited effective interventions available to public health officials in the preantibiotic era, they made important observations regarding the types of acute respiratory diseases and their apparent bacterial causes. Those officials noted that crowding greatly contributed to respiratory epidemics[12,13] and that more important than reduced floor space in sleeping quarters was the number of men placed in the same room.[13] Southerners, blacks,

and new military personnel from rural areas were thought to be at highest risk of developing pneumonia. Measles and influenza epidemics were observed to trigger epidemics of *S pneumoniae* and *S pyogenes* infections.[14,15]

Senior military officers were determined to reduce respiratory disease during the mass mobilization of personnel for World War II. Beginning in 1941, the US Department of War established the Board for the Investigation and Control of Influenza and Other Epidemic Diseases in the Army. Later, this board assembled various commissions of scientific experts and established numerous public health and research facilities to study and prevent respiratory disease.[16] These joint military and university endeavors led to many of the antibiotic and vaccine prophylaxis interventions now used in military populations (Table 38-1).

As a result of these and subsequent research efforts, today most US military personnel receive enzathine penicillin (BPG) or oral erythromycin rophylaxis, adenovirus vaccines (when available), uberculosis screening, and influenza vaccine during their first military training. This is followed by nnual influenza vaccination and periodic tuberculosis screening throughout their military careers. he pathogens recognized to cause respiratory disease among these young adults are similar to those ausing community-acquired disease among the eneral US adult population.[17–20] Most frequently, he pathogens include *S pyogenes*, *Mycoplasma neumoniae*, *S pneumoniae*, *Chlamydia pneumoniae*, denoviruses, influenza viruses, and rhinoviruses. ess frequently, military personnel also suffer infections from *Haemophilus influenzae*, *H parainfluenzae*, egionella pneumophila, *Moraxella catarrhalis*, *Bordetella ertussis*, coxsackieviruses, respiratory syncytial irus, and parainfluenza viruses. The most significant pathogens to military populations are reviewed here in more detail.

Streptococcus pyogenes

S pyogenes is a leading cause of bacterial respiratory morbidity among US military personnel. New military trainees are at particularly high risk of clinically significant infection. During the late 1940s and the 1950s, dedicated scientific teams, sponsored by Army Board Commissions, worked at a number of Army, Navy, Air Force, and Marine Corps training centers and made much progress in understanding and controlling this pathogen.

TABLE 38-1

IMPORTANT EVENTS IN THE DEVELOPMENT OF MILITARY STRATEGIES TO PREVENT EPIDEMICS OF ACUTE RESPIRATORY DISEASE

Event	Year	Reference
Streptococcus pneumoniae vaccine is effective in South Africa	1911	Maynard[a]
First US Army troops receive an *S pneumoniae* vaccine—not effective	1918	Cecil[b]
Influenza virus discovered	1933	Smith[c]
First influenza vaccine with protective results	1936	Chenoweth[d]
Daily oral sulfonamide therapy found to prevent recurrences of rheumatic fever among civilian populations	1939	Coborn[e]
US Navy administers oral sulfonamide therapy as mass prophylaxis with good success to eight large training stations that have high *S pyogenes* disease rates, but therapy-induced sulfa resistance among endemic *S pyogenes* strains	1944	Coborn[f,g]
Eaton agent is identified (later it is called *Mycoplasma pneumoniae*) and is found to cause much respiratory morbidity among military trainees	1944	Eaton,[h] Chanock[i]
First US Navy personnel receive *S pyogenes* vaccines—ineffective	1944	EUNo-22[j]
Oral penicillin therapy found to prevent rheumatic fever in civilian populations	1948	Milzer[k]
Procaine penicillin G injection therapy found to prevent rheumatic fever in military personnel with *S pyogenes* pharyngitis	1950	Denny[l]
Oral penicillin first used in US military personnel with excellent prophylaxis success against *S pyogenes*	1951	NMRU–4[m]
Benzathine penicillin G first used among civilian populations to prevent *S pyogenes* infection	1951	Stollerman[n]
Adenovirus discovered and later found to cause much respiratory morbidity among military trainees	1954	Hilleman,[o] Davenport[p]
Benzathine penicillin G used prophylactically against *S pyogenes* among large populations of US military personnel	1956	Frank[q]
Inactivated adenovirus vaccine (types 4 and 7) found effective among US military trainees	1956	Hilleman[r]
A new chlamydial pathogen is recognized (later called *Chlamydia pneumoniae*) and found to cause epidemics of respiratory morbidity among military trainees	1965	Grayston,[s] Kleemola[t]
Oral adenovirus vaccines (types 4 and 7) found effective among military trainees	1971	Gaydos[u]
Long absent, acute rheumatic fever epidemics recur among US military personnel	1987	Wallace[v]

a. Maynard GD. *An Enquiry into the Etiology, Manifestations, and Prevention of Pneumonia Amongst Natives on the Rand, Recruited from Tropical Areas.* Johannesburg, South Africa: South African Institute for Medical Research; 1913: 62–91.
b. Cecil RL, Austin JH. Results of prophylactic inoculation against pneumococcus in 12,519 men.*J Exp Med.* 1918;28:19–41.
c. Smith W, Andrewes CH, Laidlaw PP. A virus obtained from influenza patients. *Lancet.* 1933;2:66–68.
d. Chenoweth A, Waltz AD, Stokes J Jr, et al. Active immunization with the viruses of human and swine influenza *Am J Dis Child.* 1936;52:757-758.
e. Coborn AF, Moore LV. The prophylactic use of sulfonamide in streptococcal respiratory infections, with especial reference to rheumatic fever. *J Clin Invest.* 1939;18:147–155.
f. Coburn AF. Mass chemoprophylaxis: The U.S. Navy's six months' program for the control of streptococcal infections. *Naval Med Bull.* 1944;284:149–162.
g. Coburn AF. The prevention of respiratory tract bacterial infections by sulfadiazine prophylaxis in the United States Navy. *JAMA.* 1944;126:88–93.
h. Eaton MD, Meiklejohn G, Van Herick W. Studies on the etiology of primary atypical pneumonia: A filterable agent transmissible to cotton rats, hamsters, and chick embryos. *J Exp Med.* 1944;79:649–668.
i. Chanock RM, Fox HH, James WD. Epidemiology of *M. pneumoniae* infection in military recruits. *Ann N Y Acad Sci.* 1967;143:484–496.
j. Epidemiology Unit No. 22. Failure of type specific *Streptococcus pyogenes* vaccine to prevent respiratory infections *Naval Med Bull.* 1946;46:709–718.
k. Milzer A, Kohn KH, MacLean H. Oral prophylaxis of rheumatic fever with penicillin. *JAMA.* 1948;136:536–538.
l. Denny FW, Wannamaker LW, Brink WR, Rammelkamp CH Jr, Custer EA. Prevention of rheumatic fever: treatment of the preceding streptococcal infection. *JAMA* 1950;143:151–153.
m.The Personnel of Naval Medical Research Unit No. 4. *The Prophylaxis of Acute Respiratory Infections With Oral Penicillin or Chlortetracycline: Antibiotics Annual, 1953–54.* New York: Medical Encyclopedia, Inc; 1954: 123–136.
n. Stollerman GH, Rusoff JH. Prophylaxis against group A streptococcal infections in rheumatic fever patients: Use of new repository penicillin preparations. *JAMA.* 1952;150:1571–1575.
o. Hilleman MR, Werner JH. Recovery of new agent from patients with acute respiratory illness. *Proc Soc Exp Biol Med.* 1954;85:183–188.
p. Davenport FM. Influenza viruses. In: Evans AS, ed. *Viral Infections in Humans.* New York: Plenum Publishing Corp; 1984: 373–396.
q. Frank PF. Streptococcal prophylaxis in Navy recruits with oral and benzathine penicillin. *U.S. Armed Forces Med J.* 1958;4:543–560.
r. Hilleman MR. Efficacy and indications for use of adenovirus vaccine. *Am J Public Health.* 1958;48:153–158.
s. Grayston JT, Woolridge RL, Wang SP, et al. Field studies of protection from infection by experimental trachoma virus vaccine in preschool-aged children on Taiwan. *Proc Soc Exp Biol Med.* 1963;112:589–595.
t. Kleemola M, Saikku P, Visakorpi R, Wang SP, Grayston JT. Epidemics of pneumonia caused by TWAR, a new chlamydia organism, in military trainees in Finland. *J Infect Dis.* 1988;157:230–236.
u. Gaydos CA, Gaydos JC. Adenovirus vaccines in the U.S. military. *Mil Med.* 1995;160:300–304.
v. Wallace MR, Garst PD, Papadimos TJ, Oldfield EC. The return of acute rheumatic fever in young adults. *JAMA.* 1989;262:2557–2561.

Description of the Pathogen

S pyogenes is a Gram-positive coccus, or spherical bacteria, which, when grown on sheep blood agar, causes a clear zone of complete hemolysis (β-hemolysis). It is distinguished from other β-hemolytic streptococci by physiological and immunologic characteristics and by its implication as a cause of numerous acute clinical manifestations. *S pyogenes* strains are classified according to their capsular proteins, specifically T and M proteins. More than 90 unique M protein types have been identified. M types 1, 3, and 18 are associated with acute rheumatic fever, and M types 1, 3, 4, 12, and 25 are often associated with glomerulonephritis.

Epidemiology

The epidemiology of *S pyogenes* infection has been well described in military populations. Studies by military and university investigators in the 1950s demonstrate that transmission is most often by direct contact or large respiratory droplets and not commonly by fomites. The bacteria are thought to be endemic throughout the world, with perhaps some variation in the endemnicity of certain strains. Without prophylaxis, recent serologic evidence demonstrates that as many as 24% of military trainees may be infected over an 11-week period.[21]

Risk factors for serologic evidence of *S pyogenes* infection include being new to the military, crowding, lack of prophylaxis, close contact with an *S pyogenes* carrier, and close contact with a trainee not on prophylaxis.[22] A retrospective study of civilians with invasive *S pyogenes* infections suggested that Native Americans, and persons older than 65 years may be at higher risk of severe *S pyogenes* disease.[23] Active surveillance among Canadians have demonstrated that infection with human immunodeficiency virus, cancer, diabetes, alcohol abuse, and chickenpox are risk factors for invasive *S. pyogenes* disease.[24]

Pathogenesis and Clinical Findings

S pyogenes colonizes respiratory mucosal cells, causing pharyngitis and other clinical manifestations, such as fever and leukocytosis, in 36 to 72 hours. The complex interaction of cellular and extracellular *S pyogenes* products with the host immune system is not well understood, but it is recognized that immunity to *S pyogenes* is type-specific. Some patients progress to more invasive forms of infection, including streptococcal toxic shock syndrome, bacteremia, and necrotizing fasciitis. *S pyogenes*

pyrogenic exotoxins A and B and other virulence factors have been implicated in severe infection. Numerous theories regarding the interaction of host immune response and *S pyogenes* virulence factors have been postulated; however, it remains unclear why one person is severely infected by a particular strain of *S pyogenes* and another person is merely colonized with the same *S pyogenes* strain and suffers no symptoms.

S pyogenes, unlike other β-hemolytic streptococci, is implicated as a cause of numerous acute clinical manifestations, such as pharyngitis, peritonsillar abscess, pneumonia, empyema, scarlet fever, necrotizing fasciitis, myositis, bacteremia, and streptococcal toxic shock syndrome. *S pyogenes* also causes the nonsuppurative manifestations of acute rheumatic fever and glomerulonephritis. The severity of *S pyogenes* infections has changed over time. In the late 1800s, epidemics of scarlet fever were common and associated with high mortality rates.[25] Today, epidemics of scarlet fever are relatively rare.[26] In a similar fashion, acute rheumatic fever was very common during the mobilization for World War II, with 21,000 cases recorded in the US Navy alone,[27] but, until the 1980s, few cases were detected among military populations.[28,29] Changes in disease rates have been attributed to changes in the prevalence of virulent strains of *S pyogenes*.[30]

Diagnostic Approaches

Even in high-prevalence situations such as epidemics, it is difficult to clinically distinguish *S pyogenes* pharyngitis from pharyngitis caused by other pathogens. Diagnosis is best made by culture or rapid antigen detection. Generally, a rapid antigen test is accepted if it is positive, but it should be confirmed by culture if it is negative. Because a high proportion of infected military persons may not seek medical attention despite symptoms, epidemiologic studies of *S pyogenes* generally are conducted by relying on serologic tests, particularly the antistreptolysin O test. A two-dilution rise in antistreptolysin O titer is considered evidence of infection. Generally, such a rise may be detected in paired sera drawn 2 to 3 weeks apart. Other serologic tests for *S pyogenes* infection include the antideoxyribonuclease B test, the antihyaluronidase test, and a hemagglutination test (Streptozyme). Some patients with glomerulonephritis or symptoms of acute rheumatic fever may not demonstrate a rise in antistreptolysin O titer and should be evaluated further with antideoxyribonuclease B or antihyaluronidase tests before *S pyogenes* is eliminated as a cause.

Recommendations for Control

Monthly BPG injections and twice-a-day oral erythromycin have an estimated efficacy of preventing serologic evidence of infection of 45%[22] and 56%,[31] respectively.

Advances in *S pyogenes* control were first made in civilian populations just before World War II, when it was discovered that continuous antimicrobial therapy prevented recurrence of rheumatic fever. After World War II, it was learned that administering antibiotics to US military personnel with pharyngitis could reduce the incidence of acute rheumatic fever. Eventually, healthy military populations at high risk for *S pyogenes* disease were studied while being given mass antimicrobial prophylaxis against acute rheumatic fever, and this successful intervention became standard practice for crowded training populations.[27,32]

Sulfonamides were among the first antimicrobials available, and during the 1940s they were found to prevent military epidemics of acute respiratory disease.[27] Large field trials[33] of oral 0.5 to 1.0 g of sulfadiazine given daily to healthy US Navy personnel resulted in an 85% reduction in the incidence of streptococcal infections and rheumatic fever; however, daily prophylactic use caused exfoliative dermatitis and granulocytopenia in a small proportion of recipients. Bacteriostatic sulfonamide prophylaxis also often failed to eradicate *S pyogenes* from the nasopharynx of military personnel, and as soon as the therapy was discontinued, epidemics recurred. The most serious drawback occurred, however, when a Navy sulfonamide prophylaxis program reported that sulfonamide-resistant strains of *S pyogenes* had become endemic after only 1 year of routine prophylaxis.[27,34] After the failure of sulfonamides, other methods to reduce morbidity from *S pyogenes* were attempted. Military public health officials tried various environmental controls, including reductions in crowding,[13] dust suppression,[35] ultraviolet radiation,[36] and disinfectant vapors,[37] with varying degrees of success. Chlortetracycline also was tested as a mass prophylaxis agent, but it caused significant gastrointestinal side effects.[38] Military and university scientists also unsuccessfully attempted to control *S pyogenes* epidemics with inactivated, type-specific vaccines[39] (Figure 38-1).

Environmental controls, such as dust suppression by oiling floors and blankets, were largely abandoned when it was learned that penicillins were effective in the treatment and prevention of *S pyogenes* disease.[27] Oral penicillin therapy was first shown in 1948 as effective in preventing recurrent rheumatic fever in civilian populations.[40] Later, both oral and procaine penicillin G were shown to be effective in preventing rheumatic fever among healthy, high-risk military personnel; however, the drug's use in large military populations was logistically difficult because of the need for frequent dosing.[38,41,42] The development of BPG in 1951 led to its successful, large-scale testing as a prophylactic in a military population in 1956.[43] BPG's long-acting prophylactic effect, assurance of compliance, and few side effects soon made it the standard prophylactic intervention for the US Department of Defense (DoD) against *S pyogenes*, and it remains an effective intervention tool today.[27] BPG also has been used to combat epidemics of *S pneumoniae*,[44] and it seems to have a broader protective effect than can be explained by preventing *S pyogenes* disease alone.[45]

Despite the availability of antibiotic prophylaxis and surveillance programs among high-risk populations, military epidemics of *S pyogenes* continue to occur. In recent years, these epidemics have taken the form of pharyngitis and acute rheumatic fever.[22,27–29] An epidemic in 1989 of *S pyogenes* pharyngitis among Marine Corps trainees demonstrated that BPG prophylaxis for non–penicillin-allergic trainees alone might not be sufficient because unprotected penicillin-allergic recruits were shown to serve as an *S pyogenes* reservoir for reinfecting their peers.[22] This led to the Navy's adoption of oral erythromycin prophylactic therapy for penicillin-allergic recruits.[21,22]

Currently surveillance among trainees and preventive interventions vary among the military services. BPG (1.2 million units intramuscularly, once monthly) and oral erythromycin (250 mg orally, twice a day) interventions have been very effective in controlling *S pyogenes* epidemics. BPG remains effective for 2 to 4 weeks after injection. Oral erythromycin suffers from compliance problems due to its twice-daily dosing and gastrointestinal side effects. Oral azithromycin (500 mg weekly) has been shown to have an 84% efficacy in preventing *S pyogenes* infection and may be considered as an alternate therapy when an agent with a broader spectrum is desired.[31]

Reports of erythromycin-resistant *S pyogenes* isolates[46] and epidemics due to penicillin-tolerant *S pyogenes* strains[47,48] are causes for concern. Fortunately, thus far no penicillin-resistant *S pyogenes* isolates have been detected clinically; however, periodic surveillance of endemic strains among high-risk training populations should be conducted. This surveillance should contain antibiotic sensitivity testing of isolates, as well as strain typing.

The best hope for preventing *S pyogenes* disease

Adjusted Rates of Total Respiratory Diseases
27th Regiment

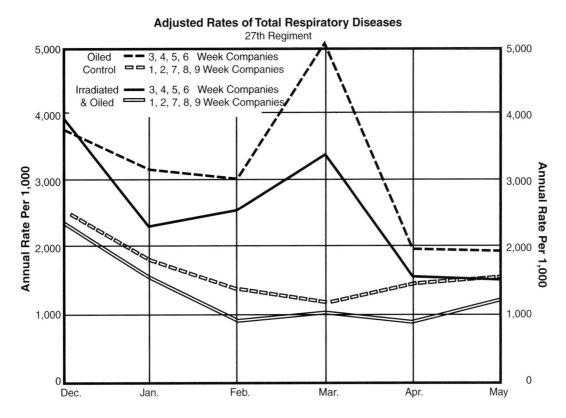

Fig. 38-1. Respiratory disease hospital admission rates by week of training and treatment groups. Dust in barracks was controlled by oiling floors and bed blankets; irradiated barracks indicates that ultraviolet radiation lamps were hung from ceilings and placed on floors. Lamps were on for 24 hours each day.
Reprinted, with permission from the *Journal of Infectious Diseases* from Miller WR, Jarrett ET, Willmone TL, Alexander H, Brown EW, et al. Evaluation of ultraviolet radiation and dust control measures in control of respiratory disease at a naval training center. *J Infect Dis.* 1948;82:86–100.

among military populations lies with the development of vaccines. Several approaches are being considered, including immunologic presentations of shared epitopes of various capsular M proteins. Vaccines, however, most likely will not be available for a number of years.

Streptococcus pneumoniae

A frequent cause of pneumonia in adults, *S pneumoniae* (pneumococcus) infections cause significant morbidity among US military populations. In the preantibiotic era, *S pneumoniae* infections could lead to large epidemics exceeding several hundred cases, particularly after influenza outbreaks. Today, epidemics caused by infection with *S pneumoniae* occur less often, but they remain a threat. Recently, an epidemic of pneumonia (128 hospitalizations) was recorded among Marine Corps trainees in southern California, triggering mass BPG and pneumococcal vaccine injections[44] (Figure 38-2).

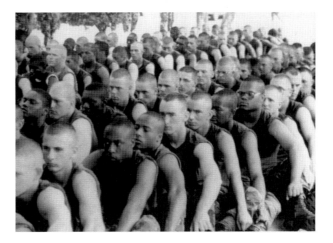

Fig. 38-2. The close and frequent person-to-person contact of trainees make military recruit training a very efficient time for respiratory pathogen transmission.
Photograph: Courtesy of Captain Gregory C. Gray, US Navy.

Description of the Pathogen

S pneumoniae is an ovoid, Gram-positive coccus that often forms distinctive pairs and chains. It grows well on sheep blood agar, causing partial hemolysis β-hemolysis), and it is distinguished from other streptococci by chemical growth inhibition and immunologic reaction. Eighty-four recognized strains or types are classified by their distinct capsular polysaccharides.

Epidemiology

S pneumoniae is spread by respiratory droplets or person-to-person contact. It is thought not to have geographical limitations, but data are sparse regarding the geographical distribution of capsular types. The incidence of disease among military personnel has not been well studied. US Navy data from 1981 to 1991 suggest that *S pneumoniae* causes approximately 12% of Navy and Marine Corps pneumonia hospitalizations, which occur at a rate of 9.5 per 100,000 person-years.[49] Because the incidence of outpatient disease is unknown and there are diagnostic difficulties identifying this pathogen, these estimates greatly underestimate its impact. Personnel at increased risk include individuals who are immunocompromised; are asplenic; or have sickle cell disease, renal disease, or diabetes mellitus. Military recruits are at high risk of *S pneumoniae* infection.

Pathogenesis and Clinical Findings

S pneumoniae is often found on the epithelium of healthy nasopharynx tissue, and its pathogenesis is not well understood. Other respiratory pathogens, especially viruses, may serve as a cofactor for invasion of local tissue by *S pneumoniae*, which if unchecked, may lead to clinical disease. Immunity is capsular, type-specific, and thought to last for years.

S pneumoniae causes various forms of pneumonia, meningitis, empyema, bacteremia, conjunctivitis, sinusitis, and arthritis.

Diagnostic Approaches

Because *S pneumoniae* is considered normal, oral bacterial flora, it is difficult to confidently diagnose infection from the oral pharynx. The accepted clinical diagnostic gold standard is bacterial culture from a normally sterile site. Blood cultures from patients with pneumonia caused by *S pneumoniae*, if studied before antibiotic administration, should be positive 20% of the time. A clinically expedient and alternative diagnostic tool for *S pneumoniae* pulmo-

nary infection is a well-prepared sputum specimen. Gram-stained sputum specimens should contain few to no squamous cells per low-powered microscopic field. The numerous serologic techniques available to assess *S pneumoniae* infection generally are confined to research institutions and involve detecting antibody to pneumococcal proteins or capsular polysaccharides. Generally, a rise in antibody titer from acute to convalescent sera is considered evidence of recent infection. Latex agglutination tests for pneumococcal antigens in urine has been found to have poor sensitivity but good specificity and are valuable when positive.[50]

Recommendations for Control

For military personnel, the 23-valent polysaccharide pneumococcal vaccine is the best protection against *S pneumoniae* infection. In 1991, the Armed Forces Epidemiological Board recommended a single dose of this vaccine be given to asplenic individuals and military personnel at bases with high prevalence of pneumonia. It is used routinely in high-risk Marine Corps trainee populations during the winter months. BPG, 1.2 million units intramuscularly, has been used to combat pneumococcal pneumonia epidemics, but it has never been evaluated for efficacy.[44] A study[31] of oral azithromycin (500 mg weekly) demonstrated an 80% efficacy of preventing serologic evidence of pneumococcal infection.

The recent rapid spread of clinically important, penicillin-resistant *S pneumoniae* strains throughout the United States and other developed countries has frustrated clinicians.[51,52] National US surveillance has demonstrated increasing prevalence of penicillin-resistant strains and increasing numbers of strains and serotypes resistant to multiple antibiotics. National public health panels have called for increased surveillance for antibiotic resistance among *S pneumoniae* isolates, careful use of antibiotics, and increased use of pneumococcal vaccine among high-risk populations.[53]

Mycoplasma pneumoniae

Long before microbiologists had distinguished agents causing acute respiratory disease, differences were noted in the clinical manifestations of pneumonias. Military personnel frequently suffered from acute pneumonia, which was milder than lobar pneumonia. Although this atypical pneumonia demonstrated significant pulmonary involvement on chest radiographs, patients lacked the high fever, pleuritic chest pain, and rigor associated with lobar pneumonia caused by *S pneumoniae*. In some

US Army camps, 85% to 90% of pneumonias were of the atypical variety.[54] The agents (or agent) causing this atypical pneumonia or primary atypical pneumonia were a matter of some debate. Often, patients with atypical pneumonia had positive cold agglutinin tests. In 1944, Eaton described his DoD-funded research, which demonstrated that a filterable agent (later named *Mycoplasma pneumoniae*) taken from patients with atypical pneumonia could cause pulmonary lesions in rats.[55] In 1961, Chanock[56] reported that *M pneumoniae* was responsible for 68% of atypical pneumonias among Marine Corps trainees and that as many as 41% of recruits had serologic evidence of infection during a 3-month training period.

Description of the Pathogen

M pneumoniae lacks a rigid cell wall and is much smaller than other bacteria. It grows very slowly on special nutrient agar, and isolation techniques most often are performed by reference laboratories. *M pneumoniae* grows on the surface of the epithelial cells that line the respiratory tract. Generally, it is not considered an agent of the nasopharyngeal flora. Due to its extracellular existence, however, it may be found in respiratory excretions weeks after clinical disease has resolved.

Epidemiology

M pneumoniae is transmitted by respiratory droplet inhalation or person-to-person contact and has a worldwide geographical distribution. Among US military populations, infection risk increases in late summer,[57] and females may be at higher risk of infection than males.[49,58,59] Certainly, crowding contributes to infection risk. Antibody to this pathogen is common among young adults. A recent study[60] demonstrated that on entry into the service, 58% of Marine trainees had evidence of previous infection with *M pneumoniae*. The prevalence and incidence of infection among US military training populations as measured by serologic antibody titer change is high, especially during outbreaks. One study[56] demonstrated seroconversion in as many as 57% of recruits during an 11-week period. Routine incidence in military training centers is more likely similar to the 6% to 8% detected among recent Marine Corps training populations during 3-month periods.[31,60]

Pathogenesis and Clinical Findings

Because of the low mortality and diagnostic difficulties, the pathogenesis of *M pneumoniae* infections has not been well determined. The pathogen adheres to epithelial cell receptors. After infection, antibodies to *M pneumoniae* surface antigens are formed, which offer protection from further infection. Many *M pneumoniae* infections evoke immunoglobulin M (IgM) autoantibody, which agglutinates human erythrocytes (cold agglutinins) and, in some cases, may trigger an autoimmunogenic mycoplasma-receptor complex.[36]

M pneumoniae infections are noted for their gradual onset of symptoms, dry cough, malaise, headache, and chills. Although some infections may be asymptomatic, *M pneumoniae* commonly causes a pharyngitis and may cause bronchopneumonia with patchy pulmonary infiltrates radiating from hilar areas. Occasionally, *M pneumoniae* may cause severe pneumonia or severe disease of the central nervous system, including meningoencephalitis, aseptic meningitis, ascending paralysis, and transverse myelitis. *M pneumoniae* also has been reported to cause various forms of cardiac disease, and numerous dermatological conditions.[61]

Diagnostic Approaches

M pneumoniae may be isolated from the nasopharynx after several weeks of incubation on special nutrient agar. For the best yield, a pharyngeal culture should be inoculated immediately into nutrient agar broth for incubation. Reference laboratories will need several weeks to isolate and identify *M pneumoniae* from clinical specimens. It is distinguished from other mycoplasmas by colony morphology, growth, and metabolic inhibition. Identification may be confirmed with serologic or molecular methods.

Clinically, the diagnosis of *M pneumoniae* infection may be presumed if the symptom complex is consistent with disease and the patient has a positive cold agglutinin test (titer ≥ 1:32 in convalescent sera). A positive test is more common with severe pneumonia. However, this test lacks sensitivity in that approximately 50% of infected patients may have a negative cold agglutinin test. The cold agglutinin test is additionally problematic in that it may be falsely positive in the presence of hematologic and hepatic diseases. Alternatively, acute *M pneumoniae* infection may be diagnosed by detecting high IgM titers specific for *M pneumoniae*[62] or by detecting *M pneumoniae*–specific nucleic acid with polymerase chain reaction assay (PCR).[63,64] Although several commercial diagnostic kits have been marketed for rapid diagnostic use in the clinical laboratory, their sensitivity and specificity have not approached that of reference laboratory serologic assays.

Two serologic tests, complement fixation assay and enzyme-linked immunosorbent assay (ELISA), have been used effectively to detect *M pneumoniae* in epidemiologic studies. Generally, these tests are performed by a reference laboratory, and a 4-fold rise in antibody titer by either method (acute symptom sera to 3- to 4-week convalescent sera) is accepted as evidence of recent infection.[62,65]

The DoD conducts no specific surveillance for *M pneumoniae* infection among military populations. The US Army's surveillance program for acute respiratory disease[45] includes morbidity from *M pneumoniae*, but only in the aggregate with that from other pathogens. At present, the DoD has no sustained *M pneumoniae* research program and no *M pneumoniae* reference laboratory. Military investigators must rely on other academic or federal laboratories for diagnostic assistance.

Recommendations for Control

Few options are available for combating *M pneumoniae* epidemics. Although several studies[66,67] have demonstrated that preexisting antibody titers against *M pneumoniae* may prevent infection and vaccine candidates were tested in the 1960s and 1970s with mixed success,[68–70] no vaccine is available. In 1965, a 10-day course of oxytetracycline was used to prevent disease in family members of patients.[59] This four-times-a-day regimen was reported to have had a prophylactic effect. This result, however, has never been validated. Navy researchers have demonstrated that weekly oral azithromycin (500 mg) has a 64% protective serologic efficacy against *M pneumoniae* among Marines, and this strategy may hold some promise.[31]

Chlamydia pneumoniae

First accepted as a new species in 1989, *Chlamydia pneumoniae* has been found to be a frequent cause of acute respiratory disease in military personnel. In Norway and Finland, *C pneumoniae* has been shown to infect as many as 56% of military recruits.[19] The agent is thought to cause approximately 8% of pneumonias in the United States.[71]

Description of the Pathogen

Like all *Chlamydia*, *C pneumoniae* is an obligate intracellular parasite, depending on its host cell for nutrients. It grows poorly on special media and is sensitive to freeze–thaw cycling.

Epidemiology

Recently recognized and difficult to diagnose, *C pneumoniae* has not been exhaustively studied. The pathogen is transmitted by person-to-person contact and respiratory droplets.[72] It has been found in many parts of the world and is thought to be both endemic and epidemic in some populations, with outbreaks lasting from 4 months to 3 years.[73] No seasonal variation in risk is apparent.[74] The prevalence of antibodies in adults is thought to average about 50%,[75,76] with a higher proportion of men having antibodies than women.[77] The pathogen is considered responsible for about 10% of pneumonias worldwide, with seroconversion peaking during teenage years, at about 10% per year.[78] Military training populations may suffer higher rates of infection. A 1989 study[60] of US Marine Corps recruits demonstrated seroconversion in 3.9% of them during an 11-week training period. Another trainee study[31] conducted in 1994 found evidence of seroconversions in 8% during a 63-day training period. Risk factors for *C pneumoniae* infection are not well defined. As military recruits seem to be at higher risk, crowding probably plays a role in transmission.

Pathogenesis and Clinical Findings

Limited data are available regarding pathogenesis caused by *C pneumoniae*. The pathogen multiplies in macrophages, various connective tissues, and smooth muscle cells.[79] A 1989 study[60] of Marines suggested that a preexisting antibody is protective against serologic evidence of infection. Evidence exists, however, that humans may be reinfected with *C pneumoniae*. Generally, reinfection results in milder disease, but among the elderly, reinfections may lead to severe disease.[80,81]

Many infections may be asymptomatic, and clinical manifestations are often insidious. *C pneumoniae* has been implicated in causing pharyngitis (often with hoarseness),[74] sinusitis, bronchitis, and lower respiratory tract infections. *C pneumoniae*–infected patients often do not have a marked fever or an elevated white blood count. Some evidence shows that *C pneumoniae* may be associated with coronary artery disease,[82] reactive airway disease,[83,84] and chronic pharyngitis.[85]

Diagnostic Approaches

Difficulties in diagnosing *C pneumoniae* infection are numerous. The pathogen is difficult to culture (sensitivity ~50%),[79] and, because of evidence of an asymptomatic carriage,[86,87] some authors argue that isolation apart from other evidence of infection may be misleading. Two serologic methods have been used to diagnose *C pneumoniae* infection among young adults: complement fixation and micro-immunofluorescence. Generally, a 4-fold rise in titer from acute to convalescent sera is considered evidence of recent infection. A high acute microimmunofluorescence IgM titer also is accepted.[88] Complement fixation is less sensitive than the microimmunofluorescence method, but the latter is technically more difficult and subject to significant reader error.[79] Neither method is widely available, and investigators must rely on reference laboratories for support. Both serologic methods may be confounded by *C trachomatis* infections, which may cause cross reactions.[79,89] Several different PCR diagnostic methods have been developed.[90,91] Dacron swabs are recommended, because other swab types may inhibit PCR technique.

Recommendations for Control

The only evidence of an effective intervention has been the data suggesting that weekly oral azithromycin (500 mg) has a 58% efficacy in preventing

serologic evidence of infection.[31] Because effective diagnostic tests are not commercially available, the DoD does not conduct routine surveillance for *C pneumoniae*. No vaccine is available.

Influenza

Before vaccines were available, influenza outbreaks could devastate a military population in a matter of weeks. A 1919 report of a 2-week outbreak of influenza in an Arkansas military camp recorded that the camp hospital received 188 to 486 influenza admissions per day, overwhelming hospital staff, who themselves had a 25% incidence of disease.[92] Despite the availability and annual use of influenza vaccine, epidemics still occur among US military populations. During 1996, a Navy ship with a 551-person crew had a 42% attack rate, although 95% of the men had recently received influenza vaccine (G.C.G., unpublished data, 2000). Viral isolates indicated that the epidemic strain was not covered by that year's vaccine (Figure 38-3).

Description of the Pathogen

Some of the most studied viruses, influenza viruses are recognized for their antigenic variation

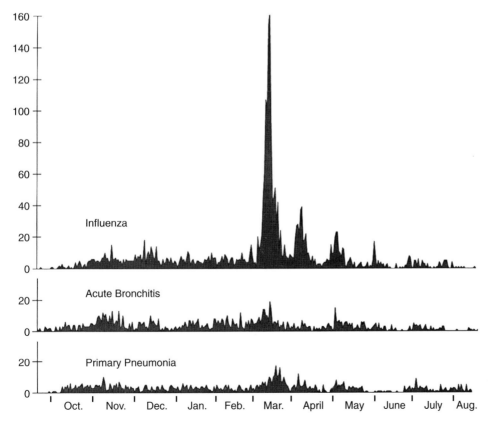

Fig. 38-3. Respiratory disease hospitalizations for influenza, acute bronchitis, and primary pneumonia at Army Camp Funston in Fort Riley, Kansas, from 20 September 1917 to 20 August 1918.
Adapted by Phil Larkins with permission from: Opie EL, Freeman AW, Blake FG, Small JC, Rivers TM. Pneumonia at Camp Funston. *JAMA*. 1919;72:114. Copyright 1919, American Medical Association.

and classified into 3 types: A, B, and C. The viruses, especially types A and B, vary their antigenic presentation and cause cyclical pandemics. Type A influenza virus is classified by the antigenic presentation of its surface glycoproteins—hemagglutinin and neuraminidase. Mutations in the genes for these glycoproteins have caused pandemics throughout recent history (1889, 1918, 1957, and 1968). A major change in glycoproteins is known as an antigenic shift, minor changes as antigenic drift. Type B influenza virus also is recognized for antigenic drift, but its antigenic variation is less than that of type A. Type C influenza virus causes sporadic disease and varies its antigenic presentation to a lesser extent than do types A and B.

Epidemiology

The influenza viruses generally are transmitted by person-to-person contact or through droplet spread from sneezing or coughing. Influenza viruses vary geographically in their antigenic makeup, and surveillance for type A variants is conducted worldwide. Surveillance information is used to anticipate epidemics and select antigenic components for vaccine production.

Influenza epidemics often are explosive and result in high mortality. The 1918–1919 influenza pandemic resulted in an estimated 20 million deaths.[93] During epidemics, more than 40% of a military population may be affected during a brief period.[94] Persons at highest risk of experiencing severe clinical symptoms from influenza infection are those with chronic cardiac, pulmonary, or renal conditions; those with diabetes mellitus or immunosuppression; pregnant women; and the elderly.

Pathogenesis and Clinical Findings

The influenza virus invades the host via the upper respiratory tract. Viral particles penetrate host respiratory epithelial cells, replicate, and infect neighboring cells. Peak viral loads are reached within 24 hours. Influenza virus is thought to remain largely in the respiratory tract. Both secretory and serum antibodies are involved in host defense against influenza virus invasion. After natural infection, immunity to influenza virus with those antigens wanes after several years.

Clinically, influenza viral infection may range in manifestations from asymptomatic or cold-like symptoms to severe pneumonia leading to death. The viruses may cause chills, fever, headache, myalgia, sore throat, backache, sneezing, anorexia, nausea, vomiting, and cough. Pneumonia is a serious complication and is often associated with concomitant secondary bacterial infections.

Diagnostic Approaches

Influenza is diagnosed by viral culture, antigen detection, or association with other laboratory-proven clinical cases. Diagnoses also may be made retrospectively in epidemiological studies by serologic assay.

Recommendations for Control

DoD-sponsored research[95,96] demonstrated the safety and effectiveness of using amantadine prophylactically to prevent influenza infection among close contacts of those infected. Today, both amantadine and rimantadine are still so used, but recent evidence suggests that viruses resistant to both drugs may emerge.[97,98]

Although vaccine work began shortly after the discovery of the influenza virus (see Table 38-1), progress was slow due to viral antigenic variation. An article on the first attempt at human influenza vaccination was published in 1936.[99] Early influenza A vaccines contained contaminants from the embryonated egg culture and caused considerable reactions. Additionally, the varying antigenic makeup of influenza isolates was not well understood, and results from early vaccine studies were mixed.

In 1943, the DoD sponsored some of the first influenza vaccine testing among military students at several US sites.[100,101] One of the earliest combined influenza A and B vaccine trials among US military students demonstrated a protective efficacy of 69% and greatly encouraged more research.[101] The DoD continued to test various types of influenza vaccines, both inactivated and attenuated,[94,102] and these studies led to the present successful strategy of altering yearly the antigenic makeup of this vaccine. Numerous public health organizations conduct surveillance for influenza infections. The focus of such surveillance is the antigenic makeup of wild viruses. Today, the military relies on a whole-cell, inactivated type of vaccine, which combines the antigenic makeup of type A and B viruses considered to be most threatening for the year ahead. This vaccine is given annually to all US military personnel.

Adenovirus

Soon after the discovery of adenovirus in 1953,[103,104] it was learned that this pathogen was an important cause of acute respiratory disease among military personnel, especially recruits.[105]

Description of the Pathogen

Adenovirus has been classified into 51 serotypes. These serotypes may have antigenically recognizable subtypes. Serotypes 4 and 7 account for most military adenovirus respiratory epidemics. Serotypes 3, 12, 14, and 21 also cause acute respiratory disease among military populations but to a lesser extent.

Epidemiology

Adenoviruses are transmitted through respiratory droplets and person-to-person contact. Adenoviruses are thought to have a worldwide distribution, and incidence rates among military trainees often have been high, especially during winter months.[107–109]

Before vaccines were developed, adenovirus infections caused 10% of US Army recruits to be hospitalized and, during winter months, explained 90% of all hospital admissions of recruits.[106] Hillman also estimated that during the winter months, adenoviruses accounted for 77% of all recruit respiratory disease.[107] Most often, adenovirus infections occurred during the first 3 weeks of recruit training,[108] and only the newest military personnel were affected.[109] However, among US Marine Corps trainees, infection was often delayed until postrecruit training.[110,111] In general, military trainees were found to be at much higher risk of infection than were similar civilian populations.

Pathogenesis and Clinical Findings

Studying adenoviruses is confounded by asymptomatic carriage and asymptomatic infection.[112,113] It is not understood why some people suffer significant clinical disease when infected and others remain asymptomatic. Some evidence indicates that adenovirus infection, when associated with infection from other respiratory pathogens, results in more severe disease.[114] The virus is thought to invade respiratory tissues and, after a several-day incubation period, to cause clinical disease and sometimes viremia. Some adenoviruses may cause prolonged infection, such as chronic pharyngitis. Evidence also suggests that latent adenovirus infection may reactivate and cause clinical disease in the immunocompromised.

Adenovirus respiratory disease often causes fever, cough, pharyngitis, and rhinitis. The infection may progress to a lower respiratory tract infection, which is generally milder than that caused by *S pneumoniae*. Adenoviruses also cause gastrointestinal symptoms, epidemic keratoconjunctivitis, and epidemic pharyngoconjunctival fever, but respiratory disease is the most common presentation among military recruits.

Diagnostic Approaches

Today, adenoviruses are detected through culture and various antigen or nucleic acid detection techniques. Culture and identification of adenovirus are relatively easy; however, serotyping traditionally requires a reference laboratory to perform neutralization tests using specific horse or rabbit antisera. In patients with symptoms, the detection of adenovirus generally is accepted as evidence of infection. Epidemiologic studies often rely on serologic evidence of infection, which is gained through several methods, including complement fixation, neutralization tests, hemagglutination-inhibition antibody tests, and ELISA tests.[115,116]

Recommendations for Control

The DoD has developed a number of adenovirus vaccines.[117,118] Early inactivated vaccines against serotypes 3, 4, and 7 were effective, given separately or in combination, in greatly reducing military recruit respiratory morbidity.[117] The inactivated vaccines suffered from production difficulties, however, and some seed virus cultures were contaminated with other viruses.[119,120] Later, live vaccines were developed for serotypes 4, 7, and 21. These vaccines caused excellent seroconversion and had few side effects when given orally as enteric-coated tablets. The success of the serotypes 4 and 7 vaccines led to their adoption by the DoD as routine preventive therapy in the early 1970s, and they remain very effective, when available.[119] Because of the infrequency of military epidemics from serotype 21 virus, the serotype 21 vaccine was not developed further or used. In addition to vaccine intervention, DoD researchers also explored prophylactically administering serum immune globulin against acute respiratory tract infection. Results of these trials were mixed; some show a protective effect but not as protective as adenovirus vaccine.[121–123]

Due largely to economic reasons, the sole manufacturer of adenovirus vaccines ceased production in 1996. The last stores of adenovirus 4 and 7 vaccines were depleted in early 1999. Subsequently, large adenoviral respiratory disease epidemics occurred among numerous US military populations,[124–127] causing costly morbidity and loss of training time. Recent serological studies demonstrate that approximately 90% of trainees enter military service are susceptible to either type 4 or type 7 adenoviral infection.[128] Despite this current and likely future morbidity and cost-benefit studies[129,130] that demonstrate large financial savings with vaccine use, at the time of this writing the Department of Defense had not yet secured a new adenovirus vaccine manufacturer.

Emerging Pathogens

With the myriad available antibiotic therapies and an assortment of effective vaccines, one might think that today's military preventive medicine personnel are well equipped to control most respiratory diseases. This might be true if pathogen-host relationships were not changing, but most certainly they are, and military populations continue to suffer from respiratory disease. In the 1980s, along with the more-virulent *S pyogenes* isolates came a newly recognized manifestation of infection, streptococcal toxic shock syndrome.[131] This syndrome and other forms of invasive *S pyogenes* infection with the same rapid tissue destruction and high mortality rates, such as necrotizing fasciitis, have caused considerable alarm among military populations. Risk factors for these rare invasive diseases have not been well identified, but available data suggest that persons with human immunodeficiency virus infection, diabetes, cancer, or varicella infection or who abuse alcohol may be at increased risk.[132]

The success of various antibiotics in controlling *S pneumoniae* and *S pyogenes* infections may soon be overshadowed by the pathogens' development of resistance to penicillin and erythromycin. Already some DoD clinicians have changed empirical therapies, and the increasing prevalence of antimicrobial resistance promises to be a continual military problem.

Some successful childhood vaccines have caused unexpected adult pathology by postponing natural infection until the adult years. Such is the case with *Bordetella pertussis*; studies[133] have shown that the childhood immunity induced by pertussis vaccine wanes in adulthood, and the proportion of US adults susceptible to infection has increased with time. A recent study[134] has shown that up to 26% of university students who report 6 or more days of cough may have evidence of acute pertussis. A similar study[135] of coughing Marine Corps trainees in 1989 demonstrated that 17% were infected. Since

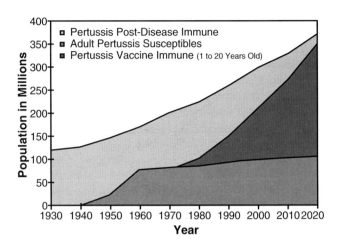

Fig. 38-4. Increasing numbers of US adults susceptible to pertussis, in millions of persons by year.
Adapted by Phil Larkins with permission of the *Pediatric Infectious Disease Journal* from: Bass JW, Stephenson SR. The return of pertussis. *Pediatr Infect Dis J.* 1987;6:141–144.

the yield of oral culture among *B pertussis* adults is poor and no good, rapid diagnostic techniques are available, recognizing such infections will be a problem for tomorrow's military clinician (Figure 38-4).

Summary

Respiratory disease remains a major cause of morbidity for today's military populations. Despite a number of preventive measures military personnel still suffer morbidity for *S pyogenes, S pneumoniae, M pneumoniae, C pneumoniae*, influenza, and adenovirus infections. Respiratory outbreaks often occur in an explosive fashion, and if the etiologic agent or agents are not easily recognized, the military preventive medicine officer may face a dilemma: wait for definitive diagnosis while the epidemic continues to build, or venture an empiric intervention that may later be judged inappropriate or expensive, and may have its own morbidity. Having an understanding of the most common pathogens, as describe din this chapter, and an understanding of their epidemiology (Table 38-2) prepares the preventive medicine officer to make good public health recommendations.

[Gregory C. Gray, MD, MPH]

MENINGOCOCCAL DISEASE

Introduction and Military Relevance

Meningococcal disease is currently an infrequent yet important problem for the military medical of-

ficer. Few, if any, infections can kill as quickly or panic the population involved so thoroughly. Despite significant gains in knowledge, the disease remains an enigma. It is caused by an exceedingly

TABLE 38-2

CHARACTERISTICS OF INFECTIOUS AGENTS TO CONSIDER DURING MILITARY EPIDEMICS

Incubation Period (d)	Organism	Epidemiologic and Clinical Clues
1-3	Influenza viruses	Very acute onset; headache, fever, malaise; onset may be followed by bacterial pneumonia; affects both veteran and new military personnel
1-3	*Streptococcus pyogenes*	Acute onset; sore and inflamed throat, fever; often associated with epidemics
1-3	*Streptococcus pneumoniae*	Frequently preceded by viral infections; acute onset; high fever, rigors; often causes lobar pneumonia; often produces a characteristic sputum
4-12	Adenovirus	Acute onset; affects new military personnel; mild disease but can cause pneumonia; affects new military personnel
6-20	*Bordetella pertussis*	Gradual onset; adults generally have cough for 7 or more days; cough is severe and with paroxysms
6-32	*Mycoplasma pneumoniae*	Gradual onset; cough, malaise, chills but no rigor, mild pneumonia; 50% with positive cold agglutinins
10-30	*Chlamydia pneumoniae*	Acute or gradual onset; pharyngitis, cough, hoarseness, fever; sputum is sparse; illness is generally mild

common, commensal organism that rarely results in symptomatic illness. The reasons for this common organism causing rare endemic disease, sporadic localized outbreaks, and periodic massive epidemics are not entirely clear. Although primarily a disease of children, adults brought together into crowded living conditions (eg, prisoners, military recruits) are at greatly increased risk of disease.

The Napoleonic armies experienced the *meningite de congelation* described by Baron Larrey in 1807. Not until 1886, however, when Weischelbaum noted the diplococcus on microscopic examination of cerebrospinal fluid of a Viennese victim, was the diagnosis of meningococcal disease well defined. Reliable rates of meningococcal disease in the US Army extend back to about 1900. Increased annual incidence of disease was clearly documented in association with military campaigns, to include the occupation of Cuba in 1907 (50/100,000) and the mobilization along the Mexican border in 1913 (35/100,000). In 1917 in association with the mobilization for World War I, rates of meningococcal disease exceeded 150/100,000 per year in the Army. As with the Mexican border mobilization, the abrupt increase in incidence was a result of epidemics in training camps and not from increased disease in seasoned, deployed troops.[136]

The last major wave of meningococcal disease to occur in the United States, both military and civilian, occurred in 1945. Significant outbreaks continued to occur at US military bases in the 1960s and 1970s, more than one of which resulted in the temporary closure of a basic training camp.[136–138]

While the use of antibiotics in the 20th century has drastically improved the outcome of meningococcal disease, case-fatality rates of 5% or more are still seen under optimal conditions. Medical research, much of it by the US armed services, has produced vaccines and drug regimens for the successful prevention of meningococcal disease. Nevertheless, meningococcal disease should remain a significant concern as long as the military assembles young adults or deploys personnel to areas of the world with high rates of meningococcal disease.

Description of the Pathogen

The responsible bacterium, *Neisseria meningitidis*, is a member of the genus *Neisseria*, which includes the closely related *N gonorrhoeae* and other bacteria found on human mucosal surfaces. The human nasopharynx is the habitat of these Gram-negative cocci measuring 0.6 to 1.0 µm in diameter. They are often seen in pairs (diplococci) with adjacent sides slightly flattened. On solid media, *N meningitidis* grows in colorless, transparent, nonhemolytic colonies. *N meningitidis* requires a degree of special handling; the organisms do not tolerate low humidity or extremes of temperature and grow best on blood-enriched media. Optimal growth occurs at 35°C to 37°C in a humid, microaerophilic atmosphere containing 3% to 10% carbon dioxide. Specimens, therefore, should be plated on warm chocolate agar and incubated in a candle jar without delay. When plating specimens obtained from nonsterile sites (eg, the nasopharynx), the use of selective media for *Neisseria* species is recommended (eg, Thayer-Martin [Martin-Lewis] medium—a chocolate agar with antibiotics added to suppress the growth of yeast and bacteria other than *Neisseria*). With this careful handling, the organism can usually be recovered within 24 hours of incubation.[139–143]

Definitive identification of genus is accomplished by analysis of the bacterial enzymes present. *Neisseria* species are identified from most other flora by the presence of cytochrome oxidase. Then, as a general rule, *N meningitis* is identified by its ability to metabolize glucose and maltose with the production of acid and its inability to metabolize sucrose or lactose.[139] Further classification of *N meningitis* is accomplished by analysis of the bacterial surface.

Based on the antigenic properties of capsular polysaccharides, at least thirteen serologic groups of *N meningitidis* (ie, A, B, C, D, E, H, I, K, L, X, Y, W-135, Z) have been designated. Historically, the majority of disease is caused by serogroups A, B, and C. The meningococcus is also found without a polysaccharide coat. Termed nonencapsulated strains, these colonies appear smooth in culture, as opposed to those colonies that produce large amounts of polysaccharide, which appear mucoid. These nonencapsulated strains have not been implicated in systemic disease and are most commonly found in the nasopharynx of asymptomatics.[140] Using sophisticated laboratory techniques, *N meningitidis* may be further classified into serotypes and subtypes based on the antigenic properties of the proteins and glycolipids in the bacterial outer membrane. This nomenclature may cause confusion because serogroup A may be called "serotype" or "type" A. The identification of serogroup is essential when planning public health strategy. In addition to differing properties of each serogroup, vaccines are available for only serogroups A, C, Y, and W-135. The identification of serotype and subtype is of particular use in the investigation of epidemics. Neither serogroup nor serotype, however, is necessary for the diagnosis or clinical management of meningococcal disease.

Epidemiology

Transmission

Transmission of the meningococci is person to person by direct contact of respiratory secretions or by respiratory droplet. The determinants of the distribution of meningococcal disease are complex and only partially understood. Colonization and infection are common; clinical disease is comparatively rare. Recovery of *N meningitidis* from the nasopharynx of healthy "carriers" is common and documented whenever sought. Most patients with symptomatic invasive meningococcal disease ("cases") are not infected by other cases, in case-to-case spread, but rather from healthy carriers.[142,144p340–345] Carriage rates are dependent on age, varying from 1% or less in infants to 20% to 40% in young adults. Increased carriage rates are associated with outbreaks; rates approaching 100% have been documented in military training camps during outbreaks.[143,145] Despite this association, carriage rates of 25% or greater are often documented in the absence of clinical disease. Additionally, while upward of 50% of military recruits have been documented as asymptomatic carriers of a pathogenic strain, the majority of carriers generally do not harbor the strain of meningococcus responsible for the disease in their midst.[142]

While carriage is responsible for the majority of disease, it is also responsible for the development of natural immunity to the meningococcus. Asymptomatic carriage and mildly symptomatic infection result in the production of protective humoral antibodies within 2 weeks, which persist at high levels for months. Immunity in the neonatal period results from transplancental transfer of humoral antibodies. In early childhood, carriage of atypical, nonpathogenic strains begins a process of recurrent sensitization and antibody production that continues throughout life.[146] These humoral antibodies are protective not only against the particular strain but also against other, but not all, strains of meningococci. Individuals who become ill generally lack effective humoral antibody against the specific pathogenic strain and become ill within the 2-week window between infection and antibody production. This explains the well-documented fact that meningococcal disease is a disease of new recruits and not seasoned service members, even when those seasoned personnel are deployed to areas of higher rates of disease. Interestingly, cases often have demonstrable, effective humoral antibody against most meningococci before infection, but it is simply not effective against the specific strain to which they succumb. To further muddy the waters, several researchers believe that induction of IgA antibody from other infections may be important in epidemic disease. This "two-bug" model postulates that induction of high levels of circulating IgA may block the action of the normally protective humoral antibodies to the capsular polysaccharide, so that disease results from invasive strains to which the individual is "immune."[145–147]

The epidemiology of *N meningitidis* has been described as serogroup specific. The US epidemics of the first half of the 20th century were due primarily to serogroup A, as is still true in developing countries, particularly in Africa.[142] Now serogroups B and C are responsible for 90% of meningococcal disease in the United States. Serogroup C has been associated with most outbreaks in older children and young adults in developed countries, while serogroup B is responsible for the majority of endemic disease, particularly that seen in infants. In the military, meningococcal disease is a disease of training camp: it is caused by serotypes A, B, or C very early in training but after that is caused mostly by serotype B.[136,148]

Geographic Distribution

The geographic distribution of meningococcal disease, as with almost all infectious diseases, has changed significantly over the past 200 years.[149] While the Napoleonic armies were experiencing the *meningite de congelation*, essentially simultaneous epidemics were documented in Geneva, Canada, New York, Ohio, and Virginia. The 19th century then experienced a succession of epidemic waves, also retrospectively attributed by most medical

historians to the meningococcus, crashing over Europe and North America. The first half of the 20th century was also marked by the propagation of several waves, generally at 5- to 10-year intervals, over the same areas. These later waves extended to include sub-Saharan Africa, now widely known as the "meningitis belt." In the second half of the 20th century, an abrupt shift in the pattern of disease occurred. Sub-Saharan Africa continued to have large epidemics, most notably in 1942 to 1951 and 1960 to 1962 and in conjunction with the hajj (the annual Islamic pilgrimage to Mecca). Meningococcal disease in the US and Europe, on the other hand, dwindled to rare endemic disease and small, sporadic outbreaks.

Incidence

For the past several decades, the annual incidence of meningococcal disease in the United States civilian population has remained in the range of 1-2/100,000, with the highest incidence of 17/100,000 found in the first year of life. Rates decline swiftly to less than 1/100,000 in the US adult civilian population.[140] The success of meningococcal vaccine use in military recruits has been striking[150] (Figure 38-5).

Case-fatality rates from invasive meningococcal disease have varied depending on the nature of the infection, the quality of the medical care, and the underlying health of those afflicted. Before any modern treatments, the mortality rate was 75% to

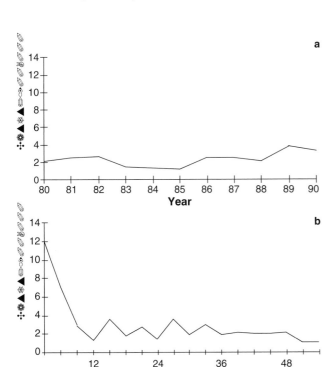

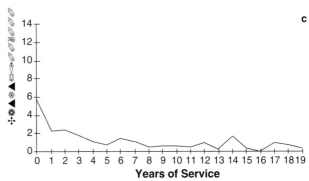

Fig. 38-5. The success of meningococcal vaccine use in military recruits has led to flat disease rates for meningococcal meningitis in US military enlisted personnel of 2/100,000 person-years from 1980 to 1990 (*a*). The higher incidence of the military enlisted population is explained entirely by a rate of 12/100,000 person-years in the first months of service (*b*). The incidence of meningococcal disease in seasoned troops mirrors that of the adult civilian population (*c*).
Source: LCDR M Ryan. Uniformed Services University of the Health Sciences, Bethesda, Md. Unpublished data.

95% or greater. In undeveloped countries and in un-treated cases, similar case-fatality rates are still en-countered. In the United States in the 1990s, the case fatality rate for meningococcal disease is between 10% and 15%.[140–142] Higher rates are seen in cases of meningococcemia without meningitis and at the extremes of age. As with many other infectious dis-eases, crowded living conditions, poor hygiene, stress, and poor nutrition are associated both with meningococcal disease and higher case-fatality rates. In addition to the groups noted above, certain other populations are more susceptible to invasive disease. Especially at risk are those with surgical or functional asplenia and those with deficiencies in the complement pathways. Cases with comple-ment deficiencies are at increased risk for re-infec-tion; many authors recommend testing all cases for such conditions. Also at increased risk are those with underlying chronic illnesses that decrease gen-eral immunocompetence, including but not limited to human immunodeficiency virus infection, ma-lignancy, alcoholism, diabetes mellitus, systemic lupus, and renal or hepatic disease.[140–144] In a recent, population-based study, two thirds of all adult cases had decreased immunocompetence due to one or more of these conditions.[151]

Pathogenesis and Clinical Findings

The pathogenesis of *N meningitidis* continues to be elucidated. The organism has pilli that adhere and gain entry into the nonciliated cells found in the nasopharynx. Once inside, the organisms are able to transmigrate to the submucosal tissues and vasculature. If the organism gains access to the bloodstream, the polysaccharide capsule thwarts the normal defense mechanism of phagocytosis. In the absence of humoral antibody allowing for the opsonization and destruction of the invading men-ingococcus, the impressive cascade of destruction begins. The rapid doubling time of the meningo-coccus coupled with a process termed blebbing, where portions of the bacterium's membrane pinch off into small sacks of endotoxin, account for the organism's ability to kill in hours. The large amounts of endotoxin interact with macrophages and other defense cells to produce cytokines, vasoactive lipids, free radicals, and tissue necrosis factor. All of these substances disrupt the vascular endothe-lium, accounting for the rash, petechia, and purpura associated with full-blown meningococcal disease. Recent research has implicated the extremely high levels of tissue necrosis factor in the destruction of

larger vessels and organs, to include Waterhouse-Friderichson syndrome, a syndrome of multi-organ failure, shock, and galloping disseminated intravas-cular coagulopathy (DIC).[140,142,143]

The result of meningococcal infection ranges from the trivial to the catastrophic. The majority of meningococcal infections are asymptomatic or sub-clinical. Significant meningococcal infection may be preceded by an unremarkable upper respiratory infection (URI) prodrome of cough, headache, and sore throat. Spontaneous resolution of mild menin-gococcal URIs (including those with *N meningitidis*–positive blood cultures) has been documented in distinctly fortunate individuals. With or without the prodrome, those not so fortunate may experience a violent onset of disease consisting of fevers spik-ing to 40°C or higher, chills, malaise, weakness, myalgias, and arthralgias. Acute systemic disease generally presents as meningitis alone, meningitis with septicemia, or septicemia alone. Very rarely (less than 5% of the time), meningococcal disease may present in a different fashion, such as an iso-lated sinusitis, septic arthritis, or chronic meningo-coccemia. In the earliest stages of the infection, the patient may appear to have an unremarkable URI (ie, headache, malaise, and slight fever—a presenta-tion all too common to any primary care physician). In a matter of hours, however, the patient appears distinctly septic; mild hypotension to profound shock may appear early or even occur at presenta-tion.[140–144] Unlike the mild prodrome, this striking presentation once seen is not likely to be forgotten. This extraordinarily rapid progression of disease is the reason that all new soldiers with URI symptoms and fever are hospitalized for observation by the US Army.[136]

The classic petechial rash of meningococcal dis-ease occurs in about three fourths of those with bacteremia. The petechial rash may be present only sparingly on the conjunctiva, soft palate, axilla, groin, wrists, or ankles. Petechia may also be in ar-eas constricted by clothing. Confusing the issue, petechia may be absent with meningococcal disease or may be present with other illnesses for different reasons (eg, on the face after violent coughing or vomiting). Additionally, the rash may begin as a fine maculopapular (morbilliform) rash and then progress to petechiae. The degree of petechial rash corresponds roughly to the degree of thrombocy-topenia and severity of disease. Accordingly, pete-chiae that coalesce into large purpuric lesions are associated with fulminant disease. Other features indicative of a poor prognosis include shock at presentation, rapid progression of petechia to purpura, fever greater than 40°C, leukopenia, and thrombocytopenia or other evidence of DIC. Especially ominous are extensive purpura, hemorrhagic bullae, or peripheral gangrene.[140,142,143]

Diagnostic Approaches

The definitive diagnosis of meningococcal disease is made with the recovery of the meningococcus from a normally sterile site, such as blood or cerebrospinal fluid (CSF). Blood cultures are positive in about 30% of those with meningitis and 70% or more of those with clinical meningococcemia.[140] Gram's stain of the CSF of those with meningitis will demonstrate purulent CSF and the Gram-negative diplococcus. Counterimmunoelectrophoresis or latex agglutination of meningococcal antigen in the CSF, serum, or urine is routinely used, although recent authors have questioned its clinical utility.[152] Gram's stain of skin lesion aspirates and the buffy coat of blood will occasionally reveal organisms but is not recommended for routine diagnosis. Other laboratory findings may be seen that are consistent with significant bacterial infection but are not specific for meningococcal disease, such as a peripheral blood leukocytosis with increase of earlier myelocytic forms (a "left shift"). The differential diagnosis of systemic meningococcal disease is not long. Systemic infection with *Haemophilus influenza* type b or streptococcus may have similar presentations, to include presentation (rarely) with a petechial skin rash. Rocky Mountain spotted fever, other rickettsial diseases, and viral diseases with morbilliform or hemorrhagic exanthems may also present similarly to meningococcal disease.[140,142,143]

Recommendations for Therapy and Control

The successful treatment of meningococcal disease does NOT wait on a definitive diagnosis.[140,142,143,153] When the diagnosis of meningococcal disease is suspected, whether from meningeal signs, evidence of septicemia, or a febrile URI with rash in a new recruit, antibiotic therapy must follow within minutes. The presumptive diagnosis of meningococcal disease is a medical emergency. The meningococcus is sensitive to a variety of antibiotics, including penicillin, third-generation cephalosporins, choramphenicol, and quinolones. Penicillin remains the drug of choice for the treatment of meningococcal disease, despite reports of relative resistance around the world (Table 38-3). In small children, clinicians must anticipate the possibility of infection with *Haemophilus influenza* type b resistant to penicillin by their initial choice of antibiotics. The successful treatment of meningococcal disease in garrison or in the field rests on the prompt initiation of antibiotics. Sophisticated life-support techniques clearly favor recovery but do

TABLE 38-3

ANTIBIOTIC TREATMENT OF MENINGOCOCCAL DISEASE IN ADULTS

Antibiotic	Dosage
Penicillin G	300,000 U/kg-d IV in divided doses q 4 h (maximum dose 24×10^6 U/d)
	or
Ampicillin	150-200 mg/kg-d IV in divided doses q 6 h (maximum dose 12 g/d)
	or
Chloramphenicol*	100 mg/kg-d IV in divided doses q 6 h (maximum dose 4 g/d)
	or
Ceftriaxone†	100 mg/kg-d IV in divided doses q 12 h (maximum dose 4 g/d)
	or
Cefotaxime†	200 mg/kg-d IV in divided doses q 4 h (maximum dose 12 g/d)

* For those severely allergic to penicillin
† For those mildly allergic to penicillin; also effective against *Haemophilus influenza* type b
kg-d: kilograms per day; IV: intravenously; q: every
Sources: Apicella MA. Meningococcal infections. In: Bennett JC, Plum F, eds. *Cecil Textbook of Medicine*. 20th ed. Philadelphia, Penn: W. B. Saunders; 1996: 1618–1622; Apicella MA. *Neisseria meningitidis*. In: Mandell GL, Bennett JE, Dolin R, eds. *Mandell, Douglas, and Bennett's Principles and Practice of Infectious Diseases*. 4th ed. New York: Churchill Livingstone; 1995: 1896–1909; Griffiss JM. Meningococcal infections. In: Isselbacher KJ, Martin JB, Braunwald E, Fauci AS, Wilson JD, Kasper DL, eds. *Harrison's Principles of Internal Medicine*. 13th ed. New York: McGraw-Hill, Inc.; 1994: 641–644.

not justify transfer of a patient with suspected meningococcal disease to a higher level of care without first administering antibiotics. Similarly, antibiotics must not be withheld in the field in an attempt to get positive blood cultures at the next level of care. Antibiotic therapy should be continued in confirmed cases for at least 7 days or for 4 to 5 days after the patient is afebrile.

The patient should be placed in respiratory isolation for the first 24 hours of treatment, with special care given to disposal of respiratory secretions. Aside from isolation and the early initiation of appropriate antibiotics, treatment of systemic meningococcal disease is supportive and will be determined by the level of sophistication of the treatment facility. Fluid resuscitation, fluid and electrolyte balance, oxygenation, and maintenance of visceral perfusion are frequent concerns. The treatment of DIC, when diagnosed, remains controversial; heparin, whole blood, cryoprecipitate, or any combination of these three have been employed with varying degrees of success. Lastly, the patient discharged after successful treatment should receive rifampin chemoprophylaxis, as intravenous antibiotics may not eliminate nasopharyngeal carriage.[140,142,143]

After the end of World War II, the US military instituted the mass use of prophylactic sulfonamides to eliminate nasopharyngeal carriage in all basic trainees. This program was quite successful in military and civilian settings for almost 2 decades until this widespread use of antibiotics lead to sulfonamide-resistant meningococci. Large outbreaks at US Army and Navy training camps in the early 1960s forced not only the temporary closure of bases but also intensive research into vaccine development.[136–138] Using the polysaccharide coats as antigens, the Walter Reed Army Institute of Research produced effective vaccines against serogroup C in 1969. In 1971, routine immunization against serogroup C was begun; other serogroups soon followed (A/C in 1978 and A/C/Y/W-135 in 1982). After the initiation of these immunizations, rates of meningococcal disease in the military fell drastically, approaching those of the civilian population (1-2/100,000)[136] (see Figure 38-5). In contrast to the success with other serogroups, an effective vaccine against *N meningitidis* serogroup B has not yet been approved for use. Interestingly, the serogroup B polysaccharide is identical in structure to a polysaccharide found in human nervous tissue and therefore is not immunogenic. Current research in this area has included using protein components of the organism's outer membrane as antigens and attempting to find similar capsular polysaccharide

antigens that might confer protection against serogroup B.[140,142,154,155]

The meningococcal vaccine is a success when given to recruits on entry to military service. What remains unclear is when, if ever, the vaccine should be repeated. As noted above, meningococcal disease has historically been a disease of training camps and not a problem for seasoned personnel even in areas of increased endemic disease. It is difficult, however, for a military medical officer to withhold a safe, proven vaccine from personnel deploying to an area with a documented epidemic of meningococcal disease. The most significant question—the duration of protection from the meningococcal vaccine—has not been answered. Several studies have demonstrated poor immunogenicity and rapid decline of detectable antibodies in children less than 4 years of age. A cross-sectional study among US Air Force personnel suggested detection of vaccine-induced antibody above prevaccination levels 10 years after immunization,[143,156] but measurement of antibody is a surrogate measurement for immunity and not infallible. Due to this and issues discussed above (eg, cases having demonstrable antibody against meningococcus before infection, the natural immunizing effect of carriage unrelated to vaccination), the actual duration of protection from meningococcal vaccine is likely to remain unknown for some time. The US military has generally erred on the side of being conservative by re-immunizing at 3- to 5-year intervals in the event of deployment to areas with documented epidemic disease. This strategy is not universal, however, as is demonstrated by the Navy's decision to forgo immunization of Marines deploying to the Persian Gulf War.[157] As with other polysaccharide vaccines, there is no immunologic memory leading to a booster effect with subsequent immunizations. Clear indications for immunization include military recruits on entry to training, patients with functional or surgical asplenia, and those with deficiencies of the complement pathways.

After the remarkable success of prophylactic sulfonamides ended, attention quickly turned to finding other effective prophylactic regimens. Rifampin was found to eliminate nasopharyngeal carriage and quickly became the drug of choice for chemoprophylaxis (Table 38-4). Rifampin use is not without its problems, however, and patients must be told to expect reddish-orange discoloration of urine, tears, feces, and sputum. Although harmless, the discoloration of tears will permanently stain soft contact lenses. More importantly, rifampin may interfere with the action of oral contraceptives. Sexu-

TABLE 38-4

PROPHYLACTIC CHEMOTHERAPY OF *NEISSERIA MENINGITIDIS* CONTACTS

Antibiotic	Dose
Rifampin	Adults: 600 mg po bid for 2 d
	Children > 1 mo: 10 mg/kg-d; divided doses po bid for 2 d
	Children < 1 mo: 5 mg/kg-d; divided doses po bid for 2 d
	OR
Ciprofloxacin	Adults: 500 mg po (single dose)
	OR
Ceftriaxone	Adults: 250 mg IM (single dose)
	Children < 15 y: 125 mg IM (single dose)
	OR
Sulfadiazine*	Adults: 1 g po q 12 h for 2 d
	Children > 2 mos: 150 mg/kg-d (not to exceed adult dose) in divided doses q 12 h for 2 d

* For use against documented sulfa-susceptible strains only; no longer manufactured in the United States
bid: two times a day, po: by mouth, kg-d: kilograms per day, q: every, IM: intramuscularly
Sources: Apicella MA. Meningococcal infections. In: Bennett JC, Plum F, eds. *Cecil Textbook of Medicine*. 20th ed. Philadelphia, Penn: W. B. Saunders; 1996: 1618–1622; Apicella MA. *Neisseria meningitidis*. In: Mandell GL, Bennett JE, Dolin R, eds. *Mandell, Douglas, and Bennett's Principles and Practice of Infectious Diseases*. 4th ed. New York: Churchill Livingstone; 1995: 1896–1909; Griffiss JM. Meningococcal infections. In: Isselbacher KJ, Martin JB, Braunwald E, Fauci AS, Wilson JD, Kasper DL, eds. *Harrison's Principles of Internal Medicine*. 13th ed. New York: McGraw-Hill, Inc.; 1994: 641–644.

ally active patients must be advised to take appropriate precautions. Unlike the sulfonamides, which may still be used in mass prophylactic campaigns against susceptible organisms, rifampin has been associated with the rapid appearance of resistant organisms and is not recommended for mass chemoprophylaxis. Ciprofloxacin and ceftriaxone may also be used for chemoprophylaxis; they share the advantage of requiring only a single dose.[140–142]

Meningococcal infection can kill a previously healthy young adult within hours of the first symptom and, in an outbreak, do this several times in the community within a few days. These qualities combine to produce a disease that truly can terrify the public. The preventive medicine officer must be informed immediately of the admission of a suspected case of meningococcal disease. Close contacts of the case, defined as household contacts and those with direct, face-to-face contact with the case, suffer an increased risk of disease several hundred times that of the general population and should receive chemoprophylaxis. An exception to this somewhat restrictive recommendation concerns children in daycare and institutionalized persons, to include military recruits. Persons in these particular high-risk groups should receive prophylaxis for even minimal contact, (eg, being present in the same daycare facility or sleeping in the same open-bay barracks).[144] Many authors recommend simultaneous immunization if the outbreak is due to a vaccine-preventable serogroup.[140,142,143] Because of the poor immunogenicity in young children, serogroup C vaccine is not recommended for those under the age of 2 years. Factors associated with increased disease, (eg, overcrowding, poor nutrition) should be remedied if possible. Investigation of the outbreak is limited to identifying contacts for chemoprophylaxis, alleviating factors associated with disease, and encouraging vigilance for the first sign of possible meningococcal disease. Screening the population using throat or nasopharyngeal cultures has not proven effective in controlling outbreaks.[144]

The public health emphasis in controlling meningococcal outbreaks should be placed on active surveillance, heightened awareness, prompt diagnosis and treatment of those ill, and effective communication to the public. The public health official must carefully convey an accurate assessment of risk to groups with varying degrees of medical sophistication. The goal is to motivate these groups sufficiently to ensure appropriate identification of contacts and heightened awareness of the early symptoms of disease without starting a panic. This being said, it is extraordinarily difficult to contain the fear in a community struck by several cases of meningococcal disease. An experience in Canada underscored again the sensitive nature of the issues in meningococcal outbreaks. In response to an outbreak in Ontario in 1991, a mass voluntary immunization campaign resulted in over 400,000 immunizations at a cost of at least US $7,000,000. Over 145,000 young adults were immunized in Ottawa alone less than a month after the first case. Debate continued for years in the medical literature as to whether the media coverage of the outbreak and the immunization campaign it engendered were appropriate.[158]

[Brian Feighner, MD, MPH]

TUBERCULOSIS

Introduction and Military Relevance

Understanding and controlling the risks posed by tuberculosis to the health of US military forces remain as relevant today as they were to preventive medicine specialists during World War I and World War II. Recruits continue to enter military service with preexisting tuberculosis infections. Military deployments and long-term assignments to regions of the world with high rates of tuberculosis infection and disease in the host population place US military personnel at increased risk for acquiring a tuberculosis infection, potentially with a multidrug-resistant organism. Militarily unique environments, such as ships and barracks, put large numbers of people together in close living and working arrangements for extended periods of time—ideal conditions for person-to-person transmission of tuberculosis. War and operations other than war, especially those requiring support for refugees, displaced persons, and prisoners of war, increase the risk for exposure to tuberculosis while requiring knowledge of tuberculosis treatment and control measures unique to those populations.

As early as 1854, tuberculosis (or phythisis pulmonalis) was recognized as a particular problem of shipboard life in the Navy.[159] During the US Civil War, the Army experienced 13,499 tuberculosis hospitalizations and 5,286 tuberculosis deaths among white soldiers, but control and treatment measures received no specific attention.[160] The Navy and Marine Corps had annual tuberculosis admission rates of 6 to 12 per 1,000 members in the 1880s.[159] By the early 1900s, the military services began to stress physical examinations as the main control measure to identify men with tuberculosis and to exclude them from military service. More than 50,000 men were excluded from Army service during World War I, yet more than 2,000 soldiers died from tuberculosis and 19 per 1,000 were hospitalized annually with tuberculosis.[161] Tuberculosis was the Army's leading cause of discharge for disability. During the war, the naval services' hospital admission rate was approximately 5 cases per 1,000 per year.[159]

Tuberculosis among military entrants remained a problem at the start of World War II. To improve tuberculosis screening of entrants, the military services had installed radiographic equipment to perform chest roentgen examinations or photofluorograms at many recruit centers in the months before the war. By the end of 1942, chest radiographs became a required part of the entrance physical examination, resulting in 1% of Army recruits being rejected for tuberculosis. During the war, the annual incidence of tuberculosis was 1.0 to 1.75 per 1,000 in the Army and 1.0 to 3.25 per 1,000 in the Navy and Marine Corps, with the higher rates occurring at the beginning and end of the war.[159,161] The higher rates at the war's end were primarily due to universal chest radiographs upon discharge, which identified many new cases of minimally active tuberculosis. While soldiers with foreign service had slightly higher rates of tuberculosis at separation processing, most new infections were probably due to exposure to fellow soldiers, not to civilians, with tuberculosis. Among US service members who had been prisoners of war, rates of active tuberculosis were 37 per 1,000 prisoners of the Japanese and 6 per 1,000 prisoners of the Germans. At the war's end, tuberculosis among displaced persons and civilians liberated from concentration camps in Germany, Italy, and Japan presented a significant challenge to military medicine[161] (see Chapter 3, The Historic Role of Military Preventive Medicine and Public Health in US Armies of Occupation and Military Government). Several Army hospitals in Germany were designated for the treatment of tuberculosis patients, while tuberculosis control programs were part of the efforts to rebuild public health infrastructures.

By 1950, routine chest radiographs of active duty members and tuberculin tests for all recruits were common practice in all services. Annual tuberculosis admission rates dropped below 1 per 1,000 sailors and Marines.[159] During the Korean War, however, 2.6% of Army casualties evacuated to the United States for care required treatment for tuberculosis. The rate of active tuberculosis among US service members who had been prisoners of the North Koreans was 1.5%.[162]

In Vietnam, US personnel had varying degrees of contact with a civilian population with a high rate of infection and disease. Almost 50% of 17- to 18-year-old Vietnamese and nearly all Vietnamese adults had tuberculin test evidence of infection; one study showed 32% of adults had radiological evidence of active infection. US military personnel experienced rates of tuberculin test conversion of 3% to 5% after 1-year assignments in Vietnam, while personnel remaining in the United States had a 1% per year conversion rate.[160]

Since World War II, there has been a downward trend in the proportion of military entrants with preexisting tuberculosis infection. A study of 1.2 million US Navy recruits from 1958 to 1969 demonstrated that 5.2% were tuberculin test reactors.[163] Among all Air Force recruits in 1964 and 1965, 4.2% were reactors using a multiple puncture test.[164] By 1990, 2.5% of 2,416 Navy recruits were tuberculin reactors with a 10-mm induration; 19.2% of foreign-born recruits and 1.6% of recruits born in the United States were reactors with 10-mm or greater induration.[165]

In the past decade, tuberculosis has maintained a low but ever-present profile in the US military. In the 1980s, an estimated 1% of sailors and Marines converted on their tuberculin tests each year.[166] Sailors participating in deployments in 1986 and 1987 involving numerous port visits in South America were diagnosed with active tuberculosis at a rate of one case per 1,000 person-years and had rates of tuberculin test reactions three times greater than the rate among sailors on other Atlantic Fleet ships.[167] Tuberculosis exposure was a concern for military personnel of all services involved in the care of refugees and displaced persons in the Caribbean region, Africa, and Southeast Asia. During 1995, approximately 40 cases of tuberculosis were reported in active duty US military personnel (Army data: Army Medical Surveillance Activity, Washington, DC; Navy data: Naval Environmental Health Center, Norfolk, Virginia; Air Force data: Armstrong Laboratories, Brooks Air Force Base, Texas).

Tuberculosis has presented a special challenge in the closed environments on ships. The most notable outbreak occurred on the destroyer USS Richard E. Byrd in 1966.[168,169] A sailor with symptomatic cavitary tuberculosis was on the ship for 6 months until he was diagnosed. There were seven secondary cases of pulmonary tuberculosis; 47% of the enlisted crew converted on their tuberculin test reactions. In 1987, a similar scenario on an amphibious ship resulted in 216 tuberculin test converters, 25% of the total crew.[170] In these shipboard outbreaks, the highest rates of tuberculin test conversion (more than 80%) were in those sailors who berthed in the same compartments as the source case.[169,170] A 1998 outbreak on an amphibious ship produced 17 cases of pulmonary or pleural tuberculosis, 171 (18.3%) tuberculin test convertors among the ship's crew, and 525 (25.2%) convertors among embarked Marines.[171] Frequently, the risk extends to the entire crew because of the closed shipboard environment and the extended exposure associated with duty at sea, which equals or exceeds that experienced by most household contacts of tuberculosis cases ashore. Exposure on shore to tuberculosis is much less intensive, but an outbreak has been documented at an isolated Army installation.[172]

Description of the Pathogen

In humans, chronic tuberculosis infection of the lungs and other organs is caused by *Mycobacterium tuberculosis* and less commonly by *M bovis*, which causes similar infections in cattle. *M tuberculosis* is a slow-growing, nonmotile bacillus, whose waxy cell wall resists decolorization by acid alcohol during staining, resulting in its "acid fast" characteristic. The waxy coat allows *M tuberculosis* to resist drying and germicides. Mycobacteria are susceptible to moist heat and ultraviolet light from both sunlight and artificial sources.

Epidemiology

Transmission

Exposure to airborne *M tuberculosis* from a person with pulmonary or laryngeal tuberculosis is the primary mode of transmission of tuberculosis. Droplet nuclei (1-5 μm diameter), produced when the infected person coughs, sings, or sneezes, dry and can remain airborne for several hours or longer. When inhaled, droplet nuclei can be carried directly to the alveoli of the lungs, where the primary infection is established. The incubation period from infection to either development of a reactive tuberculin test or evidence of a primary pulmonary lesion is 4 to 12 weeks. Unpasteurized milk can serve as the vehicle for transmission of *M bovis* from infected cows to humans.

Tuberculosis is not a highly communicable infection, but the factors affecting its spread from one person to another vary and can create localized outbreaks. Generally, only patients with pulmonary or laryngeal tuberculosis will spread infection. Communicability increases if the source case is coughing, sneezing, or singing. The presence of acid fast bacilli in sputum and cavitary disease increase communicability. Other factors include the length of time the patient has been symptomatic (especially coughing) before diagnosis, the closeness and duration of contact, and the ventilation and other environmental features of the contact space. In the United States, approximately one fifth of close contacts of a source case with active pulmonary tuberculosis will acquire a new tuberculosis infection from the exposure. Adequate treatment rapidly reduces the infectiousness of tuberculosis patients.

Geographic Distribution

Worldwide, tuberculosis causes 3 million deaths annually and is the leading cause of death among adults from a single infectious agent.[173] In 1990, there were an estimated 7.5 million cases of tuberculosis worldwide.[174] Two billion people—one third of the world's population—are infected with *Mycobacterium tuberculosis*.[173]

Incidence

Tuberculosis incidence in the United States declined to 7.4 cases per 100,000 population in 1997, the lowest rate since national surveillance began in the 1930s, but this still represents almost 20,000 new tuberculosis cases. An increasing proportion of cases (39%) was among foreign-born persons. Resistance of *M tuberculosis* isolates to isoniazid or rifampin (two first-line drugs in the treatment of tuberculosis) increased; 7.6% were resistant to at least isoniazid and 1.3% were resistant to at least isoniazid and rifampin.[175]

Pathogenesis and Clinical Findings

After inhalation, *M tuberculosis* bacilli are carried to the alveoli where they are ingested by alveolar macrophages and eventually transported to hilar lymph nodes. Most primary infections are asymptomatic, although some patients present with a primary tuberculosis pneumonia or pleurisy with effusion a few weeks after their initial infection. Once tuberculosis infection is established, the lifetime risk of developing active disease is about 5% to 10%, with the greatest risk (1% to 4%) occurring in the first year after acquiring infection. Preventive therapy significantly reduces but does not eliminate the risk of developing active disease. For more than 90% of persons infected with *M tuberculosis*, the only evidence of tuberculosis will be a reactive tuberculin test and occasionally radiographic evidence of a primary pulmonary infection, such as parenchymal scarring or calcified lymph nodes.

Reactivation tuberculosis, most commonly confined to the lungs, occurs months to years after the primary infection in up to 10% of persons with tuberculosis infections. The risk of reactivation increases in persons with immunocompromising conditions, such as human immunodeficiency virus (HIV) infection, and in those taking immunosuppressive medications. The most common presentation is one of chronic systemic and pulmonary symptoms and findings. Infiltrates and single or multiple cavities, most commonly in the upper lobes, are present on chest radiographs (Figure 38-6). Extrapulmonary presentations of tuberculosis include tuberculosis

adenitis, genitourinary infection, skeletal tuberculosis, and meningitis. Miliary tuberculosis involving multiple organs presents as a febrile wasting disease of unknown origin. Pulmonary and extrapulmonary tuberculosis are acquired immunodeficiency syndrome–defining diagnoses in HIV-infected persons.

Diagnostic Approaches

Awareness

The best tool for diagnosing tuberculosis is a high index of suspicion. Failure to suspect tuberculosis even after multiple visits to military sick call has contributed to delays in diagnosis and higher rates of new tuberculosis infections among contacts in military outbreaks.[169,170] Pulmonary tuberculosis should be suspected in per-

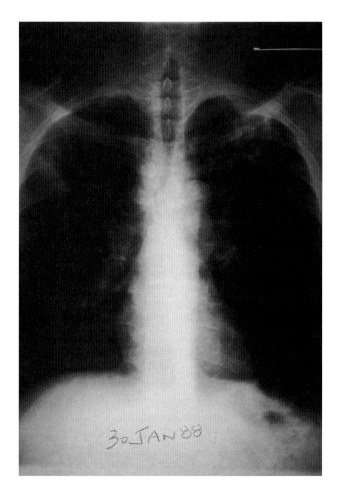

Fig. 38-6. This chest radiograph demonstrates cavitary disease characteristic of pulmonary tuberculosis. Radiograph: Courtesy of the Walter Reed Army Medical Center, Washington, DC.

sons with a productive, prolonged cough (of more than 3 weeks' duration) or in persons with fever, chills, night sweats, easy fatigability, loss of appetite, weight loss, or hemoptysis. Diagnostic suspicion should increase for persons with a history of exposure to tuberculosis or of a positive tuberculin test, persons born in foreign countries with a high incidence of tuberculosis, or persons in other high-risk groups for tuberculosis. The evaluation should include a thorough history, physical examination, chest radiograph, tuberculin test, and HIV test. A positive finding on either the tuberculin test or chest radiograph is not diagnostic of tuberculosis, while no reaction to a tuberculin test or a normal chest radiograph does not exclude a diagnosis of tuberculosis.

Culture

Demonstration of mycobacteria in sputum or another specimen is necessary to diagnose tuberculosis; a confirmed diagnosis is only possible with a positive culture for *M tuberculosis*. Smears of sputum and other specimens should be stained and examined for acid-fast bacilli. Culture examination and confirmation of *M tuberculosis* may take 3 to 6 weeks. Initial isolates on all patients should be tested for drug susceptibility.

Radiometric methods and genetic probes provide more rapid confirmation of specific mycobacteria growing in culture. To provide earlier confirmation of tuberculosis disease, enzyme-linked immuno-sorbent assays, radioimmunoassays, and chemical detection methods are being developed to identify mycobacterial antigens and other cellular products in cerebrospinal fluid, sera, and other clinical specimens.[176,177]

Tuberculin Test

A tuberculin test is the only method available to identify persons infected with *M tuberculosis* in the absence of active disease. The Mantoux method involves an intradermal injection of 0.1 mL (5 tuberculin units) of purified protein derivative tuberculin into the surface of the forearm. The injection should create a discrete wheal of the skin 6 to 10 mm in diameter. A tuberculin test is read on the second or third day after administration by measuring the diameter of induration (not erythema) transversely to the axis of the forearm and recording the measurement in millimeters. Tuberculin tests should not be administered using a jet injector.[178] While the multiple-puncture device for administering tuberculin may be useful

in screening large, low-risk populations (eg, children in low-risk communities), routine screening of such populations and use of multiple-puncture devices are discouraged.[179,180] The Mantoux method is the best method for testing military service members, health care workers, and others who will have serial screenings and for evaluating patients and contacts for evidence of tuberculosis infection. Repeat testing of uninfected persons does not sensitize them to tuberculin.[179]

Interpretation of a person's tuberculin test reaction requires combining the size of the induration with the person's risk-group information.[179,181] The most common "positive" tuberculin test reactions in a military population are:

- a tuberculin test reaction of 5 mm or larger in a person who had close contact with a patient with infectious tuberculosis,
- a tuberculin test conversion (evidence of a new infection) of a 10 mm or larger increase from the baseline tuberculin test within a 2- or 3-year period,
- a tuberculin test reaction of 10 mm or larger in foreign-born persons from countries with high prevalence rates of tuberculosis (eg, countries in Asia, Africa, Eastern Europe, and Latin America) or members of high-risk minorities, and
- a tuberculin test reaction of 15 mm or larger in any person (Table 38-5).

Those infected with *M tuberculosis* may have no reaction to a tuberculin test if they have been infected within the previous 4 to 12 weeks or if their cell-mediated immunity is suppressed.

A positive tuberculin test reaction in a person vaccinated with Bacillus of Calmette and Guérin (BCG) vaccine usually indicates infection with *M tuberculosis*. Many countries with a high prevalence of tuberculosis vaccinate infants with BCG vaccine.[179,181] While BCG vaccine is effective in preventing tuberculosis disease such as meningitis in children, its effectiveness in preventing infection and disease in adults is debatable.[181] BCG vaccine status generally should be ignored in evaluating persons for tuberculosis or in interpreting tuberculin test reactions.[179]

False-positive and false-negative tuberculin reactions can occur from improper administration or reading of the test (eg, reading erythema rather than induration, leading to a false positive; injecting too little tuberculin or injecting it subcutaneously, leading to a false negative). The most common cause of

TABLE 38-5

INDICATIONS FOR PREVENTIVE THERAPY FOR TUBERCULOSIS INFECTION

Risk Factor		Tuberculin Reaction Size (mm) Threshold
Highest Risk	Young child (< 5 y of age) who has had a recent contact with a tuberculosis-infected person[*]	0
	Immunosuppressed person with recent contact with a tuberculosis-infected person[*]	0
	Recent close contact with known tuberculosis-infected person	5
	HIV infection (known or suspected)[†]	5
	Old tuberculosis on chest radiograph	5
Increased Risk	Intravenous drug users	10
	Patients with predisposing medical condition[‡]	10
	Recent immigrants (within the last 5 y) from high-prevalence countries	10
	Medically underserved, low-income populations	10
	Residents of chronic care and correctional facilities	10
	Tuberculin test conversion within last 2 years	10
	Children younger than 4 y of age	10
	Infants, children, and adolescents exposed to adults in the highest risk categories	10
No Risk Factor		15

[*] Treat presumptively until repeat test
[†] If anergic, treat if probability of tuberculosis infection is high
[‡] Diabetes mellitus, conditions requiring prolonged, high-dose corticosteroid therapy and other immunosuppressive therapy, chronic renal failure, some hematologic disorders, certain malignancies, weight loss of 10% or more of ideal body weight, silicosis, gastrectomy, jejunoileal bypass, and chronic malabsorption syndromes
Adapted from: Centers for Disease Control and Prevention. Targeted tuberculin testing and treatment of latent tuberculosis infection. *MMWR.* 2000;49(RR-6):1–54.

a physiologic false-positive reaction is a cross-reaction with the antigens of nontuberculous mycobacteria or BCG vaccine. Physiologic false-negative reactions can occur because of anergy (eg, in the immune impaired HIV-infected person) or the "booster phenomenon."[182]

The booster phenomenon may occur in anyone who receives a tuberculin test many years after acquiring their initial infection with *M tuberculosis* or another mycobacteria or after receiving BCG vaccine. Although the reaction to the initial tuberculin test is interpreted as negative, the tuberculin antigen stimulates recall of delayed hypersensitivity to mycobacteria. A subsequent tuberculin test produces an induration of increased size (a boosted response) that may be interpreted falsely as evidence of a new infection. Use of a two-step Mantoux test is one solution to the booster phenomenon, especially in persons who will be tested periodically as part of a tuberculosis surveillance program.[182] A first tuberculin test is administered. If it is negative, a second tuberculin test is administered 1 week later. If the second test is positive, it represents a "boosted" reaction; if negative, the person is considered uninfected. The result of the second test becomes the baseline for comparison during subsequent testing. At present, the military services are not using two-step testing for recruits. Military populations with a higher risk of acquiring tuberculosis infection, such as health care workers or inmates and staff of military prisons, may benefit from two-step testing when beginning a serial screening program.

Recommendations for Therapy and Control

Drug-resistant and multidrug-resistant tuberculosis is an emerging problem in the United States and worldwide.[173–175] Tuberculosis in a military patient, especially one who is deployed, presents a challenge. Because of the characteristics of military service, potential drug-resistance patterns for the patient's isolates may not be inferred from the resistance patterns in the local population. Every attempt must be made to obtain adequate samples for culture and drug susceptibility testing before treatment is begun. Because tuberculosis is a chronic infection, it is reasonable to defer treatment (especially with an inadequate drug regimen) until the patient can be transferred to a medical treatment facility with the capabilities to collect specimens for culture and drug susceptibility testing and with the antimycobacterial agents required for an optimal drug regimen.

Therapy

For the initial, empiric treatment of tuberculosis, the preferred regimen in 1998 is four drugs: isoniazid, rifampin, pyrazinamide, and either streptomycin or ethambutol. For the first 2 months or until drug sensitivities are known, a four-drug regimen almost always guarantees that the organism will face at least two agents to which it is susceptible. This approach reduces the opportunity for the organism to develop any or any further drug resistance. Treatment continues for a minimum of 6 months with a minimum of two drugs, usually isoniazid and rifampin, if the organism is proven to be susceptible to all agents. If a patient's organism displays or develops drug resistance, the results of initial and follow-up cultures and sensitivities must determine the optimal drug regimen for each patient. A patient should always be receiving at least two drugs to which the organism is susceptible.[181,183] If the organism is resistant to isoniazid or rifampin or the treatment regimen does not contain either drug, treatment should continue for 18 to 24 months. Directly observed therapy, daily initially and eventually two to three times per week, for 6-month treatment courses is strongly recommended by the World Health Organization and the Centers for Disease Control and Prevention (CDC). Directly observed therapy improves compliance, increases the completion rate for full treatment courses, and slows the development of drug-resistant organisms.[173,181,183]

Patients should be seen at least monthly for an evaluation of their response to treatment, compliance with their drug regimen, and symptoms of adverse effects. The common adverse effects of the frequently used antituberculosis agents include:

- isoniazid—hepatotoxicity and pyridoxine-associated peripheral neuropathy,
- rifampin—gastrointestinal upset and accelerated clearance of other drugs through hepatitic microsomal enzyme induction,
- pyrazinamide—hepatotoxicity and hyperuricemia,
- ethambutol—retrobulbar neuritis, and
- streptomycin—ototoxicity.[181]

At a minimum, patients require these baseline tests: liver enzymes, bilirubin, creatinine, and complete blood and platelet count. Patients taking ethambutol require baseline tests for visual acuity and red-green color perception. If baseline results are normal, routine monitoring is not required.[181] Subsequent evaluations and monitoring are guided by symptoms, clinical assessments, and any coexistent risk factors.

A patient with suspected pulmonary or laryngeal tuberculosis should be placed in tuberculosis isolation in a private room with appropriate ventilation and other engineering controls, such as negative pressure in the room and adjoining hallways, ventilation providing at least six air changes per hour, and air exhausted directly to the outside or recirculated only after HEPA (high-efficiency particulate air) filtration. The patient should remain in the isolation room with the door closed and should cover his or her mouth and nose with a tissue when coughing or sneezing. Health care providers and visitors should wear respiratory protection when entering the isolation room. In field settings and operational environments, isolation rooms and procedures should be established as much as possible. Increasing natural ventilation and exposing patient spaces to natural ultraviolet light (sunlight) can help dilute airborne droplet nuclei and reduce the infectiousness of *M tuberculosis* in the air.[184] If a tuberculosis patient must leave the isolation room, the patient should wear a surgical mask covering the nose and mouth; attendants and other staff do not need to wear masks. Patient movements should be scheduled to minimize contact with other patients, staff, and visitors.

After a treatment regimen is begun, most patients who are infected with a drug-susceptible organisms will become noninfectious within days to a few weeks. Indications of reduced infectiousness include decreased cough, fewer acid-fast bacilli on sputum smears, and improvement in systemic signs and symptoms. The risk of transmission is low if the patient has had three negative smears of sputum collected on three separate days. Patients who remain infectious may return home and resume normal activities if their degree of infectiousness is low, ongoing contacts (eg, in the household or workplace) have already been exposed and are being monitored, and the environment is not conducive to transmission (eg, outdoors rather than indoors).[184]

If a patient with symptomatic pulmonary or laryngeal tuberculosis must be moved to another medical treatment facility, the patient should wear a surgical mask. Ground transportation is preferred; transmission of tuberculosis from a highly infectious passenger to other passengers and flight crew has been documented during a long airplane flight.[185] If air transportation is necessary, use of a rotary-wing aircraft with open doors provides excellent cabin ventilation. Transportation in fix-winged, pressurized aircraft should be avoided if possible until adequate antimycobacterial treatment has been instituted. When a symptomatic tuberculosis patient must travel by air, aircraft routing should minimize the flight time and the patient should be seated to limit contact with other passengers and crew and, if possible, be downstream in the cabin ventilation flow.

Control

Screening for tuberculosis infection in US military populations is done for several purposes. Recruits receive tuberculin tests when they arrive at recruit training for two purposes: (1) to identify the recruits with preexisting tuberculosis infection and then provide appropriate preventive therapy and (2) to establish for all recruits a baseline test result for comparison with tuberculin tests later during military service. Recruits with reactive tuberculin tests receive chest radiographs and clinical evaluations, which periodically lead to a diagnosis of active tuberculosis. Subsequent tuberculosis screening varies among and within the services. Because of the substantial risk of tuberculosis transmission in the shipboard environment, the Navy and Marine Corps require annual tuberculin testing for personnel on ships and for those assigned to deployable units. For all services, screening before and after deployments and overseas assignments is a common practice. The medical plan for an operation usually dictates the tuberculosis screening requirements based on the endemic disease threat and the nature of the military operations. A tuberculin test within 12 months of deployment is adequate for establishing the predeployment status. A tuberculin test administered 45 to 90 days after the deployment allows service members who acquired a new tuberculosis infection during the deployment to receive preventive therapy at the earliest possible opportunity. Results of postdeployment screening provide an assessment of the military-specific risk of tuberculosis exposure associated with the deployment. All of the services require annual tuberculosis screening of health care personnel. For other health care beneficiaries, the services follow CDC recommendations for screening for tuberculosis infection in population groups that experience disease and infection rates in excess of the general population.[177,179] Foreign-born spouses and other family members from most countries in Africa, Asia, and Latin America are a high-risk group; they should be screened for tuberculosis and tuberculosis infection when they enter the military health care system or immigrate to the United States.[179] For the

foreign-born person, the risk of developing active disease is highest in the first few years after arrival in the United States. In countries where tuberculosis is highly endemic, screening host-nation employees for evidence of active tuberculosis disease through tuberculin tests and chest radiograph and referring them for treatment may reduce the rate of transmission to US forces and their families.

Preventive therapy provides substantial protection against developing clinically active disease in a person infected with *M tuberculosis*—65% for a 6-month regimen with isoniazid and 70% to 90% (depending on compliance) for a 12-month regimen. The recommendations for preventive therapy and its duration vary with the person's tuberculosis risk factors, age, and size of tuberculin test reaction[179] (see Table 38-5). The two most common indications for preventive therapy of a military member are (1) close contact with a newly diagnosed infectious tuberculosis case and a tuberculin test reaction of 5 mm or larger induration and (2) recent tuberculin test converters. US Navy and Marine Corps recruits with tuberculin test reactions of 10 mm or larger receive preventive therapy (if not previously received) regardless of risk factors and age to minimize the risk of developing tuberculosis on ships.

The primary preventive treatment regimen is isoniazid daily in a dose of 300 mg (10–15 mg/kg daily for children, to a maximum dose of 300 mg/d) for 9 months. A 6-month regimen of isoniazid (at least 180 doses administered within 9 months) is also effective.[179] Children should receive 9 months of preventive therapy. The greatest barrier to effective preventive therapy is compliance,[184] which is a particular challenge in young, otherwise healthy military personnel. Directly observed therapy with twice-weekly isoniazid (15 mg/kg up to 900 mg) is an effective option to improve compliance. Preventive therapy regimens with rifampin (10 mg/kg daily, up to 600 mg/d for 4 months) or rifampin-pyrazinamide (daily for 2 months) have been shown to be acceptable alternatives for contacts of patients with isoniazid-resistant, rifampin-susceptible organisms.[179]

Before starting isoniazid preventive therapy, a history, physical evaluation, chest radiograph, and HIV test are necessary to exclude persons with current active tuberculosis, previous adequately-treated tuberculosis, previous adequately treated tuberculosis infection, or contraindications.[179] The evaluation also identifies persons requiring special precautions or monitoring. Contraindications to isoniazid preventive therapy include previous isoniazid-associated hepatitis or other severe adverse reactions and acute or unstable liver disease from any cause. Isoniazid-induced hepatotoxicity is the major adverse effect. Older studies had found that the occurrence of hepatitis increased with age: 0.3% for those 20 to 34 years of age and 1.2%, for those 35 to 49 years of age. More recent studies have demonstrated that isoniazid is well tolerated, with a lower risk for hepatic side effects. Currently, baseline liver function tests are recommended for HIV-infected persons, pregnant women and those in the immediate postpartum period, persons with a history of liver disease, daily users of alcohol, and those at risk for chronic liver disease. Although isoniazid does not appear to harm the fetus, pregnant women should generally begin preventive therapy after delivery. Concurrent therapy with pyridoxine is indicated for persons at risk of isoniazid-associated peripheral neuropathy, pregnant women, and persons with seizure disorders.[179] The interaction of isoniazid and phenytoin requires monitoring serum levels of phenytoin.

Patients on isoniazid preventive therapy should be evaluated monthly for compliance and for signs and symptoms of active tuberculosis, hepatotoxicity, or other adverse effects.[179] Failure to keep an appointment or fill a prescription indicates noncompliance and requires a follow-up contact.[184] Unexplained or persistent anorexia, nausea, vomiting, dark urine, icterus, rash, paresthesias of the hands and feet, persistent fatigue, weakness, fever, or abdominal pain (especially right upper quadrant tenderness) should prompt an evaluation, including liver function tests. Transient, mild abnormalities of liver function tests may occur in 10% to 20% of people taking isoniazid. For persons with abnormal baseline liver function tests or at risk for hepatic disease, such as daily users of alcohol, liver functions tests should be obtained monthly during preventive therapy. Isoniazid should be stopped if the aspartate aminotransferase (AST) level is three to five times the upper limit of normal or if the patient is symptomatic and has increased liver enzymes.[179]

Tuberculosis infection without evidence of active disease is not disqualifying for military service. Persons with evidence of a tuberculosis infection (a reactive tuberculin test) but without clinical or radiographic evidence of active disease are not infectious, regardless of whether they have started, completed, or never received preventive therapy. Military service members with reactive tuberculin tests without evidence of active disease are fully deployable. Upon transfer or separation, a military service member on isoniazid preventive therapy needs counseling on the importance of continuing therapy, an adequate supply of isoniazid, and ex-

plicit instructions on reporting to the military preventive medicine service or civilian public health department on arriving at the new location. The current military preventive medicine service should contact the receiving military or civilian public health office to "hand off" the military service member and minimize the opportunities for incomplete or inadequate preventive therapy.

Active tuberculosis disease is a notifiable or reportable disease in the public health reporting systems of each service, every state, and the US Public Health Service. At the unit or local level, the local military preventive medicine service should be notified as soon as tuberculosis is suspected. The preventive medicine service will initiate and conduct a contact investigation, coordinate with the civilian health department if required, and make the required notifications to the military and civilian public health surveillance systems.

A contact investigation is essential to identify others with undiagnosed tuberculosis who require treatment for their disease and who may be a source of ongoing transmission.[184] Contact investigations allow persons who have acquired a tuberculosis infection from their exposure to the source case to be identified early and given preventive therapy. Contact investigations proceed with concentric circles of tuberculin tests and clinical assessments of contacts. Close contacts, those sharing the same household or living spaces, are investigated first. Close contacts may also include work and social contacts of the case. If the level of infection (rate of tuberculin test converters) among the close contacts exceeds that expected in the general population, the investigation should expand to the next circle of contacts—those who share the same air as the case but not as frequently or as intensely as the close contacts. The investigation expands in concentric circles until the observed rate of tuberculosis infection is no greater than that expected in the general population. Most military outbreaks start with examination of the close contacts, those who share the same berthing space, barracks room, or work space. Frequently, if that assessment confirms that transmission has occurred, it is logistically easier to conduct a mass test of the remainder of the unit (eg, the entire ship's crew) than to try to discern varying levels of exposure in a population whose living, working and social arrangements may be extensively intertwined.[169,170,172] The contact investigation of a military member with tuberculosis commonly requires close coordination with the civilian public health department to ensure that nonmilitary contacts are evaluated. Special attention is required when children may have been exposed to a person with active pulmonary tuberculosis. Newly infected children can progress rapidly to active disease. They should immediately start preventive therapy even if their initial tuberculin test is nonreactive and continue preventive therapy for a total of 9 months unless a repeat tuberculin test at 3 months is negative.[179]

The Occupational Safety and Health Administration has issued detailed enforcement procedures and standards for workplaces with employees who are occupationally exposed to tuberculosis.[186] These standards apply to health care facilities, correctional institutions, and other settings. The CDC has issued specific guidelines for preventing the transmission of tuberculosis in health care facilities.[187]

Tuberculosis Control among Displaced Persons

Among refugees and displaced persons, tuberculosis incidence has been found to be two to three times greater than the incidence in the general population.[188] The World Health Organization estimates that 50% of refugees are infected with tuberculosis.[173] Among refugees and displaced persons, the effects of intense crowding, undernutrition, and stress from other diseases are superimposed on a preexisting high prevalence of tuberculosis infection and disease. Famine increases the rate of mortality from tuberculosis. In 1983, tuberculosis was the third leading cause of death in Somali refugee camps and was responsible for 25% of adult deaths.[188] Coinfection with HIV and drug-resistant tuberculosis organisms increases the complexity of diagnosing, treating, and controlling tuberculosis disease among refugees and displaced persons.[173,189]

In refugee populations, identifying and treating patients with pulmonary tuberculosis is the most effective strategy for preventing morbidity, mortality, and further transmission of infection. Chest radiographs rather than tuberculin tests are frequently the more effective screening method.[188,189] Treatment programs should use locally recognized regimens that can be continued by national or nongovernmental organizations. The World Health Organization strongly recommends the use of directly observed therapy with multidrug, short-course regimens to improve compliance and to achieve higher cure rates in the mobile refugee patients.[173] Documentation of therapy, compliance, and response to treatment (eg, serial smears) remains important. Control of tuberculosis among refugees will have a significant long-term effect but often competes with the more acute problems of diarrheal disease, measles, and undernutrition. Tuberculin tests and use of preventive therapy are not recommended in refugees or displaced persons. HIV-infected persons with normal chest radiographs may benefit from preventive therapy with isoniazid.[189] If consistent with national policy, BCG vaccination of newborns is appropriate but does not contribute to tuberculosis control among youth and adults.

Tuberculosis may pose a significant problem for prisoners of war subjected to extreme crowding, stress from other diseases, and undernutrition, especially if their confinement has been prolonged. The clinical evaluation of repatriated or liberated prisoners of war or detainees should include tuberculin testing and chest radiographs.

[David H. Trump, MD, MPH]

SEXUALLY TRANSMITTED DISEASES AND HUMAN IMMUNODEFICIENCY VIRUS INFECTION

Introduction and Military Relevance

The history of sexually transmitted diseases (STDs) and military forces is a long one. Edward IV of England invaded France in 1475 to reclaim lost provinces. In a successful attempt to buy off the enemy, Louis XI of France treated the English with royal hospitality. Louis XI provided whores, who took their own special revenge on the invaders. "Many a man was lost that fell to the lust of women, who were burnt by them; and their members rotted away and they died,"[190(p223)] claims one doleful English chronicler. Sexually transmitted diseases have been associated with the US military from its earliest campaigns. In 1778, Congress passed a resolution that military personnel afflicted with "the venereal disease" were to be fined, $10.00 for officers and $4.00 for enlisted personnel.[191]

There is no evidence to suggest US military personnel in the United States are more sexually active or have a higher STD rate than their age-matched civilian contemporaries. However, when deployed or stationed overseas, rates can increase dramatically. STD rates are closely associated with the degree of military activity, as was illustrated in the European theater in World War II.[192] In England before the Normandy invasion, US military STD rates were 35-40/1,000, falling to 5/1000 after D-day among troops in France. As US forces pushed into Europe, rates rose to 50/1000 but remained at 25/1,000 among combat troops. By September 1945, 4 months after Germany surrendered, the STD rate had risen to 190/1,000.

The Vietnam War probably provided the highest incidence of military sexual activity and STD in US forces. Sexual abstinence was statistically abnormal for unmarried personnel.[193,194] In a 1973 study on a Navy aircraft carrier, the annual rate of gonorrhea was 582/1,000 men and of nongonococcal urethritis was 459/1,000 men.[195] Although these figures reflect repeat infections in some individuals, it is sobering to consider that statistically, every crewmember had at least one case of urethritis.

Traditionally, liberty is a high-risk time for military personnel to acquire STDs. For example, during a 6-day port call in the Philippines during the Vietnam War, the average US sailor had 1.2 partners and had intercourse three times (2.5 exposures per partner). After controlling for number of exposures and partners, 8.2% of whites and 19.1% of blacks acquired gonorrhea.[196] A repeat study several years later had similar findings.[197]

Considerable anecdotal evidence indicates STD rates in the military in recent years have been far lower, less than 1% in such recent operations as Desert Shield/Desert Storm (the Persian Gulf War), Restore Hope (Somalia), Restore Democracy and Uphold Democracy (Haiti), and Sea Signal (Guantanamo Bay). In training exercises in the early 1990s, such as Cobra Gold (Thailand), rates were also reported as being down, with anecdotal reports of extensive use (or at least acquisition) of condoms. Although it is difficult to quantify this decrease, the overall conclusion that STD rates are down among military personnel overseas seems justified. Three plausible causal factors have been postulated but have no specific data to support them: (1) In some opera-

tions, such as Desert Shield/Desert Storm, interaction with the local population was severely restricted and alcohol consumption was forbidden. These restrictions were successful in reducing not just STDs but also accidents, fights, and injuries. (2) Concerted efforts to emphasize the risks of sexual activity, especially acquired immunodeficiency syndrome (AIDS), and to emphasize the use of condoms for those who insist on being sexually active seem to be working. In particular, operational medical officers report their impressions that fear of AIDS has reduced sexual activity and increased the use of condoms in areas the military population associates with AIDS, such as Africa, Haiti, and Thailand. (3) There may be a new generation of military personnel, particularly in the senior enlisted leadership positions, with a changing attitude toward sex overseas. Sexual activity, particularly with prostitutes, may no longer be as acceptable on liberty as it was during the Vietnam War.[193,194]

General Epidemiologic Issues

A discussion of the general principles of STD epidemiology will be followed by specific discussions of the STDs of military relevance. General references applicable to sexually transmitted diseases are listed in Exhibit 38-1.

Transmission

STD epidemiology is complex, and our understanding of it is rapidly changing. It is often subpopulation-specific, with age, race, and socioeconomic status being the most important determinants,[198–200]

EXHIBIT 38-1

STANDARD REFERENCES FOR SEXUALLY TRANSMITTED DISEASES

- Holmes KK, Mardh PA, Sparling PF, et al, eds. *Sexually Transmitted Diseases*. 3rd ed. New York: McGraw-Hill; 1999.

- Chin J, ed. *Control of Communicable Diseases Manual*. 17 ed. Washington, DC: American Public Health Association; 2000.

- Centers for Disease Control and Prevention. *Sexually Transmitted Diseases Clinical Practice Guidelines*. Atlanta: CDC; 1991.

- Centers for Disease Control and Prevention. Recommendations for the prevention and management of *Chlamydia trachomatis* infections, 1993. *MMWR*. 1993;42(RR-12):1–39.

- Centers for Disease Control and Prevention. 1998 guidelines for treatment of sexually transmitted diseases. *MMWR*. 1993;47(RR-1):1–128.

so pooling of STD data may obscure important differences.

In general, the epidemiology of STD differs in major respects from other communicable diseases:[201] (*a*) the populations at risk are fractions of the total community (eg, young, sexually active adults; homosexual men), (*b*) doubling the population density does not double the rate at which new infections occur, (*c*) long-term, asymptomatic carriers play an important role in perpetuating the disease, (*d*) most STDs induce no practical immunity, (*e*) the course of the infection varies greatly among individuals, and (f) STD transmission rates are characterized by considerable heterogeneity within and between different populations. These differences make STD control a uniquely challenging part of infectious disease control.

Aral and Holmes[200] point out important differences in current STD epidemiology compared to that of the classic venereal diseases: (*a*) Among educated middle- and upper-class individuals in industrialized countries, classic STDs have declined rapidly, while these same diseases have remained stable or increased among largely marginalized subpopulations, such as urban dwellers, the poor, and minorities. (*b*) Prostitution, including anonymous sex-for-drugs exchanges, has reemerged as an STD multiplier in industrialized countries. (*c*) STDs can be divided into curable bacterial STDs and incurable viral STDs, a distinction with important implications. Bacterial STD control depends on health-seeking behaviors and early diagnosis and treatment. Viral STD control depends on primary prevention through general STD education and individual counseling. (*d*) Cases of viral STDs are rapidly increasing, and reservoirs of asymptomatic viral STD cases are much larger than the number of symptomatic cases. (*e*) In developing countries, the lack of resources to identify gonorrhea and chlamydia in women make these diseases epidemiologically similar to incurable viral STDs. (f) And for the first time since the preantibiotic era, behavioral change is the most important STD prevention and control strategy.

Overseas deployment or liberty calls are the most important factors related to military STDs. Overseas deployments provide the opportunity for the largely single, male, young adult force to participate in inexpensive, readily available sexual activity in an atmosphere of numerous rationalizations for such activity. Service members involved in an exhausting exercise or deployment with a busy operational tempo feel they deserve a break, a chance to let off steam. Overseas sex is part of military culture and tradition, including rites of passage such as sexually initiating "virgins," the concept of the "geographic bachelor," and the unspoken understanding that what happens on deployment will not be talked about back home. For individuals not planning a military career, overseas deployments may be perceived as an opportunity to see the world and do something exotic before settling into conventional civilian life. And for some individuals, taking advantage of the opportunity simply to have sex as often as possible is an integral part of their personal culture. Fallacious as these rationalizations may be, they may be perceived as an integral part of military overseas culture and need to be considered in attempts to reduce STD rates. The traditional "VD lecture" is not likely to influence behavior originating in these rationalizations.

In its battle to reduce STD rates, the military has tried to determine personality risk factors for acquiring STDs. World War II–era studies[202–207] identified military personnel at risk for STDs as less intelligent or educated (non–high school graduate), abusers of alcohol, often in legal trouble (military or civilian), dissatisfied with military service, and immature, socially maladjusted individuals with inadequate personalities. Studies during the Vietnam War in Australian soldiers[193,208] failed to find any dominant personality type associated with STD acquisition or much difference between those with STDs and control subjects, but alcohol use remained an association, as did younger age, less education, presence of military legal charges, and unmarried status. Studies of US Navy and Marine Corps personnel in the years immediately following the Vietnam War reached similar conclusions.[195,197,209–212]

A Navy epidemiologist named Melton tied the increased rate of STDs in young military personnel to the risk-taking behavior associated with youth and manifested by problems such as traffic accidents, smoking, drug use, and especially peer pressure and alcohol use.[213] Risk markers were being black, being young (younger than 20 years old), being unmarried, having less than a high school education, being in pay grades E1 through E4, having served less than 1 year in the Navy, and being on their first cruise.[214,215] Levine and colleagues[216] identified the same risk markers, as well as performance marks 3.4 or lower (out of 4.0), a General Classification Score of 55 or lower, and a history of disciplinary actions. Some caution is required in interpreting these studies, since they were carried out in a era when Navy morale was widely considered to be less than optimal.

As one reviewer summarized, "The stereotypical picture of the military patient with an STD is that of a young, low-ranking, poorly educated, single male, who tends to abuse alcohol and to get into legal problems and who has usually had more than one episode of an STD."[214p92] To the extent that this stereotype is valid, there is little that is unique to the military in it; the picture is similar to those seen in many urban STD clinics. Hart,[208,217] however, veers away from the stereotype, attributing the high STD rates in his Vietnam studies to frequent intercourse with a highly infected prostitute population and "the environmental stresses of a war situation [which] produced behavior patterns which many participants would not otherwise experience."[208p546] Noting that 44% of married draftees, 56% of those over age 30, and 30% of those with more than a high school education had sex with prostitutes, he concluded that "behavior which would make one an outcast at home is considered quite normal here."[194p460] Vietnam may have been unusual in the degree of sexual activity exhibited by military personnel there, but the concept that war stress may induce increased sexual activity dates from at least World War II.[202,205,206]

In the civilian world, Rothenberg introduced the concept of STD core populations—predominantly marginalized urban, dense, low socioeconomic, ethnic, minority populations—whose behavior perpetuates disease transmission among members of the core, which in turn serves as an STD reservoir for others.[218–221] These reservoirs of STD sustain high transmission rates because of high rates of changing sex partners coupled with a high rate of endemic infection. They may also be the major source of antimicrobial resistance. Sex with members of these groups by nonmembers is an important risk factor in itself and serves to export STDs out of the reservoir. US military personnel are frequently exposed to such groups when they hire commercial sex workers (CSW) during deployments. This concept of core transmitters has been refined to suggest that local social structure may act as a barrier or facilitator to disease transmission and that this variable needs to be considered in evaluating transmission.[222] Further, STD epidemics are dynamic, moving through predictable phases.[223] With time, epidemics become localized in subpopulations characterized by progressively higher rates of sex partner change and less contact with the health care system.

Individual Risk Factors and Risk Markers. It is important to distinguish between *risk factors*, which relate to the probability of becoming infected and may be modifiable, and *risk markers*, which indicate presence of risk but no causal relationship.[200,224–241] Risk factors preeminently include sexual behaviors (eg, age at first intercourse, number of partners, rate of acquiring new partners, having casual partners,

sex preference, sex practices) and health care behaviors (eg, nonuse of condoms and other barriers, late consultation for diagnosis and treatment, nonreferral of partners, noncompliance with therapy, douching). Risk markers include marital status, race, urban residence, and lower socioeconomic status. Some variables can function as either risk factors or risk markers (eg, age, gender, smoking, alcohol use, drug abuse, other STDs, lack of circumcision, contraceptive method). Numerous studies have been done with higher-risk populations, such as STD clinic patients. The most important factors have repeatedly been found to be younger age at first intercourse, increased number of partners, casual choice of partners, and partners who themselves are at high risk for STD. Adolescents in particular attempt to minimize the effect of having multiple partners by practicing serial monogamy (ie, having sex with only partner at a time but frequently changing partners).

Commercial Sex Workers. CSWs (prostitutes, hookers, "hooks") are most common in settings of poverty, social disintegration, and a double standard of sexual behavior; they play a major role in the increase of STDs in developing countries.[242,243] A reporter summed up the relationship between CSWs and the US military using an example from the Philippines: "The base and the town share a seamy symbiosis. Servicemen have money and a need to relax. Olongapenos have flesh and a need to eat."[244(pD-8)] In countries such as Japan, the cost of CSWs is sufficiently high that few US military personnel can afford them, making such countries low risk for STDs. In most developing countries, however, commercial sex is both readily available and inexpensive. US military personnel in one country typically paid less than $20 for a night with a CSW (plus tip), and shorter encounters could be had for much less. In one African city, some CSWs charged only 50 cents. In 1995, CSWs in Thailand were charging $4.00.[245] Low prices greatly enhance the spread of STDs by removing cost as a disincentive, by requiring CSWs to have multiple partners to obtain enough money, and by allowing military personnel to have multiple partners.

In countries where US military personnel frequently visit, other factors enhance and promote their access to CSWs. Locations of CSWs are usually convenient to military personnel (an important consideration if liberty is short) and typically provide familiar amenities such as beer (often relatively inexpensive), music (often live, of good quality, and current), and fellow Americans (often friends). In short, the locations where CSWs are found may be familiar, relaxing, comfortable, inexpensive, and accessible.

Unlike the stereotype of prostitutes as hard individuals, CSWs often appear to be nice, friendly, and "clean" or uninfected. However, they are usually aggressive in going after customers, motivated by the fact that this may be the only source of income for themselves and their family, which may include a husband. The CSW may have expenses in addition to food and shelter, such as clothing and grooming or money to be paid to the bar where she works. Other job opportunities are limited or nonexistent, especially for those with minimal schooling. Manaloto and colleagues[246] studied 18 Philippine prostitutes who were positive for the human immunodeficiency virus (HIV). The women were poorly educated and came from low-income agricultural families. Returning to a low-income menial job was not attractive to them and working as a waitress or barmaid presented constant temptation to make extra money by having sex with customers.

Long practice makes CSWs persistent, aggressive, and very effective at contacting military personnel and enticing them into using their services. Liaisons are set up in numerous ways. The CSW may take the initiative in approaching a serviceman. If the serviceman voices concern about STDs, the CSW (in some countries) may honestly be able to say that she has been checked for disease at the local social hygiene clinic. Such clinics play an important role in reducing the prevalence of STDs among CSWs, particularly treatable STDs, but there is a strong economic motive to appear uninfected on examination. The CSWs achieve this by douching or taking oral antibiotics (often in subtherapeutic doses),[247] which are widely available without a prescription in developing countries.

Geographic Distribution

STDs are found worldwide. There is no evidence that the virulence or infectivity of STDs varies geographically.[248] An exception may be the HIV E clade, prevalent in Southeast Asia, which appears to be more infectious than other strains.[249] Differences in prevalence and incidence reflect such factors as the presence of STD control programs, availability of diagnostic and treatment services, population demographics, sexual behaviors, and the size of core-transmitter groups. For example, gonorrhea is more common in developing countries, while chlamydial infections are more common in the United States. This reflects the presence of effective gonorrhea control programs in the United States and their lack in developing countries.[200] In selected US cities with

vigorous chlamydia control programs (eg, Seattle), the number of chlamydial infections has declined.

Incidence

The World Health Organization estimates there are 250 million STD cases annually, including 120 million cases of trichomonas infection, 50 million of chlamydia infection, 30 million of genital warts, 25 million of gonorrhea, 20 million of genital herpes, 3.5 million of syphilis, 2.5 million of hepatitis B virus infection, 2 million of chancroid, and 11 million of HIV infection.[250] Such figures provide an overall perspective, but there is great variability among different countries and populations. For example, in the United States an estimated 4 million to 5 million persons are infected with chlamydia each year,[251] compared to approximately 600,000 reported gonorrhea cases.[252] In most developing countries, gonorrhea rates exceed chlamydia rates.

Except for HIV, the incidence and prevalence of STD in the military cannot be determined with satisfactory reliability. Most reporting systems are fragmented and passive, and they suffer from significant underreporting despite being officially required. Statistics from particular operations or exercises may be available, but they cannot be generalized. Military STD rates cannot be directly compared to civilian statistics because the military population is largely young, sexually active, single, and male. While the highest military STD rates occur among the lower-ranking enlisted personnel, in parallel with the civilian community's experience, there is little information about STD incidence rates among officers, warrant officers, and senior noncommissioned officers. Because these individuals are older and better educated—the most junior officer is at least 22 years old and a college graduate and the most junior enlisted person is typically an 18-year-old high school graduate—their rates would be expected to be lower. Additionally, a record of an STD is not career-enhancing; older individuals are more likely to be career oriented and so more motivated and better able to avoid sexual exposure or to keep their records clean. They may collude with medical personnel to treat an STD without entering it in their health record or to use a euphemism such as "urinary tract infection." Being better paid than lower-ranking service members, they may be able to obtain medical treatment outside the military system.

A study[253] conducted from 1989 to 1991 looked at 1,744 male US Navy and Marine Corps personnel on two 6-month cruises to South America and Africa. Overall, 10% of the subjects acquired an STD but only 10% of those were officers. Sexual activity on liberty was independently associated with younger age (17 to 24 years), nonwhite race, and single status. Prostitute contact was reported by 42% of the subjects, with 29% having one partner, 35% having two to three partners, and 35% having four or more partners. Enlisted personnel were more likely to have had prostitute contact than officers (43% vs. 26%). Although the overall reported rate of consistent condom use was high (but not 100%), it is not surprising that 10% of the subjects acquired an STD given the high rate of risky behavior. This study is consistent with studies showing young, nonwhite, single, military personnel have the highest risk of acquiring HIV infection and other STDs.[215,216,253–260]

Diagnostic Approaches

Several tests provide immediate information, which allows a rapid presumptive diagnosis and a prompt treatment decision. This is important because the rapidity with which military personnel can be returned to duty directly and strongly influences their willingness to come for treatment and their unit's willingness to let them go and rapid diagnosis and treatment help reduce STDs by rendering patients noninfectious. Another advantage is that these are simple tests that can be carried out under field conditions. Urethral and cervical Gram stains allow for the diagnosis of gonorrhea, nongonococcal urethritis (NGU), and mucopurulent cervicitis (MPC). The presence of Gram-negative intracellular diplococci is highly specific for gonorrhea, although the sensitivity in cervicitis is low (approximately 50% to 60%). MPC can also be presumptively diagnosed by the swab test or the cervical friability test. The leukocyte esterase test (LET) is a dipstick test that detects pyuria. It has the advantage, in males, of being noninvasive—a urethral probe is not required. It has a sensitivity of 46% to 100% and a specificity of 83% to 93% as a screen for chlamydia and gonococcal urethritis in sexually active teenage males.[261] EIA (enzyme-linked immunoassay) tests and monoclonal antibody tests for chlamydia are useful but may have somewhat limited sensitivity, especially in asymptomatic individuals and in males. A negative test result does not necessarily rule out chlamydia infection in exposed individuals. Chlamydia tests may yield false-positive results in men and women, an important concern in rape and other settings. CDC guidelines[262] discuss these issues in detail.

Bacterial culture and sensitivity tests can confirm *Neisseria gonorrhoeae* infection and determine bacterial sensitivity. The latter information can be useful for individual patients in whom antibiotic treatment fails; it can also provide population-based profiles of antibiotic susceptibility in different locations. Preventive medicine personnel should periodically arrange to collect 50 to 100 gonococcal isolates in areas where US forces deploy frequently or continuously and have them tested for sensitivity to a battery of antibiotics. Busy clinics that see large numbers of infected US personnel are ideal, but samples from CSWs seen in the local social hygiene clinic are also acceptable.

Polymerase chain reaction (PCR), ligase chain reaction (LCR), and a variety of other chlamydia tests based on DNA probe technology may make many current diagnostic techniques obsolete. They have the advantage of being rapid, specific, and capable of making a diagnosis from specimens that contain minimal amounts of pathogens. Although they are rapidly moving into commercial development, most are still research tools. Technological advancements, especially if they emphasize automation and user simplicity, could make these techniques the tools of choice for STD diagnosis. Drawbacks include the fact that these techniques are extremely sensitive to contamination, which can produce false-positive results especially in field settings, and that they are expensive for routine STD diagnosis.

Serological STD tests are used to diagnose syphilis, HIV infection, and hepatitis B virus infection. Sera can easily be obtained in a field setting and are relatively tolerant of storage conditions, although refrigeration is required. Most of these tests are not useful for immediate patient management because they cannot produce prompt results. Despite the delay in obtaining the results, they are important for population-based assessments and eventually for individual patient management. The RPR test for syphilis can provide immediate results; however, it has false-positive results. It may be appropriate to treat for presumptive syphilis on the basis of an RPR result, but, when possible, it is better to wait for a confirmatory test.

Self-treatment, particularly topical antibiotics used for genital ulcers, may interfere with the diagnosis of STDs. One study of 3,025 public STD clinic patients in the United States showed that 22% of patients self-treated, with 55% of those using a topical medication.[263] Since antibiotics can be bought without a prescription in many foreign countries, the potential for this practice interfering with STD diagnoses in military personnel is even greater, especially if the individuals belong to a unit that deals with STD among its members punitively.

Recommendations for Therapy and Control

The core roles of military preventive medicine regarding STDs are listed in Exhibit 38-2. In the absence of widespread effective methods and programs to decrease STD acquisition and transmission, the major control measure is prompt treatment that renders individuals noninfectious. Three approaches to finding infected persons are available: diagnosis and treatment of symptomatic individuals, screening of high-risk individuals, and contact tracing and partner notification.

Diagnosing and Treating Symptomatic Individuals

Diagnosis and treatment of symptomatic individuals is enhanced by a syndromic approach, that is, patient management decisions are made on the basis of symptoms and limited laboratory support, enabling rapid treatment. Advantages to this approach are many. Treatment to render individuals noninfectious occurs earlier than it would if clinicians waited for definitive laboratory results. Individuals who never return for test results have nevertheless been treated and so cannot spread their infection. (More than one third of patients in one STD clinic continued to be sexually active after becoming symptomatic or being informed they had been exposed to gonorrhea.[264]) Patients also spend less time in the clinic; this encourages individuals to come to the clinic, especially those who are not severely symptomatic.

Ensuring that individuals are seen and evaluated promptly and in a private and nonjudgmental fashion is crucial. Unless highly symptomatic, individuals are often reluctant to spend several hours being evaluated, and a service member's command will want to know the reason for any extended absence. A critical recommendation by the Centers for Disease Control and Prevention is that patients with uncomplicated STDs should be seen, diagnosed, and treated within 90 minutes.[265] The patient can be brought back later for follow-up or evaluation of an abnormal laboratory test.

In most military medical settings, service members concerned they may have an STD are seen by corpsmen, physician's assistants, or nurse practitioners, who successfully manage the bulk of STD cases without the involvement of a physician. Although this is an appropriate use of medical resources, it is necessary for the physician responsible for the STD clinic to ensure these health care providers are well trained, follow appropriate algorithms and guidelines, and know to call a physician for complicated cases. Complicated cases do occur, and aberrant treatment regimens and unnecessary steps do creep in and compromise the success of the clinic. STD clinics should use the CDC guidelines[265] for patient management and treatment, unless there are specific local reasons not to do so.

Screening

Screening may use epidemiologically identified risk factors, laboratory tests, or a combination of them. Screening can be effective in comprehensive, well-integrated, highly controlled health care systems. The usefulness of this approach is limited by the fact that several currently available diagnostic tests, particularly for chlamydia, are less sensitive

---

EXHIBIT 38-2

ROLE OF PREVENTIVE MEDICINE IN CONTROLLING SEXUALLY TRANSMITTED DISEASES

- Prevent, reduce, or ameliorate risky behavior that may result in acquiring an STD
- Interrupt transmission of STDs by ensuring that prompt diagnosis and treatment are available
- Counsel individuals who have acquired an STD how to prevent further transmission and to notify sexual partners so they may be treated
- Carry out, or arrange to be carried out, contact tracing of the sex partners of STD patients, when possible
- Collect, analyze, and disseminate epidemiologic information regarding the incidence and prevalence of STDs, including risk factors
- Collect, analyze, and disseminate antibiotic sensitivity data for bacterial STDs

STD: sexually transmitted disease

in asymptomatic individuals and that motivation to be screened may be low if the patient is asymptomatic. Adolescent males in particular are difficult to capture with screening methods.

An STD is a marker identifying an individual who has engaged in sexually risky behavior and who may have multiple STDs from current or previous liaisons. As such, the individual with an STD should also be tested for syphilis, HIV, and HBV. The individual may have acquired one of these in the past or in conjunction with the current STD. Follow-up testing for syphilis, HIV, or HBV depends on the risk for having acquired one of these diseases and, in the case of syphilis, whether the person was treated with antibiotics that would abort incubating syphilis.

Although it has never been official policy, for many years some ships' medical departments have offered members a self-screening opportunity, a "conscience check," on the way home from a deployment. Individuals who have been sexually active but are asymptomatic can be tested for syphilis and gonorrhea in an attempt to ensure they do not infect their wives or girlfriends. The yield and efficacy of this practice have never been evaluated. With the current knowledge of a broader range of STDs, the role of this practice is even more uncertain. The conscience check carries the danger of providing false reassurance if individuals do not appreciate the lower sensitivity of some tests and the inability to test in the field for some diseases. This false reassurance may evolve into a false belief that risky sexual behavior is acceptable because the medical department can catch and treat any problems before the individual returns home.

Contact Tracing and Partner Notification

It is increasingly difficult for public health and preventive medicine authorities to maintain the old model of tracking down, evaluating, and treating sex partners, generally referred to as contact tracing. This model, based on the experience with syphilis in the 1930s and 1940s, was applied to gonorrhea; it is not clear if it was effective. In recent years, numerous epidemiologic and public health changes have limited its effectiveness. These include a burgeoning population, including increasing numbers of STD cases; decreasing personnel and fiscal support for public health in general and STD work in particular; and changes in sexual activity that often make contact tracing impossible, eg, anonymous exchanges of sex for drugs or money, sex between strangers, and increased sexual activity in general. In many areas, contact tracing of sex partners may be limited to high-risk individuals, often locally defined (eg, women of child-bearing age who have been exposed to HIV).

Contact tracing may be possible when the contacts are largely within the military system, particularly within the same unit. Foreign countries that cater to sex-seeking tourists may have local social hygiene facilities and may regulate CSWs and so may allow contact tracing. But it is not clear whether impoverished countries where sex is a major industry have ever been able to follow the US-developed model for contact tracing or have interest in doing so. Preventive medicine personnel deploying overseas need to determine if such arrangements exist in popular liberty or recreation areas and make arrangements to share with the local health authorities the identities of sex partners provided by infected US military personnel. The Department of Defense uses the standard Public Health Service form CDC 73.2936S (8/91) for sexual contact reporting, as well as any required local civilian reporting form.

Contact tracing may be stymied by the inability or unwillingness of the patient to identify sex partners, as well as by other limitations. When the patient knows and can contact his or her partners, the patient must be urged to do so, a process known as *partner notification*. The health care provider should instruct the patient to tell the partner the STD diagnosis, make clear that the partner must be assumed to be infected even if the partner has no symptoms, and instruct the partner to see a health care provider for treatment.

The next crucial step after contact tracing and partner notification is epidemiological treatment (epitreatment) of sex partners, along with prompt treatment of the patient, to reduce STD transmission. All sex partners are presumed to be infected and must be promptly treated for the same diagnosis as the patient. Cultures and other tests can be obtained as appropriate, but epitreatment must be carried out when the partner is first seen, even if the partner denies symptoms or the possibility of infection, because an infected partner may go on to infect other persons. All sex contacts of patients diagnosed as having a treatable STD must receive epitreatment, using a regimen appropriate for the diagnosis. CDC guidelines[266] recommend sex partners of patients with gonorrhea, chlamydia, or nongonococcal urethritis be notified and referred for evaluation and epitreatment if they have had sex within 60 days before the onset of their symptoms or diagnosis. If the patient's last sexual contact was more than 60 days previously, the most recent sex partner should be notified and treated. Although epitreatment is emphasized, a thorough evaluation is also needed. In a Baltimore, Maryland, STD clinic, 23% of women attending as STD contacts had multiple STDs, compared to 10% of noncontacts.[267]

It is important for individuals diagnosed with nontreatable STD to be notified also. Some treatment options may be possible, for example, HBV vaccine may be offered to an uninfected partner. Notification also allows partners to determine their own situation (eg, to be tested for HIV) and then, after appropriate counseling, take steps to prevent their transmitting the infection to others. For herpes simplex virus, it is particularly important for women to know they have been placed at risk. If they become pregnant, it allows them to notify their obstetrician, who can then take steps to protect the baby from a devastating neonatal herpes infection.

Medical personnel counseling or managing STD cases should avoid identifying an individual as the source of the infection simply because that individual seems obvious or is suspected by the patient. This can be particularly sensitive and emotional when an STD occurs in an ostensibly monogamous relationship. The first priority is to identify and treat all contacts promptly. Determining who infected whom is a secondary consideration, preferably carried out with the help of an experienced sexual contact tracer and good knowledge of the epidemiology of the STD being traced. Failure to be careful in identifying the epidemiologic course of the infection or in avoiding premature conclusions may create difficulties and barriers to managing these cases and may result in legal problems for the medical staff if they inaccurately identify the source of the infection. Often it is more accurate and more appropriate simply to say that it cannot be determined who infected whom.

Prevention

When US military personnel are stationed or deployed overseas for a prolonged period, US preventive medicine personnel should try to establish an effective working relationship with local public health authorities to reduce the prevalence of STD in the core groups of transmitters, such as CSWs. The US Navy in the Philippines worked closely with the Social Hygiene Department of Olongapo City, next to the Subic Bay Naval Base, and provided technical and consultative assistance, antibiotics, and laboratory support. Gonorrhea among registered CSWs, who were examined and treated at the Social Hygiene Department clinic every other week,

had an incidence rate of 4%.[197] In contrast, unregistered CSWs, who were beyond the control of the department, had a gonorrhea rate of 40%. US Air Force personnel at nearby Clark Air Base similarly worked closely with the Social Hygiene Clinic in Angeles City. CSWs, particularly unregistered prostitutes, commonly used prophylactic antibiotics, which are available without prescription, in an attempt to protect themselves.[247] This practice offers no protection against STDs but does interfere with STD screening programs. The ability to intervene in a core group of CSWs may be limited to those STDs that can be readily diagnosed and treated by antibiotics or are vaccine preventable. However, attempts to eradicate infection by mass antibiotic treatment of all CSWs produce, at best, minor, transient reductions in STD rates.[268]

While treatment and screening are the most important step in controlling STDs, education is very important also. The challenge is to make the education more effective than the infamous "VD lectures" of the past by taking into account various behavioral factors.

Behavioral Considerations. There are no current, definitive, comprehensive data on US sexual behavior,[269] which greatly handicaps designing prevention programs. This is a critical deficiency because more than any other communicable disease, STDs are intimately and highly influenced by social behavioral factors. Data on sexual behavior come from mainly two sources whose relevance to a military population may be limited: inner city STD clinics and college campuses. A third source, prostitutes, may have relevance for the risks faced by deployed military personnel.[228]

Alcohol. Alcohol consumption promotes STD acquisition by reducing inhibitions and interfering with discrimination.[270] The relationship among alcohol, sex, and STDs was recognized far back in military experience. In World War I, under the influence of the social hygiene movement, military bases forbade the sale of any alcoholic beverages in a zone around the base extending for several miles. World War II–era studies identified alcohol use as a risk factor for STDs,[202–207] as did studies in the Vietnam War era,[193–195] a 1996 study of Thai military recruits,[245] and studies of STDs in civilians.[225,226] Attempts to reduce STDs must include education on the critical role alcohol plays in acquiring STDs and training and techniques to avoid or limit alcohol consumption.

Adolescent Risk-Taking Behavior. The majority of reported military STD cases occur among junior enlisted personnel, many of whom are still in their teens. Studies of adolescent risk-taking behavior, although only partially overlapping military personnel at the older (late teen) end of these studies, probably have considerable relevance. Adolescents tend to have unplanned, sporadic sex, and sexual activity is strongly influenced by affiliation with peers who already are sexually active.[271] The largest proportion of military personnel at risk for STDs are members of a group—adolescents and young adults—that inherently tends to take risks in all aspects of life because they perceive themselves as invulnerable. Their profession itself is risky (eg, weapons firing, parachuting, Special Forces activities) and being comfortable with risky activities may—appropriately or not—generalize to other areas of their life. Prevention efforts must take this into account.

Behavior Change and Education. Since the onset of the HIV epidemic, it has become obvious that the "one size fits all" approach to STD education and prevention is neither appropriate nor effective. Programs must be tailored to gender, race/ethnicity, culture, sexual orientation, and probably level of education and socioeconomic status, among other factors. For example, a study of 914 heterosexual individuals seen in South Carolina STD clinics (with a 41% gonorrhea prevalence) looked at recruitment of sex partners.[272] It concluded that risk reduction counseling for men should target reducing promiscuity by reducing their number of sex partners and of casual sex partners. Women, mostly monogamous and therefore facing different problems, needed counseling about care in partner selection and use of condoms with their steady sex partners.

Boyer summarizes the key qualities of a good STD intervention program for adolescents: "Programs that are likely to be most effective are those that target cognitive and behavioral skills to increase adolescents' sense of self-efficacy and enhance their ability to communicate, problem-solve, and make appropriate decisions about engaging in sexual intercourse."[273p610] Programs must go beyond simply presenting knowledge about STDs. They must impart knowledge and skills to resist peer pressure, to negotiate condom use, and to project future consequences of their behavior. Alternatives to sexual intercourse and how to decide if and when to have sex should be included. Programs that emphasize skills are more effective and need to include multi-method and multi-media approaches. Didactic information about STDs must be current and accurate. It should also emphasize that some STDs have asymptomatic periods but still may be transmissible and that some STDs are life-long and incurable. Adolescent intentions to have sex are strongly related to beliefs and motivations about sex, as opposed to knowledge about STDs.[273,274]

Physicians and other health care providers can affect the health behavior of their patients.[275–278] Patients expect health counseling from their health care deliverers and interpret the absence of such counseling as indicating the issue is not important or they are not at risk. Physicians need to emphasize harm reduction rather than absolute elimination of all risk, since the latter is usually not realistic. Particularly in the area of HIV risk reduction, insistence on a "zero defects" approach may lead to "unrealistically high standards for evaluating programs (perhaps more exacting than for clinical research), and may overlook or undermine their effectiveness."[277p1145] Arguing that condoms should not be used because they are not 100% effective is particularly pernicious.

One study[279] showed evidence that teenage sexual behavior, as measured by condom usage, average frequency of sexual intercourse, age at first intercourse, and chlamydial infection, can change. Applying the techniques proven effective in an urban STD clinic on a group of teenagers,[279] an initial study suggested this approach may be effective with Marine Corps personnel.[280] Intervention and control groups were at high risk for STDs. They were young and predominantly single, had had an average of 18 lifetime sex partners and two partners in the past 3 months, and only 9% and 14% always used condoms (49% and 42% never used condoms). About 30% had paid for sex, and about 25% had had a prior STD. The intervention, based on the Information, Motivation, and Behavioral Skills (IMB) behavior model, consisted of four 2-hour initial sessions, plus a 2-hour follow-up session, and included didactic slides, interactive group exercises, deployment-specific videos, and homework assignments. Sessions focused on STD and HIV transmission, treatment, and outcomes; perceptions of risk and self-efficacy; peer influence; the impact of alcohol and drugs; and liberty-specific risk factors. Risky behavior was significantly reduced in the intervention group: alcohol consumption (84% vs. 91%), mean number of beers per day (7 vs. 9), and number of sexual partners (none: 61% vs. 44%; more than two: 11% vs. 17%).

Education and the "VD Lecture." Traditional didactic education about STDs seems to have little effect in reducing STD incidence. Jones and colleagues[207] found no correlation between knowledge of common STDs and risk for acquiring an STD in a study of 1,885 men on an aircraft carrier. Other studies[197,281] have suggested traditional educational efforts may reduce the incidence of STDs in military personnel. Hook,[282] after reviewing the available literature, concluded it is not clear such efforts actually result in behavioral changes that decrease STD acquisition. The traditional "VD lecture" is based on the assumption that military personnel do not know how STDs are acquired and that knowledge of the nature of STDs is an effective deterrent (eg, scare tactics showing vivid pictures of genital lesions). Neither assumption seems justified, with the possible exception of fear of AIDS. The problem likely lies in an individual conviction that although STDs are a risk, someone else will be the person who acquires one.

Some didactic information may be helpful in changing behavior, notably the distinction between curable and incurable STDs; the fact that many individuals are asymptomatically infected for prolonged periods but are capable of infecting others, including spouses; and that there are no simple, reliable ways to tell when a potential sex partner is infected. All STD education programs must stress abstinence as the only sure way to avoid acquiring an STD (Plan A); however, for those who will not be abstinent, there must be a Plan B. Its foundation is the consistent, proper use of condoms. All STD educational efforts need to identify sexually risky behaviors, which should be avoided (Exhibit 38-3).

STD educational programs may indirectly reduce STD rates by sensitizing individuals to the signs and symptoms of infection, which might otherwise be overlooked or ignored. To the extent that they result in earlier diagnosis and treatment, such efforts contribute to STD control. Behavioral perceptions may provide an opportunity for behavioral change. For example, World War II studies found 12% to 36% of whites and 50% of blacks believed intercourse is necessary to maintain good health.[204,207] Only 55% of those without an STD believed masturbation was injurious to health, compared to 75% of those with an STD.[204]

Condoms. Not having condoms available results not in a lack of sexual activity but rather in sexual activity without condoms. For sexually active individuals, condoms must be available and their use promoted. As a World War I prevention poster targeting soldiers going on furlough expressed it, "NO is the best tactic; the next, PROPHYLACTIC!" Condoms should be readily available in essentially unlimited quantities, and individuals should be encouraged to take as many as they want. Condom promotion should emphasize the use of a new condom for each sex act. Boxes of condoms should be

available in numerous locations (eg, the medical clinic, bathrooms, locker rooms and gyms, galleys and mess halls, and lounges) selected to provide ready access with a degree of privacy, particularly from senior personnel. Not having condoms readily available and in large quantities markedly undermines efforts to promote safer sex practices. This lack implies condom usage is not really important (otherwise condoms would be available) and that the medical unit is not really interested in supporting the practices it urges people to follow.

Limiting the number of condoms that may be taken at one time, having individuals sign for the condoms they receive, and making individuals ask for condoms are all effective ways to discourage condom use. Any action that can be interpreted as monitoring condom usage, especially on an individual basis, should be avoided. A Navy physician once stationed himself at the gangplank of a ship tied up in a liberty port. Everyone going ashore was asked if he planned to have sex and offered a condom if the answer was affirmative. Much to the physician's surprise, few individuals admitted to this or accepted a condom. A dual authority figure— a physician and an officer—was publicly quizzing individuals about an activity not held in the highest regard by senior officers and in which they had

---

EXHIBIT 38-3

RISKY BEHAVIOR THAT PROMOTES ACQUIRING A SEXUALLY TRANSMITTED DISEASE

- Sex with prostitutes, including exchanging sex for drugs or other items
- Casual sex with strangers or casual acquaintances (eg, pick-ups, one-night stands)
- Sex with multiple partners, even if it is with only one partner at a time (serial monogamy)
- Sex between men
- Sex with an individual who uses intravenous drugs
- Sex with a partner who has multiple sex partners or who has other sex partners who use intravenous drugs
- Sex with partners who may have a sexually transmitted disease
- Sex without a condom

EXHIBIT 38-4

PROPER USE OF CONDOMS

- Use only latex condoms, not natural membrane condoms (natural membrane condoms may transmit a virus)
- Store condoms in a cool, dry place out of direct sunlight
- Do not use condoms in damaged packages or those that show obvious signs of age (eg, brittleness, stickiness, or discoloration)
- Handle condoms with care to prevent tears or punctures
- Put on the condom before any genital contact to prevent exposure to fluids that may contain infectious agents; hold the tip of the condom and unroll it onto the erect penis, leaving space at the tip to collect semen without trapping air in the tip
- Use adequate lubrication; do not use petroleum- or oil-based lubricants (eg, petroleum jelly, cooking oils, shortening, lotions) because they weaken the latex
- Replace a broken condom immediately
- Take care after ejaculation that the condom does not slip off the penis before withdrawal; hold the base of the condom while withdrawing; withdraw the penis while it is still erect
- Use a fresh condom each time; never reuse a condom

Adapted from: Centers for Disease Control and Prevention. Condoms for prevention of sexually transmitted diseases. *MMWR.* 1988;37:133–137.

---

been advised not to participate.

Medical and preventive medicine personnel need to teach condom users how to use them properly and effectively (Exhibit 38-4). Condom effectiveness has been studied by measuring two outcomes, pregnancy and STD acquisition. Pregnancy typically occurs 10% to 15% of the time over the course of a year but may be as infrequent as 2% for couples using condoms correctly and consistently. Two recent reviews[283,284] indicate condoms are effective in preventing numerous STDs, including HIV, as have other studies.[279,285–287]

The Thai government developed an active program to decrease HIV transmission among its CSWs, which included buying and distributing condoms, disciplining commercial sex establishments that did not consistently use condoms, and bluntly promoting condoms as a way to reduce HIV infection through advertising campaigns.[288] This was influenced in part by a high rate of HIV seroconversion among military recruits, largely associated with heterosexual intercourse with CSWs.[254,285] From 1989 to 1993, use of condoms by CSWs increased from 14% to 94%, and the rates of the five major STDs decreased 79%. Related studies suggest the problem of continued STD transmission may be due in part to inconsistent condom use, failure to use condoms with girlfriends (as opposed to CSWs), and alcohol use.[245,288] A subsequent study

found that HIV seroprevalence among Thai Army cohorts fell from the range of 10.4% to 12.5% (between 1991 and 1993) to 6.7% (in 1995), the proportion of men having sex with a CSW fell from 81.4% to 63.8%, and use of condoms increased from 61.0% to 92.5%.[289]

The range of effectiveness suggests condom failures are due to factors other than problems with the condoms themselves. Condom breakage rates in a variety of populations have been reported as 0.5% to 7%, with the higher figures associated with anal sex.[283] Breakage is usually due to the use of inadequate lubrication (particularly with minimal foreplay), petroleum-based lubricants (which degrade the latex), rough handling (particularly fingernail tears), or failure to leave adequate space at the tip of the condom. All these sources of "failure" are correctable by proper education in condom use and handling.

US personnel deployed overseas should not buy foreign condoms because they leak twice as much as US-made condoms.[290] The military supply system purchases the same standard condoms available to civilians.[291] Storage and transportation within the supply system may be a problem, however, so condoms should be checked for signs of deterioration from age or storage at temperature extremes.

Probably more important than mechanical factors in undercutting condom effectiveness is reluctance or inability to use them. For heterosexual men, use of drugs or alcohol is a major factor in failing to use condoms, followed by their partner not endorsing condom use.[270,292] Men were also less likely to use condoms if they reported being in love with their partners or had difficulty discussing condom usage with their partners. Women were less likely to use condoms if they were black, felt condoms decreased sexual pleasure, reported being in love with their partner, or had partners unwilling to use condoms.[270] Factors associated with condom usage included acceptance of condom advertising, perceptions of partner and peer acceptance of condoms, and effect on sexual pleasure.[293] Both the mechanical aspects of condom use and negotiating condom use with a partner can be taught to STD clinic patients, with a significant reduction of STD infections.[294] Ordering service members to use condoms is not effective, even when they are faced with possible punitive action. One half of 1,103 HIV-positive soldiers did not always use condoms, despite having been ordered to do so.[295]

Condom use by women may be particularly problematic.[296] A national survey found that overall only 41% of sexually active, never-married women aged 15 to 49 years used condoms and only 32% used them consistently.[297] Women at greater risk for STD and HIV (eg, those with larger numbers of lifetime partners) were even less likely to use condoms.[240] The perception that they might acquire AIDS did not influence condom use.[297] Negotiation of condom usage is particularly important for women, since women tend to have less control over the events of a sexual encounter, including the male partner's use of a condom. The traditional alternative suggestions that women should abstain or alter the number and selection of their partners may be less realistic for women than for men.[298,299] The so-called "female condom," approved by the Food and Drug Administration in 1993, offers a way for women to obtain greater control, but because of its price (and perhaps for other reasons which are not clear), it has not been widely accepted. Although a variety of other, female-controlled methods provide protection against some STDs,[299] Cates and colleagues[300] suggest the data are "inconclusive" regarding the absolute level of protection of spermicides against HIV and STD and recommend that both women and men who practice high-risk sex continue to use (male) condoms as their first line of defense.

It is sometimes argued that condoms should not be provided because they provide a false sense of confidence since they do not provide perfect pro-tection. This argument misses the point. A number of individuals are going to engage in risky sexual behavior, despite all efforts to dissuade them. For these individuals, even some protection is an advantage. Individuals can be taught to use condoms properly and consistently. As Roper and Curran, (then, respectively, the Director and the Director for STD Prevention at the CDC) expressed it, "Our prevention message should be clear on this point: When used correctly and consistently, condoms are highly effective; when used otherwise, they are not."[301p502]

Alternative Recreational Outlets. Social activities and recreational facilities have always been considered vital to maintaining morale and directly or indirectly to keeping STD rates down.[202,203,205,207] Ratcliffe noted higher STD rates in units without recreational or social facilities,[207] suggesting the absence of such facilities may encourage sexual activity as an antidote to boredom and frustration. It is doubtful, though, that recreational activities can totally prevent STDs or reduce them below some baseline rate. The problem was succinctly expressed in the musical *South Pacific*: "We got volleyball and Ping-Pong and a lot of dandy games; what ain't we got, we ain't got dames!" [Used with permission of the estate of Oscar Hammerstein.]

Quarantine. Particularly in the past, STD cases were sometimes "quarantined," (denied liberty until they were demonstrated to be no longer infectious) to prevent them from infecting other people. Aside from its overall impracticality, quarantine has a more pernicious effect. Faced with a possible loss of liberty, symptomatic individuals who fear they may have an STD or the worried well who have simply exposed themselves will elect not to come to sick call until the last possible day. In the meantime, they remain sexually active and infect additional people. Individuals with curable STDs should be instructed not to have sex for an appropriate period, but they are rendered noninfectious within hours using current antibiotic regimens. Quarantine should never be used. It drives symptomatic cases underground and ultimately is self-defeating.

Patients presenting with a possible STD should have at a minimum a thorough examination of the genito-rectal area, including the inguinal lymph nodes. Women should have a pelvic examination, including visualization of the cervix. This requires the patient to undress from the waist to the knees. Other areas should be evaluated depending on the patient's history and suspected disease. For example, syphilis may produce a skin rash or cranial nerve or meningeal symptoms; gonorrhea may produce a rash, joint symptoms, or pharyngitis. Evaluation of all genital ulcers should include consideration of syphilis, herpes, chancroid, and lymphogranuloma venereum. Patients should be serologically tested for syphilis, HBV, and HIV. The incubation period for HBV and HIV seropositivity is sufficiently long that a patient is unlikely to be seropositive from the current exposure. However, any STD is a marker indicating that a patient has been engaging in risky sexual behavior, and therefore the patient may be seropositive from a prior sexual exposure. Follow-up serologic testing for HBV and HIV infection should be strongly considered.

Specific Sexually Transmitted Diseases

Gonorrhea (Urethritis and Cervicitis)

Description of the Pathogen. Gonorrhea is caused by the bacterium *Neisseria gonorrhoeae*. Antibiotic resistance is a continual concern. Antibiotics of the penicillin, amoxicillin, and tetracycline types are no longer effective for most practical purposes. Spectinomycin resistance has been a problem in Asia, and quinoline resistance is a potentially emerging problem.

Epidemiology. Gonorrhea is almost always transmitted by sexual contact. Fomites are not usually considered to play a role in gonorrhea transmission. However, in an experiment at the Navy Environmental and Preventive Medicine Unit No. 2 in Norfolk, Virgina, an inflatable sex doll was inoculated in its "vagina" with a quantity of gonococci comparable to that delivered during a single sex act. The doll was maintained at room temperature under ambient conditions. Viable organisms, in sufficient numbers to infect a new partner, could be recovered for up to 24 hours. Sex toys should not be shared.

N gonorrhoeae is distributed worldwide. The rapidity of air travel from overseas deployments or exercises in high-risk areas is a particular concern to the military. Citing unpublished data, Berg reported on 28 cases of penicillinase-producing *N gonorrhoeae* (PPNG) acquired by US sailors and Marines in Southeast Asia.[214] Most (71%) had been exposed 1 to 3 days before departure; actual travel time was about 24 hours. Fifty-one percent became symptomatic the first day back in San Diego and were initially treated an average of 4.6 days after arrival. Eighteen percent had been sexually active before receiving effective treatment, an average of 12.3 days after arrival. Military deployments to Southeast Asia were possibly responsible for acqui-

sition of the HIV E clade by eight Western hemisphere military personnel, including three US Navy personnel.[302,303]

Endemic gonorrhea has been largely eradicated in Europe, but incidence rates remain high among poor and minority populations in the United States,[304] with these groups closely resembling the populations of developing countries. The US gonorrhea rate, 240/100,000 cases annually (for approximately 600,000 cases a year[251]), can be compared to a rate of 14/100,000 in Sweden,[305] but equating the United States and Europe may not be valid.[198,199,306] In the United States, gonorrhea tends to cluster in lower-economic, inner-city populations, where the rate among African-Americans is 30 times higher than among whites.[307] Studies of male military personnel have found 2% to 10% have asymptomatic gonorrhea.[213,308–310]

Pathogenesis and Clinical Findings. The incubation period in men is 3 to 7 days, and occasionally it is as long as 18 days; 10% to 20% of those infected are asymptomatic. The incubation period in women is 7 to 60 days; 50% to 80% of infected women are asymptomatic. Coinfections are highly common; 5% to 30% of men and 25% to 50% of women with gonorrhea have chlamydia, and 40% of sex partners of men with gonorrhea have chlamydia. All gonorrhea cases are presumed to be coinfected with chlamydia and are cotreated with an antichlamydial antibiotic.

Acute urethritis is the most common manifestation of gonorrhea in men. Although the classic presentation is an abrupt onset of dysuria and copious purulent discharge ("running like a river and pissing razor blades"), gonorrhea may mimic nongonococcal urethritis (NGU) or may be asymptomatic. Distinguishing gonorrhea and NGU on the basis of patient history is unreliable.

Mild cervicitis and asymptomatic endocervical infection are common manifestations in women. Endometritis, salpingitis, and pelvic peritonitis, with the subsequent risk of infertility, may also occur. All forms of female gonococcal infection are commonly minimally symptomatic. Diagnosis based only on history and physical examination will miss many cases.

Diagnostic Approaches. In men, a Gram-stained urethral smear is diagnostic for gonorrhea if it demonstrates Gram-negative intracellular diplococci. It has a sensitivity of 90% to 95% in symptomatic men and 50% to 70% in asymptomatic men; its specificity is 95% to 100%. Specimens should be obtained by inserting a calcium alginate swab about 2 cm into the urethra and leaving it there for 10 to 30 seconds. It should be withdrawn with a twisting motion, rolled (not smeared) over a glass slide, and then smeared onto a culture plate. The Gram stain can also diagnose NGU. STD laboratory personnel should be trained to report four possible Gram stain interpretations: (1) gonorrhea (presence of white blood cells and Gram-negative intracellular diplococci), (2) NGU (white blood cells without Gram-negative diplococci), (3) a nonspecific smear (cells and debris are present but in no diagnostic pattern), and (4) negative (a few epithelial cells or nothing). Ideally, the patient has not urinated for at least 4 hours before providing the urethral specimen because he may have temporarily washed out evidence of infection. If a patient with a history compatible with urethritis has a negative smear, diagnostic results may be obtained by having him return when he has not urinated for 2 to 4 hours. As a practical matter, though, taking patients as they come usually provides a diagnosis.

In women, a cervical Gram stain is 50% to 70% sensitive for diagnosing gonorrhea, with a specificity of 95% to 100%. Although a Gram stain may be useful, its relatively low sensitivity necessitates a culture. Anal cultures detect a few additional gonorrhea cases. They should be done if gonorrhea is suspected or the woman has been exposed to gonorrhea. (Women may become rectally infected from rectal intercourse or from rubbing infected secretions into the rectum.) When cervical specimens are taken for gonococcal culture, the speculum should be lubricated with only warm water to avoid the possibility of bacteriostatic agents in lubricants getting on the swab or cervix and producing a false-negative culture. Excess cervical mucus should be blotted away with a swab and then a different sterile cotton-tipped swab inserted into the cervical os. The swab should be moved from side to side for 10 to 30 seconds. It should be withdrawn, rolled on a glass slide, and then smeared on Thayer-Martin or other appropriate culture media (Exhibit 38-5).

Diagnosis and management of complicated gonococcal infections, such as disseminated gonococcal infection (arthritis-dermatitis syndrome), pelvic inflammatory disease, epididymo-orchitis, or gonococcal ophthalmia are beyond the scope of this chapter. They are prevented by the same means as uncomplicated gonococcal infections.

Recommendations for Therapy and Control. Pertinent, current CDC treatment recommendations are summarized in Exhibits 38-6 and 38-7.

Since 1994, there have been six reports of relative or high-level gonococcal resistance to ciprofloxacin, including treatment failures.[311–315] Most infections were probably acquired in Southeast Asia. A Japanese report[316] examined gonococcal isolates collected in 1992 and 1993 and compared them to those collected a decade earlier. The MIC50 (minimum concentration of antibiotic required to inhibit the growth of 50% of a collection of bacterial strains) had increased 4-fold and the MIC90 8-fold. In Baltimore, ciprofloxacin MICs in 1,846 gonococcal isolates did not increase from 1988 to late 1994,[317] which may be related to the limited use of quinolone antibiotics in that area. For now, quinolone antibiotics at recommended doses remain an acceptable treatment for gonorrhea,[318] but military personnel should be alert to the possible emergence of more widespread resistance among individuals infected in Southeast Asia.

Cotreatment of Chlamydia. Using azithromycin to treat coexisting chlamydia infections has the advantage over other antichlamydial antibiotics of much better compliance since it requires only a single dose, as opposed to 7 days of doxycycline treatment. Azithromycin powder can be dissolved to produce a suspension and administered to patients as directly observed therapy. Azithromycin has only been approved by the US Food and Drug Administration for use against proven chlamydia infections or for cotreatment of presumptive chlamydia when treating gonorrhea. Stamm and colleagues,[319] in a study of 452

EXHIBIT 38-5

CRITERIA FOR THE DIAGNOSIS OF GONOCOCCAL URETHRITIS

Suggestive Diagnosis—both:

- Evidence of mucopurulent exudate on examination

AND

- Sexual exposure to a partner known to be infected with *Neisseria gonorrhoeae*

Presumptive diagnosis—any **one** of these:

- Gram-negative diplococci on Gram stained urethral smear

- *N gonorrhoeae* cultured but not confirmed with sugar fermentation or other tests

- *N gonorrhoeae* detected by a nonculture laboratory test

Definitive diagnosis:

- *Neisseria gonorrhoeae* is both cultured and confirmed

Source: Centers for Disease Control and Prevention. *Sexually Transmitted Diseases Clinical Practice Guidelines.* Atlanta, Ga.: CDC; 1991.

EXHIBIT 38-6

TREATMENT OF URETHRITIS AND GONOCOCCAL OR CHLAMYDIA PROCTITIS IN MEN

Gonococcal Urethritis[*]

Cefixime 400 mg orally in a single dose

OR

Ceftriaxone 125 mg intramuscularly in a single dose

OR

Ciprofloxacin 500 mg orally in a single dose

OR

Ofloxacin 400 mg orally in a single dose

PLUS

Azithromycin 1 g orally in a single dose

OR

Doxycycline[†] 100 mg orally twice a day for 7 days

Nongonococcal Urethritis[‡] **and Chlamydia Urethritis**[§]

Azithromycin 1 g orally in a single dose

OR

Doxycycline[†] 100 mg orally twice a day for 7 days

Gonococcal or Chlamydia Proctitis

Regimens appropriate for gonococcal urethritis plus doxycycline 100 mg orally twice a day for 7 days.

Follow-Up and Abstention from Intercourse. Patients should be instructed to refrain from sexual intercourse until 7 days after the initiation of therapy and until all of their partners have been cured. Patients treated with a recommended regimen do not need to be seen in follow-up unless their symptoms recur. If symptoms recur, the patient should be reevaluated and retreated if there is evidence of infection. Patients who receive erythromycin may need to be reevaluated 3 weeks after completion of therapy.

Source: Centers for Disease Control and Prevention. 1998 guidelines for treatment of sexually transmitted diseases. *MMWR.* 1998;47(RR-1).

[*] Alternative single dose gonococcal regimens: Spectinomycin 2 gm IM, ceftizoxime 500 mg IM, cefotaxime 500 mg IM, cefotetan 1 gm IM, or cefoxitin 2 gm IM plus probenecid 1 gm orally. (Only cefoxitin requires probenecid.) Each of these regimens also requires antichlamydia treatment with azithromycin or doxycycline.

[†] Doxycycline can be taken with food, but Pepto Bismol, iron products, and antacids may bind with it and reduce its absorption.

[‡] Alternate nongonococcal urethritis regimens: erythromycin base 500 mg orally 4 times a day for 7 days, erythromycin ethylsuccinate 800 mg orally 4 times a day for 7 days, or ofloxacin 300 mg orally twice a day for 7 days. If only erythromycin is available but a patient cannot tolerate the erythromycin regimens just given, one of the following regimens may be used: erythromycin base 250 mg orally 4 times a day for 14 days or erythromycin ethylsuccinate 400 mg orally 4 times a day for 14 days.

[§] Alternative chlamydia urethritis regimens: erythromycin base 500 mg orally 4 times a day for 7 days, erythromycin ethylsuccinate 800 mg orally 4 times a day for 7 days, or ofloxacin 300 mg orally twice a day for 7 days.

---

men, demonstrated that a single dose of 1 gm of azithromycin was as effective as standard doxycycline treatment for NGU. An accompanying editorial,[320] a study of azithromycin for cervicitis,[321] and one for chlamydial infections in both sexes[322] argue that azithromycin, although more expensive than doxycycline, is cost effective because it prevents complicated infections and additional infections.

Treatment Failures. Preventive medicine units periodically receive reports of "ceftriaxone-resistant gonorrhea" or gonorrhea "resistant" to other antibiotics. These reports usually reflect an unacknowledged reinfection or a faulty diagnosis. Antibiotic resistance is determined in the microbiology laboratory, a resource not readily available to most field

or operational units. Such reports are, in almost all cases, actually reports of treatment failure. There are a number of possible explanations. The symptoms may represent an untreated or improperly treated chlamydia coinfection. It may be a recurrence of a simultaneous chlamydia infection, despite the patient's having taken antichlamydia medicine. If it is gonorrhea, it is almost always a reinfection, but the patient may not admit this because of the patient's belief that he or she could not be infected a second time. Reasons for this belief include an erroneous assumption that the patient's sex partner was treated simultaneously (and therefore could not reinfect the patient) or that the patient had sex with a different partner who was

EXHIBIT 38-7

TREATMENT OF CERVICITIS AND GONOCOCCAL OR CHLAMYDIA PROCTITIS IN WOMEN

Gonococcal Cervicitis[*]

Cefixime 400 mg orally in a single dose

OR

Ceftriaxone 125 mg intramuscularly in a single dose

OR

Ciprofloxacin 500 mg orally in a single dose

OR

Ofloxacin 400 mg orally in a single dose

PLUS

Azithromycin 1 gm orally in a single dose

OR

Doxycycline[†] 100 mg orally twice a day for 7 days

Mucopurulent Cervicitis

Women with mucopurulent cervicitis should be tested for *Neisseria gonorrhoeae* and *Chlamydia trachomatis* and treatment based on those test results. Empiric therapy for either or both of these entities should be considered if (a) the patient is suspected of being infected, (b) the prevalence of these infections is high in the patient population, and (c) the patient may be difficult to locate for treatment.

Chlamydia Cervicitis[‡]

Azithromycin 1 gm orally in a single dose

OR

Doxycycline[†] 100 mg orally twice a day for 7 days

Gonococcal or Chlamydia Proctitis

Regimens appropriate for gonococcal cervicitis plus doxycycline 100 mg orally twice a day for 7 days

Pregnancy. Doxycycline and erythromycin estolate are contraindicated during pregnancy. Ciprofloxacin and ofloxacin are contraindicated in pregnant and lactating women and persons less than 18 years old. Preliminary data indicate azythromycin may be safe in pregnancy, but data are insufficient to recommend its use in pregnancy. Pregnant women may be treated for chlamydia using erythomycin base, erythromycin ethylsuccinate, or amoxicillin 500 mg orally 3 times a day for 7 days. A repeat evaluation of pregnant women for chlamydia 3 weeks after completion of therapy is recommended.

Follow-up and Abstention from Intercourse. Patients should be instructed to refrain from sexual intercourse until 7 days after the initiation of therapy and until all of their partners have been cured. Patients treated with a recommended regimen do not need to be seen in follow-up unless their symptoms recur. If symptoms recur, the patient should be reevaluated and retreated if there is evidence of infection. Patients who receive erythromycin may need to be reevaluated 3 weeks after completion of therapy.

---

[*] Alternative single-dose gonococcal regimens: Spectinomycin 2 g IM, ceftizoxime 500 mg IM, cefotaxime 500 mg IM, cefotetan 1 g IM, or cefoxitin 2 g IM plus probenecid 1 g orally. (Only cefoxitin requires probenecid.) Each of these regimens also requires antichlamydia treatment with azithromycin or doxycycline.

[†] Doxycycline can be taken with food, but Pepto Bismol, iron products, and antacids may bind with it and reduce its absorption.

[‡] Alternative chlamydia cervicitis regimens: Erythromycin base 500 mg orally 4 times a day for 7 days, erythromycin ethylsuccinate 800 mg orally 4 times a day for 7 days, or ofloxacin 300 mg orally twice a day for 7 days.

IM intramuscularly

Source: Centers for Disease Control and Prevention. 1998 guidelines for treatment of sexually transmitted diseases. *MMWR.* 1998;47(RR-1).

---

thought to be uninfected (eg, a spouse). In a surprising number of these reports of antibiotic "resistance," a proper evaluation was not done at the time the patient reappeared. Instead, the medical provider simply accepted the patient's version of

what happened and retreated the patient without obtaining any laboratory tests.

True treatment failures due to antibiotic resistance are highly important sentinel events and should be investigated thoroughly. The most important action is to culture the infection and submit the gonococcal isolate for antibiotic sensitivity testing. Other steps in the investigation include reviewing the medical record and interviewing those involved to determine an accurate history of events, including which laboratory tests were done and the results. The patient should be thoroughly questioned about sexual exposures since the initial treatment, with an emphasis on identifying all sexual contacts and not simply those the patient thinks might have been the source of the infection. All contacts are presumed to be potential sources of infection and need to be evaluated accordingly.

Follow-up evaluation of uncomplicated gonococcal infections is generally not needed, because current treatment regimens based on ceftriaxone are highly effective and test-of-cure cultures are not needed. Instead, patients should be instructed to return if their symptoms persist or recur. Follow-up evaluation with test-of-cure cultures should be considered for alternative treatment regimens and particularly for patients in relationships in which all sex partnters may not be treated simultaneously, leading to possible reinfection (ping-pong infection). The patient and partners should be instructed not to have sex until 7 days after all medications have completed by everyone and the patient and partners are asymptomatic.

Gonococcal Pharyngitis

Epidemiology. Gonococcal pharyngitis can be acquired directly through oral sex.

Pathogenesis and Clinical Findings. Gonococcal pharyngitis is clinically indistinguishable from any other bacterial or viral pharyngitis. It is associated with disseminated gonococcal infection but often occurs as an isolated entity.

Diagnostic Approaches. Diagnosis is complicated by the common presence in the oropharynx of non-pathogenic *Neisseria* species, which can produce a false-positive Gram stain. Definitive diagnosis requires culture with the added step of sugar fermentation testing to identify specific *Neisseria* species. The throat swab specimen must be swabbed directly onto a Thayer-Martin culture plate. The standard culturette device used for streptococcal pharyngitis is poorly effective as a transport medium for gonococci.

Throat cultures for gonorrhea should be obtained from homosexual men with pharyngitis, individuals with pharyngitis and genital or rectal symptoms, individuals with pharyngitis and who have had recent sex contact with someone who has gonor-

rhea, and individuals engaging in risky sexual behavior whose symptoms have not responded to treatment for a "strep throat." Because eradication of *Neisseria* from the oropharynx can be difficult, two test-of-cure cultures are required, 4 days apart. Cultures must be scheduled after the patient has finished his or her antibiotic treatment for chlamydia. Although doxycycline or azithromycin may not eradicate *N gonorrhoeae*, they may have sufficient activity to cause a false-negative culture.

Recommendations for Therapy and Control. See Gonorrhea and Exhibit 38-8.

EXHIBIT 38-8

TREATMENT OF GONOCOCCAL PHARYNGITIS

Ceftriaxone 125 mg intramuscularly in a single dose

OR

Ciprofloxacin 500 mg orally in a single dose

OR

Ofloxacin 400 mg orally in a single dose

PLUS

Azithromycin 1 gm orally in a single dose

OR

Doxycycline* 100 mg orally twice a day for 7 days

Follow-up. Gonococcal pharyngitis is more difficult to treat than gonococcal infections of the urogenital and rectal areas. Few regimens reliably cure such infections more than 90% of the time. Patients should be instructed to return for reevaluation if their symptoms persist or recur. Chlamydia coinfection of the pharynx is unusual, but coinfection at genital sites sometimes occurs. Therefore treatment for both gonorrhea and chlamydia is recommended.

Pregnancy. Doxycycline is contraindicated in pregnancy; information is insufficient to recommend azithromycin in pregnancy. Ciprofloxacin and ofloxacin are contraindicated in pregnant and lactating women and persons less than 18 years old. See Exhibit 39-6 for alternate antichlamydia drugs that can used during pregnancy.

---

* Doxycycline can be taken with food, but Pepto Bismol, iron products, and antacids may bind with it and reduce its absorption.

Source: Centers for Disease Control and Prevention. 1998 guidelines for treatment of sexually transmitted diseases. *MMWR.* 1998;47(RR-1).

Chlamydia (Urethritis and Cervicitis)

Description of the Pathogen. The intracellular bacterium *Chlamydia trachomatis* causes the infection commonly referred to as "chlamydia."

Epidemiology. Chlamydia is transmitted by sexual intercourse and is found worldwide. In the United States, chlamydia infections do not appear to cluster geographically but reporting is not uniform.

In the United States, 35% to 50% of NGU cases are caused by *C trachomatis*.[144p257–261] Studies of male military personnel have found 7% to 11% have had asymptomatic chlamydia infections.[310,323] Gynecologic screening of female US Navy recruits found 10% had asymptomatic cervical chlamydial infections.[324]

Pathogenesis and Clinical Findings. In both sexes, chlamydia often occurs as a coinfection with gonorrhea, and the two conditions can mimic each other. In men, chlamydia most commonly appears as urethritis, but complications include epididymitis, infertility, and proctitis (in men practicing receptive anal intercourse). The incubation period is 7 to 10 days and asymptomatic infections are common. In women with symptomatic infections, manifestations include endocervicitis and other gonorrhea-like conditions. Complications include salpingitis, ectopic pregnancy, and proctitis. In women, the incubation period is 7 days onward (the maximum time period is not known), and more than 90% of women infected are asymptomatic.

Diagnostic Approaches. Nonculture chlamydia tests are commercially available. Most have overall sensitivities of 60% to 90%.[261] Sensitivity correlates with symptomatology and may be 100% in individuals with a profuse discharge. At the other extreme, many of these tests have not been evaluated in asymptomatic individuals, especially men; the tests' sensitivity in these individuals may be low. PCR and LCR chlamydia tests are highly sensitive and specific, especially when used in combination. They are not widely commercially available and are notorious for their sensitivity to contamination, which limits their use under field conditions. Commonly available chlamydia tests can produce false-positive results, and caution is advised when such results may have legal implications,[262] for example, in rape cases. In such cases, verification with a second test is recommended, preferably one which uses a different epitope. The CDC has developed guidelines for using and interpreting chlamydia test results,[73] which consider such factors as prevalence of chlamydia in the population of interest, patient gender, and whether a false-positive result would

have adverse effects. Serologic tests for chlamydia are not considered reliable and are not recommended.

Recommendations for Therapy and Control. Uncomplicated chlamydial infections treated with doxycycline or azithromycin do not routinely require follow-up, unless symptoms persist or recur. Retesting after 3 weeks should be considered for patients who are treated with other medications. Individuals should also abstain from sex until 7 days after completing medications (see Exhibits 38-6 and 38-7).

Chlamydia screening in men is somewhat problematic. Healthy young men rarely seek medical attention and usually avoid testing that requires a painful urethral swab. Chlamydia infections are common in sexually active young men, but the symptoms, if present, may be minimal or ignored. At least 10% are asymptomatically infected. Data on the sensitivity and specificity of nonculture chlamydia tests are limited because manufacturers may not evaluate chlamydia diagnostic tests in young men, particularly asymptomatic ones. A LET only requires a urine specimen. A positive result indicates white blood cells are present, but these may be due to gonorrhea, chlamydia, or some other infection.

Sexually active young women are also at high risk for chlamydia infection and typically have no or minimal symptoms. MPC is easily diagnosed but is insensitive as an indicator of chlamydia infection. A diagnosis of MPC is useful because it allows treatment initiation, but the diagnosis of MPC does not justify avoiding other tests. A variety of nonculture chlamydia tests are very sensitive, but have both false-positive and false-negative results. Generally accepted criteria identifying women who should be screened for chlamydia infection include any of the following:[262] (*a*) Presence of mucopurulent cervicitis, (*b*) a sexually active woman younger than 20 years old, (*c*) a woman 20 to 24 years old who either uses barrier contraception inconsistently or has either had a new sex partner or more than one sex partner in the past 3 months, (*d*) a woman older than age 24 who uses barrier contraception inconsistently and has either had a new sex partner or more than one sex partner in the past 3 months, and (*e*) a pregnant woman in a high-prevalence area for chlamydia. All screening programs should be based on local STD epidemiology, whenever possible. When a false-positive result may have adverse social, psychological, or medicolegal results, positive results should be verified with a different test.

Nongonococcal Urethritis

NGU is a urethral infection caused by any of a number of pathogens other than *N gonorrhoeae*. It is commonly diagnosed on the basis of a urethral discharge and evidence of urethral inflammation (presence of white blood cells) without making a specific etiological diagnosis. The term predates the demonstration of chlamydia as the commonest cause of NGU and originally simply meant that no organism could be identified as the cause of the infection. For practical purposes, NGU is a male infection. Women may occasionally have symptoms of a bladder infection that is chlamydial in origin. This is referred to as the "acute dysuria syndrome" or the "dysuria pyuria syndrome."

Obsolete terms for NGU are postgonococcal urethritis and nonspecific urethritis (NSU). Use of the latter term should be discouraged because it implies NGU is not a sexually transmitted disease. NGU has been attributed to beer and other alcoholic beverages, spicy foods, caffeine, masturbation, too much or too little sex, allergies, "toxins," and "strain." None of these are etiologic agents, a fact that bears emphasis because such beliefs reinforce the idea that NGU is not a sexually transmitted disease. The old practice of proscribing these agents as part of the treatment of NGU should be avoided, because doing so may undermine the credibility of medical personnel.

Description of the Pathogens. By definition, NGU is not caused by *N gonrrhoeae*, a fact that manifests itself in the absence of Gram-negative diplococci on a urethral Gram stain. NGU is caused by the intracellular bacterium *C trachomatis* or the mycoplasma *Ureaplasma urealyticum*. Herpes simplex virus, the protozoan *Trichomonas vaginalis*, and possibly *Mycoplasma genitalium* are rare causes of NGU. These latter agents should be considered when the medication prescribed to treat NGU has no effect on symptoms.

Epidemiology. NGU is transmitted in the same way as gonorrhea, and its etiological agents are distributed worldwide. Gonococcal and nongonococcal urethritis have sufficient epidemiologic overlap that all cases of gonococcal urethritis are presumed to be coinfected with chlamydia (the commonest etiological agent of NGU), and treated as such. Further, urethritis diagnosed solely on the basis of a purulent or mucopurulent discharge, a positive LET, or the demonstration of 10 WBC or greater per high power field when examining first void urine, should be treated for both gonorrhea and chlamydia. *C trachomatis* causes about 25% to 55% of NGU, although the proportion decreases with age. *Ureaplasma*

urealyticum causes up to 20% of NGU, perhaps more. *Trichomonas vaginalis* is an unusual cause of NGU in US studies, but is a more common cause in European studies. Herpes virus rarely causes NGU.

Pathogenesis and Clinical Findings. NGU is classically described as having milder symptoms than gonorrhea, with either no dysuria or dysuria described as itching or tingling. The urethral discharge is clear and mucoid, may be scanty, and may be present only on awakening in the morning. Distinguishing NGU from gonorrhea on the basic of clinical presentation is unreliable, however, since either disease can mimic the other. Asymptomatic infection is common.

Diagnostic Approaches. Although diagnostic tests are now available to identify *C trachomatis*, the most common cause of NGU, the concept of NGU is a highly utilitarian one in any setting where available lab tests may only be capable of demonstrating the presence of urethral inflammation (Exhibit 38-9). Diagnosing NGU allows the patient to be treated effectively and promptly, a key step in pre-

---

EXHIBIT 38-9

CRITERIA FOR THE DIAGNOSIS OF NONGONOCOCCAL URETHRITIS

Suggestive Diagnosis

- History of urethral discharge plus one of the following:
    - Sexual exposure to a person known to have an NGU-causing organism
    - Positive leukocyte esterase test
    - < 5 WBC per oil field on a Gram stained urethral smear[*]

Presumptive Diagnosis

- Abnormal urethral discharge

  OR

- ≥ 5 WBC per oil field on a Gram stained urethral smear[*]

  PLUS

- Exclusion of gonococci on Gram stain

---

[*]Mean of five oil fields
WBC: white blood cell
Source: Centers for Disease Control and Prevention. *Sexually Transmitted Diseases Clinical Practice Guidelines.* Atlanta: CDC; 1991.

venting the spread of infection. Recommended treatment regimens are highly active against the two agents that cause nearly all case of NGU.

Treatment. See Exhibit 38-6.

Mucopurulent Cervicitis

MPC in women may be a clinical analogue of NGU in some respects. Like NGU, it is a syndromic diagnosis based on demonstrating cervical discharge and inflammation rather than a specific etiologic agent. Its presence may allow the initiation of treatment. The etiological agents of MPC are not fully known. Both *N gonorrhoeae* and *C trachomatis* are associated with MPC, although neither organism can be demonstrated in most MPC cases. Moreover, cervical infections with these organisms may not demonstrate MPC. Most cases of MPC are asymptomatic, although cervical examination reveals a purulent or mucopurulent endocervical exudate. Some women have an abnormal vaginal discharge and vaginal bleeding (eg, after sexual intercourse).

Diagnosis. Exhibit 38-10.

Treatment. See Exhibit 38-7.

Proctitis

Description of the Pathogen. Acute sexually transmitted proctitis is most commonly caused by *N gonorrhoeae* and, especially in men who have sex with men, *C trachomatis*. *Treponema pallidum* and herpes simplex virus are also causes.

Epidemiology. These infections are most commonly acquired by receptive anal intercourse. In some cases, they may be acquired by other means (eg, digital intercourse, sex toys).

Pathogenesis and Clinical Findings. Most cases are asymptomatic or mildly and nonspecifically symptomatic (eg, rectal itching, mild discharge). Perhaps 10% of cases have anorectal pain, tenesmus, or grossly bloody discharge. Anoscopy reveals normal mucosa or nonspecific proctitis. Herpetic proctitis reveals ulcerative lesions or fissures. Syphilitic proctitis reveals chancres.

Diagnostic Approaches. Anoscopy may reveal pus, and a Gram stain may reveal white blood cells. (The Gram stain may also reveal Gram-negative diplococci in gonococcal proctitis, but this is only 30% sensitive.) Ulcerative lesions and fissures suggest herpes or syphilis. Other diagnostic tests should be obtained if available.

Treatment. If pus, white blood cells, or Gram-negative diplococci are seen, the patient should be treated as for gonococcal urethritis, plus doxycy-

---

EXHIBIT 38-10

CRITERIA FOR THE DIAGNOSIS OF MUCOPURULENT CERVICITIS*

Suggestive Diagnosis

- 10-30 WBC per oil field on a Gram stained cervical smear

PLUS

- Sexual exposure to a person known to have MPC-causing organisms

Presumptive diagnosis—any one of these

- Presence of yellow mucopurulent endocervical exudate[†]
- Swab-induced endocervical bleeding
- ≥ 30 WBC per oil field on a Gram stained cervical smear

WBC: white blood cell

* Whenever possible, women with MPC should be tested specifically for *Neisseria gonorrhoeae* and *Chlamydia trachomatis* and a treatment decision made on the basis of those test results. If there is a high local prevalence of gonorrhea or chlamydia and the woman may be difficult to locate for treatment, empiric treatment should be considered. For further details see Centers for Disease Control and Prevention. 1998 Guidelines for treatment of sexually transmitted diseases. *MMWR*. 1998;47(RR-1):1–128.

† Swab test consists of inserting a cotton swab into the cervix to obtain a specimen of endocervical mucopus. The swab is withdrawn from the vagina and held up to a dark background and examined with a bright light. The presence of yellow or yellow-green mucopus indicates a positive test.

Source: Centers for Disease Control and Prevention. *Sexually Transmitted Diseases Clinical Practice Guidelines*. Atlanta: CDC; 1991.

---

cline 100 mg orally twice a day for 7 days. Other or additional treatment should be guided by laboratory results.

Herpes

Description of the Pathogen. Genital herpes is caused by infection with the herpes simplex virus, usually type 2.

Epidemiology. HSV is transmitted by sexual contact. Because HSV can easily be inoculated on any mucous membrane or through any break in the skin, individuals with herpes labialis ("fever blisters," "cold sores") who engage in oral sex may infect their partners.

Asymptomatic shedding of HSV also occurs, although this appears to be a transient event, and relatively few virions are shed. About 1% of infected women shed asymptomatically at any time, and one study found that half of women diagnosed by culture as asymptomatic shedders noticed genital lesions *after* being informed of this.[325] Up to 75% of primary HSV genital infections may be subclinical. These and related studies have led to the conclusion that the commonest form of HSV transmission is asymptomatic.

HSV is distributed worldwide. HSV2 antibody is found in 20% to 30% of US adults and in up to 60% of those in lower socioeconomic groups or those with multiple sex partners.[144]

Pathogenesis and Clinical Findings. In first-episode symptomatic herpes, after an incubation period of 7 to 14 days, the patient experiences sensations such as tingling, itching, pain, dysuria, or vaginal discharge, which may occur almost anywhere in the genital area. Up to 4 days later, the symptoms intensify, and then multiple small clear vesicles appear, commonly described as "water blisters." These may occur on the perineum, vulva, vagina, cervix, or penis. The initial episode may be a systemic illness, particularly in patients who have never been exposed to HSV, and the patient may complain of systemic viral illness symptoms, including herpetic pharyngitis. After 24 to 48 hours, the vesicles begin to turn cloudy and change into pustules. The pustules spontaneously rupture, leaving smooth, red ulcers that are 2 to 5 mm in diameter, shallow, flat, very painful, and nonindurated. The ulcers may coalesce, forming larger irregular ulcers. After a few days, the ulcers begin to dry and crust over. First-episode genital herpes may last as long as 2 to 4 weeks, with new ulcers recurrently developing. New lesions are infectious for 7 to 12 days. First-episode herpes is commonly accompanied by bilateral tender inguinal adenopathy, sometimes sufficiently painful that the patient walks with a stooped over, bow-legged gait. A small proportion of individuals have painless ulcers.

HSV remains viable in the dorsal ganglia for the rest of the individual's life. Periodically, particularly within the first several years after the initial infection, HSV becomes active again and genital lesions recur. A large variety of factors are said to precipitate recurrences (eg, sexual intercourse, stress, fever, menstruation, birth control pills, temperature change, sunlight), and these factors vary among individuals. Most occurrences, however, appear to have no identifiable precipitating factor. Recurrences are characterized by being much milder and briefer than the initial episode, sometimes lasting less than 24 hours. In about half the cases, recurrences are signaled by premonitory paresthesias in the genital area, leg, or foot, which begin hours to 2 days before onset. Recurrent lesions are usually infectious for only a few days.

Diagnostic Approaches. Genital herpes is usually diagnosed clinically, particularly when the characteristic vesicles are present. The ulcers are typically clean, shallow, nonindurated, and painful, but descriptions of genital ulcers are at best rules of thumb. Any genital ulcer should include in its differential diagnosis herpes, syphilis, chancroid, and (less likely) lymphogranuloma venereum. A history that the ulcer began as a vesicle or that it has recurred supports a diagnosis of herpes. Herpes viral culture is the gold standard for diagnosis, with 80% to 90% sensitivity and 100% specificity,[261] but it is not readily available. Tzanck preps are made by staining a smear of fluid from the base of the vesicle or ulcer and looking for multinucleated giant cells, the remnants of epithelial cells that have fused together. It is about 60% sensitive. Both culture and Tzanck prep are more likely to be positive the earlier and more characteristic the lesions. HSV serology is generally not reliable. Only a primary episode of herpes can be serologically confirmed, by a 4-fold titer increase in acute and convalescent sera.

Recommendations for Therapy and Control. The role of anti-HSV therapy is largely limited to symptomatic treatment of initial episodes (because these tend to be significantly symptomatic and prolonged) and to control of frequent recurrences (generally defined as more than six recurrences per year). Most recurrences are too mild and transient to benefit from treatment. Acyclovir reduces viral shedding and pain and speeds healing but does not eradicate HSV. There is no evidence acyclovir provides effective prophylaxis against either acquiring or transmitting HSV (Exhibit 38-11).

Herpes produces psychological reactions out of proportion to the minimal pathological changes. Patients may deny the diagnosis, become significantly depressed and angry for long periods, complain of decreased self image and self-worth (being "damaged goods"), and spend considerable time and effort searching for alternative treatments. The health care provider needs to be supportive and should consider referring the patient to a herpes support group.

Patient education is important and needs to emphasize that there should be no sex when lesions are present, that the types and efficacies of treat-

EXHIBIT 38-11

TREATMENT OF GENITAL HERPES

First Clinical Episode of Genital Herpes[*]

Acyclovir 400 mg orally 3 times a day for 7-10 days

OR

Acyclovir 200 mg orally 5 times a day for 7-10 days

OR

Famciclovir 250 mg orally 3 times a day for 7-10 days

OR

Valacyclovir 1 g orally twice a day for 7-10 days

Episodic Recurrent Infection[†]

Acyclovir 400 mg orally 3 times a day for 5 days

OR

Acyclovir 200 mg orally 5 times a day for 5 days

OR

Acyclovir 800 mg orally twice a day for 5 days

OR

Famciclovir 125 mg orally twice a day for 5 days

OR

Valacyclovir 500 mg orally twice a day for 5 days

Daily Suppressive Therapy[‡]

Acyclovir 400 mg orally twice a day

OR

Famciclovir 250 mg orally twice a day

OR

Valacyclovir 500 mg orally once a day

OR

Valacyclovir 1 g orally once a day

Pregnancy. The safety of systemic acyclovir or valacyclovir in pregnant women has not been established. A registry of women who have received acyclovir (or valacyclovir) in pregnancy has been established. Data thus far do not indicate an increased risk for major birth defects after acyclovir treatment. The first clinical episode of genital herpes during pregnancy may be treated with acyclovir. Life-threatening maternal infections (eg, disseminated infection, encephalitis, pneumonitis, hepatitis) should be treated with intravenous acyclovir. Routine administration of acyclovir to pregnant women who have a history of recurrent genital herpes is not recommended at this time. Prenatal exposures to valacyclovir and famciclovir are too limited to provide useful information on pregnancy outcomes.

[*] Treatment may be extended if healing is incomplete after 10 days of therapy.
[†] Patients treated for recurrent herpes should be provided with either medication or a prescription to have on hand at the time of a recurrence. Treatment of recurrent herpes is most effective if started when a prodrome develops or within 1 day of the onset of symptoms.
[‡] Daily suppressive therapy with famciclovir or valacyclovir is not currently recommended for more than 1 year. Although patients have been on acyclovir suppressive therapy for as long as 6 years, annual reevaluation of the need for suppressive therapy should be conducted. Patients may adjust psychologically to the recurrences, and in many patients the frequency of recurrences decreases with time.
Source: Centers for Disease Control and Prevention. 1998 guidelines for treatment of sexually transmitted diseases. *MMWR.* 1998;47(RR-1).

ment are limited, and that infected women are at particular risk of infecting their babies. Genital herpes can infect a neonate during delivery with devastating consequences, so all pregnant women with genital herpes or who have had sex with someone who has genital herpes should be instructed to alert their obstetrician.

Individuals with active genital lesions should refrain from sex during any prodromal symptoms and until the lesions are gone. Condoms offer less protection against acquiring HSV than other STDs because lesions may be in locations not covered by the condom, but their use should be encouraged with new and uninfected partners. Because asymptomatic HSV shedding occurs between ulcerative episodes, partners may become infected even in the absence of overt lesions. Asymptomatic shedding occurs more often with HSV2 infection and within the first 12 months after infection.

Syphilis

Description of the Pathogen. Syphilis is caused by the spirochete *Treponema pallidum.*

Epidemiology. Syphilis is transmitted by direct contact with infectious lesions or fluids, usually during sexual intercourse. It can be transmitted from mother to fetus transplacentally or at delivery. It is found worldwide.

Pathogenesis and Clinical Findings. Syphilis has an incubation period of 10 to 90 days, averaging 21 days. Primary syphilis is a chancre, classically described as a clean, punched out, smooth, red, painless (unless secondarily infected) lesion, which is indurated sufficiently to feel like the cartilage in the tip of the nose. Atypical and multiple lesions are not uncommon. Chancres are typically found in the genital area and around the mouth and rectum but may appear anywhere on the body. The heal spontaneously in 3 to 6 weeks. Chancres are associated with unilateral or bilateral regional adenopathy, which is firm, discrete, moveable, and painless. The presence of any genital ulceration must put syphilis in the differential diagnosis.

Secondary syphilis is a cutaneous, systemic disease, most notable for a characteristic maculopapular rash. It occurs within 6 months of exposure, usually within 6 weeks, and often overlaps the resolving chancre in occurrence. The rash, which occurs in about one third of cases, is painless, nonpruritic, and often generalized. It may involve the mucous membranes (called a mucous patch), tends to follow cleavage lines, especially on the trunk, and has a predilection for the palms and soles. The lesions are discrete, sharply demarcated, and scaly; they are also darkfield positive, although it may require scraping the lesion to exposure serous material to demonstrate this. The eruption may last a few weeks or as long as a year. Up to 25% of untreated cas es may have a relapse of the rash, and 5% may have one to three additional relapses. Alopecia of the eyebrows and scalp occurs.

Secondary syphilis is an often protean disease, which may begin with a flu-like syndrome (eg, malaise, myalgia, headache, sore throat), with mild anemia, elevated white blood cell count and elevated sedimentation rate. There is a generalized adenopathy, with hard, rubbery, painless nodes. Splenomegaly is common, and hepatomegaly is sometimes seen. Latent syphilis is a serologic diagnosis and is divided into *early latent* (infected less than 1 year) and *late latent*.

Central nervous system disease can occur with any stage of syphilis. It may manifest itself as ophthalmologic symptoms (eg, uveitis, neuroretinitis, optic neuritis), auditory abnormalities, cranial nerve palsies, or meningeal signs and symptoms. Such patients should have a cerebral spinal fluid examination (white blood cell, protein, CSF-VDRL (Venereal Disease Research Laboratory) and be treated for neurosyphilis (Exhibit 38-12). The CSF examination should be repeated every 6 months. If the pleocytosis has not decreased after 6 months or the spinal fluid is not normal after 2 years, retreatment should be considered.

Diagnostic Approaches. Primary and secondary syphilis may be diagnosed by darkfield microscopy, using serous exudate from the chancre or condyloma lata lesions. Although sensitive and highly specific for diagnosing early syphilis, this technique is usually only available in large medical centers or dermatology clinics. Darkfield microscopy may be falsely negative if topical antibiotics have been applied to the lesion.

The majority of HIV-infected syphilitics can be diagnosed in the same manner as non-HIV infected cases. Syphilis in HIV-infected individuals may, however, take a florid and greatly accelerated course, further complicated by falsely negative serologic tests. Diagnosis in these cases may depend on Warthin-Starry staining of biopsied lesions.

Serodiagnosis of syphilis is based on two types of tests: the nontreponemal tests (ie, VDRL rapid plasma reagin [RPR]; RPR circle), which are used for screening and quantitative follow-up, and the tests for treponemal antibody. When the chancre first appears, 30% to 50% of cases are nonreactive. Patients should be retested in 1 week and at 1 and 3 months. It is important to realize that only about 60% to 90% of primary syphilis cases may be VDRL positive, with the percentage reaching 100% only when the disease has reached its secondary phase. VDRL seropositivity wanes in later stages, even without treatment.

The nontreponemal tests may be falsely negative due to the "prozone phenomenon," in which very high antibody titers overwhelm the test system. Patients highly suspected of having syphilis, particularly secondary syphilis, who have negative tests should have the test repeated with instructions to the laboratory to dilute the serum. Nontreponemal tests may also be falsely positive. The tests cross react with the organisms of yaws, endemic syphilis (bejel), and pinta. There is no way to distinguish among these entities serologically, so clinical judgment must be used. Biological false positives also occur and are divided into acute and chronic reactions. Acute biological false-positive reactions may be due to a variety of viral agents (eg, hepatitis, mononucleosis, viral pneumonia, chickenpox, measles), malaria, some immunizations, and, notably, pregnancy. Chronic false positives are due to

EXHIBIT 38-12

TREATMENT OF SYPHILIS

Primary and Secondary Syphilis and Early Latent Syphilis

Benzathine penicillin G 2.4 million units IM in a single dose

Late Latent Syphilis and Latent Syphilis of Unknown Duration

Benzathine penicillin G 7.2 million units total dose, administer as 3 doses of 2.4 million units intramuscularly at 1-week intervals

Neurosyphilis*

Aqueous crystalline penicillin G 18-24 million units a day, administered as 3-4 million units intravenously every 4 hours for 10-14 days

OR

Procaine penicillin 2.4 million units intramuscularly a day *plus* Probenecid 500 mg orally 4 times a day, both for 10 to 14 days

Penicillin Allergy. Penicillin-allergic patients with primary, secondary, or early latent syphilis should be treated with doxycyline 100 mg orally twice a day for 2 weeks or tetracycline 500 mg orally 4 times a day for 2 weeks. Patients with late latent or latent syphilis of unknown duration should be treated with doxycycline or tetracycline for 4 weeks. With any of these regimens, close follow-up is essential to ensure patient compliance. Patients with neurosyphilis who are allergic to penicillin should be desensitized to penicillin and treated with one of the penicillin regimens or treated in consultation with an expert.

Pregnancy. Doxycycline and tetracycline are contraindicated in pregnancy. Pregnant women who are allergic to penicillin should be desensitized and treated with penicillin.

Management of Sex Partners. Persons who were exposed within the 90 days preceding the diagnosis of primary, secondary, or early latent syphilis may be infected even if they are seronegative. Such patients should be treated for presumptive primary syphilis. Persons who were exposed more than 90 days before the diagnosis should be treated presumptively for primary syphilis if serologic tests are not available immediately and the opportunity for follow-up is uncertain. For purposes of partner notification and presumptive treatment of exposed persons, patients who have latent syphilis of unknown duration with high nontreponemal titers ($\geq$ 1:32) should be considered as having early syphilis. Long-term sex partners of patients who have late syphilis should be evaluated clinically and serologically for syphilis and treated on the basis of the evaluation findings. The time periods before treatment used for identifying at-risk sex partners are: (*a*) 3 months plus duration of symptoms for primary syphilis, (*b*) 6 months plus duration of symptoms for secondary syphilis, and (*c*) 1 year for early latent syphilis.

Follow-Up. Patients should be examined clinically and serologically at 6 and 12 months after treatment; more frequent follow-up may be prudent if long-term follow-up is uncertain. Patients who have signs or symptoms that persist or recur or who have a sustained 4-fold increase in a nontreponemal test titer probably failed treatment or were reinfected. These patients should be retreated after reevaluation for HIV infection. Unless reinfection is certain, a lumbar puncture should also be performed. Most experts recommend retreatment with 3 weekly injections of benzathine penicillin G 2.4 million units, unless the lumbar puncture demonstrates neurosyphilis is present. Management of patients with a coexisting HIV infection or in whom the nontreponemal titer fails to decline is beyond the scope of this chapter. Patients with latent syphilis should be evaluated with a quantitative nontreponemal serologic test at 6, 12, and 24 months.

Other Considerations. All patients with latent syphilis should be evaluated clinically for evidence of tertiary disease (eg, aortitis, neurosyphilis, gumma, iritis). Patients with syphilis and any of the following findings should have a prompt cerebrospinal fluid examination: (*a*) neurologic or ophthalmic signs or symptoms, (*b*) evidence of active tertiary syphilis, (*c*) treatment failure (titer increases 4-fold; an initially high titer [$\geq$ 1:32] fails to decline at least 4-fold; signs or symptoms attributable to syphilis develop in the patient), or (*d*) HIV infection with latent syphilis or syphilis of unknown duration.

*The procaine penicillin regimen should only be used if compliance can be assured. Some experts also give 2.4 million units IM of benzathine penicillin at the end of either of the neurosyphilis regimens.
Source: Centers for Disease Control and Prevention. 1998 guidelines for treatment of sexually transmitted diseases. *MMWR.* 1998;47(RR-1).

connective tissue diseases (a false-positive VDRL may be the earliest sign of systemic lupus erythematosus), immunoglobulin abnormalities, narcotic addiction, advanced age, malignancy, and leprosy. Biological false-positive titers are usually low. A positive test cannot be assumed to be a false positive simply because a patient has a condition that may cause a false-positive result. This is particularly true for pregnant women, because syphilis may have devastating consequences to the fetus. The serologic diagnosis should be promptly confirmed or ruled out with a confirmatory test. In cases where a confirmatory test is not readily available or the patient is unreliable, it may be necessary to treat the patient as if he or she has syphilis, in order to prevent possible disease progression and transmission to future sex partners.

The treponemal tests measure antibodies to treponema, using *Treponema pallidum* as an antigen. They are far more specific than the screening tests (although not sufficiently specific to distinguish syphilis from other treponemal infections such as yaws) but are also technically more difficult to perform and more costly. For these reasons, the treponemal tests are used to confirm positive results from the screening tests. The two tests used are the fluorescent treponemal antibody absorbed (FTA-ABS) and the microhemagglutination treponemal pallidum (MHA-TP) tests, which yield comparable results. The FTA-ABS is somewhat more sensitive than the VDRL and may be positive a few days earlier. In general, treponemal tests remain positive for life. If treatment is begun sufficiently early, however, the treponemal test will become nonreactive within 2 years in about 10% of cases.

Military field units customarily use only the rapid plasma reagin (RPR) test, often only the qualitative RPR. This can create diagnostic problems because confirmatory testing may not be readily available. This forces the health care provider to use clinical judgment in deciding whether to treat a possible case of syphilis, with accompanying implications for the accuracy of epidemiologic reporting of syphilis cases.

Recommendations for Therapy and Control. Penicillin treatment renders patients noninfectious within 24 to 48 hours. In the absence of treatment, the duration of infectiousness is variable and difficult to predict. Patients are infectious for at least a year after their initial infection and possibly for as long as 4 years. After that time, syphilis is only transmitted congenitally or by blood transfusion or blood contact. Because the VDRL test provides quantitative titers, it can be used to follow the re-

sults of treatment. Titers should be obtained at 3-month intervals for a year. During adequate treatment of primary and secondary syphilis, titers should fall 4-fold by 4 months and 8-fold by 8 months (see Exhibit 38-12).

Human Immunodeficiency Virus Infection and Acquired Immunodeficiency Syndrome

HIV has military implications that make it unique among STDs. US forces deploy to areas, such as Africa and Thailand, where HIV is highly prevalent, particularly among commercial sex workers. It is the only STD for which the US military mandates and routinely carries out screening, followed by an extensive program of support and medical treatment of those found to be infected. HIV-seropositive individuals are restricted from overseas service.

Description of the Pathogen. The human immunodeficiency virus, a retrovirus, has two types: type 1 and type 2. HIV 1 is found worldwide. HIV 2 is largely confined to western Africa.

Epidemiology. HIV infection is transmitted by sexual exposure or exposure to infected blood and is found worldwide. The combination of STDs and HIV infection has created what Wasserheit aptly termed "epidemiologic synergy,"[326] in which the interaction of these diseases promotes and enhances the spread of all of them. Diseases that cause genital ulcers increase the likelihood of acquiring HIV by providing entry portals.[327–329] Nonulcerative diseases produce inflammatory changes that may also offer opportunities for HIV acquisition.[328–331] Transmission of HIV in the opposite direction may also be enhanced because ulcers and inflammation may provide greater opportunities for virus shedding.

Studies of US Army personnel who seroconverted for HIV found these risk factors: increasing numbers of female sex partners, nonsteady partners, having sex on the first day of acquaintance, sex with prostitutes, and sex with partners who had multiple partners.[260,332] The risk perhaps was epitomized by the finding that those who had sex on first encounter with 3 or more partners had an odds ratio of 6.9 for HIV infection.

HIV infection rates are an exception among STDs in the US military in that mandatory testing, combined with a reliable laboratory test, has produced accurate incidence and prevalence information. Testing of applicants for military service between 1985 and 1989 revealed a seropositivity rate of 0.34 per 1,000 but with a marked geographic variation.[289,333] Rates were greater than 2 per 1,000 in urban areas of Maryland, New York, Texas, and the

District of Columbia. Initial testing of 1,752,191 active duty personnel who remained on active duty as of April 1988 revealed an overall HIV seroprevalence of 1.3 per 1,000. Blacks were 3.6 times and Hispanics 2.5 times as likely as non-Hispanic whites to be seropositive for HIV-1.[334] Prevalence was highest among those who were male, unmarried, and of enlisted rank. Incidence rates (per 1,000 person-years) have been less than 1. The Air Force incidence rate declined from 0.19 to 0.17 between 1987 and 1990.[254] Army rates fell from 0.77 (1985-1987) to stabilize at about 0.22 after 1988.[255,335] Navy and Marine Corps incidence rates for 1986 to 1988 were 0.69 and 0.28 respectively.[256] The Navy incidence fell from 0.55 in 1990 to 0.26 in 1995, while the Marine Corps rate fell from 0.28 to 0.11 during the same period.[336] Navy HIV infections were not associated with visits to foreign ports.[337] Rates among Army reserve personnel were comparable to those in active duty personnel.[338] The frequency of HIV testing for military personnel ranges from 1 to 3 years or more, depending on the individual service policy, the deployability of the unit, whether the unit is reserve or active duty, and other considerations such as the incidence rate. In general, rapidly deployable units are tested more frequently.

Pathogenesis and Clinical Findings. A discussion of AIDS and related management issues is beyond the scope of this book. The initial HIV infection may be asymptomatic, but an unknown proportion of individuals have an infectious mononucleosis–like illness a few weeks after the infection. This illness, particularly characterized by adenopathy, resolves quickly and is followed by seroconversion. Individuals seroconvert 6 to 12 weeks after infection, although some may require as long as 6 months. Infectivity begins about 2 weeks before seroconversion, creating a seronegative window of infectiousness. Individuals are infectious for life, although infectivity seems to be increased in the first few months of infection and in the terminal stages, when the viral burden is the greatest. Progression to deteriorating immune function, opportunistic infections, and frank AIDS requires 10 years on average but may occur as rapidly as in 1 year.

Diagnostic Approaches. Simple enzyme immunoassays (EIAs), suitable for field use, are available for diagnosing HIV. They have a relatively high rate of false-positive results and therefore require confirmation with the Western blot or another confirmatory test, which are not available in the field. Using EIAs in the field has limited practical use in the absence of a confirmatory test result. Unlike a positive RPR, which may indicate an infection that can be easily treated, there is no treatment for a putatively HIV-infected individual except counseling to avoid sexual exposure and to counteract the considerable trauma of being told he or she might have HIV infection.

Recommendations for Therapy and Control. HIV serotesting of applicants for military service began in fall 1985, with testing of active duty personnel commencing in January 1986. An organized program was implemented to obtain surveillance data on HIV infection among military personnel and in areas where they might deploy, to conduct behavioral research that might lead to reducing risky sexual behavior, and to develop HIV field tests, vaccines, and antiretroviral drugs.[339–341]

Notification of a service member that he or she is HIV positive takes place in various ways and locations, but certain common themes emerge. The matter is treated as confidential, with only the senior medical representative, the commanding officer, and a few other individuals being informed of the member's status (eg, the chaplain, the command's senior enlisted person). The reaction varies. A few members are not surprised, and some of these already know they are HIV positive from testing done outside the service. A few break down emotionally and begin crying. The majority act stunned, sometimes dramatically so. Denial is not unusual. A medical representative explains the implications of the HIV test results to the member and provides information as to what will happen next. It may be necessary to repeat this information at a later time, because the service member may not comprehend what is being said the first time. An individual may have many questions about the meaning of a positive HIV test and about AIDS. The basic information can be kept simple (Exhibit 38-13).

All services evaluate newly identified HIV-seropositive individuals at central locations. It is desirable to remove the servicemember as quickly as possible (eg, within 2 to 3 days) in case confidentiality is violated and to provide a supportive environment as quickly as possible. Suicide may be a concern. Seropositive individuals should be evaluated to determine whether suicide precautions are necessary, which may include escorting the individual to the evaluation center. Such precautions are rarely necessary, however, and are understandably resented by individuals who do not want the suicidal stigma added to the burden of being newly diagnosed as HIV-infected.

It is not necessary for field or shipboard medial units to query the HIV-infected individual as to how he or she may have been infected or by whom. This

---

EXHIBIT 38-13

WHAT TO TELL THE PATIENT ABOUT A POSITIVE HUMAN IMMUNODEFICIENCY VIRUS TEST

---

1. A positive test means you are infected with HIV, the virus that causes AIDS. You will be infected with this virus for the rest of your life.

2. You do not necessarily have AIDS now. If you had a negative test in the last few years, you probably will not develop AIDS for several years.

3. Current anti-HIV drugs are usually able to control the virus and delay the onset of AIDS for many years. They may be able to prevent you from ever getting AIDS.

4. Because you will have HIV in your body for the rest of your life, you can infect other people with this virus for the rest of your life. You can infect them by having sex with them, sharing needles with them when using drugs, donating blood, or breastfeeding your baby. What you can do about this will be explained in detail later. For now, you must not have sex with anyone or donate blood.

5. The test cannot tell us how you became infected.

6. The test cannot tell us when you became infected, except that it probably happened sometime between your last negative test and this test.

---

epidemiologic information will be obtained when the individual is evaluated to determine the extent and nature of his or her infection. The evaluation program will also assist the service member in notifying his or her sexual contacts. The evaluation programs vary but generally last 1 to 2 weeks and thoroughly evaluate the service member's health, determine the stage of HIV disease, and, if appropriate, begin anti-HIV medications. Psychological, sociological, and spiritual support is also provided for the individual and family. Detailed education and counseling is provided so the individual thoroughly understands HIV infection and AIDS, the probable course of the illness, and options regarding his or her career and other matters.

Genital Warts

Description of the Pathogen. Human papilloma virus (HPV) is the etiologic agent of genital warts (condyloma accuminata). There are over 30 strains of HPV, some of which are highly associated with cervical and other cancers.

Epidemiology. Genital warts, found worldwide, are transmitted by sexual contact. They are infectious, probably because trauma associated with sex releases virions, which are then rubbed into epithelial surfaces. By eliminating overt lesions, treatment probably reduces HPV infectiousness. However, because HPV virions are commonly present in normal skin, HPV-infected persons may infect others even in the absence of overt warts. Condoms may reduce the transmission of HPV but will not entirely prevent it. Because of the association with cervical cancer, women who have had genital warts or whose partners have had genital warts should have regular Pap smears.

Diagnostic Approaches. Diagnosis is by clinical appearance, but only a minority of infections present as overt lesions. Small lesions may require magnification to be seen.

Recommendations for Therapy and Control. Treatment removes visible, symptomatic warts but does not eradicate HPV or affect the development of cervical cancer. Removal may not decrease infectivity. Untreated, visible genital warts may resolve, remain unchanged, or increase in size and number. The numerous treatment regimens for genital warts may be divided into patient-applied (eg, podofilox 0.5% solution or gel, imiquimod 5% cream) or provider-administered (eg, cryotherapy, podophyllin resin 10%-25%, trichloracetic or bichloroacetic acid 80%-90%, surgical removal) treatments. The 1998 CDC treatment guidelines[266] should be consulted for the detailed instructions necessary to administer these treatments. The safety of podofilox, imiquimod, and podophyllin during pregnancy has not been established.

Lymphogranuloma Venereum

Description of the Pathogen. Lymphogranuloma venereum (LGV) is caused by the L1, L2, and L3 serotypes of *C trachomatis*.

Epidemiology. LGV is transmitted through direct contact with open lesions, usually during sexual intercourse. It is found worldwide and is endemic in Asia and Africa. It is more commonly diagnosed in men but that may be due to the large number of asymptomatic infections in women. In temperate climates, most cases are found in male homosexuals.[144]

Pathogenesis and Clinical Findings. The incubation period can be long and is divided into two phases. The initial period is 7 to 12 days and produces a transient papule, vesicle, or ulcer. This is painless and in 60% to 90% of the cases is never noticed. The characteristic inguinal adenitis appears from 5 to 50 days later and in two thirds of the cases is unilateral. It is firm, hard, tender, and fixed to the skin. The "groove sign" or "shelf sign," a linear depression in the adenopathy due to Poupart's ligament running between the nodes, is a helpful diagnostic sign. Systemic manifestations include chills, fever, malaise, nausea, weight loss, headache, and arthralgias. If untreated, the adenitis enlarges, becomes fluctuant, and forms multiple tracts though the skin, which may drain for months. Adenitis is seen more commonly in men than in women, by a ratio of approximately five to one. Women usually have a cervical infection, which may persist for months. Persistent urethritis, proctocolitis, and chronic ulcerations may also occur.

Diagnostic Approaches. The diagnosis of LGV is usually clinical; the presence of purple erythematous skin discoloration over the adenopathy and the development of fluctuance are helpful diagnostic signs. Serological tests for LGV are not reliable and generally should not be used. The complement fixation can be considered positive if there is a 4-fold rise in titer or a single titer of 1:64 or greater. Adenopathy and adenitis are seen in both chancroid and LGV, but chancroid is distinguished by the coexistence of an ulcer. In LGV, the ulcer occurs before the adenopathy.

Recommendations for Therapy and Control. Untreated patients may remain infectious for months; all active lesions should be considered infectious (Exhibit 38-14).

Chancroid

Description of the Pathogen. Chancroid ("soft chancre," to distinguish it from the indurated chancre of syphilis) is a genital ulcerative disease caused by *Haemophilus ducreyi*, a short, fine, Gram-negative streptobacillus. It attacks only the skin, not the mucous membranes.

Epidemiology. Chancroid is spread by contact with discharges from open lesions, usually during sexual contact. It is most prevalent in tropical and subtropical areas. It is less common in temperate zones. In tropical and subtropical areas, the incidence of chancroid may be higher than syphilis and approach the incidence of gonorrhea.[144] Women are often asymptomatic carriers, and men are much more likely to be symptomatic. Chancroid often occurs in local epidemics.

Pathogenesis and Clinical Findings. Chancroid is notable for a remarkably short incubation period,

12 hours to 3 days; 5 days is the maximum. It begins as a small macule, which quickly progresses to a pustule and then to an ulcer. The ulcer is painful, tender, soft, and rapidly growing. It is irregular, ragged, and dirty and has undermined edges and a yellow-gray membrane. When skin surfaces are opposed (eg, under the foreskin), a "kissing ulcer" develops, but this is not unique to chancroid. Over 50% of patients develop inguinal adenopathy within a week. It is usually unilateral, fixed, matted, and tender. Untreated, the inguinal nodes often evolve into a bubo, which suppurates through the skin. Constitutional symptoms are mild or absent. Patients are infectious for as long as the original ulcer is present or lymph node sinus tracts are draining, which may be months.

Diagnostic Approaches. The diagnosis is usually clinical, and, as with all genital ulcers, syphilis and HSV infection must be included in the differential diagnosis. A Gram stain of a swab from the lesion may reveal the "school of fish" appearance (curved, parallel lines of bacteria adhering to mucous strands) said to be characteristic of chancroid. Usually, however, the smear simply reveals a wide variety

---

EXHIBIT 38-14

TREATMENT OF LYMPHOGRANULOMA VENEREUM

Recommended

Doxycycline 100 mg orally twice a day for 21 days

Alternate Regimen

Erythromycin base 500 mg orally 4 times a day for 21 days

Pregnancy. Pregnant women should be treated with erythromycin.

Follow-Up. Patients should be followed clinically until signs and symptoms have resolved.

Management of Sex Partners. Sex partners of patients who have LGV should be examined, tested for urethral or cervical chlamydia infection, and treated for LGV if they had sexual contact with the patient during the 30 days preceding the onset of symptoms in the patient.

Source: Centers for Disease Control and Prevention. 1998 guidelines for treatment of sexually transmitted diseases. *MMWR.* 1998;47(RR-1).

EXHIBIT 38-15

TREATMENT OF CHANCROID

Azithromycin 1 g orally in a single dose

OR

Ceftriaxone 250 mg intramuscularly in a single dose

OR

Ciprofloxacin 500 mg orally twice a day for 3 days

OR

Erythromycin base 500 mg orally 4 times a day for 7 days

Pregnancy. Ciprofloxacin is contraindicated for pregnant and lactating women and for persons less than 18 years old. Preliminary data indicate azythromycin may be safe in pregnancy, but data are insufficient to recommend its use in pregnancy.

Follow-up. Patients should be reexamined 3 to 7 days after initiation of therapy. If treatment is successful, ulcers improve symptomatically within 3 days and objectively within 7 days after therapy. Large ulcers may require more than 2 weeks to heal; in uncircumcised men ulcers under the foreskin are slower to heal. Clinical resolution of fluctuant lymphadenopathy is slower than that of ulcers and may require drainage even if the ulcers are resolving. Needle aspiration of buboes is a simpler procedure, but incision and drainage may be preferred over multiple needle aspirations.
If no clinical improvement is evident within 3 to 7 days, the clinician should consider: (*a*) Was the diagnosis of chancroid correct? (*b*) Is the patient coinfected with another sexually transmitted disease? (*c*) Is the patient coinfected with HIV? and (*d*) Is the ulcer due to a strain of *Haemophilus ducreyi* that is resistant to the antibiotic used for treatment?

Sex Partners. Sex partners who have had intercourse with the patient during the 10 days preceding the onset of the patient's symptoms should be treated with a regimen active against chancroid even if the partner has no symptoms.

Source: Centers for Disease Control and Prevention. 1998 guidelines for treatment of sexually transmitted diseases. *MMWR.* 1998;47(RR-1).

---

of organisms in no particular pattern and is considered nondiagnostic. The organism can be cultured, but this requires a well-equipped microbiology laboratory and a highly experienced microbiologist. Consultation with the microbiologist before collecting the specimen is advisable.

Recommendations for Therapy and Control. Treatment renders the patient noninfectious in 1 to 2 weeks (Exhibit 38-15).

[S. William Berg, MD, MPH]

VIRAL HEPATITIS

Introduction and Military Relevance

Jaundice has been identified since antiquity as a problem of armies in the field and in garrison. An epidemic in 1629 in military forces in Spa, Germany, during the Thirty Years' War underscores the longstanding threat of viral hepatitis to military operations. More than 72,000 cases occurred during the American Civil War.[342] From January 1943 through March 1945, there were more than 35,000 cases of infectious hepatitis among US personnel in the Mediterranean Theater of Operations, a loss equivalent to over 2 infantry divisions.[343] During the wars in Korea and Vietnam, viral hepatitis remained a significant problem for military physicians.[344]

During World War II, two types of hepatitis were clearly recognized: (1) infectious, characterized by a short incubation period and a benign outcome, and (2) serum, characterized by a longer incubation period with longer morbidity and occasional chronic disease. These were subsequently renamed hepatitis A and hepatitis B. Ironically, recognition of hepatitis B was linked to reuse of unsterilized needles in arsenical therapy of syphilis[345] and the use during World War II of yellow fever vaccine that was stabilized with infectious human serum.[346–349] Figure 38-7 shows the incidence of jaundice cases during and immediately after World War II in the US Army.

Control of hepatitis A has been a major concern for US military forces in war and peace. Advances in sanitation, along with the discovery that immune globulin (IG) provided protection against hepatitis A[350,351] have, however, reduced the military threat of this disease in recent US military operations. The efficacy of IG was first demonstrated in an outbreak of epidemic hepatitis, which we now assume was hepatitis A, in a summer camp in 1944[350] and was confirmed in studies among US soldiers in World War II and more recently.[352–354] A large, controlled trial by the US Army during the Vietnam War determined that 5 mL of IG was as effective as 10 mL in preventing viral hepatitis.[355]

IG, though effective, is cumbersome to use. The prevalence of hepatitis A antibody has been decreasing in the general US population and hence also in the military population, putting these people at risk for hepatitis A both during and between deployments. The US Army has been very active in the development of a vaccine for hepatitis A. The first

successful cell-culture-derived, formalin-inactivated hepatitis A vaccine was developed at the Walter Reed Army Institute of Research.[356] This prototype was shown to be safe and immunogenic for humans in 1986.

Advances in trauma surgery, including increased use of blood transfusions, have led to an increasing awareness of the importance of hepatitis B and C to military medical personnel. The threat of transfusion-related hepatitis B and C for military personnel has been significantly reduced by the application of advances in basic virology, diagnostic testing, immunization, and screening of blood donors.[357] As in other segments of US society, the threat of sexually transmitted hepatitis will remain a problem for the foreseeable future.[348,358,359]

Description of the Pathogens

Table 38-6 outlines some of the characteristics of the hepatidities. Hepatitis A virus (HAV) is a member of the family *Picornaviridae* and is related to the enteroviruses and the rhinoviruses.[360] It is a nonenveloped, spherical virus 26 to 28 nm in diameter with single-stranded RNA of positive polarity. Unlike other picornaviruses, it is relatively resistant to heat, which accounts for its ease of transmission in partially cooked food.[361]

Hepatitis B virus (HBV) is an enveloped, double-stranded DNA virus of the *Hepadnaviridae* family; related viruses cause hepatitis in woodchucks and ducks.[362] The outer coat, hepatitis B surface antigen (HBsAg), is associated with intact virions (Dane particles) and other particles. The excess of antigen typically present in the blood during chronic infection is useful in diagnostic testing. It also supplies material for plasma-derived vaccines, which are no longer used in the US but are still used in other areas of the world.

Hepatitis C virus (HCV) is related to the flaviviruses, which cause dengue, yellow fever, Japanese encephalitis, but it is closer to the pestiviruses (flaviviruses of animals).[363] It is a spherical, lipid-enveloped particle ranging in size from 35 to 50 nm. The genome consists of a single-stranded RNA of positive polarity, 9.4 kilobases in size.

Hepatitis D virus (HDV) consists of a circular, single-stranded RNA molecule associated with delta antigen; this is surrounded by HBsAg. In the absence of hepatitis B infection, HDV cannot replicate. For this reason, HDV is considered a defective virus.[364]

Hepatitis E virus (HEV) is a small, round, nonenveloped virus, with properties similar to

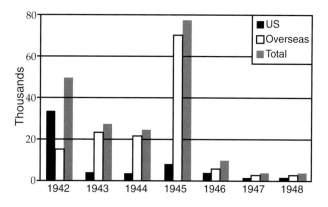

Fig. 38-7. The large number of cases of hepatitis in 1942 in the continental United Stated appears to be related to hepatitis B spread by specific lots of yellow fever vaccine containing infectious human sera, while the later rise in cases overseas primarily reflects hepatitis A contracted by US Army personnel in the European Theater of Operations.
Source: Havens WP Jr. The military importance of viral hepatitis. *U.S. Armed Forces Med J.* 1952;3:1013–1022.

TABLE 38-6

CHARACTERISTICS OF HEPATITIS VIRUSES

	Virus	Type	Distribution	Transmission	Special Characteristics
A	Picornavirus	RNA	Global	Enteric	Relatively heat resistant, vaccine preventable
B	Hepadnavirus	DNA	Global; highly endemic in Asia, Africa, Latin America	Parenteral, sexual, vertical	Chronic infection, carcinogenic, vaccine preventable
C	Flavivirus	RNA	Global	Parenteral, sexual, vertical	Chronic infection, cirrhosis, carcinogenic
D	—	RNA	Global; prevalence varies widely (highest reported prevalence: southern Italy, Africa, South America)	Parenteral	Defective virus (requires active HBV infection to replicate), unique delta antigen, vaccine preventable (HBV)
E	Calicivirus	RNA	Asia, Africa, Mexico	Enteric	Often via contaminated water, women in 3rd trimester of pregnancy especially susceptible to fulminant hepatitis
F	?	?	?	Enteric?, parenteral	Some cases may represent "silent" HBV infection by mutant HBV
G	Flavivirus	RNA	Global?	Parenteral	Post-transfusion hepatitis

those of the family *Caliciviridae.* Its genome is a single-stranded, positive-sense RNA of approximately 7.5 kilobases.[365] It infects swine, and this may play a role in the ecology of the virus.[366,367]

A candidate hepatitis F virus has been isolated from human stool and appears to be transmissible to primates.[368] Uchida and colleagues[369] believe that some cases of hepatitis F are caused by mutant hepatitis B variants with suppressed replication and HBV DNA expression.

Hepatitis G virus (HGV) is a small RNA virus, related to other flaviviruses and distantly to HCV. It is transfusion-transmissible and has a global distribution.[370] Currently there is substantial doubt regarding the role HGV plays in the pathogenesis of hepatitis. Studies[371,372] of community-acquired hepatitis and transfusion-acquired hepatitis cast doubt on the relation of HGV to disease.

Hepatitis F and G have been included here for completeness, but because they are not major causes of disease, they will not be discussed further.

Epidemiology

Hepatitis A and E (Fecal-Oral Transmission)

Hepatitis A and E are spread through fecal-oral contact. While transmission via blood contact has been described, it appears to be unusual.[373,374] Common-source foodborne and waterborne epidemics, including those caused by shellfish contaminated with human sewage, are well described. Poor hygiene and intimate contact (sexual or nonsexual) account for the spread of hepatitis A in daycare centers, among homosexuals, and in families. Spread occurs readily in households and daycare centers, although recent data suggest that, in the daycare setting, occupational exposure is uncommon under non-outbreak circumstances.[375] The risk of spread in a daycare center increases with the number of children enrolled who are younger than 2 to 3 years of age and who wear diapers. Most commonly, the adult daycare workers are symptomatic (icteric) with their disease whereas daycare attendees are frequently asymptomatic and have nonspecific disease manifestations; spread of hepatitis A frequently occurs in the daycare center before the index case is recognized. Because daycare in a military community is commonly provided by a central facility, an outbreak among young children may provoke rapid spread of hepatitis A to an active duty population.[376]

HAV is found worldwide (Table 38-7), but areas of high endemicity include Africa, Asia excepting Japan, the Mediterranean region, Eastern Europe, the Middle East, Central and South America, Mexico, and parts of the Caribbean region.

Several patterns of infection are described.[360] In developing countries with poor sanitation, infection is almost universal among children, so adults are immune; in such situations, nonimmune people

TABLE 38-7

HEPATITIS SEROPREVALENCE STUDIES IN SELECTED COUNTRIES

Country	Population Studied	HAV	HBV	HCV	Reference
Cambodia	Adults	100%	73%	6.5%	Thuring[a]
Singapore	Adults	27%	—	—	Yap[b]
Pakistan	Children	55.8%	2.97%	0.44%	Agboatwalla[c]
South Africa	White adults	50%	—	—	Sathar[d]
South Africa	Black adults	91%	—	—	Sathar[d]
Egypt	Adults	100%	66%	51%	Darwish[e]
Nicaragua	Adults	94.6%	6.5%	0%	Perez[f]
USA	Native Americans	76.2%	—	—	Shaw[g]

a. Thuring EG, Joller-Jemelka HI, Sareth H, Sokhan U, Reth C, Grob P. Prevalence of markers of hepatitis viruses A, B, C, and of HIV in healthy individuals and patients of a Cambodian province. *Southeast Asian J Trop Med Public Health*. 1993;24:239–249.
b. Yap I, Guan R. Hepatitis A sero-epidemiology in Singapore: A changing pattern. *Trans R Soc Trop Med Hyg*. 1993;87:22–23.
c. Agboatwalla M, Isomura S, Miyake K, Yamashita T, Morishita T, Akram DS. Hepatitis A, B, and C seroprevalence in Pakistan. *Indian J Pediatr*. 1994;61:545–549.
d. Sathar MA, Soni PN, Fernandes-Costa FJ, Wittenberg DF, Simjee AE. Racial differences in the seroprevalence of hepatitis A virus infection in Natal/KwaZulu, South Africa. *J Med Virol*. 1994;44:9–12.
e. Darwish MA, Faris R, Clemens JD, Rao MR, Edelman R. High seroprevalence of hepatitis A, B, C, and E viruses in residents in an Egyptian village in the Nile Delta: A pilot study. *Am J Trop Med Hyg*. 1996;54:554–558.
f. Perez OM, Morales W, Paniagua M, Strannegard O. Prevalence of antibodies to hepatitis A, B, C, and E viruses in a healthy population in Leon, Nicaragua. *Am J Trop Med Hyg*. 1996;55:17–21.
g. Shaw FE Jr, Shapiro CN, Welty TK, Dill W, Reddington J, Hadler SC. Hepatitis transmission among the Sioux Indians of South Dakota. *Am J Public Health*. 1990;80:1091–1094.

entering the community, such as military personnel, are at risk. In developed countries, fewer children are infected, and this leaves a larger pool of susceptible adults. In this setting, disease commonly occurs during breaks in either personal or communal sanitation. Epidemics may also occur in closed populations, with rapid spread and high prevalence. In addition to these age patterns, seasonal patterns have been described, with peaks in autumn or early winter in temperate climates.[377] Finally, several large groups are at higher risk for infection with HAV: workers in settings where high standards of sanitation are not met (eg, institutions for the mentally retarded, daycare centers), homosexual men, intravenous drug users, and travelers to areas with high incidence of HAV infection.

Contaminated drinking water appears to be the most prominent route of spread of hepatitis E.[378,379] Hepatitis E has a more geographically limited range than hepatitis A; originally described in India, it has been found throughout mainland Asia, Africa, and Latin America. Cases have also been reported from Italy and Spain. Of interest is the susceptibility of adults to HEV in countries with widespread childhood infection with HAV; since the mechanisms of spread are similar, it is unclear why this situation exists.[380]

Hepatitis B, C, and D (Body Fluid Transmission)

That hepatitis could be spread by intimate contact with blood or body fluids was noted in 1833, when an epidemic of jaundice occurred in Bremen among shipyard workers vaccinated against smallpox with human serum.[381] Discoveries by Blumberg in the 1960s led to the characterization of HBV as the predominant cause of bloodborne hepatitis.[382]

Hepatitis B is transmitted through blood or body fluids (eg, wound exudates, semen, cervical secretions, saliva). High levels of viremia correlate with infectivity of small inocula of blood.[383] Contracting hepatitis B through transfusion of blood or blood products, once a common mode of transmission, is now rare in the United States because of marked improvements in screening blood and blood products; the risk of HBV infection from a donor whose unit passes all screening tests is now estimated to be 1 in 63,000 (95% confidence interval, 31,000-147,000).[357] Other more common modes of transmission include sharing or reusing unsterile needles or syringes, percutaneous or mucous membrane exposure to blood or body fluids, and sexual activity. Hepatitis B infection among unvaccinated health care employees with the highest exposure to blood occurs at a rate of 1.05/100 person-years.[384] HBV is also spread efficiently by sexual contact; this is the most important source of hepatitis infection among the US military today.[358] HBV is readily transmitted vertically from mother to baby, although efforts to minimize this mode of transmission in the United States by vaccination of newborns have significantly reduced the numbers of infants infected. Hepatitis B virus can survive in the dried state for prolonged periods of time, and percutaneous contact with contaminated inanimate objects may transmit infection. Hepatitis B is not transmitted by the fecal-oral route and is found worldwide.

Unlike HAV, HBV produces chronic infections in a subset of patients. The burden of chronic disease is higher in areas where HBV infections are acquired earlier in life; a recent study[385] in China showed an overall HBV infection rate of 42.6%, with 10.3% testing positive for HBsAg. The highest risk of chronic infection occurs among infected neonates born to HBeAg-positive carrier mothers (80%-90%); of children infected before 6 years of age, chronic infection develops in about 30%. Healthy adults who become infected have a lower risk of chronic infection (< 5%); being male or having impaired immunity increases this risk.[386] Of interest, follow-up of the cohort infected by HBV-contaminated yellow fever vaccine during World War II showed a far smaller percentage of long-term carriage (0.26%).[347]

Hepatitis C

Hepatitis C is most commonly transmitted through direct contact with infected blood. In the United States, risk of transfusing blood infected with HCV has fallen to between 1 in 28,000 and 1 in 288,000 (mean: 1 in 103,000). HCV remains a significant problem among intravenous drug users. Sexual transmission of HCV appears to occur but at a much lower frequency than HBV. Sexual transmission appears likelier with longer duration of exposure to an infected partner[387] and coinfection with human immunodeficiency virus (HIV).[388] Vertical transmission also appears to occur uncommonly; the risk of transmission is proportional to the titer of HCV RNA in the mother.[389] Some health care workers are also at high risk for hepatitis C. Frequently, though, no source or risk factor can be identified. Seventy

to ninety percent of parenterally transmitted non-A, non-B hepatitis is thought to be caused by the hepatitis C virus. Hepatitis C is distributed worldwide.

Pathogenesis and Clinical Findings

Viral hepatitis spans a wide clinical spectrum, from totally asymptomatic infection (detectable by specific serologic markers) to acute fulminant hepatitis with liver failure and death. In addition, certain agents (ie, HBV, HCV, HDV) produce chronic hepatitis, with a wide variation in outcomes (from asymptomatic to chronic hepatitis, cirrhosis, and hepatocellular carcinoma). The viruses will be considered separately.

Hepatitis A

The clinical presentation of hepatitis A ranges from asymptomatic infection to fulminant hepatitis. The majority of cases are either asymptomatic or mild; there is a higher risk for more significant symptomatology in adults.[390]

In adults, the clinical syndrome of acute hepatitis A presents 15 to 50 days after infection, with a mean of 30 days.[391,392] The abrupt onset of nausea, vomiting, fever (generally low grade), and vague abdominal discomfort marks the prodromal phase. Loss of taste for food and tobacco is common.[393] Within 2 to 7 days, jaundice and dark urine occur. Serum alanine and aspartate transaminase levels rise quickly during the prodromal period, peak around the onset of jaundice, and then fall rapidly (75% per week). Serum bilirubin peaks later and falls more slowly, but in 85% of cases the period of jaundice lasts less than 2 weeks. Complete clinical recovery by 6 months is the rule.[394] Fecal viral shedding begins late in the incubation phase but before the onset of symptoms. Typically, viral shedding ceases shortly after the onset of icterus and with onset of detectable IgM serum antibody.

Occasional patients will present with a clinical picture similar to acute bacteremia, with a high fever, myalgias, shaking chills, and prostration. Prolonged cholestasis may occur.[395] Such patients have prolonged hyperbilirubinemia and a prolonged clinical course of up to 12 weeks with pruritis, fever, diarrhea, and weight loss. Cholestasis will resolve spontaneously; corticosteroids may hasten its resolution but are likely to lead to a relapse. Relapsing hepatitis occurs in 3% to 20% of adult patients with hepatitis A.[396] Relapse typically occurs 4 to 5 weeks after the acute illness and is accompanied by viral excretion in the stool.[397] The illness may last up to 40 weeks, although typically the duration is much shorter. IgM antibody to HAV persists throughout the relapse.

Fulminant hepatitis A is relatively rare, with an incidence of 1 to 8 per 1,000 clinical cases. It is more common in older adults and is characterized by rapidly deepening jaundice, hepatic encephalopathy, coma, and falling transaminase levels.[398] The fatality rate exceeds 50%.

Extrahepatic manifestations of HAV infection are rare and include evanescent rashes, transient arthralgias, arthritis, cutaneous vasculitis, and pancreatitis.

Hepatitis B

Acute hepatitis B infection in adults has a longer incubation period (40 to 180 days, average of 90 days) than hepatitis A.[399] The prodromal period may be longer also (up to 3 weeks). Hepatitis B is thought to be more severe than hepatitis A; however, this may be artifactual and based on the more common occurrence of acute hepatitis B in older individuals. During the prodrome of hepatitis B, immunologically related events such as urticaria and arthritis occur.[400]

Long-term consequences of HBV infection include chronic hepatitis, cirrhosis, and hepatocellular carcinoma. Distinguishing between chronic HBsAg carriage and chronic hepatitis relies on demonstration of necroinflammatory changes on liver biopsy. Progression to cirrhosis is more common with active chronic hepatitis but may occur even in the presence of milder histologic abnormalities.[401] Progression to hepatocellular carcinoma was described early in the understanding of HBV infection.[402] The role of HBV in the etiology of hepatocellular carcinoma is now well established. The cohort of servicemen infected with HBV from the contaminated yellow fever vaccine administered in 1942 demonstrated a small excess rate of hepatocellular cancer when compared with controls.[346]

Hepatitis C

Acute HCV infection is more indolent than the other viral hepatitides. Approximately 25% of patients are icteric, and the mortality of acute HCV infection is low (< 1%).[403] HCV infection is a rare cause of fulminant hepatitis.[404] The propensity to develop chronic HCV infection is remarkable. Whereas 2% to 5% of adult patients with HBV develop chronic infection, greater than 50% of HCV infections become chronic. Chronic infection is more likely in males, in older patients, and with larger viral

doses.[405] Chronic HCV infection is typically indolent, but despite little if any clinical symptomatology, it produces chronic hepatitis, fibrosis, and cirrhosis in many patients. Up to 25% of those infected develop cirrhosis.[406] Chronic HCV infection is also a major risk factor for developing hepatocellular carcinoma.[407]

As with HBV, HCV infection has been associated with a variety of extrahepatic manifestations. The links between HCV infection and essential mixed cryoglobulinemia,[408] membranoproliferative glomerulonephritis,[409] and porphyria cutanea tarda are strong, and it is suggested that patients with those diagnoses be screened for HCV.[410] Possible associations with other autoimmune diseases, such as Mooren corneal ulcers and autoimmune thyroiditis, also exist.

Hepatitis D

Because it cannot reproduce in the absence of active hepatitis B infection, the clinical manifestations of hepatitis D must be discussed in light of that viral infection. Acute hepatitis D infection occurs either as a coinfection with acute HBV infection or as a superinfection in a patient with chronic HBV infection;[411] the latter is more common. In cases of coinfection with HBV, the likelihood of chronic HDV infection is low (< 5%); when superinfection occurs, the risk of chronic HDV infection is 70% or more because of persistent HBsAg.[412]

Acute HDV hepatitis is clinically severe, with a mortality rate ranging from 2% to 20%.[413] The acute infection is likely to have a biphasic course and to be prolonged over months. Chronic HDV infection appears to result in a higher incidence of cirrhosis than either chronic HBV or HCV infection alone, with the majority of such patients dying of chronic liver disease. The progression to cirrhosis may be quite rapid, occurring as quickly as 2 years after infection.[414]

Hepatitis E

Clinically, HEV shares many characteristics of HAV, the other recognized enteric hepatitis virus. HEV infection has caused both epidemics and sporadic cases of acute hepatitis in developing countries.[415] Cholestasis is more pronounced than in typical HAV infection, with higher levels of serum bilirubin and alkaline phosphatase but lower levels of serum transaminases.[416] Prolonged jaundice may occur, but the disease is self-limited and does not lead to chronic hepatitis or to a carrier state. Recent studies[417] have documented that prolonged viremia and fecal shedding occur in 15% of HEV infections. This may facilitate transmission.

In the developing world, outbreaks of HEV are most commonly caused by ingestion of fecally contaminated drinking water. In contrast to hepatitis A, young adults are more frequently affected, with higher attack rates for pregnant women. The case fatality rate may be particularly high (15% to 20%) for women in the third trimester of pregnancy.[418] Vertical transmission may be seen, with significant perinatal morbidity and mortality. It is unclear how frequently this occurs.[419]

Diagnostic Approaches

In the Field

The serologic diagnosis of hepatitis A, B, C, D, and E may be made in a regional medical center, a field hospital, a regional research facility, or a forward reference laboratory worldwide.[359,420–422] Most frequently, samples are collected in the field

and transported to the regional facility for testing. Some shipboard laboratories may be able to set up commercial testing for hepatitis A, B, C, or D.

In Garrison

Viral hepatitis is suspected in the patient with typical symptoms whose liver function tests (especially serum levels of aspartate aminotransferase and alanine aminotransferase) are elevated, indicating parenchymal liver damage. The specific virus responsible for the hepatitis is distinguishable only by laboratory testing (Table 38-8), though certain epidemiologic settings and laboratory patterns may suggest a particular viral 2,000) are most characteristic of hepatitis A. Elevated alkaline phosphatase levels are not usually seen in hepatitis A and are indicative of a hepatitis-associated cholestasis. Nonspecific indicators in hepatitis A include an elevated level of total serum IgM, a mild lymphocytosis, and, occasionally,

TABLE 38-8

DIAGNOSIS OF VIRAL HEPATITIS AND THE APPROPRIATE INTERPRETATION OF IMMUNOLOGIC MARKERS

	Immunologic Marker	Interpretation				
		Ongoing/Recent Infection	Past/Resolution of Infection	Chronic Infection	Carrier State	Vaccinated
Hepatitis A	Hep A IgM	+	–	N/A	N/A	+
	Hep A IgM+IgG	+	+	N/A	N/A	+
Hepatitis B	HBsAg	+	–	+	+	–
	anti-HBc (IgG)	+	+	+	+	–
	anti-HBc (IgM)	+	–	–	–	–
	Hbe Ag	+	–	+	–	–
	anti-HBe	–	±	–	–	–
	anti-HBs	–	+	–	–	+
Hepatitis D	anti-delta IgM	+	–	–	–	N/A
	HD Ag	+	–	+	N/A	N/A
Hepatitis C	anti-HCV	±*	+	+	N/A	N/A
	HCV RNA PCR	±*	+	+	N/A	N/A
Hepatitis E	anti-HEV†	+	+	N/A	N/A	N/A

+ Marker present
– Marker absent
± Marker present or absent
* Requires 6 weeks to 9 months
† Not commercially available
PCR: polymerase chain reaction

atypical mononuclear cells on blood smear.

The specific diagnosis of hepatitis A is made based on the detection of antibody to the hepatitis A virus. The presence of hepatitis A IgM indicates ongoing or recent infection. The diagnosis of hepatitis A may be made based on a single positive specific IgM result because hepatitis A IgM is present at the time of the first rise in liver enzymes and the first clinical symptoms. Measurement of total antibody to hepatitis A (IgM plus IgG) is not useful in the diagnosis of acute disease unless a 4-fold rise in titer between acute and convalescent specimens is detected. A single positive total antibody to HAV simply indicates infection with the virus in the past.

The most commonly used specific assays for hepatitis A IgM are capture radioimmunoassays or enzyme immunoassays. These tests are highly sensitive and specific. IgM positivity may persist for 3 to 12 months following the onset of illness. False positives are rare but may be associated with administration of IG, recent transfusion, or maternal antibody transfer.

Highly specific and sensitive laboratory tests are commercially available for the multiple markers of hepatitis B infection. The pattern of positive hepatitis B markers provides not only a diagnosis of hepatitis B but often a rough estimate of the stage of the disease, the infectiousness of the patient, and the prognosis. Acute hepatitis B is characterized by positive markers for HBsAg, anti-HBc (IgG or IgM), and HBeAg. HBsAg is the most important marker for active infection since it is almost always present in acute infection. Blood or body fluids, with the exception of sweat, should be considered infectious when they are HBsAg positive. HBeAg can be detected in the serum of most patients in the early stage of infection; HBeAg disappears and anti-HBe appears during the resolution of infection. The presence of HBeAg during acute or persistent infection identifies those patients who are most infectious and in whom active viral replication is ongoing. The presence of anti-HBs either alone or with anti-HBc(IgG) is consistent with past hepatitis B infection. Alternatively, the presence of anti-HBs alone is consistent with hepatitis B vaccination. A persistently positive HBsAg accompanied by a positive anti-HBc(IgG) is found in healthy hepatitis B carriers. Patients with chronic hepatitis B display persistently positive HBsAg, anti-HBc(IgG), and HBeAg markers. (See addendum at the end of the chapter.)

The diagnosis of hepatitis D is only made in the presence of hepatitis B infection. Patients with delta antigen in the liver have antibody to delta antigen in their serum. Hepatitis D is diagnosed by a positive assay for anti-delta IgM and hepatitis D antigen, (HDAg). The presence of anti-HBc(IgM) accompanied by hepatitis D serologic markers identifies hepatitis B–hepatitis D coinfection. Coinfected chronic HBsAg carriers may be persistently positive for delta antigen.

The diagnosis of hepatitis C has been based on the detection of antibodies reactive with recom-binant proteins or synthetic peptides because hepatitis C cannot be grown in vivo to produce a sufficient quantity of viral antigen for laboratory use. HCV antibody enzyme linked immunosorbent assays (ELISAs) were developed for the screening of donated blood but have been widely used for diagnostic purposes. The first generation ELISAs were highly sensitive but poorly specific; false positives were common, particularly in populations with low prevalence of the disease. Second gener-ation ELISAs have shown improvement in both sensitivity and specificity and can make the diagnosis earlier in the infection. Nonetheless, even using second generation testing, only 70% of patients infected with hepatitis C show positive results within 6 weeks of infection.[423] Polymerase chain reaction for the detection of HCV has been developed and is being used increasingly in labor-atories, but its reliability is currently uncertain.[424]

No serologic test is commercially available now for the diagnosis of hepatitis E. The diagnosis is established by the appropriate clinical and epidemiologic characteristics, coupled with the exclusion of hepatitis A, B, C, and D, as well as other viral agents that produce a hepatitis as part of multi–organ-system involvement. Enzyme immunoassays based on recombinant hepatitis E viral proteins are being developed and appear to detect anti–hepatitis E proteins reliably.[425]

Recommendations for Therapy

Hepatitis A

The therapy and management of hepatitis A is supportive. Admission to the hospital is rarely needed; if good sanitation can be assured, patients may be managed at home or in barracks. Separate toilet facilities are needed if the patient has diarrhea or is incontinent of stool. Fulminant hepatic failure from hepatitis A is rare but may occasionally require liver transplant. No specific dietary or bed-rest restrictions have been shown to be of value. Generally, it is recommended that patients abstain from consuming alcohol.

Hepatitis B

No specific therapy has been shown to be of use in acute hepatitis B. As with hepatitis A, the duration of bed rest is dictated by the energy level of the patient. In young patients, early ambulation and mild exercise are not harmful. No dietary restrictions are of any benefit. Corticosteroids have been used in severe acute hepatitis, but controlled trials[426,427] of severe and fulminant hepatitis have shown either no benefit or a negative effect.

The therapy of chronic hepatitis B is more complex. The only agent known to have a lasting beneficial effect is interferon alpha, and hence recombinant interferon alpha is licensed in the United States for the therapy of chronic hepatitis B.[428] Interferon does suppress hepatitis B virus replication in all patients and has significant though clinically limited utility.[429] Therapy of 4 to 6 months' duration induces long-term remission in 25% to 40% of patients. Treatment is recommended for patients with persistently elevated serum levels of aminotransferases; detectable HBsAg, HBeAg, and HBV DNA in serum; chronic hepatitis as shown by liver biopsy; and compensated liver disease.[428] Suppression of hepatitis B markers may be either complete or partial and either permanent or temporary following treatment with interferon alpha. Interferon in high doses causes fever, malaise, hair loss, leukopenia, and thrombocytopenia. These effects are reversible once therapy ceases.

Agents such as prednisone, interferon gamma, thymosin, levamisole, suramin, foscarnet, didanosine, adenosine arabinoside, acyclovir, zidovudine, and fialuridine inhibit hepatitis B virus replication; however, their lackluster efficacy and toxicity have limited their use.[428,430] Ganciclovir has been shown to reduce hepatitis B virus replication after liver transplantation.[431] A number of new nucleoside analogues, such as famciclovir, lamivudine, lobucavir, and adefovir dipivoxil, show promise in the treatment of chronic hepatitis B. Of these, famciclovir and lamivudine have been studied most extensively.[428] In a preliminary trial of 32 patients with chronic hepatitis B infection, 12 weeks of lamivudine therapy were well tolerated, and daily doses of 100 mg and 300 mg reduced HBV DNA to undetectable levels. In most patients, HBV DNA reappeared after therapy was complete, but 19% of patients had sustained suppression.[432] (See addendum at the end of the chapter.)

Hepatitis C

The therapy for hepatitis C is equally complex, controversial, and unsatisfactory. In acute hepatitis C, interferon alpha appears to decrease the chronicity rate. Interferon remains the only approved therapy for chronic hepatitis C,[433] although the low rate of sustained remissions and the significant side effects have mandated a search for ways to improve the efficacy of interferon and for new and more potent agents. Therapy is recommended for patients with elevated serum aminotransferase levels, anti-HCV in serum, and chronic hepatitis as shown by liver biopsy.[428] Current research shows a general trend toward the use of interferon in combination with other agents, such as ribavirin,[434] azidothymidine,[435] or recombinant human granulocyte colony-stimulating factor (rhG-CSF).[436] The response to interferon therapy in chronic hepatitis C may depend in part not only on the dose administered but also on host factors such as the hepatitis C genotype of the infection, the levels of HCV RNA, the fibrosis score of the histologic activity index, the iron concentrations in liver tissue, and the source of the infection.[428,437] (See addendum at the end of the chapter.)

Hepatitis D

Interferon alpha has been used in the treatment of chronic hepatitis D but with marginal success. Hepatitis D virus is inhibited by interferon alpha-2b, although permanent control of the disease is not achieved.[438] In the patient with chronic hepatitis B, it is important to determine whether hepatitis D is present because patients with combined infection respond more poorly to treatment and the recommended regimen of interferon is different (higher dose given for a more prolonged time).[401]

Liver transplantation has become the treatment of choice for fulminant hepatic failure since the advent of cyclosporin A in the early 1980s. Currently more than 2,500 transplants are done annually in the United States. Approximately 7% of these patients undergo transplantation for fulminant or subacute liver failure. Sixty to ninety percent survive 1 to 2 years.[439] The decision for transplantation needs to be made before complications of the hepatic failure are present; patients with incipient hepatic failure should be referred promptly to a liver transplant center.

Recommendations for Control and Prevention

The control and prevention of hepatitis are inextricably intertwined, and both are directly related to the specific epidemiology of each agent. Patients with jaundice thought to be caused by an unidentified hepatitis virus should be placed on contact and standard (formerly known as universal) precautions pending further elucidation of the specific virus.

The advent of hepatitis vaccines has enhanced the ability to control and prevent these diseases. Hepatitis vaccines have two purposes: (1) to prevent the morbidity and occasional mortality associated with acute infection and (2) to reduce the occurrence of chronic liver disease and hepatocellular carcinoma. For the first aim, the principal targets are hepatitis A and B; for the second, the targets are hepatitis B and C. Hepatitis A and B can both be prevented by immunization. The increasing use of immunization for hepatitis A and B prevention will gradually obviate the need for IG prophylaxis.

Hepatitis A

Since hepatitis A is transmitted primarily by the fecal-oral route, good sanitation and handwashing are paramount in the control of this disease. This is especially important for food handlers, whether in garrison or in the field. Detection of the ill food handler and restriction of his or her activities are essential in prevention and control. The field offers an excellent setting for transmission of this disease via food handling if appropriate care is not exercised and the involved military personnel have not been immunized. The advent of active immunization for hepatitis A will further reduce its impact on military forces, but even so, a foodborne outbreak of hepatitis A during a field training exercise that resulted in 22 ill soldiers and more than 300 lost work days was recently described.[420] In this outbreak, the secondary attack rate was nearly 20%. The index case was a cook's aide, who complained of fatigue, anorexia, and dark urine after 12 days in the field. Poor personal hygiene, inadequate sanitation, crowded conditions, and lack of immunization (vaccine was not available at that time) all facilitated this outbreak of hepatitis A. Food handlers should be repeatedly encouraged to report illness, and a work environment should be created where food handlers are not penalized or made uncomfortable when they do so. Food handlers should be prospectively immunized against hepatitis A. As the immunization of military personnel continues, the threat of hepatitis E may be larger as US forces deploy into areas of the world where this other enterically spread pathogen is common.[440,441]

Infection with hepatitis A is endemic in developing countries. Travelers to such destinations, whether they are deploying or traveling for pleasure, should be advised to seek immunization prospectively and to take specific precautions. Only well-cooked, hot food should be ingested. Only bottled beverages should be drunk and those without ice. Eating uncooked vegetables, fruit not peeled by the consumer, and shellfish is associated with risk. Hepatitis A vaccine is now recommended for all military personnel.

Nosocomial spread of hepatitis A is rare, even when patients share the same room and toilet facilities. Standard precautions are all that is required for the hospitalized patient with hepatitis A.

Use of Immune Globulin. Before the hepatitis A vaccine, pooled IG was the mainstay of immunoprophylaxis. In the absence of prior hepatitis A vaccination, all household and sexual contacts of persons with hepatitis A should receive 0.02mL/kg of IG as soon as practical after exposure. Serologic testing of contacts is not recommended as it may delay administration of IG and add cost. The use of IG more than 2 weeks after exposure is of no benefit.

Careful handwashing and meticulous environmental hygiene are essential in a daycare setting, particularly after changing diapers and preparing or handling food. Increased education and surveillance of employees and families are necessary for interrupting an outbreak. Outbreaks of hepatitis A in such settings must be reported to local public health officials, as well as to military preventive medicine units as applicable. Currently available hepatitis vaccines are not licensed for use in children under 2 years of age. Adult care takers should be immunized prospectively against hepatitis A. Recommendations for the use of IG for an outbreak of hepatitis A in a daycare setting are complex and vary depending on the ages of the children cared for, whether they are toilet trained, whether household contacts are involved, and how long a delay has elapsed before recognition of the disease. All recommendations involve the use of IG (0.02mL/kg). For further specifics, see a standard reference.[442,443] Schoolroom exposure generally does not pose a risk for transmission, and IG administration is not indicated.

If an outbreak occurs in institutions for custodial care, such as prisons, institutions for the mentally disabled, and nursing homes, residents and staff in close contact with infected persons should receive IG (0.02 mL/kg). Emphasis should be placed on careful handwashing and good personal hygiene. Generally, immunoprophylaxis is not required in a barracks setting unless conditions of poor handwashing, hygiene, sanitation, and crowding are present and transmission is likely.

In foodborne or waterborne outbreaks of hepatitis A, generally the source is recognized too late for IG to be effective. IG may be effective if it is administered to exposed persons within 2 weeks of the last exposure to hepatitis A–contaminated food or water. Experiences in the field suggest that standard recommendations are too stringent for such settings. In the field, confirmation of a case of hepatitis A may be difficult and therefore the *presumptive* diagnosis should prompt aggressive epidemiologic investigation. When any person working in a mess tent is presumptively diagnosed with hepatitis A, aggressive use of IG is warranted if laboratory confirmation is unavailable. At a minimum, all cooks should receive IG and consideration should be given to administering IG to all who eat at the mess tent. Clinical decisions should be driven by the aggressive epidemiologic investigation. Ultimately, control and prevention in the field setting depend on good sanitation and effective vaccination of all personnel.[420]

In the absence of previous vaccination, IG prophylaxis for the prevention of hepatitis A is recommended for travelers to developing countries. Those travelers staying less than 3 months should receive 0.02 mL/kg. Those staying longer than 3 months should receive 0.06 mL/kg every 5 months. Vaccination of susceptible prospective travelers is an alternative if sufficient lead time exists. Alternatively, one dose of IG and hepatitis A vaccination may be given if no lead time exists, but this strategy may reduce the immunogenicity of the vaccine.[444]

Vaccine. Two killed-virus hepatitis A vaccines have been approved for use in the United States (HAVRIX, developed by SmithKline Beecham Pharmaceuticals, Philadelphia, Penn, and VAQTA developed by Merck & Co, West Point, Penn). Each has been shown to have protective efficacy exceeding 90% and low levels of adverse reactions in trials in children.[445,446] Within 15 days of primary injection, up to 98% of adults and 96% of children and adolescents develop protective levels of antibody against hepatitis A. See Table 38-9 for doses and administration schedules. The most

commonly reported adverse events after immunization are soreness at the injection site and headache. Research at the Walter Reed Army Institute of Research has shown that immunization by jet gun confers immunity equivalent to immunization by needle and syringe. Additionally, hepatitis A vaccine is just as effective when given with hepatitis B vaccine as it is when given alone.[447]

Hepatitis A vaccine is likely to be universally recommended for pediatric use, but its current high cost may be a problem.[448] Adults targeted for immunization include international travelers to areas of high endemicity, staff members of daycare centers and custodial institutions, military personnel, food handlers, members of population groups with a high level of endemic infection, persons whose sexual practices place them at increased risk (eg, male homosexuals, persons with multiple sexual partners), handlers of nonhuman primates, and hemophiliacs[449] and other regular recipients of blood products. Hepatitis A vaccination should replace IG for use in preexposure prophylaxis. Vaccine may be combined with IG for either postexposure prophylaxis or situations where immediate and long-term protection are required. Hepatitis A vaccination is recommended for all Department of Defense personnel[450,451]; however, the implementation of this policy is likely to be delayed by the expense. The most current recommendations for candidates for hepatitis A vaccination from the Advisory Committee on Immunization Practices are listed in Exhibit 38-16.

Hepatitis B

Standard precautions should be followed for patients with acute or chronic hepatitis B infection. Infants born to HBsAg-positive mothers should

TABLE 38-9

DOSAGE AND ADMINISTRATION SCHEDULES FOR TWO HEPATITIS A VACCINES[*]

	HAVRIX[†]	Intervals	VAQTA[‡]	Intervals
Children	2-18 y		2-17 y	
	0.5 mL or	0 and 6-12 mo	0.5 mL	0 and 6-18 mo
	0.5 mL	0,1, and 6-12 mo		
Adults	1 mL	0 and 6-12 mo	0.5 mL	0 and 6-12 mo

[*] See package inserts for updated information
[†] SmithKline Beecham Pharmaceuticals, Philadelphia, Penn
[‡] Merck and Company, Inc., West Point, Penn

EXHIBIT 38-16

CANDIDATES FOR HEPATITIS A IMMUNIZATION

For Routine Immunization

Children living in states, counties, and communities with rates that are twice the 1987-1997 national average or greater (ie, ≥ 20 cases per 100,000 population)[*]

Those at Increased Risk

Travelers to endemic regions

Men having sex with men

Users of illicit injection drugs

Persons working closely with nonhuman primates

Persons with occupational risk (eg, researchers, military personnel)

Persons with chronic liver disease

Persons who receive clotting factor concentrates

---

[*] Consideration of routine vaccination should be given for children in states, counties, and communities with rates exceeding the 1987-1997 national average (ie, ≥ 10 but < 20 cases per 100,000 population).

Source: Advisory Committee on Immunization Practices. Prevention of hepatitis A through active or passive immunization: Recommendations of the Advisory Committee on Immunization Practices (ACIP). *MMWR.* 1999;48(RR-12):1–37.

---

have maternal blood carefully removed at delivery by a gloved health care provider in addition to the subsequent administration of hepatitis B immune globulin (HBIG) and hepatitis B vaccine. The blood of these infants should be handled with standard precautions as 1% to 3% of such infants are HBsAg positive due to infection in utero.

The most effective hepatitis B immunoprophylaxis is the preexposure immunization of all susceptible individuals. Hepatitis B vaccine has been available since 1981 and is one of the most efficacious yet underutilized vaccines in the medical armamentarium. Vaccination is recommended for all infants as part of the routine childhood immunization schedule. Immunization of all adolescents is currently recommended by the American Academy of Pediatrics.[412] Universal immunization is desirable.

Postexposure prophylaxis with hepatitis B vaccine and HBIG can effectively prevent infection. HBIG provides temporary protection and is only indicated in specific instances. Hepatitis B vaccine is used for protection both before and after exposure and provides long-term protection. HBIG is prepared from plasma known to have a high titer of antibody to HBsAg and to be negative for antibodies to HIV. The initial hepatitis B vaccine was made from plasma from male homosexuals in San Francisco who were positive for HBsAg. This vac-

cine was carefully purified; at no time has there been any evidence of transmission of HIV from this vaccine. It is no longer used in the United States but is still used extensively in other countries.[452] The second generation of hepatitis B vaccines currently used in the United States is produced by recombinant DNA technology using common baker's yeast (*Saccharomyces cerevisiae*) modified to produce HBsAg in large quantities and hence HIV transmission is no longer even a theoretic issue.

The two vaccines currently in use are RECOMBIVAX (Merck & Co.) and ENGERIX-B (SmithKline Beecham Pharmaceuticals). Neither vaccine has been shown to be superior to the other when used as recommended. Three intramuscular doses are required to induce protective immunity in more than 90% of adults and 95% of adolescents, children, and infants. See Table 38-10 for doses and administration schedules. Immunocompromised and hemodialysis patients should receive larger doses. A booster dose may be given to all vaccinees 4 to 6 months after primary immunization is complete to produce higher titers and more lasting protection.[442]

High-risk candidates for hepatitis B immunization are listed in Exhibit 38-17; family members of HbsAg-positive adoptees from countries where hepatitis B is endemic are also candidates. The screening of pregnant women for evidence of

TABLE 38-10

DOSAGES AND ADMINISTRATION SCHEDULES FOR HEPATITIS B VACCINES

Population	Intervals	RECOMBIVAX[*]	ENGERIX-B[†]
Infants			
HBsAg - mother	0-2, 1-4, 6-18 mos	0.5 mL (2.5 µg)	0.5 mL (10 µg)
HBsAg + mother	birth (HBIG), 1-2 and 6 mos	0.5 mL (5 µg)	0.5 mL (10 µg)
Children			
1-10 y	0, 1-2, and 4-6 mos	0.5 mL (2.5 µg)	0.5 mL (10 µg)
11-19 y	0, 1-2, and 4-6 mos	0.5 mL (5 µg)	0.5 mL (10 µg)
Adults			
$\geq$ 20 y	0, 1-2, and 4-6 mos	1 mL (10 µg)	1 mL (20 µg)
Immunocompromised	0, 1, and 6 mos	1 mL (40 µg)	2 mL (40 µg)

[*] Merck and Company, Inc., West Point, Penn
[†] SmithKline Beecham Pharmaceutical, Philadelphia, Penn

chronic hepatitis B infection (positive HBsAg/HBe Ag) is essential and allows for the use of HBIG and hepatitis B vaccine to interrupt vertical transmission. This effort alone is expected to prevent millions of cases of hepatocellular carcinoma worldwide. The

---

EXHIBIT 38-17

CANDIDATES FOR HEPATITIS B IMMUNIZATION

For Routine Immunization

All infants

All adolescents

Those at Increased Risk

Health care workers

Clients and staff of custodial institutions

Hemodialysis patients

Patients who regularly receive blood products

Household and sexual contacts of HBsAg carriers

Travelers for more than 6 months in areas of high endemicity

Sexually active homosexual or bisexual males

Heterosexuals with multiple partners or a history of sexually transmitted diseases

---

Department of Defense mandates HBV immunization of all health care workers and those judged to be high-risk candidates.

Complex algorithms exist for the management of potential hepatitis B exposure[442,443] in health care providers following needlestick or sharps injury, but comprehensive hepatitis B immunization of all health care providers obviates their need. Today, there is virtually no rationale for health care workers not to be fully immune to hepatitis B. Hepatitis B vaccines licensed in the United States are very safe vaccines. Anaphylaxis is rare. The only contraindication to vaccine administration is hypersensitivity to yeast or another component of the vaccine.[452]

Hepatitis C

Standard precautions are indicated for the hospitalized patient with hepatitis C. Frequently a patient is found to have hepatitis C as an incidental finding in the hospital, highlighting the need for standard precautions for every hospitalized patient regardless of known or suspected diagnosis.

No immunoprophylaxis of proven benefit exists for hepatitis C. Now that screening of plasma donors and exclusion of infected persons from the donor pool is recommended in the United States, IG manufactured in this country does not contain appreciable titers of antibodies to hepatitis C, and therefore is not expected to be of any benefit. No vaccine currently exists for hepatitis C. Formulation of such a vaccine is hindered by the extensive genetic and antigenic diversity among different strains of hepatitis C and by the fact that HCV infection does not confer solid immunity against reinfection.[452]

Hepatitis D

Since hepatitis D can only be transmitted in the presence of hepatitis B infection, isolation precautions for hepatitis D are the same as those for hepatitis B. Similarly the same control and prevention methods apply. Immunization for hepatitis B will prevent acquisition of delta hepatitis. HBsAg carriers should be extremely careful to avoid exposure to hepatitis D because no immunoprophylactic measures currently exist to prevent hepatitis D superinfection.

Hepatitis E

Appropriate isolation for patients with hepatitis E is contact isolation with standard precautions routinely observed. Prevention involves good sanitation and not ingesting contaminated food or water. Passive immunoprophylaxis with IG prepared in the United States is not effective against hepatitis E. A study[453] in cynomolgus monkeys showed that immunization with a recombinant protein representing part of the hepatitis E capsid could confer immunity. This suggests that a vaccine may be developed in the future that would be useful for travelers and military persons who deploy outside the United States.

[Margan J. Zajdowicz and Thaddeus R. Zajdowicz]

ADDENDUM: ADDITIONAL DIAGNOSTIC AND UPDATED TREATMENT INFORMATION FOR HEPATITIS

Additional Diagnostic Information for Hepatitis B

Generally, patients with chronic hepatitis B display persistently positive HBsAg, anti-HBc (IgG), and HBeAg markers. Some patients with chronic hepatitis B are infected with a mutant strain of HBV, characterized by the presence of HBsAg, anti-HBc, and abnormal serum enzymes but the absence of HBeAg. This form of chronic hepatitis may sometimes be associated with more severe liver disease.

Updated Recommendations for Therapy: Hepatitis B

Because of the results in a recent study[1] among US patients showing that lamivudine administered for 1 year favorably affected liver histology, virology, and biochemical features in patients with chronic hepatitis B and appeared to be well tolerated, the drug is achieving greater popularity and is even considered by some to be the starting drug of choice. Unfortunately, long-term treatment with this drug appears to be associated with the increasing likelihood of development of mutant strains, probably necessitating extended or even life-long treatment.

Updated Recommendations for Therapy: Hepatitis C

A new form of interferon has been developed and is called pegylated interferon. This form of interferon is attached to the molecule polyethylene glycol (hence the prefix "peg") and has a delayed excretion after injection, thus maintaining a high and sustained interferon blood level. Accordingly, it is administered as a once weekly dose. First reports indicate that pegylated interferon on its own is approximately equivalent in efficacy to the combination of conventional interferon plus ribavirin.[2,3] Furthermore, preliminary reports indicate that pegylated interferon plus ribavirin is clearly superior to the prior recommended treatment regimen and is expected to be the treatment of choice for the immediate future.[4]

1. Dienstag JL, Schiff ER, Wright TL, et al, Lamivudine as initial treatment for chronic hepatitis B in the United States. *N Engl J Med.* 1999;341:1256–1263.

2. Zeuzem S, Feinman V, Rasenack J, et al. Peginterferon alfa-2a in patients with chronic hepatitis C. *N Engl J Med.* 2000;343:1666–1672.

3. Heathcote EJ, Shiffman ML, Cooksley GE, et al. Peginterferon alfa-2a in patients with chronic hepatitis C and cirrhosis. *N Engl J Med.* 2000;343:1673–1680.

4. Fried MW, Shiffman ML, Reddy RK, et al. Pegylated (40kDa) interferon alfa-2a (PEGASYS) in combination with ribavirin: Efficacy and safety results from a phase III, randomized, actively controlled, multicenter study. *Gastroenterol.* 2001;120(5, Suppl 1):A-55. Abstract 289.

Provided by Leonard B. Seeff, MD, Senior Scientist for Hepatitis C Research, National Institutes of Diabetes and Digestive and Kidney Diseases, National Institutes of Health

REFERENCES

1. Duncan LC. The days gone. The medical service in the War of 1812, III: The pneumonia epidemic of 1812–13. *Mil Surgeon.* 1933;72:48–56.

2. Love AG. A brief summary of the vital statistics of the US Army during the world war. *Mil Surgeon.* 1922;1:139–168.

3. Finland M. Recent advances in the epidemiology of pneumococccal infections. *Medicine.* 1942;21:307–344.

4. Hirsch EF, McKinney M. An epidemic of pneumococcus bronchopneumonia. *J Infect Dis.* 1919;24:594–617.

5. Opie EL, Freeman AW, Blake FG, Small JC, Rivers TM. Pneumonia following influenza (at Camp Pike, Ark.). *JAMA.* 1919;72:556–565.

6. Park JH, Chickering HT. Type I pneumococcus lobar pneumonia among Puerto Rican laborers. *JAMA.* 1919;73:183–186.

7. Nichols HJ. The lobar pneumonia problem in the Army. *N Y Med J.* 1917;106:219–223.

8. Tenney CF, Rivenburgh WT. A group of sixty-eight cases of Type I pneumonia occurring in thirty days at Camp Upton. *Arch Intern Med.* 1919;24:545–552.

9. Cecil RL, Austin JH. Results of prophylactic inoculation against pneumococcus in 12,519 men. *J Exp Med.* 1918;28:19–41.

10. Cecil RL, Vaughan HF. Results of prophylactic vaccination against pneumonia at Camp Wheeler. *J Exp Med.* 1919;29:457–483.

11. Denny FW Jr. The prophylaxis of streptococcal infections. In: McCarty M, ed *Streptococcal Infections.* New York: Columbia University Press; 1954: 176–196.

12. Gorgas WC. Recommendation as to sanitation concerning employees of the mines on The Rand made to the Transvaal chamber of mines. *JAMA.* 1914;62:1855–1865.

13. Breese BB, Stanbury J, Upham H, Calhoun AJ, Van Buren RL, Kennedy AS. Influence of crowding on respiratory illness in a large naval training station. *War Med.* 1945;7:143–146.

14. Clendening L. Reinfection with Streptococcus hemolyticus in lobar pneumonia, measles, and scarlet fever and its prevention. *JAMA.* 1918;156:575–588.

15. Hodges RG, MacLeod CM. Epidemic pneumococcal pneumonia IV. The relationship of nonbacterial respiratory disease to pneumococcal pneumonia. *Am J Hyg.* 1946;44:231–236

16. Woodward TE. *The Armed Forces Epidemiological Board: Its First Fifty Years 1940–1990.* Washington, DC: Office of the Surgeon General, US Department of the Army; 1990.

17. Amundson DE. Pneumonia in military recruits. *Mil Med.* 1994;159:629–631.

18. Holmes KK, Miller FL, Edwards EA, Johnson DW. Etiology of pneumonia in nonrecruit military personnel. *Am J Med Sci.* 1971;260:264–269.

19. Kleemola M, Saikku P, Visakorpi R, Wang SP, Grayston JT. Epidemics of pneumonia caused by TWAR, a new chlamydia organism, in military trainees in Finland. *J Infect Dis.* 1988;157:230–236.

20. Lehtomaki K, Leinonen M, Takala A, Hovi T, Herva E, Koskela M. Etiological diagnosis of pneumonia in military conscripts by combined use of bacterial culture and serological methods. *Eur J Clin Microbiol Infect Dis.* 1988;7:348–354.

21. Fujikawa J, Struewing JP, Hyams KC, Kaplan EL, Tupponce AK, Gray GC. Streptococcal prophylaxis for recruits: Efficacy of oral erythromycin in prophylaxis of streptococcal infection for penicillin-allergic military recruits: A randomized double-blind study. *J Infect Dis*. 1992;166:162–165.

22. Gray GC, Escamilla J, Hyams KC, Struewing JP, Kaplan EL, Tupponce AK. Hyperendemic *Streptococcus pyogenes* infection despite prophylaxis with penicillin G benzathine. *N Engl J Med*. 1991;325:92–97.

23. Davies HD, McGreer A, Schwartz B, et al. Invasive Group A streptococcal infections in Ontario, Canada. *N Engl J Med*. 1996;335:547–554.

24. Davies HD, McGreer A, Schwartz B, et al. Invasive Group A streptococcal infections in Ontario, Canada. *N Engl J Med*. 1996;335:547–554.

25. Katz AR, Morens DM. Severe streptococcal infections in historical perspective. *Clin Infect Dis*. 1992;14:298–307.

26. Katz AR, Morens DM. Severe streptococcal infections in historical perspective. *Clin Infect Dis*. 1992;14:298–307.

27. Thomas RJ, Conwill DE, Morton DE, Brooks TJ, Holmes CK, Mahaffey WB. Penicillin prophylaxis for streptococcal infections in the United States Navy and Marine Corps recruit camps, 1951–1985. *Rev Infect Dis*. 1988;10:125–130.

28. Wallace MR, Garst PD, Papadimos TJ, Oldfield EC. The return of acute rheumatic fever in young adults. *JAMA*. 1989;262:2557–2561.

29. Centers for Disease Control. Acute rheumatic fever among Army trainees—Fort Leonard Wood, Missouri. *MMWR*. 1988;37:519–522.

30. Schwartz B, Facklam RR, Breiman RF. Changing epidemiology of group A streptococcal infection in the USA. *Lancet*. 1990;336:1167–1171.

31. Gray GC, McPhate DC, Leinonen M, et al. Weekly oral azithromycin as prophylaxis for agents causing acute respiratory disease. *Clin Infect Dis*. 1998;26:103–110.

32. Denny FW. A 45-year perspective on the *Steptococcus* and rheumatic fever: the Edward H. Kass lecture in infectious disease history. *Clin Infect Dis*. 1994;19:1110–1122.

33. Coburn AF. The prevention of respiratory tract bacterial infections by sulfadiazine prophylaxis in the United States Navy. *JAMA*. 1944;126:88–93.

34. Coborn AF. Mass chemoprophylaxis: The U.S. Navy's six months' program for the control of streptococcal infections *Naval Med Bull*. 1944;284:149–162.

35. Loosli CG, Lemon HM, Robertson O, Hamburger M. Transmission and control of respiratory diseases in army barracks, IV: The effect of oiling procedures on the incidence of respiratory diseases and hemolytic streptococcal infections. *J Infect Dis*. 1952;19:153.

36. Miller WR, Jarrett ET, Willmon TL, et al. Evaluation of ultraviolet radiation and dust control measures in control of respiratory disease at a naval training center. *J Infect Dis*. 1948;82:86–100.

37. Personnel of the United States Naval Medical Research Unit No. 4. The use of triethylene glycol vapor for control of acute respiratory diseases in Navy recruits, II: Effect on acute respiratory diseases. *Am J Hyg*. 1952;55:202–229.

38. The Personnel of Naval Medical Research Unit No. 4. *The Prophylaxis of Acute Respiratory Infections With Oral Penicillin or Chlortetracycline: Antibiotics Annual, 1953–54*. New York: Medical Encyclopedia, Inc; 1954: 123–136.

39. Epidemiology Unit No. 22. Failure of type specific *Streptococcus pyogenes* vaccine to prevent respiratory infections. *Nav Med Bull*. 1946;46:709–718.

40. Milzer A, Kohn KH, MacLean H. Oral prophylaxis of rheumatic fever with penicillin. *JAMA.* 1948;136:536–538.

41. Stollerman GH, Rusoff JH. Prophylaxis against group A streptococcal infections in rheumatic fever patients: Use of new repository penicillin preparations. *JAMA.* 1952;150:1571–1575.

42. Denny FW, Wannamaker LW, Brink WR, Rammelkamp CH Jr, Custer EA. Prevention of rheumatic fever: Treatment of the preceding streptococcal infection. *JAMA.* 1950;143:151–153.

43. Frank PF. Streptococcal prophylaxis in Navy recruits with oral and benzathine penicillin. *US Armed Forces Med J.* 1958;4:543–560.

44. Musher DM, Groover JE, Reichler MR, et al. Emergence of antibody to capsular polysaccharides of *Streptococcus pneumoniae* during outbreaks of pneumonia: Association with nasopharyngeal colonization. *Clin Infect Dis.* 1997;24:441–446.

45. Gunzenhauser JD, Brundage JF, McNeil JG, Miller RN. Broad and persistent effects of benzathine penicillin G in the prevention of febrile, acute respiratory disease. *J Infect Dis.* 1992;166:365–373.

46. Seppälä H, Nissinen A, Järvinen H, et al. Resistance to erythromycin in group A streptococci. *N Eng J Med.* 1992;5:292–297.

47. Kim SK, Kaplan LE. Association of penicillin tolerance with failure to eradicate Group A streptococci from patients with pharyngitis. *J Pediatr.* 1985;107:681–684.

48. Dagan R, Ferne M, Sheinis M, Alkan M, Katzenelson E. An epidemic of penicillin-tolerant Group A streptococcal pharyngitis in children living in a closed community: Mass treatment with erythromycin. *J Infect Dis.* 1987;156:514–516.

49. Gray GC, Mitchell BS, Tueller JE, Cross ER, Amundson DE. Pneumonia hospitalizations in the US Navy and Marine Corps: Rates and risk factors for 6,522 admissions, 1981-1991. *Am J Epidemiol.* 1994;139:793–802.

50. Capeding MRZ, Nohynek H, Ruutu P, Leinonen M. Evaluation of a new tube latex agglutination test for detection of type-specific pneumococcal antigens in urine. *J Clin Microbiol.* 1991;29:1818–1819.

51. Breiman FR, Butler CJ, Tenover CF, Elliott AJ, Facklam RR. Emergence of drug-resistant pneumococcal infections in the United States. *JAMA.* 1994;271:1831–1835.

52. Butler JC, Hofmann J, Cetron MS, Elliott JA, Facklam RR, Breiman RF. The continued emergence of drug-resistant *Streptococcus pneumoniae* in the United States: An update from the Centers for Disease Control and Prevention's Pneumoccoccal Sentinel Surveillance System. *J Infect Dis.* 1996;174:986–993.

53. Jernigan DB, Cetron MS, Breiman RF. Minimizing the impact of drug-resistant *Streptococcus pneumoniae* (DRSP): A strategy from the DRSP Working Group. *JAMA.* 1996;275:206–209.

54. Commission on Acute Respiratory Diseases, Fort Bragg, North Carolina. Epidemiology of atypical pneumonia and acute respiratory disease at Fort Bragg, North Carolina. *Am J Pub Health.* 1944;34:335–346.

55. Eaton MD, Meiklejohn G, Van Herick W. Studies on the etiology of primary atypical pneumonia: A filterable agent transmissable to cotton rats, hamsters, and chick embryos. *J Exp Med.* 1944;79:649–668.

56. Chanock RM, Fox HH, James WD Rutekenst RR, White RJ, Senterfit LB. Epidemiology of *M. pneumonia* infection in military recruits. *Ann N Y Acad Sci.* 1967;143:484–496.

57. Edwards EA, Crawford YE, Pierce WE, Peckinpaugh RO. A longitudinal study of *Mycoplasma pneumoniae* infections in Navy recruits by isolation and seroepidemiology. *Am J Epidemiol.* 1976;104:556–562.

58. Monto AS, Bryna ER, Rhodes LM. The Tecumseh study of respiratory illness, VII: Further observations on the occurrence of respiratory syncytial virus and *Mycoplasma pneumoniae* infections. *Am J Epidemiol.* 1974;100:458–468.

59. Jensen KJ, Senterfit LB, Scully WE, Conway TJ, West RF, Drummy WW. *Mycoplasma pneumoniae* infections in children: An epidemiologic appraisal in families treated with oxytetracycline. *Am J Epidemiol.* 1967;86:419–432.

60. Gray GC, Hyams KC, Wang SP, Grayston JT. *Mycoplasma pneumoniae* and *Chlamydia pneumoniae* strain TWAR infections in U.S. Marine Corps recruits. *Mil Med.* 1994;159:292–294.

61. Cassell GH. Severe mycoplasma disease—rare or underdiagnosed? *West J Med.* 1995;162:172–175.

62. Cassell GH, Drnec J, Waites KB, et al. Efficacy of clarithromycin against *Mycoplasma pneumoniae*. *J Antimicrob Chemother.* 1991;27:47–59.

63. Williamson J, Marmion BP, Worswick DA, et al. Laboratory diagnosis of *Mycoplasma pneumoniae* infection, 4; antigen capture and PCR-gene amplification for detection of the *Mycoplasma*: Problems of clinical correlation. *Epidemiol Infect.* 1992;109:519–537.

64. Ieven M, Ursi D, Van Bever H, Quint W, Niesters HG, Goossens H. Detection of *Mycoplasma pneumoniae* by two polymerase chain reactions and role of *M. pneumoniae* in acute respiratory tract infections in pediatric patients. *J Infect Dis.* 1996;173:1445–1452.

65. Maletzky AJ, Cooney MK, Luce R, Kenny GE, Grayston JT. Epidemiology of viral and mycoplasmal agents associated with childhood lower respiratory tract illness in a civilian population. *J Pediatr.* 1971;78:407–414.

66. McCormick DP, Wenzel RP, Senterfit LB, Bean WE. Relationship of pre-existing antibody to subsequent infection by *Mycoplasma pneumoniae* in adults. *Infect Immun.* 1974;9:53–59.

67. Steinberg P, White RJ, Fuld SL, Gutekunst RR, Chanock RM, Senterfit LB. Ecology of *Mycoplasma pneumoniae* infections in Marine recruits at Parris Island, South Carolina. *Am J Epidemiol.* 1969;89:62–73.

68. Wenzel RP, Craven RB, Davies JA, Hendley J.O, Hamory BH, Gwaltney JM. Field trial of an inactivated *Mycoplasma pneumoniae* vaccine. *J Infect Dis.* 1976;134:571–576.

69. Mogabgab WJ. Protective effects of inactive *Mycoplasma pneumoniae* vaccine in military personnel, 1964–1966. *Am Rev Respir Dis.* 1968;97:359–365.

70. Smith CB, Friedewald WT, Chanock RM. Inactivated *Mycoplasma pneumoniae* vaccine. *JAMA.* 1967;199:353–358.

71. Grayston JT. *Chlamydia pneumoniae* strain TWAR pneumonia. *Ann Rev Med.* 1992;43:317–323.

72. Falsey AR, Walsh EE. Transmission of *Chlamydia pneumoniae*. *J Infect Dis.* 1993;168:493–496.

73. Grayston JT. *Chlamydia pneumoniae* (TWAR) infections in children. *Pediatr Infect Dis J.* 1994;13:675–685.

74. Thom DH, Grayston JT, Wang SP, Kuo CC, Altman J. *Chlamydia pneumoniae* strain TWAR, *Mycoplasma pneumoniae*, and viral infections in acute respiratory disease in a university student health clinic population. *Am J Epidemiol.* 1990;132:248–256.

75. Grayston JT, Campbell LA, Kuo CC, et al. A new respiratory tract pathogen: *Chlamydia pneumoniae* strain TWAR. *J Infect Dis.* 1990;161:618–625.

76. Einarsson S, Sigurdsson HK, Magnusdottir SD, Erlendsdottir H, Briem H, Gudmundsson S. Age specific prevalence of antibodies against *Chlamydia pneumoniae* in Iceland. *Scand J Infect Dis.* 1994;26:393–397.

77. Freidan HM, Brauer D. Prevalence of antibodies to *Chlamydia pneumoniae* TWAR in a group of German medical students. *J Infect.* 1993;27:89–93.

78. Cook PJ, Honeybourne D. *Chlamydia pneumoniae*. *J Antimicrob Chemother.* 1994;34:859–873.

79. Kauppinen M, Saikku P. Pneumonia due to *Chlamydia pneumoniae*: Prevalence, clinical features, diagnosis, and treatment. *Clin Infect Dis.* 1995;21:S244–S252.

80. Fang GD, Fine M, Orloff J, et al. New and emerging etiologies for community-acquired pneumonia with implications for therapy: A prospective multicenter study of 359 cases. *Medicine (Baltimore).* 1990;69:307–316.

81. Ekman MR, Grayston JT, Visakorpi R, Kleemola M, Kuo CC, Saikku P. An epidemic of infections due to *Chlamydia pneumoniae* in military conscripts. *Clin Infect Dis.* 1993;17:420–425.

82. Mendall MA, Carrington D, Strachan D, et al. *Chlamydia pneumoniae*: Risk factors for seropositivity and association with coronary heart disease. *J Infect.* 1995;30:121–128.

83. Emre U, Roblin PM, Gelling M, et al. The association of *Chlamydia pneumoniae* infection and reactive airway disease in children. *Arch Pediatr Adolesc Med.* 1994;148:727–732.

84. Emre U, Sokolovskay N, Roblin PM, Schachter J, Hammerschlag MR. Detection of anti-*Chlamydia pneumoniae* IgE in children with reactive airway disease. *J Infect Dis.* 1995;172:265–267.

85. Falck G, Heyman L, Gnarpe J, Gnarpe H. *Chlamydia pneumoniae* and chronic pharyngitis. *Scand J Infect Dis.* 1995;27:179–182.

86. Hyman CL, Augenbraun MH, Roblin PM, Schachter J, Hammerschlag MR. Asymptomatic respiratory tract infection with Chlamydia pneumoniae TWAR. *J Clin Microbiol.* 1991;29:2082–2083.

87. Hyman CL, Roblin PM, Gaydos CA, Quinn TC, Schachter J, Hammerschlag MR. Prevalence of asymptomatic nasopharyngeal carriage of *Chlamydia pneumoniae* in subjectively healthy adults: Assessment of polymerase chain reaction enzyme immunoassay and culture. *Clin Infect Dis.* 1995;20:1174–1178.

88. Grayston JT. Infections caused by *Chlamydia pneumoniae* strain TWAR. *Clin Infect Dis.* 1992;15:757–763.

89. Kern DG, Neill MA, Schachter J. A seroepidemiologic study of *Chlamydia pneumoniae* in Rhode Island. *Chest.* 1993;104:208–213.

90. Campbell LA, Melgosa MP, Hamilton DJ, Kuo CC, Grayston JT. Detection of Chlamydia pneumoniae by polymerase chain reaction. *J Clin Microbiol.* 1992;30:434–439.

91. Gaydos CA, Eiden JJ, Oldach D, et al. Diagnosis of *Chlamydia pneumoniae* infection in patients with community-acquired pneumonia by polymerase chain reaction enzyme immunoassay. *Clin Infect Dis.* 1994;19:157–160.

92. Dwinell WG. Laboratory report on epidemic pneumonia. *JAMA.* 1919;158:216–231.

93. Davenport FM. Influenza viruses. In: Evans AS, ed. *Viral Infections in Humans.* New York: Plenum Publishing Corp; 1984: 373–396.

94. Kilbourne ED. *Influenza.* New York: Plenum Medical Book Corp; 1987: 255–289.

95. Peckinpaugh RO, Askin FB, Pierce WE, Edwards EA, Johnson DP, Jackson GG. Field studies with amantadine acceptability and protection. *Ann N Y Acad Sci.* 1970;173:62–73.

96. Dolin R, Reichman RC, Madore HP, Maynard R, Linton PN, Webber-Jones J. A controlled trial of amantadine and rimandtadine in the prophylaxis of influenza A infection. *N Engl J Med.* 1982;307:580–584.

97. Hayden FG, Belshe RB, Clover RD, Hay AJ, Oakes MG, Soo W. Emergence and apparent transmission of rimantadine-resistant influenza A virus in families. *N Engl J Med.* 1989;321:1696–1702.

98. Belshe RB, Burk B, Newman F, Cerruti RL, Sim IS. Resistance of influenza A virus to amantadine and rimantadine: Results of one decade of surveillance. *J Infect Dis.* 1989;159:430–435.

99. Chenoweth A, Waltz AD, Stokes J Jr, Gladen RG. Active immunization with the viruses of human and swine influenza. *Am J Dis Child.* 1936;52:757–758.

100. Woodward TE. *The Armed Forces Epidemiological Board: The Histories of the Commissions.* Washington, DC: Office of the Surgeon General, Department of the Army, and the Borden Institute; 1994.

101. Members of the Commission on Influenza, Army Epidemiological Board. A clinical evaluation of vaccination against influenza. *JAMA.* 1944;144:982–985.

102. Francis T, Pearson HE, Salk JE, Brown PN. Immunity in human subjects artificially infected with influenza virus type B. *Am J Public Health.* 1944;34:317–334.

103. Hilleman MR, Werner JH. Recovery of new agent from patients with acute respiratory illness. *Proc Soc Exp Biol Med.* 1954;85:183–188.

104. Rowe WP, Huebner RJ, Gilmore LK, Parrott RH, Ward TG. Isolation of a cytopathogenic agent from human adenoids undergoing spontaneous degeneration in tissue culture. Proc Soc Exp Biol Med. 1953;84:570–573.

105. Hilleman MR, Werner JH, Adair CV, Dreisbach AR. Outbreak of acute respiratory illness caused by RI-67 and influenza A viruses, Fort Leonard Wood, 1952–53. *Am J Hyg.* 1955;61:163–173.

106. Hilleman MR. Efficacy of and indications for use of adenovirus vaccine. *Am J Public Health.* 1958;48:153–158.

107. Hilleman MR, Gauld RL, Butler RL, et al. Appraisal of occurrence of adenovirus-caused respiratory illness in military populations. *Am J Hyg.* 1957;66:29–41.

108. McNamra MJ, Pierce WE, Crawford YE, Miller LF. Patterns of adenovirus infection in the respiratory diseases of naval recruits. *Am Rev Respir Dis.* 1962;86:485–497.

109. Miller LF, Tytel M, Pierce WE, Rosenbaum MJ. Epidemiology of nonbacterial pneumonia among naval recruits. *JAMA.* 1963;185:92–99.

110. Bloom HH, Forsyth BR, Johnson KM, et al. Patterns of adenovirus infections in Marine Corps personnel. *Am J Hyg.* 1964;80:328–342.

111. Wenzel RP, McCormick DP, Smith EP, Beam WE. Acute respiratory disease: clinical and epidemiologic observations of military trainees. *Mil Med.* 1971;136:873–880.

112. Grayston JT, Woolridge RI, Loosli CG, Gundelfinder BF, Johnson PB, Pierce WE. Adenovirus infections in naval recruits. *J Infect Dis.* 1959;104:61–70.

113. Foy HM. Adenoviruses. In: Evans AS, ed. *Viral Infections of Humans.* 3rd ed. New York: Plenum Medical Book Co; 1989: 77–94.

114. Stille WT, Pierce W, Crawford YE. Multiple infections in acute respiratory illness. *J Infect Dis.* 1961;109:158–165.

115. Meurman O, Ruuskanen O, Sarkkinen H. Immunoassay diagnosis of adenovirus infections in children. *J Clin Microbiol.* 1983;18:1190–1195.

116. Crawford-Miksza LK, Schnurr DP. Quantitative colorimetric microneutralization assay for characterization of adenoviruses. *J Clin Microbiol.* 1994;32:2331–2334.

117. Bell JA, Hantover MJ, Heuner RJ, Looslie CG. Efficacy of trivalent adenovirus (APC) vaccine in naval recruits. *JAMA.* 1956;161:1521–1525.

118. Dudding BA, Top FH, Winter PE, Buescher EL, Lamson TH, Leibovitz A. Acute respiratory disease in military trainees: The adenovirus surveillance program, 1966–71. *Am J Epidemiol.* 1973;97:187–198.

119. Gaydos CA, Gaydos JC. Adenovirus vaccines in the U.S. military. *Mil Med.* 1995;160:300–304.

120. Gurwith MJ, Horwith GS, Impellizzeri CA, Davis AR, Lubeck MD, Hung PP. Current use and future directions of adenovirus vaccine. *Semin Respir Infect.* 1989;4:299–303.

121. Peckinpaugh RO. Hyperimmune globulin in the control of acute respiratory disease. In: *Uses of Immunoglobulins in Prevention and Therapy.* Great Lakes, Ill: Naval Medical Research Unit-4; 1971. Technical Report AD 726068: 302–307.

122. Houser H. Gamma globulin prevention of severe respiratory illness caused by adenovirus types 4 and 7. *Clin Res.* 1959;7:270–271. Abstract.

123. Rytel MW, Dowd JM, Edwards EA, Pierce WE, Pert JH. Prophylaxis of acute viral respiratory disease with gamma globulin. *Dis Chest.* 1968;6:499–503.

124. Barraza EM, Ludwig SL, Gaydos JC, Brundage JF. Reemergence of adenovirus type 4 acute respiratory disease in military trainees: Report of an outbreak during a lapse in vaccination. *J Infect Dis.* 1999;179:1531–1533.

125. Hendrix RM, Lindner JL, Benton FR, et al. Large, persistent epidemic of adenovirus type 4-associated acute respiratory disease in U.S. Army trainees. *Emerg Infect Dis.* 1999;5:798–801.

126. McNeill KM, Ridgely Benton F, Monteith SC, Tuchscherer MA, Gaydos JC. Epidemic spread of adenovirus type 4-associated acute respiratory disease between U.S. Army installations. *Emerg Infect Dis.* 2000;6:415–419.

127. Gray GC, Goswami PR, Malasig MD, et al. Adult adenovirus infections: Loss of orphaned vaccines precipitates military respiratory disease epidemics. *Clin Infect Dis.* 2000;31:663–670.

128. Ludwig SL, Brundage JF, Kelley PW, et al. Prevalence of antibodies to adenovirus serotypes 4 and 7 among unimmunized US Army trainees: Results of a retrospective nationwide seroprevalence survey. *J Infect Dis.* 1998;178:1776–1778.

129. Howell MR, Nang RN, Gaydos CA, Gaydos JC. Prevention of adenoviral acute respiratory disease in Army recruits: Cost-effectiveness of a military vaccination policy. *Am J Prev Med.* 1998;14:168–175.

130. Hyer RN, Howell MR, Ryan MA, Gaydos JC. Cost-effectiveness analysis of reacquiring and using adenovirus vaccines in US Navy recruits. *Am J Trop Med Hyg.* 2000;62:613–618.

131. Cone LA, Woodard DR, Schlievert PM, Tomory GS. Clinical and bacteriologic observations of a toxic shock-like syndrome due to *Streptococcus pyogenes*. *N Engl J Med.* 1987;317:146–149.

132. Davies HD, McGeer A, Schwartz B, et al. Invasive group A streptococcal infections in Ontario, Canada. *N Engl J Med.* 1996;335:547–554.

133. Bass JW, Stephenson SR. The return of pertussis. *Pediatr Infect Dis J.* 1987;6:141–144.

134. Mink CM, Cherry JD, Christenson P, et al. A search for *Bordetella pertussis* infection in university students. *Clin Infect Dis.* 1992;14:464–471.

135. Jansen DL, Gray GC, Putnam SD, Lynn F, Meade BD. Evaluation of pertussis infection among US Marine Corps trainees. *Clin Infect Dis.* 1997;25:1099–1107.

136. Brundage JF, Zollinger WD. Evolution of meningococcal disease in the U. S. Army. In: Vedros NA, ed. *Evolution of Meningococcal Disease.* Boca Raton, Fla: CRC Press; 1987: 5–25.

137. Gauld JR, Nitz RE, Hunter DH, Rust JH, Gauld RL. Epidemiology of meningococcal meningitis at Fort Ord. *Am J Epidemiol.* 1965;82:56–72.

138. Bristow WM, Van Peenen PFD, Volk R. Epidemic meningitis in naval recruits. *Am J Public Health*. 1965;55:1039–1045.

139. Wilfert CM, Gutman LT. *Neisseria*. In: Joklik WK, Willett HP, Amos DB, Wilfert CM, eds. *Zinsser Microbiology*. 20th ed. Norwalk, Conn: Appleton & Lange; 1992: 443–460.

140. Apicella MA. Meningococcal infections. In: Bennett JC, Plum F, eds. *Cecil Textbook of Medicine*. 20th ed. Philadelphia, Penn: W. B. Saunders; 1996: 1618–1622.

141. Apicella MA. *Neisseria meningitidis*. In: Mandell GL, Bennett JE, Dolin R, eds. *Mandell, Douglas and Bennett's Principles and Practice of Infectious Diseases*. 4th ed. New York: Churchill Livingstone; 1995: 1896–1909.

142. Griffiss JM. Meningococcal infections. In: Isselbacher KJ, Martin JB, Braunwald E, Fauci AS, Wilson JD, Kasper DL, eds. *Harrison's Principles of Internal Medicine*. 13th ed. New York: McGraw-Hill, Inc.; 1994: 641–644.

143. Fraser DW, Broome CV, Wenger JD. Meningococcal meningitis. In: Last JM, Wallace RB, eds. *Maxcy-Rosenau-Last Public Health & Preventive Medicine*. 13th ed. Norwalk, Conn: Appleton & Lange; 1992: 157–158.

144. Chin J, ed. *Control of Communicable Diseases Manual*. 17th ed. Washington, DC: American Public Health Association; 2000.

145. Broome CV. The carrier state: *Neisseria meningitidis*. *J Antimicrobial Chemother*. 1986;18(suppl A):25–34.

146. Goldschneider I, Gotschlich EC, Artenstein MS. Human immunity to the meningococcus, II: Development of natural immunity. *J Exp Med*. 1969;129:1327–1348.

147. Griffiss JM. Epidemic meningococcal disease: Synthesis of a hypothetical immunoepidemiologic model. *Rev Infect Dis*. 1982;4:159–172.

148. Wolf RE, Birbara CA. Meningococcal infections at an army training center. *Am J Med*. 1968;44:243–255.

149. Lapeyssonnie L. Milestones in meningococcal disease. In: Vedros NA, ed. *Evolution of Meningococcal Disease*. Boca Raton, Fla: CRC Press; 1987: 1–4.

150. Ryan MAK. Meningococcal disease in the United States military: 1980–1990. *Preventive Medicine & Biometrics*. Bethesda, Md: Uniformed Services University of the Health Sciences; 1995: 24.

151. Stephens DS, Hajjeh RA, Baughman WS, Harvey RC, Wenger JD, Farley MM. Sporadic meningococcal disease in adults: Results of a 5-year population-based study. *Ann Intern Med*. 1995;123:937–940.

152. Perkins MD, Mirrett S, Reller LB. Rapid bacterial antigen detection is not clinically useful. *J Clin Microbiol*. 1995;33:1486–1491.

153. Duffy TP. Clinical problem-solving: The sooner the better. *N Engl J Med*. 1993;329:710–713.

154. Sanborn WR. Development of meninigococcal vaccines. In: Vedors NA, ed. *Evolution of Meningococcal Disease*. Boca Raton, Fla: CRC Press; 1987: 121–134.

155. Diaz Romero J, Outschoorn IM. Current status of meningococcal group B vaccine candidates: Capsular or noncapsular? *Clin Microbiol Rev*. 1994;7:559–575.

156. Zangwill KM, Stout RW, Carlone GM, et al. Duration of antibody response after meningococcal polysaccharide vaccination in US Air Force personnel. *J Infect Dis*. 1994;169:847–852.

157. Hanson RK, Preventive Medicine Officer, 1st Marine Expeditionary Force. Personal communication, 1997.

158. Hume SE. Mass voluntary immunization campaigns for meningococcal disease in Canada: Media hysteria. *JAMA*. 1992;267:1833–1834,1837–1838.

159. Hanzel GD. Tuberculosis control in the United States Navy: 1875–1966. *Arch Environ Health*. 1968;16(1):7–21.

160. Guiton CR, Barrett O. Tuberculosis. In: Ognibene AJ, Barrett O, eds. *General Medicine and Infectious Diseases*. Vol 2. In: *Internal Medicine in Vietnam*. Washington, DC: Office of The Surgeon General and Center of Military History, US Army; 1982: 214–218.

161. Long ER. Tuberculosis. In: *Communicable Diseases Transmitted Chiefly through Respiratory and Alimentary Tracts*. Vol 6. In: *Preventive Medicine in World War II*. Washington, DC: Office of The Surgeon General, US Department of the Army; 1958: Chap 14.

162. Reister FA. *Battle Casualties and Medical Statistics: US Army Experience in the Korean War*. Washington, DC: The Surgeon General, Department of the Army; 1973: 3–4, 74, 90.

163. Comstock GW, Edwards LB, Livesay VT. Tuberculosis morbidity in the US Navy: Its distribution and decline. *Am Rev Respir Dis*. 1974;110:572–580.

164. Rhoades ER, Alexander CP. Reactions to the tuberculin tine test in Air Force recruits: An analysis of 193,856 tests. *Am Rev Respir Dis*. 1968;98:837–841.

165. Trump DH, Hyams KC, Cross ER, Struewing JP. Tuberculosis infection among young adults entering the US Navy in 1990. *Arch Intern Med*. 1993;153:211–216.

166. Cross ER, Hyams KC. Tuberculin skin testing in US Navy and Marine Corps personnel and recruits, 1980–86. *Am J Public Health*. 1990;80:435–438.

167. Trump DH, Lazarus AA. Tuberculosis among sailors on US Navy ships following travel to South American ports. Norfolk, Va: Navy Environmental Health Center; 1991. Typescript.

168. Houk VN, Kent DC, Baker JH, Sorensen K, Hanzel GD. The Byrd study: In-depth analysis of a micro-outbreak of tuberculosis in a closed environment. *Arch Environ Health*. 1968;16(1):4–6.

169. Houk VN, Kent DC, Baker JH, Sorensen K. The epidemiology of tuberculosis infection in a closed environment. *Arch Environ Health*. 1968;16(1):26–35.

170. DiStasio AJ, Trump DH. The investigation of a tuberculosis outbreak in the closed environment of a US Navy ship, 1987. *Mil Med*. 1990;155:347–351.

171. LaMar J, Malakooti M, Sposato J, et al. Navy-Marine Corps team tuberculosis outbreak: 26th Marine Expeditionary Unit (Special Operations Capable), USS WASP (LHD1). *Naval Med Surv Rep*. 1999;2(2):6–11.

172. Ferraris VA, Carpenter WR, Brand DR, Hollingsed MJ, Taylor BH, Montgomery SK. Mass screening for tuberculosis in an isolated US Army outpost. *Mil Med*. 1984;149:457–458.

173. World Health Organization, Global Tuberculosis Programme. *TB: Groups at Risk: WHO Report on the Tuberculosis Epidemic, 1996*. Geneva, Switzerland: WHO; 1996.

174. Raviglione MC, Snider DE, Kochi A. Global epidemiology of tuberculosis: Morbidity and mortality of a worldwide epidemic. *JAMA*. 1995;273:220–226.

175. Centers for Disease Control and Prevention. Tuberculosis morbidity—United States, 1997. *MMWR*. 1998;47:253–257.

176. American Thoracic Society, Centers for Disease Control and Prevention. Diagnostic standards and classification of tuberculosis. *Am Rev Respir Dis*. 1990;142:725–735. Published erratum: *Am Rev Respir Dis*. 1990;142:1470.

177. Centers for Disease Control and Prevention. *Core Curriculum on Tuberculosis: What the Clinician Should Know*. 3rd ed. Atlanta: CDC; 1994.

178. Wijsmuller G, Snider DE. Skin testing: A comparison of the jet injector and the Mantoux method. *Am Rev Respir Dis*. 1975;112:789–798.

179. Centers for Disease Control and Prevention. Centers for Disease Control and Prevention. Targeted tuberculin testing and treatment of latent tuberculosis infection. *MMWR*. 2000;49(RR-6):1–54.

180. American Academy of Pediatrics Committee on Infectious Diseases. Screening for tuberculosis in infants and children. *Pediatrics*. 1994;93:131–134.

181. American Thoracic Society, Centers for Disease Control and Prevention. Treatment of tuberculosis and tuberculosis infection in adults and children. *Am J Respir Crit Care Med*. 1994;149:1359–1374.

182. Centers for Disease Control and Prevention. Screening for tuberculosis and tuberculosis infection in high-risk populations: Recommendations of the Advisory Council for the Elimination of Tuberculosis. *MMWR*. 1995;44(RR-11):19–34.

183. Centers for Disease Control and Prevention. Initial therapy for tuberculosis in the era of multidrug resistance: Recommendations of the Advisory Council for the Elimination of Tuberculosis. *MMWR*. 1993;42(RR-7):1–8.

184. American Thoracic Society, Centers for Disease Control and Prevention. Control of tuberculosis in the United States. *Am Rev Respir Dis*. 1992;146:1623–1633.

185. Kenyon TA, Valway SE, Ihle WW, Onorato IM, Castro KG. Transmission of multi-drug resistant *Mycobacterium tuberculosis* during a long airplane flight. *N Engl J Med*. 1996;334:933–938.

186. Occupational Safety and Health Administration. *Enforcement Procedures and Scheduling for Occupational Exposure to Tuberculosis*. Washington, DC: OSHA; 1996. OSHA Instruction CPL 2.106.

187. Centers for Disease Control and Prevention. Guidelines for preventing the transmission of *Mycobacterium tuberculosis* in health-care facilities, 1994. *MMWR*. 1994;43(RR-13):1–132.

188. Slutkin G. Tuberculosis: The patient and the program. In: Sandler RH, Jones TC, eds. *Medical Care of Refugees*. New York: Oxford University Press; 1987: 345–363.

189. Malone JL, Paparello SF, Malone JD, et al. Tuberculosis among Haitian migrants experienced at Guantanamo Bay, Cuba. *Travel Med Intl*. 1993;11(6):21–25.

190. Desmond S. *The Wars of the Roses Through the Lives of Five Men and Women of the Fifteenth Century*. New York: Viking; 1995: 223.

191. Moore JE. *The Modern Treatment of Syphilis*. 2nd ed. Springfield, Ill: Thomas; 1947: 619.

192. Sternberg HT, Howard E. Venereal diseases. In: *Communicable Diseases Transmitted Through Contact or By Unknown Means*. Vol 5. In: *Preventive Medicine in World War II*. Washington, DC: Office of the Surgeon General, US Department of the Army; 1960: 139.

193. Hart G. Factors influencing venereal infection in a war environment. *Br J Vener Dis*. 1974;50:68–72.

194. Hart G. Psychological aspects of venereal disease in war environment. *Soc Sci Med*. 1973;7:455–467.

195. Harrison WO. Cohort study of venereal diseases. One-hundred-second Annual Meeting of the American Public Health Association and Related Organizations; 20–24 October 1974; New Orleans, La. Abstract 208–g.

196. Holmes KK, Johnson DW, Trostle HJ. An estimate of the risk of men acquiring gonorrhea by sexual contact with infected females. *Am J Epidemiol*. 1970;91:170–174.

197. Hooper RR, Reynolds GH, Jones OG, et al. Cohort study of venereal disease, I: The risk of gonorrhea transmission from infected women to men. *Am J Epidemiol*. 1978;108:136–144.

198. Piot P, Islam MQ. Sexually transmitted diseases in the 1990s: Global epidemiology and challenges for control. *Sex Transm Dis.* 1994;21(Suppl):S7–S13.

199. Coutinho RA. Epidemiology of sexually transmitted diseases. *Sex Transm Dis.* 1994;21(Suppl):S51–S52.

200. Aral SO, Holmes KK. Epidemiology of sexual behavior and sexually transmitted diseases. In: Holmes KK, Mardh PA, Sparling PF, Wiesner PJ, eds. *Sexually Transmitted Diseases.* New York: McGraw-Hill; 1990: 19–36.

201. Anderson RM. The transmission dynamics of sexually transmitted diseases: The behavioral component. In: Wasserheit JN, Aral SO, Holmes KK, eds. *Research Issues in Human Behavior and Sexually Transmitted Diseases in the AIDS Era.* Washington, DC: American Society for Microbiology; 1991: 38–60.

202. Wittkower ED, Cowan J. Some psychological aspects of sexual promiscuity: Summary of an investigation. *Psychosom Med.* 1944;6:287–294.

203. Watts GO, Wilson RA. A study of personality factors among venereal disease patients. *Can Med Assoc J.* 1945;53:119–122.

204. Brody MW. Men who contract venereal disease. *J Vener Dis Information.* 1948;29:334–337.

205. Wittkower ED. The psychological aspects of venereal disease. *Br J Vener Dis.* 1948;24:59–67.

206. Sutherland R. Some individual and social factors in venereal disease. *Br J Vener Dis.* 1950; 26:1–15.

207. Ratcliff TA. Psychiatric and allied aspects of the problem of venereal diseases in the army. *J R Army Med Corps.* 1947;89:122–131.

208. Hart G. Social aspects of venereal disease, I: Sociological determinants of venereal disease. *Br J Vener Dis.* 1973;49:542–547.

209. Jones OG, Harrison W, Hooper R, Zaidi A, et al. Personal characteristics of acquiring gonorrhea and nongonococcal urethritis. Meeting of the American Public Health Association and Related Organizations; 16–20 November 1975; Chicago. Abstract 352–H.

210. Zaidi AA, Jones OG, Reynolds GH, et al. Personal characteristics associated with risk of gonorrhea. *Summary of Papers Presented at The Joint Statistical Meetings of the American Statistical Association Biometric Society (Eastern and Western North American Regions).* Chicago: American Statistical Association Biometric Society; 1977: 260–261. Abstract.

211. Berg SW, Kilpatrick ME, Harrison WO, McCutchan JA. Cefoxitin as single-dose treatment of urethritis caused by penicillinase-producing *Neisseria gonorrhoeae. N Engl J Med.* 1979;301:509–511.

212. Lancaster DJ, Berg SW, Harrison WO. Parenteral cefotaxime versus penicillin in the treatment of uncomplicated gonococcal urethritis. Interscience Conference on Antimicrobial Agents and Chemotherapy; September 22–24 1980; New Orleans, La. Abstract 675.

213. Melton LJ. The influence of high-risk groups on the incidence of gonorrhea. *US Navy Med.* 1977;68:26–27.

214. Berg SW. Sexually transmitted diseases in the military. In: Holmes KK, Mardh PA, Sparling PF, Wiesner PJ, eds. *Sexually Transmitted Diseases.* New York: McGraw-Hill; 1984: 90–99.

215. McCreary ML. Difficulties with diagnosis and treatment of urethritis aboard ship: A possible solution. *Mil Med.* 1980;145:686–691.

216. Levine JB, Erickson JM, Dean LM. Social aspects of venereal disease aboard a US Navy destroyer. *J Am Vener Dis Assoc.* 1976;3:35–39.

217. Hart G. Social aspects of venereal disease, II: Relationship of personality to other sociological determinants of venereal disease. *Br J Vener Dis*. 1973;49:548–552.

218. Rothenberg RB, Potterat JJ. Temporal and social aspects of gonorrhea transmission: The force of infectivity. *Sex Transm Dis*. 1988;15:88–92.

219. Thomas JC, Tucker MJ. The development and use of the concept of a sexually transmitted disease core. *J Infect Dis*. 1996;174(Suppl 2):S134–S143.

220. Rothenberg RB. The geography of gonorrhea: Empirical demonstration of core group transmission. *Am J Epidemiol*. 1983;117:688–694.

221. Yorke JA, Hethcote HW, Nold A. Dynamics and control of the transmission of gonorrhea. *J Am Vener Dis Assoc*. 1978;4:51–56.

222. Rothenberg RB, Potterat JJ, Woodhouse DE. Personal risk taking and the spread of disease: Beyond core groups. *J Infect Dis*. 1996;174(Suppl 2):S144–S149.

223. Wasserheit JN, Aral SO. The dynamic topology of sexually transmitted disease epidemics: Implications for prevention strategies. *J Infect Dis*. 1996;174(Suppl 2):S201–S213.

224. Tanfer K. Sex and disease: Playing the odds in the 1990s. *Sex Transm Dis*. 1994;21(Suppl):S65–S72.

225. Anderson JE, Dahlberg LL. High-risk sexual behavior in the general population: Results from a national survey, 1988–1990. *Sex Transm Dis*. 1992;19:320–325.

226. Choi KH, Catania JA. Changes in multiple sexual partnerships, HIV testing, and condom use among US heterosexuals 18 to 49 years of age, 1990 and 1992. *Am J Public Health*. 1996;86:554–556.

227. Melnick SL, Burke GL, Perkins LL, et al. Sexually transmitted diseases among young heterosexual urban adults. *Public Health Rep*. 1993;108:673–679.

228. Centers for Disease Control. Selected behaviors that increase risk for HIV infection among high school students—United States, 1990. *MMWR*. 1992;41:231,237–240.

229. Sonenstein FL, Pleck JH, Ku LC. Sexual activity, condom use, and AIDS awareness among adolescent males. *Fam Plann Perspect*. 1989;21:152–158.

230. Rice RJ, Roberts PL, Handsfield HH, Holmes KK. Sociodemographic distribution of gonorrhea incidence: Implications for prevention and behavioral research. *Am J Public Health*. 1991;81:1252–1258.

231. Greenberg J, Magder L, Aral S. Age at first coitus: A marker for risky sexual behavior in women. *Sex Transm Dis*. 1992;19:331–334.

232. Aral SO, Schaffer JE, Mosher WD, Cates W Jr. Gonorrhea rates: What denominator is most appropriate? *Am J Public Health*. 1988;78:702–703.

233. D'Costa LJ, Plummer FA, Bowmer I, et al. Prostitutes are a major reservoir of sexually transmitted diseases in Nairobi, Kenja. *Sex Transm Dis*. 1985;12:64–67.

234. Handsfield HH, Jasman LL, Roberts PL, Hanson VW, Kothenbeutel RL, Stamm WE. Criteria for selective screening for *Chlamydia trachomatis* infection in women attending family planning clinics. *JAMA*. 1986;255:1730–1734.

235. Schachter J, Stoner E, Moncada J. Screening for chlamydial infections in women attending family planning clinics. *West J Med*. 1983;138:375–379.

236. Corey L. Genital herpes. In: Holmes KK, Mardh PA, Sparling PF, Wiesner PJ, eds. *Sexually Transmitted Diseases*. New York: McGraw-Hill; 1990: 391–413.

237. Syrjanen K, Vayrynen M, Castren O, et al. Sexual behavior of women with human papilloma virus (HPV) lesions of the uterine cervix. *Br J Vener Dis.* 1984;60:243–248.

238. Alter MJ, Antone J, Weisfuse I, Starko K, Vacalis TD, Maynard JE. Hepatitis B virus transmission between heterosexuals. *JAMA.* 1986; 256:1307–1310.

239. Dan BB. Sex and the singles' whirl: The quantum dynamics of hepatitis B. *JAMA.* 1986;256:1344.

240. Joffe GP, Foxman B, Schmidt AJ, et al. Multiple partners and partner choice as risk factors for sexually transmitted disease among female college students. *Sex Transm Dis.* 1992;19:272–278.

241. Holmes KK, Kreiss JK. Heterosexual transmission of human immunodeficiency virus: Overview of a neglected aspect of the AIDS epidemic. *AIDS.* 1988;1:602–610.

242. Day S. Prostitute women and AIDS: Anthropology. *AIDS.* 1988;2:421–428.

243. Padian NS. Prostitute women and AIDS: Epidemiology. *AIDS.* 1988;2:413–419.

244. McIntyre M. "Life Outside Subic Bay: Off Base: Troubling Trade-off Between U.S. Forces and Philippines [sic] city." *San Diego Union.* 5 November 1989, p. D-8.

245. Celentano DD, Nelson KE, Suprasert S, et al. Epidemiologic risk factors for incident sexually transmitted diseases in young Thai men. *Sex Transm Dis.* 1996;23:198–205.

246. Manaloto CR, Hayes CG, Padre LP, et al. Sexual behavior of Filipino female prostitutes after diagnosis of HIV infection. *Southeast Asian J Trop Med Public Health.* 1990;21:301–305.

247. Abellanosa I, Nichter M. Antibiotic prophylaxis among commercial sex workers in Cebu City, Philippines: Patterns of use and perceptions of efficacy. *Sex Transm Dis.* 1996;23:407–412.

248. Brunham RC, Ronald AR. Epidemiology of sexually transmitted diseases in developing countries. In: Wasserheit JN, Aral SO, Holmes KK, eds. *Research Issues in Human Behavior and Sexually Transmitted Diseases in the AIDS Era.* Washington, DC: American Society for Microbiology; 1991: 61–80.

249. Kunanusont C, Foy HM, Kreiss JK, et al. HIV-1 subtypes and male-to-female transmission in Thailand. *Lancet.* 1995;345:1078–1083.

250. Quinn TC, Cates W. Epidemiology of sexually transmitted diseases in the 1990s. In: Quinn TC, ed. *Advances in Host Defense Mechanisms.* Vol 8. New York: Raven Press; 1992: 1–37. Cited in: Quinn TC, Zenilman J, Rompalo A. Sexually transmitted diseases: Advances in diagnosis and treatment. *Adv Intern Med.* 1994;39:149–196.

251. Stamm WE, Holmes KK. *Chlamydia trachomatis* infections of the adult. In: Holmes KK, Mardh PA, Sparling PF, Wiesner PJ, eds. *Sexually Transmitted Diseases.* New York: McGraw-Hill; 1990: 181–193.

252. Centers for Disease Control. *Division of STD/HIV Prevention Annual Report 1991.* Atlanta, Ga: CDC; 1992.

253. Malone JD, Hyams KC, Hawkins RE, Sharp TW, Daniell FD. Risk factors for sexually transmitted diseases among deployed U.S. military personnel. *Sex Transm Dis.* 1993;20:294–298.

254. Warner RD, Mathis RE, Weston ME, Bigbee LR, Hendrix CW, Lucey DR. Estimates of human immunodeficiency virus (HIV) incidence and trends in the US Air Force. *Vaccine.* 1993;11:534–537.

255. Renzullo PO, McNeil JG, Wann ZF, Burke DS, Brundage JF, United States Military Medical Consortium for Applied Retroviral Research. Human immunodeficiency virus type-1 seroconversion trends among young adults serving the in the United States Army, 1985–1993. *J Acquir Immune Defic Syndr Hum Retrovirol.* 1995;10:177–185.

256. Garland FC, Mayers DL, Hickey TM, et al. Incidence of human immunodeficiency virus seroconversion in US Navy and Marine Corps personnel, 1986 through 1988. *JAMA.* 1989;262:3161–3165.

257. Cowan DN, Pomerantz RS, Wann ZF, et al. Human immunodeficiency virus infection among members of the reserve components of the U.S. Army: Prevalence, incidence, and demographic characteristics. *J Infect Dis.* 1990;162:827–836.

258. Kelley PW, Miller RN, Pomerantz RS, Wann ZF, Brundage JF, Burke DS. Human immunodeficiency virus seropositivity among members of the active duty US Army 1985–89. *Am J Public Health.* 1990;80:405–410.

259. Renzullo PO, McNeil JG, Levin LI, Bunin JR, Brundage JF. Risk factors for prevalent human immunodeficiency virus (HIV) infection in active duty Army men who initially reported no identified risk: A case control study. *J Acquir Immune Defic Syndr.* 1990;3:266–271.

260. Levin LI, Peterman TA, Renzullo PO, et al. HIV-1 seroconversion and risk behaviors among young men in the US Army. *Am J Public Health.* 1995;85:1500–1506.

261. Quinn TC, Zenilman J, Rompalo A. Sexually transmitted diseases: Advances in diagnosis and treatment. *Adv Intern Med.* 1994;39:149–196.

262. Centers for Disease Control and Prevention. Recommendations for the prevention and management of *Chlamydia trachomatis* infections, 1993. *MMWR.* 1993;42(RR-12):1–39.

263. Irwin DE, Thomas J, Leone PA, et al. Sexually transmitted disease (STD) patients' self-treatment practice prior to seeking medical care. Interscience Conference on Antimicrobial Agents and Chemotherapy; 17–20 September 1995; San Francisco. Abstract K74.

264. Upchurch DM, Brady WE, Reichart CA, Hook EW 3rd. Behavioral contributions to acquisition of gonorrhea in patients attending an inner-city sexually transmitted disease clinic. *J Infect Dis.* 1990;161:938–941.

265. Centers for Disease Control and Prevention. *Sexually Transmitted Diseases Clinical Practice Guidelines.* Atlanta: CDC; 1991.

266. Centers for Disease Control and Prevention. 1998 guidelines for treatment of sexually transmitted diseases. *MMWR.* 1998;47(RR-1):1–128.

267. Pabst KM, Reichert CA, Knud-Hansen R, et al. Disease prevalence among women attending a sexually transmitted disease clinic varies with reason for visit. *Sex Transm Dis.* 1992;19:88–91.

268. Holmes KK, Johnson DW, Kvale PA, Halverson CW, Keys TF, Martin DH. Impact of a gonorrhea control program, including selective mass treatment, in female sex workers. *J Infect Dis.* 1996;174(Suppl 2):S230–S239.

269. Ehrhardt AA. Trends in sexual behavior and the HIV pandemic. *Am J Public Health.* 1992;82:1459–1461.

270. Centers for Disease Control. Heterosexual behaviors and factors that influence condom use among patients attending a sexually transmitted disease clinic—San Francisco. *MMWR.* 1990;39:685–689.

271. Hamburg BA. Subsets of adolescent mothers: Development, biomedical, and psychosocial issues. In: Lancaster JB, Hamburg RA, eds. *School-Age Pregnancy and Parenthood: Biosocial Dimensions.* New York: Aldine De Gruyter; 1986: 115–145.

272. Aral SO, Soskoline V, Joesoef RM, O'Reilly KR. Sex partner recruitment as a risk factor for STD: Clustering of risky modes. *Sex Transm Dis.* 1991;18:10–17.

273. Boyer CB. Psychosocial, behavioral, and educational factors in preventing sexually transmitted diseases. In: Schydlower M, Shafer M-A, eds. *Adolescent Medicine: AIDS and Other Sexually Transmitted Diseases.* Vol 1, No. 3. In: *State of the Art Reviews.* Philadelphia: Hanley & Belfus; 1990: 597–613.

274. Astone J. Having sex and using condoms: Adolescents' beliefs, intentions, and behavior. *Curr Issues Public Health.* 1996;2:2933.

275. Rabin DL, Boekeloo BO, Marx ES, Bowman MA, Russell NK, Willis AG. Improving office-based physicians' prevention practices for sexually transmitted diseases. *Ann Intern Med*. 1994;121:513–519.

276. Council on Scientific Affairs. Education for health: A role for physicians and the efficacy of health education efforts. *JAMA*. 1990;263:1816–1819.

277. Stryker JS, Coates TJ, DeCarlo P, Haynes-Sanstad K, Shriver M, Makadon HJ. Prevention of HIV infection: looking back, looking ahead. *JAMA*. 1995;273:1143–1148.

278. Makadon HJ, Silin JG. Prevention of HIV infection in primary care: Current practices, future possibilities. *Ann Intern Med*. 1995;123:715–719.

279. Katz BP, Blythe MJ, Van der Pol B, Jones RB. Declining prevalence of chlamydial infection among adolescent girls. *Sex Transm Dis*. 1996;23:226–229.

280. Boyer CB, Shafer MA, Brodine SK, Shaffer RA. Evaluation of an STD/HIV intervention for deployed military men. Meeting of the International Society for STD Research; 28 August 1995; New Orleans, La. Abstract.

281. Holmes KK, Johnson DW, Trostle HJ. An estimate of the risk of men acquiring gonorrhea by sexual contact with infected females. *Am J Epidemiol*. 1970;91:170–174.

282. Hook EW. Approaches to sexually transmitted disease control in North America and Western Europe. In: Wasserheit JN, Aral SO, Holmes KK, eds. *Research Issues in Human Behavior and Sexually Transmitted Diseases in the AIDS Era*. Washington, DC: American Society for Microbiology; 1991; 269–280.

283. Cates W Jr, Stone KM. Family planning, sexually transmitted diseases, and contraceptive choice: A literature update. *Fam Plann Perspect*. 1992;24:75–84,122–128.

284. Weller SC. A meta-analysis of condom effectiveness in reducing sexually transmitted HIV. *Soc Sci Med*. 1993;36:1635–1644.

285. Weniger BG, Limpakarnjanarat K, Ungchusak K, et al. The epidemiology of HIV infection and AIDS in Thailand. *AIDS*. 1991;5(Suppl):S71–S85.

286. de Vincenzi I. A longitudinal study of human immunodeficiency virus transmission by heterosexual partners. *N Engl J Med*. 1994;331:341–346.

287. Johnson AM. Condoms and HIV transmission. *N Engl J Med*. 1994;331:391–392.

288. Hanenberg RS, Rojanapithayakorn W, Kunasol P, Sokal DC. Impact of Thailand's HIV-control program as indicated by the decline of sexually transmitted diseases. *Lancet*. 1994;344:243–245.

289. Nelson KE, Celentano DD, Eiumtrakol S, et al. Changes in sexual behavior and a decline in HIV infection among young men in Thailand. *N Engl J Med*. 1996;335:297–303.

290. Centers for Disease Control. Condoms for prevention of sexually transmitted diseases. *MMWR*. 1988;37:133–137.

291. Weiss PJ, Olson PE, Brodine SK. Navy issue condoms. *Navy Med*. 1992;83:6–7.

292. Weinstock HS, Lindan C, Bolan G, Kegeles SM, Hearst N. Factors associated with condom use in a high-risk heterosexual population. *Sex Transm Dis*. 1993;20:14–20.

293. Valdiserri RO, Arena VC, Proctor D, Bonati FA. The relationship between women's attitudes about condoms and their use: Implications for condom promotion programs. *Am J Public Health*. 1989;79:499–501.

294. Cohen DA, Dent C, MacKinnon D, Hahn G. Condoms for men, not women: Results of brief promotion programs. *Sex Transm Dis*. 1992;19:245–251.

295. Brown AE, Brundage JF, Tomlinson JP, Burke DS. The U.S. Army HIV testing program: The first decade. *Mil Med*. 1996;161:117–122.

296. Nelson EW. Sexual self-defense versus the liaison dangereuse: A strategy for AIDS prevention in the '90s. *Am J Prev Med*. 1991;7:146–149.

297. Potter LB, Anderson JE. Patterns of condom use and sexual behavior among never-married women. *Sex Transm Dis*. 1993;20:201–208.

298. Gollub EL, Stein ZA. Commentary: The new female condom—item 1 on a women's AIDS prevention agenda. *Am J Public Health*. 1992;83:498–500.

299. Rosenberg MJ, Gollub EL. Commentary: Methods women can use that may prevent sexually transmitted disease, including HIV. *Am J Public Health*. 1992;82:1473–1478.

300. Cates W Jr, Stewart FH, Trussell J. Commentary: The quest for women's prophylactic methods—hopes vs science. *Am J Public Health*. 1992;82:1479–1482.

301. Roper WL, Peterson HB, Curran JW. Commentary: Condoms and HIV/STD prevention—clarifying the message. *Am J Public Health*. 1993;83:501–503.

302. Artenstein AW, Coppola J, Brown AE, et al. Multiple introductions of HIV-1 subtype E into the western hemisphere. *Lancet*. 1995;346:1197–1198.

303. Brodine SK, Mascola JR, Weiss PJ, et al. Detection of diverse HIV-1 genetic subtypes in the USA. *Lancet*. 1995;346:1198–1199.

304. Martin DH, DiCarlo RP. Recent changes in the epidemiology of genital ulcer disease in the United States: The crack cocaine connection. *Sex Transm Dis*. 1994;21(Suppl):S76–S80.

305. Danielsson D. Gonorrhoea and syphilis in Sweden—past and present. *Scand J Infect Dis*. 1990;69:69–76.

306. Kohl PK. Epidemiology of sexually transmitted diseases: What does it tell us? *Sex Transm Dis*. 1994;21(Suppl):S81–S83.

307. Fullilove RE, Fullilove MT, Bowser BP, Gross SA. Risk of sexually transmitted disease among black adolescent crack users in Oakland and San Francisco, California. *JAMA*. 1990;263:851–855.

308. Handsfield HH, Lipman TO, Harnisch JP, Tronca E, Holmes KK. Asymptomatic gonorrhea in men: Diagnosis, natural course, prevalence, and significance. *N Engl J Med*. 1974;290:117–123.

309. Klousia JW, Tanowitz HB. Asymptomatic male gonorrhea in military personnel. *NY State J Med*. 1979;79:27–28.

310. Podgore JK, Holmes KK, Alexander ER. Asymptomatic urethral infections due to *Chlamydia trachomatis* in male U.S. military personnel. *J Infect Dis*. 1982;146:828.

311. Centers for Disease Control and Prevention. Fluoroquinolone resistance in *Neisseria gonorrhoeae*—Colorado and Washington, 1995. *MMWR*. 1995;44:761–764.

312. Tapsall JW, Limnios EA, Thacker C, et al. High-level quinolone resistance in *Neisseria gonorrhoeae*: A report of two cases. *Sex Transm Dis*. 1995;22:310–311.

313. Kam KM, Wong PW, Cheung MM, Ho NKY, Lo KK. Quinolone-resistant *Neisseria gonorrhoeae* in Hong Kong. *Sex Transm Dis*. 1996;23:103–108.

314. Tapsall JW, Phillips EA, Shultz TR, Thacker C. Quinolone-resistant *Neisseria gonorrhoeae* isolated in Sydney, Australia, 1991–1995. *Sex Transm Dis*. 1996;23:425–428.

315. Gordon SM, Carlyn CJ, Doyle LJ, et al. The emergence of *Neisseria gonorrhoeae* with decreased susceptibility to ciprofloxacin in Cleveland, Ohio: Epidemiology and risk factors. *Ann Intern Med*. 1996;125:465–470.

316. Tanaka M, Masumoto T, Kobayashi I, Uchino U, Kumazawa J. Emergence of in vitro resistance to fluoroquinolones in *Neisseria gonorrhoeae* isolated in Japan. *Antimicrob Agents Chemother*. 1995;39:2367–2370.

317. Zenilman JM. Gonococcal susceptibility to antimicrobials in Baltimore, 1988–1994: What was the impact of ciprofloxacin as first-line therapy for gonorrhea? *Sex Transm Dis*. 1996;23:213–218.

318. Handsfield HH, Whitlington WL. Antibiotic-resistant *Neisseria gonorrhoeae*: The calm before another storm? *Ann Intern Med*. 1996;125:507–509.

319. Stamm WE, Hicks CB, Martin DH, et al. Azithromycin for empirical treatment of nongonococcal urethritis syndrome in men: A randomized double-blind study. *JAMA*. 1995;274:545–549.

320. Schmid GP, Fontanarosa PB. Evolving strategies for management of the nongonococcal urethritis syndrome. *JAMA*. 1995;274:577–579.

321. Magid D, Douglas JM, Schwartz JS. Doxycycline compared with azithromycin for treating women with genital *Chlamydia trachomatis* infections: An incremental cost-effectiveness analysis. *Ann Intern Med*. 1996;124:389–399.

322. Hillis S, Black C, Newhall J, Walsh C, Groseclose SL. New opportunities for chlamydia prevention: Applications of science to public health practice. *Sex Transm Dis*. 1995;22:197–202.

323. Lavin B, Putnam S, Rockhill R, Schachter J, Oldfield E. Asymptomatic carriage of *Chlamydia trachomatis* and *Neisseria gonorrhoeae* in active duty males deployed to the western Pacific. Interscience Conference on Antimicrobial Agents and Chemotherapy; 29 September–2 October 1991; Chicago. Abstract 72.

324. Orndorff GR. Screening for *Chlamydia trachomatis* by the direct fluorescent antibody test in female navy recruits. *Mil Med*. 1991;156:675–677.

325. Langenberg A, Benedetti J, Jenkins J, et al. Development of clinically recognizable genital lesions among women previously identified as having "asymptomatic" herpes simplex virus type 2 infection. *Ann Intern Med*. 1989;110:882–887.

326. Wasserheit JN. Epidemiological synergy: Interrelationships between human immunodeficiency virus infection and other sexually transmitted diseases. *Sex Transm Dis*. 1992;19:61–77.

327. Pepin J, Plummer FA, Brunham RC, Piot P, Cameron DW, Ronald AR. The interaction of HIV infection and other sexually transmitted diseases: An opportunity for intervention. *AIDS*. 1989;3:3–9.

328. Laga M, Alary M, Nzila N, et al. Condom promotion, sexually transmitted diseases treatment, and declining incidence of HIV-1 infection in female Zairian sex workers. *Lancet*. 1994;344:246–248.

329. Aral SO. Heterosexual transmission of HIV: The role of other sexually transmitted infections and behavior in its epidemiology, prevention, and control. *Ann Rev Public Health*. 1993;14:451–467.

330. Nzila N, Laga M, Thiam MA, et al. HIV and other sexually transmitted diseases among female prostitutes in Kinshasa. *AIDS*. 1991;5:715–721.

331. Laga M, Manoka A, Kivuvu M, et al. Non-ulcerative sexually transmitted diseases as risk factors for HIV-1 transmission in women: Results of a cohort study. *AIDS*. 1993;7:95–102.

332. Brown AE, Newby JH, Ray KL, Jackson JN, Burke DS. Prevention and treatment of HIV infections in minorities in the U.S. military: A review of military research. *Mil Med*. 1996;161:123–127.

333. Burke DS, Brundage JF, Herbold JR, et al. Human immunodeficiency virus infections among civilian applicants for United States military service, October 1985 to March 1986: Demographic factors associated with seropositivity. *N Engl J Med*. 1987;317:131–136.

334. Centers for Disease Control. Prevalence of human immunodeficiency virus antibody in U.S. active duty military personnel, April 1988. *MMWR*. 1988;37:461–463.

335. McNeil JG, Brundage JF, Wann ZF, Burke DS, Miller RN, Walter Reed Retrovirus Research Group. Direct measurement of human immunodeficiency virus seroconversion in a serially tested population of young adults in the United States Army, October 1985 to October 1987. *N Engl J Med*. 1989;320:1581–1585.

336. Trump DH. Presentation to the Armed Forces Epidemiological Board Meeting; February, 26 1996; Washington, DC.

337. Garland FC, Garland CF, Gorham ED, et al. Lack of association of human immunodeficiency virus seroconversion with visits to foreign ports in US Navy personnel. *Arch Intern Med*. 1993;153:2685–2691.

338. Cowan DN, Brundage JF, Pomerantz RS. The incidence of HIV infection among men in the United States Army Reserve components, 1985–1991. *AIDS*. 1994;8:505–511.

339. Tramont EC, Burke DS. AIDS/HIV in the US military. *Vaccine*. 1993;11:529–533.

340. Kelley PW, Takafuji ET, Tramont EC, et al. The importance of HIV infection for the military. In: Wormser GP, Stahl RE, Bottone EJ, eds. *AIDS—Acquired Immune Deficiency Syndrome—and Other Manifestations of HIV Infection: Epidemiology, Etiology, Immunology, Clinical Manifestations, Pathology, Control, Treatment, and Prevention*. Park Ridge, NJ: Noyes Publications; 1987: 67–85.

341. Brown AE, Tomlinson JP, Brundage JF, Burke DS. The U.S. Army HIV testing program: The first decade. *Mil Med*. 1996;161:117–121.

342. Warren WR. The epidemiology of infectious hepatitis. *US Armed Forces Med J*. 1953;4:313–335.

343. Gauld RL. Epidemiological field studies of infectious hepatitis in the Mediterranean Theater of Operations: Clinical syndrome, morbidity, mortality, seasonal incidence. *Am J Hyg*. 1946;43:248–254.

344. Hillis WD. Viral hepatitis: An unconquered foe. *Mil Med*. 1968;133:343–354.

345. Mortimer PP. Arsphenamine jaundice and the recognition of instrument-borne virus infection. *Genitourin Med*. 1995;71:109–119.

346. Norman JE, Beebe GW, Hoofnagle JH, Seeff LB. Mortality follow-up of the 1942 epidemic of hepatitis B in the U.S. Army. *Hepatology*. 1993;18:790–797.

347. Seeff LB, Beebe GW, Hoofnagle JH, et al. A serologic follow-up of the 1942 epidemic of post-vaccination hepatitis in the United States Army. *N Engl J Med*. 1987;316:965–970.

348. Stout RW, Mitchell SB, Parkinson MD, et al. Viral hepatitis in the U.S. Air Force, 1980–89: An epidemiological and serological study. *Aviat Space Environ Med*. 1994;65(Suppl 5):A66–A70.

349. Jaundice following yellow fever vaccine. *JAMA*. 1942;119:1110.

350. Stokes J Jr, Neefe J. The prevention and attenuation of infectious hepatitis by gamma globulin. *JAMA*. 1945;127:144–145.

351. Gellis SS, Stokes J Jr, Brother GM, et al. The use of human immune serum globulin (gamma globulin). *JAMA*. 1945;128:1062–1063.

352. Krugman S. Effect of human immune serum globulin on infectivity of hepatitis A virus. *J Infect Dis*. 1976;134:70–74.

353. Aach RD, Elsea WR, Lyerly J. Gamma globulin in epidemic hepatitis: Comparative value of two dosage levels, apparently near the minimal effective level. *JAMA*. 1969;53:1623–1629.

354. Fowinkle EW, Guthrie N. Comparison of two doses of gamma globulin in prevention of infectious hepatitis. *Public Health Rep.* 1964;79:643–647.

355. Prophylactic gamma globulin for prevention of endemic hepatitis: Effects of US gamma globulin upon the incidence of viral hepatitis and other infectious diseases in US soldiers abroad. *Arch Intern Med.* 1971;128:723–738.

356. Binn LN, Lemon SM, Marchwicki RH, Redfield RR, Gates NL, Bancroft WH. Primary isolation and serial passage of hepatitis A virus strains in primate cell cultures. *J Clin Microbiol.* 1984;20:28–33.

357. Schreiber GB, Busch MP, Kleinman SH, Korelitz JJ. The risk of transfusion-transmitted viral infections: The Retrovirus Epidemiology Donor study. *N Engl J Med.* 1996;334:1685–1690.

358. Hyams KC, Krogwold RA, Brock S, et al. Heterosexual transmission of viral hepatitis and cytomegalovirus infection among United States military personnel stationed in the western Pacific. *Sex Transm Dis.* 1993;20:36–40.

359. Hawkins RE, Malone JD, Cloninger LA, et al. Risk of viral hepatitis among military personnel assigned to US Navy ships. *J Infect Dis.* 1992;165:716–719.

360. Gust ID, Feinstone SM. *Hepatitis A.* Boca Raton, Fla: CRC Press; 1988.

361. Siegl G, Weitz M, Kronauer G. Stability of hepatitis A virus. *Intervirology.* 1984;22:218–226.

362. Robinson WS, Marion PL, Feitelson M, et al. The hepadnavirus group: Hepatitis B and related viruses. In: Szumess W, Alter HJ, Maynard JE, eds. *Viral Hepatitis.* Philadelphia: Franklin Institute Press; 1982.

363. Ohba K, Mizokami M, Lau JY, Orito E, Ikeo K, Gojobori T. Evolutionary relationship of hepatitis C, pesti-, flavi-, plantviruses, and newly discovered GB hepatitis agents. *FEBS Lett.* 1996;378 (3):232–234.

364. Smedile A, Rizzetto M, Gerin JL. Advances in hepatitis D virus biology and disease. *Prog Liver Dis.* 1994;12:157–175.

365. Bradley DW. Hepatitis E virus: A brief review of the biology, molecular virology, and immunology of a novel virus. *J Hepatol.* 1995;22 (Suppl 1):140–145.

366. Balayan MS, Usmanov RK, Zamyatina NA, Djumalieva DI, Karas FR. Brief report: Experimental hepatitis E infection in domestic pigs. *J Med Virol.* 1990;32:58–59.

367. Clayson ET, Innis BL, Myint KS, et al. Detection of hepatitis E virus infections among domestic swine in the Kathmandu Valley of Nepal. *Am J Trop Med Hyg.* 1995;53:228–232.

368. Deka N, Sharma MD, Mukerjee R. Isolation of the novel agent from human stool samples that is associated with sporadic non-A, non-B hepatitis. *J Virol.* 1994;68:7810–7815.

369. Uchida T, Shimojima M, Gotoh K, Shikata T, Tanaka E, Kiyosawa K. "Silent" hepatitis B virus mutants are responsible for non-A, non-B, non-C, non-D, non-E hepatitis. *Microbiol Immunol.* 1994;38:281–285.

370. Linnen J, Wages J Jr, Zhang-Keck ZY, et al. Molecular cloning and disease association of hepatitis G virus: A transfusion-transmissible agent. *Science.* 1996;271:505–508.

371. Alter MJ, Gallagher M, Morris TT, et al. Acute non-A-E hepatitis in the United States and the role of hepatitis G virus infection: Sentinel Counties Viral Hepatitis Study Team. *N Engl J Med.* 1997;336:741–746.

372. Alter HJ, Nakatsuji Y, Melpolder J, et al. The incidence of transfusion-associated hepatitis G virus infections and its relation to liver disease. *N Engl J Med.* 1997;336:747–754.

373. Lemon SM. The natural history of hepatitis A: The potential for transmission by transfusion of blood or blood products. *Vox Sang.* 1994;67 (Suppl 4):19–23.

374. Nanda SK, Ansari IH, Acharya SK, Jameel S, Panda SK. Protracted viremia during acute sporadic hepatitis E virus infection. *Gastroenterology.* 1995;108:225–230.

375. Jackson LA, Stewart LK, Solomon SL, et al. Risk of infection with hepatitis A, B, or C, cytomegalovirus, varicella, or measles among child care providers. *Pediatr Infect Dis J.* 1996;15:584–589.

376. Benenson MW, Takafuji ET, Bancroft WH, Lemon SM, Callahan MC, Leach DA. A military community outbreak of hepatitis type A related to transmission in a child care facility. *Am J Epidemiol.* 1980;112:471–481.

377. Gregg MB. The changing epidemiology of viral hepatitis in the United States. *Am J Dis Child.* 1972;123:350–354.

378. Balayan MS, Andjaparidze AG, Savinskaya SS, et al. Evidence for a virus in non-A, non-B hepatitis transmitted via the fecal-oral route. *Intervirology.* 1983;20:23–31.

379. Skidmore SJ, Yarbrough PO, Gabor KA, Reyes GR. Hepatitis E virus: The cause of a waterborne hepatitis outbreak. *J Med Virol.* 1992;37:58–60.

380. Arankalle VA, Tsarev SA, Chadha MS, et al. Age specific prevalence of antibodies to hepatitis A and E viruses in Pune, India, 1982 and 1992. *J Infect Dis.* 1995;171:447–450.

381. Lurman A. Eine icterus epidemic. *Berl Klin Wochenschr.* 1855;22:20.

382. Blumberg BS, Alter HJ, Visnich S. A "new" antigen in leukemia serum. *JAMA.* 1965;191:541.

383. Shikata T, Karasawa T, Abe K, et al. Hepatitis B e antigens and infectivity of hepatitis B virus. *J Infect Dis.* 1977;136:571–576.

384. Hadler SC, Doto IL, Maynard JE, et al. Occupational risk of hepatitis B infection in hospital workers. *Infect Control.* 1985;6:24–31.

385. Yao GB. Importance of perinatal versus horizontal transmission of hepatitis B virus infection in China. *Gut.* 1996;38 (Suppl 2):S39–42.

386. Hyams KC. Risks of chronicity following acute hepatitis B virus infection: A review. *Clin Infect Dis.* 1995;20:992–1000.

387. Kao JH, Hwang YT, Chen PJ, et al. Transmission of hepatitis C virus between spouses: The important role of exposure duration. *Am J Gastroenterol.* 1996;91:2087–2090.

388. Eyster ME, Alter HJ, Aledort LM, Quan S, Hatzakis A, Boedert JJ. Heterosexual co-transmission of hepatitis C virus (HCV) and human immunodeficiency virus (HIV). *Ann Intern Med.* 1991;115:764–768.

389. Ohto H, Terzawa S, Sasaki N, et al. Transmission of hepatitis C virus from mothers to infants. *N Engl J Med.* 1994;330:744–750.

390. Wacker WEC, Riordan JF, Snodgrass PJ, et al. The Holy Cross hepatitis outbreak: Clinical and chemical abnormalities. *Arch Intern Med.* 1972;130:357–360.

391. Neefe JR, Gellis SS, Stokes J Jr. Homologous serum hepatitis and infectious (epidemic) hepatitis: Studies in volunteers bearing on immunological and other characteristics of the etiological agents. *Am J Med.* 1946;1:3–42.

392. Krugman S, Giles JP, Hammond J. Infectious hepatitis: Evidence for two distinctive clinical, epidemiological, and immunological types of infection. *JAMA.* 1967;200:365–373.

393. Smith FR, Henkin RI, Dell RB. Disordered gustatory acuity in liver disease. *Gastroenterology.* 1976;70:568–571.

394. Krugman S, Ward R, Giles JP. The natural history of infectious hepatitis. *Am J Med.* 1962;32:717–728.

395. Gordon SC, Reddy KR, Schiff L, Schiff ER. Prolonged intrahepatic cholestasis secondary to acute hepatitis A. *Ann Intern Med*. 1984;101:635–637.

396. Glikson M, Galun E, Oren R, Tur-Kaspa R, Shouval D. Relapsing hepatitis A: Review of 14 cases and literature survey. *Medicine (Baltimore)*. 1992;71:14–23.

397. Sjogren MH, Tanno H, Fay O, et al. Hepatitis A virus in stool during clinical relapse. *Ann Intern Med*. 1987;106:221–226.

398. Bernuau J, Rueff B, Benhamou JP. Fulminant and subfulminant liver failure: Definitions and causes. *Semin Liver Dis*. 1986;6:97–106.

399. Paul RJ, Havens WP, Sabin AB, et al. Transmission experiments in serum jaundice and infectious hepatitis. *JAMA*. 1945;128:911.

400. Gocke DJ. Extrahepatic manifestations of viral hepatitis. *Am J Med Sci*. 1975;270:49–52.

401. Fattovich G, Brollo L, Giustina G, et al. Natural history and prognostic factors for chronic hepatitis type B. *Gut*. 1991;32:294–298.

402. Sherlock S, Fox RA, Niazi SP, Scheuer PJ. Chronic liver disease and primary liver-cell cancer with hepatitis-associated (Australia) antigen in serum. *Lancet*. 1970;1:1243–1237.

403. Esteban JL, Genesca J, Alter HJ. Hepatitis C: Molecular biology, pathogenesis, epidemiology, clinical features, and prevention. *Prog Liver Dis*. 1992;10:253–282.

404. Gordon FD, Anastopoulos H, Khettry U, et al. Hepatitis C infection: A rare cause of fulminant hepatic failure. *Am J Gastroenterol*. 1995;90:117–120.

405. Iwarson S, Norkrans G, Wejstal R. Hepatitis C: Natural history of a unique infection. *Clin Inf Dis*. 1995;20:1361–1370.

406. Alter HJ, Hoofnagle JH. Non-A, non-B: Observations on the first decade. In: Vyas GN, Dienstag JL, Hoofnagle JH, eds. *Viral Hepatitis and Liver Disease*. Orlando, Fla: Grune and Stratton; 1984: 345–355.

407. Wejstal R, Widell A, Norkrans G. Hepatitis C virus infection with progression to hepatocellular carcinoma: A report of five prospectively followed patients in Sweden. *Scand J Infect Dis*. 1993;25:417–420.

408. Cacoub P, Fabiani FL, Musset L, et al. Mixed cryoglobulinemia and hepatitis C virus. *Am J Med*. 1994;96:124–132.

409. Johnson RJ, Gretch DR, Yamabe H, et al. Membranoproliferative glomerulonephritis associated with hepatitis C virus infection. *N Engl J Med*. 1993;328:465–470.

410. Gumber SC, Chpora S. Hepatitis C, a multifaceted disease: Review of extrahepatic manifestations. *Ann Intern Med*. 1995;123:615–620.

411. Hoofnagle JH. Type D (Delta) hepatitis. *JAMA*. 1989;261:1321–1325.

412. Farci P, Gerin JL, Aragona M, et al. Diagnostic and prognostic significance of the IgM antibody to the hepatitis delta virus. *JAMA*. 1986;255;1443–1446.

413. Rizzetto M, Gerin JL, Purcell RH, eds. *Hepatitis Delta Virus and Its Infection*. New York: Alan R. Liss; 1987.

414. Fattovich G, Boscaro S, Noventa F, et al. Influence of hepatitis delta virus infection on progression to cirrhosis in chronic hepatitis type B. *J Infect Dis*. 1987;155:931–935.

415. Khuroo MS. Study of an epidemic of non-A, non-B hepatitis: Possibility of another human hepatitis virus distinct from post-transfusion non-A, non-B type. *Am J Med*. 1980;68:818–824.

416. Khuroo MS, Rustgi VK, Dawson GJ, et al. Spectrum of hepatitis E virus infection in India. *J Med Virol.* 1994;43:281–286.

417. Nanda SK, Ansari IH, Acharya SK, Jameel S, Panda SK. Protracted viremia during acute sporadic hepatitis E virus infection. *Gastroenterology.* 1995;108:225–230.

418. Lok AS, Soldevila-Pico C. Epidemiology and serologic diagnosis of hepatitis E. *J Hepatol.* 1994;20:567–569.

419. Khuroo MS, Kamili S, Jameel S. Vertical transmission of hepatitis E virus. *Lancet.* 1995;345:1025–1026.

420. Rubertone MV, DeFraites RF, Krauss MR, Brandt CA. An outbreak of hepatitis A during a military field training exercise. *Mil Med.* 1993;158:37–41.

421. McCarthy MC, Burans JP, Constantine NT, et al. Hepatitis B and HIV in Sudan: A serosurvey for hepatitis B and human inmmunodeficiency virus antibodies among sexually active heterosexuals. *Am J Trop Med Hyg.* 1989;41:726–731.

422. Oldfield EC, Wallace MR, Hyams KC, Yousif AA, Lewis DE, Bourgeois AL. Endemic infectious disease of the Middle East. *Rev Infect Dis.* 1991;13(Suppl 3):S199–S217.

423. Alter MJ, Margolis HS, Krawczynski K, et al. The natural history of community-acquired hepatitis C in the United States. *N Engl J Med.* 1992;327:1899–1905.

424. Zaaijer HL, Cuypers HTM, Reesink HW, Winkel IN, Gerken G, Lelie PN. Reliability of polymerase chain reaction for detection of hepatitis C virus. *Lancet.* 1993;341:722–724.

425. Paul DA, Knigge MF, Ritter A, et al. Determination of hepatitis E virus seroprevalence by using recombinant fusion proteins and synthetic peptides. *J Infect Dis.* 1994;169:801–806.

426. Blum AL, Stutz R, Haemmerli UP, Schmid P, Grady GF. A fortuitously controlled study of steroid therapy in acute viral hepatitis, I: Acute disease. *Am J Med.* 1969;47:82–92.

427. Gregory PB, Knauer CM, Miller R, Kempson RL. Steroid therapy in severe viral hepatitis: A double-blind, randomized trial of methyl-prednisolone versus placebo. *N Engl J Med.* 1976;294:681–687.

428. Hoofnagle JH, DiBisceglie AM. The treatment of chronic viral hepatitis. *N Engl J Med.* 1997;336:347–356.

429. Wong DKH, Cheung AM, O'Rourke K, et al. Effect of alpha-interferon treatment in patients with hepatitis B e antigen-positive chronic hepatitis B: A meta-analysis. *Ann Intern Med.* 1993;119:312–323.

430. McKenzie R, Fried MW, Sallie R, et al. Hepatic failure and lactic acidosis due to fialuridine (FIAU), an investigational nucleoside analogue for chronic hepatitis B. *N Engl J Med.* 1995;333:1099–1105.

431. Gish RG, Lau JY, Brooks L, et al. Ganciclovir treatment of hepatitis B virus infection in liver transplant recipients. *Hepatology.* 1996;23(1):1–7.

432. Dienstag JL, Perrillo RP, Schiff ER, Bartholomew M, Vicary C, Rubin M. A preliminary trial of lamivudine for chronic hepatitis B infection. *N Engl J Med.* 1995;333:1657–1661.

433. Davis GL, Balart LA, Schiff ER, et al. Treatment of chronic hepatitis C with recombinant interferon alfa: A multicenter, randomized, controlled trial. *N. Engl J Med.* 1989;321:1501–1506.

434. DiBisceglie AM, Conjeevaram HS, Fried MW, et al. Ribavirin as therapy for chronic hepatitis C: A randomized, double-blind, placebo-controlled trial. *Ann Intern Med.* 1995;123:897–903.

435. Tsutsumi M, Takada A, Sawada M. Efficacy of combination therapy with interferon and azidothymidine in chronic type C hepatitis: A pilot study. *J Gastroenterol.* 1995;30:485–492.

436. Pardo M, Castillo I, Navas S, Carreno V. Treatment of chronic hepatitis C with cirrhosis with recombinant human granulocyte colony-stimulating factor plus recombinant interferon-alpha. *J Med Virol.* 1995;45:439–444.

437. Yoshioka K, Higashi Y, Yamada M, et al. Predictive factors in the response to interferon therapy in chronic hepatitis C. *Liver.* 1995;15(2):57–62.

438. Farci P, Mandas A, Coiana A, et al. Treatment of chronic hepatitis D with interferon alfa-2a. *N Engl J Med.* 1994;330:88–94.

439. Lidofsky SD. Liver transplantation for fulminant hepatic failure. *Gastroenterol Clin North Am.* 1993;22:257–269.

440. Burans JP, Sharp TW, Wallace M, et al. Threat of hepatitis E virus infection in Somalia during Operation Restore Hope. *Clin Infect Dis.* 1994;18:100–102.

441. Buisson Y, Coursaget P, Bercion R, Anne D, Debord T, Roue R. Hepatitis E virus infection in soldiers sent to endemic regions. *Lancet.* 1994;344:1165–1166.

442. Peter G, ed. *1997 Red Book: Report of the Committee on Infectious Diseases.* 24th ed. Elk Grove Village, Ill: American Academy of Pediatrics; 1997.

443. Benenson AS, ed. *1995 Control of Communicable Diseases Manual.* 16th ed. Washington, DC: American Public Health Association; 1995.

444. Green MS, Cohen D, Lerman Y, et al. Depression of the immune response to an inactivated hepatitis A vaccine administered concomitantly with immune globulin. *J Infect Dis.* 1993;168:740–743.

445. Innis BL, Snitbhan R, Kunasol P, et al. Protection against hepatitis A by an inactivated vaccine. *JAMA.* 1994;271:1328–1334.

446. Werzberger A, Mensch B, Kuter B, et al. A controlled trial of a formalin-inactivated hepatitis A vaccine in healthy children. *N Engl J Med.* 1992;327:453–457.

447. Hoke CH, Binn LN, Egan JE, et al. Hepatitis A in the US Army: Epidemiology and vaccine development. *Vaccine.* 1992;10 Suppl 1;S75–S79.

448. Bancroft WH. Hepatitis A vaccine. *N Engl J Med.* 1992;327:488–490.

449. Mannucci PM, Gdovin S, Gringeri A, et al. Transmission of hepatitis A to patients with hemophilia by factor VIII concentrates treated with organic solvent and detergent to inactivate virus. *Ann Intern Med.* 1994;120:1–7.

450. Assistant Secretary of Defense (Health Affairs). Policy for Use of Hepatitis A Virus (HAV) Vaccine and Immune Globulin (IG). Washington, DC: Department of Defense; 12 August 1996. HA Policy 96-054.

451. Armed Forces Epidemiology Meeting, February 1996.

452. Lemon SM, Thomas DL. Vaccines to prevent viral hepatitis. *N Engl J Med.* 1997;336:196–204.

453. Tsarev SA, Tsareva TS, Emerson SU, et al. Successful passive and active immunization of cynomolgus monkeys against hepatitis E. *Proc Natl Acad Sci USA.* 1994;91:10198–10202.

Chapter 39

DISEASES CONTROLLED PRIMARILY BY VACCINATION

Coleen Weese, MD, MPH; Kathryn Clark, MD, MPH; David Goldman, MD, MPH; and Paula K. Underwood, MD, MPH

MEASLES

RUBELLA

MUMPS

VARICELLA

PERTUSSIS

TETANUS

DIPHTHERIA

POLIO

C. Weese, MD, MPH; Program Manager, Occupational and Environmental Medicine Program, US Army Center for Health Promotion and Preventive Medicine, Aberdeen Proving Ground, MD 21010-5422; Formerly, Major, Medical Corps, US Army; Acting Chief, Disease Control and Prevention Division, US Army Center for Health Promotion and Preventive Medicine, Aberdeen Proving Ground, MD 21010-5422

K. Clark, MD, MPH; Infectious Disease Analyst, Armed Forces Medical Intelligence Center, 1607 Porter St., Fort Detrick, Frederick, MD 21702-5004; Formerly, Accession Medical Standards Analysis and Research Activity Coordinator, Division of Preventive Medicine, Walter Reed Army Institute of Research, Washington, DC 20307-5100

D. Goldman, MD, MPH; Director, Rappahannock Area Health District, Virginia Department of Health, 608 Jackson Street, Fredericksburg, VA 22401; Formerly, Major, Medical Corps, US Army; Command Surgeon, On-site Inspection Agency, Washington, DC 20041-0498

P.K. Underwood, MD, MPH; Colonel, Medical Corps, US Army; Preventive Medicine Staff Officer, Proponency Office for Preventive Medicine at the office of The Surgeon General, 5111 Leesburg Pike, Falls Church, VA 22041

MEASLES

Introduction and Military Relevance

Measles (rubeola) has been called "the simplest of all infectious diseases."[1] It has a relatively distinct, homogeneous, and invariant etiology and pathogenesis. A high level of infectivity and relative lack of subclinical cases have contributed to its well-characterized epidemiology. It was first described in the 7th century but was not considered distinct from smallpox until 1629.[2] In 1758, attempts to prevent it through a process similar to variolization (application of smallpox crusts to susceptibles) was performed by Home and known as morbillization; it was mildly successful but never widely practiced.[3] The epidemiology of measles was elegantly described by Panum following an outbreak in the highly susceptible population of the Faroe Islands.[4] In the prevaccine era, most cases of measles in the United States occurred in children, although outbreaks in susceptible military recruits have been well documented.[5] A vaccine licensed in 1963 eventually resulted in a 99% decrease in measles cases in the United States, although there was a relative resurgence of cases in 1989 through 1991.[6] Elimination is currently a goal in the United States and elsewhere.[6,7]

Measles has been a constant presence during military deployments. During the Civil War, the case rate per 1,000 man-years was 32.2; during World War I, it was 26.1/1,000.[2] By World War II, the disease rate in the military had dropped to 4.7/1,000, and it was 0.9/1,000 during the Vietnam era. This pattern is similar to that seen with other contagious diseases and is thought to reflect a decreased number of susceptibles left in successive cohorts as travel and urbanization became more commonplace. In 1962, 98.8% of military recruits had measurable levels of antibody to measles.[8] Even with low population susceptibility rates, however, the virus circulates in large population clusters. Thus, military recruits experienced outbreaks before widespread vaccine use.[5] This was problematic for the involved installations and, because of the high mobility of these populations, for other posts and the surrounding civilian populations as well when servicemembers went home on leave. Transmission on posts extended to daycare centers and schools. In 1979 and the first half of 1980, about 9% of the reported measles cases in the United States were military cases.[9] Subsequent to the change in policy that mandated giving measles and rubella vaccine to recruits in 1980, cases were rare among the more than 750,000-member-strong active duty Army. In 1989, though, 12 confirmed and presumptive measles cases occurred among basic trainees at Fort Leonard Wood, Missouri, where immunization was delayed until the second week of basic training. Measles can also be a problem after training ends. For deployable military personnel, the risk of acquiring measles during worldwide deployments for humanitarian assistance missions remains high, particularly in Africa and Asia.

Description of the Pathogen

The causative agent of clinical measles is the measles virus, a member of the family *Paramyxovirida* and genus *Morbillivirus;* it is closely related to the viruses of canine distemper and rinderpest.[2] It is a spherical, single-stranded RNA virus. The only known reservoir is humans.

Epidemiology

Transmission

Measles is a ubiquitous, highly contagious, seasonal disease that affects nearly every person in a given population by the age of adolescence in the absence of immunzation programs. Infection at some point in life is the rule.[2] The virus is transmitted by airborne droplet spread, by direct contact with nasal or throat secretions of infected persons, and, less commonly, by fomites. Maximal dissemination of the virus occurs during the prodromal (or catarrhal) stage. In temperate climates, infections occur primarily in the late winter and early spring.[10] Measles is endemic in large urban areas, with epidemics occurring every second or third year. In smaller communities, outbreaks are more widely spread and severe. As demonstrated by Panum, island populations can remain free of infection for variable periods.[4] On reintroduction of the virus, epidemics of the disease strike all those not affected by the last wave. Thus, although transmission usually occurs among children, outbreaks in isolated communities include many older individuals, as was documented in the Faroe Islands. Overall, it is estimated that a herd immunity of greater than 95% may be needed to interrupt community transmission.[2] Immunization of 15-month-old children produces immunity in 95% to 98% of recipients; reimmunization may increase levels to 99%.[11]

Geographic Distribution

Measles is epidemic worldwide and is often a problem when people are displaced and congregated in settings such as refugee camps. Importations contribute to transmission in the United States.[6] Isolates currently circulating in the United States are similar to strains identified in Japan and Europe. Measles activity in the Western hemisphere is currently considered low, and elimination campaigns continue in the Americas.[7]

Incidence

Prior to vaccine use in the United States, epidemics affected largely children aged 5 to 9 years.[2] Average age at infection typically correlated with the age at which susceptible children increased their contacts outside the home. With the licensure of vaccine in 1963, cases declined from 450,000 per year to less than 50,000 per year in the United States by 1968.[12] The number of cases continued to decline, although small epidemics intervened in 1971 and 1977. During the late 1970s, elimination of measles was considered an achievable goal, with fewer than 5,000 cases documented through 1985. Measles resurged nationwide from 1989 to 1991, and incidence was highest among unvaccinated preschool-aged children.[13] An estimated 55,000 cases occurred during 1989 to 1990. In communities experiencing outbreaks, immunization of children at 12 months of age was conducted to protect them, with follow-up immunization at 15 to 18 months of age because of concern over the adequacy of resultant antibody levels in that age group. Additionally, immunization campaigns were conducted to increase awareness and coverage, and cases of measles once again declined. Between 1993 and 1995, an increasing proportion of cases were reported among older age groups, representing failure to vaccinate as well as vaccine failure.[6] Serosurveys conducted with US Army recruits in 1989 demonstrated overall that only 82.8% of the sample were seropositive by commercial enzyme immunosorbent assay.[14] Younger recruits were more likely to be seronegative, representing a cohort that may have missed both immunization and naturally acquired illness due to declining rates.

In 1995, 301 confirmed measles cases were reported, representing the lowest number in a single year since measles became reportable in 1912.[6] Although the number of cases is small, it provides evidence that the second dose of measles vaccine has not been uniformly implemented in all cohorts.

Among the 96 cases who were not vaccinated, 56 were eligible for vaccine.

Worldwide, almost a million persons, mostly infants and young children, die annually from measles.[11] Poor nutrition and rapid loss of maternal antibody place infants at risk, and early exposure to the community and prolonged viral excretion result in infection. The case-fatality rates in developing countries are estimated to be 3% to 5% globally, but are commonly 10% to 30% in some localities.[1] In the spring of 2000, 2,961 cases of measles with three deaths and 68 hospitalizations occurred in the Netherlands. Although two-dose measles vaccines is recommended in the Netherlands, vaccine is not required for school attendance. The Netherlands has a large sub-population that refrains from vaccination on religious grounds. For this reason, measles epidemics occur in the Netherlands every 5 to 7 years.[15]

Pathogenesis and Clinical Findings

Measles is characterized by a prodromal fever, conjunctivitis, coryza, cough, and Koplik spots on the buccal mucosa.[10] A characteristic red, blotchy rash appears on the third to seventh day following exposure, beginning on the face, becoming generalized, lasting 4 to 7 days and sometimes ending in brawny desquamation.[1] Leukopenia is common. The incubation period from exposure to onset of fever is about 10 days, varying from 7 to 18 days; usually it is 14 days until the rash appears. Cases are infectious from the beginning of the prodromal period to 4 days after the appearance of the rash. The disease is more severe in infants and adults. Complications result from viral replication and bacterial superinfection and include otitis media, pneumonia, laryngotracheobronchitis (croup), diarrhea, and encephalitis. Subacute sclerosing panencephalitis develops very rarely (about 1 in 100,000 cases) several years after infection; over 50% of these cases have had measles diagnosed in the first 2 years of life.[10] Infection in pregnancy is not related to congenital malformations but has been associated with an increase in spontaneous abortions. The clinical course can be prolonged, severe, and fatal in the immunocompromised. The Immunization Practices Advisory Council's current recommendations include the immunization of those with human immunodeficiency virus to preclude the development of severe or potentially fatal naturally acquired measles.[16] In children who are borderline nourished, measles often precipitates acute kwashiorkor and exacerbates vitamin A deficiency, leading to blindness. In malnourished children, measles may be associated with hemorrhagic rash, protein-losing enteropathy, otitis media, oral sores, dehydration, diarrhea, blindness, and severe skin infections.[10] Children with clinical or subclinical vitamin A deficiency are at particularly high risk.

Diagnostic Approaches

Compared with other exanthematous diseases, measles infections can be diagnosed clinically with relative accuracy. A case definition of rash, cough, and fever present at the onset of rash was demonstrated to have a sensitivity of 92% and a specificity of 57%.[17] Koplik spots are pathognomonic for measles, and a diagnosis of measles should not be made if cough is absent.[18] The differential diagnosis includes exanthem subitum (roseola infantum), in which the rash appears as the fever subsides; rubella; and enteroviral infections, which have less striking rashes and generally milder illness. Rickettsial infections may have cough, but headache is more prominent. Meningococcemia may have a similar rash but no cough or conjunctivitis. Scarlet fever has a rash that is confluent, textured, and most marked on the abdomen. Serological confirmation includes complement fixation, neutralization, and hemagglutination inhibition assays.[1] Enzyme-linked immunosorbent assays for measles IgG and IgM are widely available and convenient. Classic confirmation involves an increase in antibodies between acute and convalescent specimens. The use of IgM antibody assays allows for the diagnosis from the analysis of a single acute sample, if it is taken at least 2 days after the onset of rash.

Recommendations for Therapy and Control

Therapy is supportive. There is no specific treatment.

In the prevaccine era, approximately one birth cohort of 4 million persons was infected annually. In 1985 dollars, the estimated cost of these infections was $670 milllion.[19] The low number of cases of measles and shift in age distribution in the United States highlight the effectiveness and improved implementation of the Advisory Council's recommendations to provide the first dose of measles-mumps-rubella vaccine (MMR) at 12 to 15 months of age, with a second dose to address primary vaccine failure at either 4 to 6 or 11 to 12 years of age.[16] During outbreaks, observed attack rates in those who had received measles vaccine 15 years or more before reexposure have been approximately 5% or less.[1] During 1994 and 1995, coverage with measles

vaccine was 89% among children aged 19 to 35 months, and an estimated 33% to 50% of school-aged children had received a second dose of MMR. Additionally, some states have mandated a prematiculation immunization requirement at colleges.[20]

As school requirements for second doses of MMR become the rule, the actual need for measles-rubella vaccine administration to recruits should diminish. As long as verification of vaccine status of recruits remains incomplete, however, it is a prudent practice. A second dose of MMR is recommended for health care workers and travelers. Furthermore, anyone vaccinated with a killed vaccine or a killed vaccine followed by a live vaccine within a 3-month period and anyone vaccinated between 1963 and 1967 with a vaccine of unknown type should be revaccinated.[1] Killed vaccine produced a short-lived immunity that was often associated with subsequent atypical measles—a milder but more prolonged illness.

About 5% to 15% of nonimmune vaccinees may develop malaise and fever up to 39.4°C within 5 to 12 days postimmunization and lasting 1 to 2 days but causing little disability.[10] Rash, coryza, mild cough, and Koplik spots may occasionally occur. Febrile seizures occur infrequently and without sequelae. Encephalitis and encephalopathy have been seen in approximately 1 to 3 cases per million doses distributed. The vaccine may be administered at the same time as other live vaccines and inactivated vaccines or toxoids. Contraindications include allergy to egg or neomycin, severe acute illness, and immunosuppression. Vaccination poses a theoretical risk to pregnant females, and vaccinees should be advised of the risk of fetal wastage if they become pregnant within 1 month of receiving monovalent measles vaccine or 3 months after receiving MMR.

In the event of an outbreak, vaccine given within 72 hours of exposure may provide protection.[9] If given after 72 hours, it may prolong the incubation period rather than prevent disease. Immune globulin may be given within 6 days of exposure for susceptible household members or other contacts for whom the risk is very high (eg, contacts under 1 year of age, pregnant women, immunocompromised persons) or for whom measles vaccine is contraindicated.[10] The dose is 0.25 mL/kg. For immunocompromised persons, the dose is 0.5 mL/kg up to 15 mL. Measles vaccine should be given 6 to 7 months later if there is no contraindication. Transmission to susceptible contacts often occurs before the diagnosis of the original case has been established. Isolation precautions to prevent spread, especially in hospitals or institutions that care for children, should be maintained from the seventh day after exposure until about 5 days after the rash has appeared. If vaccine is available, prompt use at the beginning of an epidemic is essential to limit spread; if vaccine supply is limited, priority should be given to young children for whom the risk is greatest. During community outbreaks, monovalent measles vaccine may be administered to 6- to 11-month olds.

Eradication of measles has been considered a fitting end to a disease confused with smallpox until 1629. Both diseases are dependent on humans for their propagation, need large human populations to sustain them, and elicit life-long immunity; neither leads to a chronic infectious state.[21] Measles vaccine has been used to reduce the incidence of the disease in the United States, Canada, Cuba, and some European countries. Elimination plans have been proposed many times, but the disease has not yet been eliminated from any large country.[11] The ineffectiveness of the vaccine for newborns and the high degree of contagion of the infection are the principal barriers to eradication of measles. The addition of "catch-up" campaigns to target all children aged 9 months to 14 years has recently been practiced in the Americas to increase coverage and, it was hoped, lead to elimination of measles by the year 2000.[7] During a 1996 meeting on global measles eradication, it was concluded that worldwide measles eradication is feasible using currently available vaccines and should be achievable worldwide within the next 10 to 15 years.[22]

[Coleen Weese]

RUBELLA

Introduction and Military Relevance

Rubella (or German measles) is a viral exantham that was recognized in the late 18th century but largely ignored until 1941, when it received dreaded notoriety because association had been made between it and congenital malformations.[23] The name German measles was popularized because German physicians distinguished it from measles, and the name rubella (little red) was given to it following an outbreak in India in 1841. Rubella is a mild febrile illness characterized by adenopathy of the head and neck, followed approximately a week later by a diffuse, punctate rash[10p435-440]; it is often indistinguishable from other mild viral exanthems. In unimmunized populations, it is largely a disease of children, who are often asymptomatic; the population of most concern is susceptible females of childbearing age. In 1941, an Australian ophthalmologist astutely observed an association between congenital cataracts and maternal rubella.[24] Rubella virus is now known to be a powerful teratogen when illness occurs during the first trimester of pregnancy, and congenital rubella syndrome (CRS) is distinguished by the classic triad of congenital cataract, heart defects, and deafness.[25] Other malformations may be seen as well. CRS patients, in addition to cataracts, congenital heart defects, and deafness, may also manifest encephalitis, microcephaly, mental retardation, autism, blindness, hepatosplenomegaly, and diabetes.[26] These cases of serious congenital disease provided the impetus to vaccine development and licensure.

Although rubella control aims primarily to prevent CRS, rubella outbreaks can disrupt military operations. In adulthood, rubella cases often occur in susceptible populations living in crowded quarters, such as university students and military personnel. Such cases represent a large proportion of the disease seen in the postvaccine era.[12p50] Serosurveys conducted among US Army recruits in 1989 demonstrated that only 85.2% had detectable rubella antibody.[14] Younger recruits were more likely to be seronegative, representing a cohort that may have missed both immunization and naturally acquired illness due to declining rates. Even with declining rates of rubella in the United States, however, susceptible recruits face risk from contact with multinational forces from countries whose immunization policies differ from the United States. In 1995, 120 German paratroopers arrived at Fort Bragg, North Carolina, to participate in a joint exercise.[27] German rubella policy immunizes only women of childbearing age. Several of the male paratroopers were incubating rubella when they arrived in the United States. Two days before the exercise, three succumbed to an illness consistent with rubella, and the entire German contingent was quarantined. Those without symptoms were given 2.0 mL of immune serum globulin to prevent further cases. Rubella IgM and IgG titers drawn on the contingent revealed that 10 of the 120 were nonimmune. Six of these became ill with rubella. Apart from the logistics of dealing with this outbreak, preventive medicine officials were faced with assessing the impact to the American troops and the wives and children who had contact with the German paratroopers. Recommendations to provide a second dose of rubella vaccine to school-age children (whether they are in kindergarten, 6th grade, or high school) or adolescents, as well as the continued policy of providing measles and rubella vaccine to recruits, should reduce the risk to US citizens from imported rubella.[16]

Description of the Pathogen

The causative agent of rubella is a virus in the genus *Rubivirus* in the family *Togaviridae*. The virus is a cubical, medium-sized (70 mm), lipid-enveloped virus with an RNA genome.[25] Humans are the only reservoir.[10]

Epidemiology

Transmission

Infection of susceptible humans follows contact with the nasopharyngeal secretions of infected people. Although other togaviruses are arthropod-borne, there is no evidence that rubella can be transmitted that way.[23] Rubella is prevalent in the winter and spring. Although most childhood infections are asymptomatic and go largely unrecognized, infection tends to occur at young ages in countries with crowded living conditions or widespread daycare use. Age at infection roughly correlates with age when congregation of susceptibles occurs. Serologic surveys indicate that most Africans are immune by their 10th birthday.[28] In unimmunized countries where crowding is not prevalent, infection may occur during the school years or while at colleges or military camps. The introduction of rubella vaccination of recruits at Lackland Air Force base in 1979 resulted in a 95% reduction in rubella cases.[29] Even in highly immunized populations, however, outbreaks may occur in such settings because of either incomplete coverage or vaccine failure.[30] While rubella is not as infectious as measles, in a closed environment such as a recruit population, all susceptibles may be infected. Herd immunity was shown to be ineffective when rubella broke out in a company of military recruits. Most had antibodies due to vaccination or prior infection at the start of the epidemic, but 100% of those susceptible were infected.[31,32] Clinical rubella and subsequent CRS has been documented during reinfection of vaccinees and naturally immune individuals, although it is a rare event.[33–35] Infants with CRS may shed virus for months after birth.[10]

Geographic Distribution

Rubella occurs worldwide at endemic levels, except in remote or island populations where epidemics occur every 10 to 15 years. This contrasts with the US interval of 6 to 9 years between major epidemics noted in the prevaccine era.[23]

Incidence

The medical and socioeconomic importance of rubella lies in its ability to produce anomalies in the developing fetus. CRS occurs in up to 90% of infants born to women who acquired confirmed rubella during the first trimester of pregnancy; the risk of a single congenital defect falls to approximately 10% to 20% when infection is acquired in the 16th week, and defects are rare when the maternal infection occurs after the 20th week of gestation.[10] In susceptible populations, rates of CRS as high as 1% of pregnancies have been documented.[36] The last major epidemic of CRS occurred in the United States in 1964 and 1965.[37] During this epidemic, it was estimated that there were 12.5 million cases of rubella, many in pregnant women. Five thousand therapeutic abortions were performed, 6,250 spontaneous abortions occurred, and an additional 2,100 babies were stillborn. CRS occurred in 20,000 infants. Of those, 11,600 were born deaf, 3,580 blind, and 1,800 mentally retarded. The cost of this epidemic has been estimated at $1.5 billion.[36] Since the licensure of the vaccine in 1969, no major epidemic has occurred in the United States. The incidence of rubella dropped to less than 1 per 100,000 while the incidence of congenital rubella syndrome has fallen to less than 0.1 per 100,000 births. Rubella incidence increased five to six times from 1990 to 1991, primarily in teenagers and young adults, but then returned to previous levels. Just less than half of the cases of known age were in individuals aged 15 and older.[12]

Pathogenesis and Clinical Findings

Rubella enters the nasopharynx, where it replicates and spreads to the local lymph nodes. Secretory IgA induced by prior disease or vaccination can block mucosal replication.[25] The incubation period for rubella is 14 to 21 days; rash typically occurs 2 weeks following exposure.[22,25] Cases are infectious 1 week before and up to 4 days after onset of the rash. During the second week, viremia occurs in the blood and can be blocked by passively or actively acquired antibody.[25] At this time, low-grade fever, malaise, and mild conjunctivitis may be present. At the end of the incubation period, a maculopapular erythemetous rash appears on the face and neck and spreads downward, fading over the next 3 days. Viremia ends with the onset of the rash. Arthralgia and arthritis are commonly observed in adults, and chronic arthritis has been reported. For unclear reasons, these complications are more common in women.[38,39]

Diagnostic Approaches

Field diagnosis of rubella is difficult and often inaccurate. Rash is not present in up to 50% of infections, and the other symptoms are relatively nonspecific.[27] The illness must be distinguished from measles, scarlet fever, mononucleosis, and other infectious exanthems and drug eruptions. Additionally, 10% to 85% of infections in various outbreaks have been inapparent.[26] Serologic confirmation of suspected cases should be sought, particularly in females of childbearing age. Such confirmation may be made by observing a 4-fold rise in titer between acute (within 7 to 10 days) and convalescent (2 to 3 weeks later) specimens via enzyme-linked immunosorbent assay, hemagglutinen inhibition, passive hemagglutination, or latex agglutination.[25] Rubella-specific IgM is quite reliable and obviates the need for multiple serum samples. Virus isolation is difficult and usually unnecessary.

Recommendations for Therapy and Control

Therapy is supportive; no definitive treatment exists.

As the goal of rubella control is the prevention of CRS, some countries have elected to immunize all adolescent girls without prescreening immune status. However, refusal rates of up to 15% in British women of childbearing years have been seen because of the concerns over the theoretical risk to the fetus.[40] It is a live virus vaccine, but no attributable increase in congenital defects in the offspring of 200 women immunized while pregnant was seen.[41] Reasonable precautions in a rubella immunization program include asking women of childbearing age if they may be pregnant and excluding those who may be, with the recommendation that those who receive vaccine not become pregnant for 3 months. Immune globulin has been used in an attempt to prevent CRS in exposed pregnant females; if any protection is incurred, however, it is incomplete at best.[42,43] The single indication for its use is a documented susceptible pregnant female who is exposed to the disease and would not consider abortion under any circumstances. The dose is 20 mL, given intramuscularly. Vaccine should not be given to anyone with an immunodeficiency or on immunosuppressive therapy, but measles-mumps-rubella vaccine (MMR) is recommended for persons with asymptomatic human immunodeficiency virus (HIV) infection and should be considered for those with symptomatic HIV infection.[10] All US military services recommend rubella immunization be given to recruits at accession.[44] The Department of Defense used to require screening of female recruits for susceptibility and pregnancy before vaccination. Susceptibility was included because of concerns about increased arthralgias and chronic rubella syndrome following vaccination in females. A 1991 Institute of Medicine report found evidence suggesting a causal association between rubella immunization and both chronic and acute arthritis.[45] The current regulation requires asking women about the possibility of pregnancy and deferring vaccine in those who are pregnant or who are unsure.[43]

The US strategy has been to immunize infants at 15 months and depend on herd immunity to protect pregnant women; postpartum vaccination is also advocated. However, rubella cases continued to occur in women of childbearing years. In 1989, the Advisory Council on Immunization Practices recommended a second dose of MMR be given to school-aged children or adolescents.[16] Until this regimen is fully implemented in successive cohorts, measles-rubella vaccination of recruits is prudent to prevent female service members and dependents from exposure and to prevent the disruption in training a rubella outbreak may cause. Other countries differ in age and sex targeted for immunization, so susceptible US service members could be exposed during multinational operations.

Mass immunization may be justified in an outbreak in a school or comparable population.[10] During an outbreak, isolation of cases to avoid contact with nonimmune pregnant women is advised; it is also recommended that contacts who may be pregnant should be tested serologically for susceptibility or early infection and advised accordingly.

[Coleen Weese]

MUMPS

Introduction and Military Relevance

Mumps is an acute communicable disease of children and young adults caused by a single strain of a paramyxovirus. The name may be related to an old English verb that means to grimace, grin, or mumble.[46] Mumps is a common cause of meningoencephalitis; other common manifestations and complications include orchitis, pancreatitis, mastitis, and oophoritis. Before widespread vaccination against mumps, the disease was associated with armies during times of mobilization. During World War I, mumps was an important cause of days lost from active duty in the US Army. Average number of days lost from duty was 18, and hospitalization occurred at a rate of 55.8/1,000 recruits.[47] In 1940, the Surgeon General of the US Army stated that next to the venereal diseases, mumps was the most disabling of the acute infections among recruits.[48] During the prevaccine era, outbreaks were more common among recruits from rural areas, who generally had not been previously exposed. Following the widespread use of vaccine, mumps cases continued to occur frequently among Soviet recruits, and an outbreak occurred among US Army troops in 1986.[49] But increased awareness that has led to increased coverage of infants with the primary series, as well as recent recommendations to require a second dose of the measles-mumps-rubella vaccine (MMR) for adolescents or younger school-aged children, should reduce cases in these populations and the spread of disease to military populations.[44,50]

Description of the Pathogen

Mumps is caused by the mumps virus, a member of the family *Paramyxoviridae* and the genus *Paramyxovirus*; it is antigenically related to the parainfluenza viruses.[48] It is an enveloped, negative-strand RNA virus that contains six major structural proteins.

Epidemiology

Transmission

Mumps is acquired by the respiratory route, and the infection is frequently accompanied by viremia, which commonly leads to organ involvement, particularly of the salivary glands. It is transmitted by droplet spread and direct contact with the saliva of an infected person. The incubation period is roughly 18 days, with a range of 12 to 25 days.[10p353–355] Virus is secreted in saliva beginning 7 days before parotitis until 9 days after it began. Exposed individuals should be considered infectious from the 12th to the 25th day following exposure, with maximum infectivity occurring 48 hours before the onset of illness. Humans are the only reservoir.

Geographic Distribution

With the exception of very isolated island groups and remote villages, mumps occurs throughout the world. It is endemic within urban populations but of somewhat irregular incidence.[51] Mumps shows slight seasonality in temperate zones, with an increase in winter and spring.

Incidence

Before widespread vaccine use, mumps most commonly afflicted school-aged children, with the highest incidence reported in children 5 to 9 years of age.[46] During World War I, cases occurred predominately among men from rural areas.[47] In the prevaccine era, serosurveys of US Army recruits demonstrate a 47% to 76% seropositivity rate.[52,53] During World War II, reported rates were only 6.9/1,000 per year, and cases were largely among personnel from rural areas.[8] An outbreak of mumps occurred in 1943 at Camp McCoy, Wisconsin, and spread slowly. It ultimately involved 1,378 cases occurring over 30 weeks, and the highest attack rate for a single company in any given week was 2.5%. The post was divided into two roughly equal groups. The attack rate in one group was 74.4/1,000 per year, whereas in the second group it was only 15.4/1,000 per year, despite the fact that both groups had ample time to mingle at clubs, theaters, and other sites. The divergence in rate was partially attributed to the geographical makeup of the two cohorts.[54]

After the licensure of mumps vaccine in the United States in 1967 and the subsequent introduction of state immunization laws, the reported incidence of mumps decreased substantially. Cases dropped 98%, from the 1968 levels of approximately 100/100,000 to an all-time low of 1.2/100,000 in 1985.[50] A number of European countries initiated MMR vaccination programs in the 1970s and 1980s.[46] Cuba has nearly eliminated mumps since it began vaccinating preschool-aged children in 1988 and achieved coverage levels above 95%.[55] Policies for providing routine vaccination of young children recommended by the Immunization Practices Advisory Committee of the Public Health Service in 1977, targeting older populations at risk, and enacting school immunization laws have contributed to the decrease in mumps incidence in the United States. From 1988 to 1993, the incidence of mumps decreased further after the number of states with immunization laws increased and the two-dose vaccination schedule for measles using MMR was initiated. However, there was a relative resurgence of mumps in 1986 and 1987, with almost 20,000 cases reported during the 2-year period. From 1988 to 1993, most cases occurred in children 5 to 14 years of age (52%) and in persons older than 15 years of age (36%).[50] This trend reflected underimmunization of the cohort born from 1967 through 1977, a period when vaccine was not administered routinely to children and the risk for exposure to mumps was decreasing.

A serosurvey of US Army recruits in 1989 found an overall seropositivity rate to mumps of 86.4%, with variation among recruits from urban, suburban, and rural backgrounds.[14] Persons from the western United States were more likely to be seronegative than others. Black, non-Hispanic recruits were more likely to be seropositive than other recruits.

The 1,692 cases of mumps reported for 1993 represents the lowest number of cases ever reported and a 99% decrease from 1968.[50] Although the incidence decreased in all age groups, the largest decrease (a greater than 50% reduction in incidence per 100,000 population) occurred in persons older than 10 years of age. Overall, the incidence of mumps was lowest in states that had comprehensive school immunization requirements and highest in states that did not.

Pathogenesis and Clinical Findings

Mumps virus is acquired through the respiratory tract with local replication there and in regional lymph nodes. Following an incubation period of 16 to 18 days, viremia occurs. At this stage, mumps most commonly presents as acute parotitis, which manifests itself as a unilateral or, more commonly, bilateral swelling of the parotid glands.[51] It may be preceded by several days of fever, headache, malaise, anorexia, and myalgia. Fever lasts from 1 to 6 days; parotid gland enlargement may last longer than 10 days. Mumps may be understood as a respiratory infection that is frequently accompanied by viremia, which commonly leads to organ involvement, particularly of the salivary glands.[46] Fifteen to twenty percent of mumps infections produce no symptoms (typically, these cases are adults), 30% to 40% of cases present with the typical parotitis (typically school-aged children), and up to 50% present as a respiratory infection (typically children under 5 years of age).[56,57] Serious complications may occur without evidence of parotitis, and some are more common in adults than children. Orchitis may occur in up to 20% to 30% of men who develop mumps.[58] Although testicular involvement can be bilateral in up to 30% of cases, sterility is thought to occur only rarely.[59] An increased risk of testicular cancer has been reported following mumps orchitis.[60] This is thought to be secondary to testicular atrophy following orchitis, as the mumps virus is not known to be oncogenic or transforming. Pancreatitis, usually mild, occurs in 4% of cases; an association with subsequent diabetes mellitus remains unproven.[61] Another concern is encephalitis, which is clinically indistinguishable from aseptic meningitis and occurs in 4% to 6% of cases.[56] Permanent sensorineural deafness may occur among children in about 1 in 15,000 cases.[62] Mastitis and oophoritis may occur in about 30% of women with mumps.

An increase in fetal death has been reported among women with mumps in the first trimester of pregnancy, although no increase in fetal abnormalities has been demonstrated.[63] Arthropathy, arthralgias, and arthritis, occasionally chronic, have been reported, more commonly in adults.[64] Nephritis, common but clinically insignificant, and myocarditis, rare but occasionally catastrophic, are other manifestations.[46]

Diagnostic Approaches

The diagnosis of mumps is usually made clinically, based on the presence of parotitis. Other viral infections, such as coxsackie virus A and lymphocytic choriomeningitis infections, can cause parotitis, and the differential diagnosis also includes suppurative parotitis, recurrent parotitis, salivary calculus, lymphadenopathy, and lymphosarcoma. One third of sporadic cases seen by family practitioners in Canada could not be confirmed serologically as mumps.[61] Virus may be readily isolated from swabs of the opening of the Stenson duct or from saliva, urine, or cerebrospinal fluid during the first 5 days of illness.[46] Historically, serological assays, including complement fixation, neutralization, and hemagglutination inhibition, have been employed to diagnose mumps.[65] Currently, enzyme-linked immunosorbent assays for mumps IgG and IgM are widely available, and they are more sensitive and specific than previous tests. The use of IgM antibody assays allows for the diagnosis of mumps from the analysis of a single acute sample; cross reactions with other paramyxoviruses do not occur.

Recommendations for Therapy and Control

There is no specific treatment for mumps, and use of immune globulin in exposed susceptibles is not recommended.[46]

Incidence rates for mumps in the United States have declined substantially since the licensure and widespread use of mumps vaccine.[50] Mathematical models of the impact of mass vaccination on the incidence of mumps predict that 85% to 90% coverage of children by the age of 2 years would be required to eliminate mumps from the United States or Western Europe.[46] However, cases continue to occur due to failure to vaccinate and vaccine failure.[66]

The mumps vaccine efficacy in clinical trials ranges from 75% to 91%.[46] The vaccine may be administered singly, as part of MMR, or with additional vaccines without impairment of antibody response or increase in side effects. Adverse reactions to the vaccine have been infrequently reported and consist most frequently of fever and parotitis.

Transient rash, pruritis, and purpura have also been reported. The population most at risk for complications of the disease is adolescents and adults, so immunization of susceptibles before the onset of adolescence is important.

US Army and Air Force recruits are given measles and rubella boosters upon entry to active duty, but mumps vaccine is recommended only for high-risk occupational groups (eg, medical care providers). The US Navy and Marine Corps routinely immunize all recruits against mumps. But outbreaks have occurred among highly vaccinated populations. Risk to susceptible military personnel would be expected to be higher during deployment to areas with lower vaccine coverage and when they have close contact with endemic populations. An outbreak occurred among US Army troops stationed in South Korea in 1986.[48] During 1989 and 1990, a large outbreak occurred among students in a primary school and a secondary school.[67] Most of the troops and the students had been vaccinated, suggesting that vaccine failure, as well as the failure to vaccinate, might have contributed to the outbreaks.

The decline in cases of mumps in recent years has made routine immunization of recruits not cost effective. The cohort most at risk is the nonimmune group that missed both naturally occurring mumps and immunization in the 1970s; this group is less likely to be problematic for the military as time passes. Additionally, the Immunization Practices Advisory Committee's two-dose recommendation should eventually reach successive cohorts, further reducing the risk. Mumps continues to pose a small risk to military populations, but this risk is expected to decrease substantially in the future with continued attention to immunization of children and adolescents.[68]

[Coleen Weese]

VARICELLA

Introduction and Military Relevance

Varicella is the primary infection caused by varicella-zoster virus. Humans are the only natural host.[10p92–97,69] The virus is worldwide in distribution; 4 million cases of varicella, or chickenpox, occur each year in the United States.[70] Approximately 9,000 cases result in hospitalization, and as many as 100 deaths have been attributed to chickenpox each year.[70,71] Military environments, with their shared living quarters and close physical contact, facilitate transmission of the virus among susceptible individuals by the aerosol route (Figure 39-1). The disease thus affects training time and readiness; often infected recruits are hospitalized just to remove them from the crowded barracks during their illness. The licensed vaccine and antiviral agents for treatment provide new intervention strategies to reduce the impact of chickenpox on the military.

Description of the Pathogen

Varicella is caused by varicella-zoster virus, a DNA virus also known as human herpesvirus 3. The virus is a member of the *Herpesvirus* group.

Epidemiology

Transmission

This generally benign disease of childhood is easily recognized because of its characteristic rash and is extremely contagious. Chickenpox is among the most highly communicable diseases in humans,

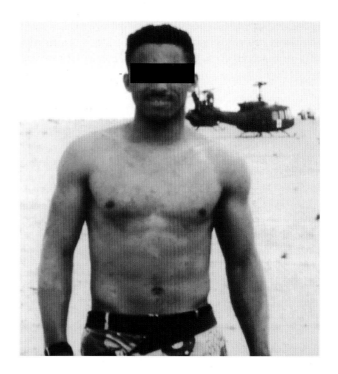

Fig. 39-1. Varicella infection in this new augmentee soldier to the 3d Armored Cavalry Regiment during Operation Desert Storm required him to be kept in an isolation tent and transported by ambulance until he was no longer infectious.
Photograph: Courtesy of Colonel Glenn Wasserman, Medical Corps, US Army.

with secondary attack rates from 70% to 90% in susceptible individuals.[10,72] Initial infection is usually symptomatic. Immunity lasts for life, but reactivation as herpes zoster can occur. Most civilian cases occur in children younger than 10 years of age.[69,72] Chickenpox is usually acquired by person-to-person contact via respiratory secretions, airborne spread, direct contact with zoster lesions, or freshly contaminated fomites. The lesions are infective until scabs have formed. The virus can also be transmitted in utero. Cases are most infectious 24 to 48 hours before the appearance of the rash and remain contagious for up to 5 days after the first vesicles appear. The average incubation period is 14 to 16 days but ranges from 10 to 20 days. Immuno-compromised patients may have a shorter incubation period and may remain communicable for longer than usual. The incubation period may be prolonged in those patients who received varicella-zoster immune globulin (VZIG).

Geographic Distribution

Chickenpox occurs in cycles of seasonal epidemics peaking in the winter and early spring in temperate zones but can occur worldwide. Infection is more common in adults in tropical climates than adults in temperate ones.

Incidence

In a sample of white, middle-class Americans, 100% were found to be immune by the age of 15, but in 810 young adults entering the US military from Puerto Rico, only 42% were seropositive.[73] The explanation for the later age of infection in tropical climates, such as Puerto Rico, the Philippines, and some Caribbean islands, is unclear but may include different population dynamics, climate, the relative heat-lability of the virus, or local protective environmental factors.[72,74]

Susceptibility to the virus among certain populations has been determined using the tools of molecular biology. National seronegativity rates in young adults in the United States have been estimated to be 6.7% from a large study of military recruits; the seronegativity rate for varicella in recruits was 8.2% by a commercial enzyme immunoassay.[75] Some protective cellular immunity may be present in persons with negative titers by enzyme immunoassay.[71] Nonwhite recruits and recruits from island nations or territories were more likely to be seronegative for varicella antibody.[75]

There was a substantial increase in the number of military hospitalizations for chickenpox from 1980 to 1988, but data from 1989 to 1995 show hospitalization rates have been declining.[74,76,77] In a review of military chickenpox admissions in the 1980s,[74] it was found that most of the persons hospitalized were new to the service. These younger service members were also more likely to be hospitalized than older personnel because otherwise they would be sent back to their barracks to recover. Soldiers with a home of record of the Caribbean islands, the Philippines, or Puerto Rico were at much increased odds of being hospitalized for varicella. An investigation done in the mid-1990s also found that those with foreign homes of record, who were junior in rank, and who were new to the service were at highest risk for hospitalization.[77]

The most common causes of death in children with chickenpox are septic complications and encephalitis, with the disease having a case fatality rate of 2 in 100,000.[10] The mortality for those 15 to 19 years old remains low at 1.3/100,000.[78] The case fatality rate in adults older than 20 years of age approaches 30/100,000, with death usually caused by varicella pneumonia.[10,78] Neonates, adults over the age of 20, the immunocompromised, persons with chronic cutaneous or pulmonary disorders, and those taking salicylates have a higher morbidity and mortality than children.

In the United States, chickenpox cases are selectively reportable and can be reported in groups instead of as individual cases. Significant underreporting is thought to occur. Notification of regional jurisdictions by local health departments can take as long as 1 year.[10] In the US Army, adult cases of varicella should be reported to the Army Medical Surveillance Activity for publication in the *Medical Surveillance Monthly Report*, published by the United States Army Center for Health Promotion and Preventive Medicine.

Pathogenesis and Clinical Findings

After varicella enters the body, the virus replicates in the oropharynx. The virus then invades local lymph nodes, blood, and viscera. After the 2- to 3-week incubation period, there is a secondary viremia and a vesicular rash that is pruritic and generalized. A single vesicular lesion scabs after 3 to 4 days as a result of host defense mechanisms.[10,79] The lesions tend to be of different ages, with all being scabbed usually by the sixth day. They are more likely to be located on covered areas of skin and in areas that are irritated. Mild fever and systemic symptoms can occur.

Complications include bacterial superinfection of the skin lesions, thrombocytopenia, arthritis, hepatitis, dehydration, encephalitis or meningitis, pneumonia, glomerulonephritis, and Reye syndrome.[69,72] Adults have an increased risk for complications of pneumonitis or encephalitis. In the immunocompromised, the course of illness can be complicated by continuing eruption of the rash, encephalitis, pancreatitis, hepatitis, and pneumonia.[69] The virus survives after the initial infection in a latent form in the dorsal root ganglia and can reactivate as shingles, typically years later under conditions of stress, trauma, malignancy, or immunosuppression.[72,79] Shingles is characterized by a unilateral vesicular eruption with a dermatomal distribution.[72] In fatal cases of varicella, intranuclear inclusions of the virus have been found in blood vessel endothelium and almost all organs of the body. In cases of encephalitis, perivenous demyelination in the brain has been described, as well as necrosis of nerve cells and meningitis.[28p801-803]

Congenitally acquired chickenpox is an uncommon syndrome consisting of skin scarring, muscle atrophy, extremity hypoplasia, low birth weight, and neurologic abnormalities. Infection of the mother in the first 16 weeks of gestation results in an estimated 2% incidence of fetal malformations.[10,72] While infection during pregnancy rarely leads to fetal death, deaths in utero can be from direct infection of the fetus with the virus or from fever and other maternal metabolic changes. Infection later in pregnancy results in fetal acquisition of protective maternal antibodies. However, maternal infection in the last 5 days of pregnancy can result in neonatal varicella, which is associated with a 30% case fatality rate.[72] With the administration of VZIG to these infants, the case fatality rate is drastically reduced, and in one uncontrolled study,[79] there were no fatalities. It does not appear that the disease is more severe in pregnant women than in other adults in the absence of pneumonia, and it is unclear whether or not it is more severe if complicated by pneumonia.

The clinical findings of varicella have some similarities to those of monkeypox and smallpox. The occurrence of monkeypox is increasing, and even though smallpox has been eradicated, it still exists as a potential biological warfare agent. Table 39-1 points out the salient differences between varicella and smallpox.

Diagnostic Approaches

Clinical diagnosis is based on the characteristic rash of varicella or dermatomal lesions of zoster. Other diagnostic options are available if necessary

TABLE 39-1

CLINICAL FEATURES OF VARICELLA AND SMALLPOX

Clinical Feature	Varicella	Smallpox
Onset	Progressive, moderate fever	Sudden, high fever; intense malaise (as in meningitis)
Rash	Appears on 2nd d, with continuing fever (in children the rash is often the first sign)	Appears on 3rd to 4th d, with transient fall of fever
	Begins on the trunk, where it will stay dense, but not on palms and soles	Begins on the face and extremities of the limbs, including palms and soles, where it will stay dense
	Macules become rapidly papular and produce clear vesicles that form crusts without going through the pustular stage	Macules require 4 to 6 d to transform into papules, vesicles, and pustules before producing scabs
	Successive crops appear during 4 to 5 d in the same area, which show lesions at different stages	Single crop only: all lesions are at the same stage in a given area
Vesicles	Soft, superficial, "tear-drop," not umbilicated	Hard, deep-seated, umbilicated; they transform into pustules with rise of fever and prostration
Crusts	Fall off rapidly, leaving temporary granular scabs	Healing is slow and leaves permanent pockmarks
Lethality	Exceptional	Case-fatality rate is 20% to 40% (Variola major)

Reprinted courtesy of the World Health Organization from Brés P. *Public Health Action in Emergencies Caused by Epidemics.* Geneva: World Health Organization; 1986.

but are not required in routine cases. The virus can be isolated from the lesions during the first 3 to 4 days. Visualizing multinucleated giant cells with intranuclear inclusions can be done using a method known as the Tzanck smear. These cells can also be visualized in herpes simplex lesions.[10,69] There are monoclonal antibodies available to diagnose the virus after immunofluorescent staining, this is a more accurate method than visualizing the giant cells.[10,14] Demonstration of viral DNA by polymerase chain reaction is also possible. Testing of acute and convalescent sera for the virus antibody (IgG and IgM) can be done using one of many available serologic tests, such the enzyme-linked immunosorbent assay (ELISA), but the tests may not be reliable in the immunocompromised. The commercial ELISA, which could be used to serologically screen populations before vaccination, has a reported sensitivity of 86.1% and specificity of 97.7%, as compared to the fluorescent antibody to membrane antigen assay (FAMA). The FAMA is a commonly used reference procedure that requires viral culture and considerable expertise to perform.[14,80]

Recommendations for Therapy and Control

No treatment is recommended for uncomplicated chickenpox in healthy children. In immunocompromised patients, treatment with intravenous acyclovir is preferred to vidarabine. Acyclovir is very effective in the immunocompromised if chickenpox is suspected; VZIG is not effective once disease is present. Oral acyclovir is recommended if the person is older than 12 years of age, has chronic cutaneous or pulmonary disorders, or is taking chronic salicylate therapy or steroids.[69] Acylovir is available for use in children, but studies have not clearly shown it has a significant effect on the rate of complications or absence from school.[70] It has been shown to be most beneficial if the drug is given within 24 hours of onset of the rash.[69,81] Because of the risk of Reye syndrome, salicylates should not be taken by individuals with varicella.

In 1995, a live attenuated vaccine for varicella was licensed in the United States. The vaccine has been shown to be safe, immunogenic, and efficacious. The most common side effects are pain and redness at the site of injection, rash, and fever.[82] Children older than 1 year of age may receive the vaccine subcutaneously in a single dose of 0.5 mL. Adolescents older than the age of 13 years and adults should receive two doses (0.5 mL each), 1 to 2 months apart.[10,83] The vaccine can be given simultaneously with MMR (measles-mumps-rubella),

DTP (diphtheria-tetanus-pertussis), OPV (oral polio virus), and *Hemophilus influenzae* vaccines.[70] Postvaccine serology in healthy people is not necessary because the seroconversion rate is high.[82] The vaccine must be kept frozen. The vaccine should be reconstituted with diluent supplied with the vaccine and then discarded if not used within 30 minutes.[70]

The chickenpox vaccine protects very well (95%) against severe disease. Protection from infection and clinical disease is lower (70% to 80%).[71] Most breakthrough cases are mild.[82] Twenty-year follow-up studies of a similar vaccine in Japan show persistent immunity after vaccination, but it is difficult to assess whether that is purely from vaccine or is also from boosting due to exposure to circulating virus in the community.[71] Examination of infants and adolescents in the United States revealed that greater than 90% of subjects had measurable antibody 5 years after vaccination.[82] Definitive duration of protection and the need for a booster is not yet defined.

The vaccine should not be given to people who are allergic to gelatin or neomycin; who have untreated tuberculosis, blood dyscrasias, leukemia, lymphoma, febrile illnesses, or most immunodeficiency conditions; or who are pregnant.[70,83] Although there are no reported cases of Reye syndrome associated with the vaccine and concomitant aspirin use, it is recommended that salicylates not be taken for at least 6 weeks after vaccination. Compared to those who experience natural chickenpox, those that receive the vaccine may be less likely to get shingles. The Centers for Disease Control and Prevention, the Advisory Committee on Immunization Practices, and the American Academy of Pediatrics currently recommend that potential vaccinees who may be exposed to pregnant women and the immunocompromised still receive the vaccine.[70] There has been one case of potentially vaccine-associated symptomatic infection documented in a pregnant woman from her vaccinated and otherwise healthy child.[71,84] Although healthy people are very unlikely to transmit virus to susceptibles after vaccination, a very small risk does exist.[84] The risk of transmission after vaccination is higher if the vaccinee develops a rash,[70,84] so vaccines who develop a rash should be isolated from susceptible individuals.

The Advisory Committee on Immunization Practices does not recommend serologic testing to confirm lack of immunity because the vaccine can be administered safely to people who have had chickenpox infection in the past.[70,85] However, the estimated cost of the vaccine, $35 per dose in 1996, along with the cost of serologic testing must also be considered.[70]

The vaccine is not being recommended for children less than 1 year of age.[10,83] All children 12 to 18 months of age should be routinely vaccinated. Persons between 18 months and 13 years of age who have not been previously vaccinated and lack a reliable history of varicella infection should receive one dose of vaccine. Selected populations of susceptible adults should be administered two doses of vaccine. These include health care workers, teachers, daycare employees, and others with potentially close and frequent contact with susceptible persons and the immunocompromised. Nonpregnant women who may become pregnant in the future should be also be vaccinated.[70] Manufacturers advise waiting at least 3 months before becoming pregnant after vaccination.[83]

According to the directive requirements for the Armed Forces Immunizations Program in November 1995, the Department of Defense policy is to administer the varicella vaccine to high-risk occupational groups and as directed by the applicable Surgeon General or Commandant, with the exception of the Marine Corps, which follows only the Commandant's recommendations.[44] The Navy and Air Force presently screen recruits using on-site rapid ELISA testing during inprocessing at basic training. Results are available within 24 hours and the 7.0% who are seronegative are vaccinated.[86] The Army is developing its policy toward screening recruits for varicella.

Relying on an individual's recall of clinical disease is one aspect of concern in varicella immunization policies. In one study, 95% of military recruits giving a history of varicella were seropositive.[75] The positive predictive value of a history of chickenpox may be lower in recruits who did not grow up in the United States. A study of US military recruits from Micronesia uncovered a positive predictive value of varicella history of only 81%.[87] A representative sample of Army basic trainees studied had a positive predictive value of 88%. Eighty-nine percent of those with a questionable history of varicella were also seropositive. Only 36% with a negative history of varicella were seronegative.[14]

Prevention other than vaccination includes keeping those who are infectious away from susceptible people, especially those at high risk in the hospital setting. The military should be especially concerned about close contact, such as in schools and military basic training. Exposed susceptibles, including health care workers, should be isolated from other susceptibles on the 8th to 21st days after the contact case develops the rash and to the 28th day if they received VZIG.[69,70] Children should be allowed to return to school or day care 6 days after the onset of their rash when all lesions are crusted over or covered, unless they are immunocompromised.[10,69] Active duty personnel and other adults should return to work according to these same guidelines.

Selected populations of exposed susceptible people need to be identified and offered VZIG. These include the immunocompromised, pregnant women, infants born to a mother who has onset of disease in the perinatal period, or premature infants (older than 28 weeks and no maternal history of varicella infection, younger than 28 weeks regardless of maternal history). VZIG should only be offered after considering the potential for significant exposure. The dose is 125 U intramuscularly for each 10 kg of body weight, with a maximum of 625 U (5 vials).[69] VZIG can prevent disease or lessen its severity if given within 96 hours of exposure, but it is not appropriate to use it as treatment once the disease has been established.

In the future, the maintenance of immunity and the need for future boosters after vaccination will become better defined. Postvaccination transmission also needs further investigation.[84] Vaccination programs should provide for those who were too old for the initial immunization campaign in children but escaped disease in childhood. The success of the immunization program in children will eventually affect the varicella seroprevalence of entering recruits and the cost-effectiveness of military vaccination strategies. Slow implementation of varicella immunization in children may for a time increase the susceptibility of incoming recruits as a result of reduced preaccession exposure. Future military policy should become more specific after incorporating economic considerations and continuing surveillance.

[Kathryn Clark]

PERTUSSIS

Introduction and Military Significance

Pertussis has been long, though erroneously, considered solely a disease of childhood. The availability of a vaccine since 1949 and the resultant 99% reduction in morbidity and mortality compared to the prevaccine era has removed pertussis from the consciousness of all but a small, specialized segment of the medical community. After the historic low of 1,010 cases reported in the United States in 1976, a cyclic (every 3 to 4 years) resurgence of cases has been noted, with a high of 6,586 cases in 1993.[88] The renewed interest and research in pertussis has revealed that adult pertussis has been underdiagnosed as well as underreported. Many feel that adults with pertussis infection represent the most significant reservoir for ongoing transmission of disease, especially to susceptible infants and children, in whom the severity of illness is greater.

Although pertussis has not yet been implicated in outbreaks of respiratory illness among military populations, it may be that it simply has not been recognized as a cause. Waning immunity in the vaccine era appears to render many young adults susceptible again at the very age most begin military service, as the last booster dose of pertussis vaccine is given before the seventh birthday and vaccine-induced immunity is thought to be absent by 12 years after the last dose. Vaccination can be viewed as both boon and curse. While surely preventing many cases of serious disease and deaths among young children, widespread immunization has left so little natural infection in the community that there is little chance for adults to be "boosted" by exposure to natural cases. Approximately one fourth of the US adult population is thus thought to be susceptible to pertussis.[89] In the 1990s, especially with licensure of acellular pertussis vaccine for children for the last two booster doses, there has been renewed interest and research into re-immunization of adults.

The knowledge that pertussis occurs with some frequency in young adults, that it is a highly contagious respiratory disease, and that a significant proportion of military recruits are likely to be susceptible make it conceivable that large outbreaks of disease could occur among barracks contacts at basic training sites. Two studies in the 1990s are pertinent to the issue of military relevance of pertussis. One hundred thirty college students (the same age group as military recruits) with a cough illness of 6 or more days were enrolled in a study to examine the prevalence of pertussis.[90] Twenty-six percent had evidence of pertussis infection. Serology detected all but one of the infections, and no cultures were positive. In the second study,[91] antibody levels of US university students were compared to German military recruits. IgA levels to four different pertussis antigens ranged from 60% to 91% among all participants and did not differ between the Americans and Germans for any of the individual antigens. Since IgA titers are thought to reflect natural infection, the authors concluded that pertussis infections are common in this age group.

A second theoretical concern for the military regarding pertussis is related to the recent shift toward increased numbers of humanitarian assistance missions, in which US forces have close, prolonged contact with host populations. Since the incidence of pertussis is roughly three orders of magnitude greater in much of the world than it is in the United States (1 per 100 vs. 1 per 100,000), exposure to the host population increases the chance of infection in young service members. Alternatively, sporadic cases in those service members whose disease may be mild enough to preclude evacuation may result in transmission of disease to a relatively highly susceptible population in the host country.

Description of the Pathogen

The causative agent of pertussis is the Gram-negative bacillus, *Bordetella pertussis*. The organism produces several cellular products responsible for its virulence and for antigen presentation to the host immune system. Pertussis toxin is an important virulence factor, mediating the attachment of the bacterium to the respiratory epithelial cells. Filamentous hemaglutinin is the other major protein product also thought to mediate attachment of the organism to the respiratory epithelial cells.[92] Both of these protein products are believed to play a role in inducing immunity after natural infection and also represent the major components of the licensed acellular vaccine for children.[93]

Epidemiology

Transmission

Pertussis is transmitted readily by contact with respiratory secretions from an infected individual spread through airborne droplets.[10p375–379,92] Up to 90% of susceptible household contacts may become infected following close contact with an index case. Indirect transmission through fomites is considered unlikely.[92] The most susceptible age groups are (*a*) infants younger than 6 months of age who have not completed the three-dose primary immunization series and who do not have passive antibody protection from mothers whose vaccine-induced immunity has waned and (*b*) adolescents and adults whose immunity has waned and who may be exposed to infected family members or close contacts.

Geographic Distribution

Pertussis is a worldwide disease problem. Vaccination policies tend to be less stringent in some other developed nations than in the United States.

Pertussis vaccination is optional in Germany[91] and Italy,[94] and the vaccine was withdrawn in Sweden in 1979.[95] The schedule in Finland is different than in the United States, with four total doses recommended and the last booster at 2 years of age.[96]

Incidence

In 1986, the World Health Organization estimated that there are 60 million new cases of pertussis each year, causing about 600,000 deaths.[97] In the United States, the incidence of pertussis has generally increased since the historic low in 1976, with the greatest number of cases since then occurring in 1993. Pertussis continues to be largely a disease of infants and children, but the percentage of cases in persons aged 10 years or older has increased from 15.1% (1977 to 1979) to 18.9% (1980 to 1989) to 28% (1992 to 1994).[88,98] The rate of complications in the older age groups, however, is significantly lower than in infants and children. Specifically, there were proportionally fewer cases requiring hospitalization or developing pneumonia, seizures, or encephalopathies in those aged 10 years or older for the years 1992 to 1994.[88] All 32 deaths occurred in children younger than 10 years of age.

One study[99] has estimated that only 11.6% of pertussis cases in the United States are reported to the Centers for Disease Control and Prevention. Coupled with the fact that the illness in adolescents and adults is milder or atypical,[89,100] it is likely that cases in the older age groups are disproportionately underreported. Other studies,[101,102] which have attempted to prospectively diagnose pertussis in adults with a prolonged cough illness, suggest that pertussis may account for 21% to 26% of these illnesses.

Pathogenesis and Clinical Findings

The clinical syndrome of pertussis is variable, but illness severity is generally greatest in the very young. After an incubation period of 6 to 20 days, the first stage of illness, known as the catarrhal stage, arises with nonspecific nasal symptoms, low-grade fever, and mild cough. This stage corresponds to the period of greatest infectivity. After 1 to 2 weeks, the paroxysmal stage begins, with the characteristic symptoms of paroxysmal cough and inspiratory whoop (Figure 39-2). Especially in young children, the paroxysms of cough may be complicated by apnea, posttussive vomiting, and hypoxia-induced encephalopathy. Pneumonia is another complication and is highly correlated with death. Bronchopulmonary pathologic findings include damage to cilia, accumulation of secretions, and

edema.[92] Adults are less likely to have paroxysms of cough or the classic whoop but are likely to present with a prolonged cough illness. Asymptomatic carriage is not a feature of this disease.

Diagnostic Approaches

Diagnosis is difficult, especially in adults. Culture of nasopharyngeal secretions has been the gold standard, but even in optimal circumstances only 80% of cultures are confirmatory.[92,103] The pertussis organism is fastidious and slow-growing, requires selective media, and must be obtained with a calcium alginate or Dacron swab. Previous immunization, use of antibiotics, or attempts to isolate the organism late in the illness all decrease the rate of recovery. Direct fluorescent antibody testing of nasopharyngeal secretions has been employed as a rapid means of diagnosis, but results have been mixed, with generally low sensitivity and specificity.[10,103] Serologic testing, using a variety of methodologies from agglutination to enzyme-linked immunosorbent assay and using either single elevated titers or paired (acute and convalescent) titers, has been employed.[92,103,104] Use of paired sera limits the applicability of the test to retrospective serosurveys in most cases. Further, because of the ubiquitous exposure to pertussis through im-

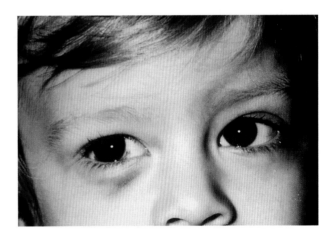

Fig. 39-2. Subconjunctival hemorrhage in pertussis occurs because the intrathoracic pressure rises sharply during violent paroxysms of coughing and leads to sudden surges in capillary pressure. In this child, the subconjunctival hemorrhage is accompanied by bleeding into the lower lid—a rarer complication. No permanent harm results, and these complications resolve rapidly.
Reprinted courtesy of Mosby-Wolfe Limited, London, UK from: Forbes CD, Jackson WF, eds. *Color Atlas and Text of Clinical Medicine.* 2nd ed. London: Mosby-Wolfe Limited; 1997: 55.

munization or natural infection, the ideal serologic test would be quantitative rather than registering the simple presence or absence of antibody. Researchers have developed a set of isotype-specific antibody responses to *B pertussis* antigens (ie, PT, FHA) for serodiagnosis of natural infection, but these are perhaps not practical except in reference laboratories.[104]

Diagnosis in a garrison environment can be accomplished with the aforementioned tools, subject to local resources. In the field or during wartime, though, reliance on clinical diagnosis is necessary because culture requires special media and direct fluorescent antibody requires special lab equipment that may not be available in forward-deployed hospital settings. It might be possible to use a single serum titer in the appropriate clinical scenario, if further study yields a quantitative titer that is judged positive and indicative of recent infection. The clinical case definition set forth by the Centers for Disease Control and Prevention consists of cough of at least 14 days' duration without other known etiology, accompanied by either paroxysms, inspiratory whoop, or posttussive vomiting.[105]

Recommendations for Therapy and Control

Erythromycin is the antimicrobial of choice for both treatment of individuals and for outbreak control. Individual patients should be treated with a 14-day course of erythromycin and are considered noninfectious after completion of 5 days of therapy. Only rarely is pertussis diagnosed early enough in the catarrhal phase to enable erythromycin to affect the clinical course; the goal of the antibiotic treatment is the eradication of the organism from the nasopharynx to interrupt transmission.[92] Close or household contacts who have not completed the vaccination series should receive a dose of vaccine as soon as possible after contact with the index case,

and all contacts, regardless of age or immunization status, should receive 14 days of prophylaxis.[10]

Prevention of pertussis is accomplished in the United States by a vaccination series consisting of five doses: three primary doses at 2, 4, and 6 months of age and boosters at 12 to 18 months and at 4 to 6 years of age. Pertussis is usually combined with vaccines against tetanus and diphtheria, as diphtheria-tetanus-pertussis (DTP) or diphtheria-tetanus-acellular pertussis (DTaP). The use of acellular pertussis vaccine has been recommended for use in the booster doses since 1991,[106] but the Advisory Committee on Immunization Practices (ACIP) has broadened its recommendations for use of acellular pertussis for the primary doses as well as the booster doses for several products licensed by the Food and Drug Administration.[107,108] The ACIP does not recommend the use of pertussis vaccine beyond the seventh birthday,[10] despite the widely recognized problem of waning immunity.

Since the availability of acellular pertussis in 1991, there has been renewed interest in testing its safety and efficacy in adult populations. Long-term immunogenicity of acellular pertussis vaccine has still not been evaluated, but preliminary research shows that it is both safe and immunogenic in the near term when administered to adults.[93,109,110] Further study is likely to yield a recommendation for a tetanus-diphtheria-acellular pertussis (TdaP) booster for adults in the future.

Because of the potential for epidemic spread in a barracks setting or aboard ship and because of the shift in the role of the military in peacetime to humanitarian missions, it seems appropriate for military personnel, particularly new recruits, Special Forces units, and Civil Affairs units, to be immunized against pertussis when acellular pertussis becomes available for use in adults.

[David Goldman]

TETANUS

Introduction and Military Relevance

Tetanus, also known as lockjaw because of its propensity to cause painful, tonic spasms of the muscles, has been and will remain an important infection from a military perspective. In the military workplace, whether it be on the battlefield or the training ground, service members will sustain wounds, exposing them to the ubiquitous spores of tetanus. Tetanus spores live in soil for many years, so the risk is ongoing and permanent.

Even though there were very few recorded cases of tetanus during the Civil War, a doctor wrote, poignantly, "On account of exposure, many wounds were gangrenous when the patients reached the hospital. In these cases delay was fatal, and an operation almost equally so, as tetanus often followed speedily."[111p30] One of the historical figures who succumbed to lockjaw was General Gladden, who was with General Bragg's command in South Carolina. He had his left arm amputated after being hit by a musket ball. Refusing convalescence, he rejoined the battle. In days, he required a second amputation, near the shoulder, but he still refused to give up command. He gave it up shortly thereafter, when he died of "lockjaw."[111]

In World War I, the case rate for tetanus was 0.16 per 1,000 wounded. The reason for the low incidence of tetanus was the universal and early administration of tetanus antitoxin as a form of passive immunization. Fifteen hundred units of tetanus antitoxin was given subcutaneously in all cases of wounds and injuries where there was the possibility of contamination with tetanus spores. A "T" was painted with iodine on the forehead of soldiers given the antitoxin at an aid station or at any point in front of the hospital station. Proof of the usefulness of antitoxin was evident in the experience of the British Army. In September 1914, their rate of tetanus was 8.6/1,000. After orders were issued to use the antitoxin, the rate fell to 1.4/1,000 by December 1914.[112p110-114]

In 1941, all US military personnel were immunized with tetanus toxoid.[113] During World War II, there were only 16 clinical tetanus cases, and only six of these died. After the toxoid was precipitated with alum or adsorbed onto aluminum salts, fewer doses were needed for effective immunization.[114]

Since the early 1990s, the US military has been increasingly involved in operations other than war, such as peacekeeping and provision of humanitarian assistance. These activities bring to bear issues in tetanus control that are especially pertinent in developing countries. Because tetanus spores are ubiquitous, it is not a matter of eliminating exposure but rather of limiting it. The issues are basic sanitation, appropriate wound care, aseptic technique during childbirth, and adequate immunization. There is precedent for military efforts in these areas. The US Army medical department made significant improvements in general sanitation measures while encamped in Cuba during the early part of the 20th century, which included decreasing the number of cases of tetanus resulting from unsanitary care of the umbilical cord in newborns.[115] Modern peacekeeping efforts provide a great opportunity to decrease the incidence of neonatal tetanus in developing countries by ensuring that pregnant women are vaccinated against tetanus.

Description of the Pathogen

Tetanus is caused by an exotoxin, called tetanospasmin, which is elaborated in wounds infected with *Clostridium tetani,* a Gram-positive, anaerobic bacillus.

Epidemiology

Transmission

The means of transmission is by introduction of tetanus spores into the body, typically through a puncture wound contaminated with soil or feces.[10p491-496] Cuts, burns, or contaminated illicit injectable drugs also create routes for infection to occur. The organism is harbored in the intestinal tract of humans, horses, and other animals. Tetanus is not communicable from person to person.

Geographic Distribution

Tetanus occurs worldwide; however, it is more prevalent in countries where immunization programs are lacking or there is difficulty in obtaining appropriate medical care. It is also found more frequently in densely populated areas with hot and damp climates where the soil is rich in fecal matter.[116]

Incidence

Almost all cases of tetanus in the United States occur in partially immunized or nonimmunized persons. Most cases occur in persons 60 years of age or older;[117] from 1989 to 1990, 58% of the 117 cases reported in the United States occurred in adults over the age of 60.[10] This is primarily due to waning immunity caused by declining antibody levels. The third national Health and Nutrition Examination Survey, a study of 10,618 people 6 years of age and older conducted from 1988 to 1991, showed that protective levels of tetanus antibody were found in 27.8% of those 70 years of age or older.[117] Lower rates of immunity were also seen in non-Hispanic blacks (68.1%) and Mexican-Americans (57.9%) in comparison to non-Hispanic whites (72.7%). A history of having served in the US military was associated with having protective levels of antibody, and male veterans had higher rates of immunity compared to female veterans. In fact, one of the risk factors for sustaining a tetanus infection for US citizens is a lack of military experience.[118] The following variables were all independent predictors of protective levels of tetanus antibody levels: male sex, non-Hispanic white race, US or Canadian birth, military service, and having some college education. Certain risk factors (ie, access to health care, poverty status, educational level of the head of the household) were not associated with immunity to tetanus.[117]

In spite of an effective vaccine, approximately 50,000 deaths from tetanus are reported per year worldwide.[118] In reality, there are many more deaths secondary to tetanus than are officially reported. Tetanus can be likened to a silent epidemic and may be the "most underreported lethal infection in the world."[119p191] After the advent of active immunization programs in the United States, the incidence declined, with 560 cases reported in 1947, 101 cases in 1974, and approximately 60 to 80 cases per year since the early 1980s.[118] These numbers reflect reported cases; underreporting of cases is also a problem in the United States. The case fatality rate varies, depending on patient age and length of incubation time. In general, the shorter the incubation period and the more extreme the age (ie, newborns, young children, the elderly), the higher the case fatality rate will be.

Pathogenesis and Clinical Findings

Once the tetanospasmin has entered the central nervous system, it binds to the ganglioside membranes of nerve synapses. This blocks release of the inhibitory transmitter from the nerve terminals, causing a generalized tonic spasticity. Spasms result from intensive afferent stimuli, which increases rigidity and causes simultaneous and excessive contraction of muscles and their antagonists.[116]

The average incubation period is 10 days, with a range from 1 day to several months, depending on the severity and location of the wound. When the period from injury to onset of symptoms is short, the illness will be more serious. Case fatality ranges from 10% to 90%. When symptoms occur within 2 or 3 days of injury, the mortality rate approaches 100%.[116] Occasionally, the presenting signs and symptoms may be nonspecific, but the most common presentation will include painful muscular contractions, especially of the masseter and neck muscles, and difficulty opening the jaw. Trismus, which may include a "risus sardonicus" or sardonic smile, may result in difficulty swallowing and irritability. Abdominal rigidity may be one of the first signs of tetanus in older children and adults. The rigidity can also occur around the site of the injury.[10] The posture of severe curving of the back upwards with the head and heels flat on the bed, or opisthotonus, is a result of tetanic spasm. Minor stimuli, such as noise or a breeze, may cause painful, tonic convulsions. Cyanosis and asphyxia may result when the respiratory muscles spasm.[120] These manifestations will increase in severity for 3 days and will remain stable for 5 to 7 days, after which

spasms will occur less frequently until they disappear altogether.[116] Complications, including death, are the result of a combination of factors. These factors include the direct results of the toxin, such as laryngospasm, which leads to impaired respiration, hypoxia, and brain damage. Vigorous therapy and prolonged bed rest can result in secondary complications such as decubitus ulcers.

In a field setting, the first symptoms of tetanus may be quite subtle, consisting only of pain and tingling at the wound site, followed by spasticity of the nearby muscle groups.[120] This is referred to as a localized tetanus. Cephalic tetanus, which can involve all cranial nerves, is seen most commonly in children and is usually associated with a chronic otitis media.

Tetanus neonatorum, a form of tetanus that affects newborns as a result of nonsanitary medical or ritualistic perinatal practices, often presents as an inability to nurse. Stiffness, spasms, convulsions, or opisthotonus are subsequently noted. The average incubation period is about a week and mortality is high.

Diagnostic Approaches

Tetanus can be insidious to diagnose because a history of an injury may be lacking. Any scenario that allows for penetration of the skin and fosters an anaerobic environment is conducive to growth of tetanus spores. Burn victims and intravenous-injecting drug addicts are examples of particularly susceptible individuals.

There are no specific laboratory tests to diagnose tetanus. Laboratory confirmation is futile, as the organism is not usually recovered from the infection site, nor is there any appreciable antibody response.[10] About one third of patients may exhibit a granulocytosis, and various fluid and electrolyte disturbances may occur.[116] Tetanus is diagnosed strictly on clinical grounds when the signs and symptoms suggest it in an individual who has not been immunized or who has let his or her tetanus immunity lapse. Therefore, the treating physician must have a heightened sense of suspicion and make inquiries about tetanus immunization history.

Recommendations for Therapy and Control

The goals of therapy for tetanus are to neutralize the toxin, to remove the source of the toxin, and to provide supportive care.[118] Patients who recover from tetanus do not develop an immune response so they also require active immunization. In addition to wound cleaning, surgical debridement (when indicated), and prophylactic antibiotics (a 7-day course of penicillin), vaccine immunoprophylaxis is necessary to prevent tetanus. This will depend on the type of wound and the history of tetanus immunizations. Patients should be asked whether they have ever received tetanus immunization, and the wound site should be characterized as to whether it is clean and minor, severe, or contaminated. If the patient cannot recall or has had less than three doses of tetanus vaccine, he or she should be given tetanus vaccine (using a combined diphtheria-tetanus-pertussis vaccine, DTP), the amount of which will vary with the age of the patient. Children younger than 7 years old should receive DTP or DTaP (a formulation with acellular pertussis). Children older than 7 years and adults should receive Td (tetanus-diphtheria). Tetanus immune globulin (TIG) provides immediate neutralization of tetanospasmin and should be administered to patients with severe or dirty wounds who are unsure of their immunization status or those with a history of having had less than three doses of tetanus vaccine. When both TIG and toxoid are given, separate sites and syringes must be used. TIG is not necessary for patients who have had a full series of tetanus immunizations. Neither is it necessary to give a booster of tetanus vaccine to patients who have previously been fully immunized, except in certain situations. If a patient has sustained a minor, clean wound and it has been more than 10 years since the last dose of tetanus vaccine, he or she should receive a Td booster. If the wound is severe or dirty or both, and it has been more than 5 years since the last dose, a booster should be given[10]

(Table 39-2).

Once tetanus is suspected, the patient should be admitted to an intensive care unit to ensure continuous monitoring capability and protection of the airway in the event of tetanus-induced laryngospasm. Aggressive therapy to inhibit generalized spasm and the treatment of autonomic instability is important.[118] Metronidazole or doxycycline can be given intravenously in large doses for 7 to 14 days. Parenteral penicillin G is an alternative treatment.[10,69p563–568,121] Tetanospasmin can be neutralized with TIG if the exotoxin has not already been fixed in the central nervous system. TIG will not ameliorate symptoms already present at the time tetanus is diagnosed.[116]

Military personnel will now usually see tetanus in the context of humanitarian assistance to non-US populations. Some of the simplest measures are also some of the most difficult to achieve in light of poverty, cultural behaviors, and lack of education. Individuals who cannot afford shoes are vulnerable to puncture wounds through their feet. The lack of control of pets and their excreta provides abundant opportunities for exposure to tetanus spores. Rituals involving abrasion or cutting provide easy access and introduction of the spores. Procedures used during childbirth, including attendance by untrained lay-midwives and use of unsterile instruments, foster tetanus infections in unimmunized pregnant women. In some cultures, mothers dress their babies' umbilical stumps with dust mixed with spider webs or dung, greatly increasing the risk for an ensuing tetanus infection unless the baby has transplacentally received passive tetanus antibody from its mother.[122]

TABLE 39-2

SUMMARY GUIDE TO TETANUS PROPHYLAXIS IN ROUTINE WOUND MANAGEMENT

History of Tetanus Immunization (doses)	Clean, Minor Wounds		All Other Wounds	
	Td[*†]	TIG	Td[*]	TIG
Uncertain or < 3	Yes	No	Yes	Yes
3 or more	No[†]	No	No[‡]	No

[*] For children less than 7 years old, DtaP or DTP (DT, if pertussis vaccine is contraindicated) is preferred to tetanus toxoid alone. For persons 7 years old or older, Td is preferred to tetanus toxoid alone.
[†] Yes, if more than 10 years since last dose.
[‡] Yes, if more than 5 years since last dose. (More frequent boosters are not needed and can accentuate side effects.)
Reprinted with permission from: Chin J, ed. *Control of Communicable Diseases Manual*. 17th ed. Washington, DC: American Public Health Association; 2000: 496. Copyright 2000 by the American Public Health Association.
TIG: Tetanus immune globulin
Td: tetanus-diphtheria

The US military has played an active role in fostering immunization programs in developing countries. Preventing tetanus neonatorum and tetanus in postpartum women is a worthy focus. (Young, nonpregnant women can also be vaccinated against rubella at the same time as receiving tetanus vaccine.) However, targeting women attending prenatal clinics will not suffice. Strategy for preventing tetanus has to be aimed at the whole population and should be tailored according to the customs and needs of the countries supported. Since tetanus spores are ubiquitous, it is important to ensure universal vaccination with adsorbed tetanus toxoid by administering a basic series of the vaccine and giving booster doses every 10 years to ensure ongoing protection.[118] If resources are limited, an initial method may be to target school-aged children for vaccination. Later, when the girls become pregnant, they will transfer tetanus antibody transplacentally to the fetus, conferring protection against neonatal tetanus.

In the US military, tetanus toxoid is administered to all active duty personnel, recruits, and reserve components. They are vaccinated as they begin their military careers, receiving a primary series of Td toxoid if they lack a reliable history of prior immunization. If they have a history of receiving Td, they will still receive a booster dose upon entry to active duty and, ideally, every 10 years thereafter.[48] During soldier readiness processing (SRP) in the Army and its equivalent in the other services and especially for targeted deployments, screening of immunization records includes checking for the date of the last Td immunization. If this has not been given within the previous 10 years, the service member is given a booster. Excessive boosting may be associated with local and systemic reactions. Both military personnel and civilians should be educated about preventive measures: routine tetanus immunization, proper care of wounds, and tetanus immunization, if indicated, after receiving a tetanus-prone wound.

[Paula K. Underwood]

DIPHTHERIA

Introduction and Military Relevance

Diphtheria is an acute bacterial infection caused by *Corynebacterium diphtheriae*. The organism elaborates a toxin that produces a characteristic patch or patches of an adherent grayish membrane with surrounding inflammation, affecting the tonsils, pharynx, larynx, nose, and occasionally other mucous membranes or skin.[10p165–170] Diphtheria gets its name from the Greek word for tanned skin or leather, which describes the nature of the membrane that is almost pathognomonic for diphtheria. The organism is spread through the respiratory route and close personal contact. Military personnel are at greater risk of contracting diphtheria when they are in crowded conditions.

Diphtheria was not distinguished from scarlet fever during the Revolutionary War. It was also called "Throat Distemper, Angina Suffocativa, Bladder in the Throat, Cyanache Trachealis, Angina Maligna, Epidemical Eruptive Miliary Fever and Angina Ulcusculosa."[123] During the Civil War, diphtheria was one of the common diseases that affected all combatants.

In 1913, Schick introduced the skin test for immunity. However, disease control in the military did not involve using the Schick test on whole units and immunizing positive reactors because of the logistical burden that would have placed on time, materials, and workload. Instead, outbreaks were prevented by testing all known contacts of cases to identify carriers. The contacts were placed into group quarantine, which allowed for early detection and treatment with antitoxin of secondary cases.[112p74–83]

By World War I, the prevailing medical opinion dismissed diphtheria as a serious threat to military operations. Disease was usually sporadic among troops but could be epidemic if the conditions were favorable. Diphtheria was the 18th cause of death and the 28th cause of lost time during World War I in the Army, but it was often difficult to differentiate tracheitis and laryngitis caused by gassing from laryngeal diphtheria.[124] Adding to the confusion were laryngeal fibrino-purulent membranes, which formed in severely gassed patients and strongly resembled diphtheric membranes.

There were three documented epidemics of diphtheria during World War I. The disease was more common among enlisted white soldiers but had a higher case fatality rate among black soldiers. Crowding of troops in trains, transports, and billeting facilitated disease spread.[112] In 2 of the 42 divisions in the American Expeditionary Forces, diphtheria became a concern. Both divisions came from camps in the United States at sites with a high prevalence of diphtheria (the 32nd Division in Camp MacArthur, Texas, and the 35th Division in Camp Doniphan, Oklahoma). Carriers were the source of infection, and the crowded conditions allowed propagation and transmission of the organism. Once the 35th Division was encamped in France, with 48 hours of close contact, a sharp increase in diphtheria admissions was noted. After troops were distributed in billets and dugouts in the Vosges Mountains, crowding decreased and the morbidity rate declined. Of 10,909 admissions for diphtheria, 2,439 complications and 107 deaths were reported. The case fatality rate for the US Army was 1.62%.[124]

During World War II, cutaneous diphtheria became a problem for military personnel in North Africa.[114] This type of indolent skin infection may act as a source of respiratory infection in others. It is more common in warmer climates.[125]

Description of the Organism

Diphtheria is caused by a Gram-positive, club-shaped bacillus. It was discovered by Kelbs in 1883, and Loeffler succeeded in growing the organism in culture in 1884.

All corynebacteria have the heat-stable O antigen. K antigens, which are heat-labile proteins in the cell wall, differ among strains of *C diphtheriae*, and these differences permit classification into a number of types. There are three morphologically different biotypes: gravis, intermedius, and mitis. There is no consistent correlation between clinical severity and specific biotype.

Epidemiology

Transmission

Humans are the reservoir. The means of transmission is person to person, from intimate physical contact with a case or an asymptomatic carrier. Because the infection can be subclinical, asymptomatic individuals can transmit the infection. There has been no clear proof of indirect transmission by airborne droplet nuclei, dust, or fomites. Cutaneous lesions are important in transmission. Also, there is evidence of outbreaks caused by contaminated milk and milk products.[125]

Geographic Distribution

In temperate climates, diphtheria occurs throughout the year but seasonal increases are seen in colder months, probably as a result of close contact indoors. In tropical and warm climates, cutaneous diphtheria is more common and is not related to the season.

In the late 1980s and continuing into the 1990s, diphtheria reemerged in all but one of the independent states of what was the Soviet Union. There is the potential for importation of cases into the United States from this region, given the ease of global travel. To date, no imported case has been reported; however, there have been imported cases in Europe.[126]

Incidence

In the past, diphtheria was a major cause of morbidity and mortality. Peaks in incidence were observed approximately every 10 years. In Massachusetts between 1860 and 1897, death rates ranged between 46 and 196 per 100,000 annually. The proportion of total deaths that were attributable to diphtheria annually ranged between 3% and 10% during the same period.[125] In the United States in 1900, more than half as many deaths were caused by diphtheria as were caused by cancer. With the introduction of diphtheria antitoxin in the early 1900s, a considerable fall in the death rate occurred, but the number of cases remained high. In 1921, more than 200,000 cases were reported, primarily among children.[127] There were only 28 cases reported in the United States between 1982 and 1991.[128]

During World War II, a major outbreak, which apparently originated in Germany, spread throughout Western Europe, and more than 1 million cases were eventually reported. Occasional widespread epidemics have occurred, notably in Austin and San Antonio, Texas, between 1967 and 1970.[125] In 1994 in the former Soviet Union, there were 47,802 cases and 1,746 deaths reported. Serological surveys for diphtheria antibodies reveal that 20% to 60% of US adults older than 20 years of age are susceptible.[126] US military recruits from Micronesia show a 39% seronegative rate for diphtheria.[87]

There has been a nearly complete disappearance of the disease in countries that have immunized widely. Ninety-six percent of school-aged children in the United States have received three or more doses of diphtheria and tetanus toxoids and pertussis vaccine.[127] A distinct and disturbing trend, though, seems to be an increasing serosusceptibility with advancing age. While diphtheria was once commonplace, it is now largely confined in the United States to adults over the age of 20 who have not obtained recommended boosting doses.[125]

Pathogenesis and Clinical Findings

Roux, one of Pasteur's assistants, and Yersin demonstrated in 1888 that the diphtheria bacillus produced a powerful toxin. Toxin production is mediated by bacteriophages. When the bacteria are infected with the corynebacteriphage that contains the gene *tox*, toxin production will occur. The toxin is identical among all the strains. The diphtheria toxin is a polypeptide with a molecular weight of approximately 58,000. The toxin has two fragments: A and B. Fragment B penetrates the cell, and toxicity is due to the disruption of cellular protein synthesis by the A fragment of the toxin.[125] Antibodies directed against the B fragment protect against infection.

The incubation period is from 1 to 6 days. Early symptoms are mild and nonspecific. Fever, if present, does not usually exceed 38°C (101°F). The patient may complain of a sore throat, and the cervical lymph nodes may be enlarged, giving rise to the so-called "bull neck." There may be a serosanguinous nasal discharge. At first, the pharynx is suffused with blood on physical exam, but about 1 day after onset, small patches of exudate appear. Within 2 or 3 days, the patches spread, become confluent, and may form a membrane that covers the entire pharynx, including the tonsillar areas, soft palate, and uvula. The membrane will take on a grayish color and is thick and firmly adherent. Efforts to dislodge it usually result in bleeding. The patient will appear very ill and may have a rapid, thready pulse. If the patient is not treated, the membrane will begin to soften after a week and will eventually slough off. Other sites may become involved, including cutaneous, vaginal, aural, and conjunctival areas. Altogether, these sites account for 2% of cases and are secondary to nasopharyngeal infection.[125]

The impact of diphtheria is largely felt by its propensity to cause complications, especially in the nervous and cardiovascular systems. Severe complications typically fall into one of three categories: acute systemic toxicity, myocarditis, and peripheral neuritis. Only toxin-producing biotypes cause myocarditis and neuritis.[127] The major complications of laryngeal diphtheria are croup and respiratory obstruction.

Bacilli that are not infected by bacteriophages can also cause disease even though they do not produce the toxin. This condition is called avirulent diphteria, and it tends to be mild.[129]

Diagnostic Approaches

An adherent, grayish membrane in the throat of a patient who is acutely ill should suggest the diagnosis. The differential diagnosis would include bacterial and viral pharyngitis, Vincent's angina, oral syphilis, candidiasis, infectious mononucleosis, acute adult epiglottis, croup, and facial nerve palsies from neurological complications of Lyme disease.[10] Diphtheria most often appears as a membranous pharyngitis. A patient with a confluent pharyngeal exudate should be suspected of having diphtheria until proven otherwise. The onset is gradual, with a steady progression through hoarseness to stridor over a period of 2 to 3 days. Material for culture should be obtained with direct visualization and is best taken from the edge or beneath the edge of the membrane. Cutaneous diphtheria may appear as a sharply demarcated lesion with a pseudomembranous base at the site of a wound. Its appearance may not be distinctive, however, and the diagnosis can only be confirmed by positive culture.[127]

Recommendations for Therapy and Control

Treatment of diphtheria is a two-step process. The first step involves the administration of diphtheria equine antitoxin. The amount of toxin produced is in direct proportion to the size of the membrane. Depending on how extensive the local lesions are, the total recommended amount of antitoxin will vary between 20,000 and 100,000 U. A higher dose of antitoxin will also be required as the interval between onset of disease and initiation of treatment lengthens.[125]

The second step of treatment is to eliminate carriage of the organism in the pharynx or nose or on the skin. It is necessary to administer a course of either penicillin (intramuscular penicillin G benzathine 600,000 U for children younger than 6 years of age or 1.2 million U for patients 6 years and older) or erythromycin (7- to 10-day course at 40mg/kg per day for children and 1 g per day for adults). Treatment should continue until there are at least three consecutive negative cultures.

If a susceptible, unimmunized patient is exposed to diphtheria but is asymptomatic, the preferred course is to obtain a throat culture, begin immunization with diphtheria toxoid, and initiate prophylaxis with either a single dose of benzathine penicillin or oral erythromycin for 7 days. Patients should be kept under observation. If they cannot be observed, they should be given 5,000 to 10,000 U of antitoxin intramuscularly and started on a course of oral erythromycin (40 to 50 mg/kg per day for 7 days, maximum 2 g per day), or be given a single intramuscular dose of benathine penicillin G (600 U for children younger than 6 years of age and 1.2 million U for patients 6 years and older).[69p230–234]

Diphtheria is a reportable infection; case reports are obligatory in most states. Measures must be taken to avoid an epidemic. Patients with pharyngeal diphtheria must be kept in strict isolation, and those with cutaneous diphtheria require contact isolation. Two cultures from the throat and nose (taken not less than 24 hours apart and not less than 24 hours after finishing antimicrobial therapy), or from skin lesions for those with cutaneous disease, must be negative for diphtheria bacilli before the isolation precautions can be discontinued. All articles used by patients need to be thoroughly disinfected. All contacts need to be kept under surveillance for 7 days, and cultures of the nose and throat should be taken to rule out asymptomatic carriage of the organism. Regardless of their asymptomatic state and their immunization history, all contacts should be given a single dose of penicillin or a 7- to 10-day course of erythromycin. If contacts of cases are employed in occupations that involve handling food or working with children who may not be immunized, the contacts should be excluded from work until they are proven not to be carriers. If contacts have been immunized, they should receive a booster dose of diphtheria toxoid. If contacts have no history of immunization, a primary series should be started, using Td, DT, DTP, or DTP-Hib vaccine, depending on each contact's age.[10]

The cornerstone of prevention remains an active immunization program. It has its roots in the work of Theobald Smith in 1907. He noted that long-lasting immunity to diphtheria could be produced in guinea pigs by injection of mixtures of diphtheria toxin and antitoxin. The presence of antibodies to the toxin ensures clinical immunity. To provide protection against diphtheria, the toxin is rendered into a toxoid by using formaldehyde to destroy the enzymatic capabilities of the toxin while allowing it to retain its immunogenicity. This concept was demonstrated by Ramon in the 1920s.[125]

By the mid-1940s, diphtheria toxoid was combined with tetanus toxoid and pertussis vaccine in the now familiar diphtheria, tetanus, and pertussis vaccine combination, called DTP. Five doses are recommended for children at ages 2, 4, 6, 15, and 18 months and at school entry before the seventh birthday. It can be safely administered with other vaccines (eg, *H influenzae* type b vaccine; hepatitis B vaccine; live, attenuated measles-mumps-rubella vaccine) without loss of efficacy. DTP contains between 10 and 20 Lf (Loeffler units) per immunizing dose of 0.5 mL. The formulation for adults, Td, contains the same amount of tetanus toxoid as does DTP, but the amount of diphtheria toxoid is reduced to 2 Lf per dose. Seventy percent or more of a childhood population must be immune to diphtheria to prevent major community outbreaks.[125] Because of the concern about the proportion of susceptible adults, it is imperative that immunity to diphtheria be sustained by booster doses of Td every 10 years.

Service members' immunization records are screened before deployments and, when indicated, the personnel receive Td boosters every 10 years.[44] With the US military's ever increasing international role in operations other than war and recent joint training missions to places such as Ukraine, where diphtheria has become epidemic, it is imperative that vaccine status be vigilantly screened and personnel be appropriately immunized.

[Paula K. Underwood]

POLIO

Introduction and Military Relevance

Polio is an enterovirus, spread person to person through the fecal–oral route. At the most severe end of the clinical spectrum, it can cause a flaccid paralysis, respiratory failure, and death; most often, though, infection is mild or asymptomatic. It is difficult today to imagine the widespread terror that polio caused in the American public in the 1940s and 1950s. Anyone, including a future president of the United States, could be stricken with polio, and parents even kept their children from public swimming pools in fear of it. Although now it has been eradicated from the Western hemisphere, polio remains a problem throughout many developing countries, especially in India and sub-Saharan Africa.

The World Health Organization's Global Poliomyelitis Eradication Initiative has reduced the number of reported cases of polio worldwide by more than 80% since the mid-1980s.[130] The goal, also ascribed to by Rotary International, the United Nations Children's Fund, and the Centers for Disease Control and Prevention, was to eradicate polio worldwide by the year 2000.[131] Certification of the complete interruption of indigenous transmission of wild polio virus is expected by 2005.[132]

Polio has not been considered an important disease in military forces primarily because 90% of the paralytic polio cases occur in persons younger than 20 years of age. During World War I, there were only 69 diagnosed cases.[112p110–114] But because of the seriousness of the disease, the probability that service members will be deployed to endemic areas, the effectiveness of the preventive measures, and the worldwide effort to eradicate polio, polio vaccination remains an important component of military preventive medicine.

Description of the Pathogen

Polio is an enterovirus, an RNA virus belonging to the family *Picornaviridae*. There are three distinct serotypes: 1, 2, and 3.

Epidemiology

Transmission

Humans are the sole reservoir of polio, and no permanent carrier state is known. Polio is transmitted by the fecal-oral route but can also be spread by direct contact with nasal and throat discharges via respiratory particles—an oral-oral route. Polioviruses are transient inhabitants of the human alimentary tract and can be detected in the throat or lower intestine.[131] Although highly contagious, most infections are subclinical. The ratio of inapparent infections to overt cases is greater than 100:1 and can be as large a difference as 1,000:1.[133] Symptomless infected persons, as well as overt cases, can spread infection.

Paralytic polio tends to appear sporadically; usually there is no clear connection among cases. Even though a family has only one case of paralytic polio, the other family members may be infected. In fact, the prevalence of infection is highest among household contacts. The virus disseminates so rapidly that by the time the first case is recognized in a family, all the susceptible family members can already be infected.[134]

Geographic Distribution

Poliovirus infection occurs worldwide, but there are some differences in seasonal patterns. It occurs year-round in the tropics, while in temperate zones it is most common during the summer and fall. This helps explain the fear in the United States of contracting polio from swimming pools.

Incidence

The virus affects all age groups, but children are more susceptible than adults because of their lack of acquired immunity. The case fatality rate is variable, but it is 5% to 10% higher in the older population.[134] There are three major epidemiological phases of poliovirus infection: endemic, epidemic, and vaccine-era.

In an endemic state, polioviruses are commonly present. New susceptibles, usually infants, provide a constant supply of individuals to maintain the infection cycle. Women of childbearing age typically possess antibodies to all three serotypes of poliovirus, and their newborns benefit from temporary passive immunity. It is estimated that in developing countries there were 20,000 to 25,000 cases of paralytic polio in 1997.[135]

At the turn of the century in the United States (the prevaccine era), there were periodic epidemics of polio. This was largely a result of the improvement in household hygiene and community standards of sanitation. Infants and young children were not being exposed as early to the polioviruses. When they did encounter the viruses, they were older and more likely to experience paralysis. The likelihood of epidemics increased because the number of susceptibles increased as the delay until exposure lengthened. In 1916, 80% of cases were in children younger than 5 years of age. From 1953 to 1954, the annual number of paralytic cases in the United States was approximately 21,000. The peak age incidence had risen to 5 to 9 years. One third of cases and two thirds of deaths were in individuals older than 15.[134]

Paralytic poliomyelitis became a notifiable disease in the United States in 1951. Case ascertainment methods have not changed since 1958, when the Centers for Disease Control and Prevention (then known as the Communicable Disease Center) began classifying cases of paralytic poliomyelitis according to criteria known as the "best available paralytic poliomyelitis case count" or BAPPCC. This count included only cases of poliomyelitis that caused permanent paralysis. These criteria omitted cases caused by enteroviruses other than polioviruses. Since 1975, cases have been classified according to criteria known as the "epidemiological classification of paralytic poliomyelitis cases" (ECPPC). This classification describes cases as epidemic, endemic, imported, or occurring in immunodeficient individuals.[136]

In the vaccine-era, polio has become a rare disease in the United States. Administration of live oral polio vaccine (OPV) has halted epidemics in progress and has greatly reduced the incidence of polio. Poliovirus vaccines have decreased by 99.9% the annual number of reported cases of paralytic polio in the United States—from 21,269 in 1954 to 6 in 1991.[137]

Recruits in basic training have been immunized against polio since the introduction of an effective vaccine in 1955. A 1989 national serosurvey of US Army recruits showed that poliovirus seronegativity rates were similar across demographic subgroups. When looking at seronegativity by birth cohort, it was apparent that seronegativity to type 3 poliovirus has not clearly lessened.[14]

The wild type of polio was officially declared eradicated from the Americas on September 29, 1994, by the International Commission for the Certification of Poliomyelitis Eradication in the Americas. The last confirmed case occurred on August 21, 1991 in Peru.[138] The few cases that occur now in the United States are related to the polio vaccine. A study[139] of cases occurring from 1973 through 1984 in the United States revealed 138 cases of paralytic poliomyelitis, of which 105 (76%) were associated with receipt of OPV. Thirty five of the cases occurred in individuals who had received OPV, 50 in contacts of OPV recipients, 14 in previously undiagnosed immunodeficient individuals, and 6 in those with no history of either receipt of OPV or contact with recent OPV recipients and were assumed to have had community contact with an OPV recipient.

An approximation is made of the frequency of paralytic polio by estimating ratios of vaccine-associated cases to net doses of OPV distributed. The overall ratio was found to be one case per 2.4 million to 2.6 million doses distributed, including cases in immunodeficient patients and cases in persons without a history of having received a recent vaccine.[130,139] Annual numbers of cases have been reduced to as few as 3 per 100 million resident population. In immunologically normal recipients, the risk of paralysis following OPV is 1 case per 6.2 million doses. The risk to close contacts of OPV recipients is 1 case per 7.6 million doses.[130]

Pathogenesis and Clinical Findings

The virus enters the alimentary tract and multiplies locally. It then appears in the throat and the stools. The virus is excreted in stools for several weeks and is present in the pharynx 1 to 2 weeks after infection. Secondary spread occurs through the bloodstream and reaches other tissues, to include the lymph nodes, brown fat, and the central nervous system (CNS).[134] The invasion of the CNS occurs several days after the virus has entered the bloodstream. By this time, antibody has already been produced and is detectable.

The incubation period is 7 to 14 days, but can range from 3 to 18 days or longer. If present, the symptoms are nonspecific at first and can include fever, malaise, headache, drowsiness, constipation, sore throat, nausea, and vomiting. This constellation of symptoms can present in any combination. Two basic patterns of illness exist: (1) a minor or abortive type and (2) a major type, which can be either paralytic or nonparalytic. Only 1% of infections result in paralysis. The paralytic-type pattern is demonstrated after several symptomless days with a reappearance of symptoms, such as reoccurrence of fever, meningeal irritation, and paralysis, 5 to 10 days later.[140] Acute flaccid paralysis, characteristic of poliomyelitis, results when there is multiplication of the virus within the CNS with subsequent destruction of motor neurons. In children younger than 5 years old, paralysis of one leg is most commonly seen, but in patients 5 to 15 years of age, weakness of one arm or paraplegia is frequent. Quadriplegia is most common in adults. About 1% of cases develop aseptic meningitis.[10p398-405]

Even many years after infection, there can be a reoccurrence of problems. Twenty-five percent of individuals who had paralytic polio in the 1940s and 1950s have had a recrudescence of paralysis and muscle wasting by the 1990s. This is referred to as post-polio syndrome and has been reported only in people who were infected during the time when wild-type poliovirus was in circulation. Patients may experience an exacerbation of their already existing weakness, or they may go on to develop new weakness or paralysis.[130] The late effects may be associated with the changes of aging and further loss of anterior horn cells, the neurons that have been depleted by an earlier poliovirus infection.[141] Alternatively, there is evidence to suggest that poliovirus can persist in postpolio patients.[142]

Diagnostic Approaches

Enteroviruses, such as poliovirus, are exceedingly common. Other enteroviruses can be found in stools of patients with symptoms resembling all but the most severe paralytic manifestations of polio. Cultures of human or monkey cells are used to recover and identify the polioviruses. Throat or rectal swabs can be used. Stool cultures yield the greatest likelihood for positive identification of the virus, but they must be collected in a timely fashion to increase the likelihood of case confirmation.[130] The virus can be found in 80% of patients during the first 2 weeks of illness. It is very difficult to isolate the virus from the cerebrospinal fluid. Neutralizing antibodies, which should be assessed for each of the three polio serotypes, are formed early; paired serum specimens show a 4-fold rise in antibody titer after 3 weeks. Cases must be clinically and epidemiologically compatible with poliomyelitis, must have resulted in paralysis, and must have a residual neurological deficit 60 days after onset of initial symptoms.[136] If a child or a young adult has any asymmetric flaccid limb paralysis or bulbar palsies without sensory loss during a febrile illness, this almost always is indicative of poliomyelitis. However, the diagnosis of polio cannot be reliably diagnosed solely on the basis of clinical presentation.[143] In reality, the only reliable method of diagnosing polio is by isolation of the virus from the stool. It is not possible to definitely distinguish polio and Guillain-Barré syndrome purely on the basis of clinical findings, because polio may have an atypical presentation.[144] Guillain-Barré may progress for up to 4 weeks, but polio usually manifests the maximum extent of paralysis within 4 days.[145] The differential diagnosis of paralytic polio also includes tick paralysis, insecticide poisoning, botulism, trichinosis, transverse myelitis, and various neuropathies.

Recommendations for Therapy and Control

Historically, quarantine was the only method of control. It was imposed for 3 weeks after the occurrence of the last diagnosed case. In 1940, Dunham's *Military Preventive Medicine*[112] noted that chemical prophylaxis (an olfactory mucosal spray of 0.5% picric acid and 0.5% sodium alum in 0.85% saline solution) was believed to be useful, but it was never proved to be effective in preventing polio.

The first polio vaccine, an inactivated polio vaccine (IPV) was developed by Jonas Salk following the successful propagation of poliovirus in tissue cultures by Enders, Weller, and Robbins. Use of IPV dramatically reduced cases of paralytic polio, from 21,269 cases in 1952 to 980 in 1961.[146] Later Albert Sabin and fellow researchers introduced the live OPV. It has been considered one of the safest vaccines in use. The first large-scale production of OPV took place in the Soviet Union, when a mass immunization campaign in 1959 and 1960 covered 77.5 million people. This resulted in a sharp decrease in incidence, from 10.6 per 100,000 in 1958 to 0.43 per 100,000 in 1963.[134] Routine use of live oral attenuated poliomyelitis vaccines was begun in many countries during the spring of 1960. OPV became a routine vaccine for childhood immunization.[147] At that time, monovalent vaccines were used, incorporating each serotype separately. The trivalent vaccine, with its mixture of three sero-

types of attenuated polioviruses, replaced this methodology in 1965 and has become the standard. Live OPV prevents paralytic polio by inducing two distinct types of antibodies: a local secretory antibody at the primary sites of virus multiplication in the alimentary tract and a humoral antibody, which prevents virus from reaching and invading the CNS. Vaccination effectively interrupts secondary spread of the virus to the CNS by induction of antibodies. Persistence of protection is clearly demonstrated by the great reductions in cases of polio in all areas of the world where OPV is used.

In 1973, the World Health Organization (WHO) established a Consultative Group on Poliomyelitis, which serves as the custodian of Sabin's attenuated vaccine strains. There are 16 manufacturers of vaccine around the world; two use human diploid cells for growing their vaccine viruses and 14 use African green monkey kidney cells. In 1978, an enhanced-potency IPV was developed and found to be more immunogenic for both children and adults than the previous formulation of IPV.[130]

Because the risk of polio has been eradicated in the Americas, the only polio cases occurring within the United States since 1979 are those secondary to receipt of the oral polio vaccine. To reduce the amount of vaccine-associated paralytic poliomyelitis (VAPP), the Advisory Committee on Immunization Practices (ACIP) changed the recommendations for polio vaccine in 1997. The recommended schedule consisted of IPV given at 2 and 4 months, followed by OPV at 12 to 18 months and 4 to 6 years. With the progression of the global polio eradication campaign, the likelihood of importing poliovirus into the United States decreased substantially. Because the sequential schedule was well accepted without any concurrent decline in childhood immunization coverage, the ACIP made new recommendations in June 1999 to go to an all-IPV schedule. This, all children should receive IPV at 2, 4, and 6 to 18 months at 4 to 6 years. Sole use of IPV in vaccination against polio carries no risk of VAPP or secondary transmission of the vaccine virus.[133]

The Global Poliomyelitis Eradication Initiative relies heavily on the use of OPV, one of the limitations of which is the need to preserve the cold chain to ensure its potency. OPV requires storage at temperatures of below 0°C (32°F). It should also not be administered to immunocompromised individuals because of their increased risk for VAPP, though the WHO does recommend its use in infants infected with human immunodeficiency virus who are subject to polio exposure. OPV is contraindicated for use in households with immunodeficient individuals, because the vaccine virus is excreted in the stool for 6 to 8 weeks and can infect the immunocompromised person. IPV is a better choice for those individuals. Other key elements of effective eradication of wild poliovirus are case detection and immediate action to eliminate foci of persistent infection with "mopping up" techniques. This involves administration of OPV to children on a house-to-house basis, then repeating the task 4 to 6 weeks later. Any child under the age of 5 years who has an acute flaccid paralysis for which no cause can be identified or any child who has a paralytic illness at any age can be considered suspected cases of polio. The WHO recommends that OPV be given concurrently with vaccines against diphtheria, tetanus, and pertussis at 6, 10, and 14 weeks of age.[147] In polio-endemic countries, an additional dose at birth is recommended.[69p465-470] It has been noted that in tropical climates seroconversion following three doses of OPV was often lower than in temperate climates. Mass administration of OPV led to a dramatic reduction in the incidence of polio in Brazil during 1980 and showed the role National Immunization Days can play in polio eradication. In spite of failed individual seroconversion, the wild poliovirus can still be eliminated with mass immunization strategies.[147]

As long as polio exists elsewhere, there will always be the risk of importation of the wild-type virus into the United States. Therefore, it is crucial not to become complacent about immunization, the only effective defense against polio.[134] Population immunity can be maintained by vaccinating children early in their first year of life.[130] At least 440,000 cases of paralytic polio have been prevented annually by the use of live OPV, according to WHO estimates.[134]

Because military personnel deploy to and live in areas of the world where polio is endemic, their risk of exposure is a real one. It is and will remain imperative to assure high levels of immunity in service members. Persons who have had a primary series of OPV or IPV and who will be exposed to polio, as might happen on military deployments, may as adults receive another booster dose of either OPV or IPV. Adults who have not previously been vaccinated with OPV should receive the IPV series prior to travel. The need for additional booster doses of either OPV or IPV has not yet been established.[130]

[Paula K. Underwood]

REFERENCES

1. Black FL. Measles. In: Evans AS, ed. *Viral Infections of Humans: Epidemiology and Control.* 3rd ed. New York: Plenum; 1989: 451–469.

2. Markowitz LE, Katz SL. Measles. Plotkin SA, Mortimer EA, eds. *Vaccines.* 2nd ed. Philadelphia: W.B. Saunders; 1994: 229–276.

3. Enders JF. Francis Home and his experimental approach to medicine. *Bull Hist Med.* 1964;38:101–112.

4. Panum PL. Observation made during the epidemic of measles on the Faroe Islands in the year 1846. *Med Classics.* 1939;3:839–886.

5. Crawford GE, Gremillion DH. Epidemic measles and rubella in Air Force recruits: Impact of immunization. *J Infect Dis.* 1981;144:403–410.

6. Centers for Disease Control and Prevention. Measles—United States, 1995. *MMWR.* 1996;45:305–307.

7. de Quadros CA, Olive JM, Hersh BS, et al. Measles elimination in the Americas: Evolving strategies. *JAMA.* 1996;275:224–229.

8. Black FL. A nationwide survey of US military recruits, 1962, III: Measles and mumps antibodies. *Am J Hyg.* 1964;80:304–307.

9. Kelley PW. *Susceptibility to Measles and Rubella Among US Army Recruits: A Seroepidemiologic Analysis of Risk Factors, Temporal Trends, and Disease Control Policy Options.* Baltimore, Md: Johns Hopkins University; 1994. Dissertation.

10. Chin J, ed. *Control of Communicable Diseases Manual.* 17th ed. Washington, DC: American Public Health Association; 2000.

11. Centers for Disease Control and Prevention. Recommendations of the International Task Force for Disease Eradication. *MMWR*. 1993;42(RR-16):14–18.

12. Centers for Disease Control and Prevention. Summary of notifiable diseases, US, 1994. *MMWR*. 1994;43:1–80.

13. National Vaccine Advisory Committee. The measles epidemic: The problems, barriers, and recommendations. *JAMA*. 1991;226:1547–1552.

14. Kelley PW, Petruccelli BP, Stehr-Green P, Erickson RL, Mason CJ. The susceptibility of young adult Americans to vaccine-preventable infections: a national serosurvey of US Army recruits. *JAMA*. 1991;266:2724–2729.

15. Centers for Disease Control and Prevention. Measles outbreak—Netherlands, April 1999-January 2000. *MMWR*. 2000;49:299–303.

16. Centers for Disease Control and Prevention. Recommended childhood immunization schedule—US, 1995. *MMWR*. 1995;44(RR-5):4–5.

17. Ferson MJ, Young LC, Robertson PW, Whybin LR. Difficulties in clinical diagnosis of measles: Proposal for modified clinical case definition. *Med J Aust*. 1995;163:364–66.

18. Behrman RE, Vaughan VC. *Nelson Textbook of Pediatrics*. Philadelphia: W.B. Saunders; 1988.

19. White CC, Koplan JP, Orenstein WA. Benefits, risks, and costs of immunization for measles, mumps, and rubella. *Am J Public Health*. 1985;75:739–744.

20. *American Medical News*. 1994;24–31(Oct):20.

21. Boyden SV, ed. *The Impact of Civilization on the Biology of Man*. Toronto: University of Toronto Press; 1970.

22. Centers for Disease Control and Prevention. Recommendations from a meeting on the feasibility of global measles eradication. *MMWR*. 1996;45:891–892.

23. Horstmann DM. Rubella. In: Evans AS, ed. *Viral Infections of Humans: Epidemiology and Control*. 3rd ed. New York: Plenum; 1989: 617–631.

24. Gregg NM. Congenital cataract following German measles in the mother. *Trans Ophthalmol Soc Aust*. 1941:3:35–46.

25. Plotkin SA. Rubella. In: Plotkin SA, Mortimer EA, ed. *Vaccines*. 2nd ed. Philadelphia: W.B. Saunders; 1994: 303–336.

26. Ingalls TH. Rubella—epidemiology, virology, and immunology: The epidemiology of rubella. *Am J Med Sci*. 1967:253:349–356.

27. United States Army Center for Health Promotion and Preventive Medicine. Rubella outbreak in German troops at Fort Bragg. *Morbidity Surveillance Monthly Report*. 1995;1(2):2.

28. Centers for Disease Control and Prevention. Recommendations of the International Task Force for Disease Eradication. *MMWR*. 1993;42(RR-16):14–18.

29. Crawford GE, Gremillion DH. Epidemic measles and rubella in Air Force recruits: Impact of immunization. *J Infect Dis*. 1981;144:403–410.

30. Vaananen P, Makela P, Vaheri A. Effect of low-level immunity on response to live rubella virus vaccine. *Vaccine*. 1986;4:5–8.

31. Horstman DM, Leibhaber H, LeBouvier GL, Rosenberg DA, Halstead SB. Rubella infection of vaccinated and naturally immune person exposed in an epidemic. *N Engl J Med*. 1970;283:771–778.

32. Brody JA. The infectiousness of rubella and the possibility of reinfection. *Am J Public Health*. 1966;56:1082–1087.

33. Forrest JM, Menser MA, Honeyman MC, Stout M, Murphy AM. Clinical rubella eleven months after vaccination. *Lancet*. 1972;2:339–400.

34. Northrop RL, Gardner WM, Geittmann WF. Rubella reinfection during early pregnancy: A case report. *Obstet Gynecol*. 1972;39:524–526.

35. Morgan-Capner P, Burgess C, Ireland RM, Sharp JC. Clinically apparent rubella reinfection with a detectable rubella specific IgM response. *Brit Med J*. 1983;286:1616–1624.

36. Alford CA, Griffiths PD. Rubella. In: Remington JS, Klein JO, eds. *Infectious Diseases of the Fetus and the Newborn Infant*. Philadelphia: W.B. Sanders; 1983.

37. National Communicable Disease Center. *Rubella Surveillance*. Washington, DC: United States Department of Health, Education, and Welfare: June 1969. Report 1.

38. Fraser FR, Cunninghan AL, Hayes K. Rubella arthritis in adults: Isolation of virus, cytology, and other aspects of infection. *Clin Exp Rheumatol*. 1983;1:287–291.

39. Moriuchi H, Yamasaki S, Mori K, Sakai M, Tsuji Y. A rubella epidemic in Sasebo, Japan in 1987 with various complications. *Acta Paediatr Jpn Overseas Ed*. 1990;32:67–75.

40. Peckham CS, Marshall WC, Dudgeon JA. Rubella vaccination of schoolgirls: Factors affecting vaccine uptake. *Brit Med J*. 1988;297:760–761.

41. Enders G. Rubella antibody titers in vaccinated and non-vaccinated women and the results of vaccination during pregnancy. *Rev Infect Dis*. 1985;7(Suppl):S103–S107.

42. Plotkin SA, Cochran W, Leindquist J, Schaffer D. Congenital rubella syndrome in late infancy. *JAMA*. 1967;200:435–441.

43. Siber GR, Werner BG, Halsey NA. Interference of immune globulin with measles and rubella immunization. *J Pediatr*. 1993;122:204–211.

44. Departments of the Air Force, Army, Navy, and Transportation. *Immunizations and Chemoprophylaxis*. Washington, DC: DoD; 1995. Air Force Joint Instruction 48-110, Army Regulation 40-562, BUMEDINST 6230.15, CG COMDTINST M6230.4E.

45. Institute of Medicine. *Adverse Effects of Pertussis and Rubella Vaccines*. Washington, DC: National Academy Press; 1991.

46. Feldman FA. Mumps. In: Plotkin SA, Mortimer EA, ed. *Vaccines*. 2nd ed. Philadelphia: W.B. Saunders; 1994: 471–491.

47. Brooks H. Epidemic parotitis as a military disease. *Med Clin North Am*. 1918;2:493–505.

48. Parran T. Health and medical preparedness. *JAMA*. 1940;115:49–51.

49. Arday DR, Kanjarpane DD, Kelley PW. Mumps in the US Army 1980–1986: Should recruits be immunized? *Am J Public Health*. 1989;79:471–474.

50. Centers for Disease Control and Prevention. Mumps Surveillance—United States, 1988–1993. *MMWR*. 1995;44(SS-3)1–14.

51. Feldman FA Mumps. In: Evan AS, ed. *Viral Infections of Humans: Epidemiology and Control*. 3rd ed. New York: Plenum; 1989.

52. McGuinness AC, Gall EA. Mumps at army camps in 1943. *War Med*. 1944;5:95–104.

53. Liao SJ, Benenson AS. Immunity status of military recruits in 1951 in the United States, II: Results of mumps complement fixation tests. *Am J Hyg*. 1954;59:273–281.

54. McGuiness AC, Gall EA. Mumps at Army camps in 1943. *War Med*. 1944;5:95–104.

55. Krugman S, de Quadros C. *Eradication of Measles, Rubella, and Mumps in Cuba: Report of a Technical Advisory Group*. Washington, DC: Pan American Health Organization; 1989.

56. Falk WA, Buchan K, Dow M, et al. The epidemiology of mumps is Southern Alberta, 1980–1982. *Am J Epidemiol*. 1989;130:736–749.

57. Cooney MK, Fox JP, Hall CE. The Seattle Virus Watch, VI: Observations of infections with and illness due to parainfluenza, mumps, and respiratory syncytial viruses and *Mycoplasma pneumoniae*. *Am J Epidemiol*. 1975;101:532.

58. Werner CA. Mumps orchitis and testicular atrophy, I: Occurrence. *Ann Intern Med*. 1950;32:1066–1074.

59. Werner CA. Mumps orchitis and testicular atrophy, II: A factor in male sterility. *Ann Intern Med*. 1950;32:1075–1086.

60. Swerdlow AJ, Huttly SR, Smith PG. Testicular cancer and antecedent diseases. *Br J Cancer*. 1987;55:97–103.

61. Sultz HA, Hart BA, Zielezny M, Schlesinger ER. Is mumps virus an etiologic factor in juvenile diabetes mellitus? *J Pediatr*. 1975;86:654–656.

62. Hall R, Richards H. Hearing loss due to mumps. *Arch Dis Child*. 1987;62:189–191.

63. Philip RN, Reinhard KR, Lackman DB. Observations on a mumps epidemic in a "virgin" population. *Am J Hyg*. 1959;69:91–111.

64. Gordon SC, Lauter CB. Mumps arthritis: A review of the literature. *Rev Infect Dis*. 1984;6:338–344.

65. Ukkonen P, Vaisanen O, Penttinen K. Enzyme-linked immunosorbent assay for mumps and parainfluenza type 1 immunoglobulin G and immunoglobulin M antibodies. *J Clin Microbiol*. 1980;11:319–323.

66. Anderson RM, Crombie JA, Grenfell BT. The epidemiology of mumps in the UK: A preliminary study of virus transmission, herd immunity and the potential impact of immunization. *Epidemiol Infect*. 1987;99:65–84.

67. Wharton M, Cochi SL, Hutcheson RH, Bistowish JM, Schaffner W. A large outbreak of mumps in the postvaccine era. *J Infect Dis*. 1988;158:1253–1260.

68. Erickson RL. Of mumps and men. *Walter Reed Army Institute of Research Communicable Disease Report*. 1990;1(2):6–9.

69. Pickerling LK, ed. *2000 Red Book: Report of the Committee on Infectious Diseases*. 25th ed. Elk Grove Village, Ill: American Academy of Pediatrics; 2000: 624–638.

70. Centers for Disease Control and Prevention. Prevention of varicella: Recommendation of the Advisory Committee on Immunization Practice (ACIP). *MMWR*. 1996;45(RR-11):1–36.

71. Plotkin SA. Varicella vaccine. *Pediatrics*. 1996;87:251–253.

72. Sweard JF, Wharton M. Varicella and herpes zoster. In: Wallace RB, ed. *Maxcy-Rosenau-Last Public Health and Preventive Medicine*. Stamford, Conn: Appleton & Lange; 1998: 117–123.

73. Longfield JN, Winn RE, Gibson RL, Juchau SV, Hoffman PV. Varicella outbreaks in Army recruits from Puerto Rico: Varicella susceptibility in a population from the tropics. *Arch Intern Med*. 1990;150:970–973.

74. Gray GC, Palinkas LA, Kelley PW. Increasing incidence of varicella hospitalizations in United States Army and Navy personnel: Are today's teenagers more susceptible? Should recruits be vaccinated? *Pediatrics*. 1990;86:867–873.

75. Streuwing JP, Hyams KC, Tueller JE, Gray GC. The risk of measles, mumps, and varicella among young adults: A serosurvey of US Navy and Marine Corps recruits. *Am J Public Health*. 1993;83:1717–1720.

76. Rubertone MV. Chief, Army Medical Surveillance Activity, US Army Center for Health Promotion and Preventive Medicine, Written Communication, 1997.

77. Herrin VE, Gray GC. Decreasing rates of hospitalization for varicella among young adults. *J Infect Dis*. 1996;174:835–838.

78. Zaia JA, Grose C. Varicella and herpes zoster. In: Gorbach SL, Bartlett JG, Blacklow NR, ed. *Infectious Diseases*. Philadelphia: W.B. Saunders; 1992: 1101–1111.

79. Gershon AA. Chickenpox, measles, and mumps. In: Remington JS, Klein JO, ed. *Infectious Diseases of the Fetus and Newborn Infant*. Philadelphia: W.B. Saunders; 1995: 565–591.

80. Demmler GJ, Steinberg SP, Blum G, Gershon AA. Rapid enzyme-linked immunosorbent assay for detecting antibody to varicella-zoster virus. *J Infect Dis*. 1988;157:211–212.

81. Choo DC, Chew SK, Tan EH, Lim MK, Monteiro EH. Oral acyclovir in the treatment of adult varicella. *Ann Acad Med Singapore*. 1995;24:316–321.

82. Clements DA, Armstrong CB, Ursano AM, Moggio MM, Walter EB, Wilfert CM. Over five-year follow-up of Oka/Merck varicella vaccine recipients in 465 infants and adolescents. *Pediatr Infect Dis J*. 1995;14:874–879.

83. Oka/Merck Vaccine Division. Varivax (Varicella Virus Vaccine Live). 1995. Package insert.

84. Reef S, Centers for Disease Control and Prevention, Oral Communication, 1996.

85. Kuter BJ, Ngai A, Patterson CM, et al. Safety, tolerability, and immunogenicity of two regimens of Oka/Merck varicella vaccine (Varivax) in healthy adolescents and adults. *Vaccine*. 1995;13:967–972.

86. Ryan M. Great Lakes Naval Training Center, Great Lakes, Ill, Oral Communication, 1997.

87. Withers BG, Kelley PW, Pang LW, et al. Vaccine-preventable disease susceptibility in a young adult Micronesian population. *Southeast Asian J Trop Med Public Health*. 1994;25:569–574. Published erratum: *Southeast Asian J Trop Med Public Health*. 1995;26:198.

88. Centers for Disease Control and Prevention. Pertussis—United States, January 1992–June 1995. *MMWR*. 1995;44:525–529.

89. Herwaldt LA. Pertussis in adults: What physicians need to know. *Arch Intern Med*. 1991;151:1510–1512.

90. Mink CM, Cherry JD, Christenson P, et al. A search for *Bordetella pertussis* infection in university students. *Clin Infect Dis*. 1992;14:464–471.

91. Cherry JD, Beer T, Chartrand SA, et al. Comparison of values of antibody to *Bordetella pertussis* antigens in young German and American men. *Clin Infect Dis*. 1995;20:1271–1274.

92. Hodder SL, Mortimer EA Jr. Epidemiology of pertussis and reactions to pertussis vaccine. *Epidemiol Rev*. 1992;14:243–267.

93. Edwards KM, Decker MD, Graham BS, Mezzatesta J, Scott J, Hackell J. Adult immunization with acellular pertussis vaccine. *JAMA*. 1993;269:53–56.

94. Binkin NJ, Salmaso S, Tozzi AE, Scuderi G, Greco D, Greco D. Epidemiology of pertussis in a developed country with low vaccination coverage: The Italian experience. *Pediatr Infect Dis J.* 1992;11:653–661.

95. Isacson J, Trollfors B, Taranger J, Zackrisson G, Lagergard T. How common is whooping cough in a nonvaccinating country? *Pediatr Infect Dis J.* 1993;12:284–288.

96. He Q, Viljanen MK, Nikkari S, Lyytikainen R, Mertsola J. Outcomes of *Bordetella pertussis* infection in different age groups of an immunized population. *J Infect Dis.* 1994;170:873–877.

97. Muller AS, Leeuwenburg J, Pratt DS. Pertussis: Epidemiology and control. *Bull World Health Organ.* 1986;64:321–331.

98. Centers for Disease Control and Prevention. Resurgence of pertussis—United States, 1993. *MMWR.* 1993;42:952–953,959–960.

99. Sutter RW, Cochi SL. Pertussis hospitalizations and mortality in the United States, 1985–1988: Evaluation of the completeness of national reporting. *JAMA.* 1992;267:386–391.

100. Cromer BA, Goydos J, Hackell J, Mezzatesta J, Dekker C, Mortimer EA. Unrecognized pertussis infection in adolescents. *Am J Dis Child.* 1993;147:575–577.

101. Rosenthal S, Strebel P, Cassiday P, Sanden G, Brusuelas K, Wharton M. Pertussis infection among adults during the 1993 outbreak in Chicago. *J Infect Dis.* 1995;171:1650–1652.

102. Wright SW, Edwards KM, Decker MD, Zeldin MH. Pertussis infection in adults with persistent cough. *JAMA.* 1995;273:1044–1046.

103. Onorato IM, Wassilak SG. Laboratory diagnosis of pertussis: The state of the art. *Pediatr Infect Dis J.* 1987;6:145–151.

104. Meade BD, Mink CM, Manclark CR. Serodiagnosis of pertussis. *Proceedings from the Sixth International Symposium on Pertussis.* Bethesda, Md: Department of Health and Human Services, United States Public Health Service; 1990: 322–329. DHHS (FDA) 90–1164.

105. Wharton M, Chorba TL, Vogt RL, Morse DL, Buehler JW. Case definitions for public health surveillance. *MMWR.* 1990;39(RR-13):26–27.

106. Centers for Disease Control. Pertussis vaccination: Acellular pertussis vaccine for reinforcing and booster use—supplementary ACIP statement: Recommendations of the Immunization Practices Advisory Committee (ACIP). *MMWR.* 1992;41(RR-1):1–10.

107. Centers for Disease Control and Prevention. Pertussis vaccination: Use of acellular pertussis vaccines among infants and young children: Recommendations of the Immunization Practices Advisory Committee (ACIP). *MMWR.* 1997;46(RR-7):1–25.

108. Centers for Disease Control and Prevention. Use of diphtheria toxoid-tetanus toxoid-acellular pertussis vaccine as a five-dose series: Supplemental recommendations of the Immunization Practices Advisory Committee (ACIP). *MMWR.* 2000;49(RR-13);1–8.

109. Englund JA, Glezen WP, Barreto L. Controlled study of a new five-component acellular pertussis vaccine in adults and young children. *J Infect Dis.* 1992;166:1436–1441.

110. Shefer A, Dales L, Nelson M, Werner B, Baron R, Jackson R. Use and safety of acellular pertussis vaccine among adult hospital staff during an outbreak of pertussis. *J Infect Dis.* 1995;171:1053–1056.

111. Straubing HE. *In Hospital and Camp: The Civil War Through the Eyes of Its Doctors and Nurses.* Harrisburg, Penn: Stackpole Books; 1993: 30–32.

112. Dunham GC. *Military Preventive Medicine.* 3rd ed. Harrisburg, Penn: Military Service Publishing Company; 1940: 110–114.

113. Wassilak SG, Orenstein WA, Sutter RW. Tetanus toxoid. In: Plotkin SA, Mortimer, Jr. EA, eds. *Vaccines.* 2nd ed. Philadelphia: W.B. Saunders; 1994: Chap 4.

114. Benenson AS. Immunization and military medicine. *Rev Infect Dis.* 1984:6:1–12.

115. Gillett MC. *The Army Medical Department 1865–1917.* Washington, DC: Center of Military History, US Army; 1995: 251.

116. Beaty HN. Tetanus. In: Petersdorf RG, Adams RD, Braunwald E, Isselbacher KJ, Martin JB, Wilson JD, eds. *Principals of Internal Medicine.* 10th ed. New York: McGraw Hill; 1983.

117. Gergen PJ, McQuillan GM, Kiely M, Ezzati-Rice TM, Sutter RW, Virella G. A population-based serologic survey of immunity to tetanus in the United States. *N Engl J Med.* 1995;332:761–766.

118. Groleau G. Tetanus. *Emerg Med Clin North Am.* 1992:10:351–360.

119. Steinglass R, Brenzel L, Percy A. Tetanus. In: Jamison DT, ed. *Disease Control Priorities in Developing Countries.* Washington, DC: World Bank; 1993.

120. Craig GK. *U.S. Army Special Forces Medical Handbook.* Boulder, Colo: Paladin Press; 1986: 176.

121. Gilbert DN, Moellering Jr RC, Sande MA. *The Sanford Guide to Antimicrobial Therapy.* 28th ed. Vienna, Va: Antimicrobial Therapy, Inc.; 1998: 44.

122. Juan G. Jaramillo-Angel, MD, MPH, Personal Communication, 1997.

123. Wilbur CK. *Revolutionary Medicine 1700–1800.* Chester, Conn: The Globe Pequot Press; 1980.

124. Weed FW, ed. *Communicable and Other Diseases.* Vol 9. In: *The Medical Department of the United States Army in the World War.* Washington DC: US Government Printing Office; 1928: 233–261.

125. Mortimer EA Jr. Diphtheria toxoid. In: Plotkin SA, Mortimer, Jr. EA, eds. *Vaccines.* 2nd ed. Philadelphia: W.B. Saunders; 1994.

126. Centers for Disease Control and Prevention. Diphtheria acquired by U.S. citizens in the Russian Federation and Ukraine—1994. *MMWR.* 1995;44:237,243–244.

127. Centers for Disease Control and Prevention. Diphtheria, tetanus, and pertussis: Guidelines for vaccine prophylaxis and other preventive measures, recommendation of the Immunization Practices Advisory Committee (ACIP). *MMWR.* 1985;34:405–426.

128. Centers for Disease Control and Prevention. Respiratory diphtheria caused by *Corynebacterium ulcerans*—Terre Haute, Indiana, 1996. *MMWR.* 1997;46:330–332.

129. Rocha H. Diphtheria. In: Beeson PB, McDermott W, Wyngaarden JB, eds. *Cecil Textbook of Medicine.* 15th ed. Philadelphia: W.B. Saunders; 1979.

130. Centers for Disease Control and Prevention. Poliomyelitis prevention in the United States: Introduction of a sequential vaccination schedule of inactivated poliovirus vaccine followed by oral poliovirus vaccine: Recommendations of the Advisory Committee on Immunization Practices. *MMWR.* 1997;46(RR-3):1–25.

131. Hull HF, Burmingham ME, Melgaard B, Lee JW. Progress toward global polio eradication. *J Infect Dis.* 1997;175(suppl 1):S4–S9.

132. Cochi SL, Hull HF, Sutter RW, Wilfert CM, Katz SL. Commentary: The unfolding story of global polio eradication. *J Infect Dis.* 1997;175(suppl 1):S1–S3.

133. Centers for Disease Control and Prevention. Poliomyelitis prevention in the United States: Updated recommendations of the Advisory Committee on Immunization Practices (ACIP). *MMWR*. 2000;49(RR5):1–22.

134. Melnick JL. Live attenuated poliovirus vaccines. In: Plotkin SA, Mortimer EA Jr, eds. *Vaccines*. Philadelphia: W.B. Saunders: 1994: Chap 7.

135. The Global Polio Eradication Initiative. Fact sheet: Polio eradication initiative at a glance. http://whqsabin.who.int:8082/fact.htm. Accessed 1/2/99.

136. Kim-Farley RJ, Bart KJ, Schonberger LB, et al. Poliomyelitis in the USA: Virtual elimination of disease caused by wild virus. *Lancet*. 1984;2:1315–1317.

137. US Department of Health and Human Services. *Clinician's Handbook of Preventive Services*. Washington, DC: US Government Printing Office; 1994: Chap 16.

138. Centers for Disease Control and Prevention. Certification of poliomyelitis eradication—the Americas, 1994. *MMWR*. 1994;43:720–722.

139. Nkowane BM, Wassilak SG, Orenstein WA, et al. Vaccine-associated paralytic poliomyelitis: Unites States: 1973 through 1984. *JAMA*. 1987;257:1335–1340.

140. Dowdle WR, Birmingham ME. The biologic principles of poliovirus eradication. *J Infect Dis*. 1997;175(suppl 1):S286–S292.

141. Johnson RT. Late progression of poliomyeltis paralysis: Discussion of pathogenesis. *Rev Infect Dis*. 1984;6(suppl 2):S568–S570.

142. Colbere-Garapin F, Duncan G, Pavio N, Pelletier I, Petit I. An approach to understanding the mechanisms of poliovirus persistence in infected cells of neural or non-neural origin. *Clin Diagn Virol*. 1998;9:107–113.

143. Tangermann RH, Aylward B, Birmingham M, et al. Current status of the global eradication of poliomyelitis. *World Health Stat Q*. 1997;50:188–194.

144. Gear JH. Nonpolio causes of polio-like paralytic syndromes. *Rev Infect Dis*. 1984;6(suppl 2):S379–384.

145. Hughes RA, Rees JH. Clinical and epidemiologic features of Guillain-Barre syndrome. *J Infect Dis*. 1997;176(suppl 2):S92–S98.

146. Sutter RW, Cochi SL. Poliomyelitis. Wallace RB, ed. *Maxcy-Rosenau-Last Public Health and Preventive Medicine*. 14th ed. Stamford, Conn: Appleton & Lange: 1998: 123–125.

147. Ward NA, Milstien JB, Hull HF, Hull BP, Kim-Farley RJ. The WHO–EPI initiative for the global eradication of poliomyelitis. *Biologicals*. 1993,21:327–333.

Chapter 40

PRINCIPLES OF INFECTION CONTROL AND PREVENTION DURING MILITARY DEPLOYMENT

BRENDA ROUP, RN, PhD AND PATRICK W. KELLEY, MD, DrPH

B. Roup, RN, PhD, Lieutenant Colonel, Nurse Corps, US Army (retired); Nurse Consultant in Infection Control, Maryland Department of Health and Mental Hygiene, Baltimore, Maryland 21201; Formerly: Chief, Infection Control Service, Walter Reed Army Medical Center, Nurse Consultant in Infection Control, Office of the Army Surgeon General, 5109 Leesburg Pike, Falls Church, VA 22041

P.W. Kelley, MD, DrPH, Colonel, Medical Corps, US Army; Director, Division of Preventive Medicine and the Department of Defense Global Emerging Infections Surveillance and Response System, Walter Reed Army Institute of Research, Silver Spring, MD 20910-7500

INTRODUCTION

Long-established concepts of infection control, plus those that have achieved prominence since recognition of the bloodborne human immunodeficiency virus (HIV), pose challenges even to fixed health care facilities in peacetime. Medical care under deployed conditions, especially in combat, stretches the feasibility of infection control approaches, yet patients and their providers still deserve the best care that the circumstances allow. During deployments, uncommon and unique infection control hazards must be appreciated by providers who normally work in well-equipped and well-staffed fixed facilities. On the battlefield, infection control must extend from semi-fixed facilities through rapidly mobile units to the warfighter. Medical personnel must recognize that mass casualty situations under fire, biological warfare, challenging logistics, care of non-US patients, natural environmental hazards, and exotic infectious diseases call for innovative adaptations of the US fixed-facility model of infection control. Though much research remains to be done and doctrine to be written, prudent and creative application of basic principles can help achieve successful infection control in the field setting.

Prevention and control of infection in military medical settings is in some respects more important during deployment than it is during more stable operations, such as occur in military hospitals in the United States. Infections that not only cause needless morbidity and mortality and threaten the well-being of other warfighter-patients also put a drain on what may be an already over-taxed health care and medical evacuation system. If key health care providers must be placed under isolation because they have been exposed to diseases such as Crimean-Congo hemorrhagic fever or Lassa fever, health care can be compromised for many current and future patients. Provider anxiety over potential exposure to bloodborne pathogens can also affect performance.

Infection control challenges in the deployed setting may be compounded by higher rates of antibiotic resistance in many overseas settings; greater susceptibility to common infectious diseases such as rubella, mumps, and varicella among some patients from allied forces; the greater possibility of transmissible infections such as tuberculosis among local-hire workers; logistic delays; and bloodborne

pathogens. Biological warfare involving a transmissible agent such as smallpox would dwarf any previous infection control concern. These scenarios may be well beyond those envisioned by current US occupational safety standards. Infection control problems arising on deployments may reach back to US-based fixed facilities. The growing emphasis on rapid medical evacuation may result in the importation into the United States of infection control problems, such as previously unknown drug-resistant organisms or exotic emerging infections.

In the civilian sector, the amount of attention paid to controlling the spread of infection in medical facilities is related broadly to the level of general health care. This, in turn, depends on the country's degree of development. At one end of the spectrum, infection control and prevention practices may be ignored by the lower-echelon health care worker; the practices are simply left up to the initiative and concern of individual physicians and nurses. At the other end of the spectrum are facilities that practice all of the Northern American or European models of infection control, complete with surveillance activities and outcome measures.

Since deployment may occur anywhere in the world and since other cultures and geographic areas pose different challenges in infectious disease prevention, general concepts will be the focus of this chapter. Instituting infection control and prevention practices during deployment will present varying levels of difficulty and require varying levels of creativity, depending on the mission, geographic area, logistical support, and beliefs of the local people about health and medicine. Local people who are hired to work for the military medical unit may not understand why certain practices are mandated; they may also be a source of infection or contribute to transmission themselves if, for example, they have undetected tuberculosis or continue to work (to produce income) while they have an enteric illness. Major educational efforts may be necessary for such personnel, with particular attention paid to cultural misunderstandings concerning the transmission of infectious diseases. The challenge to the military medical system while under deployment conditions is not only to improvise in incorporating practices familiar to the US-based practitioner but also to bridge this gap between those practices and local circumstances.

ELEMENTS OF AN INFECTION CONTROL PROGRAM

An effective infection control and prevention program for military and nonmilitary personnel in

a deployed environment should be based as much as possible on the same elements and principles that guide such programs in garrison. Because of the austerity of the deployed environment, though, common sense and creativity may be needed to adjust to the situation at hand. Health care workers must first understand that while infection control principles remain the same, the infection control threat under deployed conditions may be different and more complicated than normal. Health care workers at all levels need to be educated concerning how a deployment scenario may call for particular and even unfamiliar infection control emphases. For example, patient-to-patient transmission of a vector-borne infection such as dengue would not typically be an issue in the controlled environments of a US hospital, but bednets may be essential to protect staff and patients if mosquitoes are present in a deployed hospital with viremic dengue patients.

Infection control encompasses those policies, procedures, and concepts necessary to minimize the transmission of infectious diseases in the health care setting. Successful infection control programs usually have an active multidisciplinary infection control committee; proactive surveillance; effective methods for isolating patients and specimens that pose a risk to others; an occupational health program; policies regarding antibiotic use, aseptic technique, and facility sanitation; and access to at least basic microbiological laboratory support. The underpinning of a successful program is regular education and communication. Infection control must be given emphasis and responsible personnel to be successful.

Infection control policies have to address both facility-acquired and community-acquired infections. Facility-acquired infections, also known as nosocomial infections, are generally defined as those infections that are neither present nor incubating at the time of admission to a facility but develop 48 to 72 hours afterward, unless the infection is clearly related to a procedure or exposure that occurred within the first 48 to 72 hours of hospitalization. Criteria for defining such infections have been outlined by the Centers for Disease Control and Prevention (CDC) and should be used by military personnel.[1] Community-acquired infections are generally considered to be all infections that arise from exposures outside the facility. In this chapter, "facility" refers to any setting in which patients are treated, including hospitals, clinics, or forward treatment areas.

According to Meers,[2] the problems of facility-transmitted infections in developing or war-ravaged countries are 2-fold. The first is communication between the medical personnel and patients. The second is the spectrum of diseases. Some community-acquired infections that are viewed as major problems in the United States are seen as minor problems or everyday occurrences in other nations and cultures (eg, tuberculosis, hepatitis). This can also be true of infections that are transmitted within the facility. An understanding of local attitudes towards infections and infectious diseases may be crucial to the successful prevention of infections in a deployed environment.

THE INFECTION CONTROL COMMITTEE

While most infection control committees are focused on and based in hospitals, on deployment infection control must be addressed at levels extending from the warfighter to supporting hospitals in the United States. This requires layers of infection control management tailored to the size and circumstances of the deployment. For this reason, there is no single model for how to manage infection control efforts in the deployed setting. Individuals should be formally appointed to manage this function.

The committee has several key functions; it formulates theater-specific infection control policies, oversees surveillance activities, develops appropriate medical education, and evaluates the program. This group should also, recognizing resource limitations, advise medical commanders on what infection control programs and settings deserve the highest priority. The frequency of meetings will depend on the maturity of the theater and the complexity of the

medical care system being put into place. Efficiency may require meetings by individuals responsible for specific parts of the health care continuum. Membership on the infection control committee, and any subcommittees, should reflect the expertise of clinicians (to include medics), clinical nurses, preventive medicine and environmental science officers, an epidemiologist or a surveillance nurse, the pharmacist, medical regulators involved with moving patients, and laboratorians.

The committee should develop appropriate medical education for all medical personnel, but special emphasis should be placed on education for nurses because of their intense contact with patients and implementation of standard procedures. The committee can also help clinicians in the theater by researching and reporting local antibiotic-resistance patterns. Another important educational focus should be the avoidance of occupational injuries from contaminated sharps and medical waste. Nonclinicians who may find themselves involved in patient care (eg, first aid and triage personnel, litter carriers) should be taught how to protect themselves from bloodborne infections. Regular feedback of infection control information, including surveillance data, to supported facilities is desirable.

SURVEILLANCE

If a military unit will be stationary for some period of time, a program for nosocomial infection surveillance should be instituted. Ideally, the deployed unit will already have in place policies and procedures for such a program and will only need to implement them. Since microbiological laboratory support may be minimal, if it is present at all, other information about patients (eg, unexplained fevers, new rashes, purulent drainage from wounds) will need to serve as markers for the possible spread of nosocomial infection. Considering that resources are often constrained in the deployment setting, a role of the infection control committee will likely be to prioritize surveillance efforts. This may involve targeting specific high-risk facilities or wards, rotating surveillance of lower-risk wards, and focusing on infections associated with the highest mortality (eg, bacteremia, pneumonia).

One individual should be designated to perform surveillance "rounds" of the patients in the medical treatment facility at least once a week, using patient records, written or oral nursing reports, and pharmacy and laboratory records as primary sources of data and clues as to which patients have nosocomial infections. For example, more scrutiny might be given to those whose records show suggestive antibiotic prescriptions, intravenous catheter sites, wound dressing changes, or abnormal

---

EXHIBIT 40-1

CASE DEFINITION FOR SUSPECTED EBOLA HEMORRHAGIC FEVER

The following case definition may be useful for surveillance in an area at recognized risk for the emergence of Ebola hemorrhagic fever.

Anyone presenting with fever and signs of bleeding such as:

- Bleeding of the gums
- Bleeding from the nose
- Red eyes
- Bleeding into the skin
- Bloody or dark stools
- Vomiting blood
- Other unexplained signs of bleeding

Whether or not there is a history of contact with a suspected case of Ebola

OR

Anyone living or deceased with:
- Contact with a suspected case of Ebola

AND

- A history of fever, with or without signs of bleeding

OR

Anyone living or deceased with a history of fever

AND

three of the following symptoms:

- Headache
- Vomiting
- Loss of appetite
- Diarrhea
- Weakness of severe fatigue
- Abdominal pain
- Generalized muscle or joint pain
- Difficulty swallowing
- Difficulty breathing
- Hiccups

OR

Any unexplained death in an area with suspected cases of Ebola

Source: Centers for Disease Control and Prevention. *Infection Control for Viral Hemorrhagic Fevers in the African Health Care Setting.* Atlanta: CDC; 1999.

fever curves. Such a program in a deployed unit would not give primary emphasis to the compilation of reports and the calculation of infection rates, although that would be useful information for future deployments, but would rather gain early information on the possible nosocomial clusters or epidemics and prioritize appropriate measures to halt the spread of infection to uninfected patients. The individual performing infection surveillance may also monitor compliance with the military unit's infection control policies and procedures during the course of rounds, possibly using a previously developed checklist.

Surveillance at the point of admission (eg, aid station, clinic, hospital) for patients with certain syndromes or specific diagnoses is indicated. In certain scenarios, the admission of patients who potentially have highly transmissible conditions must be anticipated so that these cases can be isolated rapidly and environmental contamination minimized. Staff involved with the admission process must be alerted to the medical threat for the region and kept informed of up-to-date medical intelligence. It is advisable to have training sessions and standard operating procedures so that patients with conditions such as active tuberculosis and viral hemorrhagic fevers are recognized promptly and safely isolated. Exhibits 40-1 and 40-2 outline case definitions, developed for use in Africa, that may be useful for identifying at the time of presentation patients who may have Ebola fever or Lassa hemorrhagic fever.

The military practice of medical evacuation through echelons of care complicates infection control surveillance since patients may acquire infections in one location and manifest them at another echelon thousands of miles away. The dynamic ebb and flow of casualties further complicates recognition of changes in the rate of infections. Feedback mechanisms should be developed to inform the theater surgeon of clusters or epidemics in evacuated personnel that might have come from theater exposures.

EXHIBIT 40-2

CASE DEFINITION FOR SUSPECTED LASSA HEMORRHAGIC FEVER

Unexplained fever at least 38°C (100.4°F) for 1 week or more

AND

One of the following:

- No response to standard treatment for most likely cause of fever (malaria, typhoid fever)
- Readmitted within 3 weeks of inpatient care for an illness with fever

AND

One of the following:

- Edema or bleeding
- Sore throat and retrosternal pain or vomiting
- Spontaneous abortion following fever
- Hearing loss following fever

Source: Centers for Disease Control and Prevention. *Infection Control for Viral Hemorrhagic Fevers in the African Health Care Setting.* Atlanta: CDC; 1999.

OCCUPATIONAL HEALTH FOR DEPLOYED HEALTH CARE WORKERS

Health care workers in the deployed setting may face particular challenges because of patient care requirements in austere, combat conditions and contact with injured or ill local persons. Care of wounded US forces poses obvious risks, but care of personnel from other countries can be more hazardous. In many overseas areas, prevalence rates of chronic hepatitis B virus carriage exceed 5%.[3] This explains why any member of the military medical departments who could potentially be involved with not only patient care but also triage and patient transport should be fully immunized. In some parts of the world, the HIV infection rates in soldiers exceed 30%.[4] The US military health care system must be prepared to handle a higher risk to health care personnel of inadvertent exposures to HIV and other bloodborne pathogens than would be the case in a typical military fixed facility. Currently recommended prophylactic antiretroviral regimens must be immediately available for use (Table 40-1).[5] US military health care workers should also anticipate the greater possibility of exposure to agents such as measles, rubella, mumps, varicella, hepatitis A, and polio. Whereas the furlough of a susceptible health care provider exposed to varicella in peacetime may be an inconvenience, in a deployed setting such a loss can have a major impact on unit performance. If immunity is in doubt, the health care worker should be screened and, if indicated, immunized. Childhood and military

TABLE 40-1

BASIC AND EXPANDED HIV POSTEXPOSURE PROPHYLAXIS REGIMENS[*]

Regimen Category	Application	Drug Regimen
Basic	Occupational HIV exposures for which there is a recognized transmission risk	4 wk (28 d) of both zidovudine 600 mg every day in divided doses (ie, 300 mg twice/d, 200 mg three times/d, or 100 mg every 4 h) and lamivudine 150 mg twice/d
Expanded	Occupational HIV exposures that pose an increased risk for transmission (eg, larger volume of blood and/or higher virus titer in blood)	Basic regimen plus either indinavir[†] 800 mg every 8 h or nelfinavir 750 mg 3 times/d[*]

[*]These drug recommendations are current as of August 2000. Because these regimens changed rapidly, the reader is urged to check with the Centers for Disease Control and Prevention for the most up-to-date recommendations at www.cdc.gov.
[†]Idinavir should be taken on an empty stomach and with increased fluid consumption (ie, drinking six 8 oz glasses of water throughout the day); nelfinavir should be taken with meals.
Source: Centers for Disease Control and Prevention. Public Health Service guidelines for the management of health-care worker exposures to HIV and recommendations for postexposure prophylaxis. *MMWR*. 1998;47(RR-7):1–28.

immunization practices are now associated with high rates of immunity to most of these agents in US forces. However, these agents remain common in some parts of the world. Many members of multinational coalitions, even from some developed countries, are susceptible to some of these agents due to differences in immunization practice.[6]

The likelihood of a US military health care worker being exposed to tuberculosis is significant in certain refugee situations and may necessitate respiratory protection and predeployment and postdeployment screening.[7] The military health care system should also be prepared to provide prophylaxis in the event of exposures to meningococcal and other infections. In addition to these measures, thorough education on basic items such as the need for frequent handwashing and the use of barrier equipment remains central to proper occupational health in the deployed setting.

THREE LEVELS OF INFECTION CONTROL

An infection control program in the deployed setting should be based on three levels of control. First is the prevention of transmission of infection through the faithful practices of handwashing, aseptic technique, and sanitation. Second is the control of sources of contamination by disinfection or sterilization of articles. Third is the protection of uninfected patients and health care workers through the appropriate and judicious use of isolation of patients who have infections, through proper specimen handling, and through the use of other measures such as immunization.

Control Level 1: Sanitary Practices

The first level of control in an infection control program during deployment is the prevention of transmission by thorough handwashing, aseptic technique, and sanitation.

Handwashing in a deployed setting may require creativity but must be enforced. Handwashing is the most single important element in the prevention of infection.[8] It not only prevents transmission of infection between patients but, if done conscientiously, prevents health care workers from becoming casualties themselves. There are at least four methods of providing handwashing facilities in a deployed setting, assuming that the deployed unit is not in a fixed facility with running water.

Handwashing

The preferred handwashing facility in a deployed unit would be a portable sink, in which a foot pump or other pump supplies running water. The second method would be a Lyster bag, or some method of suspending 5-gal cans of water, which would also serve as a source of running water. The third choice would be to use alcohol-based handwashing towelettes that are individual and disposable or alcohol-based disinfectant waterless hand foams or lotions. This may be the most practical approach for medics and others with very limited resources at their disposal. It should be noted, however, that blood, dirt, and any organic material should be removed with water before using waterless cleaners. There is a problem with this third choice, however, if a residue from the towelettes, foams, or lotions accumulates on the hands. Then the use of soap and water becomes mandatory. The last resort would be a basin of water in which some type of antiseptic (eg, povidine-iodine, chlorhexidine) has been added, accompanied by a basin of clear water for rinsing. It should be emphasized, however, that this "bird bath" is an absolute last resort. As suboptimal as this method is, it will at least remove blood, dirt, and organic matter from the hands, thus allowing personnel to then use a waterless hand antiseptic. The "bird bath" contents, however, need to be changed frequently, perhaps hourly, to prevent the buildup of organic material in the water. Those allergic to the antiseptic may be precluded from using this method.

All of these methods require that three items be available: a water source, soap or antiseptic, and a method of drying the hands. For the lack of a paper towel or other drying material, busy health care workers may dry their hands on their clothing. If supplies of disposable paper towels are interrupted, a cloth "roller towel" could be used for hand drying but only if each person has a clean, unused area on the towel on which to dry their hands.

Various types of soap should be available to the deployed unit. For general patient care, a plain, non-antimicrobial soap can be used. Such a soap can be in almost any form, (ie, bar, leaflets, liquids, powders). Detergent-based products may contain very low concentrations of antimicrobial agents used as preservatives. If bar soap is used, small bars that can be changed frequently and soap racks that promote drainage should be used to minimize microbial growth. Before invasive or surgical procedures, an antimicrobial handwashing agent should be used. Such agents should contain alcohol, povidine-iodine, or chlorhexidine.

Aseptic Technique

Aseptic technique is the next step in this basic level of control. Anything that is used on what is considered a sterile body cavity must be sterile—free of all bacteria and spores. Anything that is used on a body cavity that is normally contaminated with environmental organisms must be at least clean or disinfected.

Aseptic technique is generally divided into two categories: clean technique and sterile technique.[9] Both types must be employed in a deployed environment to the extent possible. Clean technique refers to practices that reduce the number of microorganisms or prevent or reduce transmission of organisms from one person or place to another. It includes handwashing using soap and friction and cleaning patient-care areas from areas requiring the highest level of cleanliness to less-critical areas. Clean technique also refers to the use of physical barriers, such as gloves and gowns, to prevent contact with microbes.

Sterile, or surgical, technique refers to practices designed to render and maintain objects and areas maximally free of microorganisms. This includes such practices as skin antisepsis before the skin is broken for a procedure. It also includes the concept of barriers (eg, sterile drapes, gowns, and gloves used during surgical procedures). In general, clean technique is employed to prevent the transmission of infection from patients to personnel and other patients, and sterile technique is used to prevent the transmission of infection to patients.

Sanitation

Effective sanitation is essential to the control of infections of any type in any setting and is itself a type of clean technique. Removal of microorganisms from environmental surfaces and from equipment and supplies that could transmit them to patients or from personnel to patients is basic to infection prevention. Florence Nightingale wrote:

> The only way I know to remove dust, the plague of all lovers of fresh air, is to wipe everything with a damp cloth. And all furnishings ought to be so made as that it may be wiped with a damp cloth without injury to itself....[10(p89)]

Miss Nightingale's triumphs during the Crimean War have been well-chronicled.[11] She convincingly demonstrated that safe food and water and a clean environment could result in a major decrease in death rates in a military hospital. Those practices are no less important during deployment today than they were at the British military hospital in Scutari, Turkey, during the 1850s.

Sanitation in deployed medical units will generally be accomplished by housekeeping personnel, very probably employed from the local population. Such personnel may have to be taught an appreciation for the level of sanitation needed for a health care area. Housekeeping operations will be directed toward safety and the reduction of direct and indirect transmission of infection from environmental sources. Improper housekeeping can actually spread pathogenic organisms.

There are several basic housekeeping principles that need to be followed. First, some type of disinfectant-detergent should be used for all cleaning, if it can be obtained. At the minimum, plain soap should be used. Second, all horizontal surfaces should be cleaned at least daily and when obviously soiled. Third and finally, all cleaning performed in a facility should employ the "damp-cleaning" method, that is, the materials used to clean the furniture, floors, and other surfaces should be wet with the disinfectant-detergent solution or soap before they are applied to the item being cleaned.

Control Level 2: Disinfection and Sterilization

The second level of infection prevention and control in a deployed environment is the reduction of contamination through the proper disinfection and sterilization of articles. In such an environment, the luxury of presterilized, disposable supplies and equipment may not be available. Consequently, some types of reusable equipment that can be processed by the deployed unit should be maintained. Examples include bedpans and urinals that can be decontaminated and reused.

Spaulding[12] recommends a rational approach to disinfection and sterilization of patient care items, which should be workable for military units during deployment. Spaulding divides the disinfection of patient care items into three categories: critical, semicritical, and noncritical. A basic principle of this method is that all items must be cleaned with some type of soap or detergent and water before being subjected to the next level of processing. The most efficient sterilization process or chemical disinfectant will not work unless the item is cleaned of all organic matter beforehand.

Critical items are those that must be sterilized because they enter a body cavity that is normally sterile. This category includes surgical instruments, urinary and intravascular catheters, and intravenous needles. If presterilized items are not available on deployment, some type of local sterilization procedure must be employed, such as treatment with a chemical sterilizing agent (eg, 2% gluteraldehyde, 6% stabilized hydrogen peroxide). Such sterilizing agents may be available locally or may be brought in from another geographic area. Twenty percent hydrogen peroxide is widely available, and can be diluted to 6%. Cleaning must precede the treatment, and contact time and temperature of the sterilizing solution must be as recommended by the manufacturer. Deployed units that have steam sterilization capability, such as autoclaves or sterilizers, should use them for items such as surgical instruments.

In a deployed setting, there may be situations in which logistics is unable to resupply the military unit with sterile, disposable supplies, such as intravascular tubing or indwelling urinary catheters. There are currently no US government guidelines for the resterilization or reprocessing of such items. It is recommended that rather than attempting resterilization, such devices should be left in place and not routinely changed, as they are in US-based facilities. The possibility of contamination would probably be much greater if reprocessing were attempted using inadequate methods than if the devices were simply left in place until the supply flow was reestablished.

Semicritical items are objects that come in contact with skin or mucous membranes that are not intact. Examples of items in this category would include respiratory equipment, anesthesia equipment, gastrointestinal endoscopes, and thermometers. These objects should, if possible, be free of all microorganisms with the potential exception of bacterial spores. Semicritical items require disinfection, preferably using a chemical such as 2% gluteraldehyde. Wet pasteurization is another method that can work well in a deployed setting. It is hot water disinfection at temperatures below 100°C and involves exposing the equipment to 75°C water for 30 minutes.[9]

Noncritical items are those that come in contact with intact skin and mucous membranes. Examples of these items are bedpans, blood pressure cuffs, crutches, bed rails, linens, food utensils, and furniture. In contrast to critical and semicritical items, most noncritical items can simply be cleaned where they are used and do not need to be transported to a central processing area. Any safe, hospital-approved disinfectant-detergent solution will be adequate to clean these items. If questions arise regarding methods of sterilization or decontamination of items, the military unit's operating room or central supply personnel should be consulted.

Control Level 3: Isolation Procedures

Isolation technique may be difficult in a deployed environment, and creativity may be necessary to solve the problem of disease transmission from a patient to others. The CDC has recommended a two-tiered system of isolation techniques that should function well in a deployed environment.[8]

Standard Precautions

The first tier of this system is termed "standard precautions." The term indicates that every patient who enters a military health care facility of any kind be treated as if he or she were carrying a pathogen that is transmitted through contact with mucous membranes, broken skin, blood, excretions, or body fluids (eg, HIV, a hepatitis virus).[8] Additional precautions may be indicated depending on the specific diagnosis. Standard precautions are designed to reduce the risk of transmission of microorganisms from both recognized and unrecognized sources of infection in facilities. The standard precautions system consists of several basic principles, which should be used by all military health care providers (Exhibit 40-3). These principles address where appropriate and practical the wearing of gloves, gowns, masks or facial protection, eye protection, patient placement, transport of infected patients, care of linen and dishes, routine cleaning, and waste disposal. Some type of barrier "kit" that includes gloves, masks, eye protection, and gowns should be available in all settings, to include military vehicles that transport patients and those that respond to mass casualty situations.

Gloves are worn for three important reasons. First, gloves are worn to provide a protective barrier and prevent gross contamination of the hands when touching blood, body fluids, secretions, excretions, mucous membranes, and nonintact skin. Second, they are worn to reduce the likelihood that microorganisms present on the hands of personnel will be transmitted to patients during invasive or other patient care procedures that involve touching a patient's nonintact skin or mucous membranes. Third, gloves are worn to reduce the likelihood that hands of personnel contaminated with microorganisms from a patient or article will transmit these microorganisms to another patient. Wearing gloves does not replace the need for handwashing because gloves may have small unnoticeable defects or be torn during use, thus allowing hands to become contaminated. Hands may also become contaminated during the removal of gloves. Gloves must be changed between patient contacts.

Whether latex or vinyl gloves are to be used will generally depend upon the task to be performed.[13] Both types protect the health care worker from blood and body fluids. Latex is more flexible than vinyl and, since it conforms to the hands, allows more freedom of movement. Latex gloves have a network of lattices that allow them to reseal tiny punctures automatically, a feature not found in vinyl gloves. Therefore, latex gloves should be used in the following situations: (*a*) when flexibility is needed, such as in phlebotomy, (*b*) when performing tasks that may cause stress on the glove, such as when handling sharp instruments or tape, and (*c*) when the exposure to pathogens may be unknown,

---

EXHIBIT 40-3

KEY ELEMENTS OF STANDARD PRECAUTIONS

Wash hands with soap (preferably antimicrobial) before and after contact with a patient's blood, body fluids, or contaminated items

Wear clean, thin gloves if there will be contact with blood, body fluids, mucous membranes, or broken skin and change gloves between patients and procedures

Use a mask, eyewear, and a gown if splashes or sprays of body fluids are likely

Handle needles and other sharp instruments safely

Routinely clean and disinfect frequently touched environmental surfaces

Clean and disinfect soiled laundry safely

Isolate patients whose blood or body fluids are likely to contaminate surfaces or other patients

Minimize invasive procedures to avoid the potential for injury or accidental exposure

Source: Centers for Disease Control and Prevention Infection Control Practices Advisory Committee. Guidelines for isolation precautions in hospitals. *Am J Infect Control.* 1996:24:24–51.

such as in surgical, labor and delivery, and disaster areas. For tasks that are unlikely to stress the glove material, vinyl gloves may be worn. Such tasks would typically be performed in outpatient and psychiatric settings.

One problem that may be faced during deployment is the possibility of having to wash or otherwise reprocess disposable latex or vinyl gloves. This problem may arise when supplies of gloves are interrupted. At least one study[14] has examined the ability of three different handwashing agents to reduce bacteria inoculated on gloves. Both 4% chlorhexidine and 70% ethyl alcohol were more effective in removing the bacteria from the gloves than nonantibacterial soap and water. None of the agents, however, removed all of the organisms. Clearly, the optimal practice is to use disposable gloves once and discard them.

For standard precautions, various types of gowns and protective apparel are worn to provide barrier protection and reduce opportunities for transmission of microorganisms to health care personnel and other patients. Gowns or aprons are worn to prevent contamination of clothing and protect the skin of personnel from blood or body fluids. Ideally, disposable gowns with a fluid-resistant front should be used. In a deployed setting, however, such gowns may not be available. Gowns that can be laundered can be used, perhaps with a plastic apron worn underneath. As with other infection control practices in such an environment, ingenuity may be necessary. In some cases, health care workers with an acute, unanticipated need for barrier protection have improvised using plastic trash bags in place of aprons and boots. Gowns and gloves should be changed after dealing with infective material. Nondisposable items, such as respirator masks, should be disinfected after each use. Removal of contaminated aprons, gloves, and other supplies should be done in such as way as to avoid self-contamination or contamination of others or the environment.

Various types of masks, eye protection, face shields, and caps need to be worn when the possibility of splashing of blood, oral secretions, or body fluids exists. A mask that covers both the nose and mouth with goggles or a face shield will provide protection of the health care worker's eyes, nose, and mouth. A surgical mask that fits snugly over the nose and mouth is generally worn to provide protection against the spread of infectious large-particle droplets that are transmitted by close contact and generally travel only short distances (up to 1 m) from infected patients who are coughing or sneezing, such as those with influenza.

Transmission-based Precautions

The second level of precautions that the CDC recommends is for patients with known or suspected highly transmissible or epidemiologically important infectious diseases. These precautions, termed transmission-based precautions, are used in addition to standard precautions. They include airborne precautions, droplet precautions, and contact precautions. Exhibit 40-4 and Tables 40-2 and 40-3 detail the conditions and type of precautions needed for selected militarily-relevant infectious diseases.

Airborne Precautions. Airborne precautions are designed to reduce the risk of airborne transmission of infectious agents, such as measles, varicella (including disseminated zoster), and tuberculosis. Airborne transmission occurs by dissemination of either airborne droplet nuclei (5 μm or smaller) that remain suspended in the air for long periods of time or by dust particles that contain the infectious agent. Microorganisms carried in this manner can be widely dispersed by air currents and may become inhaled by a susceptible host in the same area as the source patient or one a long distance away, depending on environmental factors.

Obviously, the institution of these precautions in a deployed setting can be difficult. Negative pressure rooms will generally not be available, but the placement of a patient with an airborne disease in a small tent (or sealed-off area in a tent) in which the air will not be circulating to other patients and staff is imperative. Tents or other movable facilities can be configured to allow a private area for patients with a transmissible airborne infection.

Some type of respiratory protection must be worn when entering the room or area of a patient with a known or suspected infectious respiratory disease. If the patient has measles or varicella, those who are susceptible to those diseases should not enter the room. It is important to remember that while US service members likely either have natural or vaccine-induced immunity to infections such as these, allied personnel and local-hire workers may have a significantly different pattern of susceptibility.

An area of major concern and controversy has been the selection of respiratory protection equipment for prevention of the transmission of tuberculosis, a disease that may well be present during deployment. Although its efficacy was unproved, a surgical mask was traditionally worn for isolation precautions in hospitals when patients were known or suspected to be infected with microorganisms spread by the airborne route of transmission. The

---

EXHIBIT 40-4

SYNOPSIS OF TYPES OF PRECAUTIONS AND PATIENTS REQUIRING THE PRECAUTIONS[*]

Standard Precautions
For all patients

Airborne Precautions (In Addition to Standard Precautions)

For patients known or suspected to have serious illnesses transmitted by airborne droplet nuclei (eg, measles, varicella [including disseminated zoster][†], tuberculosis[‡])

Droplet Precautions (In Addition to Standard Precautions)

For patients known or suspected to have serious illnesses transmitted by large-particle droplets (eg, invasive *Haemophilus influenzae* type b disease, invasive *Neisseria meningitidis* disease, pharyngeal diphtheria, mycoplasma pneumonia, pertussis, pneumonic plague, streptococcal [group A] pharyngitis, pneumonia, adenovirus[†], influenza, mumps, parvovirus B19, rubella)

Contact Precautions (In Addition to Standard Precautions)
For patients known or suspected to have serious illnesses easily transmitted by direct patient contact or by contact with items in the patient's environment:

- Gastrointestinal, respiratory, skin, or wound infections or colonization with multidrug-resistant bacteria

- Enteric infections with a low infectious dose or prolonged environmental survival (eg, *Clostridium difficile,* respiratory syncytial virus, parainfluenza virus, enteroviral infections in infants and young children)

- Skin infections that are highly contagious or that may occur on dry skin (eg, cutaneous diphtheria); herpes simplex virus (neonatal or mucocutaneous); impetigo; major (noncontained) abscesses, cellulitis, or decubiti; pediculosis; scabies; staphylococcal furunculosis in infants and young children; zoster (disseminated or in the immunocompromised host)[†]

- Viral/hemorrhagic conjunctivitis

- Viral hemorrhagic infections (Ebola, Lassa, or Marburg)[*]

---

[*]Not a complete listing
[†]Certain infections require more than one type of precaution
[‡]See Centers for Disease Control and Prevention. Guidelines for preventing the transmission of *Mycobacterium tuberculosis* in health care facilities. *MMWR.* 1994;43(RR-13).
Source: Centers for Disease Control and Prevention Infection Control Practices Advisory Committee. Guidelines for isolation precautions in hospitals. *Am J Infect Control.* 1996:24:24–51.

CDC currently recommends that respiratory protection equipment used by health care workers caring for tuberculosis patients should meet the following two basic standards: (1) the ability to filter particles of 1 μm in the unloaded state with a filter efficiency of greater than 95% and (2) the ability to fit the different facial characteristics of personnel.[15] This second recommendation generally means that at least three sizes of masks should be available. Logistic personnel should be able to determine if the masks available meet these minimum requirements. If such masks are not available in a deployed environment, a surgical mask that fits snugly over the nose and mouth should be worn when entering the tent or area where a tuberculosis patient is housed. If the patient must leave the tent or area for any reason, he or she must wear the mask. In fact, it may also be prudent for any patient suspected of having active tuberculosis to wear a mask at all times, even inside the tent because of the difficulty in maintaining negative pressure in that setting.

Droplet Precautions. The next sublevel of isolation precautions is used for diseases that are spread through droplets. Droplet infection is distinct from airborne transmission, and such infections as meningitis, diphtheria, pertussis, influenza, mumps, and rubella are spread in droplets. All of these infectious diseases may be present in a deployed setting. Droplet transmission involves contact of the conjunctivae or the mucous membranes of the nose

TABLE 40-2

TYPE AND DURATION OF PRECAUTIONS NEEDED FOR SELECTED INFECTIONS AND CONDITIONS

Infection/Condition	Precaution Type
Acquired immunodeficiency syndrome	Standard
Amebiasis	Standard
Anthrax, pulmonary	Standard
Arthropod-borne viral encephalitides	Standard/screening
Arthropod-borne viral fevers (eg, dengue, yellow fever)	Standard/screening
Brucellosis	Standard
Campylobacter, cholera, and *Escherichia coli* O157:H7	Standard if continent
Chickenpox	Airborne and Contact
Clostridium perfringens (gangrene)	Standard
Diphtheria, cutaneous	Contact
Enteroviral infections	
Adults	Standard
Infants and young children	Contact
Hantavirus pulmonary syndrome	Standard
Hemorrhagic fevers (eg, Ebola, Lassa)	Contact
Hepatitis, viral	Standard if continent
Influenza	Droplet
Malaria	Standard with screens
Measles (rubeola)	Airborne
Meningitis (*Neisseria meningitidis*)	Droplet
Multidrug-resistant organisms, infections, colonization	
Gastrointestinal	Contact
Respiratory (except pneumococcal)	Contact
Skin (eg, wound, burn)	Contact
Mumps	Droplet
Mycoplasma pneumoniae	Droplet
Pertussis	Droplet
Plague, bubonic	Standard
Plague, pneumonic	Droplet
Rabies	Standard
Rickettsial fevers, tick-borne	Standard
Rubella	Droplet
Strongyloidiasis and hookworm	Standard
Tuberculosis, pulmonary/laryngeal (confirmed or suspected)	Airborne
Zoster in a normal patient	Standard with immune health care workers

Source: Centers for Disease Control and Prevention Infection Control Practices Advisory Committee. Guidelines for isolation precautions in hospitals. *Am J Infect Control*. 1996:24:24–51.

or mouth of a susceptible person with large particle droplets containing microorganisms. Droplets are generated from the infected person or carrier during talking, coughing, and sneezing. Transmission involves close contact, because the droplets usually do not remain suspended in the air and generally travel at most a meter.

Droplet precautions also require that the patient

TABLE 40-3

CLINICAL SYNDROMES OR CONDITIONS WARRANTING ADDITIONAL EMPIRIC PRECAUTIONS TO PREVENT TRANSMISSION OF EPIDEMIOLOGICALLY IMPORTANT PATHOGENS PENDING CONFIRMATION OF DIAGNOSIS

Clinical Syndrome or Condition[*]	Potential Pathogens[†]	Empiric Precautions
Diarrhea		
Acute diarrhea with a likely infectious cause in an incontinent or diapered patient	Enteric pathogens[‡]	Contact
Diarrhea in an adult with a history of recent antibiotic use	*Clostridium difficile*	Contact
Meningitis	*Neisseria meningitidis*	Droplet
Rash or exanthems, generalized, etiology unknown		
Petechial/ecchymotic with fever	*N meningitidis*	Droplet
Vesicular	Varicella	Airborne and Contact
Maculopapular with coryza and fever	Rubeola	Airborne
Respiratory infections		
Cough/fever/upper lobe pulmonary infiltrate in an HIV-negative patient or a patient at low risk for HIV infection	*Mycobacterium tuberculosis*	Airborne
Cough/fever/pulmonary infiltrate in any lung location in an HIV-infected patient or a patient at high risk for HIV infection	*M tuberculosis*	Airborne
Paroxysmal or severe persistent cough during periods of pertussis activity	*Bordetella pertussis*	Droplet
Respiratory infections, particularly bronchiolitis and croup, in infants and young children	Respiratory syncytial or parainfluenza virus	Contact
Infection with Multidrug-resistant Microorganisms		
History of infection or colonization with multidrug-resistant organisms	Resistant bacteria	Contact
Skin, wound, or urinary tract infection in a patient with a recent hospital stay in a facility where multidrug-resistant organisms are prevalent	Resistant bacteria	Contact
Skin or Wound Infection		
Abscess or draining wound that cannot be covered	*Staphylococcus aureus*, group A streptococcus	Contact

[*]Patients with the syndromes or conditions listed below may present with atypical signs or symptoms (eg, pertussis in neonates and adults may not have paroxysmal or severe cough). The clinician's index of suspicion should be guided by the prevalence of specific conditions in the location, as well as clinical judgment.
[†]The organisms listed here are not intended to represent the complete, or even most likely, diagnoses, but rather possible etiologic agents that require additional precautions beyond Standard Precautions until they can be ruled out.
[‡]These pathogens include enterohemorrhagic *Escherichia coli* O157:H7, *Shigella,* hepatitis A virus, and rotavirus.
Source: Centers for Disease Control and Prevention Infection Control Practices Advisory Committee. Guidelines for isolation precautions in hospitals. *Am J Infect Control.* 1996:24:24–51.

be placed in a private tent or area or with another patient who has the same diagnosis. If this is not possible, the patient should be placed at least 1 m from other patients. Health care workers should wear a mask when working within 1 m of the pa-tient. If transport of the patient is necessary, the patient should be masked.

Contact Precautions. All other infections and infectious diseases, whether facility- or community-acquired, may be contained through the next sublevel of precautions, contact precautions. Contact precautions are designed to reduce the risk of transmission of infections that are spread through direct or indirect contact, such as on health care workers' hands or on fomites (eg, patient-care articles). Contact precautions should be used with patients who have conditions such as diarrhea or skin or wound infections.

Direct-contact transmission involves skin-to-skin contact and physical transfer of microorganisms to a susceptible person from an infected person. Such transmission may occur while turning a patient, giving a patient a bath, or performing other care activities that require close physical contact. Patients who have direct physical contact with each other may also serve as a source of infection. This might happen when convalescent patients help with nursing tasks. The use of gloves is necessary; the use of gowns may also be necessary. Devices for use in mouth-to-mouth resuscitation can be helpful in reducing those associated direct-contact risks.

Patient Isolation and Placement

Appropriate patient placement is an important component of isolation precautions, especially for enteric or respiratory conditions or other conditions requiring contact isolation. As mentioned previously, creativity in using the facilities at hand may be necessary. Of course, the most desirable situation for persons with these types of conditions would be a private accommodation with toilet facilities. Under field conditions, this is not an absolute requirement. For example, if tents are the only housing facilities available, a tent with patients with the same airborne-transmitted diseases should be placed downwind of the main patient-care facility. Sharing of rooms or areas by patients with the same known or suspected diagnosis at the same stage of the disease, also known as cohorting, is especially useful during enteric outbreaks. Grouping respiratory patients with infections due to different etiologies should be avoided to reduce the risk of cross-infections. In the case of patients with a communicable respiratory disease, careful use of exhaust fans may help keep contaminated air from flowing back into common patient-care areas by creating a negative pressure. Signs should be posted indicating the presence of an infectious disease risk and the precautions to be taken for those entering the area. The excreta of individual patients with enteric diseases are normally disposed of in a sanitary sewer and this is usually considered safe, but disinfection may be desirable during an outbreak when the quantity

of agents placed into the environment is larger. As in the United States, medical waste should be handled and disposed of appropriately on deployment to avoid infecting others or contaminating the environment.

For some conditions, such as viral hemorrhagic fevers, strict or high-level contact isolation may be indicated. The US standard calls for private negative pressure rooms with anterooms equipped with sinks. Exhaust passes through high-efficiency filters. In the field, such approaches may not be easily achieved short of using plastic-film patient isolators. These isolators have interior spaces below atmospheric pressure, HEPA (high efficiency particulate air) filters for exhaust air, and a lock system for bagging and removing contaminants. As an alternative to an isolator, the medical personnel should be clothed in special suits to provide a microbiological barrier. In addition, these patients should be housed separately from others in another building or at least in a place with separate air flow. For nonmilitary personnel, it may be possible to approach the desired level of isolation by having patients cared for in their homes by trained personnel equipped with protective equipment.

The highest level of personal protection measures, including disposable clothing and microbiological masks, is indicated for strict contact isolation situations. Although the CDC recommends that personnel with known or suspected viral hemorrhagic infections be handled with contact precautions, US military units may be placed under political pressure from foreign governments to severely isolate, and possibly evacuate, such patients. Concern for troops or other personnel succumbing to infectious diseases could initiate the mobilization of the high-containment Aeromedical Isolation Team based at the US Army Medical Research Institute of Infectious Diseases at Fort Detrick, Md. High-containment isolation provides a means by which medical personnel can be physically separated from the patient by a microbiological barrier. The Aeromedical Isolation Team, using the Vickers Patient Isolation System (Figure 40-1), provides such a barrier by enclosing the patient in a negatively pressurized transparent plastic envelope and filtering the exhausted air. Facilities in the form of half-suits or glove-sleeves are provided in the envelope walls of each isolator so patient care procedures can be carried out without breaking the microbiological barrier. The patient could then be safely transported to a facility with the capability of caring for patients with such infectious diseases.

As noted, care of viral hemorrhagic fever patients

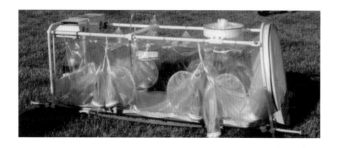

Fig 40-1. The Vickers Patient Isolation System
Photograph: Courtesy of Brenda Roup.

necessitates proper clothing. This would include a scrub suit (or a similar inner layer), a thick set of gloves over a thin set, rubber boots or overshoes if the floor is soiled, a surgical or disposable gown with long sleeves and cuffs, a plastic apron, a HEPA-filter or other biosafety mask, a cotton head covering, and eye protection.[16] Personnel with cuts or broken skin on their hands should refrain from direct contact with these patients. After use, protective clothing should be removed carefully and according to a written standard operating procedure to avoid contamination of the provider or environment. The clothing should be disinfected or laundered appropriately. Gloves, boots, and aprons can be disinfected with 1:100 bleach solution. If possible, providers should

shower before putting on street clothes.

Decontamination of sewage, disinfection of excreta, and terminal disinfection of patient-care spaces are also indicated for high-level isolation situations, such as with viral hemorrhagic fever patients. Health care providers involved with the care of these patients should be under medical surveillance.

Moving Patients

Limiting the movement and transport of infected patients and ensuring that they leave their tents or areas only for essential purposes reduces the opportunities for transmission of infections in health care facilities. When patient transport is necessary, whether the patient is having a procedure in another area or is being evacuated from the facility, it is important that risk-appropriate barriers are worn or used by the patient to reduce the opportunity for transmission of microorganisms. The barriers used will depend on the route of transmission of the disease. It is also crucial that the personnel in the area to which the patient is to be taken be notified of his or her impending arrival and the special precautions to be used. Patients must also be informed of their responsibilities to prevent the transmission of infections, such as wearing masks.

VECTOR-BORNE DISEASE CONTAINMENT

Vector transmission, while generally not a problem in US-based facilities characterized by screens and central air conditioning, may be a problem during deployment. Standard precautions are recommended for patients with such infections, whether within or outside of the treatment area. Mosquitoes, which transmit various types of encephalitis and dengue fever, as well flies, ticks, fleas, lice, and mites, can be problematic and spread diseases from person to person. For example, patients viremic with the dengue virus during US military operations in Haiti in the 1990s were recognized as a potential threat to other patients in the same treatment facility. Such basic procedures as keeping tent flaps or doors closed and using mosquito bednets that have been impregnated with an insecticide such as permethrin should assist with halting the spread of these and other vector-borne diseases.

HANDLING OF LINEN, SHARPS, SPECIMENS, AND TERMINAL CLEANING

The risk of disease transmission from soiled linen is usually small, even in a deployed setting, if it is handled, transported, and laundered in a manner that avoids the transfer of microorganisms to patients, personnel, and the facility environment. Sanitary and common sense storage and processing of clean and soiled linen will usually be adequate. Laundry practices that include hot water (71°C [160°F] and above), vigorous washing action, and a laundry detergent will remove soil and mi-

croorganisms, to include scabies, lice, and the hemorrhagic fever viruses. Placing linen from patients in two bags, commonly known as "double bagging," is not usually necessary, unless the linen is soiled with blood or body fluids and has the potential to leak through the original bag.[9] In caring for patients deserving strict contact isolation, though, linens and contaminated protective clothing should be placed in a bag in the patient's room, the exterior of the bag decontaminated with hypochlorite in an anteroom, and then the decontaminated bag placed into another bag before being taken into clean common space. Hands should also be washed in the transition zone between the patient's room and the clean area. Instruments, such as blood pressure cuffs, for patients in strict isolation should only be used for that one particular patient.

Whatever the infectious disease, no special precautions are needed for decontaminating dishes, glasses, cups, or eating utensils. Either disposable or reusable dishes and utensils may be used for patients on isolation precautions. The combination of hot water and a detergent is sufficient to decontaminate such articles.

The tent or area and furniture of a patient who has been placed on some type of isolation precautions may be cleaned using the same procedures used for other patients. No special "airing" of the area or special procedures need to be used in most cases. However, for surfaces potentially contaminated with excreta, blood, or respiratory tract secretions, thorough cleaning and disinfection is indicated. Enterococci are especially prone to survive on inanimate objects for a long time. Facility waste should be disposed of in accordance with US and local laws.

Sharps safety should be maintained, and sharps should be disposed of in some type of rigid container at the point of use. If possible, sharps containers should be made of a rigid plastic that will not allow the sharps to penetrate the container. The disposal containers may be placed between each patient's bed or secured in some manner to the bed to facilitate rapid and safe disposal. When potentially contagious patient specimens are transported, placement in properly labeled, clear double plastic bags is indicated. To prevent contamination, the outer bag should only be handled with clean hands or a new pair of gloves.

HANDLING OF CADAVERS

A persistent myth is that cadavers pose a serious risk of starting epidemics if they are not buried or burned promptly. This is particularly true after natural disasters. Although dead bodies have been associated with the transmission of certain infections that were present before death, dead bodies resulting from a natural disaster usually do not pose a high priority public health threat. The handling of patients who have died of known or suspected infectious diseases should not present difficulties, but there are several principles to remember. The first is protection for the health care worker while preparing the body. Gloves and gowns, at a minimum, should be worn because of the opportunity for contact with blood and body fluids. The health care worker should also wear a mask if the patient was infected with a respiratory disease when he died. After preparation, the cadaver should be carefully identified as having had an infectious disease, and that disease should be written on the identification tags attached to the body.

According to the CDC, patients who have died as a result of a hemorrhagic fever virus should be handled with contact precautions. Those preparing the body should wear protective clothing as indicated for those working in the patient care isolation area. During the preparation of the body, it and the surrounding area should be sprayed with a 1:10 bleach solution. After placing the body in the body bag, the bag should also be sprayed with this solution and placed in a sealed, leakproof coffin. The coffin exterior should be disinfected and rinsed if contaminated. Those handling the body bag should be suitably protected. The body should then be transported safely for deep burial (at least 2 m deep).[16]

FUTURE RESEARCH

Much infection control doctrine for the deployed setting remains to be written. Considerable research remains to be done regarding the best ways of mitigating risk to combat lifesavers, medics, other health care providers, and patients. Studies should assess the proper role of "waterless" disinfectants in settings where recommended bloodborne precautions cannot be adequately implemented. New diagnostics should be tested and placed far forward to facilitate earlier diagnosis, not only for the benefit of the patient but also to protect those in the patient care and evacuation system. More effective diagnostic algorithms should be tested and employed to rapidly identify patients who should be segregated. Questions about when an exposed health care provider should be put into isolation and when he or she should be given prophylactic medications need to be addressed.

SUMMARY

Each deployed military medical unit, whether a hospital, clinic, or forward treatment area, must ensure that all personnel are familiar with the unit's infection control policies and procedures. Such an orientation should include the location and procurement of equipment and supplies necessary to accomplish required infection control activities. The principles of infection control and prevention in a deployed setting are the same wherever the deployment may be. The institution of the three levels of control should ensure that community-acquired infections are not transmitted to other patients and that facility-acquired infections are kept to a minimum. If logistical support fails or is interrupted, cleanliness in all things is still the goal.

REFERENCES

1. Garner J, Jarvis W, Emori G. CDC definitions for nosocomial infections. *Am J Infect Control*. 1988;16:128–140.

2. Meers PD. Infection control in developing countries. *J Hosp Infect*. 1988;11:406–410.

3. Centers for Disease Control and Prevention. Protection against viral hepatitis: Recommendations of the Immunization Practices Advisory Committee (ACIP). *MMWR*. 1990;39(RR-2):1–26.

4. National Intelligence Council. *The Global Infectious Disease Threat and Its Implications for the United States*. January 2000:53.

5. Centers for Disease Control and Prevention. Public Health Service guidelines for the management of health-care worker exposures to HIV and recommendations for postexposure prophylaxis. *MMWR*. 1998;47(RR-7):1–28.

6. Adams MS, Croft AM, Winfield DA, Richards PR. A outbreak of rubella in British troops in Bosnia. *Epidemiol Infect*. 1997;118:253–257.

7. Kortepeter MG, Krauss MR. Tuberculosis infection after humanitarian assistance, Guantanamo Bay, 1995. *Mil Med* 209;166:116–120.

8. Centers for Disease Control and Prevention Infection Control Practices Advisory Committee. Guidelines for isolation precautions in hospitals. *Am J Infect Control*. 1996:24:24–51.

9. Association for Professionals in Infection Control and Epidemiology. *APIC Infection Control and Applied Epidemiology: Principles and Practices*. St. Louis: C.V. Mosby; 1996.

10. Nightingale F. *Notes on Nursing*. Toronto, Ontario: Dover Publications; 1860.

11. Cook E. *Life of Florence Nightingale*. Vol 2. London: Macmillan; 1913.

12. Spaulding EH. Chemical disinfection of medical and surgical materials. In: Laurence CA, Block SS, eds. *Disinfection, Sterilization, and Preservation*. Philadelphia: Lea and Febiger; 1968.

13. Korniewicz DM, Kirwin M, Larson E. Do your gloves fit the task? *Am J Nurs*. 1991;91:38–40.

14. Doebbeling MD, Pfaller MA, Alison K, Houston BS, Wenzel RP. Removal of nosocomial pathogens from contaminated gloves. *Ann Intern Med*. 1988;109:394–398.

15. Centers for Disease Control and Prevention. Guidelines for preventing the transmission of *Mycobacterium tuberculosis* in health care facilities. *MMWR*. 1994;43(RR-13).

16. Centers for Disease Control and Prevention. *Infection Control for Viral Hemorrhagic Fevers in the African Health Care Setting*. Atlanta: CDC; 1999.

MILITARY PREVENTIVE MEDICINE: MOBILIZATION AND DEPLOYMENT
Volume 2

Section 7: Preventive Medicine Efforts Following Disasters

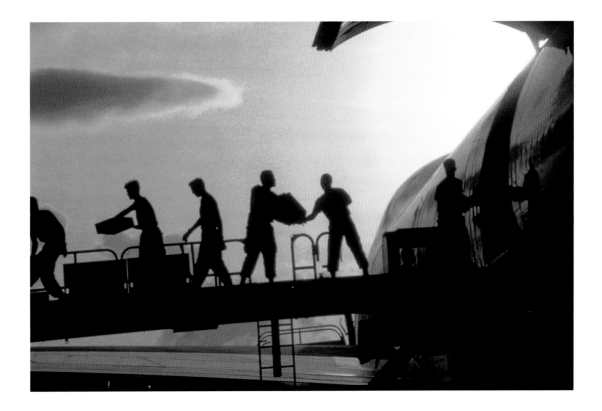

Airmen unload boxes of MREs (Meals Ready To Eat) for victims of Hurricane Marilyn. The hurricane hit the US Virgin Islands in September 1995. The role of military organizations in operations other than war is long and distinguished. As the issue of homeland defense evolves, it is likely that the mission of both Active and Reserve Component units will encompass some of the new challenges the United States faces.

Department of Defense Photograph: Defense Visual Information Center photo identification number DFST9805176.

Chapter 41

THE CHALLENGE OF HUMANITARIAN ASSISTANCE IN THE AFTERMATH OF DISASTERS

TRUEMAN W. SHARP, MD, MPH; FREDERICK BURKLE, MD, MPH; AND KENT L. BRADLEY, MD, MPH

T.W. Sharp, MD, MPH, Commander, Medical Corps, US Navy; Formerly: Preventive Medicine Officer, Headquarters, US Marine Corps, 2 Navy Annex, Washington DC 20380-1775; Currently: Officer in Charge, US Navy Medical Research Unit No. 3, PSC 452, Box 5000, FPO AE 09835-0007

F. Burkle, MD, MPH, Captain, Medical Corps, US Naval Reserve; Deputy Assistant Administrator, Bureau for Global Health, US Agency for International Development, Washington, DC 20523

K.L. Bradley, MD, MPH, Lieutenant Colonel, Medical Corps; Division Surgeon, 7th Infantry Division, Ft. Carson, CO 80913

INTRODUCTION

Military forces of the United States and other developed nations are sometimes called on to cope with the aftermath of the entire spectrum of disasters, from natural events to complex humanitarian emergencies (Table 41-1). While the appropriate roles of military forces in the post-Cold War world and in coping with disasters are controversial, it is likely that the military will always play some role in coping with disasters.

This section provides background on the causes and consequences of disasters and the potential roles of military preventive medicine personnel. This chapter focuses on basic definitions, concepts, and future challenges for the growing discipline of disaster medicine. The next three chapters, numbers 42

to 44 (Military and Public Health Aspects of Natural Disasters, Complex Emergencies, and Public Health Perspectives Related to Technological Disasters and Terrorism, respectively) describe the public health consequences of different types of disasters: natural, complex, and technological. Chapter 45, The International Humanitarian Response System, and Chapter 46, Domestic Disaster Response: FEMA and Other Governmental Organizations, describe the intricacies of the US domestic and international disaster response systems and Chapter 47, Nutritional Assessment and Nutritional Needs of Refugee or Displaced Populations, describes nutritional aspects of humanitarian relief operations. All chapters highlight issues relevant to the military.

DISASTERS AND DISASTER MEDICINE

Disaster is a broad term that has been defined in several different ways.[1,2] One commonly used definition is "...events of environmental disruption or destruction that can be of sudden or gradual onset,

TABLE 41-1

SELECTED US MILITARY DISASTER OPERATIONS FROM 1990 THROUGH 1996

Operation	Type of Disaster
Fiery Vigil Philippines, 1990	Volcano
Provide Comfort Northern Iraq, 1991	Complex emergency
Sea Angel Bangladesh, 1991	Tropical cyclone
JTF Andrew Florida, 1992	Hurricane
Restore Hope Somalia, 1992	Complex emergency
JTF Hawaii Hawaii, 1992	Hurricane
Support Hope Rwanda, 1993	Complex emergency
Uphold Democracy Haiti, 1994	Complex emergency
Joint Endeavor Bosnia, 1996	Complex emergency

JTF: Joint Task Force

and that are severe enough to overwhelm the resources of the affected community and necessitate outside assistance."[1(p422)] An alternate definition is "...an event that exposes the vulnerability of individuals and communities in such a way that their lives are directly threatened, or sufficient harm has been done to their community's economic and social structures to undermine their ability to survive."[2(p13)] Both definitions emphasize the catastrophic nature of disasters and the need for externally provided assistance.

Disasters may be categorized in different ways. Some authors have differentiated between natural disasters (such as typhoons) and man-made disasters (such as war). Others have grouped disasters into sudden-onset events (such as earthquakes) and long-term situations that develop over months or years (such as refugee crises). Technological disasters, which are events such as the Chernobyl nuclear accident that involve major exposures to chemicals or radiation, are often placed in another category. Terrorist actions involving conventional explosives or weapons of mass destruction are regarded as an increasingly important type of disaster.[3,4]

Any categorization scheme is somewhat arbitrary and may oversimplify the interaction of many factors. For example, a disaster in Durunka, Egypt, in 1994 combined elements of both natural and technological phenomena. Torrential rains led to severe flash-flooding, which disrupted fuel depots located in flood-washed ravines. Fuel-contaminated water flooded downstream villages and caught on fire. The majority of the 580 deaths that occurred were not due to drowning but to burning fuel.[5] Also, some disasters can be difficult to categorize. Land mines may be considered as a technological disaster or as an aspect of conflict. Natural disasters are often part of the dynamic of conflict and complex emergencies. The 1971 India-Pakistan war and subsequent refugee crisis was triggered in large part by a cyclone when the disruption caused by this natural event exacerbated political unrest. A severe drought was the principal catalyst for the civil war and humanitarian crisis in Somalia from 1991 to 1992.[6]

While the term "disaster" invokes connotations of the forces of nature to many, the hand of humans is found in almost all disasters. What is identified as the disaster, even when it is a natural event, is often better understood as a trigger event that exposes underlying societal problems. Virtually every famine since 1977 has been the result of underdevelopment, armed conflict, inadequate economic and social systems, failed governments, and other man-made factors.[3,7]

The term "complex emergency" (also complex humanitarian emergency or conflict-related complex emergency) was coined to refer to disasters that involve an intricate interaction of political, military, economic, and natural factors and that have armed conflict as a central feature.[8] These types of disasters have been increasingly common since the end of the Cold War. Victims are usually large populations or specific ethnic groups or cultures; armed conflict against these groups is almost always a critical factor.[9] Somalia in 1992 is an example in which civil violence was the most visible, proximate cause of the disaster, but years of underdevelopment, governmental failures, superpower intervention, ethnic conflict, drought, and famine all contributed substantially to the situation.

To provide a basic approach to the subject of disasters, this section will consider three basic types of disaster: natural, complex, and technological (Table 41-2). Some events that could be considered disasters, such as a disease outbreak, are considered in other chapters.

The discipline of disaster medicine is rapidly evolving. Disaster medicine has its roots in the emergency activities undertaken in the immediate aftermath of natural disasters, but the discipline is

TABLE 41-2

CATEGORIES OF DISASTERS*

Natural

    Flood

    Tropical cyclone

    Hurricane

    Earthquake

    Tornado

    Volcano

    Tsunami

    Drought

Complex

    Civil conflict

    War

    Famine

    Mass migration or displacement of people

Technological

    Explosions

    Fires

    Chemical Exposures and Spills

    Radiation Exposures

    Terrorist Actions

*This is not a comprehensive list of all disasters.

evolving to include other types of disasters. This chapter will use a broad definition for disaster medicine: "The study and collaborative application of various health disciplines—eg, pediatrics, epidemiology, communicable diseases, nutrition, public health, emergency medicine, social mending, community care, international health—to the prevention, immediate response and rehabilitation of the health problems arising from disaster, in cooperation with other disciplines involved in comprehensive disaster management."[10(p23–24)]

PREVENTIVE MEDICINE IN DISASTERS

One way to understand disasters, especially complex emergencies, is as catastrophic public health crises. Disasters often involve serious damage to preventive and curative medical systems and to important public health infrastructure, such as water treatment systems and sanitation networks. Disasters also may affect the public health through disruption of other segments of society, such as the

police, judiciary, communications networks, transportation systems, agricultural production, and markets.

In the aftermath of disasters, interventions that are the most urgent, that save the most lives, and that are the most cost-effective are often basic public health measures. Military medical personnel, particularly those in preventive medicine, may be able to make substantial contributions after disasters by organizing immunization campaigns, reestablishing water treatment systems, investigating outbreaks, providing basic sanitation, controlling disease vectors, and implementing other fundamental public health programs.[3–5,11–13]

Another important role for preventive medicine personnel is using the tools of epidemiology to gather critical information. In the aftermath of disasters, sound information is always needed to develop relief priorities and strategies and to identify vulnerable populations. Rapid assessments, targeted surveys, and surveillance are essential for effective disaster response.[14,15] Preventive medicine personnel have unique skills in collecting needed data and using those data to develop objectives and strategies for disaster response.

Although some aspects of disasters and disaster response are well understood, there is still much to be learned. The tools of preventive medicine—epidemiology and biostatistics—are also useful in conducting research to better understand the causes of disasters and their management.[16–18] In addition to helping with the immediate response, documentation of the principal causes of morbidity and mortality in disasters and of the effectiveness of relief measures through well-conceived epidemiologic studies is essential.

Preventive medicine personnel can be of great assistance in planning and preparation for disasters. Important activities in this domain include preparing disaster contingency plans, devising standard medication and supply lists, organizing disaster response medical teams, developing early warning systems, and helping plan better infrastructure engineering.[19–21]

Preventive medicine personnel may become involved in a myriad of activities that are beyond their usual realm. Organizing feeding programs for a malnourished population, developing standardized treatment protocols to be used by health workers in refugee camps, or establishing rehydration centers during a diarrhea epidemic are just a few examples.[21–23] Preventive medicine personnel could also become involved in investigating and documenting human rights abuses.[24]

Finally, preventive medicine personnel are the best advocates for the public health agenda in disaster response.[12,25] Because preventive medicine personnel are trained to see the big picture and to understand "health" in a broader context, they are in a unique position to see important consequences of a disaster and to work across disciplines in helping to develop and coordinate the most effective response. Military medical officers must advise line commanders on the best roles for the military in disaster response. Preventive medicine personnel in particular are well situated to understand what the military can and cannot contribute to relief efforts. When line commanders, who may become focused on security issues or other aspects of a response, lose sight of critical public health needs, preventive medicine personnel can have a powerful voice in focusing relief priorities.[11,26,27]

THE MAGNITUDE OF DISASTERS

Natural Disasters

Each week there is at least one natural disaster in the world of sufficient magnitude to require the assistance of the international community.[5] In the 1970s and 1980s, natural disasters affected at least 800 million people and caused more than 3 million deaths.[28] The incidence of natural disasters appears to be rising, and the number of highly vulnerable persons in disaster-prone areas, particularly in the developing world, is at least 70 million and growing.[29] Large populations are vulnerable to disasters in at least 60 countries, many of which are in the tropics. The devastating tropical cyclone in Bangladesh in 1991, in which more than 100,000 persons were killed, illustrates the potential impact of natural disasters on a vulnerable population in the developing world. Historically, the US military has responded to many natural disasters domestically and internationally.

Complex Disasters

The number of armed conflicts in the world has increased dramatically since World War II[30] (Figure 41-1). Between 1980 and 1997, more than 150 major armed conflicts were waged.[31] Complex emergencies are inextricably linked with violence; the number of complex emergencies has increased in parallel with the increase in war. Whereas in the late 1970s there were approximately 5 complex emergencies per year, by the late 1980s there were 10 to 15 per year, and by the late 1990s there were 25 to 30 each year.[8]

Armed conflict and its related complex humanitarian emergencies have profound effects on civilian populations,[30–34] particularly since most armed conflict occurs in the developing world (Figure 41-2). Some estimate that in many conflicts for every death of a combatant there are eight to nine deaths among civilians.[31,32] Toole and Waldman have described the

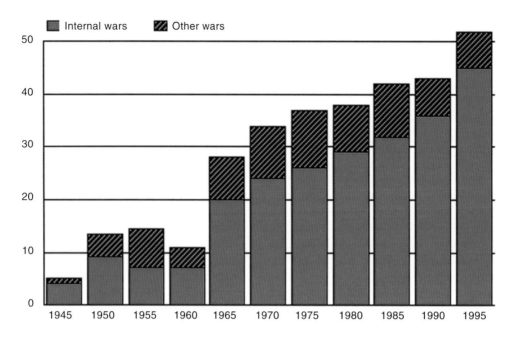

Fig. 41-1. Increase in Armed Conflicts and Internal Wars since World War II. This figure shows the dramatic increase in armed conflict overall, and particularly in internal conflicts, since the end of World War II. Most armed conflict since World War II has not involved the militaries of two nations fighting each other but, rather, has been strife within the borders of a sovereign country. The combatants in internal wars have typically been less clearly defined groups than national armies. They have usually been factions based on ethnic, cultural, or tribal affiliations, and many have had shifting allegiances. Some factions have acted essentially as a form of organized crime, attempting simply to control valuable resources. Prominent examples of internal wars in the 1990s were the conflicts that occurred in Somalia, Rwanda, and the former Yugoslavia. Adapted with permission from: International Federation of Red Cross and Red Crescent Societies. *World Disasters Report, 1992.* Dordrecht, The Netherlands: Martinus Nijhoff Publishers, 1992. Additional data from: Sollenberg S, Wallensteen P. Armed conflicts, conflict termination, and peace agreements, 1989-96. *J Peace Res.* 1997;34:339-358.

insidious cycle of armed confrontation, famine, and population displacement.[33,34] In 1980 there were approximately 5 million refugees in the world; as a consequence of this cycle, though, by the mid-1990s there were approximately 23 million refugees and 25 million internally displaced persons (those who have fled their homes but who have crossed no international boundaries).[33] Thus, roughly 1 in 110 persons in the world was a refugee or was displaced from his or her home. As demonstrated by operations in Somalia, Rwanda, Haiti, and the former Yugoslavia, the US military has been drawn increasingly often into these situations.

Technological Disasters

The rapid and unregulated industrialization of much of the world and the misuse of technologies are increasingly recognized phenomena.[3,5,35,36] The extensive environmental pollution in former Soviet bloc nations, the nuclear reactor accident at Chernobyl, and the toxic gas leak at Bhopal, India, are examples of disasters resulting from industrial pollution and industrial accidents. While an important issue in the industrialized world, this is also an urgent concern in much of the developing world, where industrial growth often far exceeds necessary regulatory laws and safety practices.

The sarin gas attack in the Tokyo subway system and the Oklahoma City bombing, both in 1995, demonstrate how weapons technologies in the hands of terrorists have the potential to become massive disasters.[36–39] The potential for terrorist actions has increased markedly since the collapse of the Soviet Union and the ensuing dissemination of technologies for building weapons of mass destruction. The US military has critical capabilities for coping with both technological disasters and terrorism and increasingly is seen as having an important role in responding to these incidents.

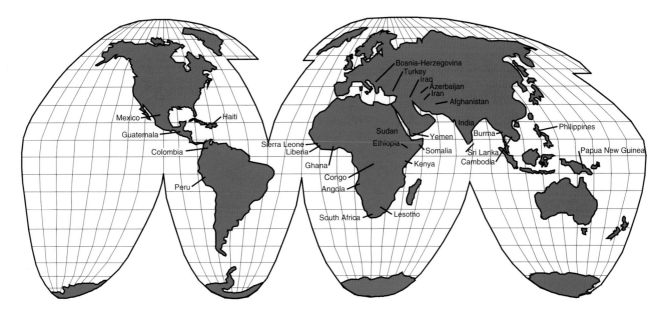

Fig. 41-2. Worldwide Conflicts, mid-1994. This figure shows the countries in the world in 1994 in which significant armed conflict was occurring. The fact that approximately one in five countries overall was at war is notable for the extent of armed conflict worldwide, as well as the fact that most conflict was taking place in the tropical developing world. Wars in the former Yugoslavia and former states of the Soviet Union were exceptions to this general trend. Data source: Fitzsimmons DW, Whiteside AW. *Conflict, War and Public Health.* London: Research Institute for the Study of Conflict and Terrorism, 1994. Study 276.

THE CONSEQUENCES OF DISASTERS

Every disaster is unique, and the consequences of each one will vary considerably by person, place, and time. In part this is because different types of disasters have very different effects. Whereas an earthquake often causes many immediate trauma deaths and usually does not result in food shortages, a flood typically causes few immediate deaths and disrupts food production and distribution networks.[3] Similar events that occur in different environments can have very different consequences. An earthquake in Armenia has a markedly different impact than an earthquake in southern California because the extent of the development, the local building codes, the population density, and the local response capabilities are different. One refugee population may be devastated by measles while in another, in which vaccination coverage has been high, diarrhea may be the most important cause of morbidity and mortality.[21,22,40]

Within any given disaster, relief needs can evolve considerably over time.[23] Some authors have described the phases of natural disasters, such as an impact phase, post-impact phase, and recovery phase, to discuss the importance of understanding how relief needs change.[41] In the impact phase after earthquakes, for example, there may be an urgent need for trauma services, but deploying trauma hospitals that will arrive 4 or 5 days after the earthquake is fruitless and wasteful.[3]

It can be difficult to delineate clear phases of a complex disaster. Because the crisis is usually the result of many years of complicated and deeply rooted problems, events do not progress in a clear, linear fashion. Nevertheless, relief needs in complex emergencies change substantially over time as well. For example, priorities for refugees who have just arrived in a location—usually shelter, food, water, and basic medical care—are likely to be different from what this population needs a few months after a camp has been established, such as family planning, medical care for chronic problems, and rehabilitation.[22,23]

The health effects of a disaster can vary considerably by location. De Ville de Goyet describes the different spatial zones of a natural disaster to illustrate the severity of effects in relation to the epicenter of an earthquake.[41] In hurricanes, the devastation can be quite unevenly distributed across an affected area.[3,42]

Within a particular disaster, certain subpopulations may be more vulnerable, have fewer biological or social reserves to fall back on, and have less access to help. Women and children, particularly small children, typically experience much increased morbidity and mortality.[21,22] In Rwanda, for example, it was shown that refugee-camp children living in households headed by single women had a significantly higher risk of malnutrition because they had less access to food and other relief services.[43] Ethnic, religious, or cultural groups may be particularly vulnerable. In Somalia, certain unarmed agriculturally based clans who were not participants in the fighting were particularly devastated by the civil conflict and had extremely limited access to emergency relief services. Even adults and adolescents, who are the most capable segments of the population, require special attention in some circumstances.[44]

ASSESSING AND RESPONDING TO DISASTERS

A critical first task for disaster responders is assessing rapidly what has occurred so as to determine urgent needs and relief priorities for that unique situation. The importance of rapid assessments has been increasingly recognized, and the science of conducting these assessments has developed considerably.[14,15,42] Although good assessments may not be the norm, it is widely recognized that in the absence of sound early assessments, relief efforts can easily be misguided and inappropriate.

After initial assessments, targeted surveys and specific investigations can be of much value in answering more focused questions.[45] In addition, standardized surveillance and health information systems need to be established (or re-established) after disasters to continually assess and monitor the needs of the affected population[22] (Figure 41-3). Relief efforts should be modified accordingly as critical data become available. In the absence of mechanisms to constantly evaluate the health of the target population, priorities may become skewed and resources may be inappropriately directed or even wasted.[46] There are many examples in the disaster medicine literature of how early information collection has been a critical factor in successful disaster response.[43,45,47,48]

Emergency assistance following a disaster is often thought of as providing the basic necessities, such as food, water, shelter, medical care, and agricultural supplies, to save lives in the immediate aftermath of a devastating event. This is a key aspect of disaster response, but disaster response is often much more than this. According to the United Nations High Commissioner for Refugees, the "aim of humanitarian assistance is to sustain dignified life, to strengthen local institutions' efforts to relieve suffering and build self-reliance, and to assure that the first step is taken towards reconstruction, rehabilitation and development."[27(p1)] This definition emphasizes the importance of viewing disaster response in a broader and more long-term context. Therefore, disaster relief often must consider long-term development and must involve many realms, such as political, economic, social, security, and human rights, among others.

Relief needs may vary substantially in different cultural situations. Food items appropriate for one population may not be appropriate for another. For example, potatoes donated to the displaced Kurds in northern Iraq remained uneaten because potatoes are not a part of the normal Kurd diet. Sanitation practices can also vary markedly. Latrines inadvertently built facing Mecca were not used by Muslim Kurds.

In addition to cultural sensitivity, international relief responders must be careful to involve local personnel in relief efforts. Although this seems obvious, much emergency relief is conducted by outside groups who presume that they know best and that they must do everything for the "helpless" victims. In fact, disaster-affected populations are not helpless victims. The most effective disaster relief gives local personnel themselves the means to recover and rebuild.[49]

PROGRESS IN DISASTER RESPONSE

In 1975, Dr. Michael Lechat noted that disaster relief could be described as "the crisis dominated convergence of unsolicited donations of mobile hospitals, time expired drugs, medical students volunteering for disaster safaris, and vaccines for diseases with zero incidence."[50(p845–846)] Fortunately, the knowledge and practice of disaster response has progressed considerably.

Since the publication of the first textbook on disaster medicine in 1984,[51] there has been an explosion in research into and knowledge about disaster relief. Many articles have been published in the peer-reviewed scientific literature, and there are many excellent technical manuals, textbooks, guide-

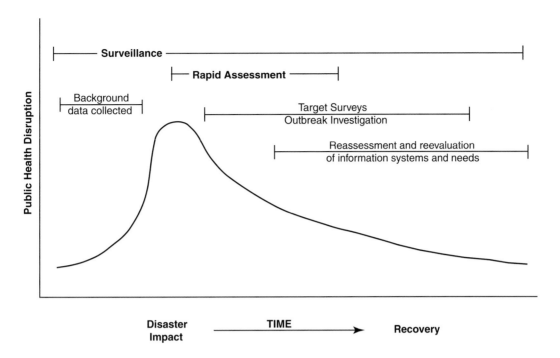

Fig. 41-3. Information Gathering in a Sudden-onset Disaster. This figure illustrates when information should be collected in a sudden-onset disaster. Ideally, certain background information is collected and archived before a disaster strikes, such as baseline rates of diarrheal diseases or malnutrition. Baseline data is needed for comparison to make sense of information collected after the disaster has occurred. Once disaster has struck, rapid assessments of the situation should be undertaken, followed quickly by focused surveys and outbreak investigations as they are needed. Ideally, surveillance systems are in operation before the disaster and are either continued or reestablished after the event. If not, surveillance should be started or modified as soon as possible after the disaster to gather data on appropriate medical outcomes. As conditions stabilize, assessments of information needs and information collection practices should take place to improve information gathering and adjust to changing circumstances.

books, and other publications[22,23,27] that address not only clinical aspects of disaster-related medical problems but also public health issues, supplies, logistics, program management, and other important aspects of disaster response.

There is much evidence that improved understanding of the consequences of disasters and disaster relief has lead to improved practice since the 1970s.[33,34,43] The development and implementation of the Federal Disaster Response Plan[52] has greatly facilitated appropriate and coordinated relief efforts in the United States (see Chapter 46: Domestic Disaster Response: FEMA and Other Governmental Organization). This plan identifies the many different disaster response organizations in the United States and how they are to work together in a crisis. Internationally, the Pan American Health Organization has made enormous strides in preparing for and coping with natural disasters in the Western hemisphere. Most major UN agencies and nongovernmental organizations have also developed much-improved response capabilities.[6] Nongovernmental

organizations have also made major strides in improving their capabilities to respond to disasters.[6]

The 1994 civil war in Rwanda was an unprecedented and overwhelming complex emergency by any standard. By the third week of international intervention, however, much critical information had been obtained through rapid assessments, targeted surveys, and standardized surveillance. The most important relief measures, such as potable water, measles immunizations, vitamin A supplementation, standardized treatment protocols, and community outreach programs, were implemented based on good information and sound practices while other less-effective interventions were curtailed. During the relief efforts in Rwanda, a very high level of cooperation and coordination among the majority of governmental, nongovernmental, and military relief efforts was achieved.[43] There were clearly still substantial problems in the response to this disaster, but it nevertheless exemplified much of the progress that has been made.

CHALLENGES IN DISASTER RELIEF

Despite the advances made in the knowledge and practice of disaster relief, many challenges remain. The number of disaster-affected persons in the world continues to increase, and the numbers of disasters and disaster-affected persons will probably continue their almost exponential rise.[5,29,33]

Alternative Approaches

Focusing only on the acute, emergency response to an event once it has occurred is inadequate and, some argue, even detrimental. Early warning systems and early intervention strategies that may prevent

---

EXHIBIT 41-1

THE PREVENTION PARADIGM APPLIED TO DISASTERS

Complex Emergencies	Natural Disasters

Primary Prevention (action taken before the disaster to avoid or minimize adverse effects)

• Establish and maintain sound public health programs, including surveillance	• Conduct risk analysis of natural threats
• Foster development overall and within health sector	• Promote safe engineering and building practices
• Promote disarmament and demilitarization	• Foster development overall and within health sector
• Promote democracy and democratic institutions	• Develop early warning and rapid evacuation systems
• Develop disaster contingency plans and public health early warning systems	• Develop disaster contingency plans

Secondary Prevention (actions taken when the disaster is imminent or in its early stages)

• Perform public health assessments and early interventions as indicated	• Implement early warning and rapid evacuation
• Use diplomatic and/or military pressure or intervention	• Implement contingency plans
• Conduct advocacy to alert decision-makers and public	

Treatment (actions taken during or after the disaster to treat the effects)

• Conduct rapid assessments, targeted surveys, and outbreak investigations	• Conduct rapid assessments, targeted surveys, and outbreak investigations
• Undertake peacemaking or peacekeeping interventions	• Provide emergency relief services
• Provide emergency relief services	
• Conduct advocacy to alert decision-makers and public	

Tertiary Prevention (actions taken post-disaster to prevent further ill effects)

• Stabilize peace	• Rehabilitate society, economy, and health systems
• Rehabilitate society, economy, and health systems	• Resume development
• Resume development	
• Demobilize militaries	
• Dearm and clear landmines	
• Strengthen democratic institutions	

crises from being so severe are important in coping with complex emergencies as well as natural disasters.[6,43,46,53] With the dramatic rise in complex emergencies, the resources devoted to emergency response has increased markedly in the past few years. At the US Agency for International Development, for example, the dramatic shift in funds from long-term development programs to disaster response may, ironically, serve to exacerbate the threat and consequences of disasters by sapping funds that otherwise would be used for infrastructure improvement and disaster preparedness.[53,54] A true preventive approach would call for better development strategies, preventive diplomacy, and early conflict resolution. Once a crisis has occurred and emergency relief efforts have been begun, increased resources should be devoted to the stabilization, rehabilitation, and development of the affected communities (Exhibit 41-1). Without this, a society can plunge back into a catastrophe, as occurred in Somalia.

How limited emergency response resources are allocated around the world is a concern. Some observers argue that particularly during the Cold War, but still today, populations who receive relief often have been chosen on the basis of political agendas rather than true need. The media can play a critical role in determining which crises receive public attention. In general, government-controlled areas instead of rebel-controlled areas, refugees instead of internally displaced persons, and regions of interest to the major powers instead of regions less strategically valuable receive more international assistance.[53] Thus some have argued that the international community needs improved mechanisms to determine who merits international aid.[55]

Coping with Violence

Many humanitarian emergencies today are inextricably linked with violence.[31,32,56-60] Fighting is waged between various factions, many of whom do not recognize or follow international humanitarian law. Unfortunately, as has been well described regarding Cambodia and the Sudan, the provision of humanitarian relief can easily be perceived as a partisan act or it can be overtly manipulated for the benefit of certain warring factions.[7,46,59] Many humanitarian organizations are struggling with how to work with "predator" states (those governments that exist to prey on their own population) or amoral warlords while providing impartial and neutral humanitarian aid.

In some emergencies, the greatest public health threat may be violence. In the former Yugoslavia,

for example, many more people were killed by shelling and shooting than by food shortages and disease.[60,61] The provision of traditional humanitarian relief can be largely ineffective in such circumstances; the most effective humanitarian relief would be enforcing and keeping the peace.[32,57,60,61]

Provision of relief is dangerous for humanitarian workers. As of 1996, more than 1,000 relief workers had been killed in the former Yugoslavia. The International Committee of the Red Cross has had over 35 workers killed between 1992 and 1997.[62] Relief organizations are struggling with how to operate in insecure environments without having to resort to arms themselves or depend on military forces to protect them.

Improved Strategic Planning and Coordination

In domestic disaster response, local, state, federal, civilian, and military agencies must work together. Internationally, United Nations agencies, nongovernmental organizations, the International Committee of the Red Cross, local officials, and militaries must cooperate. The diversity of the many participants in humanitarian assistance has been both a blessing and a curse. The independence, autonomy, and flexibility of some relief agencies, particularly the nongovernmental organizations, have been critical in many situations, but the lack of overall strategies and poor coordination among the various participants have hampered many relief efforts.[9,53] There is a need for much-improved strategic planning, coordination, and cooperation among the major responders.[63] Without an overarching strategy that most participants support, it is impossible to address the almost intractable causes and consequences of complex disasters. Within the United States, the Federal Response Plan and related efforts have improved domestic disaster response coordination substantially. While progress has been made on the international scene, much more work needs to be done.

Improved Emergency Response

Even though much of the science of good relief is well delineated, problems still remain in implementing effective emergency relief programs. Despite a massive international relief effort in northern Iraq during the Kurdish refugee crisis, many deaths occurred due to preventable diarrheal disease. This was in large part a failure to implement basic environmental health interventions and diarrhea control programs early enough in this crisis.[45] The Goma (Zaire) Epidemiology Group reported after the Rwanda refugee crisis that there is an urgent need for more intensive and focused training of relief workers in the prevention and management of diarrheal diseases and other essential relief programs, such as measles immunization, public health surveillance, community outreach, and nutritional rehabilitation.[43]

Recent emergencies have fueled considerable discussion about how relief workers are trained and whether there should be standards of practice or even some type of certification for relief workers. Disaster medicine is still in its infancy as a recognized field of medical practice, and its training lacks uniformity and a curriculum that covers the range of knowledge needed to cope with disasters.[20,64,65] Many relief workers, although well-intentioned, are often recruited and sent out on short notice with little preparation or training. In many disasters, responders are also burdened with large quantities of unneeded and unwanted supplies.[66,67] Well-intentioned but inappropriate relief supplies actually hinder rather than help relief efforts.

Need for Research

Despite many advances in the discipline of disaster medicine, much research is still needed to better elucidate the health effects of disasters and ensuing medical needs. Much disaster planning and response is based on anecdotal reports, which are sometimes valuable but are often sources of nonuniform, nonobjective, and nonspecific data. An improved understanding of the epidemiology of disasters is clearly needed so that more appropriate choices can be made about relief supplies, equipment, and personnel.[20,68] Many questions still remain about the role and effectiveness of different interventions. An example is the considerable discussion following the Rwanda crisis on the best use of new cholera vaccines in emergency situations.[69] Research is needed to develop standardized and valid assessment tools, reliable surveillance programs, low-technology environmental health interventions, and more effective intervention strategies.[20,34]

Very little work has been done to evaluate the cost-effectiveness of various relief efforts. Only rarely have relief organizations or the military been held accountable for the money they spend in relief efforts, but measuring outcomes and effectiveness of relief interventions is increasingly demanded by donors, politicians, and commanders. The cost-benefits of investing in emergency response, as opposed to prevention, conflict resolution, and development, are not well delineated.[53,70]

New Threats: Land Mines, Laser Weapons, and Terrorists

One of the most pressing and overwhelming challenges ahead is coping with land mines.[71–74] The 100 million to 200 million land mines that are in the ground in more than 65 countries, with almost no records of their location, are a massive public health emergency.[60] Many mines have been placed as instruments of terror in areas of no military strategic value. Livestock, herders, and children are at great risk. Mines are not only immediately devastating to victims but also impose tremendous burdens in the rehabilitation of survivors. In Cambodia, approximately 1 in 250 persons is a land-mine amputee. The health care system of Cambodia is overwhelmed with caring for and rehabilitating these victims.[72] Other places, such as Eritrea, Afghanistan, Egypt, and the former Yugoslavia, have literally millions of land mines in place.[60]

An emerging concern is the development of laser weapons as a weapon of terror. The technology of lasers for military use on the battlefield has progressed markedly since 1980. Because lasers have now become lightweight and portable and require only low-energy sources to operate, it is possible for an individual to carry a small laser rifle that is silent, is easily hidden, and has the potential to permanently blind large numbers of persons indiscriminately. Protection against these weapons is very difficult. Although such blinding weapons have not yet been employed, some fear they will appeal to some military commanders and terrorists alike.[75]

Terrorism itself is not new. What is new, however, is that terrorists today have unparalleled access to highly destructive weapons. Conventional explosives, nuclear devices, and chemical and biological weapons are all potential terrorist weapons. Information on how to construct bombs and weapons of mass destruction is readily available through public libraries and the Internet. The materials to build most weapons are available from a variety of commercial sources. Some observers have argued that terrorism is appealing to many groups unable to achieve their goals by conventional military or political means, and the world is unprepared to cope with the increasing threat posed by terrorist actions.[76–78]

Vulnerable Populations

The unique concerns of women, particularly those who are pregnant or lactating, are an important focus of disaster relief. Epidemiologic studies[22,43] document that in some disasters women have less access to medical care and other relief services. And while data are limited, pregnancy, sexually transmitted diseases, sexual abuse, and human immunodeficiency virus infection are believed by some investigators to be common issues in many disaster-affected populations, especially refugees and internally displaced populations.[79–81] Few relief programs have yet addressed these issues.

The special problems of children have been increasingly recognized. Children are more vulnerable than adults to many of the adverse health effects of disasters, such as malnutrition and infectious diseases. Additionally, the plight of unaccompanied children in Rwanda illustrated a problem common to many complex emergencies.[82] The psychological impact of disasters on children has only just begun to be documented but is clearly profound. The appalling practice of using children as soldiers in many countries of the world is a crisis of unprecedented proportions.[83,84]

International Humanitarian Law

Relief workers face many difficult challenges in the realm of international humanitarian law. Under current law, internally displaced persons and nondisplaced persons do not have the same right to protection as those who cross international borders and thereby become refugees. The provisions of international humanitarian law that were written principally to deal with conflict between sovereign nations are difficult to apply to conflicts that occur within a country's borders.[85–87] Contradictory interpretations of the Geneva Conventions and how they apply to complex emergencies have complicated some relief efforts.[46]

Recent disasters in Rwanda, Somalia, and the former Yugoslavia are characterized by profound human rights abuses, such as torture and genocide. Issues of education of combatants regarding international humanitarian law, enforcement of humanitarian laws, and prosecution of war criminals remain extremely difficult but critical problems.[87]

Using Information Technologies

How to best use information technologies is an important issue in disaster relief. Epidemiologists and other responders have used computers to gather and analyze data rapidly. Disaster responders are also learning to take advantage of global positioning systems, electronic mail, and satellite and cellular phones. They are learning to use computers to improve management of other aspects of relief efforts, such as the Pan American Health Organization's computer program that helps manage relief supplies.[88] Computer-based models have been developed that predict environmental effects of natural disasters.[89] A variety of bulletin boards and home pages on the Internet have been established to facilitate training and information exchange, such as the Federal Emergency Management Agency's website at http://www.fema.gov. Computers and distance-learning technologies are increasingly used in training of relief workers, but their full potential has yet to be understood or reached.[90–92]

Expanding Professional Boundaries

Preventive medicine is fundamentally concerned with improving and protecting health. Accomplishing this after disasters requires a multi-disciplinary approach that may go well beyond usual preventive medicine practice. Preventive medicine personnel are likely to become involved with logistics, communications, triage, evacuation, and other areas. The preventive medicine professional may have to work closely with a confusing variety of local, state, federal and international agencies. Wasley notes that in the aftermath of natural disasters, epidemiologists must work not only with health care personnel but also with engineers, seismologists, meteorologists, sociologists, and anthropologists.[5] In complex emergencies, the media, politicians, human rights organizations, local health officials, and other militaries may be added to the list. Preventive medicine personnel involved in a complex emergency must expand their professional boundaries to effect the greatest good in disaster-affected populations.[25]

MILITARY INVOLVEMENT IN DISASTERS

Disaster relief is not a new mission for the military forces of the United States or for many other developed nations. Gaydos[93] describes many of the reasons military forces often become involved in humanitarian assistance, such as the ready availability of highly capable forces, the similarities between traditional military missions and disaster response,

and the training opportunities.

Military forces of many nations are likely to continue to play a role in disaster response both within their own countries and abroad. As the problem of responding to the use of chemical or biological agents grows, some militaries are likely to have a particular role in this area, given their unique capabilities.[37–39,94] Subsequent chapters in this section describe in more detail many of the important considerations of using military forces in various types of disaster response.

In regard to the military's response to complex emergencies, the predominant and most devastating type of disaster in the post–Cold War era, the Kurdish relief effort in 1991 was in many respects a watershed. In this crisis, the militaries of the United States and a number of other developed countries were called on to deal with over half a million displaced persons, a formidable problem. However, conditions were almost perfect for a successful military intervention.[95] The US military and other participating militaries were quickly able to establish a safe haven in northern Iraq. With security established, the military filled what was then an important void in the international humanitarian response system by organizing and orchestrating relief efforts on the ground. Solutions to the crisis, primarily establishing security, providing emergency relief, and then facilitating the return of the displaced persons to their homes, were attained in a short period of time.

Based on this success, the militaries of developed nations were regarded by many as critical future participants in responding to the marked increase of complex emergencies in the post–Cold War world. Outside military intervention in complex emergencies was viewed as a solution to security issues, as well as a way to provide critical emergency logistical support in dangerous or remote areas.[9] The initial wave of enthusiasm for military intervention in complex emergencies was quickly tempered, however, by events in Somalia in 1993 when a number of US peacekeeping personnel were killed. In addition, there were serious problems with coordination between the military and the relief organizations, which, in contrast to the situation in Kurdistan, had been in Somalia for many years prior to military intervention.[96,97] Other large international relief missions that followed the Kurdish crisis, such as those in the former Yugoslavia and in Rwanda, in which relief problems were also much more complex, perhaps even intractable, also showed that using military forces in a humanitarian role would not always be so easy.

How the military best fits into international humanitarian response remains an area of much discussion and controversy. Military forces clearly have many positive attributes in the emergency provision of humanitarian services. In addition to providing security, which sometimes may be their most important contribution, militaries can add critical transportation assets, logistics expertise, command and control systems, deployable medical facilities, and intelligence capabilities.[9,26]

Military forces have significant constraints as well. Some have questioned the effectiveness of using military forces for humanitarian relief.[98] There is little evidence to show that much is accomplished for the often tremendous amounts of money and resources expended to deploy servicemembers. Using a medical organization that is staffed, trained, and equipped to support combat operations for a humanitarian mission can be problematic. Military medical staff are often ill-trained and equipped to cope with disaster relief situations.[26] Line commanders may not fully appreciate the public health issues in disaster response or their solutions. Some have argued that the use of armed forces is fundamentally incompatible with and may even be detrimental to accomplishing humanitarian objectives.[98] Armed forces usually support only some factions in the conflict or will be perceived as supporting only certain interests,[43] which can make neutral, impartial relief problematic. Some have argued that the use of military force in complex emergencies is symptomatic of a failure of political will, and while it may offer a respite, military intervention is unlikely to result in long-term solutions.[97,98]

The US government and military must resolve a number of difficult issues. Other nations face similar dilemmas. One of the most important is the role of military forces in the post–Cold War era, and whether armed forces should embrace disaster relief and humanitarian assistance as one of their principal missions. If humanitarian assistance is indeed a core mission, strategies to determine which crises warrant intervention need to be elaborated. Much effort has been expended in developing mechanisms for the military to work effectively with other relief agencies.[99,100] The Federal Response Plan is an excellent template for the role of the military in domestic disaster response. On the international scene, though, how military forces relate to other disaster responders and where they fit into an overall disaster response architecture are still contentious issues. In addition, as the military continues to downsize and resources to support more traditional combat missions are increasingly limited, there will continue to be problems regarding adequate staffing, training, and equipment for these missions.

SUMMARY

The world of disasters and disaster relief is quite complex. The military preventive medicine officer involved in these types of efforts must understand not only the public health consequences of disasters but also the intricacies of the existing disaster response systems, the challenges facing disaster responders, and the US military's role in this often chaotic environment.

REFERENCES

1. Lechat MF. The epidemiology of disasters. *Proc R Soc Med*. 1976;69:421–426.

2. International Federation of Red Cross and Red Crescent Societies. *World Disasters Report 1993*. The Netherlands: Martinus Nijhoff Publishers;1993.

3. Noji ED, ed. *Public Health Consequences of Disasters*. New York: Oxford University Press; 1997.

4. Sidel VW, Onel E, Geiger HJ, Leaning J, Foege WH. Public health responses to natural and human-made disasters. In: Last JM, Wallace RB, eds. *Maxcy-Rosenau-Last Public Health and Preventive Medicine*. 13th ed. Norwalk, Conn: Appleton and Lange; 1992: 1173–1186.

5. Wasley A. Epidemiology in the disaster setting. *Curr Issues Public Health*. 1995;1:131–135.

6. Chen LC, Rietveld A. Human security during complex emergencies: rapid assessment and institutional capabilities. *Med Global Survival*. 1994;1:156–163.

7. Macrai J, Zwi AB. Food as an instrument of war in contemporary African famines: a review of the evidence. *Disasters*. 1992;16:299–321.

8. Office of Foreign Disaster Assistance. *OFDA Annual Report FY 1992*. Washington, DC: US Agency for International Development; 1992:42.

9. Burkle FM. Complex, humanitarian emergencies, I: concepts and participants. *Prehospital Disaster Med*. 1995;10(1):36–42.

10. Gunn SWA. *Multilingual Dictionary of Disaster Medicine and International Relief*. Dordrecht, The Netherlands: Kluwer Academic Publishers; 1990:23–24.

11. Moore GR, Dembert ML. The military as a provider of public health services after a disaster. *Mil Med*. 1987;156:303–305.

12. Perrin P. Strategy for medical assistance in disaster situations. *Intl Rev Red Cross*. 1991;284:494–504.

13. Binder S, Sanderson LM. The role of the epidemiologist in natural disasters. *Ann Emerg Med*. 1987;16:1081–1084.

14. Lillibridge SR, Noji EK, Burkle FM. Disaster assessment: the emergency health evaluation of a population affected by a disaster. *Ann Emerg Med*. 1993;22:1715–1720.

15. Toole MJ. The rapid assessment of health problems in refuge and displaced populations. *Med Global Surveillance*. 1994;1:200–207.

16. Vis HL, Goyens P, Brasseur D. Rwanda: the case for research in developing countries. *Lancet*. 1994;344:957.

17. Waeckerle JF, Lillibridge SR, Burkle FM, Noji EK. Disaster medicine: challenges for today. *Ann Emerg Med*. 1994;23:715–718.

18. Toole MJ, Waldman RJ. Prevention of excess mortality in refugee and displaced populations in developing countries. *JAMA*. 1990;263:3296–3302.

19. Staes C, Orengo JC, Malilay J, Rullan J, Noji E. Deaths due to flash floods in Puerto Rico, January, 1992: implications for prevention. *Intl J Epidemiol.* 1994;23:968–975.

20. Glass RI, Urrutia JJ, Sibony S, et al. Earthquake injuries related to housing in a Guatemalan village. *Science.* 1977;207:734–738.

21. Glass RI, Craven RB, Bregman DJ, et al. Injuries from the Wichita Falls tornado: implications for prevention. *Science.* 1980;207:734–738.

22. Centers for Disease Control and Prevention. Famine-affected, refugee, and displaced populations: recommendations for public health issues. *MMWR.* 1992;41(RR-13):1–76.

23. Burkholder BT, Toole MJ. Evolution of complex disasters. *Lancet.* 1995;346:1012–1015.

24. Geiger HJ, Cook-Deegan RM. The role of physicians in conflicts and humanitarian crises. *JAMA.* 1993;270:616–620.

25. Burkle FM. Complex, humanitarian emergencies: medical liaison and training. *Prehospital Disaster Med.* 1995;10:43–47.

26. Sharp TW, Yip R, Malone JD. U.S. military forces and emergency international humanitarian assistance: observations and recommendations from three recent missions. *JAMA.* 1994;272:386–390.

27. United Nations High Commissioner for Refugees. *A UNHCR Handbook for the Military on Humanitarian Operations.* Geneva: United Nations High Commissioner for Refugees; 1994: 1.

28. National Research Council. *Confronting Natural Disasters: an International Decade for Natural Disaster Reduction.* Washington, DC: National Academy Press; 1987: 1–67.

29. United States Mission to the United Nations. *Global Humanitarian Emergencies, 1996.* New York: ECOSOC Section of the United States Mission to the United Nations; 1996.

30. International Federation of Red Cross and Red Crescent Societies. *World Disasters Report 1995.* The Netherlands: Martinus Nijhoff Publishers; 1995.

31. Sivard RL. *World Military and Social Expenditures 1993.* Washington, DC: World Priorities; 1993.

32. Fitzsimmons DW, Whiteside AW. *Conflict, War, and Public Health.* London: Research Institute for the Study of Conflict and Terrorism; 1994. Conflict Study 276.

33. Toole MJ. Mass population displacement: a global public health challenge. *Infect Dis Clinics North Am.* 1995;9:353–365.

34. Toole MJ, Waldman RJ. Refuges and displaced persons: war, hunger and public health. *JAMA.* 1993;270:600–605.

35. Koplan JP, Falk H, Green G. Public health issues from the Bhopal chemical disaster. *JAMA.* 1990;260:2795–2796.

36. Bertuzzi PA. Industrial disasters and epidemiology. *Scand J Work Environ Health.* 1989;15:85–100.

37. Sidel VW. Weapons of mass destruction: the greatest threat to public health. *JAMA.* 1989; 262:680–682.

38. Sidell FR. Chemical agent terrorism. *Ann Emerg Med.* 1996;28:223–224.

39. Mobley JA. Biological warfare in the twentieth century: lessons from the past, challenges for the future. *Mil Med.* 1995;160:547–553.

40. Aghababian RV, Teuscher J. Infectious diseases following major disasters. *Ann Emerg Med.* 1992;21:362–367.

41. de Ville de Goyet C, Lechat MF. Health aspects in natural disasters. *Trop Doct.* 1976;6:152–157.

42. Hlady WG, Quenemoen LE, Armenia-Cope RR, et al. Use of a modified cluster sampling method to perform rapid needs assessments after Hurricane Andrew. *Ann Emerg Med.* 1994;23:719–725.

43. Goma Epidemiology Group. Public health impact of Rwandan refugee crisis: what happened in Goma, Zaire, in July, 1994? *Lancet.* 1995;345:339–344.

44. Collins S. The need for adult therapeutic care in emergency feeding programs. *JAMA.* 1993;270:637–638.

45. Yip R, Sharp TW. Acute malnutrition and high childhood mortality related to diarrhea. *JAMA.* 1993;270:587–590.

46. Cobey JC, Flanagin A, Foege WH. Effective humanitarian aid: our only hope for intervention in civil war. *JAMA.* 1993;270:632–634.

47. Marfin AA, Moore J, Collins C, et al. Infectious disease surveillance during emergency relief to Bhutanese refugees in Nepal. *JAMA.* 1994;272:377–381.

48. Elias CJ, Alexander BH, Sokly T. Infectious disease control in a long term refugee camp: the role of epidemiologic surveillance and investigation. *Am J Public Health.* 1990;80:824–828.

49. Cuny F. From Disasters to Development. New York: Simon and Schuster; 1979.

50. Disaster epidemiology. *Lancet.* 1990;336:845–846.

51. Burkle FM. *Disaster Medicine.* New Hyde Park, NY: Medical Examination Publishing; 1984.

52. Roth PB, Gaffney JK. The Federal Response Plan and Disaster Medical Assistance Teams in domestic disasters. *Emerg Med Clinics North Am.* 1996;14:371–382.

53. Minear LM. The international relief system: a critical review. Presented at the Parallel National Intelligence Estimate on Global Humanitarian Emergencies; Washington, DC; September, 1994. Unpublished material presented in duplicated form by the Humanitarianism and War Project, Brown University.

54. US Agency for International Development. *Public Health Crisis Prevention, Mitigation, and Recovery: Linking Relief and Development.* Washington, DC: USAID; 1996. A report prepared for the US Agency for International Development. SARA Contract Task Order 263.

55. Weisbrodt D. Additional comments: humanitarian intervention and the erosion of national sovereignty. In: *Refugees in the 1990s: New Strategies for a Restless World.* Minneapolis: American Rescue Committee; 1993.

56. Manoncourt S, Doppler B, Enten F, et al. Public health consequences of the civil war in Somalia, April 1992. *Lancet.* 1992;340:176–177.

57. Toole MJ, Galson S, Brady W. Are war and public health compatible? *Lancet.* 1993;341:1193–1196.

58. Flanagin A. Somalia's death toll underlines challenges in post-cold war world. *JAMA.* 1992;268:1985–1987.

59. Shawcross W. *The Quality of Mercy.* New York: Simon and Schuster; 1984.

60. Centers for Disease Control and Prevention. Status of public health—Bosnia and Herzegovinia, August-September 1993. *MMWR.* 1993;42:973,979–983. Published errata: *MMWR.* 1994;43:110 and *MMWR.* 1994;43:450.

61. Mann J, Drucker E, Tarantola D, McCabe MP. Bosnia: the war against public health. *Med Global Survival.* 1994;1:130–146.

62. Perrin P. Personal communication, International Committee of the Red Cross, 1997.

63. Lee K, Collinson S, Walt G, Gilson L. Who should be doing what in international health: a confusion of mandates in the United Nations? *BMJ.* 1997;35:10–18.

64. Lillibridge SR, Burkle FM, Noji EK. Disaster mitigation and humanitarian assistance training for uniformed service medical personnel. *Mil Med.* 1994;159:397–403.

65. Perrin P. Training medical personnel: HELP and SOS course. *Intl Rev Red Cross.* 1994;284:505–512.

66. Cobey JC. Donation of unused surgical supplies: help or hindrance? *JAMA.* 1993;269:986–987.

67. de Ville de Goyet C. Post disaster relief: the supply management challenge. *Disasters.* 1993;17:169–171.

68. Lillibridge S. Disaster medicine: current assessment and blueprint for the future. *Acad Emerg Med.* 1995;Dec:1068–1076.

69. World Health Organization. *The Potential Role of New Cholera Vaccines in the Prevention and Control of Cholera Outbreaks during Acute Emergencies: Report of a Meeting.* Geneva: WHO; 13–14 Feb 1995.

70. Burkle FM, McGrady KAW, Newett SL, et al. Complex, humanitarian emergencies: measures of effectiveness. *Prehospital and Disaster Med.* 1995;10:48–56.

71. Strada G. The horror of land mines. *Sci Am.* 1996;274:40–45.

72. Stover E, McGrath R. *Land Mines in Cambodia—The Coward's War.* Boston: Physicians for Human Rights; 1991.

73. Ascherio A, Biellik R, Epstein A, et al. Deaths and injuries caused by landmines in Mozambique. *Lancet.* 1995; 346:721–724.

74. Coupland RM, Korver A. Injuries from antipersonnel mines: the experience of the International Committee of the Red Cross. *BMJ.* 1991;303:1509–1512.

75. International Committee of the Red Cross. *Blinding Weapons.* Geneva: ICRC; 1994.

76. Federal Bureau of Investigation. *Terrorism in the United States, 1994.* Washington, DC: FBI; 1995.

77. Laquer W. Postmodern terrorism. *Foreign Affairs.* 1996;75:24–36.

78. Yeskey K. Susceptibility to Terrorism. Presented at the First Harvard Symposium on the Medical Consequences of Terrorism. April 24–25, Boston.

79. Reproductive freedom for refugees. *Lancet.* 1993;341:929–930.

80. Swiss S, Giller JE. Rape as a crime of war—a medical perspective. *JAMA.* 1993;270:612–615.

81. Heise LL, Raikes A, Watts CH, Zwi AB. Violence against women: a neglected public health issue in less developed countries. *Soc Sci Med.* 1994;39:1165–1179.

82. Dowell SF, Toko A, Sita C, Piarroux R, Duerr A, Woodruff BA. Health and nutrition in centers for unaccompanied refugee children: experience from the 1994 Rwandan refugee crisis. *JAMA.* 1995 273:1802–1806.

83. United Nations Children's Fund. *The State of the World's Children.* New York: Oxford University Press; 1996.

84. United Nations Children's Fund. *Children in War: A Guide to the Provision of Services.* New York: Oxford University Press; 1992.

85. International Committee of the Red Cross. *The Geneva Conventions of August 12, 1949.* Geneva: ICRC; 1981.

86. International Committee of the Red Cross. *Protocols Additional to the Geneva Conventions of August 12, 1949.* Geneva: ICRC; 1977.

87. International Committee of the Red Cross. *International Humanitarian Law.* Geneva: ICRC; 1993.

88. Pan American Health Organization. *Supply Management Project in the Aftermath of Disasters: User's Manual.* Washington, DC: PAHO; 1994.

89. Malilay JM, Quenemoen LE. Applying a geographic information system to disaster epidemiologic research: Hurricane Andrew, Florida, 1992. In: *Proceedings of the 1993 Conference on Stimulation for Emergency Preparedness and Management.* Washington, DC, March 29–April 1, 1993.

90. Kramer JM, Cath A. Medical resources and the Internet: making the connection. *Arch Intern Med.* 1996;156:833–842.

91. Houtchens BA, Clemmer TP, Holloway HC, et al. Telemedicine and international disaster response. *Prehospital Disaster Med.* 1993;8:57–66.

92. Llewellyn C. The role of telemedicine in disaster medicine. *J Med Sys.* 1995;19:23–28.

93. Gaydos JC, Luz GA. Military participation in emergency humanitarian assistance. *Disasters.* 1994;18:48–57.

94. Sharp TW, Brennan RJ, Keim M, et al. Medical preparedness for a terrorist incident involving chemical and biological agents during the 1996 Atlanta Olympic Games. *Ann Emerg Med.* 1998;32:214–223.

95. Minear L, Weiss TG, Campbell KM. Humanitarianism and War: Lessons Learned from Recent Armed Conflicts. Providence, RI: Institute for International Studies, Brown University; 1991. Occasional Paper No. 8.

96. Weiss TG. A research note about military-civilian humanitarianism: more questions than answers. *Disasters* 1997;21(2):95–117.

97. Center for Naval Analysis. *Military Support to Complex Humanitarian Emergencies: From Practice to Policy.* Alexandria, Va: CNA; 1995. Proceedings of the Annual Conference, October 26–27, 1995.

98. *World Disasters Report, 1995: Humanitarians in Uniform?* Geneva: International Federation of Red Cross and Red Crescent Societies; 1995:60.

99. Seiple C. *The U.S. Military Relationship and the Civil Military Operations Center in Times of Humanitarian Intervention.* Carlisle, Penn: Peacekeeping Institute, US Army War College; 1996.

100. *Multi-Service Procedures for Humanitarian Assistance Operations.* Langley AFB: US Atlantic Command Sea–Air Application Center; 1994.

Chapter 42

MILITARY AND PUBLIC HEALTH ASPECTS OF NATURAL DISASTERS

JOSE L. SANCHEZ, MD, MPH and STEVE HOROSKO III, PhD

J.L. Sanchez, MD, MPH, Colonel, Medical Corps, US Army; Medical Epidemiologist and Military Chief, Department of Global Epidemiology and Threat Assessment, US Military HIV Research Program, 13 Taft Ct. Suite 200, Rockville, MD 20850; Formerly: Manager, Epidemiology Services Program, US Army Center for Health Promotion and Preventive Medicine, Aberdeen Proving Ground, MD 21010-5403

S. Horosko III, PHD, Lieutenant Colonel, Medical Service Corps, US Army; Preventive Medicine Staff Officer, Office of the Surgeon General, XVIII ABN Corps, Fort Bragg, NC 28310

INTRODUCTION

The involvement of the US military in providing disaster relief is an original intent of the Constitution and is defined in Titles 10 and 32 of the US Code.[1] Humanitarian disaster relief efforts date back to the pre–Civil War era, when Congress in 1847 approved the loan of naval vessels for transport of supplies to the victims of the Irish potato famine.[2] Army troops were subsequently used in the administration and maintenance of stockpiles of food, clothing, and tents during domestic relief operations. After the turn of the 20th century, the Army also assumed a role in the conduct of sanitation and vaccination programs in the United States and its territories.[2] Since 1972, the military has been actively involved in conducting medical, logistic, operational, and command and control functions during emergency humanitarian relief after major natural disasters. Examples include earthquakes

(Peru, 1970; Nicaragua, 1972; Guatemala, 1976), floods (Sudan, 1988; Venezuela, 1999), windstorms (Bangladesh, 1970, 1991; Sri Lanka, 1978; Florida, 1992, 1995; Hawaii, 1992; Central America 1998-1999), and volcanic eruptions (Philippines, 1990).[3,4]

Since the Persian Gulf War in 1991, the US military has deployed smaller contingents more frequently in peacekeeping operations and civilian assistance missions. For example, on a typical day in April 1996, as many as 41,000 US Army soldiers were deployed on temporary duty to as many as 59 separate locations in the United States and overseas in support of foreign humanitarian assistance missions.[5] Clearly, there is an ever-increasing need for military preventive medicine and other medical personnel to know about the specific needs that arise in domestic or international natural disaster relief operations.

MILITARY ROLE AND RESPONSIBILITIES

In the event of a natural disaster, the military may be tasked to provide assistance (Figure 42-1). In either a domestic or international scenario, military support to civil authorities is the responsibility of the Department of Defense, not the individual services. In international scenarios, the Department of State will request assistance through its coordinating agency, the Office of Foreign Disaster Assistance, which coordinates all military and civilian operations.[1] Military forces will be under the com-

a
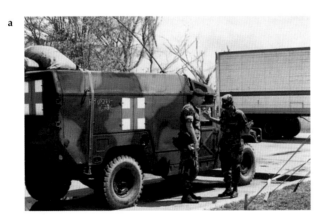

b
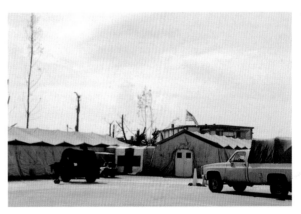

Fig. 42-1. The military is unique in its ability to get rapidly deployable medical systems to the site of a disaster quickly. After Hurricane Andrew struck southern Florida in August 1992, destroying hospitals and clinics as well as homes and schools, military units responded by moving needed medical infrastructure to the area. (**a**) This is a front line ambulance (FLA) that was driven to southern Florida by members of the 82nd Airborne Division, Fort Bragg, North Carolina. It transported victims to medical treatment facilities such as (**b**) this Air Force Air Transportable Hospital, which was set up close to the previously existing military hospital of Homestead Air Force Base. This transportable hospital was set up within a few days of Hurricane Andrew's landfall. US Army photographs.

mand of the Commander in Chief (CINC) responsible for the US military units' activities within that theater of operations. The CINC may establish a Joint Task Force (JTF) to provide the necessary response in the disaster area. The JTF Commander will have the responsibility, in turn, to deploy US forces to the area. The JTF Commander will rely on the JTF Surgeon to direct and coordinate the medical response. Routinely, all military preventive medicine (PVNTMED) assets will be subordinate to the JTF PVNTMED structure and will report to the JTF Surgeon. On occasion, however, PVNTMED personnel or teams will provide direct assistance to a civilian lead agency, usually local public health officials.

The JTF Surgeon will first focus on immediate lifesaving efforts and distribution of emergency resources through host-nation and international relief organizations, as well as through the host-nation's military. A Humanitarian Assistance Survey Team is normally deployed within 12 hours of the CINC's notification. The team's mission is to assess mortality, injury and illness, dislocation or displacement of persons, and disruption of governmental and national infrastructure. Within 48 to 72 hours, direct relief operations will start in the affected area. At the same time, a Civil–Military Operations Center directed by the US military will be established to provide security and humanitarian assistance in the field in coordination with the United Nations (UN), non-governmental and private volunteer organizations, and the local military.[1] See Chapter 45, The International Humanitarian Response System, for a further explanation of the roles of these organizations in disaster relief.

In the absence of a large-scale military PVNTMED deployment or when military PVNTMED professionals are involved in a disaster response only as consultants, the chain of command is not as clear. It is essential, however, that one individual, preferably the senior military officer present, coordinate the military response with the local government agency responsible for the relief effort.[6]

TYPES OF NATURAL DISASTERS

Disasters are catastrophic events that overwhelm a community's emergency response capability and threaten the public health and the environment.[7] Natural disasters are a major cause of premature death, impaired health status, and diminished quality of life.[8] It is estimated that between 1977 and the mid-1990s, 3 million people have been killed by natural disasters, 820 million others have been adversely affected, and property worth $25 billion to $100 billion has been damaged.[9,10] It was estimated that the US government spent an average of $1 billion per week in 1994 as a result of natural disasters.[11]

The natural disasters to be considered in this chapter can be subdivided into (*a*) climatological (ie, weather-related) disasters, such as windstorms, tornadoes, and floods (including associated landslides and avalanches), and (*b*) geophysical disasters, such as earthquakes, tsunamis, and volcanic eruptions (Table 42-1). These two types of disasters are generally of sudden onset and pose unforeseen, serious, and immediate threats to public health. Other disasters requiring external assistance but that are predictable and slowly developing in nature will not be considered here.[9,12] These include droughts, which are often associated with famine and desertification, and wildfires, which can sometimes be caused by natural forces such as lightning, extreme heat, earthquakes, or volcanic eruptions.

Windstorms

Windstorm-related events cause an average of 30,000 deaths and $2.3 billion in damages worldwide each year.[9] Severe tropical storms (called hurricanes if they are located in the Atlantic Ocean, Caribbean Sea, and eastern Pacific Ocean; typhoons in the western Pacific; and cyclones in the Indian Ocean), tornadoes, blizzards, and other storms affect man-made structures and agricultural areas in every country of the world (Figure 42-2). About 15% of the world's population is at risk from tropical storms. Tornadoes are notorious in the midsection of the United States, with some reaching wind speeds of 500 kph (300 mph). As many as 700 to 1,000 strike that area every year, causing an average of 80 deaths per year.[9,13]

Floods

Flooding, generally the result of torrential rains and other factors such as poor farming practices, deforestation, and urbanization, was responsible for more than 63% of the federally declared disasters in the United States from 1965 to 1985. Floods are the most commonly occurring natural disaster worldwide. In the United States alone they cause an average of 140 deaths per year. Their impact is long-term because of (*a*) damage to human settlements,

TABLE 42-1

MAJOR NATURAL DISASTERS AND ASSOCIATED MORTALITY

Type		Country (Yr)	No. of Deaths
Climatological			
	Windstorms	East Pakistan (1970)	300,000
		Bangladesh (1991)	140,000
		East Pakistan (1963–1965)*	10,000–30,000 ea
		India (1971)	10,000–25,000
		India (1977)	20,000
		Bangladesh (1988)	15,000
		Hong Kong (1906)	10,000
		USA—Galveston, Texas (1900)	> 6,000[†]
		USA—Florida; Louisiana (1992)	50[‡]
	Tornadoes	USA—Illinois; Indiana; Missouri (1925)	689
	Floods/Landslides	China (1887)	900,000
		China (1969)	> 50,000
		USA—9 Midwest states (1993)	50[§]
Geophysical			
	Earthquakes	China (1556)	830,000
		India (1737)	300,000
		China (1976)	240,000
		China (1920)	200,000
		Japan (1923)	143,000
		USSR (1948)	100,000
		Italy (1908)	75,000
		China (1932)	70,000
		Peru (1970)	70,000
		Iran (1990)	40,000
		Armenia (1988)	25,000
		Iran (1978)	25,000
		Guatemala (1976)	23,000
		USA—Anchorage, Alaska (1964)	131
		USA—Loma Prieta, California (1989)	62
		USA—Northridge, California (1994)	60[¶]
	Tsunamis	Indonesia (1883)	36,000
		Japan (1933, 1946, 1983, 1995)*	1,000–5,000 ea
	Volcanic eruptions	Martinique (1902)	38,000
		Colombia (1985)	25,000
		Sicily (1669)	20,000
		Guatemala (1902)	6,000
		Indonesia (1919)	5,200

*Four separate events are shown
[†]Deadliest natural disaster in US history
[‡]Costliest hurricane disaster, Hurricane Andrew, in US history ($32 billion)
[§]Costliest flood disaster in US history ($10 billion)
[¶]Costliest natural disaster in US history ($40 billion)
Data sources: (1) Sharp TW, Yip R, Malone JD. US military forces and emergency international humanitarian assistance: observations and recommendations from three recent missions. *JAMA.* 1994;272:386–390 (2) Sidel VW, Onel E, Jack Geiger H, Leaning J, Foege WH. Public health responses to natural and human-made disasters. In: Last JM, Wallace RB, eds. *Maxcy-Rosenau-Last Public Health and Preventive Medicine.* 13th ed. Norwalk, Conn: Appleton & Lange; 1992: 1173–1186 (3) National Research Council Advisory Committee on the International Decade for Natural Hazard Reduction Report. *Confronting Natural Disasters: An International Decade for Natural Hazard Reduction.* Washington, DC: National Academy Press; 1987: 1–60 (4) Lechat MF. Disasters and public health. *Bull World Health Organ.* 1979;57:11–17 (5) National Geographic Society. *Raging Forces: Earth in Upheaval.* Washington, DC: National Geographic Society; 1995 (6) Disasters. *The World Book Encyclopedia.* Chicago: World Book Inc.; 1988: D225.

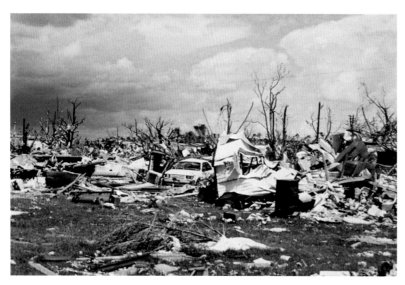

Fig. 42-2. Devastation of a mobile home park in southern Florida by Hurricane Andrew in August 1992. This level of destruction presented a range of problems to rescue workers, from navigating streets with no street signs or traffic lights to dealing with broken water and gas lines, downed electrical lines, and lots of debris. US Army photograph.

(*b*) forced evacuation or migration of large numbers of people, (*c*) damaged crops and food stocks, (*d*) erosion of large areas of land, and (*e*) loss of vital irrigation systems that have been washed away. The Mississippi River flood of 1993, the costliest flood disaster in US history, caused an estimated $10 billion in damages. Landslides, which often follow floods, cause an estimated $1 billion to $2 billion in economic losses and 25 to 50 deaths each year in the United States.[13]

Earthquakes and Tsunamis

Earthquakes have the potential for causing the greatest human losses of all natural disasters. Dangers associated with earthquakes include other phenomena, such as surface faulting, landslides, and tsunamis. Tsunamis are large ocean waves generated by the earth's motion occurring in the ocean's bottom, which cause damage by inundation, wave impact on structures, and coastal erosion. At least 35 countries, mostly located in the Pacific region's "Rim of Fire," face a high probability of earthquakes or tsunamis. Scientists estimate that there are some 500,000 detectable quakes worldwide each year. Of these, 1,000 are capable of causing significant damage. The extent of damage depends on three main factors: the quake's magnitude, its proximity to populated urban areas, and the population's degree of preparation.[13]

Volcanic Eruptions

Volcanic eruptions have killed more than 266,000 people in the past 400 years.[9] There are, on average, 50 volcanoes erupting above sea level each year.[13] Eruptions have immediate catastrophic effects through ash falls, surges of lethal gas, blasts, mudflows (also known as lahars), and lava flows. Fatalities occur in approximately 5% of all eruptions. Very large eruptions can also cause worldwide climatic changes and agricultural disruption, as was illustrated by the eruptions of Mount St. Helens in Washington State (1980) and Mount Pinatubo in the Philippines (1991).

IMPACT OF DISASTER PREPAREDNESS PLANS

Early warning systems allow the population to prepare, especially in cases of windstorms and tsunamis. It is important that early warning systems be in place to foster early evacuation and proper sheltering of communities threatened by these types of disasters. The timing of the warning is all-important; the earlier the notification, the more effectively the evacuation can be conducted, even if this means false alarms are given. The development of Doppler radar technology in the 1980s has helped tremendously in preventing problems associated with windstorms in the United States and the Caribbean region.[12] An adequate predisaster preparedness plan, such as the one in California, has limited the mortality of recent earthquakes in Loma Prieta (1989, 62 deaths) and Northridge (1994, 60 deaths).[14] Also reasons for decreased mortality and morbidity in the United States after natural disasters are the availability of pre-determined evacuation routes, a National Disaster Medical System (see Chapter 46,

Domestic Disaster Response: FEMA and Other Governmental Organizations) for medical regulating of casualties, and government and private agencies with dedicated resources for disaster relief, facilitated by the Disaster Relief Act of 1974.[9] There is no question that vital preparedness programs and public awareness in the United States have been major fac-

tors in reducing mortality rates after natural disasters since 1982.[15] Similarly, the countries of Latin America and the Caribbean (with assistance from the Pan American Health Organization) have also developed health preparedness plans and training that have greatly improved the response to natural disasters in the region.

SURVEILLANCE

A basic knowledge of the types of illnesses and injuries caused by natural disasters is essential to determine appropriate relief resources on-site, such as supplies, equipment, and personnel.[16,17] A knowledge of the phases of a disaster is also useful. Disasters have three phases: the impact phase, which includes 2 to 3 days after the event; the relief phase, which is an indeterminate amount of time when active relief activities are ongoing; and the rehabilitation phase, during which life and disease rates start to return to normal. Epidemiologic surveillance is the tool used to evaluate the distribution and determinants of disaster-related deaths, illnesses, and injuries in the population affected. Surveillance efforts also tend to separate into three types: (1) immediate ("quick and dirty") assessment, (2) short-term assessment, and (3) ongoing medical surveillance (Table 42-2). An explanation of each follows.

Immediate Assessment

This "quick and dirty" type of surveillance involves the rapid collection of information immediately after (within 2 to 3 days) the impact phase of a disaster to help define the geographic extent of the disaster, the major problems occurring before and immediately after the disaster, and the number of people affected. In this initial survey, quantifiable but not highly technical information is collected by the military PVNTMED health officer in charge. An aerial survey by helicopter is an ideal means of obtaining part of this information. Census data can be obtained from local health and disaster assistance centers. This will provide a rough estimate of the population living in the disaster-stricken area—the denominator or population at risk. The measurement of total and age-specific mortality is useful to quickly evaluate the severity of the impact phase of a disaster.[12] Hospitals, clinics, and morgues may be able to provide estimates of numbers and types of known deaths and injuries that have occurred within 2 to 3 days after the event.[8,19] Background, or baseline, data can be collected from reporting

medical treatment facilities (MTFs) and practitioners in the area to help define disease and injury patterns existent before the disaster.[19]

Monitoring patterns of visits to health care sites after a disaster is a vital part of surveillance. The number of deaths or injuries usually peaks in the first 3 to 4 days, which is the impact phase. Morbidity usually returns to baseline after 1 to 2 weeks during the relief phase (more quickly for earthquakes, more slowly for other natural disasters). The medical needs after the impact phase is over are related to normal, baseline medical conditions and emergencies, not to disaster-associated trauma. Except in the case of earthquakes, the number of disaster casualties requiring medical attention immediately after the impact is usually low in relation to the number of deaths.[12] Major earthquakes can produce a very high number of deaths compared to the number of injuries (ie, a high disease-to-injury ratio) during the impact phase. The evaluation of the need to deploy field emergency MTFs or mobile surgical hospitals by the military has to be done immediately after impact, based on initial estimates of morbidity, because these facilities are of less practical use later, during the relief phase.

Short-term Assessments

This type of surveillance involves a more systematic and detailed method of collecting data and should result in more reliable and refined estimates of damages, condition of shelters and health care facilities, water and food supply, and nutritional status of the affected population. The measurement of total, age-specific, and cause-specific morbidity rates, as well as the death-to-injury ratio, are more reliable parameters to evaluate the postimpact severity and are significant in the planning of the need for relief supplies, personnel, and equipment. Other health-related outcomes that are useful for planning include the bed occupancy rate, the area-specific injury rates, the proportional morbidity rate (ie, percentage of visits for each cause), and the average duration of stay in the hospital.[12,15,20,21] It is

TABLE 42-2

EPIDEMIOLOGIC METHODS USED IN THE ASSESSMENT OF NATURAL DISASTERS

Type of Method	Characteristics

1. Immediate Assessment	Is rapid, superficial, "quick and dirty" (look and listen)
	Is conducted preferably within 2 to 3 d of impact
	Defines geographical extent of disaster
	Defines major health problems encountered (deaths and injuries)
	Estimates number of people affected (denominator)
	Assesses roughly
	   - availability of shelter facilities
	   - access to potable water
	   - current level of sanitation
	   - status of health care infrastructure
	   - level of communications network
	   - status of transportation systems

2. Short-term Assessment	Uses more systematic and detailed methods (surveys, questionnaires)
	Is conducted within the first week after impact, then every 1 to 2 wks as necessary
	Uses cluster, modified cluster, or random sampling methods
	Determines number of deaths and injuries by age and sex
	Assesses in a more complete fashion
	   - damage to buildings, public utilities, roads, transport, and communication systems
	   - condition of shelters, schools, public buildings, and health facilities
	   - condition of water and food supply
	   - type and number of medical personnel, equipment, and supplies in area
	   - nutritional status of affected population

3. Ongoing Medical Surveillance	Is longer-term monitoring of disaster-associated problems Starts as soon as possible after impact Is run by local workers at each site Monitors daily the visits to health care facilities categorized by age, sex, location, and diagnostic or symptom group Daily monitoring of number of beds available and deaths Is established early at MTFs, DMATs, shelters, tent cities, camps, food distribution centers, and daycare centers Serves as excellent source of reports or rumors of problems that may need to be investigated Allows analysis of data for critical evaluation of relief efforts and cost-effectiveness of emergency response measures

MTF: medical treatment facility
DMAT: disaster medical assistance team

important to remember, however, that for these health outcomes to be evaluated appropriately, comparisons have to be made with baseline (ie, predisaster) experiences.

This assessment preferably should be conducted by mobile teams of 2 to 3 people who sample the disaster-stricken area by dividing it into discrete clusters and survey a sample of homes within each cluster.[22,23] Teams from the Centers for Disease Con-

trol conducted rapid health assessments, in a good example of this approach, immediately after Hurricane Andrew in southern Florida and Louisiana.[23] The information requested in these surveys should be as brief and concise as possible. These assessments may take only a few hours to administer and collect or they may take a few days. The data should be compared with predisaster, baseline data and the results summarized in a report to be sent to either the JTF Surgeon or the local government agencies responsible for the relief effort or to both.

Ongoing Medical Surveillance

The basic principles of epidemiologic surveillance after disasters are no different from those applied in other settings.[16,24] Ongoing medical disaster surveillance is directed at monitoring disaster-associated problems and determining the effects that relief activities have on these problems. It should start as soon as possible after impact and concurrently with emergency care of casualties. It should continue throughout the relief and rehabilitation phases. The initial setup of this early warning system to detect outbreaks of infection or diseases or an increase in certain types of injuries is of fundamental importance. An active surveillance system, consisting of in-depth monitoring of selected conditions at existing MTFs by mobile, field-deployed, military medical teams, will be necessary. Ideally this would involve assessment teams that are familiar with the particular types of disaster areas affected, as well as local customs. Ideally, assessment teams should be available on stand-by in risk areas or disaster-prone countries where the US military has a presence. In practice, however, this effort will usually be limited to the use of selected, local workers at each MTF and other reporting sites (eg, shelters, tent cities, camps, food distribution centers, daycare centers) and disaster medical assistance teams who will monitor conditions of interest.

EPIDEMIOLOGIC ASSESSMENT TEAMS

The concept of a deployable epidemiologic assessment team was pioneered in the early 1980s at the Walter Reed Army Institute of Research in Washington, DC, and repeatedly tested during peacetime deployments throughout the world. Quickly fielding an epidemiologic assessment team with initial medical assets and under the direct control of the JTF Surgeon is an absolute necessity. Military health experts who should participate as part of this assessment team include: (*a*) public health physicians, (*b*) epidemiologists, (*c*) emergency or family practice physicians, (*d*) community or public health nurses, (*e*) environmental health, sanitary engineering, or entomology officers, (*f*) public health technicians, and (*g*) data entry clerks. Additional consultants from nongovernmental organizations, private volunteer organizations, the Pan American Health Organization, the World Health Organization, the UN Children's Fund, the Centers for Disease Control and Prevention, or the country affected should also be included as necessary.

Some basic information must be obtained immediately after arriving in the area. Maps of the affected area will be necessary, preferably showing streets, airports, and MTFs. The location of tent cities, camps, schools, clinics, hospitals, military medical units, disaster medical assistance teams, and civilian relief agencies need to be plotted and posted for easy access by team members at all times. Lists, including phone numbers, of all involved agencies should be obtained as early as possible and a compendium of points of contact in each location should be made for the use of team members and other JTF medical and logistics personnel. Checking this information with the JTF operations section ensures completeness and accuracy.

Certain methods should be followed to help ensure the reliability and timeliness of the data gathered. The disaster area should be divided into blocks or segments. Population centers (eg, tent cities, camps, shelters) should be emphasized first in the start-up of surveillance efforts. Data should be collected using simple, preformatted, standardized forms. A list of symptom and diagnostic categories should be created a priori, and data should include total numbers in each of these categories by age groups, sex, and reporting location. It is also important to be able to separate medical visits by civilians from those by military personnel. Samples of reporting forms can be found in the surveillance chapter of this textbook (Chapter 31, Disease and Nonbattle Injury Surveillance Outcome Measure for Force Health Protection). Initially, monitoring should be done daily; it should encompass facilities such as clinics, hospitals, tent cities, camps, shelters, disaster medical assistance teams, food distribution centers, daycare centers, and all military MTFs in the area. After 2 to 3 weeks, frequency of reporting can be decreased to two to three times per week, eventually decreasing to a standard of no less than once a week on return to baseline conditions, which usually occurs during the rehabilitation phase. The transition of medical surveillance responsibilities from the military to the local civilian health authorities should be done in a step-by-step fashion, preferably with an overlap of 1 to 2 weeks.

DISEASE CONTROL

Communicable Diseases

Risk

The risk of communicable disease outbreaks after natural disasters is very low. Epidemics are likely only if a new pathogenic agent is introduced, transmission of preexisting pathogens is increased, or susceptibility of the population is increased.[25] The introduction of new pathogens after a natural disaster is a rare occurrence.

Increased transmission or susceptibility can occur because of several factors. These include (*a*) malnutrition (as in the case of measles outbreaks in refugee populations),[26] (*b*) massive population movements, which cause increases in crowding and concomitant increased risk of infection with respiratory pathogens by person-to-person transmission (eg, meningitis, tuberculosis, viral respiratory pathogens), and (*c*) deterioration of environmental and personal hygiene, causing increased risk of waterborne and foodborne diseases (eg, cholera, shigellosis, hepatitis).[27–29] Additionally, the increased breeding of disease vectors can cause outbreaks of vector-borne diseases such as malaria (eg, Haiti, 1963[30]; Guayas River Basin, Colombia, 1982-1985[31]). The contamination and breakdown of the potable water supply can lead to outbreaks of typhoid fever (Puerto Rico, 1956[32]; Mauritius, 1980[32]), balantidiasis (Truk District, Trust Territories of the Pacific, 1971[32]), hepatitis (Dominican Republic, 1979[33]), and giardiasis (Utah; 1983[34]; Washington State, 1980[35]). Lastly, increased contact with water and contamination of water sources with human or animal waste and waterborne pathogens, such as leptospira and hepatitis E, often occurs following floods (Portugal, 1967[36]; Brazil, 1975[32,37]; Nicaragua, 1995[38,39]; Vietnam, 1994[40]; Nepal, 1995[41]; Puerto Rico, 1996[42]).

There is a higher probability of waterborne epidemics after floods and windstorms than other natural disasters because of contamination of surface water by run-off and contamination of piped water supplies by cross-connections (typhoid fever and diarrheal diseases early, hepatitis A and E later). Also, because of direct contact with accumulated surface water, leptospirosis and skin infections could represent a problem in endemic areas. The potential for increased vector breeding and vector contact because of destruction of housing in windstorms and floods can result in epidemics of dengue (within 2 to 4 weeks) and malaria (within a few months). There can be a higher risk for acute respiratory illnesses, measles, and gastrointestinal illnesses in shelters, tent cities, daycare centers, feeding centers, and refugee camps because of overcrowding, lower levels of sanitation, and possible importation of endemic diseases into these locations. Finally, recent global climatic changes are beginning to exert a role in the acceleration and resurfacing of infectious diseases following major natural disasters.[43]

Control

Attempts to control communicable diseases should focus principally on improving personal and environmental hygiene and providing clean food and water. Other preventive measures of secondary importance include chemoprophylaxis, vaccination, early treatment of infectious patients, and isolation of infectious patients. Massive immunization campaigns, although sometimes popular with political authorities and the public, are often of only short-term benefit and should be undertaken only on the basis of sound epidemiologic evidence.[33] Examples of vaccinations that may be indicated include: (*a*) measles vaccine in crowded camps and refugee populations at risk, (*b*) meningococcal meningitis and typhoid fever vaccines for early control of outbreaks in specific populations at high risk, (*c*) tetanus toxoid for minor trauma victims, and (*d*) rabies diploid cell (inactivated) vaccine for animal bite victims in areas with ongoing rabies transmission. The use of any of the oral cholera vaccines, although debatable, may be considered during acute emergencies, such as natural disasters and refugee crises, or before impending cholera outbreaks in populations at risk.[44,45] Giving chemoprophylaxis to close contacts may be advisable during epidemics of meningococcal meningitis, cholera, or shigellosis. Chemoprophylaxis may also be indicated for high-risk groups in areas with significant threats of leptospirosis (eg, during or immediately following floods) or malaria (eg, following an influx of refugees from endemic areas). The most important element for the control of communicable diseases after natural disasters, however, is the establishment of effective surveillance.

Malnutrition

Another major disaster-related problem, especially in developing countries, is malnutrition (see

Chapter 47, Nutritional Assessment and Nutritional Needs of Refugees or Displaced Populations). Malnutrition affects populations in many ways, principally by direct effects on the population's level of immunity and fertility potential.[12] It also causes higher rates of morbidity and mortality from diseases such as measles, acute respiratory infections, tuberculosis, and diarrheal diseases, especially in the very young (under 4 years old), nonimmune, susceptible age groups.[46] The military can play a major role in securing transport and availability of food supplies, especially to remote, rural areas, as was the case during Operation Restore Hope in Somalia (1992–1993).[3] The role of malnutrition is especially important when addressing refugee or displaced populations and superimposed disasters, such as acute diarrheal disease following Bangladesh cyclones or measles, cholera, and shigella following droughts in Ethiopia and Somalia. It is in these situations that provision of potable water, adequate nutritional supplementation, and vaccines is especially crucial. These measures are the most effective ones in reducing mortality among disaster victims, especially young children.[46,47]

Psychological Effects

The mental health effects of disasters can be significant, especially in urban areas and during civil unrest or war. Psychological symptoms common during the immediate postdisaster period include intrusive thoughts, emotional numbness, difficulty concentrating, anxiety episodes, depression, and, in some cases, shock syndrome.[48] In most cases, the majority of people quickly adapt. Sociological studies[49] in the postdisaster period document that within 30 minutes of a major disaster, up to 75% of healthy survivors will be engaged in rescue activities. Affected populations have also proved remarkably effective at rapidly reestablishing the basic microenvironment in which they can survive. For example, after the 1976 earthquake in Guatemala, as many as 50,000 families had relocated to improvised dwellings within the first 24 hours.[50] Delayed, long-term effects, such as posttraumatic stress disorder syndrome, are directly related to the intensity of the event (eg, loss of life, destruction of property) and are more common in females and in those without access to social support systems, such as relatives and close friends.[51,52]

Quick adaptive response and low-level violent behavior by the affected persons are the norm after most natural disasters. Previous "disaster experience" has been shown to be of greater value than any other human factor in decreasing the risk of adverse mental events, as well as death or injury, during a natural disaster.[53] This is nowhere more evident than in the populations of the US Virgin Islands and Puerto Rico, who are frequently exposed to the threat of hurricanes. In addition, social support systems have been found to be more important than the actual magnitude or severity of the event in helping the individual cope with the situation.[54]

The loss of life or property can cause a significant amount of stress in relief workers already overburdened by disaster-associated job responsibilities. Role conflicts and acute stress reactions are more likely to occur in these workers.[55] Losses after the main disaster (eg, loss of loved ones) can precipitate mental crises in already stressed disaster workers and victims.

Neuropsychiatric casualties will require specialized triage and both psychological stress intervention and long-term support.[56] Emergency mental health services should be delivered and supervised by practitioners in the field as soon and as far forward as possible. This is analogous to the military's forward treatment and return-to-duty concept of combat stress management. This task is best managed by mental health intervention (also known as combat stress control or CSC) teams, a number of which are a part of major deployable military medical units.[57]

Long-term Illnesses

Available, but limited, data collected among disaster-affected populations in developed countries seem to point to certain associations with long-term morbidity and mortality following major disasters. Significant increases in mortality from all causes and from malignant diseases, as well as an increase in reporting of surgical conditions and hospitalizations, was noted in a study of flood victims in Bristol, England, in 1968.[58] Similarly, Melick[59] and Logue[60] conducted two long-term follow-up studies in the Wyoming Valley in Pennsylvania from 1975 to 1977 after the floods caused by Hurricane Agnes (1972) and found more health problems were reported among flood victims and their close relatives than unaffected people. Flood victims also experienced more stress from major life events after the floods. A 35% increase in rates of leukemia, lymphoma, and spontaneous abortion, beginning about 2 years after the floods, was also noted in the river valley areas of southern New York State that were affected by the flooding caused by

Hurricane Agnes.[61] There also is some evidence in the literature to support a disaster–stress association with cancer.[21] Recently, the mortality of residents on Kauai, Hawaii, was examined after Hurricane Iniki struck in September 1992; the overall mortality rate during the 12-month period after Iniki was found to be elevated, especially the rate of deaths related to diabetes mellitus.[62] The extent and types of long-term or chronic illnesses seen after a natural disaster can vary, however, and accurate generalizations to developing countries cannot be made.

DEATH AND INJURY

Patterns and Mechanisms

The degree to which disasters, regardless of their location, cause death and injury varies within and between disaster types; the predominant causes of death and injury will also depend on the region or country where the disaster occurs.[63] The main distinction is between earthquakes, which frequently cause large numbers of deaths and severe injuries, and other types of disasters (Table 42-3). Earthquakes generally cause deaths through the collapse of dwellings and other structures, as well as by secondary fires. They tend to cause more serious problems when they happen at night because sleeping people become trapped inside their homes, especially those people occupying upper floors of apartment buildings.[64,65] Injuries tend to be orthopedic in nature; "crush syndrome" has been reported after many earthquakes.[66] Death-to-injury ratios have ranged from a low of 1:3 to 1:4 (Guatemala, 1976[67]; Italy, 1980[68]) to as high as 3:1 (Armenia, 1988[69]).

Tsunamis, floods, and landslides may cause large numbers of deaths, especially in urban, coastal areas and in areas where large segments of the population live around major rivers, such as the Yellow River in China (see Table 42-1). Usually there are deaths but few, if any, severe injuries after these events. For example, the great storm surge that struck East

TABLE 42-3

HEALTH AND ENVIRONMENTAL EFFECTS OF NATURAL DISASTERS

	Earthquakes	Volcanoes	Tsunamis	Floods	Hurricanes	Tornadoes
Deaths	Few-Many*	Few-Many	Many	Few	Few-Many†	Few
Injuries						
Severe	Many*	Few-Many	Few	Few	Few†	Few
Mild	Many	Few	Few	Few	Many	Few-Many‡
Outbreak risk	Minimal	Minimal	Minimal	Moderate§	Moderate§	Minimal
Damage	Great*	Great	Great	Variable	Great†	Great
Food scarcity	Rare	Variable	Common	Common	Rare	Rare
Migration	Rare¶	Common	Common	Common	Rare	Rare

*Depending on pre-earthquake existence of a seismic building code and intensity
†Depending on location (ie, greater in coastal urban areas) and storm intensity
‡Depending on tornado path, pre-impact warning, and type of housing
§Risk of direct contact waterborne diseases (leptospirosis, skin infections) and diarrheal illnesses in first 2 weeks, vector-borne illnesses and hepatitis A and E afterwards; increased risk of person-to-person transmission in overcrowded settings
¶Significant population movements to marginal zones may occur in heavily damaged urban areas (eg, Nicaragua, 1972)
Sources: (1) Sidel VW, Onel E, Jack Geiger H, Leaning J, Foege WH. Public health responses to natural and human-made disasters. In: Last JM, Wallace RB, eds. *Maxcy-Rosenau-Last Public Health and Preventive Medicine*. 13th ed. Norwalk, Conn: Appleton & Lange; 1992:1173–1186 (2) Blake PA. Communicable disease control. In: Gregg MB, ed. *The Public Health Consequences of Disasters*. Atlanta: Centers for Disease Control; 1989: 7–12. (3) Pan American Health Organization. *A Guide to Emergency Health Management after Natural Disaster*. Washington, DC: PAHO; 1981. Emergency Preparedness and Disaster Relief Coordination Program Scientific Publication No. 407 (4) Llewellyn CH. Public health and sanitation during disasters. In: Burkle FM, Sanner PH, Wolcott BW, eds. *Disaster Medicine: Application for the Immediate Management and Triage of Civilian and Military Disaster Victims*. New York: Medical Examination Publishing; 1984: 132–161 (5) Western K. *The Epidemiology of Natural and Man-made Disasters: the Present State of the Art*. London: London School of Hygiene and Tropical Medicine, University of London; 1972. Dissertation.

Pakistan (now Bangladesh) in 1970 killed an estimated 300,000 people, approximately 20% of the population in affected areas. Injuries, however, were largely limited to cuts and bruises.[70] An individual who is caught by the flooding waters drowns; one who is not, survives, usually uninjured.

Windstorms cause deaths and injuries in developed countries, but, unlike in developing countries, rarely on a large scale. The wind is not the biggest killer; more important is the flooding due to the storm surge that usually accompanies a windstorm, especially in coastal areas of developing countries where there is no adequate warning system in place. The East Pakistan cyclone of 1970 is an example.[71] This phenomenon is also illustrated by Hurricanes Hugo (1989), Andrew (1992), Marilyn (1995), and Opal (1995), which affected Puerto Rico, the Bahamas, and southeastern United States. Although only 128 deaths were reported in those four hurricanes (41, 50, 10, and 27, respectively), hundreds of injuries, especially minor cuts and bruises during the relief phase, were reported.[20,72–76] Most of the deaths were preventable, occurred during the impact phase, and were mainly due to drowning, electrocution, and asphyxiation and burns from home fires. In some cases, the incidence of heart attacks has also increased after major hurricanes and is mainly attributed to physical exertion of older people during the clean-up process.[74–76]

Like other windstorms, tornadoes cause deaths and injuries in modest numbers when compared with earthquakes. The leading causes of death during tornadoes are craniocerebral trauma and crushing wounds of the chest and trunk.[77,78] These are most often caused by high-speed, flying debris.

Fractures are the most common type of nonfatal injury, involving mostly the lower extremities (35%), head (25%), upper extremities (16%), and thorax, vertebrae, and pelvis (8% each). Contusions, lacerations, and other soft-tissue injuries are also frequent, with a subsequent increased risk of secondary sepsis complications from wound contamination.[78,79]

Human and Socioeconomic Factors

The very young and the very old are at increased risk of death and injury during earthquakes and flash floods.[12] In East Pakistan in 1970, those younger than 4 years and older than 60 years who could not escape the flooding were at increased risk.[70] Likewise, during the Guatemalan earthquake in 1976, the death rates in the 5- to 9-year-old age group and the over-60 age group were found to be higher, suggesting that they got trapped inside collapsed brick and adobe homes. It appears also that parents took preferential care of the very young and more defenseless children.[80] For some disasters, such as tornadoes,[81] floods, and cyclones,[70] females have been found to be at increased risk. By comparison, males tend to be at increased risk of minor injuries during the clean-up period (Figure 42-3).

Socioeconomic level appears to be inversely related to risk; the poorest and least educated are the worst prepared for the disaster before impact and have less access to medical care after impact. This is especially true in rural areas. Other special high-risk groups include alcoholics, physically and mentally disabled persons, and older persons with chronic medical conditions. Studies of victim behavior during floods have suggested an association between alcohol con-

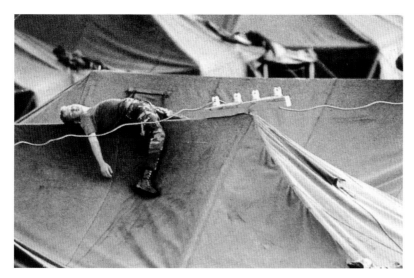

Fig. 42-3. In this photograph, Marines are putting up tents and stringing electrical wire as part of the military's response to Hurricane Andrew in southern Florida in August 1992. The need of the community was so great that military rapid-response personnel worked long hours at physically demanding jobs. This exhausted Marine fell asleep on top of a tent he had just helped to erect and next to a high voltage electrical wire. Risk of injury for rescue personnel, especially those doing heavy manual labor, is serious and often discounted in the push to alleviate the suffering of victims of a disaster. US Army photograph.

sumption and mortality.[82] Other studies of tornado victims have indicated that older people are less likely to heed evacuation warnings.[81,83]

Physical, Environmental, and Geographic Factors

Improper building techniques, the introduction of newer, cheaper building materials (such as concrete), and the inappropriate use of these materials in construction have resulted in high mortality rates after earthquakes in certain areas of the world (eg, Mexico City, 1985; Armenia, 1988). In certain areas, such as Iran, eastern Turkey, and Central America, the practice of building unframed rock and earth houses and the use of insufficiently reinforced adobe walls has resulted in high casualty rates.[15,49,80] By comparison, more strict seismic building codes in California have resulted in significantly lower mortality rates.[14] The construction of elevated shelters and physical barriers in flood- and cyclone-prone areas has been recently proven to be very effective in reducing morbidity and mortality in areas such as Bangladesh[53] and Japan.[9]

Perhaps the best example of government involvement in the prevention of disaster casualties can be found in Japan and its implementation of disaster-mitigation measures for typhoons, tsunamis, floods, and landslides in 1958. There was a consequent marked reduction in mortality and property damage (pre-1958 vs. post-1958).[9] Another example of the positive effect of disaster-mitigation measures, such as improved building codes, can be seen in southern Florida. Although Hurricane Andrew was one of the strongest recorded hurricanes to make landfall in the United States, only 50 deaths were attributed to that storm.[14]

There is an increased risk of serious or fatal injuries for people inside vehicles during flash floods and tornadoes.[81,84] Conversely, there is a documented decreased risk of injury during tornadoes for people inside buildings, especially in basements.[81,83] The intensity and duration of the disaster is directly related to the amount of damage; location of the disaster is also important as higher damage is sustained in populated, urban, and coastal areas.

ENVIRONMENTAL HEALTH

Preventive medicine plays a key role in the relief effort, as natural disasters can disrupt the ecological balance and so cause outbreaks of disease. Measures to ensure needed sanitation and pest management must be planned before and implemented as soon as possible after the occurrence of a disaster. Organizational and educational efforts and other public health measures to help victims avoid disease outbreaks are important aspects of preventive medicine support.

Natural disasters cause considerable deterioration of environmental conditions. Disruption of environmental health services commonly occurs, particularly in services such as potable water and waste disposal systems. When waste disposal systems are disrupted and general sanitation levels decrease, the contamination of food and water supplies and the proliferation of insect and rodent pests increase the risk of disease.

The sudden creation of areas of high population density, such as camps for displaced persons, causes additional public health concerns. The lack of proper shelter, water, soap, detergent, and basic cleaning and washing facilities makes it difficult to maintain usual standards of personal hygiene and often results in outbreaks of diarrheal disease and vector-borne diseases in areas where they were prevalent before the disaster.[17,30–32,34,35]

Initial Environmental Health Assessment

During the immediate impact phase, there are five major environmental health issues that need to be addressed promptly: safe drinking water, shelter, human waste disposal, personal hygiene, and vector-borne disease avoidance.[17,85] The specific objective of emergency measures is to restore environmental health conditions and services to whatever levels existed before the disaster occurred, regardless of judgments about predisaster quality.[17] It is counterproductive to solve chronic problems by giving sophisticated aid that the local government cannot sustain. If the local professionals and facilities are unable to continue a procedure after relief organizations withdraw, that procedure should probably not be started.

To assist in solving these problems, a PVNTMED team should be deployed to the disaster area as soon as possible after military assistance has been requested. Areas of expertise on this team should include epidemiology and public health, entomology, environmental health, sanitary engineering, veterinary medicine, civil affairs, and occupational health and toxicology.

The US Army, Navy, and Air Force all deploy specialized units or teams to provide preventive medicine support to contingency operations. Army PVNTMED detachments provide preventive medicine support and consultation in the areas of entomology, field sanitation, sanitary engineering, and epidemiology.[18] The Navy forms contingency preventive medicine or vector control teams from supporting Navy Disease Vector Ecology and Control Centers and Navy Environmental and Preventive Medicine Units. These teams become part of the Mobile Medical Augmentation Readiness Team and are tailored to the needs of each contingency operation. The mission and capabilities of these teams are similar to those of the Army units described above. The US Air Force support for contingency operations may be provided by Prime BEEF (Base Engineer Emergency Force). Capabilities of this team include field sanitation and hygiene, general pest management, and specialized aerial pesticide spraying.

Water

Sources and Storage

The first priority in a disaster-stricken area is to ensure an adequate supply of drinking water, followed by water for personal hygiene. During the initial on-site assessment, all potential local sources of potable water need to be investigated. The assistance of local authorities in this assessment is very important, as is the advice of a sanitary engineer or water system specialist familiar with the host country conditions. Daily water supply requirements for relief operations (eg, temporary shelters and camps), is 15 to 20 L per person for eating and drinking purposes.[17,19,86] Greater amounts are required in field hospitals and mass feeding centers.

Drinking water should be obtained from operational water distribution systems, if possible, and from undamaged private sources (eg, breweries, dairies, wells).[17] These same private sources can also be contacted for the use of their trucks to transport bulk volumes to refugee camps or centers. Tanks used for storing and transporting drinking water must be free of and protected against contamination. Gasoline, chemical, or sewage trucks or containers should not be adapted to hold drinking water. All water sources and water produced from existing facilities should be tested by PVNTMED personnel before use. Bulk water treatment and distribution is a quartermaster responsibility. PVNTMED personnel should assist in selecting sources of water and establishing water points.

They should also advise both the quartermaster and the engineer groups and perform water quality assessment functions.

Multi-liter containers should be provided to store and distribute water. These containers should be easily transportable and have a means to prevent recontamination during storage. A study in Bolivia, for example, demonstrated that 20-L plastic containers with screw-top lids and a spigot were ideal for preventing recontamination of treated water.[87] Similar containers were also used successfully during Operation Uphold Democracy (1994–1995) relief efforts in Haiti.

Disinfection

Residual concentration of chlorine in the water distribution system should be increased after a disaster. For drinking water under normal field conditions, the US military requires a chlorine residual of 5 ppm (5 mg/L) after a 30-minute contact time.[88] Under emergency conditions, the JTF Surgeon or senior medical authority may authorize reduced chlorine residuals and decide which water quality standards apply: the Department of Defense's, the World Health Organization's, or some other agency's. In a disaster situation, a large quantity of reasonably safe water may be preferable to a smaller amount of very pure water. Water quality standards vary; the Pan American Health Organization recommends at least a 1 ppm residual after 30 minutes.[17] The United Nations High Commissioner for Refugees recommends a minimum of 0.2 ppm residual.[89] The rationale is that if the chlorine content of water is much above 0.5 ppm, people may prefer drinking untreated water. One way to avoid over-chlorinating drinking water is to check that the water is free of a chlorine residual before starting chlorination efforts. PVNTMED personnel should check public water supplies daily to ensure an adequate chlorine residual is maintained.

If water supplies in the disaster area are not being chlorinated because chlorination systems within the distribution networks are not functioning, water must be disinfected in small quantities. This can be accomplished by boiling the water or by adding agents in the form of pills, powder, or solution (Table 42-4). For boiling water, the US military recommends keeping the water at a rolling boil for 5 to 10 minutes. The United Nations High Commissioner for Refugees recommends boiling water for 1 minute for every 1,000 m of altitude above sea level.[89] In general, boiling water for 1 minute will

TABLE 42-4

EMERGENCY DISINFECTION OF SMALL VOLUMES OF WATER

Disinfectant	Techniques	Contact Time
Calcium Hypochlorite 70% CaOCL$_2$ (powder)	Add 1 heaping tsp (7 g) to 8 L water for stock solution of 500 ppm (500 mg/L). Add stock to water in proportion of 1 part to 100 parts water for a 5 ppm (5 mg/L) concentration.	30 min
Sodium Hypochlorite 5% NaOCL (liquid)	Household bleach usually contains 5% chlorine. Add 2 drops bleach per liter water (double the dose if water is very cold or cloudy).	30 min
Halazone tablets (4 mg or 160 mg)	Chlorine tablets. Add one 4 mg tablet per L water. One 160 mg tablet is added to 40 L water (double the dose if water is very cold or cloudy).	30 min
Iodine Tablets	Add one to 1 L water (double the dose if water is very cold or cloudy).	30 min
Tincture of Iodine (2% solution)	Common household tincture of iodine. Add 5 drops of tincture of iodine to 1 L clear water (double the dose if water is very cold or cloudy).	30 min
Potassium permanganate KMnO$_4$ (powder)	Dissolve 40 mg KMnO$_4$ in 1 L warm water for stock solution. This solution will disinfect approximately 1 m^3 (250 gal) of water. This method is seldom used because of the long contact time required.	24 hr
Heat	Boil water for 5 to 10 min. This requires extra effort to protect water, as boiling provides no residual protection from recontamination.	N/A

ppm: parts per million
Sources: (1) Pan American Health Organization. *A Guide to Emergency Health Management after Natural Disaster*. Washington, DC: PAHO; 1981. Emergency Preparedness and Disaster Relief Coordination Program Scientific Publication No. 407 (2) US Dept of the Army. *Occupational and Environmental Health: Sanitary Control and Surveillance of Field Water Supplies*. Washington, DC: DA, 1986. Technical Bulletin MED 577.

kill most disease-causing bacteria and viruses. In areas where protozoal and helminthic diseases are endemic, longer boiling times are necessary.[90] The availability of adequate fuel and containers for boiling needs to be kept in mind.

Individual water purification methods should only be considered during an emergency for disinfecting small quantities of drinking water in limited and controlled populations, on an individual basis, and for only 1 to 2 weeks.[17] PVNTMED personnel should determine the chlorine residual before any form of disinfectant is distributed to individual users. Providing tablet, powder, or liquid disinfectants to individual users should be considered only when distribution can be coupled with a strong health education campaign teaching people how to use the disinfectants properly. Additionally, PVNTMED personnel will need to provide follow-up instruction and supervision to ensure proper and continued use of the disinfectants. There is potential for misuse of these disinfectants, especially with children.

Human Waste

An acceptable and practical system for the disposal of human waste should be a primary consideration. Improper disposal not only leads to the contamination of food and water supplies, it also attracts flies and other disease-carrying pests. The waste disposal system must be developed in cooperation with the refugees or local population and be culturally appropriate. Expert advice should also be sought from a sanitary engineer who is familiar with the habits of the refugees or inhabitants of the disaster area.[17]

Two main factors will affect the choice of a toilet system: the traditional sanitation practices of the users and the physical characteristics of the area, including the geology, rainfall, and drainage.[89] Once these considerations have been taken into account, the cleanliness of the latrines and their accessibility will determine whether they are used. Users must be trained in latrine upkeep. Frequent on-site visits by PVNTMED personnel will help ensure latrines are maintained properly.

Latrines should be placed where needed in relocation camps, relief worker settlements, and areas of dense population where facilities have been destroyed. There are many simple options that, if properly constructed and maintained, will meet all public health requirements. Examples of different types of field latrines suitable for disaster relief operations are shown in Table 42-5. The ideal latrine confines excreta; excludes insects, rodents, and animals; prevents contamination of the water supply; provides convenience and privacy; and remains clean and odor-free.[90]

Waste Water

Waste water is created by personal hygiene and food preparation activities. Sources of waste water should be localized as much as possible, and drainage should be provided. Water allowed to stand will soon become malodorous, provide breeding sites for insect pests (especially mosquitoes and filth flies), and become an additional source of contamination of the environment. Soakage pits or trenches can be used for the collection of bath and wash water. This same system equipped with a grease trap can also be used for the collection of liquid kitchen waste.

Solid Waste and Dust

Uncontrolled accumulation of solid waste (garbage) and improper disposal increases the risk of diseases spread by insects and rodents. An effective garbage disposal system using burial or incineration must be provided.[88] Garbage burial sites should be located at least 30 m from any potable water source and at least 50 m downwind from camps. Open burning of garbage on-site should be avoided; incinerators should be used to burn garbage.

Solid waste disposal containers in tent camps should be waterproof, insect-proof, and rodent-proof. The waste should be covered tightly with a plastic or metal lid. A 50-L waste receptacle should be provided for every 10 families (25 to 50 persons). The containers should be placed throughout the site such that no dwelling is more than about 15 m away from one. The weight and shape of containers must also be kept within the limits that can be conveniently

TABLE 42-5

TYPES AND CHARACTERISTICS OF LATRINES SUITABLE FOR DISASTER RELIEF OPERATIONS

Type	Characteristics
Shallow trench latrine	A quick-action solution; cheap and easy to construct. Should only be used a few days. Approximately 30 cm wide, 1 m deep. Excreta covered with soil after each use.
Deep trench latrine	Easy to construct. Can be used for a few months. Appropriate for tent camps. Approximately 2 m deep, 80 cm wide. Recommended length for 100 persons is 3.5 m. Requires a structure providing a seat or squatting hole with lid. Trench should be fly-proofed.
Pit latrine	Most common worldwide. Appropriate for tent camps. Consists of a superstructure for privacy and a squatting hole or seat above a hole in the ground. Can be used by individual families or in clusters as communal facilities. Pit should be about 1 m across, and more than 2 m deep.
Chemical latrine	Self-contained, expensive to maintain. Includes a holding tank with chemical additives. Contents must be pumped out daily for disposal in a conventional sanitary waste water system.
Burn-out latrine	Used when soil is hard, rocky, or frozen and when sufficient fuel is available for burning (a mixture of 1 part gasoline with 4 parts diesel oil is effective). Also suitable in areas with high water tables. Oil drums, cut in half, can be used to collect the waste. A structure that has a seat with a fly-proof, self-closing lid is required.

Sources: Pan American Health Organization. *A Guide to Emergency Health Management after Natural Disaster*. Washington, DC: PAHO; 1981. Emergency Preparedness and Disaster Relief Coordination Program Scientific Publication No. 407. United Nations High Commissioner for Refugees. *Handbook for Emergencies*. Geneva: UNHCR; 1982.

handled by the collection crew. The collection of garbage from the containers should take place regularly, daily if possible.

Large amounts of dust carried in the air can be harmful to human health by irritating eyes, respiratory systems, and skin and by contaminating food and water.[89] The best preventive measure is to stop the destruction of vegetation around the site. Dust control can be achieved by spraying roads with water (especially helpful around health facilities and feeding centers), limiting traffic, and banning traffic from certain areas, if necessary.

Hazardous Substances and Medical Waste

Hazardous wastes include chemical, biological, flammable, explosive, and radioactive substances, which may be solid, liquid, or gaseous.[90] Handling of hazardous substances may be a significant public health problem during and after certain disasters. The advice of an industrial hygienist may be necessary to handle such waste safely. The treatment and disposal of medical waste requires special attention. Needles, scalpels, and materials contaminated with infectious waste are especially dangerous. Medical waste should be treated separately; as much of it as possible should be burned without delay. The designated burning area should be fenced to prevent unauthorized access.

Management of the Dead

Suitable arrangements for the management of the dead are required from the start of any natural disaster that causes a refugee emergency.[89] The mortality rate after a refugee influx will probably be higher than under normal conditions. The health hazards associated with unburied bodies are minimal, especially if death resulted from trauma. However, bodies must be protected from rodents, animals, and birds. Additionally, bodies decomposing in wells and streams can cause gastroenteritis in those that drink the water.

Dead bodies have the potential to create social problems, which must be delicately addressed by public health authorities. Every effort should be made to treat bodies with respect. Whenever possible, the customary method of disposal should be used, and the traditional practices and rituals should be allowed. Burial is the simplest and best method of disposal if it is acceptable to the community and physically possible. The necessary

space for burial will need to be taken into account when planning the site, particularly in crowded conditions. Cremation may be used, but it can require large amounts of fuel and is not required as a public health measure. Before burial or cremation, bodies must be identified and the identification and cause of death recorded, if possible. This is important for disease control, registration, and tracing. Procedures must be in place to assure the care of orphaned minors who are left without appropriate care.[89]

Shelter

Natural disasters can result in the sudden creation of areas of high population density, such as camps for displaced persons. These persons need temporary public shelter that will not lead to further deterioration of public health or the environment. The site selection, planning, and provision of shelter require expertise and must be closely integrated with the planning of other services, especially water and sanitation.[89] It is important that PVNTMED specialists work closely with engineers, experts from the Pan American Health Organization and the World Health Organization, and local authorities early in the process to select refugee camp locations.

Existing public buildings, such as schools, churches, and hotels, are good choices as temporary shelters because they will likely have their own washing and toilet facilities that are usually sufficient for emergency purposes. If existing buildings are used as shelters, the recommended floor space is 3.5 m² per person.[17] Overcrowding can have serious health implications.

If tent cities or camps are necessary to accommodate the evacuees, the requirements are more complex. Sites should be chosen that have adequate drainage and are away from mosquito breeding areas, refuse dumps, and commercial and industrial zones. The layout of the site should meet the following specifications:[17,19,86]

- 3 m² of floor space per person,
- 10-m–wide roads between tents, minimum distance of tents to road of 2 m,
- Minimum distance between tents of 8 m, and
- 4 hectares (10 acres) of land per 1,000 persons.

Tent camps should be subdivided into a community service area and a residential area. The residential area should be further subdivided into clusters around personal service areas, which contain cooking and washing facilities and latrines. This subdivision is important because personal service areas used by relatively few persons are more likely to be self-maintained.

Safe water, food, and basic sanitation facilities must be available in all camps for displaced persons. Sanitation teams that provide such services and educate camp dwellers should be designated for each campsite.[17] Teams can be composed of volunteers, but they must be supervised by an environmental health technician. Teams should develop sanitation regulations for the sites and educate the residents about basic sanitation measures.

Water distribution points should be located in the camp so that families are not required to carry water for more than 100 m. These points should be located in the community service center and in the center of each residential area. Multi-liter containers for carrying water should be made available to camp residents.

Characteristics of tent camps, such as a high density of people, combustible shelter materials, and individual cooking fires, make them vulnerable to major fires.[89] The most effective preventive measure is the proper spacing and arrangement of tents to provide fire breaks. Other measures include allowing individual fires only in specific areas and having an alarm system, fire-fighting teams, and plans prepared. Residents must also take proper precautions in storing and using fuels and other highly flammable materials.

Food Sanitation

The availability and distribution of food may be disrupted after a natural disaster. Food can become contaminated, especially in mass feeding centers, by flood waters, insects, rodents, and unsanitary handling. Degradation of food products results from power outages that disrupt refrigeration; contact with water; and purposeful adulteration. The use of outdated stocks can also be a problem.

Bulk distribution of food is not always necessary in a disaster area. Food becomes a problem only if local stocks are destroyed or if the road system is so disrupted that normal distribution patterns break down. Available food supplies should be located and inspected by a qualified health specialist. It is important to try to provide familiar foodstuffs to refugees and displaced persons. Priority should be given to the consumption of uncontaminated perishable food, particularly if the food supply originates in areas where there have been power outages. The health specialist should also inspect all damaged places of food production and distribution before food is prepared and distributed. Food storage and preparation at mass feeding facilities should also be closely supervised.

To avoid health problems related to contaminated food, the public should be informed about proper food preparation and handling measures and which foods are the most likely to be safe. Local public health personnel should be used to the fullest extent possible to educate those affected, particularly refugees. Military food supplies may not be suitable for refugees, and their use may unintendedly cause detrimental results.[3] During disaster relief operations, US military forces will initially rely on the field ration Meal, Ready-to-Eat (MRE). These high-calorie, highly salted rations may be potentially dangerous to malnourished persons, especially children.[3] Recently, the Department of Defense has been involved in developing an MRE designed for humanitarian relief purposes. Its use in this scenario remains to be defined, however.

Personal Hygiene

Personal hygiene is obviously more difficult during emergencies, especially in densely populated areas such as refugee camps. As such, the potential for diseases associated with poor personal hygiene rises. Diarrheal diseases are very common in developing countries, and the added stress and relatively poor environmental services in refugee camps accentuate the problem. Public health workers should inform disaster-stricken populations about personal hygiene practices that will lessen the potential for disease. Trained and respected individuals from the refugee community should be more effective than outsiders in communicating health-related issues to their own people.[89]

Adequate cleaning and bathing facilities are critical for displaced persons to practice good hygiene, and local customs will dictate specific policies. Generally, however, there should be separate washing blocks for men and women.[17] One wash basin should be provided for each 10 people or a 3-m, double-edged wash bench for every 50 persons. Approximately 70 cm of wash bench should be fabricated for each wash basin. One shower head should be available for every 30 to 50 persons. For washing clothes, washtubs and clotheslines are necessary and scheduling of some sort will be required.

Insect and Rodent Control

By altering the environment, disasters may increase the transmission of diseases that already exist in a region. This may be due to the movement of large numbers of people, resulting in overcrowding in some areas and poor sanitation; the disruption of routine vector control programs; or the alteration of the distribution of vector species.[85,91] The increased risk of transmission of vector-borne diseases must be seriously considered after all natural disasters.

Pest control in a disaster situation is difficult, and physical barriers, such as screens, may be the best immediate measure.[89] The most effective method of controlling pests over the long term is to practice preventive measures, such as proper sanitation, garbage disposal, and food storage. Pest problems need to be explained to the affected populace, who need to be educated on the significance of pest control efforts, especially those with which they may not be familiar.

All pest or vector control activities should be supervised by an entomologist, preferably one with disaster experience and familiarity with local conditions before the disaster. Specialist advice about and supervision of all chemical pest control measures are essential. Detailed recommendations for the selection, application, and use of pesticides in field situations worldwide can be found in the US Department of Defense *Contingency Pest Management Pocket Guide*.[92] This guide is a concise reference to pesticides available through military supply channels (National Stock Numbers are listed) and designated for contingency use by one or more of the armed services. It contains information on pesticide uses, dosages, application methods, dilution formulas, and dispersal equipment; surveillance, trapping, and safety equipment; personal protective equipment against disease vectors; air transport of pesticides that do not meet transport requirements; and US military points of contact overseas who can provide information on vector-borne disease control in their areas of the world.

An additional source of information on vector control is the Pan American Health Organization publication, *Emergency Vector Control After Natural Disasters*.[91] This guide provides technical information necessary for evaluating the need for disease vector and rodent control following natural disasters, information for initiating immediate and postdisaster control measures, and guidelines for planning and carrying out surveillance and control programs against specific vectors under austere conditions.

An increased incidence of animal bites, especially dog bites, may occur as neglected strays come into close contact with persons living in temporary shelters. A program for the elimination of stray dogs should be considered, especially in areas where rabies is endemic.

SUMMARY

The role of the US military in providing assistance following major natural disasters is a role for which PVNTMED personnel need to be trained.[18] Familiarity with the procedures to follow in such support operations is critical to the successful accomplishment of the mission. The primary mission of PVNTMED personnel or units will continue to be to support US, allied, and coalition forces. However, involvement in a wide range of activities in support of the local or host-nation populace will also be required. Definition (a priori) of the military's roles and responsibilities and delineation of unit preparedness plans are necessary to respond to such contingencies in a timely and efficient manner. PVNTMED personnel serving in both operational and garrison units may also be called on to assist units in the preparation of disaster preparedness plans or to provide direct support during these types of missions. It is with this in mind that we have written this chapter. The Recommended Readings, which follow the references, may be helpful to PVNTMED personnel during disaster assistance deployments.

REFERENCES

1. Burkle FM, Frost DS, Greco SB, Petersen HV, Lillibridge SR. Strategic disaster preparedness and response: implications for military medicine under Joint Command. *Mil Med*. 1996;161:442–447.

2. Navy Environmental Health Center. Public Health Aspects of Disaster Management. 28th Navy Occupational Health and Preventive Medicine Workshop. Norfolk, Va; 1986.

3. Sharp TW, Yip R, Malone JD. US military forces and emergency international humanitarian assistance: observations and recommendations from three recent missions. *JAMA*. 1994;272:386–390.

4. Lillibridge SR, Burkle Jr FM, Noji EK. Disaster mitigation and humanitarian assistance training for uniformed service medical personnel. *Mil Med*. 1994;159:397–403.

5. Willis GE. On the road again...and again and again. *Army Times*. 1996;July1:12–14.

6. Moore GR, Dembert ML. The military as a provider of public health services after a disaster. *Mil Med*. 1987;152:303–307.

7. Waeckerle JF, Lillibridge SR, Burkle Jr FM, Noji EK. Disaster medicine: challenges for today. *Ann Emerg Med*. 1994;23:715–718.

8. Sidel VW, Onel E, Jack Geiger H, Leaning J, Foege WH. Public health responses to natural and human-made disasters. In: Last JM, Wallace RB, eds. *Maxcy-Rosenau-Last Public Health and Preventive Medicine*. 13th ed. Norwalk, Conn: Appleton & Lange; 1992: 1173–1186.

9. National Research Council Advisory Committee on the International Decade for Natural Hazard Reduction Report. *Confronting Natural Disasters: An International Decade for Natural Hazard Reduction*. Washington, DC: National Academy Press; 1987: 1–60.

10. SAEM Disaster Medicine White Paper Subcommittee. Disaster medicine: current assessment and blueprint for the future. *Acad Emerg Med*. 1995;2:1068–1076.

11. Subcommittee on Natural Disaster Reduction, National Science and Technology Council Committee on the Environment and Natural Resources. *Final Report*. Washington, DC: NSTC; Nov 7, 1994.

12. Lechat MF. Disasters and public health. *Bull World Health Organ*. 1979;57:11–17.

13. National Geographic Society. *Raging Forces: Earth in Upheaval*. Washington, DC: National Geographic Society; 1995.

14. Wasley A. Epidemiology in the disaster setting. *Curr Issues Public Health*. 1995;1:131–135.

15. Lechat MF. Updates: the epidemiology of health effects of disasters. *Epidemiol Rev*. 1990;12:192–198.

16. Glass RI, Noji EK. Epidemiologic surveillance following disasters. In: Halperin W, Baker EL, eds. *Public Health Surveillance*. New York: Van Nostrand Reinhold; 1992:195–205.

17. Pan American Health Organization. *A Guide to Emergency Health Management after Natural Disaster*. Washington, DC: PAHO; 1981. Emergency Preparedness and Disaster Relief Coordination Program Scientific Publication No. 407.

18. US Dept of the Army. *Preventive Medicine Services*. Washington, DC: DA; 1998. Field Manual 8-10-17.

19. Lillibridge SR, Noji EK, Burkle Jr FM. Disaster assessment: the emergency health evaluation of a population affected by a disaster. *Ann Emerg Med*. 1993;22:1715–1720.

20. Lee LE, Fonseca V, Brett K, et al. Active morbidity surveillance after Hurricane Andrew—Florida, 1992. *JAMA*. 1993;270:591–594.

21. Logue JN, Melick ME, Hansen H. Research issues and directions in the epidemiology of health effects of disasters. *Epidemiol Rev*. 1981;3:140–162.

22. Malilay J, Flanders WD, Brogan D. A modified cluster-sampling method for post-disaster rapid assessment of needs. *Bull World Health Organ*. 1996;74:399–405.

23. Centers for Disease Control. Rapid health needs assessment following Hurricane Andrew—Florida and Louisiana, 1992. *MMWR*. 1992;41:685–688. Published erratum: *MMWR*. 1992;41:719.

24. Gregg MB. Surveillance and epidemiology. In: Gregg MB, ed. *The Public Health Consequences of Disasters*. Atlanta, Ga: Centers for Disease Control; 1989: 3–4.

25. Seaman J. Epidemiology of natural disasters. In: Klingberg MA, ed. *Contributions to Epidemiology and Biostatistics*. Vol 5. Basel, Switzerland: S. Karger; 1984: 1–177.

26. Toole MJ, Waldman RJ. Refugees and displaced persons: war, hunger, and public health. *JAMA*. 1993;270: 600–605.

27. Centers for Disease Control and Prevention. Morbidity and mortality surveillance in Rwandan refugees—Burundi and Zaire, 1994. *MMWR*. 1996;45:104–107.

28. Bioforce. Cholera in Goma, July 1994. *Rev Epidemiol Sante Publique*. 1996;44:358–363.

29. Goma Epidemiology Working Group. Public health impact of Rwandan refugee crisis: what happened in Goma, Zaire, in July, 1994? *Lancet*. 1995;345:339–344.

30. Mason J, Cavalie P. Malaria epidemic in Haiti following a hurricane. *Am J Trop Med Hyg*. 1965;14:533–539.

31. Moreira-Cedeño JE. Rainfall and flooding in the Guayas River Basin and its effects on the incidence of malaria 1982–1985. *Disasters*. 1986;10:107–111.

32. Blake PA. Communicable disease control. In: Gregg MB, ed. *The Public Health Consequences of Disasters*. Atlanta, Ga: Centers for Disease Control; 1989:7–12.

33. de Ville de Goyet C. Maladies transmissibles et surveillance epidemiologique lors de desastres naturels. *Bull Organ Mondiale Sante*. 1979;57:153–165.

34. Centers for Disease Control. Outbreak of diarrheal illness associated with a natural disaster—Utah. *MMWR*. 1983;32:662–664.

35. Weniger BG, Blaser MJ, Gedrose J, Lippy EC, Juranek DD. An outbreak of waterborne giardiasis associated with heavy water runoff due to warm weather and volcanic ashfall. *Am J Public Health*. 1983;73:868–872.

36. Simoes J, Fraga de Azevedo J, Maria Palmeiro J. Some aspects of the Weil's disease epidemiology based on a recent epidemic after a flood in Lisbon (1967). *An Esc Nac Saude Publ Med Trop (Lisbon)*. 1969;3:19–32.

37. Research Center on Disaster Epidemiology (CRED). An epidemiological study of the impact of floods on communicable diseases: case studies in flood prone areas of Santa Catarina and São Paulo, Brazil. Brussels, Belgium: CRED, 1989. CRED Working Document No. 79.

38. Zaki SR, Shieh WJ, the Epidemic Working Group at the Ministry of Health in Nicaragua. Leptospirosis associated with outbreak of acute febrile illness and pulmonary haemorrhage, Nicaragua, 1995. *Lancet*. 1996;347:535–536.

39. Bia FJ. Symposium: leptospirosis—a re-emerging disease. *TMA Update*. 1998;8:5–7.

40. Hau CH, Hien TT, Tien NT, et al. Prevalence of enteric hepatitis A and E viruses in the Mekong River delta region of Vietnam. *Am J Trop Med Hyg*. 1999;60:277–280.

41. Clayson ET, Innis BL, Myint KS, et al. Detection of hepatitis E in infections among domestic swine in the Kathmandu valley of Nepal. *Am J Trop Med Hyg*. 1995;53:228–232.

42. Sanders EJ, Rigau-Perez JG, Smits HL, et al. Increase of leptospirosis in dengue-negative patients after a hurricane in Puerto Rico in 1996. *Am J Trop Med Hyg*. 1999;6:399–404.

43. Patz JA, Epstein PR, Burke TA, Balbus JM. Global climate change and emerging infectious diseases. *JAMA.* 1996;275:217–223.

44. World Health Organization. The Potential Role of New Cholera Vaccines in the Prevention and Control of Cholera Outbreaks During Acute Emergencies: Report of a Meeting. Geneva: WHO; 1995. Document No. CDR/ GPV/95.1.

45. Waldman RJ. Cholera vaccination in refugee settings. *JAMA.* 1998;279:552–553.

46. Centers for Disease Control. Famine-affected, refugee, and displaced populations: recommendations for public health issues. *MMWR.* 1992;41:1–76.

47. Center for Public Health Surveillance, Somalia. Results of morbidity, mortality, nutritional, and vaccine assessment-cluster survey of Johwar, Somalia. Report of February 1993.

48. Burkle FM Jr. Triage of disaster-related neuropsychiatric casualties. *Emerg Med Clin North Am.* 1991;9:87–105.

49. Lechat MF. The epidemiology of disasters. *Proc R Soc Med.* 1976;69:412–426.

50. Davis I. Housing and shelter provision following the earthquakes of February 4th and 6th 1976. *Disasters.* 1977;1:82.

51. Garrison CZ, Weinrich MW, Hardin SB, Weinrich S, Wang L. Post-traumatic stress disorder in adolescents after a hurricane. *Am J Epidemiol.* 1993;138:522–530.

52. Shore JH, Tatum EL, Vollmer WM. Evaluation of mental effects of disaster, Mount St. Helens eruption. *Am J Pub Health.* 1986;76(3 Suppl):76–83.

53. Noji EK, Sivertson KT. Injury prevention in natural disasters: a theoretical framework. *Disasters.* 1987;11:290–296.

54. Lin N, Simeone RS, Ensel WM, Kuo W. Social support, stressful events, and illness: a model and an empirical test. *J Health Soc Behav.* 1979;20:108–119.

55. Lima BR. Primary mental health care for disaster victims in developing countries. *Disasters.* 1986;10:203–204.

56. World Health Organization, Division of Mental Health. Psychosocial consequences of disasters: prevention and management. Geneva: WHO, 1992: 7–39.

57. Ritchie EC, Ruck DC, Anderson MW. The 528th Combat Stress Control Unit in Somalia in support of Operation Restore Hope. *Mil Med.* 1994;159:372–376.

58. Bennet G. Bristol floods 1968: controlled survey of effects on health of local community disaster. *Br Med J.* 1970;3:454–458.

59. Melick ME. *Social, Psychological and Medical Aspects of Stress-related Illness in the Recovery Period of a Natural Disaster.* Albany, NY: State University of New York at Albany; 1976. Dissertation.

60. Logue JN. *Long-term Effects of a Major Natural Disaster: the Hurricane Agnes Flood in the Wyoming Valley of Pennsylvania, June 1972.* New York, NY: Columbia University: 1978. Dissertation.

61. Janerich DT, Stark AD, Greenwald P, Burnett WS, Jacobson HI, McCusker J. Increased leukemia, lymphoma, and spontaneous abortion in Western New York following a flood disaster. *Public Health Rep.* 1981;96:350–356.

62. Hendrickson LA, Vogt RL. Mortality of Kauai residents in the 12-month period following Hurricane Iniki. *Am J Epidemiol.* 1996;144:188–191.

63. Seaman J. Disaster epidemiology: or why most international disaster relief is ineffective. *Injury.* 1990;21:5–8.

64. De Bruycker M, Greco D, Lechat MF. The 1980 earthquake in Southern Italy—morbidity and mortality. *Int J Epidemiol.* 1985;14:113–117. Published erratum: *Int J Epidemiol.* 1985;14:504.

65. De Bruycker M, Greco D, Annino I, et al. The 1980 earthquake in southern Italy: rescue of trapped victims and mortality. *Bull World Health Organ.* 1983;61:1021–1025.

66. The 1988 earthquake in Soviet Armenia: implications for earthquake preparedness. *Disasters.* 1989;13:255–262.

67. de Ville de Goyet, del Cid E, Romero A, Jeannee E, Lechant M. Earthquake in Guatemala: epidemiologic evaluation of the relief effort. *Bull Pan Am Health Organ.* 1976;10:95–109.

68. Alexander D. Death and injury in earthquakes. *Disasters.* 1985;9:57–60.

69. Lindley D. US team returns with insights into Armenian earthquake. *Nature.* 1989;337:107.

70. Sommer A, Mosley WH. East Bengal cyclone of November, 1970: epidemiological approach to disaster assessment. *Lancet.* 1972;13:1029–1036.

71. French JG. Hurricanes. In: Gregg MB, ed. *The Public Health Consequences of Disasters.* Atlanta, Ga: Centers for Disease Control; 1989:33–37.

72. Centers for Disease Control. Update: work-related electrocutions associated with Hurricane Hugo—Puerto Rico. *MMWR.* 1989;38:718–720,725.

73. Centers for Disease Control. Medical examiner/coroner reports of deaths associated with Hurricane Hugo—South Carolina. *MMWR.* 1989;38:754,759–762.

74. Centers for Disease Control. Preliminary report: medical examiner reports of deaths associated with Hurricane Andrew—Florida, August 1992. *MMWR.* 1992;41:641–644.

75. Centers for Disease Control and Prevention. Injuries and illnesses related to Hurricane Andrew—Louisiana, 1992. *MMWR.* 1993;42:242–243,249–251.

76. Centers for Disease Control and Prevention. Deaths associated with Hurricanes Marilyn and Opal—United States, September-October 1995. *MMWR.* 1996;45;32–38.

77. Bakst HJ, Berg RL, Foster FD, Raker JW. The Worchester County tornado: medical study of the disaster. Washington, DC: National Research Council, Committee on Disaster Studies; 1954.

78. Hight D, Blodgett JT, Croce EJ, Horne EO, McKoan JW, Whelan CS. Medical aspects of the Worchester tornado disaster. *N Engl J Med.* 1956;254:267–271.

79. Sanderson LM. Tornadoes. In: Gregg MB, ed. *The Public Health Consequences of Disasters.* Atlanta, GA: US Department of Health and Human Services, Public Health Service, Centers for Disease Control; 1989:39–49.

80. Glass RI, Urrutia JJ, Sibony S, Smith H, Garcia B, Rizzo L. Earthquake injuries related to housing in a Guatemalan village. *Science.* 1977;197:638–643.

81. Glass RI, Craven RB, Bregman DJ, et al. Injuries from the Wichita Falls tornado: implications for prevention. *Science.* 1980;207:734–738.

82. Staes C, Orengo JC, Malilay J, Rullan J, Noji E. Deaths due to flash floods in Puerto Rico, January 1992: implications for prevention. *Int J Epidemiol.* 1994;23:968–975.

83. Centers for Disease Control. Tornado disaster—Kansas, 1991. *MMWR.* 1992;41:181–183.

84. French JG. Floods. In: Gregg MB, ed. *The Public Health Consequences of Disasters.* Atlanta, Ga: Centers for Disease Control; 1989:69–78.

85. Horosko S 3rd, Robert LL. US Army vector control (preventive medicine) operations during Operation Restore Hope, Somalia. *Mil Med*. 1996;10:577–581.

86. Llewellyn CH. Public health and sanitation during disasters. In: Burkle FM, Sanner PH, Wolcott BW, eds. *Disaster Medicine: Application for the Immediate Management and Triage of Civilian and Military Disaster Victims*. New York: Medical Examination Publishing; 1984: 132–161.

87. Quick RE, Venczel LV, Gonzalez O, et al. Narrow-mouthed water storage vessels and in-situ chlorination in a Bolivian community: a simple method to improve drinking water quality. *Am J Trop Med Hyg*. 1996;54:511–516.

88. US Dept of the Army. *Occupational and Environmental Health: Sanitary Control and Surveillance of Field Water Supplies*. Washington, DC: DA; 1986. Army Technical Bulletin MED 577.

89. United Nations High Commissioner for Refugees. *Handbook for Emergencies*. Geneva: UNHCR; 1982.

90. Salvato, JA. *Environmental Engineering and Sanitation*. 3rd ed. New York: John Wiley and Sons; 1982.

91. Pan American Health Organization. *Emergency Vector Control after Natural Disasters*. Washington, DC: PAHO; 1982.

92. Defense Pest Management Information Analysis Center. *Contingency Pest Management Guide*. Washington, DC; DPMIAC: 1998. Technical Information Manual (TIM) No. 24.

RECOMMENDED READINGS

Pan American Health Organization. *Epidemiologic Surveillance After Natural Disasters*. Washington DC: PAHO; 1982.

Pan American Health Organization. *Environmental Health Management After Natural Disasters*. Washington DC: PAHO; 1982.

Pan American Health Organization. *Emergency Vector Control after Natural Disasters*. Washington DC: PAHO; 1982.

United Nations High Commissioner for Refugees. *Handbook for Emergencies*. Geneva: UNHCR; 1982.

Benenson AS, ed. *Control of Communicable Diseases Manual*. 16th ed. Washington, DC: American Public Health Association; 1995. US Dept of the Army Field Manual 8-33.

US Defense Pest Management Information Analysis Center. *Contingency Pest Management Guide*. Washington, DC: DPMIAC; 1998. Technical Information Memorandum (TIM) No. 24.

US Defense Pest Management Information Analysis Center. *Military Pest Management Handbook*. Washington, DC: DPMIAC; 1994.

US Dept of the Army. *Preventive Medicine Specialist*. Washington, DC: DA; 1986. Army Field Manual 8-250.

US Dept of the Army. *Field Hygiene and Sanitation*. Washington, DC: DA; 2000. Army Field Manual 21-10.

US Dept of the Army. *Unit Field Sanitation Team*. Washington, DC: DA; 2000. Army Field Manual 21-10-1.

US Dept of the Army. *Occupational and Environmental Health: Sanitary Control and Surveillance of Field Water Supplies*. Washington, DC: DA; 1986. Army Technical Bulletin MED 577.

Chapter 43

COMPLEX EMERGENCIES

TRUEMAN W. SHARP, MD, MPH

T.W. Sharp, Captain, Medical Corps, US Navy; Officer in Charge, US Naval Medical Research Unit 3, PSC452, Box 5000, FPOAE 69835-0007

INTRODUCTION

In the post–Cold War era, much of the world's population is deeply affected by armed conflicts and their closely related complex humanitarian emergencies (see Chapter 41, The Challenge of Humanitarian Assistance in the Aftermath of Disasters). Through the first half of the 1990s, over 30 armed conflicts raged.[1,2] Primarily as a result of this armed violence and its consequences—famine, destruction, population displacement, epidemic diseases—complex humanitarian emergencies occurred in 23 countries, including Somalia, Rwanda, Bosnia and Herzogovina, Liberia, Sudan, Mozambique, and Afghanistan.[3] Because of these situations, almost 1% of the world's population, approximately 41.5 million people, were either refugees or displaced from their homes (Figure 43-1). Many millions more had not fled their homes but were also profoundly affected by these crises.[4]

Each complex emergency is unique, with its own causes and dynamics; however, many of these situations follow a somewhat predictable sequence of events.[5] A brief review of the evolution of a complex emergency will give a sense of many of these disasters. The place is usually a developing nation with many fundamental problems, including widespread poverty and a politically repressive, corrupt, and tenuous government. Political instability, the persecution of certain minorities, and human rights abuses lead to unrest and violent insurrection against the government. Further repression in turn breeds more violence and the development of a well-armed anti-government faction, often more than one. Escalating armed confrontation leads to extensive damage to social infrastructure, economic collapse, and deterioration of medical services. This is followed by population displacement as people seek safety and food. The medical treatment facilities that survive are typically understaffed and undersupplied and are overwhelmed by trauma victims. Preventive programs and routine medical care may cease to exist, which leads to extensive communicable disease outbreaks. In extreme cases, such as in Somalia and Liberia, that part of the economy involved in producing, transporting, and marketing food is totally destroyed, which causes severe food shortages and their devastating consequences. Widespread human rights abuses and callous manipulation of international relief efforts occur, which exacerbates the conflict. Schools, police, courts, and other basic institutions of society may cease to function altogether. Violence and a vicious anarchy reign. The international community often recognizes these situations and attempts to intervene only once they have reached an advanced stage.

Between 1990 and 1997, the US military was involved in complex emergencies in northern Iraq, Somalia, Rwanda, Haiti, and Bosnia and Herzegovina. The military in the post–Cold War world is likely to continue to become engaged in places where conflicts and complex emergencies occur—this will

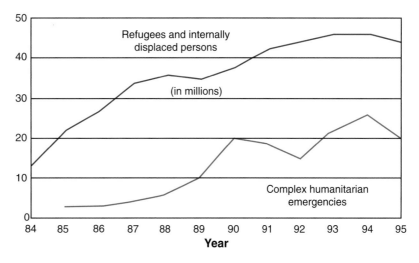

Fig. 43-1. Complex Emergencies, Refugees and Internally Displaced Persons, 1983-1995. There have always been complex humanitarian emergencies but in the late 1980s and early 1990s, the number of these emergencies increased markedly worldwide. Concomitantly, there was a rapid rise in the number of refugees and internally displaced persons, almost all of whom were victims of complex humanitarian emergencies. Intervening in post–Cold War emergencies of this type has been extremely difficult because of the almost intractable political, economic, social, legal, logistical, and security issues involved and because the large numbers of refugees and internally displaced persons have severely strained limited humanitarian relief resources. Data sources: (1) Office of Foreign Disaster Assistance. *Annual Report FY 1995.* Washington, DC: US Agency for International Development, 1996: 10 and (2) the United States Mission to the United Nations. *Global Humanitarian Emergencies, 1996.* New York: United States Mission to the United Nations, 1996: 5.

probably be unavoidable.[6,7] The specific roles the military will play in these missions and to what extent the military will engage in humanitarian assistance missions in the post–Cold War era are not clear (see also Chapter 45, The International Humanitarian Response System and the US Military).[8–11] The diversity of missions in the 1990s shows that those missions can assume many different forms, from providing security to providing emergency medical care.

Preventive medicine personnel who become involved in complex emergencies are entering dangerous and confusing territory. It is a formidable challenge to understand what the mission is, who is in charge, what plans have been made, what resources are available, what the scope of responsibilities is, and who are the many other organizations involved. When military medicine has been called on to provide health services directly to civilian populations in complex emergencies, preventive medicine has usually played a pivotal role because so much of the relief revolves around public health concerns. Even in operations in which military forces do not provide direct medical services, preventive medicine has been relevant because whatever the military does is likely to have significant repercussions on the overall relief effort and public health. If, for example, the military is tasked to provide only logistical support to international relief agencies, military commanders still need advice on the scope of the disaster, public health consequences, relief priorities, relief procedures, and other public health–related matters to make sound decisions.

This chapter provides a three-part framework for understanding and coping with the public health aspects of complex emergencies. The first section describes the critical information needed to make effective health interventions and how this information can be obtained. The second describes the principal causes of morbidity and mortality in complex emergencies. The third lists the ten most important basic relief priorities.

This chapter provides only a basic framework because responding to complex emergencies can seem as complex as the emergency itself. The details of program implementation and the specifics of clinical management of common disease problems, such as malnutrition, malaria, and diarrheal diseases, are beyond the scope of this chapter. Many other important dimensions of complex emergencies—political, social, cultural, and economic—are also beyond this chapter's purview. Other chapters in this book and other published resources discuss these topics in detail.[12–21] Excellent practical guides on public health needs in complex emergencies have been published by the Centers for Disease Control and Prevention (CDC), the International Committee of the Red Cross (ICRC), and Medicins sans Frontieres.[5,13–15] Also of note, military publications address doctrine and operational aspects of humanitarian assistance operations.[22–24] Institutions such as the Centers for Naval Analysis in Alexandria, Va, and the US Army Peace Institute in Carlisle Barracks, Penn, also have published a number of relevant reports on humanitarian assistance and, specifically, the role of the military in it.[25,26]

CRITICAL HEALTH INFORMATION IN COMPLEX EMERGENCIES

One of the most important roles for military preventive medicine in complex emergencies is to interpret the essential public health data that characterize the crisis and to use that information to help establish and guide the most appropriate relief measures. Conducting effective relief operations without timely, reliable, accurate, and integrated health information is extremely difficult, if not impossible. The history of disaster medicine has innumerable examples of well-intentioned but inefficient, inappropriate, and counterproductive relief efforts undertaken in the absence of good information.[27,28]

Gathering and using information in the setting of a complex emergency is a formidable task. Complex emergencies are dangerous, confused, and chaotic; good data are rarely readily accessible. Collecting sound epidemiologic data presents many methodological and logistical challenges.[29–31] Collecting information requires dedicated resources, but commanders and key decision makers may view data collection as an unnecessary luxury and a waste of limited assets. Once data are obtained, they must be analyzed, sometimes in austere field conditions. Then, and this is very important, timely information and recommendations must be disseminated to decision makers in a format that they can understand and use.[32]

Principal Tools

The principal methods of gathering data in complex emergencies are obtaining available background health data and then conducting rapid assessments, targeted surveys, standardized surveillance, and special investigations. While the basic underlying principles of collecting and using data are well described in many articles and textbooks, unique techniques and procedures have been developed for disasters and complex emergencies.[28]

Background data on a population in crisis, and on the areas to which it has migrated, are useful to interpret the current health situation and to plan appropriate relief interventions. For example, a population that has had prolonged food scarcity before a crisis may have little capacity to cope with sudden food deprivation. Or a population from a nonmalarious area moving into an endemic area, as has occurred in refugee crises in southeast Asia, will probably have many cases of malaria. Knowing this background should focus relief planning accordingly.

Background data are available from many sources (Table 43-1). The CDC, the World Health Organization (WHO), the United Nations (UN) Children's Fund, and the World Bank are examples of governmental organizations with information describing immunization status, nutrition status, endemic diseases, and other basic health parameters of affected populations. Various US Government agencies, such as the Central Intelligence Agency and the State Department, also have materials on other countries that are relevant to health.[33] Local governments, refugee leaders, and local health care

TABLE 43-1

VARIOUS SOURCES OF BACKGROUND DATA AND INFORMATION ON DISASTERS, CONFLICT, AND COMPLEX EMERGENCIES*

Agency	Telephone Number and Internet Address
US Agency for International Development	(202) 647-4000; http://www.info.usaid.gov
Bureau for Humanitarian Response and the Office for Foreign Disaster Assistance	(202) 647-8924; http://www.info.usaid.gov/hum_response/
OFDA Field Operations Guide for Disaster Assessment and Response	http://www.info.usaid.gov/hum_response/ofda/fog/foghme.htm
Centers for Disease Control and Prevention	(404) 639-3311; http://www.cdc.gov
CDC International Emergency and Refugee Health Unit	(770) 488-1033
Federal Emergency Management Agency	(202) 647-8924; http://www.fema.gov/
US Committee for Refugees	(202) 347-3507; http://www.refugees.org
Interaction	(202) 667-8227; http://www.interaction.org/ia/
Armed Forces Medical Intelligence Center Bulletin Board	(301) 619-7574; (800) 325-0195 (sysop 3883)
United Nations	(212) 963-1234; http://www.un.org
UN Children's Fund	(212) 326-7000; http://www.unicef.org
UN Development Program	(212) 963-1234; http://www.undp.org
UN High Commissioner for Refugees	(212) 963-6200; http://www.unhcr.ch
UN Office for the Coordination of Humanitarian Affairs (ReliefWeb)	(212) 963-6821; http://www.reliefweb.int/
World Health Organization	41-22-791-2111; http://www.who.ch
International Committee of the Red Cross	(212) 599-6021; http://www.icrc.org
CIA Publications and Handbooks	http://www.odci.gov/cia/publications/pubs.html
The Carter Center	(404) 331-3900; http://www.emory.edu/CARTER_CENTER
Project Ploughshares	(519) 888-6541; http://watserv1.uwaterloo.ca/~plough/
Center for Excellence in Disaster Management and Humanitarian Assistance†	(808) 433-7035; http://coe.tamc.amedd.army.mil/

* This is not a comprehensive list but has most major resources. Other resources can be found through links on the Internet. The ReliefWeb in the UN Department of Humanitarian Affairs allows access to much useful data, such as the *World Factbook*, country-specific immunization coverage, and other health statistics.
† This sight has an excellent source:"Disaster-related Web pages."

providers can sometimes provide much valuable information. Many nongovernmental organizations, particularly those that specialize in long-term infrastructure building, also have data on countries where they work. Often data can be found in published medical literature.

Within the military, the Armed Forces Medical Intelligence Center can be a particularly valuable resource. Its CD-ROM, "Medical Environmental Disease Intelligence and Countermeasures," reviews in detail the health situation in almost every country in the world.[34] The military intelligence community is also a good resource for information on political conditions, culture, local militaries, and other issues relevant to understanding health conditions.[35]

Despite these many resources, however, background health data can require substantial effort to obtain, and often there is not much time. Background health information, particularly for areas in the developing world, is likely to be fragmented,

outdated, or incomplete. Also, refugees and displaced persons may come from marginalized groups, which are not well characterized and may have worse health status than general statistics would indicate. Thus, applying background data in the conditions of a complex emergency may be problematic.

Rapid Assessments

Most relief agencies conduct rapid health assessments before intervening in a crisis. Rapid assessments characterize the emergency needs of the situation quickly but accurately, ensure that the type of assistance provided will be appropriate, alert the international community to the severity of the situation, and enable relief to be targeted to the most vulnerable populations.[36] The types of information typically collected in a rapid assessment are shown in Exhibit 43-1. Although background information

---

EXHIBIT 43-1

BASIC INFORMATION NEEDED IN A RAPID HEALTH ASSESSMENT*

Background Information: usual population demographics, normal health status, immunization coverage, indigenous diseases, usual diet and food situation, maps

Population Profile: current size of population, location, age and sex distribution, household organization and size

Health Situation: rates and causes of morbidity and mortality by age and sex, crude mortality rate

Food Availability and Nutritional Status: available food supplies (indigenous and external), accessibility, evidence of acute malnutrition or micronutrient deficiencies

Water: current use, availability, local sources

Shelter and Fuel: availability, sources

Environmental Conditions: climate, terrain, disease vectors, waste disposal

Local Infrastructure: airports, seaports, roads, communications, electricity, trucking, warehousing

Local Belief and Customs: health beliefs, food preferences, sanitary habits

Other Responders: indigenous capacities, external groups present, organization of relief efforts, services being provided

Political Situation: reasons for crisis, historical factors, host-nation position, external influences, underlying ethnic and cultural issues, underlying resource issues

Security Situation: armed factions, level of banditry, availability of weaponry

---

*For more details on information to be collected and on methodologies of conducting rapid assessments, please consult these references: Centers for Disease Control and Prevention. Famine-affected, refugee, and displaced populations: recommendations for public health issues. *MMWR*. 1992;41(RR-13); United Nations High Commissioner for Refugees. *Handbook for Emergencies*. Geneva: UNHCR; 1982; Office of Foreign Disaster Assistance. *Field Operations Guide for Disaster Assessment and Response*. Version 2.0. Washington, DC: US Agency for International Development; 1994 (also available on the Internet, see Table 43-1); Toole MJ. The rapid assessment of health problems in refugee and displaced populations. *Med Global Surveillance*. 1994;1:200–207.

can be helpful, there is no substitute for "examining the patient" directly. In recent years, the rapid assessment has been recognized as a distinct type of study with unique methodologies. In a rapid assessment of Kampuchean refugees in Thailand[39] conducted within 2 weeks of their arrival, malnutrition and malaria were identified as major health problems. This information was not anticipated. It proved to be essential in characterizing the nature and extent of health problems in this population and helped refocus relief efforts toward these issues. There are many examples in the literature of the use of rapid health assessments, as well as examples of misguided relief efforts when they were not conducted.[14(p23–25),28,37–39]

Teams exist in the military specifically to assess disaster situations, such as the Humanitarian Assistance Survey Teams at some major US military commands. Ad hoc assessment teams can also be constructed, as in the Kurdish refugee crisis in northern Iraq in 1991: a medical team from US European Command and units from the US Army Special Operations Command performed health assessments of the Kurds.[40] In Operation Sea Angel in Bangladesh in 1993, the military collaborated with other agencies, principally a Disaster Assistance Response Team from the US Office of Foreign Disaster Assistance, to obtain information on the damage caused by a cyclone.[41] In a complex emergency, many other assessments are likely to be conducted, so finding and using the results of surveys conducted by others can be an efficient way of obtaining needed information. Practical matters such as team composition, communications, travel arrangements, and language barriers are critical concerns.[20,36]

Targeted Surveys and Special Studies

Targeted surveys and special studies usually follow initial, rapid assessments. These investigations delve into issues for which more detailed information is needed. Figure 43-2 illustrates typical causes of mortality in refugee situations for which more detailed information would be useful in designing effective interventions. Typical areas of more-intensive investigation are nutritional status, immunization coverage, disease outbreaks, and rates and causes of morbidity and mortality. Surveys and special studies benefit from more focus and time than is possible with a rapid assessment. However, the

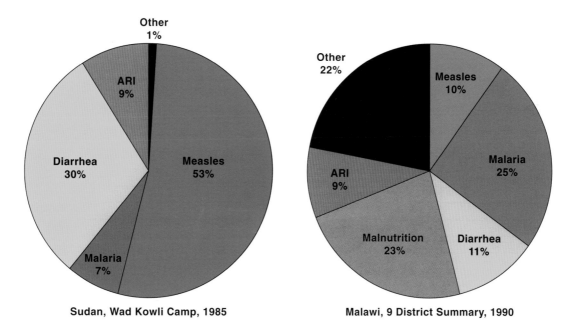

Sudan, Wad Kowli Camp, 1985   Malawi, 9 District Summary, 1990

Fig. 43-2. Causes of Mortality in Refugee Situations. These two pie graphs show common profiles of mortality in displaced populations during complex humanitarian emergencies. Common and usually preventable communicable diseases typically predominate, and young children are usually the most affected. Of note, the principal causes of death in Malawi were malnutrition and malaria, whereas in the Sudan measles and diarrhea predominated. This illustrates that while the same culprits may be important in many crises, their relative contributions can be very different. These types of data must be collected to characterize the causes of morbidity and mortality accurately, and relief efforts should be based on this information. Adapted from: Centers for Disease Control and Prevention. Famine-affected, refugee and displaced populations: recommendations for public health issues. *MMWR.* 1992;41:8–9.

WEEKLY SURVEILLANCE REPORTING FORM

Site: _____   From: _____/_____/_____   To: _____/_____/_____

I. Population
A. Total population at beginning of week:
B. Births: _____   Deaths: _____
C. Arrivals: _____   Departures: _____
D. Total populations at end of week: _____
E. Total Population < 5 years of age: _____

II. Mortality

Reported cause of death	0-4 Years		5 + Years		Total
	Males	**Females**	**Males**	**Females**	
Diarrheal disease					
Respiratory disease					
Malnutrition					
Measles					
Malaria					
Other/unknown					
Total					
Total < 5 years			XXXXXXXXXXXXXXXXX		

AVERAGE TOTAL MORTALITY RATE _____
(Deaths/10,000 Total Population/day averaged for week)

AVERAGE UNDER-FIVE MORTALITY RATE _____
(Deaths/10,000 Under-fives/day averaged for week)

III. Morbidity

Primary Symptoms/Diagnosis	0-4 Years		5 + Years		Total
	Males	**Females**	**Males**	**Females**	
Diarrhea/dehydration					
Fever with cough					
Fever with chills/malaria					
Measles					
Trauma					
Suspected hepatitis					
Suspected cholera					
Suspected meningitis					
Other/unknown					
Total					

IV. Comments

_____
_____
_____
_____

need to collect epidemiologically sound data must still be balanced against the need to have information quickly. As with rapid assessments, a body of methods has evolved to support the unique requirements of surveys in disaster settings. For example, the 30-cluster survey, which is a technique first used in the smallpox eradication campaign to conduct rapid and valid population sampling, is a commonly used technique that allows a team to collect accurate data on a large population in just a few days.

There are also many examples of surveys and special studies in the literature.[14,28,36,42,43] For example, a retrospective, population-based household survey[43] conducted in Kabul, Afghanistan, documented very high death rates in a population devastated by civil war. War trauma and various preventable infectious diseases (eg, measles, diarrhea, acute respiratory infection) were shown to be the main causes of death. Basic public health measures and actions to stop hostilities were shown to be the most urgent health needs. In the Kurdish refugee crisis[42] and in Somalia,[44–47] US military preventive medicine personnel worked closely with civilian agencies to conduct nutritional surveys, mortality surveys, and investigations of malaria, hepatitis, and dysentery in civilian groups. The results documented causes of morbidity and mortality and were used to refine relief efforts.

Surveillance

Establishing regular, standardized surveillance is a critical component of a health information system in a complex emergency. Whereas rapid assessments and surveys usually focus on a specific point in time, surveillance allows the ongoing, real-time monitoring of critical health parameters. Disease conditions for which surveillance is conducted in complex emergencies are shown in a typical weekly surveillance form (Figure 43-3). Surveillance has contributed substantially to relief efforts in a number of complex emergencies.[14,28,48] For example, a basic surveillance system was established by inter-national relief workers helping Bhutanese refugees in Nepal. This system enabled health workers to identify and manage outbreaks of malaria, dysentery, Japanese encephalitis, and measles.[48] In northern Iraq and Bangladesh, the US military contributed to efforts to establish and maintain surveillance systems.[40,41] The information derived from surveillance enabled decision makers to focus on documented problems rather than on hearsay. During the Kurdish refugee crisis, rampant diarrhea, which was by far the predominant cause of mortality, was initially unrecognized. Once identified, civilian and military officials concentrated on providing oral rehydration salts and other more-appropriate relief supplies.[40,42]

Conducting surveillance in conditions of armed conflict is particularly difficult.[29–31] Efforts in Lebanon and the former Yugoslavia suggest that surveillance during conflict is best accomplished by rebuilding and supporting indigenous capabilities rather than attempting to impose a new external system.[29–31]

Crude Mortality Rate

To gauge and follow the health status of a population affected by a complex emergency, certain basic indicators are commonly used. The crude mortality rate (CMR) is often cited as the most specific indicator of the health status of a population.[14,36] A CMR not only indicates the current health state of a population but also provides a baseline against which the effectiveness of relief programs can be measured.

The CMR is usually expressed as the number of deaths per 10,000 population per day. In a developing country, the usual baseline CMR is 0.4-0.6/10,000 per day. A CMR greater than 1 is considered elevated and greater than 2 is an emergency situation calling for urgent relief action.[14,36] Table 43-2 shows CMRs from some recent complex emergencies.

Depending on the circumstances, the CMR can be estimated from rapid assessments, surveys, special investigations, or routine surveillance. To esti-

◀———————————————————————————————————

Fig. 43-3. A Weekly Surveillance Reporting Form for Refugees or Displaced Persons in a Complex Humanitarian Emergency. Surveillance is a critical aspect of dealing with a complex humanitarian emergency. Reliable data are needed to monitor the public health vital signs of the affected population so that health problems are rapidly identified and appropriate relief measures implemented. Every situation demands the collection of different data in a somewhat different way at different time intervals. This form, however, provides a useful template for collecting information on most of the health outcomes of importance in the acute phases of a disaster during which people have been displaced. In a disaster situation, the desire for detailed data must be balanced against the need for an information collection system that provides what is really needed in a simple, straightforward, and practical way. Source: Centers for Disease Control and Prevention. Famine-affected, refugee and displaced populations: recommendations for public health issues. *MMWR*. 1992;41:42–3.

TABLE 43-2

CRUDE MORTALITY RATES IN SELECTED REFUGEE AND DISPLACED POPULATIONS, 1990–1994

Country of Origin	Country of Asylum	Year	CMR
Liberia	Internally displaced	1990	2.4
Iraq (northern provinces)	Internally displaced	1991	4.2
Somalia	Kenya	1992	7.4
Somalia	Internally displaced	1992	17.0
Burma (Myanmar)	Bangladesh	1992	1.6
Sudan	Internally displaced	1993	7.6
Burundi	Rwanda	1993	3.0
Rwanda	Burundi	1994	9.0
Rwanda	Zaire	1994	59-94

CMR: crude mortality rates
Data Sources: (1) Defense Intelligence Agency. *Bosnia Country Handbook*. Washington, DC: DIA; 1996, (2) Centers for Disease Control and Prevention. Famine-affected, refugee, and displaced populations: recommendations for public health issues. *MMWR*. 1992;41(RR-13):23–25, and (3) Smith CR. *Angels from the Sea: Relief Operations in Bangladesh, 1991*. Washington, DC: History and Museums Division, Headquarters, US Marine Corps; 1995: 9–27.

mate the CMR, a reasonable estimate of a denominator is needed. As was found in Goma, Zaire, however, obtaining an estimate of population size can be very difficult. Despite much attention to this issue, in that crisis the denominator was ultimately judged to be within the range of 500,000 to 800,000 persons; a more precise estimate was not possible.[49]

Many different techniques are used to estimate population size, most relying on some kind of simple sampling scheme.[13,14,17,18] Population estimates can be highly politicized as displaced populations and some relief groups may have an interest in larger numbers while some governments may promote smaller estimates. Some within and outside the military have suggested that the powerful technology of the US military intelligence community and other military technologies, such as satellite imagery, may be of great value in locating and accurately counting displaced populations. These clearly could have an important role in some situations.

Obtaining the numerator, the number of deaths, can be a problem as well. Techniques used for counting deaths in a crisis include counting new plots in graveyards, counting burial shrouds sold, and interviewing local religious leaders and civil authorities. In some situations, the number of deaths may be very hard to quantify. For example, families that receive a food ration for every family member may be very reluctant to report a death. (Often food rations will be continued in order to encourage reporting.) In some cultures, individuals may be very reluctant to report deaths to outside authorities for religious or cultural reasons. In the chaos of Goma, Zaire, where there was no way to dig graves in the volcanic rock, epidemiologists were able to quantify death rates by counting the bodies left by the roadside.[49] This is one example of how methods can be devised on the scene to collect data.

Nutritional Surveys

Another important focus of information collection in an emergency is nutritional data, specifically evidence of acute malnutrition or acute micronutrient deficiencies. In the nutritional survey, anthropomorphic measures of a random sample of children between 6 months and 5 years of age (the most vulnerable group) are taken to assess the nutritional state of the population overall. Either weight-for-height is measured or a mid–upper arm circumference (MUAC) is taken (see Chapter 47, Nutritional Assessment and Nutritional Needs of Refugee or Displaced Populations).

The nutritional status of the population is typically expressed as the prevalence of wasting in the children measured, as determined by low weight-for-height or small MUAC. A prevalence of wasting of greater than 8% is considered severe and of greater than 10% is critical.[50] The percentage of children with edema, which indicates severe malnutrition, can also be a useful indicator. Indicators of specific micronutrient deficiencies, such as xerophthalmia from vitamin A deficiency, can be important as well. Considerable literature is available on nutritional surveys and the specific methods used to conduct them.[13,14,42,50] Part of the Epi Info[51] software package is a nutrition module that allows rapid data entry and analysis.

While many humanitarian workers focus on nutritional surveys in the emergency phase of a crisis, the occurrence of malnutrition is the result of what are usually complex and long-standing food problems. Techniques exist to evaluate food production, availability, accessibility, security, stores, markets, and distribution;[13,14,50] these techniques can also provide critical information for relief efforts and may predict a food crisis before malnutrition becomes apparent.

An Effective Health Information System

Obtaining data is only half of the battle. Data must be translated into usable information and disseminated to those who need to know.[13,14,32] Information is powerful only if it is used effectively. A commander or a regional supervisor, for example, may need only key statistics that bear on a major programmatic decision. A survey that shows that a low percentage of persons in a particular camp are immunized against measles supports a decision to devote resources to an emergency immunization campaign. Reports going back to headquarters in Washington, DC, should stress items of interest to senior commanders. A graphical representation of escalating crude mortality rates in certain regions may provide the basis for redirecting support or perhaps even redefining the mission. Care providers on the front lines of a crisis may be interested in simple graphs showing recent trends in local febrile illness, such as a sudden increase in malaria, so they can develop local treatment protocols.

A successful health information system requires substantial proactive effort and, sometimes, clever marketing to use and disseminate information effectively. Exhibit 43-2 lists the steps in developing a health information system. Of note is that a health information system is dynamic and must be tailored for the situation. A sound system includes the ongoing evaluation of the system itself to ensure that it is effective and meeting the needs of the decision makers.

As a rule, information should be carefully scrutinized in a complex emergency. Data of poor quality or obtained by questionable methods are often readily available, and they can easily be misinterpreted and misused. For example, if a clinic reports that 25% of children are malnourished based on the self-selected clinic population and this was interpreted as the extent of malnutrition in the population overall, a highly skewed view of the situation would result.

Boss and colleagues[52] reviewed 23 surveys conducted in Somalia between 1991 and 1993. A wide diversity of methods and reporting procedures was used. Despite much effort to obtain needed information in this crisis, the differences in study objectives, designs, parameters measured, methods of measurement, definitions, and analyses prevented decision makers from making the most effective use of the data. Those conducting surveys in complex emergencies should define clear study objectives, use standard sampling and data collection methods, and ensure precise, written documentation of objectives, methods, and results.

EXHIBIT 43-2

STEPS IN DEVELOPMENT OF AN EFFECTIVE HEALTH INFORMATION SYSTEM

---

1. Assign primary responsibilities for coordinating and operating the health information system (HIS)

2. Define HIS objectives

3. Identify specific data to be collected and measures to be used

4. Establish chains of information transmission

5. Develop case definitions

6. Develop data collection forms

7. Train personnel and field-test system

8. Develop methods of data entry and analysis

9. Develop feedback mechanisms

10. Evaluate regularly and adapt HIS as needed

Data source: Centers for Disease Control and Prevention. Famine-affected, refugee, and displaced populations: recommendations for public health issues. *MMWR.* 1992;41(RR-13).

The findings of field studies will have to be carefully explained to decision makers and the media, all of whom may not readily understand the meaning of the data collected and the data's limitations. In southern Sudan, where security problems prevented access by relief workers to the population at large, nutrition and mortality assessments were intrinsically biased because they could only be conducted in areas where food was being distributed. Inappropriate use of this information led to misunderstandings of the relief needs and to misreporting of the situation.[36]

Ideally, an information system is an integrated and coordinated effort. Responsibilities for reporting, analyzing, and disseminating data should be clear. This can be hard to accomplish in the chaos of complex emergencies. In relief efforts in Goma, Zaire, the UN High Commissioner for Refugees successfully established an integrated health information system involving many other agencies and the coalition military forces.[49] Similarly, in Bosnia and Herzegovina, the WHO worked closely with other agencies and with indigenous persons to collect and use health information.[31] These unprecedented efforts in complex emergencies led to a much better understanding of morbidity and mortality patterns and thus to improved decision making about relief efforts.

PRINCIPAL CAUSES OF MORBIDITY AND MORTALITY

Much work has been done to elucidate the causes of death and dying in both the combatants and the civilian victims of complex emergencies. The combatants in situations of armed conflict often experience very high rates of injury and death because of the type of fighting going on, the weapons available, and the lack of medical care to treat the wounded.[53]

In some complex emergencies, however, the preponderance of morbidity and mortality (up to 90% of deaths) occurs in civilians.[54–56] This is the result of many complex and interrelated factors, including violence, destruction of the food economy, destruction of the health system, population displacement, poverty, and infectious disease. In some refugee camps in Somalia (1991 and 1992), for example, an estimated 74% of children younger than 5 years of age died.[57] This was the result of malnutrition, communicable disease, and other problems stemming from the ongoing violence.[58]

The ICRC, which provides much of the casualty care in complex emergencies, has published information on the subject of the war-wounded and their management.[13,59] Dealing with war trauma is beyond the scope of this textbook, but preventive medicine personnel should consider that violence and trauma are an important aspect of complex emergencies. Indeed, in some complex emergencies, violence has been the greatest threat to the public health.[43,53–56,60,61]

Civilians may find themselves in the way of the fighting, but in some complex emergencies, intentional humans rights violations and outright genocide are the most important causes of violent death. In the former Yugoslavia, as many as 250,000 civilians were killed in the late 1980s and early 1990s;

many were targets of warring factions.[60] In Rwanda, perhaps as many as a million people were killed by violence in civil disturbances and massacres in 1994.[49] In Cambodia in the late 1970s, an estimated 4 million to 6 million people died under the Khmer Rouge regime; most of the deaths were from violent causes.[62] Land mines are an enormous cause of morbidity and mortality among civilians during and after many complex emergencies[63] (see Chapter 41, The Challenge of Humanitarian Assistance in the Aftermath of Natural Disasters).

Understanding the causes of violence and how they can be prevented is a major public health concern. Preventive medicine personnel could become involved in planning health services and allocating limited health resources. For example, the ICRC, using an epidemiologic approach to casualty management, has reevaluated how it provides surgical care in situations of conflict and how the effectiveness of providing surgical services compares to other health interventions.[64,65]

Aside from violence, the principal causes of death among refugees and displaced persons have been childhood diseases, such as the primarily preventable communicable diseases measles, diarrheal disease, acute respiratory infection, and malaria.[14,66–70] Other infectious diseases, such as meningococcal meningitis, are occasionally important. Protein energy malnutrition and specific micronutrient deficiencies have been critical cofactors of mortality in many crises.[71–73] Figure 43-2 shows typical causes of death in two refugee situations. In many crises, certain groups have been more vulnerable. Excess mortality in complex emergencies is typically greatest in the 1- to 14-year-old age groups and in women.[14,66,67]

TEN CRITICAL EMERGENCY RELIEF MEASURES

Although every complex emergency is different and the relative priority of emergency health interventions varies, there is a fundamental core of urgent relief measures. The ten essential emergency relief measures discussed below are adapted from a report of a WHO conference.[74] During this meeting, a group of experienced relief experts decided on the key priorities in providing emergency relief for refugees and displaced persons, excluding measures to contain violence. The measures are not listed in any particular order because their relative importance will change depending on the situation. It is unusual, however, for another measure to crack into this core group during the emergency phase of a relief operation.

Rapidly Assess the Health Status of the Affected Population

Effective relief depends on characterizing the situation with timely and sound public health data.

Establish Disease Surveillance and a Health Information System

The ongoing monitoring of important diseases and the use of this information for public health action is critical in designing and running effective relief efforts.

Immunize Against Measles and Provide Vitamin A in Situations of Food Shortage

Measles in children has been shown repeatedly to be a major, and often the most important, cause of death in refugees and displaced persons. Measles outbreaks can be explosive and have caused thousands of deaths in just a few weeks. Studies among refugees show that large measles outbreaks can occur even if vaccine coverage rates exceed 80%. Therefore, measles immunization campaigns must be accorded the highest priority.[75] They should not be delayed until measles cases are reported or until other vaccines become available. Measles deaths occur primarily in young children, but children as old as 14 to 15 years have been affected.[66–73,75]

The most common nutritional deficiency in refugee and displaced populations is lack of vitamin A.[72,76] Deficiency of this vitamin has been shown to be an important cause of mortality in measles cases and of mortality from all causes. Vitamin A supplementation is cheap and easy. Thus, mass administration of vitamin A at the same time as measles vaccination can be an important adjunct intervention to reduce the consequences of measles infection, particularly in malnourished populations.

In selected situations, vaccination against diphtheria, pertussis, tetanus, polio, tuberculosis, meningococcal meningitis, or cholera may be appropriate. But rarely, if ever, will these interventions be as important as immunization against measles. These other immunizations usually become considerations after the emergency phase has passed.[14,67–74,76]

The US military has a number of logistic capabilities to assist in emergency vaccination campaigns. Military commanders must be careful, however, not to support unnecessary campaigns, as has been done in the past,[77] or fail to support needed programs in a timely fashion. In northern Iraq, an urgent measles vaccination campaign for the Kurds was delayed unnecessarily.[40] Also commanders must realize that although US service members receive many vaccinations, few in the armed forces have much experience with the technical aspects of mounting an emergency vaccine campaign in the field in another population. Furthermore, the military may not have critical supplies readily available, such as pediatric vaccine formulations or equipment for an extended cold chain.[9]

Institute Diarrhea Control Programs

Diarrheal diseases are often a principal cause of morbidity and mortality in complex emergencies.[13,14,66,68–71,78] Common pathogens such as rotavirus and *E coli* are often important causes of diarrhea outbreaks, but *Vibrio cholera* and drug-resistant *Shigella* species have also caused devastating outbreaks. Prevention of all types of diarrhea involves providing good sanitation, clean water, and adequate personal hygiene. Simple emergency measures to prevent diarrhea include organizing chlorination brigades, isolating defecation fields, and providing soap.[79,80] Simple measures such as providing soap are inexpensive and can substantially reduce person-to-person disease transmission.

In some situations, though, and particularly in the emergency phases of a relief effort, preventive measures may not be feasible or effective. The critical intervention in coping with diarrheal disease then becomes preventing mortality through effective case management. Sound case management of diarrheal disease, even in cholera epidemics, can reduce case fatality rates to less than 1%.[79,80]

Effective case management of diarrhea is based primarily on providing fluid replacement through aggressive oral rehydration therapy. Intravenous fluid replacement and antibiotics are used selectively and according to protocols relevant to the situation. While these concepts are easy to understand, experience has shown that effective diarrhea treatment programs require substantial organization and numerous personnel with experience and training. In northern Iraq in 1991, for example, the abundance of rehydration salts and enthusiastic medical providers was not enough in the absence of effectively run rehydration centers.[42] Effective case management of cholera and dysentery was also problematic in Rwanda in 1994.[49]

Choosing an appropriate antimicrobial to treat cases during diarrhea outbreaks can be difficult. In Rwanda, *Shigella dysenteriae*, which was causing a devastating outbreak, demonstrated extensive resistance to the commonly available antimicrobials.[49] The US military had a large stockpile of ciprofloxacin, to which the bacteria were shown to be highly sensitive. Many relief groups, however, did not want an expensive and "high-tech" drug to become widely used, in part because ciprofloxacin resistance might develop. Ultimately, the US military collaborated with relief agencies to use ciprofloxacin in a controlled manner under agreed upon protocols.

An important component of diarrhea control programs is developing community outreach programs to seek out cases that may not present to treatment facilities. Education of the community, particularly mothers, on the use of oral rehydration therapy, the importance of continuing breast feeding, and the importance of personal hygiene is also a priority. Active case finding, surveillance, and outbreak investigation are essential in determining the causes of the outbreak.

While medical personnel deployed on military missions certainly may participate in diarrhea control programs, military commanders and care providers must appreciate that the approach to diarrhea management in a complex disaster is different from the approach that would be followed in the military setting. Military care providers may not have the necessary training or supplies, such as oral rehydration salts, to treat large numbers of diarrhea cases effectively.

Provide Elementary Sanitation and Clean Water

Many of the diseases that occur in the setting of a complex emergency are to a great extent the consequence of poor environmental conditions. Water is often in short supply and of poor quality. There are limited means to dispose of waste. Vectors of communicable diseases may be prevalent. The means for basic personal hygiene may be lacking.[13,14,79–82]

Addressing these environmental health issues, particularly providing potable water, usually is a very high priority. Water needs are frequently underestimated. Only 3 to 5 L of potable water per day must be consumed for short-term survival, but people need at least 15 to 20 L per day for cooking, cleaning, medical care, and, sometimes, important ritual purposes. In some situations, such as when people are active in a hot environment, water needs are even greater. Medical facilities require much more water, usually at least 100 L per patient per day.[81]

Environmental issues are often very difficult to resolve because they require considerable resources and technical expertise. Providing potable water to a group of refugees, for example, may require experienced engineers who can locate the best sources of water, whether from the ground, the surface, or a spring. Expertise, such as how to construct a proper well and select the appropriate pump, is needed to access the source. The characteristics of a water distribution system are important because they can greatly influence the way water is accessed and therefore used; if people have a difficult time obtaining water, they will use it sparingly.[83] Assessing and maintaining water quality is a critical aspect of a water program.[84] Local water may be a limited resource and local political considerations may be critical in its access and use. Cultural considerations can also be important factors in how water is accessed and used by the local population.[85]

The technical skills and other considerations in waste disposal, vector control, and personal hygiene can be equally complex. Some relief organizations focus on environmental health issues but most do not. The technical challenges and lack of donor appeal of environmental issues remain major problems.

The military clearly has resources and expertise in environmental health; environmental health officers, entomologists, and other preventive medicine specialists have made many contributions to relief efforts in the past. In 1994 in Goma, Zaire, for example, US forces helped provide and distribute clean water. What is appropriate for supporting US service members, though, may not be appropriate for a humanitarian emergency. Some relief officials were critical of military efforts in Rwanda that relied on more technically difficult and slow purification techniques (primarily the reverse osmosis water purification unit) rather than simpler and more expedient chlorination techniques. Some officials argued that using chlorine and teaching refugees to use it themselves would have been more effective.

Provide Adequate Shelter, Clothes, and Blankets

Shelter is a basic human need. The provision of the basic means to be protected from the elements—sun, rain, and cold—is a high priority. The WHO recommends that each person in a refugee camp have at least 30 m² of total area, with 3.5 m² of that for housing.[86] Also, in populations with nutritional deficits, substantial energy can be expended simply in trying to keep warm. So some have argued that in certain situations distributing shelter, clothes, and blankets may be more economical than distributing food.[87]

As with environmental interventions, there is a substantial body of knowledge that deals with the technical considerations of emergency housing.[13,20,86,87] The selection of the specific sites for shelter, the layout of camps, and the type of materials used in construction are all important issues. Camps constructed in poor locations and with inadequate design can accelerate communicable disease transmission. Other factors to consider are the local availability of materials, the economic level of development of the population, the social habits, the local customs, and the political context.

The decision to provide shelter can have significant long-term consequences. Simple shelters provided on an emergency basis may unintentionally evolve into a permanent camp and end up attracting more refugees to the site. Many of these issues may become faits accomplis before reasoned decisions can be made by relief officials. Refugees are often forced by circumstances into poor locations that would never have been chosen by relief workers who had been given the opportunity to make decisions based on health and safety.

In sum, military officials must be cautious when providing housing. Although materials may be available and shelter may be a high-priority issue, tents or other such items should not be reflexively supplied if they are unnecessary or inappropriate for the situation.

Ensure Food Supplies Are Adequate and Reach Intended Recipients

One of the hallmarks of complex emergencies is a shortage of food. Thus, providing at least 2,000 kcal per day per person is an essential priority in emergency situations. While it is often uncertain how many people actually die of starvation during complex emergencies,[87] acute malnutrition has been shown to be a critical underlying cause of much morbidity and mortality.[13,14,17–20,50,73] There are many ways of providing emergency food relief. General food rations can be distributed widely to the population, perhaps in exchange for work or school attendance. General food rations consist of nutritionally balanced basic commodities that are appropriate to the situation and culture. Selective or supplemental feeding programs target food for certain high-risk persons, such as malnourished children, tuberculosis patients, or lactating mothers. This food may be distributed as rations to take home or can be provided at feeding centers, such as "soup kitchens." Therapeutic or rehabilitative feeding can be provided for significantly malnourished persons as a medical intervention and is usually given on an inpatient basis through assisted eating, nasal-gastric tube, or intravenous line.

The mechanics of managing food distribution and feeding programs are often complex. For example, an intensive rehabilitative program for severely malnourished children must have mechanisms to identify patients in the affected population. To some extent, patients may be self-referred, but often they must be proactively sought through clinic referrals and community outreach workers. Protocols and procedures must be developed to screen patients and determine who is eligible. Refeeding is labor-intensive and requires care providers with training and experience.[50] Patients typically have other aggravating illnesses and infections, such as malaria, that can complicate refeeding efforts. After discharge, follow-up programs must exist to prevent relapse. Sometimes family interventions are needed to counteract the social context that was a factor in the malnutrition. For example, in some cultures one child may be singled out to be deprived so that the other children may survive. The management of other food distribution programs can be complicated also and requires technical skills and experience.

Food programs have not always been successful, due in part to formidable problems of logistics, security, and distribution. Food aid can be highly politicized and food relief misused. Food supplies must be nutritionally balanced and culturally appropriate, and there has been much debate about the appropriate number of calories and the best content of food rations. Remarkably, micronutrient deficiencies have occurred in populations relying on donated food.[72]

The causes of food shortages are complex and may involve disruption of harvests, collapse of markets, lack of distribution systems, manipulation of food supplies by warring factions, and many other factors. Thus, an emergency feeding campaign must not only provide food urgently and effectively, but also begin to address the root problems of the crisis. Supplying seeds and agricultural implements may, in the long run, be as important as supplying emergency food.

There are a number of agencies that specialize in managing the "food pipeline" to emergency situations: the procurement, processing, shipping, and storing of bulk food. The World Food Programme is the principal international agency. In the United States, some of the principal agencies include Care, Catholic Relief Services, World Vision, and Feed the Children. On the scene of an emergency, other agencies, such as the ICRC and private volunteer organizations, often assume responsibility for actually distributing food and for administering feeding programs.

Military relief providers should be sensitive to the many facets and complexities of food relief. The US military has used the Meal, Ready to Eat (MRE) on occasion for emergency food relief, sometimes by dropping them from the air into inaccessible areas. While MREs may be better than nothing in an extreme crisis, they are a highly imperfect solution.[9] Humanitarian MREs have been developed that are designed to be culturally appropriate and nutritionally balanced for almost any population (see Chapter 47, Nutritional Assessment and Nutritional Needs of Refugee or Displaced Populations). These could have a limited but very important niche in military relief efforts.

Establish Appropriate Curative Services

Establishing curative medical services that follow standard treatment protocols, are based on essential drug lists, and provide basic coverage to the community as a whole are usually a high priority in complex emergencies. Providing acute medical care is one of the most visible and understandable aspects of a relief operation, and experience has shown that many external medical providers are willing to volunteer in an emergency. In fact, one of the hallmarks of emergency relief is the dispatch of medical teams from developed countries to treat sick victims. However, what medical care is actually needed should be carefully considered before providing curative services; noble intentions may not necessarily translate into effective action.

Substantial experience shows that medical care in emergency situations should be based on simple standardized protocols. The WHO and other organizations have developed basic, easily adaptable, field-tested protocols for managing diarrheal disease, respiratory infection, febrile illness, and other common problems.[13,14,18,79,80,89] Underlying these basic protocols are basic essential drug and supply lists.[90]

Using standard protocols and basic supplies assures that the care provided will be appropriate and allows the most efficient use of limited resources. Following basic protocols enables physician assistants, nurses, and community health workers to provide effective medical care without time-consuming and overly technical interventions. This allows care to be delivered that is appropriate for the population and the same level of care to be sustained after the military and other outside relief workers depart. The management of relief supplies has been a very difficult problem in many disaster efforts; using essential drug and supply lists helps assure that logistic resources are devoted to needed items.

Medical providers must be prepared to treat the conditions they will face. Volunteer providers from sophisticated hospitals in developed nations may not be well trained in dealing with the common problems of refugees or in using basic protocols and techniques appropriate to the situation. They may be called on to use drugs and techniques that are no longer used in their countries. In many emergencies, field hospitals or specialty teams have been deployed when basic primary care that reaches a large number of the population was what was needed.[27,28]

Military medical teams are highly capable and rapidly deployable to isolated and austere locations. Military medicine certainly has much to offer in times of crisis[11,91]; however, military medicine may not be well prepared or well supplied to handle some emergency situations. A battalion aid station, for example, that is designed primarily to stabilize trauma cases in US combat troops and evacuate them is poorly equipped, staffed, and supplied to handle diarrhea and respiratory illness in children or other common problems of displaced persons. Medical teams deployed to complex emergencies may have to be staffed and supplied quite differently than when they are supporting military operations.[9,92] Training medical personnel before they arrive in the field on the management of common health problems may be necessary.

Organize Human Resources

Community health experts are essential in assuring that medical care in an emergency is truly community-based and oriented toward primary care.[13,18,85] While it is easy to focus on clinics and hospitals, community health workers are the means by which health services actually reach much of the population. An effort should be made to ensure there is one community health expert for every 1,000 individuals in the target population.

Relief will only be effective if it is based on the needs and idiosyncrasies of the local cultures. Outside relief personnel may know little about local food preferences, sanitary mores, social customs, indigenous medical practices, and other such issues. A food program, for example, that provides culturally inappropriate commodities will not succeed. Community health experts will have insights into these matters that can profoundly effect the delivery of health services.

The access that community health experts have to the community can be critical. They are essential in communicating with local leaders, who play a central role in the success or failure of relief programs. If local leaders do not support an urgent measles vaccination program, for example, few people will participate. There can be many barriers to seeking medical care in an emergency, some practical and some cultural. Community health experts are often able to locate those in need. In northern Iraq, severely malnourished and dehydrated children were sometimes kept in a dark corner of their shelter and were not brought into the clinic unless the community health expert actively sought them out.[42]

Those from outside the affected population who are providing relief may tend to see aid recipients as helpless victims, but disaster-affected populations have a wealth of human resources. In fact, those affected by disasters are usually very anxious to help themselves and only lack the means. Community health experts are the key to mobilizing indigenous resources into relief efforts. The US military needs to understand these issues and what relief agencies are trying to achieve with community health experts.

Coordinate Activities of Local Authorities and Relief Agencies

A hallmark of a complex emergency is the complex response. Many agencies and organizations—governmental and private, civilian and military, indigenous and external—become involved. Without effective cooperation and coordination, time, energy, money, supplies, and most importantly lives may be lost. This extremely important issue is covered in detail in Chapters 41, The Challenge of Humanitarian Assistance in the Aftermath of Disasters; 45, The International Humanitarian Response System and the US Military; and 46 Domestic Disaster Response: FEMA and Other Governmental Organizations.

PRISONERS OF WAR AND OTHER DETAINEES

Enemy prisoners of war, retained persons, and civilian internees are protected under international humanitarian law, the Law of War, and the US military's Uniformed Code of Military Justice.[93–97] They state that all persons captured, detained, interned, or otherwise held in armed conflicts must receive humanitarian care and treatment. The stress of combat or other factors never justifies inhumane actions.

From a preventive medicine point of view, all detained persons must be provided with sanitary living conditions, food, water, and access to necessary medical care. Preventive medicine personnel are likely to be involved in planning for detained persons and assuring that these basic conditions are met. The Persian Gulf War is a recent example of this type of preventive medicine involvement; during and after the ground war, preventive medicine personnel were largely responsible for managing

thousands of Iraqi prisoners. Of additional note is that sick and wounded detainees are eligible for repatriation to their home country or neutral territory. Also, detained medical personnel must be granted facilities and the means to provide medical care to fellow detainees. Preventive medicine personnel may therefore have to work with detained providers to medically screen new arrivals, contain disease outbreaks, run vaccination campaigns, or provide other medical services.

The ICRC has special responsibilities in regard to detained persons. The ICRC regularly conducts missions all over the world to assess, monitor, and assist war prisoners and other detained persons. Under international humanitarian law, representatives from the ICRC have the right to be closely involved in any activities the military undertakes involving detained persons, and they exercise that right.

SUMMARY

Complex humanitarian emergencies are a tragic but inescapable part of our world. US military forces will continue to be involved in at least some of these

crises. Whatever the specific mission, preventive medicine personnel have the potential to play a major role in shaping both military and overall relief efforts through understanding and interpreting critical health information for commanders.

Most experience to date in complex emergencies comes from crises in the developing world, principally Africa. At the time of this writing, major complex emergencies are ongoing or pending in very different environments. The crisis in the former Yugoslavia has focused attention on trauma and human rights abuses as public health issues. The severe food shortages and declining health situation in North Korea may lead to a complex emergency in a more developed country in which, because of the repressive political regime, people stay at home and do not become displaced. This may lead to different patterns of morbidity and mortality and the need for different intervention strategies. The continued massive influx of persons into cities throughout the world and the extensive environmental damage in former Iron Curtain countries are other factors that could put a different face on future complex emergencies. Thus, while the principles enumerated above will remain important, preventive medicine personnel dealing with future complex emergencies will have to understand and cope with the unforeseen.

REFERENCES

1. Sivard RL. *World Military and Social Expenditures 1996.* Washington, DC: World Priorities; 1996: 7.

2. Stockholm International Peace Research Institute. *Yearbook 1996.* Uppsala, Sweden: Uppsala University; 1996: 15–22.

3. United States Mission to the United Nations. *Global Humanitarian Emergencies, 1996.* New York: United States Mission to the United Nations; 1996.

4. US Committee for Refugees. *World Refugee Survey 1996.* Washington, DC: Immigration and Refugee Services of America; 1996: 4–7.

5. Toole MJ. Complex emergencies: refugee and other populations. In: Noji E, ed. *The Public Health Consequences of Disasters.* New York: Oxford University Press, 1996: 419–442.

6. Committee on the Navy and Marine Corps in Regional Conflict in the 21st Century. *The Navy and Marine Corps in Regional Conflict in the 21st Century.* Washington, DC: National Academy Press; 1996: 27–39.

7. Marine Corps Intelligence Activity. *Threats in Transition, Marine Corps Mid-Range Threat Estimates 1995–2005.* Quantico, Va: MCIA; 1995.

8. Burkle FM Jr, Frost DS, Greco SB, Peterson HV, Lillibridge SR. Strategic disaster preparedness and response: implications for military medicine under joint command. *Mil Med.* 1996;161:442-447.

9. Sharp TW, Yip R, Malone JD. US military forces and emergency international humanitarian assistance: observations and recommendations from three recent missions. *JAMA.* 1994;272:386–390.

10. Sharp TW, Malone JD, Bouchard JF. Humanitarian assistance from the sea. *Proceedings of the U.S. Naval Institute.* 1995;121:70–75.

11. Gaydos JC, Luz GA. Military participation in emergency humanitarian assistance. *Disasters.* 1994;18:48–57.

12. United Nations High Commissioner for Refugees. *A UNHCR Handbook for the Military on Humanitarian Operations.* Geneva: UNHCR; 1994.

13. Perrin P. *Handbook on War and Public Health.* Geneva: International Committee of the Red Cross; 1996.

14. Centers for Disease Control and Prevention. Famine-affected, refugee, and displaced populations: recommendations for public health issues. *MMWR.* 1992;41(RR-13).

15. Medicins sans Frontieres. *Refugee Health: An Approach to Emergency Situations.* London: MacMillan; 1997.

16. United Nations Children's Fund. *Children in War: A Guide to the Provision of Services.* New York: Oxford University Press; 1992.

17. United Nations High Commissioner for Refugees. *Handbook for Emergencies.* Geneva: UNHCR; 1982.

18. Sandler RH, Jones TC, eds. *Medical Care of Refugees.* New York: Oxford University Press; 1987.

19. Desenclos JC, ed. *Clinical Guidelines, Diagnostic and Treatment Manual.* Paris: Medicins sans Frontieres; 1990.

20. Office of Foreign Disaster Assistance. *Field Operations Guide for Disaster Assessment and Response.* Version 2.0. Washington, DC: US Agency for International Development; 1994. (Also available on the Internet, see Table 43-1), Various Sources of Background Data and Information on Disasters, Conflict, and Complex Emergencies.

21. Lillibridge SR, Sharp TW. Public health issues in disasters. In: Last JM, Wallace RB, eds. *Maxcy-Rosenau-Last Public Health and Preventive Medicine.* 14th ed. Norwalk, Conn: Appleton and Lange; 1997: 1171–1175.

22. *Joint Task Force Commanders Handbook for Peace Operations.* Ft. Monroe, Va: Joint Warfighting Center; 1995.

23. *Expeditionary Forces Conducting Humanitarian Assistance Missions.* Norfolk, Va: Surface Warfare Development Group; 1995. Fleet Marine Force Operational Handbook OH 1–24.

24. *Multi-service Procedures for Foreign Humanitarian Assistance Operations.* Langley Field, Va: US Atlantic Command Air-Land-Sea Application Center; 1994.

25. Lamon KP. *Training and Education Requirements for Humanitarian Assistance Operations.* Alexandria, Va: Center for Naval Analysis; 1996.

26. Dworken JT. *Military Relations with Humanitarian Relief Organizations: Observations from Restore Hope.* Alexandria, Va: Center for Naval Analysis; 1993.

27. Seaman J. Disaster epidemiology: or why most international disaster relief is ineffective. *Injury.* 1990;21(1):5–8.

28. Noji EK. Disaster epidemiology. *Emerg Med Clin North Am.* 1996;14:289–300.

29. Armenian HK. In wartime: options for epidemiology. *Am J Epidemiol.* 1986;124:28–32.

30. Armenian HK. Perceptions from epidemiologic research in an endemic war. *Soc Sci Med.* 1989;28:643–647.

31. Weinberg J, Simmonds S. Public health, epidemiology and war. *Soc Sci Med.* 1995;40:1663–1669.

32. Gregg MB. Communicating epidemiologic findings. In: Gregg MB, ed. *Field Epidemiology.* New York: Oxford University Press; 1996: 130–151.

33. Central Intelligence Agency. *World Factbook 1996.* Washington, DC: CIA, Office of Public and Agency Information; 1996. (Also available on the Internet, see Table 43-1), Various Sources of Background Data and Information on Disasters, Conflict, and Complex Emergencies.

34. Armed Forces Medical Intelligence Command. *Medical Environmental Disease Intelligence and Countermeasures.* Fort Detrick, Md: AFMIC; 1996. CD-ROM disk.

35. Defense Intelligence Agency. *Bosnia Country Handbook.* Washington, DC: DIA; 1996.

36. Toole MJ. The rapid assessment of health problems in refugee and displaced populations. *Med Global Surveillance.* 1994;1:200–207.

37. Lillibridge SR, Noji EK, Burkle FM Jr. Disaster assessment: the emergency health evaluation of a population affected by a disaster. *Ann Emerg Med.* 1993;22:1715–1720.

38. Tailhades M, Toole MJ. Disasters: what are the needs? How can they be assessed? *Trop Doct.* 1991;21(suppl 1):18–23.

39. Glass RI, Cates W Jr, Nieburg PN, et al. Rapid assessment of health status and preventive-medicine needs of newly arrived Kampuchean refugees, Se Kaeo, Thailand. *Lancet.* 1980;1:868–872.

40. Centers for Disease Control. Public health consequences of acute displacement of Iraqi citizens—March–May 1991. *MMWR.* 1991;40:443–447.

41. Smith CR. *Angels from the Sea: Relief Operations in Bangladesh, 1991.* Washington, DC: History and Museums Division, Headquarters, US Marine Corps; 1995: 9–27.

42. Yip R, Sharp TW. Acute malnutrition and high childhood mortality related to diarrhea. *JAMA.* 1993;270:587–590.

43. Gessner BD. Mortality rates, causes of death, and health status among displaced and resident populations of Kabul, Afghanistan. *JAMA.* 1994;272:383–385.

44. Sharp TW, DeFraites RF, Thornton SA, Burans JP, Wallace MR. Illness in journalists and relief workers during international relief efforts in Somalia, 1992–93. *J Travel Med.* 1995;2:70–76.

45. Sharp TW, Thornton SA, Wallace MR, et al. Diarrheal disease among military personnel during Operation Restore Hope, Somalia, 1992–1993. *Am J Trop Med Hyg.* 1995;52:188–193.

46. Wallace MR, Sharp TW, Smoak B, et al. Malaria among U.S. troops in Somalia. *Am J Med.* 1996;100:49–55.

47. Burans JP, Sharp TW, Wallace M, Longer CP, Hyams KC. The threat of hepatitis E virus in Somalia during Operation Restore Hope. *Clin Infect Dis.* 1994;18:80–83.

48. Marfin AA, Moore J, Collins C, et al. Infectious disease surveillance during emergency relief to Bhutanese refugees in Nepal. *JAMA.* 1994;272:377–381.

49. Goma Epidemiology Group. Public health impact of Rwandan refugee crisis: what happened in Goma, Zaire, in July, 1994? *Lancet.* 1995;345(8946):339–344.

50. Arbelot A, ed. *Nutrition Guidelines.* Paris: Medicins sans Frontieres; 1995.

51. *Epi Info.* Version 6.0. Atlanta: Centers for Disease Control and Prevention; 1995.

52. Boss LP, Toole MJ, Yip R. Assessments of mortality, morbidity, and nutritional status in Somalia during the 1991–1992 famine: recommendations for standardization of methods. *JAMA.* 1994;272:371–376.

53. Garfield RM, Neugut AI. Epidemiologic analysis of warfare, a historical review. *JAMA.* 1991;266:688–692.

54. Fitzsimmons DW, Whiteside AW. *Conflict, War, and Public Health.* London: Research Institute for the Study of Conflict and Terrorism; 1994. Conflict Study 276.

55. Leaning J. When the system doesn't work: Somalia 1992. In: Cahill KM, ed. *A Framework for Survival: Health, Human Rights, and Humanitarian Assistance in Conflicts and Disasters.* New York: HarperCollins; 1993:103–120.

56. Mann J, Drucker E, Terantola D, McCabe MP. Bosnia: the war against public health. *Med Global Survival.* 1994;1:130–146.

57. Moore PS, Marfin AA, Quenemoen LE, et al. Mortality rates in displaced and resident populations of central Somalia during the 1992 famine. *Lancet.* 1993;341:935–938.

58. Manoncourt S, Doppler B, Enten F, et al. Public health consequences of the civil war in Somalia, April 1992. *Lancet.* 1992;340:176–177.

59. Coupland RM, Parker PJ, Gray RC. Triage of war wounded: the experience of the International Committee of the Red Cross. *Injury.* 1992;23:507–510.

60. Toole MJ, Galson S, Brady W. Are war and public health compatible? *Lancet.* 1993;341:1193–1196.

61. Flanagin A. Somalia's death toll underlines challenges in post-cold war world. *JAMA.* 1992;268:1985–1987.

62. Shawcross W. *The Quality of Mercy.* New York: Simon and Schuster; 1984.

63. Strada G. The horror of land mines. *Sci Am.* 1996;274:40–45.

64. Coupland RC. Epidemiologic approach to surgical management of the casualties of war. *BMJ.* 1994;308:1693–1697.

65. Perrin P. Strategy for medical assistance in disaster situations. *Intl Rev Red Cross.* 1991;284:494–504.

66. Toole MJ, Waldman RJ. Prevention of excess mortality in refugee and displaced populations in developing countries. *JAMA.* 1990;263:3296–3302.

67. Toole MJ. Communicable diseases and disease control. In: Noji E, ed. *The Public Health Consequences of Disasters.* New York: Oxford University Press; 1996: 80–100.

68. Toole MJ. Communicable disease epidemiology following disasters. *Ann Emerg Med.* 1992;21:418–420.

69. Howard MJ, Brillman JC, Burkle FM Jr. Infectious disease emergencies in disasters. *Emerg Med Clin North Am.* 1996;14:413–428.

70. Aghababian RV, Teuscher J. Infectious diseases following major disasters. *Ann Emerg Med.* 1992;21:362–367.

71. Shears P. Epidemiology and infection in famine and disasters. *Epidemiol Infect.* 1991;107:241–251.

72. Toole MJ. Micronutrient deficiencies in refugees. *Lancet.* 1992;339:1214–1216.

73. Yip R. Famine. In: Noji E, ed. *The Public Health Consequences of Disasters.* New York: Oxford University Press; 1997: 305–335.

74. World Health Organization. *The Potential Role of New Cholera Vaccines in the Prevention and Control of Cholera Outbreaks during Acute Emergencies: Report of a Meeting, 13-14 Feb 1995.* Geneva: WHO; 1995: 3–5.

75. Toole MJ, Steketee RW, Waldman RJ, Nieburg PI. Measles prevention and control in emergency settings. *Bull World Health Organ.* 1989;67:381–386.

76. Nieburg P, Waldman RJ, Leavell R, Sommer A, DeMaeyer EM. Vitamin A supplementation for refugees and famine victims. *Bull World Health Organ.* 1988;66:689–697.

77. Byrd T. Disaster medicine: toward a more rational approach. *Mil Med.* 1980;145:270–273.

78. Centers for Disease Control and Prevention. Health status of displaced persons following civil war—Burundi, December 1993–January 1994. *MMWR.* 1994;43:701–703. Published erratum: *MMWR.* 1995;44:654.

79. World Health Organization. *Treatment and Prevention of Acute Diarrhea: Practical Guidelines.* 2nd ed. Geneva: WHO; 1989.

80. World Health Organization. *Guidelines for Cholera Control.* Geneva: WHO; 1992.

81. Pan American Health Organization. *Environmental Health Management after Natural Disasters.* Washington, DC: PAHO; 1982: 3–8. Scientific Publication 432.

82. Pan American Health Organization. *Emergency Vector Control after Natural Disasters.* Washington, DC: PAHO; 1982: 8–18. Scientific Publication 419.

83. Cairncross S, Feachem R, eds. *Environmental Health Engineering in the Tropics*. 2nd ed. New York: John Wiley and Sons; 1993: 111–147.

84. World Health Organization. *Guidelines for Drinking Water Quality*. 2nd ed. Geneva: WHO; 1993: 131–142.

85. Whyte A. *Guidelines for Planning Community Participation Activities in Water Supply and Sanitation Projects*. Geneva: World Health Organization; 1986.

86. World Health Organization. *Health Principles of Housing*. Geneva: WHO; 1989.

87. Rivers JPW. The nutritional biology of famine. In: Harrison GA, ed. *Famine*. London: Oxford Scientific Publications, 1988: 87–95.

88. Hansch S. *How Many People Die of Starvation in Humanitarian Emergencies?* Washington, DC: Refugee Policy Group; 1995: 9–16. Working paper.

89. World Health Organization. Clinical management of acute respiratory infections in children. *Bull World Health Organ*. 1981;59:707–716.

90. World Health Organization. *The New Emergency Health Kit*. Geneva: WHO; 1993: 1–43.

91. Coultrip R. Medical aspects of U.S. disaster relief. *Mil Med*. 1974;139:879–883.

92. Yeskey KS, Llewellyn CH, Vayer JS. Operational medicine in disasters. *Emergency Med Clin North Am*. 1996;14:429–438.

93. US Department of the Army. *Enemy Prisoners of War, Civilian Internees, Retained Personnel, and Other Detainees*. Washington, DC: DA; 1996. Army Regulation 190-8.

94. International Committee of the Red Cross. *The Geneva Conventions of 12 August 1949*. Geneva: ICRC; 1995.

95. International Committee of the Red Cross. *Protocols Additional to the Geneva Conventions of 12 August 1949*. Geneva: ICRC; 1977.

96. International Committee of the Red Cross. *International Humanitarian Law*. Geneva: ICRC; 1993.

97. Vollmar LC. Development of the laws of war as they pertain to medical units and their personnel. *Mil Med*. 1992;157:231–235.

Chapter 44

PUBLIC HEALTH PERSPECTIVES RELATED TO TECHNOLOGICAL DISASTERS AND TERRORISM

SCOTT R. LILLIBRIDGE, MD and RICHARD J. BRENNAN, MBBS, MPH

S.R. Lillibridge, *Director, Center for Biosecurity and Public Health Preparedness, University of Texas Health Science Center at Houston School of Public Health, PO Box 20186, Houston, TX 77225; Formerly, Office of Global Health, Centers for Disease Control and Prevention, Atlanta, Georgia*

R.J. Brennan, *Director, Health Unit, International Rescue Committee, 122 East 42nd Street, New York, NY 10168, (212) 551-3019; Formerly, Visiting Scientist, National Center for Environmental Health, Centers for Disease Control and Prevention, Atlanta, Georgia*

INTRODUCTION

Disasters are catastrophic events characterized by urgent requirements for relief resources, technical expertise, and other vital services to assist the stricken population.[1] The public health demands associated with disaster response usually focus on the emergency needs of large populations.[2] Technological disasters are events that result from the unexpected release of hazardous materials, including fuels, chemicals, explosives, nuclear materials, and biological pathogens, during their manufacture, storage, transportation, or distribution. Technological disasters may be characterized by explosions, fires, chemical contamination, toxic plumes, radiation exposure, or infectious disease outbreaks.[3,4] (Table 44-1) Many segments of a community's vital infrastructure, such as transportation routes, communications, and water systems, can be affected. The frequency of such disasters is increasing, particularly as societies with limited experience in occupational safety and emergency medical systems rapidly industrialize.[5,6]

Adverse health effects associated with technological disasters include thermal burns, inhalation injury, blast injury, psychological trauma, and illness and injury due to contamination with chemical, radiological, or biological agents.[4,7–9] Long-term environmental considerations following technological disasters may include contamination of surface water, the water table, the soil, and the food chain.[4,10,11] The resulting biological effects from such environmental exposures may not be apparent until years later, when members of the exposed population present with subtle impairments of the nervous system or immune system.[12–15]

Terrorism has been defined as the use or threat of violence to sow panic in a society, to weaken or overthrow its leaders, and to bring about political change.[16] Although the common forms of terrorist acts, such as bombings, assassinations, and hostage taking, have important political and security implications for a nation, the public health impact of these incidents is usually minimal. They are not covered in this chapter. Unfortunately, new, more lethal technologies have made it possible for terrorists to target larger segments of the population.[17–19] Some authors have used the term weapons of mass destruction to convey the public health impact from chemical, biological, or nuclear weapons designed specifically for the purpose of attacking populations.[20]

From the public health perspective, acts of terrorism

TABLE 44-1

A FEW EXAMPLES OF MAJOR INDUSTRIAL DISASTERS

Date	Place	Event	Result
9/21/1921	Oppau, Germany	Explosion at a nitrate manufacturing plant destroyed plant and nearby village	561 deaths; > 1,500 persons injured
4/16/1947	Texas City, Texas	Explosion in freighter being loaded with ammonium nitrate	561 deaths; much of city destroyed
7/28/1948	Ludwigshafen, Federal Democratic Republic of Germany	Vapor explosion from dimethyl ether	209 deaths
7/10/1976	Seveso, Italy	Chemical reactor explosion released 2,3,7,8-TCDD	100,000 animals killed; 760 people evacuated; 4,450 acres contaminated
2/25/1984	Cubatao, Sao Paulo, Brazil	Gasoline leak from a pipeline exploded and burned nearby shanty town	> 500 deaths
11/19/1984	San Juan Ixtaheupec, Mexico City, Mexico	5,000,000 L of liquefied butane exploded at a storage facility	> 400 deaths; 7,231 persons injured; 700,000 evacuated
12/03/1984	Bhopal, India	Release of methyl isocyanate from pesticide plant	> 2,000 deaths; 100,000 persons injured

Reprinted from: Centers for Disease Control. *The Public Health Consequences of Disasters 1989*. Atlanta, Ga: US Dept of Health and Human Services, Public Health Service, CDC; 1989.

with such agents may be considered "intentional" technological disasters. But whether a disaster results from the accidental disruption of an industrial process or from a calculated terrorist act involving weapons of mass destruction, many of the same emergency public health skills will be required for successful response for the stricken population.[21] A multidisciplinary approach that includes professionals such as toxicologists, chemists, microbiologists, laboratorians, industrial hygienists, health physicists, physicians, and epidemiologists will generally be required to mount an effective response to such hazards. This chapter reviews the public health management of technological disasters, focusing on civilian population needs rather than on those of military personnel, although military personnel are often involved in addressing public health and medical contingencies in civilian populations. Chemical, biological, and radiological warfare and the appropriate medical countermeasures involving military personnel are covered in Chapters 27, Chemical Warfare Agents; 28, Biological Warfare Defense; and 29, Medical Response to Injury from Ionizing Radiation.

RISK FACTORS FOR TECHNOLOGICAL DISASTERS

In civilian populations, people from lower socioeconomic levels may be at greater risk from technological disasters because of their more limited access to emergency services and because of the frequency with which hazardous industrial sites are located near low-income residential areas.[22,23] The lack of effective urban zoning regulations and enforcement policies designed to maintain geographic separation between residential communities and industrial sites contributes to this problem.[24] Developing countries are at particular risk for technological disasters. This is largely due to industrial safety problems, including the inability to ensure the proper use of new technology, the underdevelopment of occupational health and the general public health infrastructure, the lack of prehospital emergency medical services, and, in some cases, civil unrest.[25] Nonmedical occupational groups at risk during the emergency response to technological disasters include plant workers, emergency responders, media representatives, and law enforcement officials.

PLANNING FOR TECHNOLOGICAL DISASTERS IN A CIVILIAN ENVIRONMENT

One of history's worst technological disasters involved a nighttime chemical release in the city of Bhopal, India, on 3 December 1984. The toxic agent was methyl isocyanate (MIC) vapor, which was vented into the atmosphere because of a combination of operator error and malfunctioning safety systems within a local chemical plant.[6] MIC is an intermediate product in the manufacture of carbamate pesticides. The toxic plume of MIC covered an area of 40 km^2 and extended 8 km beyond the factory.[26] Because proper warning and evacuation guidance were delayed, many victims first became aware of the disaster as they were overcome by MIC. More than 2,500 people in the adjacent community may have died, and 200,000 people were affected by the chemical release.[8,27] Thousands of victims sought urgent medical assistance, overwhelming local medical services.

The magnitude of the Bhopal disaster exposed a number of vulnerabilities associated with the release of a hazardous agent within a minimally prepared civilian population. In particular, basic disaster management strategies, such as informing the community of the types and quantities of the chemicals stored on the site and ensuring the emergency notification of the nearby population, were incomplete.[8,26] Consequently, many medical personnel and public health officials were unaware of the appropriate treatment options during the initial phase of the emergency response. In addition, poor initial documentation of patients' clinical status, inadequate laboratory sampling, and incomplete epidemiologic studies further limited longer-term relief initiatives and exposure studies.[27,28] Unfortunately, such deficiencies in emergency response activities for technological disasters are widespread in both developed and less-developed countries.[21]

An effective response to disasters such as Bhopal requires the development of a comprehensive and effective local strategy to manage the risk of disasters. It is a collaborative process that requires cooperation between government agencies, private organizations, and the community. Key objectives of disaster planning include the clarification of the capabilities, roles, and responsibilities of the agencies involved and the strengthening of emergency networks. Public health response considerations should be incorporated into local, regional, state, and national disaster plans to ensure the health of populations at risk. For technological disasters, such considerations will include rapid assessment, community notification, mass decontamination, mass vaccination or other medical management, evacuation procedures, and public health surveillance. Disaster plans, including the public health components, should be tested regularly in exercises to evaluate their effectiveness, train personnel, and improve the overall emergency response. Activities to assess and mitigate local risks should be integrated into a program of ongoing disaster management.

During domestic disasters, the US military provides important support as part of the National Disaster Medical System (see Chapter 46, Domestic Disaster Response: FEMA and Other Governmental Organizations).[29] The United States has a well-developed Federal Disaster Response Plan, in which public health professionals play a key role. This system is supported by the involvement of 26 federal agencies, including the Department of Defense, the Department of Veterans Affairs, the Federal Emergency Management Agency, and the Department of Health and Human Services. Unfortunately, many developing countries lack these resources for national disaster response. Within the United Nations system, a number of agencies and organizations may be able to assist such countries following a technological disaster by providing important technical information and services. Some of these agencies are listed in Exhibit 44-1. Military medical officers may need to coordinate relief operations with these organizations within contingency situations involving civilian populations.

As part of their responsibility to protect populations from the effects of industrial disasters, public health professionals should facilitate communication between local clinical services (eg, hospitals,

---

EXHIBIT 44-1

UNITED NATIONS ORGANIZATIONS OR PROGRAMS THAT MAY PROVIDE ASSISTANCE FOLLOWING TECHNOLOGICAL DISASTERS

Food and Agricultural Organization

Industrial Development Organization

International Labour Organization

International Programme for Chemical Safety

United Nations Environment Programme

World Health Organization

World Meteorological Organization

---

ambulance services), occupational health professionals at the industrial site, and members of the surrounding community.[30] Other technological disaster mitigation activities for public health officials and preventive medicine officers may include the following: (a) establishing warning systems to alert nearby communities of a toxic agent release, (b) determining minimal threshold concentrations of toxic chemicals, biological agents, or radiation that would require the community to evacuate in the event of a release, (c) coordinating evacuation activities following a hazardous release, (d) coordinating medical care and appropriate referral destinations for patients exposed to hazardous materials, and (e) ensuring the appropriate collection and laboratory analysis of specimens.[6,8]

ASSESSMENTS OF PUBLIC HEALTH AFTER A TECHNOLOGICAL DISASTER

Following the release of a chemical or radiological agent, the adverse health effects associated with that agent may appear rapidly within the population, focusing early attention by health authorities on the task of identifying the responsible toxin or toxins. Public health mitigation procedures, such as evacuation, sheltering in place, and decontamination, can often be initiated quickly, in some cases even without precise knowledge of the hazard. The health effects of other technological disasters, however, may present more insidiously. For example, an infectious disease outbreak secondary to the accidental or deliberate release of a biological agent may be detected only after an unusual infection or clinical presentation has been diagnosed by a phy-

sician or identified by routine surveillance activities or an epidemiologic investigation.[4,31]

At other times, it may be unclear if a disease outbreak is due to a chemical or a biological agent. For example, a 1996 disease outbreak in Haiti characterized by fever and renal failure in children was initially believed to be caused by an infectious agent.[32] However, the cause of these deaths was ultimately determined to be poisoning by di-ethylene glycol–contaminated paracetamol, which had been used to control fever in children.[33] The final diagnosis and subsequent public health interventions may have been delayed because of the lack of consideration of a toxic agent. The important lesson learned was the need to consider from the outset the possibility that a chemical or other toxic agent may be responsible for any unusual epidemic. Public health personnel use assessment tools to evaluate the situation and gain the knowledge they will need to make appropriate decisions.

In an emergency, public health assessments of the affected population are used to determine the nature and magnitude of the emergency, the extent or risk of injury to the population, the availability of local resources, and the need for external resources to mitigate the adverse health effects. Several methods of data collection are used during the rapid assessment, including a review of data available through local and government sources, a visual inspection of the affected area, interviews with key informants, and, occasionally, rapid surveys. Results of a well-conducted rapid assessment can be used to formulate public health recommendations and to determine appropriate patient care, such as evacuation, mass decontamination, and administration of antidotes. Established epidemiologic methods used to investigate public health emergencies in a community can be adapted to provide rapid assessment of populations exposed to nuclear, chemical, and biological agents.[34,35] Key operational assessment issues follow.

Obtaining an Accurate History

During the emergency response to a population affected by a technological disaster, the need to rapidly obtain an accurate history of the unfolding disaster cannot be overemphasized. This information should include a review of the type of agent or agents released; clinical presentations; existing laboratory data (eg, human, animal, environmental); and how chemical, biological, or radiological agents were detected or confirmed in the community. These data assist greatly in quickly determining the need for emergency public health interventions, such as evacuation, sheltering in place, pharmacological prophylaxis, or treatment. Often, a basic estimate, such as the number of people killed or ill, is sufficient basis on which public health officials can estimate the magnitude of the event, organize the initial assessments, and determine emergency response options. This information may also alert responders of the need to deploy specialized laboratory equipment and technical teams and to coordinate the transfer of hazardous samples to reference laboratories. After the initial assessment, regular surveillance measures should be instituted and are discussed later in this chapter.

Determining Appropriate Levels of Personal Protective Equipment

Regardless of the cause of the disaster, responders working in a contaminated area, or "hot zone," will require personal protective equipment to protect their skin, eyes, and airways. In most developed countries, occupational guidelines exist to protect workers in stable workplaces from environmental and infectious exposures. When faced with a rapidly unfolding emergency caused by an unknown chemical, biological, or radiological hazard, it is necessary to ensure that responders have the appropriate protective equipment and training.[36] Limitations of physical performance and sensory input due to this equipment can be extreme and require consideration during the planning and coordination process of any assessment mission. Emergency personnel required to wear protection equipment may also be at risk of certain physical and psychological stresses, including dehydration, heat exhaustion, and claustrophobia.

Assessing Clinical Presentations

Some clinical syndromes associated with human exposure to certain biological, chemical, and radiological agents may suggest a specific etiology long before confirmatory laboratory tests are completed. A case definition describing the key clinical and other diagnostic features of an environmental illness or injury should be established early. It may be modified later as more information becomes available. Confirming an increase in the incidence or prevalence or both of a disease or environmental illness may be problematic without baseline public health surveillance information. Some events (eg, an outbreak of pulmonary anthrax, or a case of smallpox) are so unusual, however, as to overwhelmingly suggest the presence of a nonnatural event, such as biological terrorism.

Laboratory Evaluation of the Affected Population

Biological specimens from victims (eg, blood, hair, urine, skin) may be required to determine the type of environmental exposure. Portable monitoring and analytical instruments may assist with the identification and quantification of human exposure from environmental hazards under field conditions. Coordination of the safe and efficient transfer of human samples from the field to appropriate reference laboratories is a key component of the emergency response activities following a technological disaster. This may require cold chain technology to maintain refrigeration or consideration of chain of custody issues as part of an ongoing criminal investigation.

Laboratory Evaluation of the Environment

Specimens of air, water, soil, and munitions should be taken for laboratory analysis. In addition to the identity of the agent, the following information will be important for the public health assessment and response: the quantity of the agent released, the method of its release, the time and location of its release, whether the release is continuing, the prevailing weather conditions, and the location of citizens at risk.[37] In the setting of a chemical, infectious, or nuclear plume, such information can be combined with information from other databases (eg, regional maps, population census) to provide a computer model of the likely path of the plume and an estimate of the population at risk.[38]

Analyzing Data

Data collected from field investigations should be rapidly analyzed to provide information on affected persons and the characteristics of their illnesses. Clinical and laboratory data may be used to refine case definitions further. Information related to the timing of the onset of illness helps investigators detect trends in incidence or prevalence rates. In dealing with the exposure of the population to an unidentified environmental or infectious agent, it may be useful to plot epidemic curves, to compare attack rates in cases and controls, or to represent cases graphically on maps. The information derived from these exercises may help determine a possible etiological agent, other risk factors for the illness, the source of exposure, and the mechanism of exposure. Timely and accurate analysis of the data may help in the rapid development of rational public health and clinical recommendations. Regular surveillance should be instituted as soon as possible to provide reliable information about the changing situation and the effectiveness of interventions.

SURVEILLANCE

Public health surveillance has been described as the ongoing, systematic collection, analysis, and interpretation of important health data.[39] In general, these data are used in planning, implementing, and evaluating public health programs. Following a technological disaster, however, surveillance data can be used to estimate the magnitude of adverse health outcomes, identify groups at increased risk of adverse outcomes, detect epidemics or smaller outbreaks, evaluate public health interventions, and identify research needs.[40]

Surveillance activities usually begin as soon as immediate life-threatening conditions (eg, fire, explosions, chemical spills, plumes) are controlled and after contaminated patients have received appropriate emergency care.[41] In an infectious disease emergency, increased surveillance may be a component of the initial operational public health response to the epidemic. Appropriate surveillance following a technological disaster requires active pursuit of important public health information, such as the collection of clinical data from workers, emergency responders, and community members; the abstraction of information from treatment facilities; the evaluation of medical examiner reports for cause-of-death information; and a review of laboratory results from clinical and technical facilities.[42–44]

Surveillance tasks for health officers also include the institution of disease and injury registries to follow exposed individuals for the appearance of illness or injury over time. Such registries facilitate the recognition of adverse health effects within an exposed population and will suggest directions for long-term population-based studies.[45] For example, victims exposed to radiation may require follow-up for many years to detect complications such as thyroid cancer.[46,47] Individuals from populations sustaining chemical exposures may not present with clinical illness for many years. Table 44-2 lists a number of chemicals that have known late-presenting health effects.[48] In addition to medical illness, psychological complications such as post-traumatic stress disorder, depression, anxiety, somatization, and alcohol abuse have been documented following technological disasters.[8,22,49] Mental health surveillance and outreach programs may be useful in identifying psychological trauma among survivors of and emergency responders to technological disasters.[49] As the situation unfolds and more surveillance data become available, more extensive epidemiologic studies may be undertaken; some of the methods commonly used are discussed below.

TABLE 44-2

EXAMPLES OF LONG-TERM MEDICAL CONSEQUENCES AFTER EXPOSURE TO SELECTED CHEMICALS

Category	Example	Agent
Carcinogenic	Liver cancer	Vinyl chloride
Teratogenic	Cerebral palsy syndrome	Organic mercury
Immunological	Abnormal lymphocyte function	Polybrominated biphenyls
Neurological	Distal motor neuropathy	Triorthocresyl phosphate
Pulmonary	Parenchymal damage	Methyl isocyanate
Hepatic	Porphyria cutanea tarda	Hexochlorobenzene
Dermatological	Chloracne	Polychlorinated biphenyls

Sources: (1) Baxter PJ. Review of major chemical incidents and their medical management. In: Murray V, ed. *Major Chemical Disasters— Medical Aspects of Management*. International Congress and Symposium Series No. 155. London: Royal Society of Medicine Services Limited, 1990: 7–20. (2) Douidar SM, Shaver CS, Snodgrass WR. Hepatotoxicity from hazardous chemicals. In: Sullivan JB, Krieger GR, eds. *Hazardous Materials Toxicology, Clinical Principles of Environmental Health*. Baltimore: Williams & Wilkins, 1992: 109–123. (3) Shields PG, Whysner JA, Chase KH. Polychlorinated biphenyls and other polyhalogenated aromatic hydrocarbons. In: Sullivan JB, Krieger GR, eds. *Hazardous Materials Toxicology, Clinical Principles of Environmental Health*. Baltimore: Williams & Wilkins, 1992: 748–755.

EPIDEMIOLOGIC STUDIES

It is estimated that a complete hazard assessment is available for less than 7% of the most widely used chemical substances,[48] but well-conducted environmental epidemiologic studies can help elucidate adverse health effects following exposures. Case-control studies are useful when the disease or injury is rare. Finding appropriate controls may be difficult, though, when years have passed since the exposure or when confounding influences, such as smoking and increasing age, are present. Case series reports are also useful if there is a limited number of patients but may not be as representative of the effect being studied as better designed studies. In addition, exposure levels may be difficult or impossible to estimate in both case-control and case series studies. Consequently, such studies may not present convincing evidence that a specific chemical exposure is associated with a particular adverse health outcome. Cross-sectional studies may provide an estimate of disease prevalence, but the incidence of a medical condition following an environmental exposure cannot be determined. Cohort studies, while limited in their value when the adverse health outcome under investigation is relatively rare, may be extremely helpful when focusing on high-risk populations such as victims or emergency responders.[50]

One of the major challenges of epidemiologic studies following a technological disaster is quantifying levels of exposure within the population and the environment. Postdeployment epidemiologic investigations of US service members following the Persian Gulf War were hampered by the fact that investigators were often unable to determine preexposure levels of certain toxins or chemicals within the deployed populations. In addition, during the investigation of "agent smoke," the general name given to the byproducts of the burning oil wells in Kuwait that may have contributed to illness among service members, many of the potentially offending chemicals under investigation were volatile organic compounds that are rapidly eliminated from the body. Therefore, any blood samples used to determine serum levels of these compounds would primarily reflect exposure from the preceding day. Exposures at other times may have been significantly higher or lower and would not have been documented by such a sampling methodology.[51]

The difficulties in establishing accurate exposure histories highlight the potential benefit of early involvement of laboratory and epidemiologic services with specialized environmental or toxicological capabilities in protecting service members' health. Baseline toxicological exposure information, such as that derived from physical examinations, serological tests, and mental health screening among those deployed to areas where serious environmental exposures might be encountered, is now being collected on a trial basis during selected deployments. Factors to consider when attempting to quantify a person's or population's level of exposure following a technological disaster include the onset of exposure, the duration of exposure, the route of exposure (eg, inhalation, ingestion, contact with the skin), and in some cases the distance from the source of the release.[52,53]

PUBLIC HEALTH RESPONSE TO TERRORISM

Recent events have demonstrated that in addition to conventional weapons, terrorists now have access to chemical, biological, and, perhaps, radiological materials.[17,18,31,54–57] The sarin vapor release on March 29, 1995, in Tokyo highlighted the insidious nature of terrorism in an urban center using a weapon of mass destruction capable of harming tens of thousands of citizens. Members of the Aum Shinrikyo religious sect coordinated multiple releases of the nerve agent within the city's subway system.[17] The US medical delegation dispatched to Tokyo from the Centers for Disease Control and Prevention (CDC) determined that more than 5,000 people were affected, 12 of whom ultimately died.[58] Although the overall response by the Japanese emergency services was commendable, a number of deficiencies were recognized. These related to assessment issues, the use of personal protective equipment by prehospital and hospital personnel, and therapeutic strategies. Areas identified as needing better planning for the mitigation of the health consequences of such terrorist chemical releases are listed in Exhibit 44-2. Many of these points parallel those from disaster management recommendations for dealing with other, more common hazardous materials.

Consequence management in the health sector refers to those activities designed to control and mitigate the harmful health effects of terrorism on the population. Public health approaches to emergency management, such as evacuation and mass vaccination, become increasingly important when terrorists use the technology of destruction to threaten whole communities. Preparedness for terrorist attacks using weapons of mass destruction has become an important focus for both health professionals and security forces.[31,55,56]

Operational tasks for preventive medicine officers after a chemical, biological, or radiological release include instituting measures to reduce exposures within the population and measures to mitigate the effects of known exposures. Measures to reduce exposure include the use of a public warning and information system to inform the community about the nature of the problem and the actions they can take to protect themselves (eg, retreat to sealed rooms, evacuate, use gas masks).[38,54] Potential means of notifying the public include sirens, loud speakers, radio, television, and door-to-door home visits. Potential mitigation procedures include mass decontamination, vaccination, medical prophylaxis, distribution and use of antidotes, and development of medical treatment strategies.[17,18,38]

During some disasters, the deployment of specialized medical or laboratory teams in operational support of civilian populations may be required. Although the Ebola hemorrhagic fever outbreak in Zaire in 1994 is thought not to have been the result of terrorism, the event exposed some of the limitations in the civilian medical sector's ability to respond to technological disasters involving biological agents. Such limitations included difficulties in fielding a proper containment laboratory, coordinating medical logistics, and evacuating relief workers who contract the virus. Interagency cooperation between the CDC and components of the Department of Defense (eg, the US Army Medical Research Institute of Infectious Diseases) mitigated some of these

---

EXHIBIT 44-2

IMPORTANT EMERGENCY RESPONSE PLANNING ISSUES THAT WERE IDENTIFIED FOLLOWING THE SARIN VAPOR RELEASE IN TOKYO, 1995

Chemical agent detection

Toxicological information dissemination

Environmental epidemiology

Personal protective equipment training

Decontamination procedures training

Emergency medical services enhancement

Source: Lillibridge SR. Sarin vapor attack on the Japanese subway system: Report of the US Medical Delegation to Japan. Atlanta: Centers for Disease Control and Prevention; April 1995. Trip Report.

TABLE 44-3

ASSESSMENT UNITS COLLOCATED AT THE SCIENCE AND TECHNOLOGY CENTER, ATLANTA, GEORGIA, DURING THE 1996 OLYMPICS

Type of Assessment	Assessment Unit
Biological Assessment	Centers for Disease Control and Prevention[*]
	Environmental Protection Agency[*]
	Food and Drug Administration[*]
	Navy Medical Research Institute
Chemical Assessment	Agency for Toxic Substances and Disease Registry[*]
	Centers for Disease Control and Prevention[*]
	Environmental Protection Agency[*]
	US Army Research and Materiel Command Treaty Verification Laboratory
	US Coast Guard Atlantic Strike Force
Radiological Assessment	Centers for Disease Control and Prevention[*]
	Environmental Protection Agency[*]
	Food and Drug Administration[*]

[*]Selected technical staff, or laboratories, or both

deficiencies and contributed to successful management of the emergency public health issues associated with the Ebola outbreak. In addition, US military health personnel were successfully integrated into the World Health Organization and the CDC outbreak investigation teams, providing important epidemiologic, laboratory, and technical support.

During the 1996 Olympics in Atlanta, the multidisciplinary Science and Technology Center was established to manage the public health consequences of an act of terrorism involving weapons of mass destruction.[59] The Center, which was located at the CDC, was charged with coordinating rapid assessment and public guidance in the event of a terrorist attack with a nuclear, chemical, or biological agent. Multiple federal agencies and components of the Department of Defense were collocated at the Science and Technology Center (Table 44-3). Personnel and assets from other federal agencies, such as the Department of Energy, the US Marine Corps Chemical Biological Incident Response Force (CBIRF), the US Army Medical Research Institute of Infectious Diseases, the US Army Medical Research Institute for Chemical Disease, and the US Army Technical Escort Unit, were staged throughout Atlanta to support the overall federal emergency response to a terrorist incident. Coordination of all federal assets was organized through the Federal Bureau of Investigation as the lead US agency in combating terrorism. Military medical personnel provided the critical liaison between the civilian medical community and the military tactical response units that had been deployed in support of health consequence management.

The experience in Atlanta demonstrated that an all-hazards approach to rapid assessment involving chemical, biological, or radiological terrorism and to the development of public health recommendations requires significant planning and interagency coordination. Activities that required daily review included appropriate collection of samples, procedures for alerting the civilian population, appropriate routing of specimens to reference laboratories, rapid development of public health advice following an event, and development of the method by which agencies would report their results to an appropriate coordination point of the lead agency.

SUMMARY

Technological disasters, whether caused by accidents or terrorism, are becoming increasingly common,[5,60] and the environmental or infectious consequences of these events may not stop at the borders of the nation immediately affected.[47] Urgent preventive medicine responsibilities associated with technological disasters include rapidly assessing and quantifying chemical and radiological exposure levels and, given the new developments related to the potential for biological terrorism, detecting infectious disease outbreaks within the population.[4] These investigations may require skills from many allied health fields, such as pathology, laboratory science, toxicology, and environmental and occupational health. No single civilian institution or military unit offers the range of skills and equipment required to mitigate the adverse health effects in service members, as well as in civilian populations. Recent events have shown that the need for organizational collaboration will likely increase, if not become indispensable, as new and complex technical threats are identified.

REFERENCES

1. Lillibridge SR, Noji EK, Burkle FM Jr. Disaster assessment: the emergency health evaluation of a population affected by a disaster. *Ann Emerg Med.* 1993;22:1715–1720.

2. Perrin P. Training medical personnel: HELP and SOS course. *Intl Rev Red Cross.* 1994;284:505–512.

3. Sanderson LM. Toxicologic disasters: natural and technologic. In: Sullivan JB, Krieger GR, eds. *Hazardous Materials Toxicology: Clinical Principles of Environmental Health.* Baltimore: Williams and Wilkins, 1992: 326–331.

4. Meselson M, Guillemin J, Hugh-Jones M, et al. The Sverdlovsk anthrax outbreak of 1979. *Science.* 1994;266: 1202–1208.

5. Glickman TS, Golding D, Silversman ED. Acts of god and acts of man—recent trends in natural disasters and major industrial accidents. Washington, DC: Center for Risk Management, Resources for the Future; 1992. CRM92–02.

6. Lillibridge SR. Industrial disasters. In: EK Noji, ed. *Public Health Consequences of Disasters.* New York: Oxford University Press, 1997: 354–372.

7. Williams D. Chernobyl, eight years on. *Nature.* 1994;371:556.

8. Mehta PS, Mehta AS, Mehta SJ, Makhijani AB. Bhopal tragedy's health effects: a review of methyl isocyanate toxicity. *JAMA.* 1990;264:2781–2787.

9. Hamit HF. Primary blast injuries. *Ind Med Surg.* 1973;42:14–21.

10. Manchee RJ, Broster MG, Melling J, Henstridge RM, Stagg AJ. *Bacillus anthracis* on Gruinard Island. *Nature.* 1981;294:254–255.

11. Manchee RJ, Broster MG, Anderson IS, Henstridge RM, Melling J. Decontamination of *Bacillus anthracis* on Gruinard Island? *Nature.* 1983;303:239–240.

12. Centers for Disease Control. Preliminary report: 2,3,7,8-tetrachlorodibenzo-p-dioxin exposure to humans—Seveso, Italy. *MMWR.* 1988;37:733–736.

13. Centers for Disease Control. Follow-up on toxic pneumonia—Spain. *MMWR.* 1981;30:436–438.

14. Andersson N. Technological disasters—towards a preventive strategy: a review. *Trop Doct.* 1991;21(suppl 1):70–81.

15. Straight MJ, Kipen HM, Vogt RF, Maler RW. *Immune Function Test Batteries for Use in Environmental Health Field Studies.* Atlanta: Agency for Toxic Substances and Disease Registry, 1994.

16. Laqueur W. Postmodern terrorism. *Foreign Affairs.* 1996;September/October:24–36.

17. Okumura T, Takasu N, Ishimatsu S, et al. Report on 640 victims of the Tokyo subway sarin attack. *Ann Emerg Med.* 1996;28:129–135.

18. Sidell FR. Chemical agent terrorism. *Ann Emerg Med.* 1996;28:223–224.

19. Mobley JA. Biological warfare in the twentieth century: lessons from the past, challenges for the future. *Mil Med.* 1995;160:547–553.

20. Sidel VW. Weapons of mass destruction: the greatest threat to public health. *JAMA.* 1989;262:680–682.

21. Lillibridge SR, Burkle FM, Waeckerle J, et al. Disaster medicine: current assessment and blueprint for the future. *Acad Emerg Med.* 1995;2:1068–1076.

22. Le Claire G. *Environmental Emergencies—A Review of Emergencies and Disasters Involving Hazardous Substances over the Past 10 Years.* Vol 1. Geneva: United Nations Environmental Programme, United Nations Centre for Urgent Environmental Assistance; 1993. Report.

23. International Federation of the Red Cross and Red Crescent Societies. *World Disaster Report 1993.* Norwell, Mass: Kluwe Academic Publishers; 1993: 48.

24. Noji EK. Public health challenges in technological disaster situations. *Arch Pub Health.* 1992;50:99–104.

25. Lillibridge SR, Noji EK. Industrial preparedness, Bombay, India: World Environmental Center—Centers for Disease Control and Prevention Emergency preparedness visit of March 1993. Atlanta: Centers For Disease Control and Prevention; 1993. Trip Report.

26. Bhopal Working Group. The public health implications of the Bhopal disaster. *Am J Public Health.* 1987;77:230–236.

27. Andersson N. Disaster epidemiology: lessons from Bhopal. In: Murray V, ed. *Major Chemical Disasters—Medical Aspects of Management.* London: Royal Society of Medicine Services Limited, 1990: 183–195. International Congress and Symposium Series No. 155.

28. Koplan JP, Falk H, Green G. Public health lessons from the Bhopal chemical disaster. *JAMA.* 1990;264:2795–2796. Erratum published in *JAMA.* 1991;265:869.

29. Federal Emergency Management Agency. *The Federal Response Plan.* Washington, DC: FEMA; 1997.

30. Leonard RB, Calabro JL, Noji EK, Leviton RH. SARA (Superfund Amendments and Reauthorization Act), Title III: implications for emergency physicians. *Ann Emerg Med.* 1989;18:1212–1216.

31. Stephenson J. Confronting a biological Armageddon: experts tackle prospect of bioterrorism. *JAMA.* 1996;276:349–351.

32. Selanikio J. Personal communication, 1997.

33. Centers for Disease Control and Prevention. Fatalities associated with ingestion of diethylene glycol-contaminated glycerin used to manufacture acetaminophen syrup—Haiti, November 1995–June 1996. *MMWR.* 1996;45:649–650.

34. Barss P. Epidemic field investigation as applied to allegations of chemical, biological or toxin warfare. *Politics and Life Sciences.* 1992;February:5–22.

35. Willems JL. Difficulties in verifying the use of chemical weapons and the implications: some brief case studies. *Physicians for Social Responsibility Quarterly.* 1991;1:201–206.

36. National Institute for Occupational Safety Health, Occupational Safety and Health Administration, US Coast Guard, Environmental Protection Agency. *Occupational Safety and Health Guidance Manual for Hazardous Waste Site Activities.* Washington, DC: Dept of Health and Human Services; 1985. NIOSH Publication No. 85-115.

37. Leffingwell SS. Public health aspects of chemical warfare agents. In: Somani SM, ed. *Chemical Warfare Agents.* San Diego: Academic Press, 1992: Appendix I.

38. Borak J, Callan M, Abbot W. *Hazardous Materials Exposure: Emergency Response and Patient Care.* Englewood Cliffs, NJ: Prentice-Hall, 1991.

39. Thacker SB, Berkelman RL. Public health surveillance in the United States. *Epidemiol Rev.* 1988;10:164–190.

40. Wetterhall SF, Noji EK. Surveillance and epidemiology. In: Noji EK, ed. *The Public Health Consequences of Disasters.* New York: Oxford University Press, 1997: 37–64.

41. Falk H. Industrial/chemical disasters: medical care, public health and epidemiology in the acute phase. In: Bourdeau P, Green G, eds. *Methods for Assessing and Reducing Injury from Chemical Accidents.* Chichester, Great Britain: John Wiley and Sons; 1989: 105–114.

42. Glass RI, Noji EK. Epidemiologic surveillance following disasters. In: Halperin WE, Baker E. *Textbook of Public Health Surveillance.* New York: Van Nostrand Reinhold; 1992: 195–205.

43. Baron RC, Etzel RA, Sanderson LM. Surveillance for adverse health effects following a chemical release in West Virginia. *Disasters.* 1988;12:356–365.

44. Parrish RG, Falk H, Melius JM. 1987 industrial disasters: classification, investigation and prevention. *Recent Advances in Occupational Health.* 1987;3:155–168.

45. Dhara VR, Kriebel D. The Bhopal gas disaster: it's not too late for sound epidemiology. *Arch Environ Health.* 1993;48:436–437.

46. Henshaw DL. Chernobyl 10 years on. *BMJ.* 1996:312;1052–1053.

47. Balter M. Children become the first victims of fallout. *Science.* 1996:272;357–360.

48. Baxter PJ. Review of major chemical incidents and their medical management. In: Murray V, ed. *Major Chemical Disasters—Medical Aspects of Management.* London: Royal Society of Medicine Services Limited, 1990: 7–20. International Congress and Symposium Series No. 155.

49. Gerrity ET, Flynn BW. Mental health consequences of disasters. In: Noji EK, ed. *The Public Health Consequences of Disasters.* New York: Oxford University Press; 1997: 101–121.

50. Piantadosi S. Epidemiology and principles of surveillance regarding toxic hazards in the environment. In: Sullivan JB, Krieger GR, eds. *Hazardous Materials Toxicology: Clinical Principles of Environmental Health.* Baltimore: Williams and Wilkins, 1992: 61–64.

51. Etzel RA, Ashley DL. Volatile organic compounds in the blood of persons in Kuwait during the oil fires. *Int Arch Occup Environ Health.* 1994;66:125–129.

52. Centers for Disease Control. Dermatitis among workers cleaning the Sacramento River after a chemical spill—California. *MMWR.* 1991;40:825.

53. Agency for Toxic Substances and Disease Registry. *ATSDR Public Health Assessment Guidance Manual.* Chelsea, Mich: Lewis Publishers; 1992: 2.1–2.8.

54. Goldsmith JR. Prevention, gas masks, and sealed rooms: a public health perspective. *Public Health Rev.* 1992–93;20:342–346.

55. Goldsmith MF. Preparing for the medical consequences of terrorism. *JAMA.* 1996;275:1713–1714.

56. Freeh LJ. Statement before the House Committee on International Relations. Hearings on Russian organized crime. April 30, 1996.

57. Bentura S. "Chechen leader threatens Moscow with nuclear terrorism." Agence France Presses English Wire Service. November 8, 1991.

58. Lillibridge SR. Sarin vapor attack on the Japanese subway system: report of the US Medical Delegation to Japan. Atlanta: Centers for Disease Control and Prevention; April 1995. Trip Report.

59. Ember L. FBI takes lead in developing counterterrorism effort. *ChemEngineering News*. November 4, 1996: 10–16.

60. Inside the mind of the terrorist. *The National Times*. 1996; August:10–13.

Chapter 45

THE INTERNATIONAL HUMANITARIAN RESPONSE SYSTEM AND THE US MILITARY

ANDREW S. NATSIOS, MPA

A.S. Natsios, *Lieutenant Colonel, US Army Reserve (Retired); Administrator, US Agency for International Development, Ronald Reagan Building, Washington, DC 20523-1000*

This chapter is adapted from: Natsios AS. The international humanitarian response system. *Parameters*. Spring 1995:68–81. © Copyright 1995 by Andrew S. Natsios.

INTRODUCTION

The chaos spreading through many countries in the developing world has drawn together an unusual, sometimes incompatible, assortment of organizations to respond to these multiplying crises. Each year from 1978 to 1985 saw an average of five complex humanitarian emergencies, the term used in the disaster discipline for these crises (see Chapter 43, Complex Emergencies); by contrast, there were 17 in 1992, 20 in 1993, and 25 in 1997. The increase in these emergencies appears to be one of the few clear patterns in the post–Cold War world.

Virtually the entire international emergency response system is a post–World War II phenomenon; part of it was in its infancy but most of it was not even conceived of at the time of the Marshall Plan. For those who work in the relief discipline, it seems a small miracle that the existing system works as well as it does, given the conflicting mandates of the responding organizations, the enormous complexity of the problems addressed, and the organizational incongruities that have emerged in the years since the United States helped Europe recover from World War II.

This chapter examines the existing humanitarian response system—made up of private voluntary organizations (PVOs), the International Committee of the Red Cross (ICRC), and United Nations (UN) agencies—through which the international community responds to these emergencies. Understanding the cultures and operational habits of this triad of organizations and the manner in which each interacts with the others is crucial for anyone who tries to work with them but particularly for military personnel. A civilian US government agency, the Office of Foreign Disaster Assistance (OFDA) in the US Agency for International Development (USAID), coordinates US responses to foreign disasters and so is another major participant in these efforts. Examples of how the US military has fit into this complex system are taken from missions in the 1990s.

PRIVATE VOLUNTARY ORGANIZATIONS AND THE US MILITARY

What is known in the United States as a PVO is known in Europe and the rest of the world as a nongovernmental organization. A PVO is a private, nonprofit organization that specializes in humanitarian relief and development work in the Third World and, increasingly, in formerly communist countries. American PVOs employ more than 100,000 people in developing countries. In 1996, they received $4.8 billion in private revenue and $1.4 billion in public revenue from USAID.[1] They communicate with the public through newsletters and magazines whose aggregate circulation is in the millions.

Most American PVOs, although private by charter, accept grants of federal money from the USAID. For a PVO to remain eligible to receive such grants or food aid, it must by law raise at least 20% of its total income from private sources. While the proportion of a PVO's income from the US government, whether in the form of cash grants or food aid, varies according to its corporate strategy, some PVOs raise so little private funding that they are dangerously close to this 20% limit. A few PVOs accept no USAID money so they can maintain their distance from the government, whose policies they find objectionable.

The PVO suspicion of US government influence extends to the military as well. When President Bush ordered US military forces to Kurdistan in June 1991, several PVOs, particularly European ones, refused to cooperate with them. Kurdistan became a seminal experience for American PVOs as it showed them that they could work together productively with US forces in a humanitarian emergency, something that even organizations not opposed to close association with the military had doubted.

To paraphrase management expert Chester Barnard, the US military and American PVOs are unalike in every important way.[2] Indeed, it is difficult to imagine two more dissimilar cultures. The military is highly disciplined, hierarchical, politically and culturally conservative, and tough; it has a mission to defeat the enemy. American PVOs are generally independent, resistant to authority, politically and culturally liberal (with the exception of some Christian PVOs), and sensitive and understanding; they have a mission to save lives. Because military missions tend to be explicit and tangible, the military sometimes fails to appreciate all the subtleties of humanitarian mission statements, where objectives can be implicit and intangible.

PROFILE OF THE PRIVATE VOLUNTARY ORGANIZATION CULTURE

Goals and Personnel

All PVOs have ideologies and missions based, to some degree, on each organization's private donor base and institutional history. Many are firmly on the ideological left, others are more centrist, still others are on the right. PVO comfort levels in working with the US military decline as one moves from right to left on that spectrum. Nearly all PVOs share a devotion to the concept of sustainable development in any country or region in which they operate. They share an aversion to quick fixes, which they believe military operations tend to emphasize. Their own painful experiences through 4 decades in the field have taught them that real development is a slow, difficult process. One political value all PVOs share is a robust internationalism; there are no isolationists in these organizations.

PVOs tend to recruit former Peace Corps workers, religiously committed activists in the faith-based PVOs, and young people with graduate degrees in development economics and public health. Most get the bulk of their operational training on the job; there are few equivalents to military doctrine or field manuals to describe how a particular program is to be run. Where PVO doctrine does exist, it is developed from generally shared experiences and responses, is seldom written down, and is not always followed uniformly. Field experience in the culture of PVOs is comparable to combat experience in the military: a badge of honor, accorded the highest respect.

Types

PVOs are a diverse group and may be divided into those that attempt to influence public policy and remain focused on advocacy work and those that manage projects in the field and remain focused on operational issues. Most large PVOs do both because they have realized that thoughtless or pernicious behavior (whether government policy, donor attitudes, or developing country demands) can quickly undo generally well-conceived and well-implemented community development work.

Advocacy and operational groups both have their weaknesses. PVOs that only advocate tend to have a limited understanding of field realities in the developing world. They tend to be governed by ideological preconceptions rather than pragmatic appraisals of what works. PVOs that exclusively operate in the field can go only so far in criticizing public policy before their workers and programs are threatened by government officials intolerant of criticism.

Some PVOs specialize by sector, such as health, education, or economic development. A few do only relief work, others only development. Some do both, particularly the larger PVOs, such as the three largest in the United States: Care, Catholic Relief Services, and World Vision. Since the Ethiopian famine of 1985, a body of scholarship has developed suggesting that well-conceived relief work should be designed with developmental components and that good development work should include disaster prevention and mitigation measures to reduce the need for relief in disaster-prone areas. Agricultural development programs in drought-prone areas, for example, should include drought-resistant crop varieties and water conservation measures.[3]

Although most PVOs of US origin employ indigenous staff to manage their programs, some remain Western in their leadership, culture, and standards. In most developing countries, there is an array of indigenously organized and managed PVOs that do relief and development work, sometimes forming partnerships with Western PVOs to meet common objectives. While many of these indigenous groups run fine programs, some are suspect in their operational capacity, professionalism, and accountability. Their reputation, good or bad, usually precedes them.

The assumption that Western PVOs can be trusted and Third World PVOs cannot is both unfair and simplistic. Such an assumption, all too easy to make during planning, can endanger a mission if it is used to support operational decisions. In Somalia in the early 1990s, the UN and, before it, the United States gave short shrift to Somali PVOs, with unfortunate consequences. When the battle was joined with General Aideed, Somali PVOs might have rallied support for the international presence in the country. Instead, the UN received little help from the more responsible elements of Somali society that were represented by local PVOs.

Funding Pressures

The fundraising imperative, which provides insight into their sometimes curious behavior, operates to some degree in all PVOs. PVOs must communicate with the American people, either through electronic media or direct mail solicitation, to raise funds. Income increases significantly when paid advertisements are combined with coverage of the PVO's work on national television and radio news programs. The more dramatic and heart-wrenching the scenes and reports of disaster in the developing world, the more income PVOs can expect from their solicitations. As well, the donors to the PVOs expect to see public recognition of their role in media reports of the success of "their" PVO.

In spite of their nonprofit nature, PVOs need to compete—less so than private businesses, perhaps, but compete they must. The quality of their field programs affects their capacity to win government grants, and their public visibility affects their private contributions. The interest of PVOs in telling their stories to the news media is not so much a case of large ego (though that is sometimes there, too) as it is of survival. US government personnel who take public credit for a response to a complex emergency must understand that PVOs find that annoying; an organization's financial health can be affected by military or other government public affairs announcements. Conversely, a carefully tailored series of such announcements, emphasizing the teamwork involved in success, would go a long way to reassuring many PVOs, their workers, and their donors that young Americans, in and out of uniform, were together helping those in need.

Chain of Command

PVOs have chains of command just as the military does; the chains are not as disciplined or explicit, though, and they inevitably contribute to tensions between the PVO field staff and the central staff at headquarters. Differing policy or operational concepts within the same PVO usually occur because each level in the hierarchy responds to a different agenda and a different set of pressures. Headquarters considers donor concerns, budget limitations, and the worldwide institutional consequences of a given policy. The field staff focus on the human need in a particular village, where they struggle daily to overcome operational difficulties and chaotic work-

ing conditions so they can alleviate suffering and save lives.

Security Issues

PVOs will likely already be anywhere in the world where a humanitarian crisis exists when US or other military forces arrive and will generally be there when military forces depart. (Kurdistan in 1991, which did not have any PVOs, was an exception to this rule.) Military action can create animosity in the indigenous population that will eventually affect the PVOs, who have little or no security and so are very vulnerable when conflict erupts. The PVOs can be perceived at worst as Western or at best as foreigners from the same tribe or clan that produced the troops. The World Vision headquarters in Baidoa, Somalia, was bombed in February 1994 by a Somali militia leader annoyed with UN peacekeepers over an issue unrelated to World Vision policies or operations. And in an example of why PVOs are suspicious of military efforts, when the staff injured in the bombing needed UN peacekeeper help to get to a medical facility, the help was late and hesitant.

PVOs do not rely on guards (whom they seldom employ) or on weapons (which they virtually never carry themselves) for their security. They rely on two aspects of their culture to keep them safe from violence. The first is the importance of the work they do for the community. Even after Somalis as a group had turned violently against the UN presence in Somalia, they continued to request expansion of foreign PVO programs in their country. The second is their perceived nonpartisanship. Many PVOs find it difficult to remain neutral in conflicts that are inherently political (eg, the Cambodian or Rwandan genocides), but it is essential to their security in such conflicts. So when military forces, whether under the flag of the UN or the United States, are perceived to be supporting one side in a conflict, PVOs are at increased risk of violence.[4]

INTERNATIONAL COMMITTEE OF THE RED CROSS

The ICRC, founded in 1863, is by far the oldest humanitarian relief organization. It is also the largest such organization, with 6,300 employees worldwide and a budget of $608 million in 1993.[5] It specializes in conflicts and it and UN Office of the High Commissioner for Refugees are the only relief organizations with a mandate under international law, a fact which ICRC's managers, called delegates, frequently cite. Of all humanitarian in-

stitutions, it is the most doctrinally developed. It has an elaborate system of rules for functioning in conflicts, which work well most of the time and which its delegates can recite in their sleep.

While the ICRC is part of the International Red Cross movement, it has a tenuous and sometimes acrimonious relationship with the International Federation of Red Cross and Red Crescent Societies, the "United Nations" of the Red Cross national offices. The ICRC, the Federation, and the UN agencies described later in this chapter are international organizations; they are not PVOs.

Mission

The ICRC is the most focused international aid organization, using its authority under the Geneva Conventions to gain access to the vulnerable in conflicts where other relief agencies have difficulty. It does no development work—a strength in that its mission is clearly focused and a weakness in that it does not address root causes of an emergency. Its focus is on family reunification, delivery of messages between family members separated by a conflict, protection of civilians and prisoners of war, and humanitarian relief for those most severely affected. It is the most expensive relief organization, given the high cost of living of its largely Swiss staff and the cost of the high standards it sets. It is the only organization primarily funded through annual contributions from donor governments and national Red Cross and Red Crescent Societies; those funding sources relieve it of the requirement to solicit funds from the public (although it does some modest fundraising among the Swiss public). The US government for many years has been by far its largest donor.

How It Operates

The ICRC's impressive performance in chaotic situations may have less to do with its age, budget, size, and doctrine and more to do with the fact that it is run by the Swiss, whose culture values both discipline and order. An ICRC program is fairly predictable programmatically and in terms of quality wherever it is to be found, a claim that few PVOs or UN agencies can make. Little is left to chance or human discretion in ICRC operations. Conflicts by their nature are chaotic; consequently, any organization that can impose a modest degree of order in a conflict has an immediate operational advantage. The ICRC is the relief organization with the most in common with the military; it is also the one least likely to have much to do with the military. This apparent paradox can be traced to its operating doctrine, which calls for absolute political neutrality in all conflicts. ICRC doctrine places a premium on voluntary adherence to international law by contestants. The very presence of peacemaking forces with an aggressive mandate means ICRC persuasion has been replaced by armed force, even if that

force operates under the UN banner. Only on direct order from ICRC headquarters will delegates even converse with any military force, let alone work with them.

The ICRC will not work in a conflict unless both sides agree in writing to complete transparency in standard operating procedures. This means in practice that all sides of the conflict will get prior notice of each relief flight and each convoy, including travel routes, cargo descriptions, and times of departure and arrival. In Somalia it also meant getting approval from the clan elders for each region in which the ICRC operated. Indeed, until Somalia the ICRC never employed armed guards or drove in convoys protected by military forces. In fact, it was doctrinal heresy for the ICRC to use force to protect its operations and to work closely with the military. The change was caused by the chaos in the countryside rather than a deliberate change in ICRC doctrine.

The Red Cross symbol appears on every vehicle, building, and piece of equipment the ICRC employs, not so much for its public relations value (though it does not hurt), but because in conflicts this symbol has become associated with the neutrality provided for in the Geneva Conventions. The ICRC's desire to protect this symbol led at one point to an extended debate with US representatives over whether the US flag or the Red Cross would appear on US Air Force planes delivering ICRC relief food—donated by the US government and the European Community—to famine-ravaged Somali cities during Operation Restore Hope in 1992 and 1993. The Red Cross won.

Staff

The ICRC was until the early 1990s entirely staffed by Swiss nationals. It has served in some respects as their version of the US Peace Corps, an outlet for the altruistic and adventurous instincts of Swiss youth that is also open to older people. The pathological levels of violence encountered at various times in the post–Cold War world, however, have dramatically increased the fatality rate of ICRC delegates, as well as the psychological problems of staff traumatized by the atrocities they sometimes witness. The Liberian civil war reached such brutal levels in 1992 and 1994 that the ICRC withdrew twice and several delegates required psychiatric hospitalization. These conditions have caused fewer young Swiss to volunteer, and, for the first time in its 150-year history, the ICRC has resorted to hiring non-Swiss staff.

THE UNITED NATIONS

Some in the disaster relief community blame the UN for most failed responses to complex humanitarian emergencies. While some of this blame is properly directed, much is not. The UN has been held accountable for work it was not staffed to do until the mid-1990s. It has also been held responsible for some work it will never be able to perform, given two different realities: its nature as an institution and the fact that the permanent members of the Security Council and many developing countries do not want it to be involved in certain types of interventions.

Organizational Structure

The UN is not one institution, centrally managed, with a hierarchical organizational structure. The UN General Assembly and Security Council together resemble the US Congress, with the Secretary General representing the Speaker of the House more than the President. The Secretary General presides rather than rules.

Four nearly autonomous UN agencies provide most of the operational support and services required to respond to a complex humanitarian relief situation. They also are voluntary agencies; countries are not assessed fees for their operation but instead contribute what they wish. The four agencies are the United Nations Office of the High Commissioner for Refugees (UNHCR), which has responsibility for refugees and, in practice, for internally displaced people; the World Food Program (WFP), which provides food for people affected by droughts and civil wars and for UNHCR-mandated refugee camps; the United Nations Children's Fund (UNICEF), which specializes in medical, educational, and job training support for women and children; and the United Nations Development Program (UNDP), which has responsibility for development assistance, usually through country governments. In addition, the Office for the Coordination of Humanitarian Affairs (OCHA), part of the Secretary General's staff, conducts the negotiations needed to bring humanitarian support through conflict lines and provides a modicum of coordination among the four UN agencies, to the extent that any of the four UN agencies wishes to be coordinated. It is one of the great ironies of the UN system that its least important and badly run work is supported by assessment, while its better work is funded voluntarily through these agencies. A half dozen other

UN agencies claim an operational role, but they are more modest players.

The four agencies, resembling feudal barons, only nominally report to the Secretary General. They are in fact quite independent of the Secretary General and of each other, obtaining their resources and political support from donor countries whose representatives sit on their independent governing boards. All assiduously cultivate their bases of political support in their home countries. While the Secretary General has a hand in appointing the leaders of each of these agencies, few have ever been removed by the Secretary, nor does the Secretary control their budgets, staffing, or policy. Until 1994, they did not report to the General Assembly in any managerially significant way, nor did they get policy guidance from it. In Somalia, the field directors of these agencies reported to their headquarters in New York, not to the director of UN humanitarian operations located in Somalia. The UN Security Council in 1994 approved a little-noticed but significant managerial reform of the governance of UN specialized agencies. Under the reforms, the Economic and Social Council of the UN has budget and policy review authority over all specialized agencies, the first time such authority and oversight has been vested in a membership body of the UN.

Humanitarian Relief Operations

These four UN agencies had little operational capacity in the 1980s but instead provided money to the governments of developing countries to do the work through indigenous government ministries. UNHCR's refugee camps in many countries were managed through the ministries of the host government or under grant agreement with PVOs. It is only since the end of the Cold War and the rise of the complex emergency as a painful fact of international life that the agencies have hired staff with operational skills and experience. The quality remains uneven in 1997, the depth limited.

These UN agencies have used four models for coordinating humanitarian relief operations with varying degrees of success. In the first model, the Secretary General assigns leadership in a particular disaster to one of the four agencies. In Bosnia (1992-present) it has been UNHCR, in the southern African drought (1992) it was the World Food Program, and in Sudan (1989-present) and Kurdistan it has been UNICEF. The second model, successfully employed in Angola (1992-1996), vests leadership in OCHA.

The third model, used in Somalia from 1992 to 1994, had no lead agency. Instead, the UN Secretary General, Boutros Boutros-Ghali, created a new, hybrid entity not tied to any of the UN agencies. The UN military, political, and humanitarian section heads reported to the Special Representative of the Secretary General, who reported directly to the Secretary General. The Somalia experience suggests that this last model, however much preferred by the Secretary General, is unmanageable. The Secretary General and his staff were incapable of centrally supporting extended field operations in Somalia. The procurement, personnel, contracting, and budgeting systems of the four UN agencies, however weak, are greatly superior to those of the UN Secretariat in New York.

The fourth model was the norm before 1989. Seldom followed now except in smaller natural disasters, it called for the country director of UNDP to act as the chief UN officer in any country affected by a major disaster. UNDP's lack of experience and interest in complex emergencies has made this traditional model inefficient.

Constraints on Reform

All of the models reflect the vagaries of UN personnel policy, which mixes skilled and dedicated career international bureaucrats with friends of those whose votes in the General Assembly or on governing boards are important to the agency bureaucrats. The size of this latter group is debatable, but it is certainly not representative of the average operational UN staff in the specialized agencies. Within the UN as a whole, though, there is no functional personnel system, there are no career ladders, and promotions based on merit are not the norm. The newer, operationally skilled employees are too often contractors with limited career opportunities. The personnel system still reflects the much less rigorous demands of an earlier era, when the permanent members of the Security Council did not want a robust UN system. It is arguable whether this situation has much changed in the 1990s.

Because of the institutional weaknesses of the position of the Secretary General and the feudal structure of the UN system, humanitarian emergency activities, ranging from routine coordination to development of comprehensive and integrated strategy, are difficult to plan and implement. In late

1990, led by the Nordic bloc nations and supported by the United States, donor countries proposed and the General Assembly approved reforms that created the OCHA, which is managed by one of 17 Under Secretaries General. But the role that OCHA can play in complex emergencies is affected by its limited statutory authority and the byzantine bureaucratic politics of the UN system.

Developing countries were quite unenthusiastic about the reforms that created OCHA and strengthened the UN's operational capacity in complex emergencies: some of their governments were causing the problems that the reforms were meant to address. Third World elites and intellectuals suspected that the OCHA reforms would advance the case for humanitarian interventionism, which some of them perceived to be a form of Western neocolonialism masquerading as altruism. They feared that the changes promised to unleash meddling, do-gooder PVOs and donor aid agencies whose roots are sometimes found in the colonial affairs offices of contributing countries. The protection of national sovereignty in nation-states with weak national identities, some of which govern using police-state tactics, is a central concern in these states' policy formation processes. Indeed, the issue of sovereignty threatens the very foundation of states. Consequently, to secure approval of the OCHA reforms, the reformers diluted the language of the resolution to ensure OCHA had no independent authority to intervene in a nation-state, even if for humanitarian reasons. Given its real mandate, OCHA has done reasonably well, particularly as it has matured organizationally, but its work reflects modest incremental improvements to the old system, not breakthroughs in innovative organization or management.

The UN will always be held hostage to some degree by the governments it serves. In its assessments of impending famines, for example, crop estimates are heavily influenced by local ministries of agriculture, whose estimates are sometimes politicized and frequently suspect. The agricultural production figures used to judge food aid requirements for the southern African drought in 1992 were based on such estimates, most of which turned out to be significantly overstated. The effect of the distortion was a significant overcommitment of food aid in Mozambique. In 1990 the Bashir government in Sudan refused to acknowledge a massive drought during its critical early months. When the government finally did report drought conditions, under intense international pressure, it overestimated food requirements. When the UN promptly publicized the Sudanese numbers, its credibility suffered.

Even with the UN's institutional weaknesses, however, the international community needs the UN when responding to a humanitarian crisis. No sovereign state alone has the UN's legal and moral sanction to intervene, its coordinating authority, its peacekeeping troops (however constrained by their home governments), its diplomatic good offices, and its financial and staff resources.

DONOR-GOVERNMENT AID AGENCIES

The final component of this complex system is represented by donor-government aid agencies. In the United States, that function is fulfilled by the OFDA in USAID. OFDA is charged under the Foreign Assistance Act of 1961 with coordinating all US government assistance in foreign disasters. It operates under a unique and jealously guarded provision of law—the so-called "notwithstanding" provision. This allows OFDA to act quickly in a disaster situation, notwithstanding many of the procedural, administrative, and bureaucratic requirements of the federal government and irrespective of other policy measures restricting US assistance to particular countries (eg, sanctions against military aid, economic support funds, or development assistance). Because it is exempt from prohibitions on US government assistance to certain countries, OFDA can provide life-saving relief assistance to people suffering the effects of natural or man-made disasters anywhere that the State Department has declared a disaster. OFDA, with expenditures of approximately $190 million a year and a staff of 25 regular and 25 contract employees, has a simple, focused mission: save lives and reduce human suffering through relief and rehabilitation interventions.[6] It is not authorized to do development or reconstruction work.

OFDA projects itself into disasters either indirectly, through grants to PVOs, the ICRC, or UN agencies, or through direct operational intervention using its Disaster Assistance Response Teams (DART). These teams have the authority to spend money in the field, and with their satellite telephone capacity, they can order additional staff, equipment, and logistical capacity from the OFDA office in Washington. Their daily situation reports to USAID and State Department leadership can shape US policy. Early in the Kurdish emergency, for example, the only reports that the Secretary of State and the Deputy Secretary of State received on what was actually happening in the field were situation reports from OFDA.

Because of their technical expertise in relief, rapid contracting capacity, and long experience in emergencies and in giving grants to other actors, OFDA officers have influence that, even if unofficial, extends throughout the response system. OFDA is perhaps the only element of the international humanitarian relief system that can call meetings, get quarreling groups to work together, and draft strategic plans that other organizations will take seriously. Frequently when the UN is either not present in the field or its contracting mechanisms are too slow, OFDA will fill the gap and hand operations over to the UN later. In 1993, the European Community created an office modeled after OFDA, the European Community Humanitarian Office (ECHO), that attempts to provide them with a similar operational capacity in emergencies.

WORKING TOGETHER

The relief response institutions—the PVOs, ICRC, and UN, in conjunction with OFDA and ECHO—make up the system used by the international community to respond to complex humanitarian emergencies. The challenge in the system is that many of the institutional players do not like or trust one another. The PVOs quarrel quietly among themselves and publicly with the UN. The UN does not often deal with the ICRC, which keeps to itself and protects its prerogatives. Much of this distrust is understandable. It results from the ambiguous or overlapping organizational mandates; the stresses of working in combat where relief workers are regularly kidnapped, wounded, or killed; the competition for scarce private or donor-government resources; the lack of experience in dealing with each other; and the turf issues over geographic and sectoral (eg, food security, health, sanitation) focus.

Fortunately, coordination and cooperation are improving rather than declining as the humanitarian relief system matures. In spite of its decentralized character, the system does function, though it is more effective when competent and skillful leaders manage the response in the field. Experience in the early 1990s suggests, not surprisingly, that the quality of this leadership can profoundly affect the competence with which the relief response is managed and whether it ultimately succeeds or fails. As in most organizations, leadership does make a difference.

How well this humanitarian response system works with military forces in peacekeeping operations, whether or not the forces operate under the UN banner, is determined by the quality of military and civilian leadership and the leaders' familiarity with the humanitarian response structure. The only part of the US military force structure prepared by doctrine, training, experience, and personnel recruitment policy to deal with these organizations is the Civil Affairs Branch of the Army. Unfortunately, commanders and military planners often include a civil affairs function in a humanitarian relief operation only as an afterthought, if at all. Both PVO and UN managers have repeatedly commented how well they could work with US forces if they could deal with civil affairs officers instead of combat commanders.

Civil Affairs

The greatest strength of the civil affairs organization is also its greatest weakness, that except for a small, overextended, active duty battalion at Ft. Bragg, NC, all civil affairs assets are in the Army's reserve components. The strength derives from the recruitment of professionals in the civilian world who generally are not found in the active force; these specialists readily understand civilian humanitarian agencies. The weakness lies in their reserve status and in the low opinion that some individuals in the active force have of the reserves. Interservice rivalry in Somalia aggravated the already-present friction between the active and reserve forces and tended to weaken the US relief effort.

The way in which civil affairs units were employed in the Persian Gulf War and in Somalia was counterproductive in the former instance and nearly catastrophic in the latter. In Rwanda, Haiti, and Bosnia, the US humanitarian assistance effort included a robust civil affairs component, which reduced incidents significantly and increased contacts of the military with the civilian population. The requirement for civil affairs units in all humanitarian operations is becoming more apparent, so much so that commanders could be judged negligent if they fail to integrate them into operational plans. In a complex humanitarian emergency, a civil affairs unit is a powerful force multiplier; in a UN peacekeeping operation, a civil affairs company could be worth an infantry battalion.

Who Is in Charge?

Perhaps the most consistently difficult lesson for US military forces to learn is that unlike their role in combat, they are not in charge of managing the response to a complex humanitarian emergency. US forces in Europe, apparently unfamiliar with the disaster relief discipline, attempted to write an operations plan for Kurdistan that was impractical and slowly paced. Once commanders were directed to let field staff from USAID take the lead with the ICRC and PVOs (the UN had not yet arrived), the situation improved.

The unfortunate reality is that usually no one is in charge in a complex humanitarian emergency, a situation which is unlikely to change in the foreseeable future. The notion that if any institution is in charge it should be the UN is by no means universally acknowledged among relief responders. It would also be challenged within the UN by agencies that do not want their rivals in the system to be in charge if they can not be. UN performance up to the mid-1990s has not matched its mandate, and, until it does, the UN cannot assume an undisputed leadership position in disaster relief operations. When the military, which is trained to deal with chaos, steps in to fill this vacuum, it can be perceived to be usurping the prerogatives of other agencies. Training and practice in humanitarian operations with PVOs and UN agencies can overcome such misperceptions.

The Military's Capabilities

The two most important capabilities the military brings to any emergency response remain logistics and security; these are areas in which relief organizations can never match the military's expertise but find they increasingly need during complex emergencies. When the military focuses on what it does best, it serves well; when it is required to do nation-building and development, complex disciplines about which it knows relatively little, it can do more harm than good.

The military must learn to live and work with the other humanitarian actors described in this chapter. The US military now finds itself committed to a doctrine of cooperative engagement with humanitarian agencies in which the military contributes three key proficiencies: security; logistics; and limited, temporary assistance in providing food, water, and medicine when humanitarian organizations are unable to cope with a life-threatening emergency event. The military should not attempt to replace or dominate humanitarian organizations, nor should it be directed to undertake nation-building activities. Projects such as port and road reconstruction, which the military sometimes undertakes as part of its own transportation requirement, should be of short duration and sustainable without its ongoing attention.

SUMMARY

A reasonable person might conclude that there will be more, rather than fewer, humanitarian relief operations in the years ahead. The planner's paradox is that no single source of support in such operations—the PVOs, ICRC, UN, or national assistance offices—is organized, trained, or equipped to perform all of the functions necessary to relieve human suffering in complex emergencies. With military forces in the asset pool, many more capabilities become available to overcome suffering. Success in such operations will be determined by the degree to which all of the players can step outside of their individual cultures and value systems, surrender some of their autonomy, and seek the best in those with whom they must solve the problems of a complex humanitarian emergency. Planning, training, exercises, application of operational lessons learned—all these can contribute to improved understanding and eventually improved execution of relief responses when millions of lives may be at risk.

REFERENCES

1. US Agency for International Development, Bureau for Humanitarian Response, Private and Voluntary Cooperation. *Report of American Voluntary Agencies Engaged in Overseas Relief and Development Registered with the U.S. Agency for International Development.* Washington, DC: USAID; 6.

2. Chester Barnard. *The Functions of the Executive.* Cambridge, Mass: Harvard University Press; 1968.

3. *Rising from the Ashes: Development Strategies in Times of Disasters* Boulder, Colorado, and Paris: Westview and UNESCO Press; 1989.

4. International Federation of the Red Cross. *Code of Conduct for the International Red Cross and Red Crescent Movement and NGOs in Disaster Relief.* Geneva: IFRC; 1994.

5. International Committee of the Red Cross. *International Committee of the Red Cross Annual Report 1993.* Geneva: ICRC; 273, 277.

6. US Agency for International Development, Office of Foreign Disaster Assistance. *Office of Foreign Disaster Assistance Annual Report for Fiscal Year 1993.* Washington DC: OFDA; 1994: 57.

Chapter 46

DOMESTIC DISASTER RESPONSE: FEMA AND OTHER GOVERNMENTAL ORGANIZATIONS

Kevin S. Yeskey, MD, FACEP

K.S. Yeskey, *Captain, US Public Health Service; Director, Office of Emergency Preparedness and Response, US Department of Homeland Security, Washington, DC 20528*

INTRODUCTION

The United States has been and remains susceptible to natural and technologic disasters. Hurricanes, earthquakes, floods, and tornadoes have caused significant loss of life and property damage. Accidents involving hazardous materials occur with regularity, causing evacuation of populations and exposure to victims. As coastal regions and areas surrounding flood plains and fault lines become more populous, the risk of large-scale injury and death increases.[1] Additionally, the threat of widespread release of hazardous materials, accidentally or intentionally, remains significant. The US federal government, through its various departments and their respective agencies, is responsible for providing assistance to state and local governments in their response to disasters. The Federal Response Plan (FRP) is the means by which the government assigns agency responsibility for the various components of the disaster response.[2] The National Disaster Medical System (NDMS), a component of the FRP, has been created to direct the medical response to domestic disasters. It is important that military medical personnel understand their role in this intricate yet immense system because they have played a successful part in many recent domestic disasters and so will probably be called on again.

EVOLUTION OF DOMESTIC DISASTER RESPONSE

Historically, domestic disaster response has been fragmented and uncoordinated.[3] Federal agencies were not integrated into an overall national system of response. The Defense Production Act of 1950 authorized the President to establish performance priorities and allocate resources to promote the national defense. In the 1960s, local civil defense organizations were the primary means of managing the aftermaths of disasters. Volunteer organizations, mainly the American Red Cross, augmented the local response by running temporary shelters and providing food.

The Civilian–Military Contingency Hospital System was developed in 1980 by the Department of Defense (DoD) in recognition of the possibility that large numbers of casualties from an overseas conflict could overwhelm the military's hospital capacity. This system utilized volunteer private hospitals that promised inpatient beds to back up the combined medical systems of the DoD and the Veterans Administration. Although the system was never deployed, it served as the model for the NDMS.

In 1979, the Federal Emergency Management Agency (FEMA) was established to develop a national plan for responding to a catastrophic domestic disaster. FEMA was also tasked with providing a mechanism for the continuity of government in the event of a domestic nuclear strike. But as the Cold War ended in the late 1980s, FEMA's emphasis was shifted from continuity of government toward the coordination of the federal government's response to domestic disasters. In 1981, the Emergency Preparedness Mobilization Board was created to establish policy and programs to improve the nation's preparedness for a catastrophic disaster. One of the key laws guiding the government response is the Robert T. Stafford Disaster Relief and Emergency Assistance Act (Public Law 93-288, as amended), which allows the federal government to respond to disasters by giving assistance and protecting the public health, safety, and property.

THE FEDERAL EMERGENCY MANAGEMENT AGENCY

By executive order (12148, Federal Emergency Management, July 20, 1979), the director of FEMA has the authority and responsibility to coordinate and oversee the federal response during declared disasters. Coordination is provided by FEMA through the FRP in support of agencies at national, regional, and field levels (Figure 46-1). At the initiation of a federal response, the FEMA director appoints a Federal Coordinating Officer (FCO) who assumes command of the overall coordination and allocation of federal resources. The FCO works closely with the officials from the affected states to establish needs and priorities. The FCO ensures that, in accordance with the FRP, federal resources are made available to the state and that the appropriate federal agencies provide those resources. The FCO's responsibilities include administration and logistics, information and planning, response operations, and recovery operations (Figure 46-2).

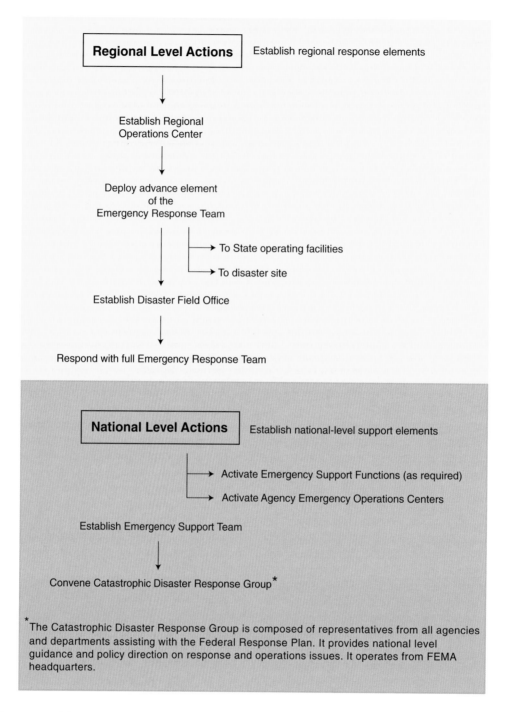

Fig. 46-1. Sequence of Actions Taken To Establish Response Activities on the Regional and National Levels. Source: Federal Emergency Management Agency. *The Federal Response Plan.* Washington DC: FEMA; 1997.

FEMA not only coordinates the response activities but also assists the states before disasters strike. FEMA has training programs for disaster planners and responders to improve the local response capability. FEMA also assists states in the recovery phase of a disaster. Recovery programs within FEMA include Individual Assistance (eg, temporary housing, grants and loans to individuals and businesses), Public Assistance (eg, debris clearance, repair of utilities) and Hazard Mitigation (eg, measures to lessen the impact of future disasters).

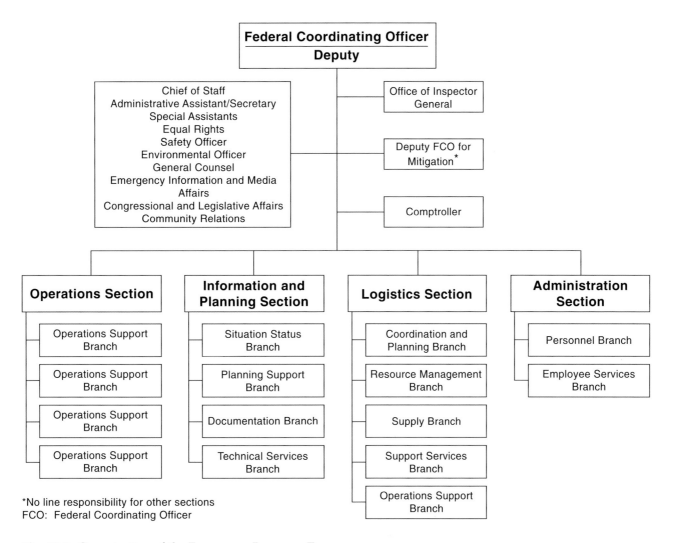

Fig. 46-2. Organization of the Emergency Response Team.
Source: Federal Emergency Management Agency. *The Federal Response Plan.* Washington DC: FEMA; 1997.

THE FEDERAL RESPONSE PLAN

The FRP was developed in 1992 as a means of delineating the federal responsibilities for disaster response under the authorization of the Stafford Act. The FRP has been tested and refined since it was written.[4–8] A variety of natural disasters of significance have resulted in the activation of the FRP since its inception. By incorporating the lessons learned from each disaster, in a relatively short time the FRP has been significantly improved and refined.

Scope

The FRP describes the mechanisms by which the federal government mobilizes its resources to aug-ment state and local disaster response efforts. Through the FRP, federal response is designed to be systematic, coordinated, and effective. The FRP establishes policy, describes a concept of operations for interagency response, assigns and coordinates agency responsibilities based on function, and iden-tifies specific actions to be taken by participating agencies.

The FRP assists in the efforts to save lives, pro-tect public health and safety, and protect property. It does not address recovery assistance, even though this often occurs concurrently with response efforts. In those cases where national security is at risk, the FRP includes national security authorities in the response. The FRP is an "all hazards" plan, meaning that regardless of the nature of the disaster, the FRP uses a single mechanism to respond. The "all hazards" concept increases the odds that the response will be more effective than a separate plan for each type of disaster because of established nature of the federal agency relationships, the ability to activate a response quickly, and the ability to utilize common resources.

There are several assumptions made in the FRP. Foremost is that the FRP will be coordinated with individual state response plans. The FRP will augment the state response, but it is not a substitute for a state plan.[9] It is also understood that components of the FRP will need to be activated quickly and deployed rapidly to minimize morbidity and mortality. If an imminent disaster can be reasonably predicted, advanced deployment of federal assets may be approved. Finally, the federal response requires a rapid needs assessment performed in the immediate postdisaster period. FEMA uses this assessment to coordinate the activation of the Emergency Support Functions (ESFs) and ensure that the response is more directed, effective, and fiscally efficient. All FRP efforts are built on these assumptions.

Terrorism Incident Annex

The Terrorism Incident Annex of the FRP addresses the federal response to a terrorist event within the United States. This annex is based in Presidential Decision Directive 39, which establishes policy to reduce vulnerability to terrorism; respond to terrorist events; and enhance capacity to prevent, detect, and manage the consequences of terrorism. A delineation between crisis management and consequence management is made in the directive. Crisis management is defined in the annex as "measures to identify, acquire, and plan the use of resources needed to anticipate, and/or resolve a threat or act of terrorism"[2] and is the primary responsibility of the federal government. The Department of Justice is the lead federal agency responsible for crisis management, with the Federal Bureau of Investigation responsible for the operational response. Consequence management is referred to as "measures to protect public health and safety, restore essential government services, and provide emergency relief to governments, businesses, and individuals affected by the consequences of terrorism."[2] FEMA is designated as the lead federal agency for consequence management. State and local governments have primary responsibility for this response.

The health and medical components of the consequence management are coordinated through ESF No.

8 and are managed by the Department of Health and Human Services (DHHS). DHHS enhanced its response through the development of Metro-politan Medical Response System (MMRS) teams, which maintain specialized equipment and supplies to perform extrication, decontamination, and initial medical treatment of chemical and biological casualties. The MMRS teams are considered local assets and are available to respond immediately. DHHS has also developed four National Medical Response Teams, which are located regionally and can be rapidly deployed in response to a chemical or biological terrorist event. They can also be predeployed, as needed. These teams provide decontamination and medical management augmentation of local assets.

The DoD has a role in consequence management. In 1999, the DoD established the position of Assistant to the Secretary of Defense for Civil Support as the focal point and coordinator for DoD's consequence management. DoD also created the Joint Task Force-Civil Support (JTF-CS), which is the primary DoD command and control headquarters for domestic consequence management. JTF-CS is designed to respond on-site and provide military support to the lead federal agency and to provide life-and-limb-saving support to local responders.

The National Guard and Reserves also have roles in domestic consequence management. Army and Air National Guard personnel staff 10 Weapons of Mass Destruction Civil Support Teams, which can provide medical and technical assistance to local responders. Each team consists of 22 full-time, specially trained personnel. These teams will perform their mission primarily under the command and control of the state governor (through the adjutant general of the state).

The Federal Radiological Emergency Response Plan

There is a specific federal plan to manage radiological emergencies. The Federal Radiological Emergency Response Plan (FRERP) evolved from perceived inadequacies in federal plans used to respond to the Three Mile Island nuclear power plant accident in 1979. In June 1980, the National Contingency Plan became law, and it outlined a coordinated response by federal agencies to protect the public health and safety in the event of a commercial nuclear power plant accident. In 1982, the Federal Radiological Monitoring and Assessment Plan was developed, and its expanded scope included all radiological emergencies. In 1996, it was replaced by the FRERP.

The FRERP delineates the federal government's response to a peacetime radiological emergency that may have potential or actual consequences within the United States. It provides a concept of operations, outlines relevant policy, and specifies authorities and responsibilities of those federal agencies that may have a role in a radiological emergency. Like the FRP, the FRERP recognizes state, local, and tribal preeminence. The FRERP identifies the Lead Federal Agency (LFA) specific to the type of radiological event. The LFA is responsible for coordination of the federal response. The Department of Energy, DoD, National Aeronautics and Space Administration, Environmental Protection Agency, and Nuclear Regulatory Commission can all be the LFA, depending on the scenario.

The FRERP can be employed without Stafford Act declaration or activation of the FRP. The LFA has overall coordination of the federal response to the emergency, and FEMA will use the FRP to coordinate any nonradiological support. Under a Stafford Act declaration, the LFA coordinates the radiological response while FEMA coordinates the overall federal response to assist the affected state.

Emergency Support Functions

The FRP consists of twelve ESFs, which describe the most likely types of assistance needed. Each ESF is directed by a primary agency and supported by secondary agencies, based on the authority, the resources available, and the capabilities in the functional area. The ESFs are the mechanisms through which federal assistance is directed. It is important to note that ESFs may be activated individually or in limited numbers or in their entirety, based on need. The twelve ESFs and their responsible agencies are listed in the Figure 46-3. Twenty-six federal agencies and the American Red Cross have responsibilities under the ESFs.

IMPLEMENTING THE FEDERAL RESPONSE PLAN

Activation of the FRP begins a sequence of events that ultimately results in federal assistance to the affected area. After a disaster occurs, the state governor must request that the President declare the affected area a federal disaster area. The President, after making the declaration, then assigns the FEMA director as the overall coordinator of the federal response. Various regional and national activities may occur, as is outlined in Figure 46-1. The FEMA director may activate all or part of the plan based on the situational requirements. At the onset of a declared disaster, the FEMA director appoints a federal coordinating officer (FCO). Near the site of the disaster, a disaster field office is established to serve as the primary field office for the FCO, the state emergency manager (or representative), and the ESF representatives. An advance emergency response team is sent by the FEMA regional office to the affected area to perform an initial needs assessment, as well as to provide early on-site coordination of the federal response. In multi-state disasters, this arrangement is repeated in each state.

THE NATIONAL DISASTER MEDICAL SYSTEM

The NDMS was established as the medical component of the federal disaster response.[10,11] It is a joint venture among the DoD, Department of Health and Human Services, Department of Veterans Affairs, and FEMA. The US Public Health Service oversees the NDMS and is responsible for mobilizing medical resources when the system is activated. The NDMS provides medical assistance to disaster areas, evacuates patients from the disaster site, and develops a nationwide network of hospitals to accept patients from a catastrophic disaster.

Disaster Medical Assistance Teams

The essential component of NDMS is the Disaster Medical Assistance Team (DMAT), which is based on the military's medical clearing company.[12] The DMATs are medical teams deployed to perform forward stabilization of casualties, definitive medical care, and evacuation. DMATs consist of volunteer civilian medical professionals organized locally but coordinated through the NDMS. When the NDMS is activated under the FRP, these civilian volunteers become federalized, thus permitting them to practice medicine in any state. Deployed team size ranges from 30 to 50 members, usually with 3 to 5 physicians, 8 to 12 nurses, 5 to 10 emergency medical technicians, 2 to 4 pharmacists, 1 to 2 lab technicians, and 4 to 8 ancillary personnel.[13] Standardized supply and pharmaceutical packages have been developed for the DMATs. There are no organic transportation or security assets within the DMATs. Logistical support for the teams is provided through mission support teams (which are also part of the NDMS), whose purpose is to provide re-supply, equipment, transportation, and communications.

Emergency Support Function / Organization	1 Transportation	2 Communications	3 Public Works and Engineering	4 Firefighting	5 Information and Planning	6 Mass Care	7 Resource Support	8 Health and Medical Services	9 Urban Search and Rescue	10 Hazardous Materials	11 Food	12 Energy
USDA	S	S	S	P	S	S	S	S	S	S	P	S
DOC		S	S	S	S	S	S			S		
DOD	S	S	P	S	S	S	S	S	S	S	S	S
DOEd					S							
DOE	S		S		S		S	S		S		P
DHHS			S		S	S	S	P	S	S	S	
DHUD						S						
DOI		S	S	S	S					S		
DOJ					S			S		S		
DOL			S				S		S	S		
DOS	S									S		S
DOT	P		S		S	S	S	S	S	S	S	S
TREAS	S				S							
VA			S			S	S	S				
AID								S	S			
ARC					S	P		S			S	
EPA			S	S	S			S	S	P	S	
FCC		S										
FEMA	S	S		S	P	S	S	S	P	S	S	
GSA	S	S	S		S	S	P	S	S	S		S
NASA					S							
NCS		P			S		S	S				S
NRC					S					S		S
OPM							S					
SBA					S							
TVA	S		S									S
USPS	S					S		S				

P: Primary agency; responsible for management of the Emergency Support Function
S: Support agency; responsible for supporting the primary agency
USDA: US Department of Agriculture; DOC: Department of Commerce; DOD: Department of Defense; DOEd: Department of Education; DOE: Department of Energy; DHHS: Department of Health and Human Services; DHUD: Department of Housing and Urban Development; DOI: Department of the Interior; DOJ: Department of Justice; DOL: Department of Labor; DOS: Department of State; DOT: Department of Transportation; TREAS: Treasury Department; VA: Department of Veterans Affairs; AID: Agency for International Development; ARC: American Red Cross; EPA: Environmental Protection Agency; FCC: Federal Communications Commission; FEMA: Federal Emergency Management Agency; GSA: General Services Administration; NASA: National Aeronautics and Space Administration; NCS: National Communications System; NRC: Nuclear Regulatory Commission; OPM: Office of Personnel Management; SBA: Small Business Administration; TVA: Tennessee Valley Authority; USPS: US Postal Service

Fig. 46-3. Emergency Support Function Assignment Matrix: Primary and secondary support responsibilities by Agency under the federal response plan.

Medically Related Emergency Support Functions

The medically related ESFs include ESF No. 8, "Health and Medical"; ESF No. 9, "Urban Search and Rescue"; and ESF No. 6, "Mass Care." The scope of responsibilities in ESF No. 8 is listed in the Exhibit 46-1. The US Public Health Service, through its Office of Emergency Preparedness, has primary responsibility for all of the 16 items listed. In addition to managing the acutely injured and ill, another major function of ESF No. 8 is restoring the public health infrastructure. Crucial partners with the Department of Health and Human Services (the parent organization of the US Public Health Service) in the operations of ESF No. 8 are the Centers for Disease Control and Prevention (CDC) and the DMATs. In addition to performing hazards assessment and vector control assistance, the CDC will, on request, provide medical epidemiologists to perform needs assessments and health surveillance during the acute and recovery phases. The DMATs fill the vital role of augmenting patient care in the disaster area. DMATs perform patient triage, resuscitation and stabilization, inpatient care, and patient evacuation. Specialty DMATs also can provide surgical care. Mortuary services and victim identification are provided by Disaster Mortuary Services Teams. Federal health and medical resources are coordinated through the NDMS, which will be discussed in detail later.

Mass Care (ESF No. 6) is coordinated through the American Red Cross. Mass Care encompasses shelter, feeding, disaster welfare information (eg, death notification, help in locating relatives), and distribution of emergency relief items. The American Red Cross personnel may provide emergency first aid to residents of Red Cross temporary shelters, but patients requiring more extensive care will be treated by local medical resources or the DMATs. Because of the relatively crowded living conditions, health surveillance, food safety, and reliable sanitation facilities must be major priorities to prevent disease outbreaks.

Urban Search and Rescue (ESF No. 9) can be activated when victims are trapped in collapsed structures. Urban search and rescue teams maintain medical resources for initial treatment of trapped victims; however, it is expected that these teams will turn over extricated victims to DMATs or to local medical care. Since victims of building collapse are often seriously injured, coordination with other medical services is essential for effective urban search and rescue operations.

EXHIBIT 46-1

SCOPE OF RESPONSIBILITY: EMERGENCY SUPPORT FUNCTION NUMBER 8, HEALTH AND MEDICAL SERVICES

1. Assessment of health and medical needs
2. Health surveillance
3. Medical care personnel
4. Health and medical equipment and supplies
5. Patient evacuation
6. In-hospital care
7. Food, drug, and medical device safety
8. Worker health and safety
9. Radiological hazards
10. Chemical hazards
11. Biological hazards
12. Mental health
13. Public health information
14. Vector control
15. Potable water, wastewater and solid waste disposal
16. Victim identification, mortuary services

Source: Federal Emergency Management Agency. *The Federal Response Plan.* Washington DC: FEMA; 1992.

The Military's Role

The military's role in domestic disaster response is directed through the Secretary of the Army. The Directorate of Military Support is the lead agent for civil emergency relief operations. The DoD Directive 3025.1 "Military Support to Civil Authorities" of 1997 outlines DoD policy on assistance to the civilian sector during disasters and other emergencies. This act limits DoD support to those resources that are not otherwise needed for DoD to conduct its primary defense mission. After a disaster is declared, a Defense Coordinating Officer is appointed to serve in the field as the DoD point of contact for requests of military assistance. The Defense Coordinating Officer should be familiar with DoD assets and how to identify and access such assets quickly. There is no formal training available for this position, but those familiar with logistics and supply are well suited for this assignment. The DoD has an FRP-defined role in all the ESFs. The advantages of military forces detailed by Sharp and colleagues for an international response also apply to a domestic response.[14]

EXAMPLES OF THE SYSTEM AT WORK

The FRP and NDMS have been activated and deployed to respond to a wide variety of situations since 1989, including hurricanes, earthquakes, and floods. The lessons learned from each experience have improved responses to subsequent disasters. The DMAT concept was given its first real challenge in the 1989 Hurricane Hugo response. Two DMATs were deployed to the Virgin Islands to provide care. The military's deployable medical system (DEPMEDS) facility was used as the temporary medical facility. The DEPMEDS facility can provide advanced medical and surgical services and radiological and laboratory diagnostics; it can also support a large number of inpatients in a field setting. Several items of note came from this deployment. The first is that the DMAT concept did work in the austere setting. Military support in the form of security, transportation, and medical evacuation were necessary for the concept's success.[4] The other significant factor in this activation was the time it took to get the DMAT in place. Almost 2 weeks passed before the island government requested assistance and the DMATs were deployed. This resulted in a perceived limitation of the effectiveness in this mission.[4]

Hurricane Andrew was at the time (1992) the most expensive natural disaster to affect the United States. It destroyed or seriously damaged over 75,000 homes and created over 160,000 homeless people with significant increases in medical needs.[7,13] The hurricane affected southern Florida and Louisiana. The FRP had been implemented shortly before Andrew struck, but many were not familiar with the plan. Additionally, activation of the plan was delayed for several days. Criticism of the federal response to Hurricane Andrew was summarized in a General Accounting Office report,[13] which contended that the FRP lacked provisions for postdisaster assessment, did not have the mechanisms in place for timely response, and was unable to provide mass care for such a large-scale event. The GAO concluded that the DoD should be given a larger role in domestic disaster response, that FEMA and other federal agencies should have greater authority in responding, and that state and local governments' capacities to respond should be enhanced.

Three weeks after Hurricane Andrew's landfall in Florida, Hurricane Iniki struck the island of Kauai. DMATs were deployed within 24 hours. Medical teams there noted that, as in other disasters, delivery of basic primary care consumed most of the medical assets.[4–6,15] The General Accounting Office report praised the federal response in Hawaii, primarily for its timeliness, but also for the plan's flexibility in meeting the island's needs.[13]

The 1993 floods in the midwestern United States did not cause a need for acute medical care; however, the magnitude of the flooding and the vast area affected by the floods posed unique problems for the federal responders. Although no DMATs were deployed, members of federal teams worked very closely with state officials and state health departments, assisting them in managing potable water outages, sanitation problems, and other preventive medicine problems. This slow-developing, prolonged disaster permitted local, state, federal, and DoD personnel to work cooperatively and to develop insights into each agency's response capabilities.

The Northridge, Calif, earthquake of 1994 resulted in activation of the FRP. Using the lessons learned from Hurricane Andrew, rapid activation of the FRP provided a timely medical response. Medical assets deployed and provided care with an emphasis on community outreach. Rather than setting up fixed facilities, DMATs remained relatively mobile and went into the affected communities to provide care to those who were unable or unwilling to leave their property and belongings. The timeliness, responsiveness, and flexibility of the response restored credibility to FEMA.

Another significant event has altered the planning of the federal response to disasters. The terrorist bombing of the Alfred P. Murrah Building in Oklahoma City, Okla, in April 1995 has resulted in a far greater emphasis on planning for a domestic terrorist attack. The threat is considered to include conventional weapons, as well as chemical and biological weapons. Plans include mitigation to limit consequences (eg, shatter-resistant windows) and further development of multiple rapid-response teams trained in the management of chemical or biological injuries.

EFFORTS FOR THE FUTURE

Since the inception of a coordinated federal response to domestic disasters, planning has been constantly refined, based on a wide variety of ex-

periences. Despite differences in these disasters, several concepts remain crucial to a federal response. First, local governments and states must be prepared to manage the disaster response until federal assets can be mobilized.[3,9,16,17] The need for training and research on all levels has been articulated.[3,17] The basics of epidemiology, planning, medical response in a disaster setting, and public health are curriculum components that have been suggested.[18,19] This training needs to include uniformed personnel as well.[20] Response time needs to be shortened as much as possible for improved effectiveness. Current national plans include predeployment of assets when the disaster can be reliably predicted.

Many also argue the need for disaster research. Epidemiologic research regarding the types of injuries caused by specific types of disasters may aid in the determination of the response needed.[17,21,22] Specific areas, such as standard methodologies for needs assessments, casualty estimations, and triage, require more research. Burkle and colleagues[23] have developed the concept of "measurements of effectiveness" as a method of assessing the success of a disaster response. They propose that their yardsticks serve as a unifying mechanism for the various components of a disaster response.

SUMMARY

It is clear from experience, in both international and domestic areas, that the US military has many valuable assets necessary for disaster response.[24] Domestically, the military is a major participant in the FRP and has provided outstanding support in recent disaster responses. The expertise provided by the military in the areas of command and control, communications, field operations, logistics, and preventive medicine are in great demand during a domestic disaster.

Activation of the FRP results in a complex series of activities designed to augment the local and state capabilities in times of domestic disasters. Coordination of federal assets is directed by FEMA, and responsibility for providing those assets is delegated to a variety of federal agencies. Field-level coordination is provided by representatives of the ESFs located at local and regional emergency operations centers. The DoD maintains the expertise in the areas of command, control, communications, field operations, logistics, and preventive medicine, all of which are in great demand during a domestic disaster. As a result, the DoD provides support to each of the ESFs. DoD assets are made available through the Directorate of Military Support and then coordinated on a regional level by the Defense Coordinating Officer. Since the issuance of the FRP in 1992, the military has provided outstanding assistance in responding to domestic disasters. Disaster specific training for military personnel has been recommended as a means of improving the military's response capabilities.

REFERENCES

1. Auf der Heide E. *Disaster Response: Principles of Preparation and Coordination.* St. Louis: CV Mosby Company; 1989.

2. Federal Emergency Management Agency. *The Federal Response Plan.* Washington DC: FEMA; 1997.

3. Lillibridge SR, Burkle FM Jr, Waeckerle J, et al. Disaster medicine: current assessment and blueprint for the future. *Acad Emerg Med.* 1995;2:1068–1076.

4. Roth PB, Vogel A, Key G, Hall D, Stockhoff CT. The St Croix disaster and the National Disaster Medical System. *Ann Emerg Med.* 1994;20:391–395.

5. Henderson AK, Lillibridge SR, Salinas C, Graves RW, Roth PB, Noji EK. Disaster Medical Assistance Teams: providing health care to a community struck by Hurricane Iniki. *Ann Emerg Med.* 1994;23:726–730.

6. Alson R, Alexander D, Leonard RB, Stringer LW. Analysis of medical treatment at a field hospital following Hurricane Andrew. *Ann Emerg Med.* 1993;22:1721–1728.

7. Quinn B, Baker R, Pratt J. Hurricane Andrew and a pediatric emergency department. *Ann Emerg Med.* 1994;23:737–741.

8. Lillibridge SR, Conrad K, Stinson N, Noji EK. Haitian mass migration: Uniformed Service medical support, May 1992. *Mil Med.* 1994;159:149–153.

9. Witt JL. National disaster plans crucial; local practitioner readiness essential. *Acad Emerg Med.* 1995;2:1021–1022.

10. Mahoney LE, Reu TP. Catastrophic disasters and the design of disaster medical care systems. *Ann Emerg Med.* 1987;16:1085–1091.

11. Moritsugu, KP, Reutershan, TP. The National Disaster Medical System: a concept in large-scale emergency medical care. *Ann Emerg Med.* 1986;15:1496–1498.

12. Mahoney LE, Whiteside DF, Belue HE, Moritsugu KP, Esch VH. Disaster Medical Assistance Teams. *Ann Emerg Med.* 1987;16:354–358.

13. US General Accounting Office. *Disaster Management Improving the Nation's Response to Catastrophic Disasters.* Washington, DC: GAO; July 1993. GAO/RCED- 93–186.

14. Sharp TW, Yip R, Malone JD. US military forces and emergency international humanitarian assistance: observations and recommendations from three recent missions. *JAMA.* 1994;272:386–390.

15. Yeskey K, Cloonan C. Disaster relief efforts. *Ann Emerg Med.* 1992;21:344. Letter.

16. Waeckerle JF. Disaster planning and response. *N Engl J Med.* 1991;324:815–821.

17. Waeckerle JF, Lillibridge SR, Burkle FM Jr, Noji EK. Disaster medicine: challenges for today. *Ann Emerg Med.* 1994;23(4):715–718.

18. Benson M, Koenig KL, Schultz CH. Disaster triage: START, then SAVE- a new method of dynamic triage for victims of a catastrophic earthquake. *Prehospital Disaster Med.* 1996;11:117–124.

19. Kampen KE, Krohmer JR, Jones JS, Dougherty JK, Bonness RK. In-field extremity amputation: prevalence and protocols in emergency medical services. *Prehospital Disaster Med.* 1996;11:63–66.

20. Lillibridge SR, Burkle FM Jr, Noji EK. Disaster mitigation and humanitarian assistance training for uniformed service medical personnel. *Mil Med.* 1994;159:397–403.

21. Disaster epidemiology. *Lancet.* 1990;336:845–846. Editorial.

22. Binder S, Sanderson LM. The role of the epidemiologist in natural disasters. *Ann Emerg Med.* 1987;16:1081–1084.

23. Burkle FM Jr, McGrady KAW, Newett SL, et al. Complex, humanitarian emergencies: III, measurements of effectiveness. *Prehospital Disaster Med.* 1995;10(1):48–56.

24. Gumby P. Somalia operations just one of many demands on US military medicine. *JAMA.* 1993;269:11–12.

Chapter 47

NUTRITIONAL ASSESSMENT AND NUTRITIONAL NEEDS OF REFUGEE OR DISPLACED POPULATIONS

Patricia A. Deuster, PhD, MPH, LN; Anita Singh, PhD, RD; Peggy P. Jones, MS, RD, LD

P.A. Deuster, Director, Military and Emergency Medicine, Uniformed Services University of the Health Sciences, 4301 Jones Bridge Road, Bethesda, MD 20814

A. Singh, Food and Nutrition Service, US Department of Agriculture, OANE, Room 1014, 3103 Park Center Drive, Alexandria, VA 22302

P.P. Jones, Major, Medical Service, US Army; Nutrition Care Division, General Leonard Wood Army Community Hospital, Fort Leonard Wood, MO 65473

INTRODUCTION

Over 30 million persons are refugees or displaced due to war, civil strife, natural disasters, and other similar events.[1,2] Such social disruptions have the potential to increase morbidity and mortality and, in many cases, require varied relief programs to provide public health assistance.[2] A critical public health issue encountered during such disturbances is a food shortage. Food shortages during conflicts can result from deliberate targeting of local food production and distribution, manipulation of relief supplies, interference by political groups, inadequate organizational controls, destruction of food sources, and other such actions.[3,4] In almost all cases, a direct consequence of food shortages is malnutrition among the targeted population, and children are among the most susceptible to malnutrition and nutritional insults.[1,5–7] All of these issues must be considered when nutritional support is to be provided.

Physicians, epidemiologists, preventive medicine and public health specialists, and nutritionists and dietitians routinely participate in peacetime and war-related humanitarian relief efforts worldwide. Integrated teams of health care providers are required to ensure efficient assessments and rapid implementation of assistance programs. In addition, registered dietitians and nutritionists are key players in humanitarian missions and disaster relief efforts, particularly when an assessment of available food resources and malnutrition prevalence is needed.[8–12]

The US military has both the integrated teams and the experience to assist displaced populations during social disruptions. The military is increasingly called on to render assistance and humanitarian aid during disaster situations, international crises, regional conflicts, and civic assistance programs.[8,9,12–14] Recent efforts by the US military have included disaster assistance after hurricanes and humanitarian aid in Haiti, Panama, Somalia, Bosnia, the Kwajalein Atoll in the Pacific Ocean, the Kurdish homelands in northern Iraq, and Kosovo.[7,8,14–17] For example, following hurricane Marilyn in St. Thomas, Virgin Islands, US servicemembers were deployed for disaster assistance to reestablish patient and personnel feeding in hospitals.[18] In many international humanitarian assistance missions, military personnel have been involved with conducting baseline evaluations and nutritional screenings and assessments, developing emergency food plans, monitoring plans that have been implemented, and monitoring changes in mortality through follow-up surveillance.[8,9] In virtually all assistance efforts, nu-

tritional support has been a major focus, and lessons learned from those efforts can develop into new approaches for future humanitarian missions.

The main objective of nutritional support for refugee or displaced populations is to supply sufficient energy so they can maintain adequate levels of the essential nutrients to sustain life. Timely introduction of nutritional support can make the difference between success and failure of such specialized missions. Humanitarian nutrition-assistance responses are determined by the type and complexity of the emergency and based on an understanding of the resources, socioeconomic characteristics, and specific needs of the population.[19,20] Table 47-1 describes four types of emergencies or conditions wherein nutritional support or assistance may be needed and the characteristics of each.

One of the key reasons for providing nutritional assistance during these emergency situations is the association between nutritional status and mortality.[21] The inseparable link between malnutrition and mortality reflects a nutritionally induced decrease in host resistance that leads to an increased susceptibility to infectious diseases among malnourished individuals. Other factors that may contribute to increased mortality among displaced populations include poor sanitation, poor water quality, increased transmission of infectious disease through crowding, and unexpected environmental changes.[22,23]

When possible, an assessment of the nutritional needs, food habits, and dietary practices of the population is recommended before introducing nutritional support. In all cases, careful planning of how relief activities and nutritional support might be implemented is critical. Despite differences in food choices and dietary practices, which vary throughout the world, the basic nutritional needs of populations are quite similar. Differences in the amounts of specific nutrients needed are primarily due to age, sex, size, physical activity, and physiology. Thus, basic needs as well as specific nutritional needs must be considered when assessing the overall condition in a deployed setting. Initial assessments of the population, to include their nutritional status and the availability of food, are important so that timely interventions can be started. The objective of this chapter is to present an overview of how to assess the nutritional status of a population under conditions of deployment and determine the type and extent of nutritional support required.

TABLE 47-1

CHARACTERISTICS, RESPONSES AND MODES OF RESPONSE FOR FOUR TYPES OF EMERGENCIES.[*]

Emergency Type	Characteristics	Action Needed	Intervention Mode
Rapid Onset	Triggered by a natural event (eg, flood, earthquake, epidemic) or high-intensity war; predictable in some cases; can affect both stable and displaced populations; mass temporary displacement; destruction of public utilities and infrastructure	Meet basic needs (food, water, shelter, and health); reduce mortality and morbidity; control health problems; best done by local governments but may need military assistance	Rapid assessment of acute situation; prioritization of health and nutrition needs; definition of options for intervention; support to health services; establishment of best possible surveillance system to monitor progress
Slow Onset	Triggered by natural disaster (eg, drought, livestock loss from drought) and lasts several years; effect is widespread and variable depending on vulnerability; leads to disposal of assets; migration; increased nutrition and disease burdens on humans and livestock	Meet basic needs (food, water, shelter, and health); reduce impact on production and income losses; improve food security; reestablish livelihood systems, including employment-based safety nets	Assessment of and responses to declining resource base and food insecurity; rapid assessment approaches; prioritization of health and nutrition needs; definition of options; establishment of surveillance to prioritize needs; cross-sectional surveys to establish needs
Permanent Emergencies	Most common; due to socio-economic structural problems that cause poverty; characterized by hunger, environmental stress, and social unrest; migrations; increased nutrition and disease burdens on humans and livestock	Meet basic needs (food, water, shelter, and health); reestablish livelihood systems, including employment-based safety nets	Assessment of and responses to declining resource base and food insecurity; rapid assessment approaches; prioritization of health and nutrition needs; definition of options; establishment of surveillance to prioritize needs; cross-sectional surveys to establish needs
Complex Emergencies	Combination of the above but with an emphasis on civil strife or insecurity that affects the local population, displaced persons, and groups responding to the emergency; affects large populations over large areas; populations may be internally displaced or refugees	Security; basic needs (food, water, shelter, and health); reestablish livelihood systems; human capital development; community capacity building; conflict mediation	Assessment of and responses to declining resource base and food insecurity; rapid assessment approaches; prioritization of health and nutrition needs; definition of options; establishment of surveillance to prioritize needs; cross-sectional surveys to establish needs

[*]In all emergencies, military personnel should seek all available information, get access to nongovernmental organizations, local structures, and government resources; be impartial and work with local experienced staff where possible; provide logistical capacity, communications, and simple standardized epidemiologic procedures; and work to decentralize power. In rapid onset emergencies, personnel must also be ready to provide flexible and short-term planning perspectives.
Adapted from Dept of the Army. *Army Medical Field Feeding Operations*. Washington, DC: DA. FM 8-505. In press.

NUTRITIONAL ASSESSMENT

The nutritional status of a previously well-fed population is likely to remain within normal limits during the first 1 to 2 weeks following an acute food disruption. In situations where conditions continue to deteriorate, a nutritional assessment of the population may be necessary. A general nutritional assessment of the population at risk serves to establish the degree and type of malnutrition present and the requirements for other resources, such as water and sanitation, to relieve the situation. The initial assessment also establishes a baseline for the affected population that can be used for comparison over time in the evaluation process, not only for the nutritional status of the population but also for the impact of various relief efforts. Special attention should be paid to vulnerable groups, including children younger than 5 years of age, pregnant and lactating women, the elderly, and members of specific ethnic or religious groups. These vulnerable groups can also be evaluated over time to determine the impact of various interventions. For example, the United Nations Children's Fund conducted a 3-year prospective study to assess the effects of war and economic sanctions on the nutritional status of children in Baghdad.[1] The percentage of children with mild-to-severe malnutrition increased following the imposition of sanctions before the Persian Gulf War (from 21% pre-war with no sanctions to 29% pre-war with sanctions), and the proportion increased markedly during the war with sanctions (to 43%).

In addition to evaluating specifics of the population, assessing the environment and infrastructure in which the affected population lives is important for identifying underlying problems. Such assessments are useful for determining the origin (if unknown) and severity of the nutritional crises. Identifying social or community institutions and governmental and nongovernmental organizations that may be available to help reestablish the infrastructure is invaluable for establishing assistance responses. Although a nutritional assessment can provide valuable information about the health status of a displaced population, a watchful eye and careful management of potentially disruptive events should be considered, whenever possible, to avert an emergency food crisis.[23]

Both overall and nutritional assessments consist of a two-phase information gathering process that uses interviews, group discussions, observation, and surveys.[5] The first phase is a general evaluation to obtain a global picture of the problem and the need for rapid intervention. This includes determining the reasons for the specific crisis (eg, war, famine, natural disaster), the size and general status of the population, the environmental conditions, the existence and organization of food distribution activities, a crude estimate of available food and resources, and the activities of local or international organizations that can provide assistance. The sec-ond phase encompasses four basic activities: data collection, problem analysis, reporting, and follow-up.[24] Onsite data collection should take place, as well as the collection of background data from officials in the local government, United Nations (UN) agency officials, or relief personnel from other humanitarian agencies. Background data include

- Population demographics, in particular the total refugee or displaced population by age and sex, average family or household size, and at-risk groups (eg, children younger than 5 years of age, pregnant and lactating women, disabled or wounded persons, the sick, the elderly),
- Geographical features of the area,
- Weather and climate patterns,
- Agricultural and economic conditions,
- Health conditions and infectious diseases endemic to the area,
- Ethnic or tribal conflicts
- Types of assistance available from other organizations, and
- Logistical support.[5,21,25]

This information can provide a more comprehensive overview of the situation. Once background information has been gathered, a sample survey should be conducted to determine the specific and immediate nutritional needs of the population. Such a field assessment may be the single most important step in assessing the overall situation; simply observing selected families will not provide a fair estimate. Data collection from field site visits should include the following information: nutritional status of the population; culturally acceptable foods; availability and type of foods consumed; mortality rates and causes; availability of water; availability of wood, cooking utensils, and other necessities for food preparation; shelter; and logistics.

Selecting the Sample and Collecting Data

When a survey is to be conducted and data collected for an estimate of malnutrition, the population must be clearly defined. The data collected during the survey can provide a reasonable estimate of the health and nutritional status of the population of interest. Typically, a survey involves obtaining anthropometric measures on children (usually between 6 and 59.9 months of age) from a sample of families because measures on this age group have been shown to be reflective of the whole population.[24,26] The anthropometric measures obtained can then be compared to a reference or cutoff value to define the degree of malnutrition within the population. If the population is relatively small, with only 400 to 500 children, all children should be evaluated. For larger populations, various sampling procedures can be used. These procedures include simple random sampling, systematic random sampling, and cluster sampling.[27] Random sampling and systematic sampling procedures require a sampling base—either a list of individuals or a geographical organization—that allows each individual or family an equal chance of being surveyed. Cluster sampling is used in larger populations for which only estimates of the number of people are available so the other two methods cannot be used. For cluster sampling, the population is grouped into identifiable units from which a sample estimate may be obtained. For example, clusters could be individual villages or camps. Within each cluster, a predetermined number of children is selected and they are then surveyed. Because children within a cluster tend to have similar nutritional status, the size of the cluster sample must be large enough to override this inherent bias. This is usually accounted for by using a sample size twice that of the systematic random sampling.[5,27] In all cases, the choice of sampling will be determined by the conditions in the field. An example of a data collection form for a cluster sample survey is presented in Figure 47-1.

Although there are many ways to conduct sample surveys, the World Health Organization and Medecins Sans Frontieres have published detailed guidelines for rapid nutritional assessment in the field.[27,28] These publications provide appropriate standards for assorted measures, examples of sampling and sample size determination, approaches to data analysis and interpretation, and discussions on other issues critical to nutritional assessments and humanitarian assistance endeavors. The primary steps include determining the following:

- Basic information on demography, geography, and population to be assessed,
- Index measure to be assessed and whether specific groups need to be evaluated,
- Sampling methods to be used,
- Age groups to be included,
- Sample size,
- Indicators to be used,
- Personnel, equipment, and resources needed,
- Number of people to be evaluated per day,
- Training status of field workers and supervisory controls,

- Standards to be used and data analysis procedures, and
- Responsibility for logistics.

Before conducting an assessment, it should be recognized that anthropometric data alone can be misleading, especially when malnutrition levels are high due to infection or low due to death or emigration. If many of the severely malnourished children have already died or if families with very sick children have been able to leave the area, then the prevalence of acute malnutrition will be underestimated. These are important issues to consider. Certain high-risk groups are more vulnerable to malnutrition and micronutrient deficiencies,[29] so questions should be asked to determine recent changes within these vulnerable subgroups. Familiarity with the clinical diagnosis of classic nutrition-related illness, such as kwashiorkor (a severe form of protein-energy malnutrition), marasmus (wasting from lack of food and protein), xerophthalmia (night blindness caused by vitamin A deficiency), scurvy (vitamin C deficiency), beri-beri (thiamine deficiency), is helpful in determining the duration of a nutritional program. Factors such as the amount and type of foods and animals available and supplies of water and fuel should also be noted. If there have been food shortages for an extended period, many people may already be malnourished and special foods or food programs will be needed to refeed them.

Nutritional Indicators

Children between 6 and 59.9 months of age are the ones on whom anthropometric measures should be obtained for nutritional assessments because of their extreme vulnerability to nutritional insults.[5,27,28] A variety of different anthropometric indexes can be used, but each one has inherent limitations. The most commonly used index for acute malnutrition and recent weight loss in nutritional assessments is the weight-for-height ratio.[15,21,23,26,30,31] Based on numerous population surveys, the weight-for-height measure is the most reliable index of acute malnutrition for famine and emergency situations. The weight-for-height index is indicative of current status, is a good predictor of immediate mortality risk, is sensitive to rapid changes, and can be used for monitoring the course of recovery from malnutrition.[5,15,23,27] However, if edema (the clinical sign of kwashiorkor) is present in a child, then the weight-for-height index should not be used. Edema, typically pitting edema on the upper surface of the foot,

CLUSTER DATA FORM

Cluster N⁰:_____   Village/Section:_____

Date of Survey: ____/____/____   Team Number:_____

First birth date to be included: ____/____/____

Last birth date to be included: ____/____/____

Birth date after which children should be measured standing:____/____/____

N⁰	Birth date	Age in months	Sex 1 = M 0 = F	Weight in kg or g	Height in cm or mm	Edema 1 = Yes 0 = No	MUAC	Other	Other
1	/ /								
2	/ /								
3	/ /								
4	/ /								
5	/ /								
6	/ /								
7	/ /								
8	/ /								
9	/ /								
10	/ /								
11	/ /								
12	/ /								
13	/ /								
14	/ /								
15	/ /								
16	/ /								
17	/ /								
18	/ /								
19	/ /								
20	/ /								

MUAC = mid–upper arm circumference

Fig. 47-1. A Data Collection Form for a Cluster Sample.
Reprinted with permission from: Arbelot A, ed. *Nutrition Guidelines.* Paris: Medecins Sans Frontieres; 1995.

is a major risk factor for mortality in children and is always indicative of severe, acute malnutrition.[32] Thus, the presence of edema should be carefully noted. Basic equipment for gathering weight-for-height index measurements includes a length board, non-stretch tape measures, a 25-kg hanging spring scale, rope, weighing pants, a standard weight (10 kg) to calibrate and check the scale, questionnaires,

---

EXHIBIT 47-1

PROCEDURES FOR EVALUATING MID–UPPER ARM CIRCUMFERENCE

---

1. Seat the child comfortably in the mother's lap

2. Select the child's bare right arm for measurement

3. If the child is not in a shortsleeved shirt, roll the sleeve up; do not measure arm circumference over clothing

4. Let the child's arm hang down loosely with the arm bent at the elbow in a 90° angle

5. Make a mark at a point halfway between the tip of the shoulder (acromial process of the scapula) and the tip of the elbow (olecranon process of the ulna)

6. Draw a horizontal line on the back of the arm 1 cm (0.5 in.) above the midpoint; use a felt-tipped marker

7. Let the child's arm hang down loosely, circle the tape measure around the arm, and pull it snugly but not too tightly

8. Read arm circumference to the nearest 0.1 cm and record reading on the survey form (see Table 47-2)

Adapted from: Intertect. *Assessment Manual for Refugee Emergencies*. Washington, DC: Bureau for Refugee Programs, Dept of State; 1985.

---

data sheets, clipboards, tables, a calculator, a computer, and pencils.[20,27,28] The general method for weighing is to zero the scale daily, place weighing pants on the child, attach the pants to the scale, and suspend the child in the pants from the scales. To measure length, shoes are removed and a child younger than 2 years of age is placed face up on the board with feet flat against the fixed board and head near the movable measuring piece. Children older than 2 years are measured standing, using vertical measuring equipment.[27]

Another index, which has been used frequently when measures of height and weight are not possible, is the mid–upper arm circumference (MUAC). This is the most simple measure and provides a rapid indicator of wasting.[15,21,26,28,30,31] The accessories needed for determining MUAC are a tape measure, data sheets, clipboards, and pencils. Exhibit 47-1 provides a detailed, step-by-step procedure for measuring MUAC. The MUAC is often used when rapid assessments are needed, such as when large numbers of children need to be screened for feeding programs.[15] Although it has been suggested that there is minimal change in the normal arm circumference of children between 6 and 59.9 months of age, the common cutoff (12.5 or 13 cm) can result in an age bias.[23] As such there is not yet agreement on what the definitive cutoff value should be.[15,26,30,31] For this reason and because of the inherent mea-surement error with MUAC, this measure may have limited use in determining the prevalence of malnutrition.

Other measures include the weight-for-age index, which is an index of both chronic and acute malnutrition depending on the age of the child, and the height-for-age index, which reflects chronic malnutrition.[21,26,30,31] With all of these measures, differences between individual measurers can be considerable and these differences can bias the data.

Mortality Information

When possible, crude mortality rates should be calculated because they are critical indicators of health status. The Centers for Disease Control and Prevention recommends calculating a crude mortality rate over a short period of time, usually less than a month.[2,21] If the number of deaths over a given number of days can be determined and the size of the population is known, then a daily crude mortality rate can be estimated. Deaths per 10,000 per day or deaths per 1,000 per month are the preferred rates. Ideally, they are age-, sex-, and cause-specific rates because such measures indicate the need for interventions for specific subgroups. Even a crude estimate can prove helpful. The appropriate denominator must be used, however, and this requires an understanding and accounting of the population dynamics.[15] During a survey, a log of all deaths should be maintained whenever possible, and surveillance systems should be set up in the community to record both recent and new deaths. Death rates are also used as criteria for nutritional interventions by relief agencies, and crude mortality rates are very helpful for tracking changes over time.

Mortality rates for refugees and displaced populations during various stages of a crisis have been reported to have ranged from 2.8 to 21.3 for the Kurds in northern Iraq,[7] from 7.3 to 67.1 in Somalia,[15-17] from 10 to 59 in Rwanda,[33] and from 5.4 to 8.0 in Sudan (all ranges are per 10,000 per day).[2] A crude mortality rate of 0.5 per 10,000 per day is not unusual in African countries during nonemergency times. As such, a crude mortality rate of more than 1 per 10,000 per day or a mortality rate of more than 4 per 10,000 per day in children younger than 5 years old has been suggested to be of extreme concern. When the crude rate falls below 1 per 10,000 per day, this is an indication that the emergency phase is over.[21] Whenever possible, the overall and infant expected (or baseline) crude mortality rates for the area should be obtained.

Data and Problem Analysis

Once the survey form has been completed, the data need to be evaluated, expressed in a standardized format, and compared to reference tables. Most data can be analyzed with simply a pen, paper, and calculator, but portable computers can be very helpful. In particular, *Epi Info*,[34] a word processing, database, and statistics system for personal computers, can be extremely useful for analyzing data in the field. It contains specific programs for nutritional anthropometry and a questionnaire that can be modified to suit specific needs. The anthropometric data collected can be compared to growth reference curves recommended by the World Health Organization (WHO) for international use. Thus the proportion of children with malnutrition can be determined, as well as the trends in mortality, morbidity, and nutritional status.

Data can be expressed in many ways, but the most common are as a percentile, a Z-score, and a percent of the median relative to reference tables.[28] (One exception is the MUAC: the actual values are used and no calculations are required.) When data are expressed as a percentile, the 50th percentile is the weight that divides the population into two equal parts and represents the median. Similarly,

10% of the children would fall below the weight designated by the 10th percentile. Given the percentiles of the reference population, one can compare the distribution of weights from the survey and the proportion below a given percentile. For example, if the cutoff point is the 5th percentile, then one would determine the proportion of children in the sample population whose weight is below the cutoff point for the 5th percentile.

Although percentiles are used in many countries, the WHO and other organizations recommend using the Z-scores.[27,28] The weight-for-height index of a child expressed in a Z-score represents the difference between the observed weight and the median weight of the reference population in standard deviation units:

$$\text{Weight-for-Height Index} = (\text{Observed Weight} - \text{Median Weight}) \div \text{Standard Deviation}$$

For example, if a child measured 9.2 kg and 80 cm and the reference tables give a median weight of 10.8 kg and a standard deviation of 0.87 kg for a child of that height, then the weight-for-height index expressed in a Z-score for this child would be

$$(9.2 - 10.8) \div 0.87 = -1.84.$$

Once critical indicators have been expressed in a standardized format, the data can then be used to determine the percent of children with malnutrition. Also needed are an estimate of the total population and the number of children under 5 years of age as a percent of the total. Table 47-2 presents the cutoff points typically used when the anthropometric data of children are being analyzed, and Figure 47-2 provides a sample form for calculating the degree of malnutrition. These should be used as guidelines and should be based on the population being evaluated. However, the global acute malnutrition rate, which combines moderate and severe malnutrition, and the severe acute rates are critical markers for deciding on the need for or type of intervention.[5,28] A weight-for-height value 2 standard deviations below the mean or 80% of weight-for-height by the National Center for Health Statistics standards are typically considered indicators of wasting or acute malnutrition[23]; a value 3 standard deviations below would indicate severe wasting.[15,23,32] During non-emergency conditions, 3% to 6% of children worldwide have low weight-for-height values, and although prevalence rates of 5%

TABLE 47-2

CUTOFF POINTS MOST OFTEN USED TO DEFINE ACUTE MALNUTRITION BY VARIOUS INDICATORS*

Nutritional Status (level of malnutrition)	W/H Z Score	W/H% of Median	MUAC
Moderate Acute	-3 < W/H < -2	70% < W/H% < 80%	110 mm < MUAC < 125 mm
Severe Acute	W/H < -3 or edema	W/H% < 70% or edema	MUAC < 110 mm or edema
Global Acute	W/H < -2 or edema	W/H% < 80% or edema	MUAC < 125 mm or edema

*W/H: weight-to-height ratio; MUAC: mid–upper arm circumference
Reprinted with permission from: Arbelot A, ed. *Nutrition Guidelines*. Paris: Medecins Sans Frontieres; 1995.

to 10% can indicate increased malnutrition,[23] such prevalence rates are not unusual in African populations.[32] For MUAC measurements, values between 110 and 125 mm are usually equivalent to 2 standard deviations below the mean and less than 110 mm is consistent with 3 standard deviations below the mean.[28] Given these references, a 20% prevalence of wasting or a MUAC of less than 125 mm would be a high prevalence and indicate a serious situation.[32] Although additional information should be carefully examined and the data gathered should be compared with data obtained by other health staff in the area, nutritional assistance programs are usually implemented when a prevalence above 20% has been noted.

Other pertinent information to be gathered includes the number of cases of nutritionally related illnesses, specifically kwashiorkor and marasmus. If the presence of specific vitamin- or mineral-deficiency illnesses is suspected, this should be documented by medical personnel during the assessment.[28] Additionally, the amount, types, and location of available food, the implementation of supplemental feeding programs (to be discussed later), and the level of physical activity must all be determined.

Reporting of Results and Follow-Up Activities

A formal report should be prepared soon after completion of the survey. The report should include stated objectives, a description of the survey methodology, the sampling frame and types of data collected, a presentation and interpretation of the results, and recommendations. A clear description of the sample and the distribution of its characteristics should be included. The data can be presented in tables—if possible with appropriate confidence intervals—according to specific population characteristics (eg, age, sex), but the data should also be compared with other groups for an interpretive analysis. For example, malnutrition rates from previous surveys can be compared so that trends can be inferred. It is imperative that the report have a set of recommendations and realistic actions that can be taken to alleviate the problems, because only then can various actions be considered and appropriate ones implemented. Documentation of ongoing health issues is critical for demonstrating program effectiveness and efficacy and program effects on the displaced population. Such efforts are critical for modifying less-than-effective procedures in future efforts.

FOOD ASSISTANCE PROGRAMS FOR EMERGENCY SITUATIONS

States of emergency resulting from natural disasters or outbreaks of hostilities commonly cause a disruption of food supplies and acute food shortages in civilian communities that had been adequately nourished. Interruption of civilian markets and food supply channels may cause food shortages in any community, even ones with adequate overall food stockpiles. And when families and individuals have been forced to leave their usual food sources, finding food becomes a matter of survival.

In fact, Hansch[35] found that the major activities of all refugee populations involved some aspect of food. In a survival setting, providing adequate energy to minimize wasting of body mass is the prime consideration. From a psychological perspective, though, the knowledge that food is available, no matter how limited the quantities, is important.[19]

The military, in conjunction with other governmental agencies and possibly nonprofit organizations as well, will often be called on to provide nutritional

Location _____   Site _____   Date _____

Total Refugee Population at Site _____

Total Number of Children From Whom Random Sample was Taken _____

Surveyor's Name/Organization _____

Normal (A)	B	C	D
No Edema and Index > -2 Z-Scores	Edema[*]	Index < -2 Z-Scores	Index < -3 Z-Scores
Record the number of cases above. These numbers are used below for statistical purposes.			
Total Sample = A + B + C + D			
% Malnutrition = (B + C + D) x 100 / (A + B + C + D)			
% Global Acute Malnutrition = (C + D) x 100 / (A + B + C + D)			
% Severe Malnutrition = (B + D) x 100 / (A + B + C + D)			
Other Observations			

Index = Weight-for-height index
[*]Children with edema should not be included in Z-Score columns.

Fig. 47-2. A Form for Quantifying Malnutrition from the Weight-for-Height Index and Edema. Adapted with permission from Arbelot A, ed. *Nutrition Guidelines*. Paris: Medecins Sans Frontieres; 1995.

assistance during emergency situations. These occasions may arise when local government officials seek aid from local commanders or when a state of martial law is declared and the military is directed to assume civil functions. Military activities can range from providing medical, technical, and administrative advice to setting up and managing mass feeding programs. This can mean determining the kinds, amounts, and sources of foods and fuel needed, as well as providing the personnel and

equipment necessary for food preparation and distribution.[20] The duration of this type of assistance is usually short, and emphasis is placed on maintaining nutritional status through adequate energy and protein intakes, on ensuring availability of potable water, and on boosting morale.

Food assistance programs vary, depending on the needs of the population, the military mission, the resources, and the current emergency situation. The assessment of the population should show a clearly demonstrated need for nutritional assistance, and the overall objectives of a food assistance program should also be clear before action is taken.[36] Food assistance can be provided in several ways, including onsite mass feeding programs, general food distributions, and selective feeding programs.

Onsite mass feeding programs are usually for those whose homes have been destroyed, for relief workers, or for transients. Military personnel may become involved in this type of program when they work with camp personnel to provide nutritional support for refugee camps. This type of feeding is often the first approach in emergencies of short duration and is meant to be an interim measure only.

General food distributions are also designed to provide food to refugees or displaced populations for survival over the short term, but the food is provided to the families to take home. The overriding objective is to make food available and accessible through the provision of a ration that meets the basic nutrient requirements and suits the cultural customs of the affected population.[20]

Selective feeding programs can be of several types, including therapeutic and supplemental. Therapeutic feeding programs are always designed to reduce the mortality of severely malnourished children younger than 5 years of age and other vulnerable populations; when possible, such programs should be located near a health facility. These programs can be labor intensive: the first phase requires medical diagnoses and a 24-hour care unit to ensure nutritional and medical treatment of those identified at highest risk. The second phase, which commences when complicated cases are brought under control, still provides nutritional rehabilitation but fewer meals are provided and those meals are more calorically dense and consist of local foods. Vitamin supplements are provided during this phase if needed. A therapeutic feeding program is an effective treatment for severe protein energy malnutrition, but such programs require specific resources and a medically trained staff to be optimally successful.[5,28]

In contrast to the therapeutic feeding program, the supplemental feeding program is designed to provide high-quality foods, usually in the form of a ration, as a supplement to the daily diet.[5] There are two types of supplemental programs: targeted and blanket.[5,28] Targeted supplementary programs are designed to provide medical follow-up and reduce the percentage of children (primarily those younger than 5 years of age) who are moderately malnourished. Many of the children will be coming out of a therapeutic program. The blanket supplementary feeding program is designed to prevent further deterioration of malnutrition and mortality by providing all vulnerable groups with a food supplement. The vulnerable groups include children younger than 5 years of age, pregnant and lactating women, the elderly, and individuals with specific medical needs.[28] As the objective of blanket programs is to minimize the prevalence of malnutrition and mortality rates, a large proportion of the population may qualify for assistance. This program is considered only a temporary measure, however, and should be suspended when the area's general food supply is restored.[5]

Supplemental rations for feeding programs can be provided in one of two forms: wet and dry.[5,28,36] The distribution of rations is typically determined by the type of ration appropriate for the particular situation. Wet rations refer to food that is prepared and distributed at designated sites once or twice a day. This type of ration program is often used for highly vulnerable populations, when fuel and cooking utensils are scarce, or when there are security issues involved in getting rations to the homes intact. Dry rations refer to food that is distributed in bulk without prior cooking; preparation and consumption are off-site, usually in the home. The assumption is that the food will be shared by all family members. Dry ration feeding programs are generally easier to coordinate, and they keep the responsibility for food preparation and feeding in the home.

The seriousness of the situation will dictate the type of food assistance program (See Figure 47-3). For more detailed descriptions of feeding programs and supplemental rations, *Nutrition Guidelines*[28] and *Refuge Health: An Approach to Emergency Situations*,[5] both published by Medecins Sans Frontieres, should be consulted.

Energy Requirements

Although limited information on the level of energy and protein required to sustain life in developing countries is available, the WHO and other governing bodies have developed guidelines. The guidelines are for planning purposes and are used with groups based on age, height, and physiological state (eg, activity level, pregnancy, lactation). Currently two levels of support have been identified: (1) the emergency subsistence level—an energy level of 1,500 kcal per day for the average person, which is expected to maintain survival for several weeks, but lower levels may result in starvation and death and (2) the temporary maintenance level—an energy level of 1,800 kcal per day for the average

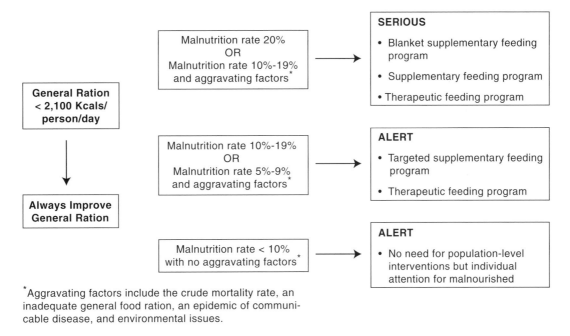

Fig. 47-3. General Guidelines for Implementing Nutritional Assistance Programs. Reprinted with permission from Arbelot A, ed. *Nutrition Guidelines*. Paris: Medecins Sans Frontieres; 1995.

person, which should sustain work for several months but may result in weight loss.

These guidelines have been useful, but in 1995 the Committee on International Nutrition, responding to a request by the US Agency for International Development, developed an estimated mean per capita energy requirement (EMPCER) that could be used to expedite food relief when information on the population was limited. Such an estimate would be useful in planning the food energy requirements in emergency situations.[37] On careful review of the available scientific and technical literature and after discussions among experts in the field, the committee presented methods for estimating the energy requirements of refugees and displaced populations. The committee, composed of members of the WHO, the UN High Commission for Refugees, the UN Children's Fund, and the World Food Programme, recommended the EMPCER be set at 2,100 kcal per day, with modifications depending on sex, weight, height, and energy expenditure.[37]

Many international agencies have been using a value of 1,900 kcal per day and other relief organizations may have different standards, but the Committee on International Nutrition believed that 1,900 kcal per day, based on biological principles, was too low. It was also acknowledged that various factors would influence this estimate, with physical activity exerting the greatest impact. If the population

is known to engage in more than light activity, the total energy recommendation increases by 100 kcal per day for moderate activity and 400 kcal per day for heavy activity. Other factors the committee considered important include recovery from malnutrition, environmental temperatures, and adult body size. If the average height and weight of the adults is greater than the averages set forth in the assumptions, a higher energy intake value should be used. In cold weather, the energy recommendation increases as mean temperature decreases so, for example, the EMPCER increases by 100 kcal per day at 15°C, 200 kcal at 10°C, and 300 kcal at 5°C.[37]

Humanitarian Rations

Humanitarian rations are available for refugee populations, and guidelines and sample food rations have been prepared by the World Food Programme and the Office of the UN High Commissioner for Refugees. The rations are intended to supplement local food products or, when necessary, meet all the basic nutritional requirements. Food rations may be provided by a variety of sources, including host governments, nongovernmental organizations, and the international community at large. The World Food Programme publishes guidelines for calculating food rations for refugees, which can be found at their website: www.wfp.org/OP/

TABLE 47-3

LEVELS OF ENERGY-PROVIDING NUTRIENTS IN HUMANITARIAN RATIONS

Nutrient	Grams	Energy (kcal)	Percentage of Total Energy
Fat	40-75	360-675	10-30
Protein	50-70	200-280	10-15
Carbohydrate	≥ 345	≥ 1380	≥ 60

index.htm.

Suitability of the rations is a critical issue. The chosen ration should provide a variety of basic food items, with the staple food being one the target population is accustomed to. Basic food items include cereals, flours or grains, oil, and a source of protein; the source of protein must be familiar. Complementary food items, such as fresh meat or fish, vegetables, fruit, fortified cereal blends, sugar, condiments, salt, and spices may be included as well, if available. If humanitarian assistance rations are required, both basic and complementary foods should be provided at a minimum level of 2,100 kcal per person per day,[37] unless a more accurate estimate of the population's specific energy needs can be obtained.

Within the US Government, the Office of the Assistant Secretary of Defense, Humanitarian and Refugee Affairs, saw a need for ways to feed large groups of refugees or displaced persons. The result was the development of Humanitarian Rations, rations packaged to tolerate environmental extremes and designed to meet the nutritional requirements of any specific cultural group. As of 1999, two specific humanitarian rations had been developed: the Humanitarian Daily Ration (HDR) and the Humanitarian Pouched Meal (HPM). These rations are available through the US Government and have been used in humanitarian missions. Tables 47-3 and 47-4 present the amounts of energy-providing nutrients, vitamins, and minerals required in the HDR.

The HDR is similar in concept to the military's Meal, Ready-to-Eat in that it was designed as one day's complete food supply; it has a minimum of two entrees, which can be eaten either cold or hot (warming the meal is preferable). The components of the HDR have been carefully chosen so that the various rations do not contain items prohibited for cultural or religious reasons but do provide the nutritional requirements established for moderately malnourished individuals. Prohibited products, which include beef, pork, poultry, fish, other animal products and by-products, and ethyl alcohol, cannot be included or used in preparing or processing the ration components. Although dairy products can be used, they are permitted only in amounts that are easily digested by lactose-intolerant individuals.[36] Exhibit 47-2 presents the contents of one HDR menu: each day's menu provides no fewer than 2,200 kcal, with 10% to 13% of calories from protein, 27% to 30% from fat, and no less than 60% from carbohydrate. An accessory packet is provided with each meal. The shelf life of the HDR is 36 months from the time of placement in the meal bag when stored at 80°F. As of 1999, five different menus are available, but they are updated regularly based on customer responses and situational or cultural demands.

The HPM is similar to the HDR in that it is ready to eat, cold or hot, but it contains only one entree with complementary components and so provides

TABLE 47-4

LEVELS OF VITAMINS AND MINERALS NECESSARY TO MEET THE REQUIREMENTS FOR HUMANITARIAN RATIONS

Micronutrient	Amount	Micronutrient	Amount	Micronutrient	Amount
Vitamin A	750 μg RE[*]	Folate	150 μg	Phosphate	1,000 mg
Vitamin C	60 mg	Vitamin B_6	2 mg	Magnesium	300 mg
Vitamin D	10 μg	Vitamin B_{12}	6 μg	Zinc	15 mg
Thiamin	1.5 mg	Iron	25 mg	Calcium/Phosphorous	1:1
Riboflavin	1.7 mg	Calcium	1,000 mg	Iodine	0.5 mg
Niacin	5.5 mg/1,000 kcal				

*retinol equivalents

EXHIBIT 47-2

ONE DAY'S SAMPLE MENU FOR THE HUMANITARIAN DAILY RATION

A	B	C
Lentils and Vegetables	Lentil Stew	Lentil Stew
Beans with Potatoes	Peas in Tomato Sauce	Red Beans and Rice
Crackers	Vegetable Biscuits	Biscuits
Flat Bread	Jam	Vegetable Crackers
Peanut Butter	Peanut Butter	Peanut Butter
Raisins	Fruit Bar	Strawberry Jam
Apple Fruit Bar	Fruit Pastry	Fruit Bar
Accessory Packet*	Shortbread Cookies	Fruit Pastry
	Accessory Packet*	Shortbread
		Accessory Packet*

*Accessory Packet contents: red pepper, pepper, salt, sugar, spoon, matches, towelette (alcohol-free), and napkin

Source: Defense Supply Center Philadelphia website: www.dscp.dla.mil/subs/rations/rations.htm

---

only 967 kcal; the same percentage of calories is derived from protein, fat, and carbohydrate as the HDR. This particular ration was designed to be a supplement to ongoing food programs that are unable to provide adequate nutrients and calories. The shelf life of the HPM is 12 months at 80°F. Further information on humanitarian rations can be found at the website www.dscp.dla.mil/subs/rations/rations.htm.

Issues with Food Assistance Programs

Food assistance programs require considerable effort in terms of personnel, organization, logistics, and resources. For these programs to be organized and effective, a number of issues should be considered: the total number of beneficiaries, the duration of feeding programs, the kind and amount of food and fuel required, the degree to which food can be provided from indigenous sources, and the level of military support required to accomplish the mission.

Specific considerations include finding willing donors, ensuring well-planned organization of the food acquisition and distribution process, formulating an equitable distribution system, determining and registering those families entitled to or requiring rations, and organizing a regular monitoring system.[5] Once these issues have all been considered and decisions have been made, the appropriate food items and supplies need to be made available.

When the program is in place, a surveillance system to monitor and document program efficiency and effectiveness should be initiated. Procedures for monitoring selective feeding programs and general food distribution programs will differ, but individuals with specific needs should be followed up, no matter which program they are in.[20] Specific issues to consider in selective feeding programs include registration, attendance indicators, health indicators (eg, weight, growth charting, edema evaluation, food needs and intake), mortality rates, and malnutrition prevalence. Children should be remeasured after a month to document changes in anthropometric indexes, and recipients should be queried about the availability, quality, and quantity of the food. Such information will allow for an evaluation of the program's implementation and its impact.

There are a variety of factors that can compromise the efficiency and effectiveness of general food distribution programs. Monitoring at some level needs to be done for these potential problems: food diversion, gaps in the supply of food, food losses during distribution, inadequacy of ration nutrient content, poor organization, failure to coordinate logistics adequately, and problems with food preparation.[5]

Since food aid has value, food diversion is common. Households may exchange part of the ration for essential items such as shelter or firewood. Another type of food diversion occurs when groups in power inequitably control distribution and access to food. Food distribution sites should be inspected, since this allows the methods and timing of distribution to be assessed and ensures that food is actually being distributed equitably, both during and after the emergency phase. Additional assessments of food supplies, including food production, exports, imports, and storage and usage rates, should be conducted before and after the intervention. If the infrastructure of the country or region has been affected, movement of food and supplies to the affected population areas may be restricted. An example of this occurred in Iraq during the Persian Gulf War when the country's normal food distribution system collapsed, resulting in restricted access to necessary food items.[1] Finally, rationing of food under extreme situations may be necessary to minimize overconsumption and ensure that food supplies will last over prolonged periods. Despite the wide range of potential problems, food distribution programs continue to serve refugee and displaced populations and meet their needs in times of distress.

In addition to the feeding programs, Yip and colleagues[7] note that a safe water supply, sanitation measures, and a diarrhea-control program are often critical aspects of any relief mission. Thus, personnel experienced in various aspects of public health should be consulted. Military dietitians and nutritionists should be included in planning and implementing nutrition relief efforts so that logistical decisions can be coupled with the nutritional assessment.

This is an ever-expanding field with world events determining what the best approaches to nutritional assessments and feeding programs are. The military has served and will continue to serve a critical role. Integrated teams who understand the science, social science, public health, and cultural issues will be needed to deal with the urgent crises faced by the increasing numbers of natural and political emergencies. Fortunately, excellent resources for humanitarian assistance nutrition programs and other public health issues during emergency situations are available.[1,5,23,28]

SUMMARY

There are a myriad of factors that must be considered and addressed during humanitarian assistance or disaster relief missions due to war, civil strife, natural disasters, and other such events. In many cases, assessment and analysis of the emergency situation, using information on increased morbidity and mortality rates, indicate that nutritional support programs are critical. Nutritional support in the form of population screening efforts, assessments, surveys, and nutritional interventions is a critical element of any type of relief mission. Such activities are often combined efforts between military units and national and international relief organizations because diverse skills are required to provide for those in need. Military personnel are uniquely qualified to support humanitarian efforts; they have been involved in such operations throughout history and have the public health specialists, clinical dietitians, epidemiologists, medical professionals, and logistical and support services necessary for both advance planning and day-to-day operations. In particular, dietitians and nutrition care personnel, in conjunction with other health care providers, have the expertise to identify and implement nutrition programs that will interrupt the course of malnutrition, disease, and death. Victims of any crisis must have food to obtain energy, not only to survive but also to rebuild.

REFERENCES

1. Levy BS, Sidel VW, eds. *War and Public Health*. New York: Oxford University Press; 1997.

2. Toole MJ, Waldman RJ. Prevention of excess mortality in refugee and displaced populations in developing countries. *JAMA*. 1990;263:3296–3302.

3. Cobey JC, Flanagin A, Foege WH. Effective humanitarian aid: our only hope for intervention in civil war. *JAMA*. 1993;270:632–634.

4. Macrae J, Zwi AB. Food as an instrument of war in contemporary African famines: a review of the evidence. *Disasters*. 1992;16:299–321.

5. Medecins Sans Frontieres. *Refugee Health: An Approach to Emergency Situations*. London: MacMillan; 1997.

6. Toole MJ, Waldman RJ. Refugees and displaced persons: war, hunger, and public health. *JAMA*. 1993;270:600–605.

7. Yip R, Sharp TW. Acute malnutrition and high childhood mortality related to diarrhea: lessons from the 1991 Kurdish refugee crisis. *JAMA*. 1993;270:587–590.

8. Cashman TM, Hassell LH, Barker AJ, Funderburk LK. Operation Tropic Refuge: the East Wood Rescue. *Mil Med*. 1994;159:723–729.

9. Craig MJ, Morgan WA. The Army dietitian in Panama: military hospital feeding and humanitarian efforts during Operation Just Cause. *Mil Med*. 1996;161:723–725.

10. Hodges PA, Lyon JM. Perspectives on history: Army dietetics in southwest Asia during Operation Desert Shield/ Desert Storm. *J Am Diet Assoc*. 1996;96:595–597.

11. Hodges PA. Perspectives on history: Army dietetics in the European, North African, and Mediterranean theaters of operation in World War II. *J Am Diet Assoc*. 1996;96:598–601.

12. Kemmer T, Podojil R, Sweet LE. US Army dietitians deploy in support of Cobra Gold: a humanitarian mission. *Mil Med*. 1999;164:488–494.

13. Outram Q. Cruel wars and safe havens: humanitarian aid in Liberia 1989-1996. *Disasters*. 1997;21:189–205.

14. Rumbaugh JR. Operation Pacific Haven: humanitarian medical support for Kurdish evacuees. *Mil Med*. 1998;163:269–271.

15. Boss LP, Toole MJ, Yip R. Assessments of mortality, morbidity, and nutritional status in Somalia during the 1991-1992 famine: recommendations for standardization of methods. *JAMA*. 1994;272:371–376.

16. Manoncourt S, Doppler B, Enten F, et al. Public health consequences of the civil war in Somalia, April, 1992. *Lancet*. 1992;340:176–177.

17. Moore PS, Marfin AA, Quenemoen LE, et al. Mortality rates in displaced and resident populations of central Somalia during 1992 famine. *Lancet*. 1993;341:935–938.

18. Thomas CT. Personal Communication, 1995.

19. Davis A. What is emergency public health? MSF-Holland. March 1995. Mimeo draft. Cited by Cogill B. Nutrition in emergency situations. Presented at Nutrition Support for Combat Casualties and Humanitarian Missions Course; January 1997; San Antonio, Tex.

20. Dept of the Army. *Army Medical Field Feeding Operations*. Washington, DC: DA. FM 8-505. In press.

21. Centers for Disease Control and Prevention. Famine-affected, refugee, and displaced populations: recommendations for public health issues. *MMWR*. 1991;41(RR13).

22. Shears P. Epidemiology and infection in famine and disasters. *Epidemiol Infect*. 1991;107:241–251.

23. Yip R. Famine. In: Noji EK, ed. *The Public Health Consequences of Disasters*. New York: Oxford University Press; 1997.

24. Intertect. *Assessment Manual for Refugee Emergencies*. Washington, DC: Bureau for Refugee Programs, Dept of State; 1985.

25. Food and nutrition. In: UN High Commissioner for Refugees. *Handbook for Emergencies. Part One: Field Operations*. Geneva: UNHCR; 1982: Chap 8.

26. Simmonds S, Vaughan P, Gunn SW, eds. *Refugee Community Health Care*. New York: Oxford University Press; 1983.

27. World Health Organization Regional Office for the Eastern Mediterranean. *Field Guide on Rapid Nutritional Assessment in Emergencies*. Geneva: WHO; 1995

28. Arbelot A, ed. *Nutrition Guidelines*. Paris: Medecins Sans Frontieres; 1995.

29. Toole MJ. Micronutrient deficiencies in refugees. *Lancet*. 1992;339:1214–1216.

30. Quinn VJ. User's Manual for Conducting Child Nutrition Surveys in Developing Countries. Ithaca, NY: Cornell Food and Nutrition Policy Program; 1992.

31. Centers for Disease Control. *A Manual for the Basic Assessment of Nutrition Status in Potential Crisis Situations*. 2nd ed. Atlanta: CDC; March 1981.

32. World Health Organization. *Report on the Nutrition Situations of Refugee and Displaced Populations*. Geneva: WHO; 1996. ACC/SCN No. 18.

33. Dowell SF, Toko A, Sita C, Piarroux R, Duerr A, Woodruff BA. Health and nutrition in centers for unaccompanied refugee children: experience from the 1994 Rwandan refugee crisis. *JAMA*. 1995;273:1802–1806.

34. Epi Info. Version 6. Atlanta: Centers for Disease Control and Prevention; 1994.

35. Hansch S. Diet and ration use in Central American refugee camps. *J Refugee Studies*. 1992;5:300–312.

36. Sanghvi TG. *Supplement on Emergency Rations: Commodities Reference Guide*. Draft. Washington, DC: US Agency for International Development; 1993.

37. Allen LH, Howson CP, eds. *Estimated Mean Per Capita Energy Requirements for Planning Emergency Food Aid Rations*. Washington, DC: Institute of Medicine, National Academy Press; 1995.

MILITARY PREVENTIVE MEDICINE:
MOBILIZATION AND DEPLOYMENT
Volume 2

Section 8: Postdeployment

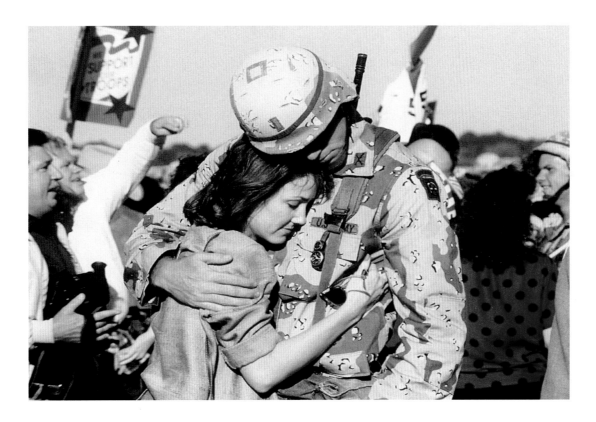

The medical and psychological effects of deployment do not necessarily dissipate once the deployment is over. Service members and their families make significant, though incompletely understood, sacrifices during deployment and may need to make major readjustments after the deployment ends. This is not a new phenomenon, but it has been much better illuminated in the wake of the Persian Gulf War.

Department of Defense Photograph: Defense Visual Information Center photo identification number DDST9209054.

Chapter 48

PSYCHOLOGICAL ASPECTS OF DEPLOYMENT AND REUNION

JAMES E. MCCARROLL, PhD, MPH; KENNETH J. HOFFMAN, MD, MPH; THOMAS A. GRIEGER, MD; AND HARRY C. HOLLOWAY, MD

J.E. McCarroll; Colonel (Retired), MS, US Army; Research Professor, Department of Psychiatry, Uniformed Services University of the Health Sciences, 4301 Jones Bridge Road, Bethesda, MD 20814-4799

K.J. Hoffman; Colonel, Medical Corps, US Army; Medical Director, Population Health Programs, Office of the Assistant Secretary of Defense (Health Affairs)/TRICARE Management Activity, 5111 Leesburg Pike, Falls Church, VA 22041

T.A. Grieger; Captain, Medical Corps, US Navy; Associate Professor, Department of Psychiatry, Uniformed Services University of the Health Sciences, 4301 Jones Bridge Road, Bethesda, MD 20814-4799

H.C. Holloway; Colonel (Retired), Medical Corps, US Army; Professor of Psychiatry, Department of Psychiatry, Uniformed Services University of the Health Sciences, 4301 Jones Bridge Road, Bethesda, MD 20814-4799

INTRODUCTION

A deployment is a military operation in which the service member is sent from the home station, usually as a part of a military unit, to a distant location to accomplish a special mission. Routine training is not included in this definition. Families are not permitted to accompany him or her. Both deployment and reunion are often stressful for service members and their families. An increased knowledge of the stresses of predeployment, deployment, and reunion will help commanders and medical personnel develop preventive measures to counter them. In this chapter we present a brief history of deployments in the post–Cold War environment and give illustrations of the stressors in four of the most prominent recent ones: the Persian Gulf War, Somalia, Haiti, and Bosnia. We present and discuss deployment issues that affect service members and family members and the command and medical actions that might be taken to prevent or ameliorate them.

THE NATURE OF CURRENT MILITARY OPERATIONS

Military Operations from World War II to the Post–Cold War Environment

There have been substantial modifications in the nature of military operations since World War II, with a broadened spectrum of experiences for service members and their families. World War II typified the long-duration war in which there were peaks and valleys of combat intensity. Massive numbers of personnel, ships, and aircraft were engaged in battle theaters throughout the world. Soldiers, sailors, and Marines were involved for the duration of the war or until a wound or other medical or psychiatric condition required their evacuation.

The Korean and Vietnam wars were more limited in scope, even though the Korean War involved large-scale land and air campaigns, and the Vietnam War lasted longer than World War II. The overall mission, politically and militarily, in both these latter conflicts was less clearly defined than it was in World War II. Both represented combat phases of the much-longer global Cold War between the United States and its allies and the Soviet bloc of nations. The desire to limit the spread of communism was balanced by the fear of extensive involvement in a land war against the communist superpowers. Ground efforts were limited geographically and bombing missions for aircraft were tightly controlled.

Politically, the Cold War was marked primarily by postures of conventional warfare, wars of national liberation, terrorist groups of various ideological commitments, and nuclear deterrence. The world was roughly divided into a Western bloc plus Japan and other Pacific nations; a Communist block that included the Soviet Union, the Warsaw Pact nations, and the People's Republic of China; and third-world countries, many of which varied in their alliances between the Western and Communist blocs. Militarily, it was characterized by global deployment.

Large numbers of US personnel were assigned to installations in Europe and Asia to preclude overt aggression by Communist forces. The US Navy and Air Force developed and deployed highly advanced weapons platforms. Deployments could generally be planned and careers scheduled around deployment cycles, particularly in the Navy. Even though separation from families and the high tempo of training took their toll, there was seldom a direct threat of loss of life and limb, as compared with war.

With the fall of the Soviet Union and the collapse of the Warsaw Pact in 1989, multiple areas of regional instability became the focus of US political leadership. The military forces of the United States have taken on new missions and roles that challenge the capabilities and ingenuity of service members and their military and civilian leaders. Much of the deployment effort is now shared by active duty and reserve units, which are often activated and deployed for several months. Differences in training, experience, and equipment between active duty and reserve units and the short-notice activation of units have proved highly disruptive to both the military and family environments.

Current US National Strategy

The National Security Strategy for the United States was outlined in a White House publication.[1] The United States must be able to respond to crises, such as threats to vital national interests. These interests are of broad, overriding importance to the survival, safety, and vitality of the nation, and they affect both national well-being and the character of the world. Among these are humanitarian crises, natural disasters, and manmade disasters or gross violations of human rights that demand action. For the foreseeable future, the United States and its allies must be able to deter and defeat large-scale cross-border aggression in two distant theaters with overlapping time frames. This scenario includes the rapid defeat of initial enemy advances, victory against an enemy that may use unconventional approaches, and successful transitions from multiple small-scale contingencies to major wars.

The second group of threats are transnational and involve terrorism, international crime (eg, trafficking in drugs and illegal arms), environmental damage, and intrusions into information infrastructures. They have filled the vacuum left by the fall of the Soviet Union and the end of the Cold War. The third group of threats is composed of smaller-scale contingencies, operations which fall short of major-theater warfare, including humanitarian assistance, peacekeeping missions, disaster relief, maintenance of no-fly zones, reinforcement of key allies, and limited strikes and interventions.

The current period is also characterized by political disagreements between various political groups and branches of the US government concerning national strategic goals. These disagreements create distinctive problems for the military that receives its orders from the Executive Branch, but its funding from the US Congress that may or may not support the strategic goals established by the president. Such conflicts have obvious implications for the welfare of the service member, since the success of a particular mission often depends on unity of purpose to support the deployment.

Environmental, Psychological, and Moral Factors in Operational Stress

With the diversity of military missions in the modern era, a systematic method is needed to accurately predict, assess, and minimize their negative psychological aspects. One approach is to categorize the various types of risks. Environmental factors include weather, geography, terrain, ease of communication, noise, availability of adequate food and shelter, presence or threat of disease, and toxins or fear of toxins (eg, chemical and biological agents). Psychological factors encompass those individual and interpersonal aspects of situations to which individuals and units respond negatively. Moral factors relate to the individual's or unit's overall sense of the rightness or worth of the campaign. These environmental, psychological, and moral factors affect individual and unit performance. Similar concepts appear in the discussion of the environment of combat in Army Field Manual 100-5, *Operations*.[2]

Environmental Factors

Environmental risks can be assessed based on known or predictable conditions of deployment, although adequate intelligence about local conditions is often lacking. The tempo of operations will affect sleep, hygiene, nutrition, hydration, and fatigue. The degree to which military personnel are affected by the environment may depend on their sensitivity to its influences. Age, physical fitness, presence of medical or psychiatric illnesses, and response to medications (including prophylactic medications) can affect sensitivity. The effect of the environment can be modified by equipment deployed with the forces to counter such threats. Unfortunately, unanticipated negative consequences of equipment and systems failures can result in another source of environmental risk. A commander's desire to avoid any harm to personnel can result in excessive use of personal protective equipment. This may increase the negative impact of environmental factors and actually create casualties.

Psychological Factors

Psychological factors operate at individual and group levels. Each service member has a unique history of experiences that set the framework for the perception and interpretation of current experiences. Successful relationships and positive performances build confidence and resiliency, while broken trusts and failures lead to isolation and pessimism. Units have a collective character that is formed over time. Appropriate communication, respect, and mutual support build team spirit and cohesion. Active, realistic training and prior success in combat build unit confidence and initiative. Frequent reorganizations, rapid turnover of personnel, and limited communication lead to behavior that is not cohesive. Limited training and assignment to operations in which the mission is poorly defined and success difficult to measure will erode the confidence of the unit.

Moral Factors

The military services provide a means to accomplish the political goals and strategies of national leadership. Clausewitz described the trinity of the military, political leadership, and the people. He believed that there must be an alignment of the three to ensure success in war. In most instances, the leaders are attuned to the moral tone of the nation and

TABLE 48-1

ENVIRONMENTAL STRESSES AND MITIGATING FACTORS

Environmental Stress	Mitigating Factors
Weather: heat, cold, rain, mud	Shelter, proper clothing, warming tents, rotation of personnel
Toxins: biological and chemical weapons	Available MOPP*, education briefings concerning actual threat
Disease: airborne, insect vector, direct contact	Prophylaxis if available, repellents, barrier protection, education about prevention and briefing about actual threat
Weapons systems	Armor, dispersion, training to respond, briefings on actual threat

*Mission-oriented protective posture

TABLE 48-2

PSYCHOLOGICAL STRESSES AND MITIGATING FACTORS

Psychological Stress	Mitigating Factor
Personal fears and doubts	Briefings regarding actual threats, training in realistic environments, "buddying" new personnel with seasoned veterans
Lack of effective communication	Education at all levels on appropriate means of passing information, encouraging initiative within proper bounds of rank and respect
Poor unit cohesion	Leadership, limit changes in personnel and routine, train in environment and conditions likely to be encountered, foster cohesion through additional team-building events, such as organized sports
Sleep deprivation	Forced rest periods, noise attenuation, sleep hygiene education
Casualties of boredom: substance abuse, reckless behaviors, sexual promiscuity	Maintain active training schedule (even when deployed), provide clear limits to behavior and apply appropriate and uniform punishment for infractions

their use of military forces is seen as good. When this occurs, the people of the nation are supportive of the service members at many levels, from personal support of family members to positive national media coverage.

At times, military and political goals may be unclear or poorly stated. In many instances, goals may seem mutually exclusive. For example, it may seem correct to help preserve the internal security of another country and yet undesirable to use deadly force to stop civilians or paramilitary personnel whose views differ from those of the national leader. It is the nature of the US democracy to question the goals of its leadership, which may lead to questions of whether the nation is engaged in a worthwhile and morally correct endeavor. Once this occurs, the support for the military forces may diminish. Some portion of media coverage may speak out against military actions, family members may question the need for the hardship of separation and the threat of death or injury, and individual service members may begin to doubt their role in the operation. These factors have a direct effect on the psychological well-being of individuals and units. This creates the potential for shifting political support for most any strategic initiative. For example, during the Vietnam War changes in policies par-

alleled changes in US public opinion and support for the war between 1963 and 1973.[3]

This background provides examples of contexts for performing a situational assessment of environmental, psychological, and moral factors likely to affect individual and unit performance within the myriad of possible operational assignments. Quantification of the degree and duration of stress can be balanced against positive factors that provide for resiliency and endurance. Lists of some environmental stresses and mitigating factors are provided in Table 48-1 and some psychological stresses and mitigating factors in Table 48-2. A commander's impact on moral factors may vary with rank and with operational contingencies. Commanders must be aware of the influence of moral factors in determining their impact on the service member and the family.

STRESSORS IN MAJOR DEPLOYMENTS IN THE 1990s

Many persons involved in the diverse US military operations of the 1990s have described a variety of stressors that affected the health of individuals assigned to those operations. In the discussion that follows, elements of stress are identified as environmental, psychological, or moral. Although there are persistently similar themes in these operations, some were unique, and the surveillance systems and nomenclature used to identify and track them were as varied as the missions themselves.

The Persian Gulf War: Operations Desert Shield (Aug '90–Jan '91) and Desert Storm (Jan–Mar '91)

Environmental

Some of the commonly reported stressors of this conflict were the rapid and unexpected activation of the operation, exposure to Scud missile attacks, anticipation of possible chemical or biological attacks, austere living conditions, environmental pollution, and instantaneous media coverage of the war.[4]

Psychological

Major psychological stressors for those in the French Army were serving under the United Nations banner, imposed passivity in the face of the rules of engagement (no ripostes), not being able to distinguish allies from the enemy, difficulty of communications, discomfort, lack of security, the inability to change the complex social problems, and the threat of attack with chemical weapons.[5] The major sources of chronic psychological stress reported by US forces were long duty days, extensive time spent in chemical protective clothing, lack of sleep, crowding, lack of privacy, physical work load, boredom, and lack of contact with family.[6] Directly experienced stressors were the danger of being killed or wounded, being fired on by the enemy, and seeing dead bodies. The threat of weapons of mass destruction was more stressful than actual events. This was understandable since few service members had any actual contact with the enemy. In addition to these stressors were the need for special immunizations and prophylactic drugs to protect against chemical and biological agents. The use of such measures may create uncertainty on the part of the service member regarding their potential health effects.

Moral

The US force that deployed was well-equipped and had a good sense of mission, a low frequency of disciplinary problems, and a high degree of cohesion. Alcohol and other drugs of potential abuse were not factors in this conflict because of Islamic laws forbidding their use in Saudi Arabia, where most US personnel were located.[7] There was also a high level of support from home, and a large number of mental health personnel were available for consultation in the theater.

Somalia: Operations Restore Hope (Dec '92–May '93) and Continue Hope (May '93–Mar '94)

Environmental

Disease is rampant in Somalia. The extent of disease, however, was unknown because of the lack of a medical establishment that could collect reliable epidemiologic information. Service members faced a lack of sanitation, diverse insect populations, a hot and humid climate, and large numbers of seriously ill Somalis.[8] In such a situation, there should be cooperative efforts among command, preventive medicine, and mental health personnel to solve operational problems. For example, some Marines in Somalia perceived insect repellent use as ineffective and unpleasant because it caused dust to cake on their skin and showers were not available.[9] Limitations of the agents (in this case, insecticide) and human responses to those limitations can be a problem in such an environment. Command monitoring of such behavioral aspects of a primarily preventive medicine problem should be a priority.

Psychological

The mission lacked clear policies for redeployment or recreational leave, and people faced austere, dangerous working conditions and the challenges of working with personnel with different languages, customs, and work methods.[10] Adherence to preventive policies and programs can also be affected by the operational environment. For example, Marines did not use their bed nets (suspended on poles above their cots) because the apparatus made them bigger targets. Psychological factors and preventive medicine policies also intersected when it was noted that service members forgot to take doxycycline (an

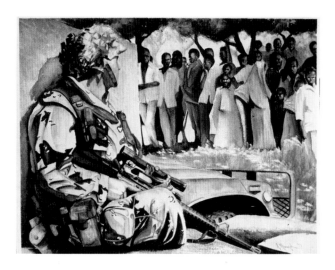

Figure 48-1. "On Watch, Somalia" by Jeffrey Manuszak. Security operations in a deployed environment may require service members to interact with, work with, and challenge people of different cultures, who may speak a different language and have unfamiliar customs. This may be particularly difficult, as in Somalia, when hostile actions had been taken toward US military personnel. Art: Courtesy of Army Art Collection, US Army Center of Military History, Washington, DC.

antimalarial drug) because of too little sleep and irregular schedules.[9]

Moral

Toward the end of the mission, public support for the US military's role in Somalia had eroded.[10] Personnel were confined to compounds, sorrowful over the deaths of 26 of their comrades in an ambush in downtown Mogadishu, resentful of an ill-defined mission, angry at some Somalis, homesick, and bored (Figure 48-1). Additional stressors were the lack of a return date and poor communication with home.[10,11]

Haiti: Operation Uphold Democracy (Sep '94–Apr '95)

Environmental

In Haiti, many US military personnel had to live in tents and cope with heat, insects, rodents, and tarantulas. Commanders tried to increase the supply of hot food, showers and latrines, laundry and recreational facilities, and air conditioning. There were significant risks to personnel of sexually transmitted and diarrheal diseases. There was also the

need to use insecticides because malaria and dengue fever were considered health risks for the US personnel assigned to Haiti[12] (Figure 48-2).

Psychological

The passive posture forced on US personnel after they had been prepared for a combat invasion may have played a role in the number of early psychiatric presentations. There were 233 psychiatric visits and 15 air evacuations among 20,000 US personnel during the first 4 months in Haiti.[13]

Moral

It was difficult to gauge the public tolerance for this mission. There was relief that a combat invasion was avoided, but there was not any apparent enthusiasm for the mission, either. It seems that public interest in a deployment rapidly fades as the media discontinues its coverage.

Bosnia: Operation Joint Endeavor (Dec '95–Present)

As of 2000, the US deployment to Bosnia has taken on additional missions, such as the return of refugees displaced by the civil war. There is no end in sight to this deployment, so additional characteristics are bound to appear in the future.

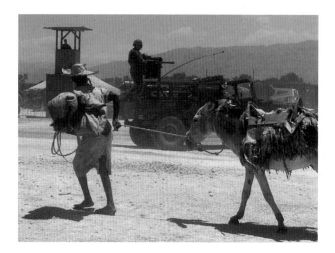

Figure 48-2. US military operations often take place in the midst of local cultural activities. A Haitian man leads a donkey past US Army soldiers providing security for US Navy Seabee Engineers as they build a road and bridge in the outskirts of Port-au-Prince, Haiti. US Army photograph.

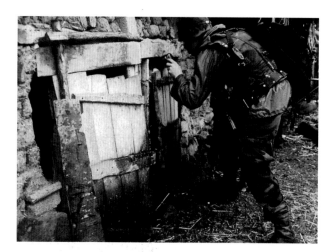

Figure 48-3. Deployed service members often must face dangerous tasks for which they might have had little or no training. Because conflict in the town of Zitinje in Kosovo had been high, US Army soldiers were required to search every home, animal pens not excluded, and confiscate any automatic weapons found.
US Army photograph by SPC Daniel Ernst.

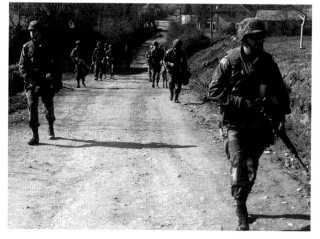

Figure 48-4. US Army soldiers in Bosnia may be asked to perform civil affairs missions and other missions for which they may not have been trained. US Army soldiers patrol through a village of Donje Dubrave near Tuzla, Bosnia, to assess the attitude of the local people and to gather information.
US Army photograph.

Environmental

In Bosnia, the 20,000 troops of the United Nations Implementation Force faced environmental risks from severe cold and wet weather, poor roads, and undetected land mines.[14] They also faced health threats from poisonous snakes and spiders, environmentally related diseases, and foodborne, waterborne, and insect-borne disorders[15] (Figure 48-3).

Psychological

Some personnel specifically referred to the monotony of their existence.[16] The most frequently cited stressor was the unclear length of the deployment.[17] The initial reports from Bosnia detailed many personal difficulties, such as loneliness, and the stress of dealing with environmental factors. These included mud, cold, rain, snow, fog, unheated latrines and showers, prefabricated quarters heated by kerosene heaters (which require an all-night fire guard), and wearing protective clothing and battle gear weighing approximately 45 pounds in some duty areas (Figure 48-4).

Moral

US forces, as a part of a North Atlantic Treaty Organization mission, were sent to Bosnia on 20 December 1995 to enforce the Dayton Peace Accords and to help return refugees to their homes. It was announced that the mission would last 1 year.[18] As of 2000, US personnel are still deployed there. Only time will tell the effect of public opinion on the mission and personnel stationed there.

PSYCHOLOGICAL EFFECTS OF PREDEPLOYMENT, DEPLOYMENT, AND REUNION ON THE SERVICE MEMBER

It is hard to separate the factors that affect service members and those that affect the family. While there some factors that affect only the service member and some only the family, distinctions are somewhat arbitrary and most of what affects the service member will also affect the family.

Predeployment

When notified of a deployment, the individual must be prepared to move rapidly from a normal work, training, and home environment to a distant theater of operations. Commanders are usually not well informed about the time parameters of deployments. Often, criticism and suspicion of commanders begins early when the soon-to-be-deployed do not know how long they will be away. Commanders are sometimes suspected of holding back information or lying. Departures are often delayed again and again; multiple good-byes are stressful and a bad way to leave home. Frequently, the national leadership is not helpful. Leaders may state that the deployment will begin and end on a certain date only to change the mission and its time frame as political and policy factors change. Such changes have important implications for the morale and stress level experienced by personnel and their families.

Specific policies and treatment procedures should be in place before deployment. As the reality of the deployment evolves, medical and psychiatric recommendations will need to be modified to deal with special situations and difficulties that will emerge. The need to institute preventive measures can meet resistance from command, individual service members, and caregivers. This is particularly true when psychiatric and behavioral issues are involved. Medical staff officers advising the highest levels of military leadership must be of appropriate rank, experienced in both the military and medicine, and trusted by the leadership.

Unit readiness should be known before deployment. Elements of unit readiness include determining if units have (*a*) been assigned appropriate personnel for their assigned authorizations, (*b*) trained well and regularly together, (*c*) reduced the number of individuals with significant medical profiles, and (*d*) have on file current family support plans. Each of these topics can be measured with existing data using personnel and unit readiness evaluation systems.

Depending on Department of Defense, service-specific, and mission-specific policies and needs, some individuals may be excluded from the deployment. All profiles that limit individuals from full duty should be reviewed. The potential need for mental health consultation and services should be anticipated, and the location and capability of mental health assets known.

Unfortunately, the outcome of deployments depends on tactical and political factors unknown at the time of deployment. Even if all the factors cited above are optimal, success is not assured. Commanders must face multiple demands at times of deployment. The requirement to act rapidly with limited logistical resources may require the commander to accept greater risk than special staff officers consider desirable.

The state of predeployment readiness will affect how a unit adapts to the new environment. Many education and training programs are available and should be used before notification of a deployment. From a psychological perspective, stress-relief plans should be considered by commanders for service members since almost all deployments have had long periods of waiting. Waiting and boredom go together and create unnecessary stress. Each deployed service member should have a plan to prevent boredom. Unit leadership responsible for assuring regular work schedules should also allocate resources and plan time for rest and recreation. This includes supplying reading and military-specific course material, organizing recreational excursions, encouraging sporting events, regular unit training schedules (eg, establishing rifle and pistol ranges), and physical fitness training.

All personnel (including medical staff) should be fully trained in as realistic an operational environment as possible. People should expect to work in austere and sometimes rugged environments. Such conditions will require equipment, technology, and treatment approaches appropriate to the conditions. The capacity to develop work-arounds and to use field-expedient solutions is critical to achieving success. Because the medical doctrines and terminology of the services often differ, an essential component of predeployment training is addressing differences in doctrine and equipment of the US services and those of its allies and the host country. Operational failures that result from inadequate or unrealistic training can raise anxiety and uncertainty to the level of major stressors. By taking the steps noted above, this can be prevented.

Deployment

Commonly Identified Stressors

There are a number of stressors that are common in almost any deployment. Many of the stressors that were identified by Menninger[19] during World War II are still present: uncertainty, separation, privations, bombing in noncombat areas, isolation, climate, danger, fatigue, and differences in status and privilege among ranks and services. Other stressors are the length of the deployment, the degree of security (which may not allow adequate communication with family members or friends), boredom, and interruption of future plans (Figure 48-5).

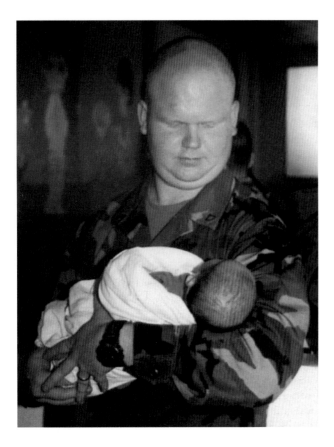

Figure 48-5. A soldier returns from a deployment to see his newborn son for the first time. Deployed service members often complain of missing births, deaths, and other important events in the lives of their family members. US Army photograph.

Phases of Deployment

Deployment may be thought of as occurring in three phases: an arrival period lasting days to weeks, a middle period that goes on for most of the deployment, and a terminal period that starts when service members are notified of their return date. Each period creates stresses on the service member that may affect the service member and last for a variable length of time. In addition, concerns about service and personal matters (eg, finances, unit procedures, career advancement, the future of one's life) do not disappear on deployment.

Passage of Time During Deployment

Time is a prominent issue in the prevention as well as the development of psychiatric disability in deployment and war. During World War II, personnel served for the duration of the war. During the

Vietnam War, each tour was limited to 1 year (actually 13 months within the draft period of 2 years of active duty) and, because of this rotation policy, each individual experienced his or her own early, middle, and late portion of deployment. Within the year in Vietnam, characteristic patterns of stress were interpreted based on the time in country. For example, Morris[20] described the phases of time for 225 noncombatant psychiatric patients in Vietnam, referred for treatment at Cam Ranh Bay, an Air Force field hospital in a secured area. Referrals were most frequent during the initial adjustment period, around the end of the first month. Separation from families was the most important precipitating factor (Figure 48-6). A second wave of referrals was seen between the fourth and sixth months, and this was called the "over the hump" phenomenon because these psychiatric problems tended to disap-

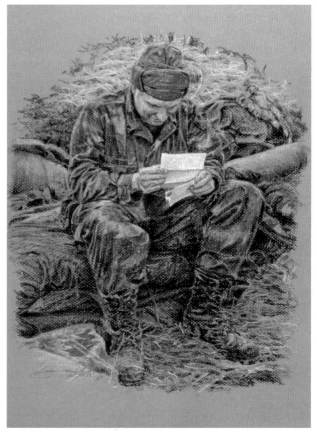

Figure 48-6. "Two Minutes at Home" by SSG Brian Fairchild. In spite of modern communication media, such as e-mail and cell phones, a letter from home is still the most valued form of support to deployed service members. Art: Courtesy of Army Art Collection, US Army Center of Military History, Washington, DC.

pear once personnel reached the midpoint of their tours. The service members participated in a kind of social ritual involving the parceling of time. Each parcel was a landmark; the person could aim for it and so reduce tension and renew the sense of hope. This served as an apparently effective way to cope with everyday stress.

Pincus and Benedek[17] observed that once soldiers were alerted for deployment to Bosnia they were already "psychologically deployed." Their sense of being "truly" deployed changed once they were on the ground in Europe and again when they crossed the Sava River and saw the destruction that had been caused by the war.

People pay attention to and use time differently in ways that may or may not be helpful. Time boundaries are often unclear in operational circumstances, and stages of deployment are but rough indicators of psychological processes that may or may not occur in service members and family members.

Deployment Stresses for Women

Chapter 18, Health Care for Women in Mobilization and Deployment, provides an extensive discussion of health issues for military women who may deploy. This chapter will detail only issues of women exposed to combat and other trauma. A discussion of military women as single parents is covered under the section on children in this chapter.

During fiscal year 1991, active duty female soldiers made up 9.1% of the US Army. It was reported that 49,950 women were deployed to the Persian Gulf during Operations Desert Shield and Desert Storm.[21] The large numbers of active duty and Reserve component women that are likely to be deployed will require the military services to consider new policies for social and operational interactions of men and women and provide additional health care resources for women. For example, elements of privacy for housing may impact on unit cohesion.

The exposure of women to combat trauma is by no means new (Figure 48-7). Women are also exposed to high levels of trauma, particularly in modern warfare where battle lines not clearly defined. Of the traumatic experiences of women in the Persian Gulf War, among the most prominent are Major Cornum's experiences as a prisoner of war[22] and the Scud missile attack that produced female casualties.[23] There were five reported deaths of women from hostile causes in the Persian Gulf War.[24]

Among troops returning from the Persian Gulf War, Army females were more symptomatic than males in response to certain war zone stressors, at least during the immediate postdeployment phase[25] (Figure 48-8). Because certain variables were not

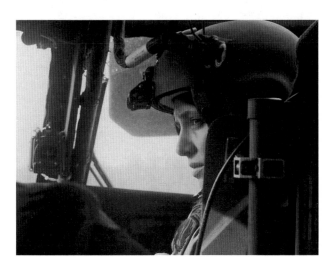

Figure 48-7. US Army women are assigned to some aviation units. Aviation missions are an important part of peacekeeping duties. In this photo, a female US Army officer prepares to fly a route reconnaissance mission over the city of Brcko, Bosnia.
US Army photograph by SPC Ricardo Gordon.

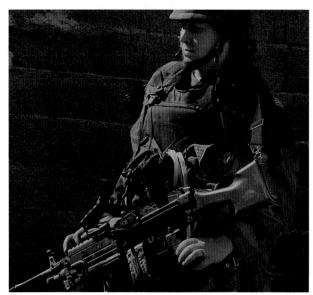

Figure 48-8. Military women must often carry weapons and perform the same duties as men. This soldier is on perimeter security duty with her M249 Squad Assault Weapon during a cordon and search mission in the village of Ugljare, Kosovo.
US Army photograph by SSG Milton H. Robinson.

controlled, such as prior sexual and criminal victimization experiences and sexual harassment during the deployment, these results should be interpreted cautiously. Some war zone stressors are likely to affect men and women differently as the nature of deployment missions continues to evolve. As women have more medical complaints and seek medical care more in civilian life than men, it should not be surprising that they would do so in military life.

In addition to the trauma of exposure to combat is the risk of interpersonal violence and sexual harassment.[26] Deployed military women were found to have higher rates of sexual and physical assault and sexual and verbal harassment than were typically found in civilian or peacetime military populations.[27] Sexual assault had a larger impact on post-traumatic stress disorder (PTSD) than combat exposure, and frequency of physical sexual harassment predicted PTSD symptomatology. However, the level of combat exposure was particularly low compared with Vietnam and the effects of combat and other stressors may differ across contexts.

The effect of deployment on spousal abuse has also been a matter of concern for the military. In a study of active duty Army personnel, a small increase was found in the probability of severe self-reported aggression for men and women who had deployed in the past year compared with those who had not deployed, and the increase was positively related to the length of deployment. The rate of severe aggression was from 3.7% to 4.1% for no deployment and increased to 5% for a deployment of 6 to 12 months. Thus, it was not solely the deployment that accounted for the severe aggression, but the longer the deployment the more likely the severe aggression becomes.[28]

During the Persian Gulf War, a significant number of mothers were deployed for the first time in American history, although there is no accurate count of these women.[29] A study[30] of deploying Navy mothers found higher levels of anxiety and parenting stress in women anticipating deployment than those who had recently returned. Single mothers reported more separation anxiety, less family cohesiveness, and less family organization than did married mothers. Maternal adjustment to a husband's deployment can vary with the type of deployment. For a routine deployment, maternal depression was highest at predeployment and progressively decreased at middeployment and postdeployment. For mothers whose husbands were deployed to the Persian Gulf War, significantly more depression was reported at predeployment and middeployment than at postdeployment, and

more dysphoria was reported at predeployment than at middeployment or postdeployment. There has been very little recent research on the deploying single fathers and their children, although one study[31] found that single Air Force fathers adapted well to separation.

Prior War Zone Experience

Prior deployment experience, particularly to a combat zone, can have significant effects on an individual. In some cases, an individual may be "inoculated" or "sensitized." Inoculation occurs when an experience provides an individual the opportunity to become more resistant to stress, such as by learning new skills and overcoming personal fears, an attitude of "I can take it." Sensitization is the opposite. The individual has suffered because of a prior experience. It is not wise to assume that just because an individual has had deployment or combat experience that the person will do well or will assist others. Experienced individuals can provide useful positive leadership, but in some cases, they may become liabilities by providing a negative message to the inexperienced that their lives will be ruined by their deployment experience or that they will never return home. These messages can have an effect on the morale of others, particularly younger, inexperienced personnel.

In some cases, earlier trauma can influence the reaction to the current conflict, or symptoms might actually be a result of that prior conflict and not the current one at all. A review of the records of medical discharges for PTSD given by the Army to soldiers who served in the Persian Gulf War found that 35% of these soldiers had also served in Vietnam.[32] About one-half of this group developed PTSD in anticipation of deployment to the Persian Gulf and, presumably, exposure to a combat environment. Also, soldiers with prior Vietnam service had odds ratios for PTSD that were between 5 and 24 when compared with soldiers without Vietnam service. These results indicated that for some service members with prior war experience, the threat of another exposure is sufficient to exacerbate existing symptoms or provide a new episode of PTSD. However, it should be noted that some literature indicates that risk of later PTSD is not increased by trauma but is increased by having had symptoms of PTSD. Victims of a motor vehicle accident with a history of PTSD were 8.02 times more likely at 1 month and 6.81 times more likely at 3 months to have PTSD than those without a history of PTSD.[33]

Coping With Deployment: A Navy Example

On war ships, the tempo of maintenance, drills, and standing watch keep the crew busy. On hospital ships, in contrast, there are extensive periods when the medical staff has little or nothing to do. Yerkes[34] described the stressors and coping strategies of the personnel unexpectedly assigned to the naval hospital ship USNS *Comfort* during its deployment to the Persian Gulf in August 1990 (Figure 48-9). The deployment of large numbers of medical personnel to sea duty was unusual at that time. Thus, most of the personnel were not used to working as a team and new rules had to be worked out. Multiple ship failures contributed to a lack of confidence in the ship and to feelings of helplessness and defenselessness. Information and mail were both slow and sporadic. The ship traveled alone for most of its trip. The prevalent feeling of abandonment led to personal interpretations of events. Feelings of grief were also seen due to personal losses such as loss of loved ones, coworkers, well-habituated shore positions, and physical security. The duration of the deployment was unknown, and there was no established rotation date.

Coping strategies included a variety of psychological defenses: humor (including pranks, songs, and stories), overeating, overexercising, and overworking. Group identification, after it formed, helped people feel that they were not alone. Space, time, and symbols such as different uniforms created boundaries. Some individual creativity was discouraged in favor of group norms. Some specific strategies recommended to help the crew adapt in future deployments included immediate assignment to a berthing and work center to create a sense of belonging, a visible administrative command, a flexible chain of command, training to foster an individual's sense of competency, and support for individuality and creativity as long as it does not interfere with group norms.

Stresses Encountered Before the Return Home

Some soldiers were frustrated at the perceived unfairness of their failure to return home following the end of the ground phase of the Persian Gulf War.[35] Some feared that they had been forgotten and were being left in Saudi Arabia. Among the presenting complaints were lethargy, suicidal and homicidal ideation, irritability, and nostalgia. In some cases, the symptoms became worse as a return date became more firm. This was described as "finish line fever," which may be a variation on or another name for short-timer's syndrome.

Substance Abuse

Drug and alcohol abuse must be considered as potential problems in any deployment. In the Vietnam War, drug abuse developed as a significant military and societal problem. It had not been anticipated and was, for a period, treated as a psychiatric problem. From 1960 until the Tet offensive of 1968, there was an extremely low rate of psychiatric casualties. As American involvement in combat intensified from 1966 through 1968, this rate relatively remained low but began to rise in late 1969.[36] Much of this rise in psychiatric casualties was based on drug abuse. Drug abusers were sometimes placed in the psychiatric category of character and behavior disorders. By 1971, a full-scale heroin epidemic had been recognized in Vietnam as well as in the United States.[37–39] The availability of relatively pure, cheap heroin made it the drug of choice. There was a difference of opinion about whether the increase in drug abuse was due to military duty in

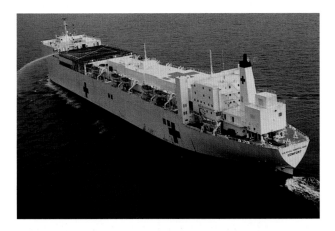

Figure 48-9. The hospital ship USNS Comfort (T-AH-20) is a large ship, about the size of a supertanker, with 12 operating rooms and a 1,000-bed capacity. The ship can be activated and crewed within 5 days, often by personnel who do not know each other. A vessel this large can present the command with problems of lack of cohesion among the crew as well as feelings of vulnerability when she travels unaccompanied by combat navy vessels. Unlike warships, on which the crew is constantly training and conducting maintenance, the medical crews of the hospital ships have long periods of boredom when the ship is not actually receiving casualties from ashore. US Army photograph.

Vietnam or was a minor problem and unrelated to the US presence there.[40] Studies demonstrated that combat units were no more likely to have a high percentage of drug abuse (measured by positive urinalyses on leaving Vietnam) than support units. However, by about August 1970, senior commanders recognized that heroin use by their personnel was a serious problem.[41] One of the major responses to the drug epidemic in Vietnam was to institute a urinalysis screening program for service members leaving Vietnam, and drug treatment programs were initiated throughout the service worldwide to handle increasing problems of drug and alcohol abuse.[38]

These factors demonstrate the influences of the overseas context but also indicate that trends in behavior found their most basic roots in American cultural behavior. Control of the illegal drug use in Vietnam required the combined efforts of many branches of the military services, including commanders, law enforcement and treatment agencies, and personnel to plan, administer, and evaluate the urinalysis program, perform epidemiological surveys, and conduct drug abuse education programs. It also encompassed major research efforts in Vietnam and the United States.[41] Prudence requires that military medical personnel be prepared for future drug and alcohol abuse problems that will create their own unique challenges in a deployed environment. Various programs to provide alternative behaviors should be provided (eg, hobby shops, USO [United Service Organizations] entertainment and tours, sports competitions, and physical fitness facilities).

Surveillance During Deployment

A mental health surveillance system is needed to enhance the capability of current surveillance methods so that an assessment of psychosocial factors is possible. A targeted psychosocial assessment can produce recommendations to counter effects of stressors. These countermeasures can later be assessed for effectiveness. Results can be compared with the lessons of other deployments and a classification of stressors and countermeasures developed. Such a model should involve both preventive medicine and behavioral science personnel, blending the traditionally medical with the psychological. Such a model should be more effective in preserving the health of service personnel than either approach alone.

A surveillance procedure to monitor injuries, diseases, and accidents, as well as psychosocial problems (eg, substance abuse, low unit cohesion), may help highlight specific commands or units that are under greater stress and would benefit from psychiatric consultation (Figure 48-10). During the arrival period, personnel are likely to be affected by the loss of the familiar home and work environment, cultural change, jet lag, and sleep disturbances. During the middle phase of the deployment, surveillance should include outcome review of medically evacuated patients to determine if there are particular types of complaints or behaviors that are likely to result in an individual being evacuated. It is then critical to establish whether patients wishing to return home consciously or unconsciously developed a particular symptom pattern (sometime called an "evacuation syndrome") to achieve an acceptable escape from the stressors of deployment. If such a situation develops, it will be necessary to determine the appropriateness of medical evacuation policy guidelines. In the terminal phase of the deployment, once service members know they are going home, vigilance on the part of service members, command, and the medical staff becomes especially important. It has been anecdotally noted that this is a time when some service members become careless and may be more prone to injuries and preventable disease.

An example of a clinical mental health monitoring effort was undertaken in Somalia by an Army combat stress control unit, a corps-level asset that

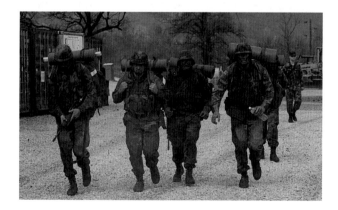

Figure 48-10. These soldiers are performing a "spur ride." The event is a tradition throughout cavalry units in the US Army. Spur candidates run around the camp to different events at Camp Demi in Bosnia. The purpose of the event is to build teamwork and confidence in the officers. Such activities are often important elements in building and maintaining unit cohesion.
US Army photograph.

supplements the division mental health section.[42] During predeployment, the stress control unit attempted to forecast the types of cases they would see and the types of medications they would need. They had expected to find service members traumatized by seeing starving children or dead bodies. Instead, they found stresses similar to those of low-intensity guerrilla warfare: changing rules of engagement, shooting incidents in which US personnel fired on Somalis, threats of violence, crowd control, and removing weapons from Somalis. They worked with preventive medicine personnel to visit the battalion aid stations, offered to see patients, and provided classes and consultations. This system provided an informal method of mental health surveillance. Classes focused on delineating the stresses on the soldiers, their reactions, and coping methods. Differences were found in the morale of the troops as the mission progressed and different stressors operated at different times. Among those encountered were environmental (eg, heat, sun, wind, noise), operational (eg, restricted travel, restricted missions), and personal stresses (eg, separation from home, boredom, ethical questions, lack of communication with home). Importantly, they also described the differences between psychiatric evacuations and attempted administrative actions that would have used the medical system, if possible, to remove unwanted service members from Somalia.

Reunion

There has been less research on the reunion phase of deployment than on the predeployment phase and the deployment itself. Many have written about the problems that service members have on their return, and the psychological and somatic symptoms that some suffer. There has been little focus on the less-symptomatic aspects of deployment and reunion, such as how individuals integrate their experiences (particularly of war and combat) into their own development in a positive way. Returnees should be advised to keep an open mind and not be committed to the outcome they have anticipated. Soldiers returning from Vietnam were advised to anticipate difficulties they might have in coping to help them reintegrate with families and integrate into new military units.[43]

With the ready availability of airlift from distant locations to home, reunion can now occur very quickly. Even after the end of World War II, though, it appeared that military personnel were also quickly being returned home. Menninger noted that after

the end of World War II, men were "catapulted"[19p365] back into civilian life. Even weeks on a ship returning home were short when compared with years in a war zone. Many had readjustment problems and needed to dissipate hatred, envy, and resentment.[44] During a combat deployment, fighting men endured the hell they were in by idealizing people and situations at home. The reality of their home situation was obscured by long separation. Both loved ones and veterans needed extra patience and understanding to weather the period of "factual refocusing."[19p367]

Postwar Physical and Psychological Symptoms

Somatic and stress symptoms may occur following deployment. A small percentage of war veterans have experienced somatic syndromes.[45] These have been associated with a variety of descriptive names depending on the conflict and most prevalent symptom. After the US Civil War, Da Costa's syndrome was noted; in World War I, effort syndrome; in World War II, battle fatigue, combat exhaustion, or operational fatigue; following the Vietnam War, post-Vietnam syndrome; and following the Persian Gulf War, as yet unexplained illnesses. These syndromes have been described as characterized by fatigue, shortness of breath, headache, disturbed sleep, and impaired concentration. Regardless of the name of the syndrome or pattern of symptoms, their lists look more alike than different, and they suggest a common core of symptoms associated with war-related medical and psychological stress.[45]

Depressive disorders were a significant problem for enlisted personnel returning from Vietnam. One quarter had some depressive symptoms, with 7% meeting criteria for an affective disorder. One third of those who had a psychiatric diagnosis had received psychiatric care since their return.[46] A 3-year follow-up study[47] of a randomly selected sample of 571 Vietnam veterans and 284 matched civilian controls provided some evidence that the depression found 1 year after combat was transient and that the effect of combat as a predictor of depression diminished over time. It should be noted that almost all studies of Vietnam veterans suffer from limitations imposed by the course of the war itself. During the last phase of the war, combat exposure was limited and morale was deteriorating, both in Vietnam and in the United States. Hence, studies of veterans who served in Vietnam at different times are difficult to interpret in terms of the impact of their experience in Vietnam and are difficult to compare with studies of combat veterans of other operations such as the invasion of Panama in 1989 or the Persian Gulf War. This is particularly true since the formal psychiatric diagnostic classification system was in the process of radical change during the 1970s. In 1980, the diagnosis of PTSD was introduced into the 3rd edition of the *American Psychiatric Associations' Diagnostic and Statistical Manual, (DSM-III)* as a result of a complex interaction between clinical experience, and political pressure.[48]

Postwar Readjustment

Bey[49] wrote of the psychological adjustment of the service member to Vietnam as well as the return home. He is one of the few authors who noted the difficulty personnel had in returning home, breaking bonds with fellow service personnel in Vietnam, missing friends, and feeling estranged at home. He attributed cases of adjustment depression to these types of losses, suggested that this reaction be treated as normal, and encouraged talking about and working through the relinquishing of ties with wartime friends. The camaraderie that helps to maintain closeness within a unit can sometimes be a later source of grief.[50] Extraordinary bonds that have been made have to be broken. Following the Persian Gulf War, readjustment was seen as easy because of three factors: (1) the low number of casualties, which resulted in less strain than if there had been mass casualties, (2) the support of the American people, and (3) the lack of drugs of abuse and alcohol in the theater.[50]

Reunion Briefings

Some Navy ships have a reunion briefing, generally conducted by the chaplain. The chaplain is likely to emphasize possible changes in family dynamics. This may include how a spouse has changed, the management of finances, and the disciplining of children. The sailor can then focus on the impact of newly gained family independence and changes in children's rewards and punishment.[51]

Readjustment of Female Veterans

The readjustment of female veterans has received little attention. Structured interviews were conducted between 1983 and 1985 with 50 female nurses who served in Vietnam from 1965 to 1973.[52] In the year immediately after the war, 12% reported minimal reactions, 8% had major emotional reactions including alcoholism and severe depression, while 80% had mixed reactions. Forty percent had high levels of involuntary intrusive thoughts, and 32% had avoidant behaviors. In subsequent years, including the time of the interviews, the group with an initially high level of intrusive thoughts (40%) had declined to 22%, and the level of avoidance declined from 32% to 14%. Those nurses who continued to have the highest levels of PTSD reported that they experienced an intense personal and professional year in Vietnam and faced poorly effective social networks at home. This study indicated that while nurses did not undergo the battlefield trauma experienced by men in the field, their experiences of witnessing trauma produced the same need to talk about the war as other veterans had and that the "toughness" that they developed to have been a veneer to cope with the stresses of the situation.

Shared Experiences and Memories

Memories of deployments or wars are often portrayed as a source of negative memories. The memories that are cited are often related to the development of PTSD or other forms of distress. Certainly, traumatic experiences that occur during war can result in PTSD; however, most who serve do not develop PTSD. Many memories of these experiences are positive. There were many descriptions of positive experiences in the Persian Gulf War and later US military operations.[29,53–56] Humor has kept up many spirits during difficult times in the military.[57] Informal "group therapy" sessions held by military physicians that allowed people to vent their frustrations and anxieties were important, as was group support from peers and from home.[58]

PSYCHOLOGICAL EFFECTS OF PREDEPLOYMENT, DEPLOYMENT, AND REUNION ON FAMILY MEMBERS

Spouses

There are many factors that determine family responses to deployment.[59] Among these are the deployment itself, as well as family, spouse, and child factors. Deployment factors include its length and frequency and whether it is a wartime or peacetime deployment. Family factors include the age and sex of children, parental attitudes, availability of social supports, history of coping skills and adaptability, and past experiences with separation.

Predeployment preparations can often isolate the family from the service member quickly. Many operational deployments occur on short notice. Unscheduled deployments are considered more stressful than scheduled ones.[60] Unscheduled (and sometime scheduled) deployments often require an intense period of unit preparation, which gives the service member less time for personal and family preparation for the impending absence. There are often additional training requirements that can keep the service member in the field for long periods of time and some that require the unit to temporarily relocate to another installation for special training. Most spouses adapt well to the stress of deployment.[59] Stresses in families, however, can lead to clinical problems that must be addressed by the health care system. A spouse's role becomes that of a single parent and decisions are made by that person rather than by the departed spouse or the couple. New skills must be learned and new responsibilities shouldered by the spouse and the family left behind. The relationships with children can change when children challenge discipline and have to fulfill some parental roles.

During the Persian Gulf War, both younger and older spouses of Army soldiers experienced high levels of emotional discomfort, albeit for different reasons.[61] There was a perception that available family support services favored younger spouses and ignored the problems of older spouses. Spouses rated their expectation of what the Army should provide them while their spouses were deployed and their use of and satisfaction with 15 different types of community services before and during the deployment. Groups with the highest level of distress also had the highest ratings of expectations of the Army and the highest unsatisfactory ratings of the use of support services.

After the war, spouses of junior enlisted soldiers who remained on active duty were less likely to have had unrealistic expectations of the Army than the spouses of those soldiers who left active duty. For mid-level noncommissioned officers, the main predictor of retention was the spouse's wish that the soldier stay in the Army.[62] In some cases, these expectations of spouses may be impossible to correct, but it does underscore the importance of commanders providing accurate information to families before, during, and after a deployment. It is important to avoid statements that will lead to unrealistic expectations.

A survey was conducted of 378 wives of enlisted Army soldiers deployed to Somalia for 2 to 5 months.[63] Changes in marital satisfaction and four stressors that could have affected the wives during the deployment were investigated: pregnancy, death of a friend or relative, loneliness, and difficulty communicating with the husband. The effects of the various difficulties were less stressful in terms of their impact on marital satisfaction than is often assumed, even for marriages that might be considered relatively unstable. The investigators concluded that being stressed during a husband's deployment was not necessarily enough of a problem to detract from marital satisfaction.

Family support groups have become a regular feature of the military services.[59] When a service member deploys, the spouse (usually a wife) is encouraged to participate in a spouses' support group, which is often affiliated with the rear detachment of the unit. This rear detachment can facilitate contact between members of the deployed unit and the families and perform valuable advocacy services for the spouses. We do not know of any research or reports on support groups that have included husbands of deployed service members.

Bey and Lange[64] interviewed 40 spouses whose husbands had deployed to Vietnam and described the stresses of these women. A wide variety of different stressors were described during the time before deployment, the deployment phase, and following the husband's return. When the husband received orders to deploy, they described feelings of numbness, shock, and disbelief even though they knew logically that the husband would receive orders. They noted increasing distance between themselves and their husbands as the time for departure neared. During the separation, wives complained of their awkward social situation. Friendship and even contact with men was often viewed negatively and as infidelity by some. They described themselves as estranged from others who had little empathy for their plight. Those who were in a "waiting wives" group were an exception. Most said that these groups helped to alleviate stress but at other times increased it. The social situation of the civilian milieu also increased their stress in that the commonly held view was that the war was stupid and futile. Those who expressed their discomfort through somatic complaints were sometimes rebuffed by the medical staff who saw them as demanding but physically well. Failure of the medical professional to appreciate the problems created by deployments for these spouses can needlessly serve as an additional stressor.

Reunion can eliminate some stressors, but it often creates additional ones.[59] Adjustments required during separation are often undone after reunion, sometimes not to everyone's satisfaction. New skills and independence manifested by spouses and children may not be appreciated by and may actually be seen as threatening to the returning service member. The discipline of children can be a particularly difficult adjustment area for families. Children may also find it difficult to include the returning parent into relationships formed with the remaining parent.

Children

Parental deployment puts additional stresses on children that often are not recognized by the parent.[59] Constancy of the relationship with the departed parent is broken, children can blame themselves for the parent's absence, and they can be angry at the military for taking the parent away. Symptoms in children may depend on their stage of development, but some of the most frequent complaints are abdominal, followed by sleep disturbance, headaches, decreased motor activity, withdrawal, moodiness, and school phobia.

Internalizing (distress that is directed inward) and externalizing (distress that is directed outward) behaviors of children were compared for children of fathers on routine deployment and the deployment to the Persian Gulf War. For children whose fathers were deployed during peacetime, both internalizing and externalizing behaviors declined from predeployment to postdeployment but stayed high throughout for children whose fathers were deployed to the Persian Gulf War.[65] In a study of 1,601 children of soldiers deployed to the Persian Gulf War, questionnaires were completed by the parent who stayed at home with the child.[66] Sadness was commonly reported, but few parents considered their children had problems severe enough to warrant counseling. In a review of the literature on the military family, brief father absences (less than 1 to 2 years) were associated with temporary emotional and behavioral symptoms in family members, primarily wives and sons.[67]

SURVEILLANCE RESEARCH DURING DEPLOYMENT

Surveillance Research in the Baltic States

When psychiatric illness or disturbance is infrequent, a surveillance system that uses only case counts will not be satisfactory for determining the psychological status of those deployed. Another mental health and behavior surveillance system, one in which behavioral scientists interview, give paper-and-pencil surveys, and observe individuals, was used on the Bosnia deployment.[68] Data were collected on approximately 300 soldiers on a 6-month deployment to Croatia in November 1992, a second group of approximately 200 soldiers deployed to Croatia in March 1993, and an Army infantry unit in Macedonia in July 1993 on a border patrol mission. Topics covered in the surveys included sources of stress, physical and mental health outcomes (including morale), and individual and organizational factors that might influence responses to stress. Extensive studies of a subgroup provided examples of the stressors service members faced at each stage of the deployment.

The major stress factor in the predeployment phase was uncertainty about who was going and when and getting to know peers and leaders. During the middeployment phase, one critical stress factor was boredom due to lack of meaningful work in the hospital. Other stressors included restrictions by command about outreach programs and a perceived lack of support from rear echelon support elements. The key stressors of the late-deployment period were concerns about the future location of the unit after they returned (some units were moved and some de-activated after the conflict) and whether the service members would have to move their families. Analysis of the stress factors produced a set of stressors and countermeasures (Table 48-3). The major stressors identified were isolation, ambiguity, powerlessness, boredom, and threat. Countermeasures included steps recommended for leaders to reduce these stressors. This report provides one model for the development of hypotheses and analyses in deployment research.

Post-Bosnia Medical and Psychological Surveillance

The national leadership would like to have better knowledge of the medical status of service personnel before and during deployments. With the support of the Congress, the Department of Defense is attempting to implement a screening program in which service members departing from Bosnia receive a medical fact sheet and a physical examination, including a personalized review of any findings (see Chapter 49, Medical Issues in Redeployment).

Changes in health status are documented in a service member's medical record. The follow-up should be scheduled within 30 days of returning to the United States, and within 90 days personnel should receive a Mantoux tuberculin test and undergo psychological testing.[69] As a part of the Bosnian rotation, extensive screening programs for medical and mental health conditions are being put in place. Screening takes place before new personnel join the implementation force, during the deployment, and as they pull out to return to their home base. This should provide the Department of Defense with information on the health status of its personnel that could be used to investigate postdeployment health problems. This is an attempt to avoid the lack of data for investigations in the past as happened with Agent Orange in the Vietnam War and the controversial Persian Gulf War illnesses.[70] It is essential that a surveillance system should also track illegal drug and alcohol abuse.

Psychometric Tests and Epidemiology

Part of the difficulty in understanding the relationships between stress and either distress or illness in psychiatric epidemiology is that of defining what is a case.[71,72] Symptom measures on questionnaires do not constitute a diagnosis and may be misleading. While symptoms of depression do not necessarily constitute a case of depression, many questionnaires attempt to measure symptoms of depression, anxiety, and PTSD because ignorance of the etiology of many psychiatric illnesses makes symptoms the defining criteria.[73] This situation results in problems relating to sensitivity and specificity, problems quite familiar to those who have used urinalysis to identify drug abusers.[74] Since psychiatric diagnosis carries stigma, false positives are particularly undesirable. Thus the development of truly effective psychiatric surveillance programs continues to be a considerable technical challenge.

TABLE 48-3

PSYCHOLOGICAL ISSUES IN PEACEKEEPING OPERATIONS

	Stressors	Countermeasures
ISOLATION	Physically remote locations	Give accurate and useful information—what to expect
	Communication problems	Provide briefings by those who have been there
	Multiple units in task force	Encourage use of e-mail, phone, fax
	Individuals cross-attached	Conduct team-building exercises
AMBIGUITY	Mission not clear	Give clear definition of mission
	Command structure confusion	Hold frequent meetings, "commander calls" to provide information and answer questions
POWERLESSNESS	Rules of engagement restrictions	Explain and justify rules of engagement
	Limited activity/productivity	Provide education and self-development options
	Foreign culture and language	Provide classes on host culture, language
	Relative deprivation: "double standards"	Assure fair access to goods and services, explain discrepancies honestly
BOREDOM	Repetitive, monotonous routine	Use creative training programs
	Shortage of professional work	Establish personnel exchange programs with other forces
	Lack of meaningful work	Self-development and education programs
THREAT OR DANGER	Threat to life or limb	Provide sound training, equipment, policies
	Mines, snipers, disease	Keep soldiers informed about physical threat
		Offer regular debriefings

Adapted from: Bartone PT, Adler AB. A model for soldier psychological adaptation in peacekeeping operations. *Proceedings of the 36th Annual Conference of the International Military Testing Association.* Rotterdam, The Netherlands; 1994: 33-40. As cited in: US Army Medical Research Unit-Europe, Walter Reed Army Institute of Research. A Model of Psychological Issues in Peacekeeping Operations. WRAIR; 18 March 1996. Research Report #23.

COMMAND AND MEDICAL CONSULTATION

One of the primary duties of a special staff officer is to educate the commander in the area of the staff officer's expertise. Among the major tasks of medical staff officers throughout predeployment, deployment, and reunion are assessment and consultation. Consultation in a military environment is the process of providing advice to commanders and members of the commander's staff on issues that affect the health and performance of military personnel in their organization.[75] Thus, the unit of consultation is the group and not the individual.

Consultation is a two-way street, one that involves interchange between the consultant and the commander, staff, service members, and families. Without such interchange, the consultant is likely to have little understanding of the unit and its problems, and the likelihood of the consultant's advice being followed will depend in some degree on the confidence the command has in the consultant. Such confidence is based on the development of a mutually satisfactory relationship. To be deserving of command support, the medical officer must have a deep understanding of the relevant biomedical and behavioral risk factors associated with the deployment being planned and the overall military mission. The primary mission of the medical officer and other special staff officers is to build this understanding with the line officers.

The appropriate outcome of the consultation process is the incorporation of the medical and psychiatric recommendations in a form that can be supported by the commander as elements within operation plans. Such plans involve complex systems that will require those medical and psychiatric recommendations to interact with other technical requirements.

Infectious Diseases

Infectious diseases that are endemic in the deployment area but rare in the United States are a significant threat to military forces. Deployments will almost always require the medical staff to recommend procedures to prevent or lessen the effects of problems with infectious disease and biological and chemical agents. Sometimes this advice will entail that the service members take prophylactic medications. There are significant psychological factors that will inhibit adherence with medical recommendations and policies. To achieve better acceptance of medical advice and compliance to its requirements, those providing the advice must understand the psychological factors underlying the resistance or acceptance of medical recommendations. Frequently, this is based on a lack of understanding of the technical basis of the medical recommendations. Failure to appreciate limitations of preventive programs may result in angry and disappointed commanders and will promote resistance to further medical recommendations.

The use of negative reinforcements or punishment to assure compliance may produce complicated aggressive behaviors and destructive actions. To support a program that is geared to available resources and assure compliance, is it critical that the intervention being recommended be well understood in terms of both intended effects and side effects. Such programs require careful scientific monitoring to assure they are effective and cost-efficient.

Chemical and Biological Agents

The medical and military responses to chemical and biological warfare are complex. Physicians must be responsible for the diagnosis and treatment of the psychiatric and organic consequences associated with biological weapons. They and other medical professionals must provide reassurance and care required to maintain morale in the presence of such a threat. One of the most important roles of physicians is to assist the leadership, whether military or civilian, in considering the psychological and social impact of terrorist or military attacks on US military personnel or populations. Primary prevention efforts by all concerned are critical in preventing panic, counterproductive responses, and demoralization in the attacked community.[76] Examples of counterproductive actions would be the inappropriate use of unproven drugs, inappropriate vaccination that results in acute side effects but provides minimal protection, and inappropriate evacuation and quarantine. Risk communications plans (see next section) must be developed so that the population threatened may be accurately and effectively informed concerning the nature of the risk and appropriate responses.

Prophylactic Medications

If they have the expertise, mental health and preventive medicine consultants must advise commanders how to effectively communicate the risks and benefits associated with using vaccines and prophylactic agents.[77] This information must be provided to service members before and during the deployment phase of an operation, as well as at the homecoming and long afterward. If the mental health and preventive medicine consultants do not have specific training in risk communication, it would be appropriate for them to advise the commander on how to find such expertise. Risk communication requires great care in the use of language that is accurate and can be understood by the service member.[78]

Risk communication must be interactive. Those instituting programs must understand what information the subject population requires and how they understand the information. It is sometimes difficult for those who have knowledge of risks to communicate those risks to service members in such a way that the risks and benefits are understood and supported. Risk communication should help to explain to service members that they are not being used for experimental purposes or otherwise being put at more risk from the drug than they would be from the enemy or the environment. One of the goals of risk communication should be to create confidence in service members that the command has a true concern about their health and well-being. It is likely that risk communication will occur in an environment in which the media may report material incorrectly or in a way that would undermine such confidence. Service members who lack confidence in the intervention may later attribute a variety of later problems to having received a medication or vaccine, regardless of the safety profile of that medication or procedure.

PREVENTION AND TREATMENT OPTIONS

Preventive Interventions

The Institute of Medicine proposed a prevention model for mental health disorders in 1994 that encompasses three echelons of prevention interventions: universal, selective, and indicated.[79] Universal interventions can be performed by many individuals and are considered appropriate for everyone. Interventions can include education programs that provide information about the environment, principles of leadership, or the purpose of specific deployments.

As deploying units are identified, members may be assumed to be at higher risk for developing a mental health problem. Selective interventions may be aimed at the groups at highest risk for potential adverse outcomes. A variety of mental health and general health care providers may become engaged in this effort. Interventions may include creation of family support groups, stress management lectures, suicide prevention lectures, and routine informational debriefings after missions. When such programs are designed, however, measures of need and effectiveness should be developed at the same time. Studies documenting the positive and adverse effects of programs would also be welcome.

Indicated interventions are appropriate for individuals who have been specifically identified as being at high risk of developing a new or recurrent mental disorder but are without a clinically active illness. These may include individuals with diagnosed-but-stable disorders or with significant family, occupational, or drinking problems. These problems may predispose the individual toward developing a diagnosable disorder or experiencing a recurrence of a mental disorder, and early intervention may avert the occurrence or worsening of the disorder. Early intervention is a key concept behind the traditional treatment intervention of military psychiatry. There is a need for additional research concerning the effectiveness and cost of such early interventions.

The best possible working group of available personnel should assess risk and design interventions that will minimize distress and disability. Such a group might consist of preventive medicine officers, flight surgeons, psychiatrists and other physicians, psychologists, social workers, chaplains, staff planners, enlisted leadership, and commanders. The programs should encourage cohesion, social support, and information about the mission; it should generally deal with needs reported by ordinary service members and their immediate supervisors. Once an individual's problem reaches the threshold of a diagnosable psychiatric condition, physicians and mental health personnel should become involved in the direct care of that patient.

Training of Medical Professionals

It is likely that inexperienced personnel will be in positions of responsibility in future deployments, as they have been in the past. Inexperienced medical personnel may be in regions in which they will have little familiarity with endemic diseases. These physicians may not have been exposed to extreme violence or its consequences. All staff personnel will be called on to develop some understanding of the effect of the local culture on deployed service members. They would also be required to understand how service members affect the local culture. Reservists called to active duty may have little opportunity to become familiar with these issues. Regardless of service members' level of experience, each new deployment brings its own problems. Part of the primary prevention function among the medical community involves educating each other and the development of flexible doctrine and policy that can be applied to other situations. This is particularly true of joint operations where there are significant differences in the professional jargon and nomenclature of equipment between the services, which can sometimes make even basic communication difficult.[75] Increasing the amount of training in joint operations will make this less of a risk. Currently, the US military medical departments have joint medical training for medical students at the Uniformed Services University of the Health Sciences and for residents, hospital staff, and field units. In addition, the medical evacuation chain has always been a joint service operation. It will be important, however, for Reservists to be included in joint training or to make special efforts to teach them in such procedures as soon as they are involved in preparation for deployment or in deployment itself.

Booklets, Pamphlets, Training Manuals, and Models

During recent deployments, the Headquarters, Department of the Army has prepared a number of information-transmitting media for soldiers and their families. Some of them are only a few pages and are made to fit in the pocket of field gear (for example, titles include *Stress Dimensions in Military Operations Other Than War*, *When the Mission Requires Recovering Human Dead Bodies*, and *Critical Event Debriefing* and others). Other examples of material created for such training are the Army's relocation and deployment books, a course for organizing family support groups during the soldier's absence. The US Army Community and Family Support Center, a headquarters element of the Army staff, in 1995 prepared a series of books for families called Operation READY (Resources for Educating About Deployment and You) to prepare soldiers and families for deployment. There are six binders entitled Pre-deployment Ongoing Readiness, Family Assistance Center, Family Support Group Advanced Training, Post-deployment Homecoming Reunion, Army Readiness Handbook, and Children's Workbook. They were distributed Army-wide with five training videos. In addition to these Army publications, commercial firms have published a wide variety of self-help pamphlets for children and spouses.

Peebles-Kleiger and Peebles[60] described a model of peacetime deployment used by the Navy for family education and intervention before, during, and after the Persian Gulf War. This model was based on an "emotional cycle" of adjustment to the various phases of deployment. They cautioned against using a peacetime model for wartime deployments because wartime deployment is unexpected, disruptive, and hazardous and involves the anticipation of trauma, which increases the level of stress.

The development of educational materials is often based on specific models or theoretical constructs. While models can be useful for conceptualizing knowledge about stresses, vulnerabilities, and interventions, they can be limiting in that they do not take account of the diversity of individual differences and situations. Some models overemphasize the risk factors for negative outcomes of individuals and pay less attention to possibilities of personal gains that come from coping with stress. Rutter has provided thoughtful discussion of the interplay of adversity, risk, and resilience in individuals at various stages of life.[80] In his view, risk factors operate in a variety of different ways, and people respond to adversity based on their own personal history, their own stage of development, and the external circumstances. Resilience may thus reside in the social context as well as in the individual. While he notes that there is some knowledge of what the risk and protective factors are, we have little understanding of the processes they reflect or how to use them to increase resilience. The processes by which interventions work are largely untested.

It is Department of Defense policy to implement combat stress control (CSC) policies.[81] CSC is seen largely as a preventive activity and attempts to foster cooperation between preventive medicine and the mental health disciplines (see Chapter 16, Combat Stress Control and Force Health Protection). Army field manuals address issues of combat stress and provide the Army doctrine for mental health operations in the field at the unit level, for separate combat stress control detachments, and for leaders.[82,83] The US Marine Corps combat stress doctrine is published in US Marine Corps Fleet Marine Force Manual 4-55 (13 April 1992).

Debriefing as a Preventive Mental Health Strategy

The group interview technique that is commonly known as a debriefing has become popular in a variety of military situations, particularly following exposures to traumatic events. It is hoped that debriefing after a traumatic event will help to prevent future psychiatric disorders, such as PTSD and other forms of distress. As the Department of Defense directive states, CSC unit personnel "will evaluate units after exceptionally stressful events and conduct Critical Event Debriefings, as indicated."[81]

There are now numerous references in the military medical literature to situations in which some form of debriefing has been used.[13,84–91] Debriefings seem to be uncritically accepted in today's military as necessary and beneficial. Toward the end of the Persian Gulf War, debriefings were extensively provided as a preventive measure.[35] It is important to note, though, that documentation of the efficacy of debriefing and other recommendations and interventions is generally lacking. The inference is sometimes drawn that PTSD is the most common outcome of stress, which also has not been proven. Other outcomes, such as acute stress disorder, dissociative disorders, adjustment disorder, depression, anxiety, and substance abuse disorders, are often not even considered.

There is a limited theoretical basis for debriefing in the prevention of psychiatric disorders. Application of debriefing around events described as "critical" can be misleading in a number of ways to the practitioner, the subject, and the commander. First, although there are many events that are called critical, there are always other issues that are also important and deserve attention, such as an event or policy that has affected unit morale. Second, the implication for some will be that once the preventive debriefing has been held, there is no further need to worry about the longer-term effects of the critical event. Such beliefs could lead the subject or the practitioner to overlook symptoms that develop later. Third, there is no standard evaluation technique by which to judge the effectiveness of the procedure.

There is a growing body of literature on this subject that includes controversy about the efficacy of the procedure. Psychological debriefing following a traumatic event does not, in itself, guarantee that its recipients will suffer no future psychological disturbances. Studies of group debriefing after extreme events have failed to show a significant long-term effect of this technique, but the heterogeneity of the interventions studied and the length of time between debriefing and its assessment may make a proper evaluation of findings difficult.[92] Israeli soldiers were provided a historical group debriefing within 72 hours after having been exposed to combat. Anxiety, self-efficacy, and combat evaluation were measured before and immediately after the sessions. Debriefing was followed by a reduction in anxiety, an improvement in self-efficacy, and an increase in homogeneity of the group. The investigators concluded that the effects of the debriefing might have been attributable to enhanced group cohesion or to the beneficial effects of the debriefing.

A study of 62 British soldiers who served in the Persian Gulf War, found evidence suggestive of PTSD in 50% of them following debriefing.[93] British body handlers reported subjective benefit from debriefings but had no fewer symptoms compared with those who were not debriefed. In addition, critical incident stress debriefing and management teams could be a hindrance to first responders in biological and other disasters.[94]

Among the values of the debriefing, as practiced by Shalev[95] and Koshes and colleagues[96] are the opportunity of the debriefer to hear the perspective and experiences of those participating in the group interview and the opportunity of the participants to hear the thoughts, feelings, and descriptions of events provided by others in the group. Shalev provides a good discussion of the goals of psychological debriefing and Koshes and colleagues provide examples. Debriefing limited numbers of key personnel may serve as an assessment tool in determining possible problem areas regarding unit morale, cohesion, and function. Instructing commanders to perform debriefing in a fact-finding, lessons-learned format will also foster unit cohesion and a sense of mission. Whenever possible, unit self-reliance should be encouraged rather than unit reliance on external mental health resources.

There are many other activities that are appropriate for victims instead of or in addition to a debriefing. McDuff illustrated the value of a recovery environment for victims in several different hostage-release scenarios.[97] The postcaptivity environment should attempt to promote cohesiveness within the victim group, isolate the victims from external groups, promote abreaction, and provide an opportunity for rest. Interventions may help by restoring the sense of power to the victim and reducing feelings of isolation, of helplessness, and of being dominated. These procedures provide a structured termination process for the group, which may help in the individual's long-term recovery.

Use of Psychotropic Medications

Use of psychiatric medications in a deployment setting is controversial among military psychiatrists, and there are differences in medication policies among the services. With few exceptions, Navy and Marine Corps personnel will not be deployed when taking psychiatric medications. Frequently, these units are widely dispersed and psychiatric follow-up is not routinely available. Army personnel are more frequently deployed while taking these medications. The Army routinely deploys in greater mass and with more substantial medical support, to include psychiatric services. Mental health services at the division level are frequently augmented by combat stress detachments, which may provide some capability for monitoring service members taking psychotropic medications.

The need for antipsychotic or mood stabilizing medications is an indication of severe or chronic psychiatric illness, which generally should not be managed in a deployment setting. On a case-by-case basis, a service member who chronically uses anxiolytic or stimulant agents should be evaluated by a psychiatrist before deployment. Short-term use of benzodiazepines or other soporific agents may

be indicated in restoring normal sleep patterns disrupted by irregular schedules and sleep deprivation,[98] but they can interfere with prophylactic medication schedules.[9] Training personnel in how to manage other disruptions to work-rest cycles and other operational problems on an individual and a unit basis without medications is an important consideration for future operations. Clinicians have frequently been tempted to use psychotropic medications to aid individuals distressed by combat. The use of antipsychotic agents such as chloropromazine was common in Vietnam. We do not know the consequence of this usage, but given our knowledge of the effect of these drugs on performance, it is unlikely that anyone would recommend their use in a combat setting today. At present, there is little data that would justify the use of these agents in the combat context. There is a need for research on the impact of psychotropic drugs on military and combat performance.

THE NEED FOR RESEARCH ON REUNION ISSUES

Research on the stresses of homecoming following deployment is needed. This topic covers a variety of issues. First among these is the need to determine the expectations of service members or their families before reunion. Reunion briefings and other materials prepared to assist people in this phase have been developed, based on a general theory of stress that includes a myriad of possible symptoms. It would be helpful to know what stresses service members, spouses, and children expect to face, the stresses that they actually face, and how they cope.

The number of studies in this area on women, whether single or married, mothers or childless, is

very limited. Research should investigate the different deployment and homecoming experiences of men and women, as well as women's adjustment, coping strategies, health care utilization, morbidity, and mortality.[99] The long-term adjustment of the deployed female veteran has been little researched except in nurses.

The material referenced for this chapter has been almost exclusively based on active duty military personnel. In the future, it will be important to develop a better understanding of the stressors that confront Reservists who deploy. Finally, long-term follow-up of deployed service members and their families has not been carefully studied.

SUMMARY

The preventive medicine officer should work with the military mental health community to prepare for and successfully accomplish the deployment mission in the post–Cold War environment. The medical mission includes the preparation of the service member, the family of the service member, and the military unit for the three phases of deployment.

Deployments today tend to be unexpected, rapid, and of uncertain duration and have a mission that shifts as the deployment unfolds. The deployment environment in the 1990s developed during an era of shrinking military resources and increasing demands on service members and their families. The services are truly doing more with less. Military

medical resources have not escaped the overall cuts. The result is a thinly spread, largely inexperienced force that is not always deployed as a unit but often as individuals or in small groups. The result is a unit in which cohesion must be constructed during an operation only to be lost when the mission is completed or individuals are rotated out. Finally, the battlefield has changed to include the high likelihood of the use of chemical and biological agents and information technology and new classes of weapons, such as lasers and smart munitions, that can deliver increased firepower more accurately. This means that smaller and smaller military units may be fighting on a very fluid and very deadly battlefield.

Military deployments have the potential to be widely dispersed over the earth's surface. This means service members face unfamiliar, severe environmental challenges and exotic diseases on a scale for which the US civilian medical community may be unprepared. The stress on all military medical practitioners is high as they contend with preventing and treating illness and injury.

Much of the published literature consists of case reports or case series that have not been developed on solid epidemiologic, sociological, or anthropological principles. Most articles convey the medical reporter's snapshot of a specific deployment or tour of duty. As cases are described diagnostically, there is a tendency to rely on psychological scales or tests for which predictive values are erroneously considered equal to test sensitivity or specificity.

The effects of deployments on the family of the service member continue to be studied, and the services have developed a wealth of preventive and support practices to help spouses and children. A lingering problem, however, is the hesitance, particularly of younger spouses, to use the supports available. Family structures are constantly changing, and families who live off the installation are particularly difficult to find and attract to on-installation services.

Studies of how leadership interacts with preventive medicine practices are essential to a good operational outcome. Commanders face challenges such as working in a multinational environment, serving as ambassadors to the local population, using vaccines and pharmaceuticals to prevent morbidity and mortality, being involved in political decisions, and having their decisions reviewed by politicians. These requirements are very demanding of a commander's time and energy, but coordination of national political goals with military goals is essential in many deployments. That such requirements exist at all is controversial, but a commander should expect to spend considerable time and energy on such issues, particularly as they may affect the morale of the command.

The importance of support of service members and their families will continue to be of the greatest importance to the leadership of the military services. The spirit of pride and accomplishment demonstrated by military personnel in the post–Cold War environment has been exemplary. Continued support by the national leadership, the media, the US public, commanders, and families have also been crucial to the military forces. All these elements support unit cohesion, a cornerstone of deployment readiness and mission accomplishment.

This chapter has been designed to illustrate the depth of information that is published while attempting to link psychological and social issues to the traditional practice of preventive medicine. The integrated disciplines have the potential to develop a solid bio-psycho-social picture of the behavioral and social risks that confront service members and families. In this way, the affect education, training, and deployment have on health status can be tracked and environmental, psychological, and moral factors considered. At some later point, these factors may be embedded in a medical record system that directly feeds surveillance systems, such that researchers can understand the exposures and measure outcomes. Such a system does not exist today but should be considered critical to the military mission.

Acknowledgment

The authors would like to express their appreciation to Jennifer Erk for her reading and commentary on the many drafts of this manuscript.

REFERENCES

1.   The White House. *A National Security Strategy for a New Century*. Washington, DC: The White House; May 1997.

2.   Department of the Army. *Operations*. Washington, DC: DA; 1993. US Army Field Manual 100-5.

3.   Young MR. *The Vietnam Wars: 1945–1990*. New York: HarperCollins; 1991.

4.   Sutker PB, Uddo M, Brailey K, Allain AN. War-zone trauma and stress-related symptoms in Operation Desert Shield/Storm (ODS) returnees. *J Social Issues*. 1993;49:33–49.

5. Doutheau C, Lebigot F, Moraud C, Crocq L, Fabre LM, Fabre JD. Stress factors and psychopathological reactions of UN missions in the French Army. *Int Rev Armed Forces Med Svcs.* 1994;1/2/3:36–38.

6. Stretch RH, Bliese PD, Marlowe DH, Wright KM, Knudson KH, Hoover CH. Psychological health of Gulf War-era military personnel. *Mil Med.* 1996;161:257–261.

7. Gunby P. Service in strict Islamic nation removes alcohol, others drugs from major problem list. *JAMA.* 1991;265:560,562.

8. Gunby P. Somalia operation just one of many demands on US military medicine. *JAMA.* 1993;269:11–12.

9. Ledbetter E, Shallow S, Hanson KR. Malaria in Somalia: lessons in prevention. *JAMA.* 1995;273:774–775.

10. Gunby P. Could late spring bring an end to US military medicine's "New World Order" role in Somalia? *JAMA.* 1994;271:92–96.

11. Hall DP, Cipriano ED, Bicknell G. Preventive mental health interventions in peacekeeping missions to Somalia and Haiti. *Mil Med.* 1997;162:41–43.

12. Trofa AF, DeFraites RF, Smoak BL, et al. Dengue fever in US military personnel in Haiti. *JAMA.* 1997;277:1546–1548.

13. Hall DP. Stress, suicide and military service during Operation Uphold Democracy. *Mil Med.* 1996;161:159–162.

14. Gunby P. Military medicine has NATO role in Balkans. *JAMA.* 1996;275:24.

15. Gunby P. Military medicine offers support on land, sea, and in the air for US Bosnia peace enforcers. *JAMA.* 1996;275:507.

16. Gunby P. Military physicians face new challenges as Bosnia peacekeeping effort lengthens. *JAMA.* 1997;277:617–618.

17. Pincus SH, Benedek DM. Operational stress control in the former Yugoslavia: A joint endeavor. *Mil Med.* 1998;163:358–362.

18. Gunby P. Military medicine's role continues in Bosnia. *JAMA.* 1996;276:1370.

19. Menninger WC. *Psychiatry in a Troubled World.* New York: MacMillan; 1948.

20. Morris LE. "Over the Hump" in Vietnam: Adjustment patterns in a time-limited stress situation. *Bull Menninger Clin.* 1970;34:352–362.

21. Murphy F, Browne D, Mather S, Scheele H, Hyams KC. Women in the Persian Gulf War: Health care implications for active duty troops and veterans. *Mil Med.* 1997;162:656–660.

22. Cornum R, as told to Copeland P. *She Went to War.* Novato, Calif: Presidio Press; 1992.

23. Perconte ST, Wilson AT, Pontius EB, Dietrick A, Kirsch C, Sparacino C. Unit-based intervention for Gulf War soldiers surviving a SCUD missile attack: Program description and preliminary findings. *J Trauma Stress.* 1993;6:225–238.

24. Department of Defense, Washington Headquarters Services, Directorate for Information Operations and Reports, Statistical Information Analysis Division. Worldwide US Active Duty Military Deaths (Table 13). Washington, DC: DoD; 2000. http://web1.osd.mil/mmid/casualty/table13.htm (Accessed on 5/9/00)

25. Wolfe J, Brown PJ, Kelley JM. Reassessing war stress: exposure and the Persian Gulf War. *J Social Issues.* 1993;49:15–31.

26. Wolfe J. Abuse and trauma in women: broadening the social context. *Am Psychol.* 1990;45:1386.

27. Wolfe J, Sharkansky EJ, Read JP, Dawson R, Martin JA. Sexual harassment and assault as predictors of PTSD symptomatology among U.S. female Persian Gulf War military personnel. *J Interpersonal Violence*. 1998;13:40–57.

28. McCarroll JE, Ursano RJ, Liu X, et al. Deployment and the probability of spousal aggression by U.S. Army soldiers. *Mil Med*. 2000;165:41–44.

29. Hoogendorn RK. Deployed to Desert Storm: The first 40 hours. *J Emerg Nurs*. 1991;17(4):26A–29A.

30. Keller ML, Herzog-Simmer PA, Harris MA. Effects of military-induced separation on the parenting stress and family functioning of deploying mothers. *Mil Psychol*. 1994;6:125–138.

31. Bowen GL. Single fathers in the Air Force. *Social Casework*. 1987;68:339–344.

32. McCarroll JE, Fagan JG, Hermsen JM, Ursano RJ. Posttraumatic stress disorder in U.S. Army Vietnam veterans who served in the Persian Gulf War. *J Nerv Ment Dis*. 1997;185:682–685.

33. Ursano RJ, Fullerton CS, Epstein RS, et al. Acute and chronic posttraumatic stress disorder in motor vehicle accident victims. *Am J Psychiatry*. 1999;156:589–595.

34. Yerkes SA. The "Un-comfort-able:" Making sense of adaptation in a war zone. *Mil Med*. 1993;158:421–423.

35. Garland FN. Combat stress control in the post-war theater: Mental health consultation during the redeployment phase of Operation Desert Storm. *Mil Med*. 1993;158:334–338.

36. Colbach EM, Parrish MD. Army mental health activities in Vietnam: 1965-1970. *Bull Menninger Clin*. 1970;34:333–342.

37. Baker SL. Drug abuse in the United States Army. *Bull New York Acad Med*. 1971;47:541–549.

38. Baker SL. Present status of the drug abuse offensive in the Armed Forces. *Bull New York Acad Med*. 1972;48:719–732.

39. Robins LN, Davis DH, Nurco DN. How permanent was Vietnam drug addiction? *Am J Public Health Suppl*. 1974;64:38–43.

40. Char J. Drug abuse in Viet Nam. *Am J Psychiatry*. 1972;129:123–125.

41. Holloway HC. Epidemiology of drug dependency among soldiers in Vietnam. *Mil Med*. 1974;139:108–113.

42. Ritchie ED, Ruck DC, Anderson MW. The 528th Combat Stress Control Unit in support of Operation Restore Hope. *Mil Med*. 1994;159:372–376.

43. Borus JP. Reentry, 3: Facilitating healthy readjustment in Vietnam veterans. *Psychiatry*. 1973;36:428–439.

44. Kupper HI. *Back to Life: The Emotional Adjustment of Our Veterans*. New York: L.B. Fischer; 1945: 125. Cited in: Menninger WC. *Psychiatry in a Troubled World*. New York: MacMillan; 1948.

45. Hyams KC, Wignall FS, Roswell R. War syndromes and their evaluation: From the U.S. Civil War to the Persian Gulf War. *Ann Intern Med*. 1996;125:398–405.

46. Helzer JE, Robins LN, Davis DH. Depressive disorders in Vietnam returnees. *J Nerv Ment Dis*. 1976;163:177–185.

47. Helzer JE, Robins LN, Wish E, Hesselbrock M. Depression in Viet Nam veterans and civilian controls. *Am J Psychiatry*. 1979;136(4B):526–529.

48. American Psychiatric Association. *Diagnostic and Statistical Manual of Mental Disorders*. 3rd ed. (DSM-III). Washington, DC: APA; 1980.

49. Bey DR. The returning veteran syndrome. *Medical Insight*. 1972;4(7):42–49.

50. Bennett PJ. Desert Storm: one Army nurse's experience in a forward surgical unit during the ground offensive. *J Emerg Nurs.* 1991;17:27A–34A.

51. Mateczun JM, Holmes EK. Return, readjustment, and reintegration: The three R's of family reunion. In: Ursano RJ, Norwood AE, eds. *Emotional Aftermath of the Persian Gulf War.* Washington, DC: American Psychiatric Press; 1996.

52. Norman EM. Post-traumatic stress disorder in military nurses who served in Vietnam during the war years 1965-1973. *Mil Med.* 1988;153:238–244.

53. Garnett CF. Remembering Desert Storm. *Nursing.* 1991;21:127.

54. Kelly PJ. On the home front: a reservist's Desert Storm experience. *J Emerg Nurs.* 1991;17:42A–44A.

55. Rhoads J. Desert Shield nurse: firsthand account. *J Emerg Nurs.* 1991;17:46A–47A.

56. Forster E. Deployment to Haiti: an emergency nurse's story. *J Emerg Nurs.* 1996;22:160–161.

57. Melini J. From "June Cleaver" to active duty. *J Emerg Nurs.* 1991;17:39A–41A.

58. Ross C. Desert Storm nursing. *Aviat Space Environ Med.* 1995;66:596–597.

59. Blount BW, Curry A Jr, Lubin GI. Family separations in the military. *Mil Med.* 1992;157:76–80.

60. Peebles-Kleiger MJ, Kleiger J. Re-integration stress for Desert Storm families: Wartime deployments and family trauma. *J Traumatic Stress.* 1994;7:173–194.

61. Rosen LN, Westhuis DJ, Teitelbaum JM. Patterns of adaptation among Army wives during Operations Desert Shield and Desert Storm. *Mil Med.* 1994;159:43–47.

62. Rosen LN, Durand DB. The family factor and retention among married soldiers deployed in Operation Desert Storm. *Mil Psychol.* 1995;7:221–234.

63. Schumm WR, Bell DB, Knott B, Rice RE. The perceived effect of stressors on marital satisfaction among civilian wives of enlisted soldiers deployed to Somalia for Operation Restore Hope. *Mil Med.* 1996;161:601–605.

64. Bey DR, Lange J. Waiting wives: Women under stress. *Am J Psychiatry.* 1974;131:283–286.

65. Keller ML. Military-induced separation in relation to maternal adjustment and children's behaviors. *Mil Psychology.* 1994;6:163–176.

66. Rosen LN, Teitelbaum JM, Westhuis DJ. Children's reactions to Desert Storm deployment: Initial findings from a survey of Army families. *Mil Med.* 1993;158:465–469.

67. Jensen PS, Lewis RL, Xenakis SN. The military family in review: Context, risk, and prevention. *J Am Acad Child Psychiatry.* 1986;25:225–234.

68. Bartone PT, Adler AB. A model for soldier psychological adaptation in peacekeeping operations. *Proceedings of the 36th Annual Conference of the International Military Testing Association.* Rotterdam, The Netherlands; 1994: 33–40. As cited in: US Army Medical Research Unit-Europe, Walter Reed Army Institute of Research. *A Model of Psychological Issues in Peacekeeping Operations.* WRAIR; 18 March 1996. Research Report #23.

69. Gunby P. Medical support of troops in Bosnia includes screening for problems when homeward bound. *JAMA.* 1997;277:779.

70. Gunby P. Military medicine's role continues in Bosnia. *JAMA.* 1996;276:1370.

71. Wing JK, Mann SA, Leff JP, Nixon JM. The concept of a "case" in psychiatric population surveys. *Psycholog Med.* 1978;8:203–217.

72. Williams P, Tarnopolsky A, Hand D. Case definition and case identification in psychiatric epidemiology: review and assessment. *Psycholog Med*. 1980;10:101–114.

73. Kendell RE. What is a case? Food for thought for epidemiologists. *Arch Gen Psychiatry*. 1988;45:374–375.

74. Rothberg JM, Holloway HC, Nace EP. An application of stepwise discriminant analysis to the characterization of military heroin dependents, illicit drug users, and psychiatric patients. *Int J Addict*. 1976;11:819–830.

75. McCarroll JE, Jaccard JJ, Radke AQ. Psychiatric consultation to command. In: Jones FD, Sparacino LR, Wilcox VL, Rothberg JM, eds. *Military Psychiatry: Preparing in Peace for War*. Washington, DC: Office of the Surgeon General, Department of the Army and Borden Institute; 1994: 151–170.

76. Holloway HC, Norwood AE, Fullerton CS, Engel CC Jr, Ursano RJ. The threat of biological weapons: Prophylaxis and mitigation of psychological and social consequences. *JAMA*. 1997;278:425–427.

77. Slovic P. Perception of risk. *Science*. 1987;236:280–285.

78. Kraemer HC, Kazdin AE, Offord DR, Kessler RC, Jensen PS, Kupfer DJ. Coming to terms with the terms of risk. *Arch Gen Psychiatry*. 1997;54:337–343.

79. Mrazek PJ, Haggerty RJ, eds. *New Directions and Definitions in Reducing Risks for Mental Disorders*. Washington, DC: National Academy Press; 1994: 19–32.

80. Rutter M. Resilience: Some conceptual considerations. *J Adolescent Health*. 1993;14:626–631.

81. Department of Defense. *Combat Stress Control Programs*. Washington, DC: DoD; February 23, 1999. DoD Directive 6490.5.

82. Department of the Army. *Combat Stress Control in a Theater of Operations: Tactics, Techniques, and Procedures*. Washington, DC: DA; 1994. US Army Field Manual 8-51.

83. Department of the Army. *Leader's Manual for Combat Stress Control*. Washington, DC: DA; 1994. US Army Field Manual 22-51.

84. Applewhite L, Dickens C. Coping with terrorism: the OPM-SANG experience. *Mil Med*. 1997;162:240–243.

85. Armfield F. Preventing post-traumatic stress disorder resulting from military operations. *Mil Med*. 1994;159:739–746.

86. Dobson M, Marshall RP. Surviving the war zone experience: Preventing psychiatric casualties. *Mil Med*. 1997;162:283–287.

87. Fitzgerald ML, Braudaway CA, Leeks D, et al. Debriefing: A therapeutic intervention. *Mil Med*. 1993;158:542–545.

88. Jiggets SM, Hall DP Jr. Helping the helper: 528th Combat Stress Center in Somalia. *Mil Med*. 1995;160:275–277.

89. Pichot T, Rudd D. Preventative mental health in disaster situations: "Terror on the autobahn." *Mil Med*. 1991;156:540–543.

90. Young SA, Holden MS. The formation and application of an overseas mental health crisis intervention team, part I: Formation. *Mil Med*. 1991;156:443–445.

91. Young SA, Holden MS. The formation and application of an overseas mental health crisis intervention team, part II: Application. *Mil Med*. 1991;156:445–447.

92. Shalev AY, Peri T, Rogel-Fuchs Y, Ursano RJ, Marlowe, D. Historical group debriefing after combat exposure. *Mil Med*. 1998;163:494–498.

93. Deahl MP, Gillham AB, Thomas J, Searle MM, Srinivasan M. Psychological sequelae following the Gulf War: Factors associated with subsequent morbidity and the effectiveness of psychological debriefing. *Br J Psychiatry.* 1994;165:60–65.

94. Simon JD. Biological terrorism: Preparing to meet the threat. *JAMA.* 1997;278:428–430.

95. Shalev AY. Debriefing following traumatic exposure. In: *Individual and Community Responses to Trauma and Disaster: The Structure of Human Chaos.* Ursano RJ, McCaughey BG, Fullerton CS, eds. New York: Cambridge University Press; 1994: 201–219.

96. Koshes RJ, Young SA, Stokes JW. Debriefing following combat. In: Jones FD, Sparacino LR, Wilcox VL, Rothberg JM, Stokes JW, eds. *War Psychiatry.* Washington, DC: Office of The Surgeon General, US Department of the Army and Borden Institute; 1995: 271–290.

97. McDuff DR. Social issues in the management of released hostages. *Hosp Community Psychiatry.* 1992;43:825–828.

98. Caldwell JA Jr. A brief survey of chemical defense, crew rest, and heat stress/physical training issues related to Operation Desert Storm. *Mil Med.* 1992;157:275–281.

99. Ursano RJ. Trauma, stress and health: Military women in combat, deployment and contingency operations: Recommendations. Bethesda, Md: Department of Psychiatry, F. Edward Hebert School of Medicine, Uniformed Services University of the Health Sciences; 1996.

Chapter 49

MEDICAL ISSUES IN REDEPLOYMENT

Sterling S. Sherman, MD, MPH

S.S. Sherman, Commander, Medical Corps, US Navy; Head, Threat Assessment Department, Naval Environmental and Preventive Medicine Unit No. 5, 3235 Albacore Alley, San Diego, CA 92136

INTRODUCTION

Problems related to the health of military personnel returning home after serving abroad are varied and not easily solved. Veterans expect and deserve recognition for the sacrifices that they have made in service to their country. The expected health effects of a deployment and the normal occurrence of diseases among veterans often blend with the hazards of the war zone to blur the line between expected and unexpected health events among veterans. Because of this, veterans and their health may become a focus of national discussion and inquiry. When this occurs, the most influential triad will be—as it always has been—the veterans, their elected representatives, and the military medical community. Other interested parties will be families of veterans,

the press, other coalition forces, and the scientific community. The general public angst that can occur during and after a major military action often leads to suspicion of the military establishment. In this atmosphere, it can be difficult to establish the cause of service member health problems. As an outgrowth of this, some of the ties between health problems and military service will be tenuous, if not specious. The military's primary response to this situation and to its responsibility to safeguard the health of service members is the redeployment medical plan. While risk communication teaches that perception is reality, the task of the military medical officer is to prepare the redeployment medical plan so that its reality shapes perception.

HISTORICAL PERSPECTIVES ON RECURRING ISSUES IN REDEPLOYMENT

Throughout the long history of warfare, there have been medical problems associated with the redeployment of military personnel to their home country. In the United States, these problems have included such psychiatric manifestations as "nostalgia" in the Civil War,[1] shell shock in World War I,[2] and post-traumatic stress disorder in the Vietnam War.[3] Other problems have included "gas lung" after World War I and the question of that condition's association with the subsequent development of tuberculosis.[4] After the Vietnam War, veterans and scientists became concerned that the wide use of herbicides might have contributed to a number of postdeployment medical problems.[5] A similar argument has been made that a possible multiple chemical sensitivity or new clinical syndrome (from the combined use of anti–biological warfare vaccinations and anti–nerve agent medications or exposure to insect repellents, pesticides, or chemical warfare agents) may have resulted in the protean manifestations of Persian Gulf War illnesses.[6-10]

Surviving Battle Trauma

War affects the returning population of veterans and society not just by disease but also in another way: disability. Historically, most of those seriously injured during combat died on the field of battle or in the forward aid stations near the line of battle. Beginning with the Civil War, advances in medical and surgical practice resulted in greater numbers of veterans surviving to return home with amputations or other medical problems. In 1865 assistance to refugees, freed slaves, and veterans of the Civil

War became the duty of the Bureau of Refugees, Freedmen, and Abandoned Lands within the War Department.[11] This responsibility grew out of the Congressional requirement in 1862 that the Army provide prostheses to veterans below the rank of captain. From this program developed the military's, and ultimately military medicine's, greatly expanded and improved mission of postwar care of veterans.

Combat Stress

Psychological issues, though incompletely understood, have always been important in returning veterans and are addressed more fully in Chapter 48, Psychological Aspects of Deployment and Reunion. Practical experience with combatants has shown that the immediate treatment veterans receive is an important factor in their likelihood of developing long-term psychiatric morbidity. The simple measures employed since World War I, illustrated by the PIE acronym (proximity, immediacy, expectancy) or the expanded BICEPS (brevity, immediacy, centrality, expectancy, proximity, simplicity), remain effective guidelines for the treatment of acute combat stress reactions. Use of these principles to return the majority of service members to duty quickly decreases long-term morbidity as manifested in chronic post-traumatic stress disorders.[12] Since the military has been unable to develop an efficient method to "screen out" all personnel who are at increased risk for combat stress reactions, medical providers must be ever vigilant to minimize this postdeployment problem.

Infectious Disease

The potential for infectious disease is another redeployment medical issue. There has long been great concern, particularly relating to tropical diseases and diseases with longer incubation periods, of introducing or reintroducing these illnesses into the United States.[13-16] All countries recognize the potential for disease transmission given the ease of international travel and have established various quarantine measures to help prevent transmission of diseases and vectors of concern. During the great plague pandemic of the 14th century, the Venetians established a council of three men that was to supervise and safeguard the public health of the city. Over time, the Venetians and other cities adopted a 40-day isolation period for ships, goods, and persons, hence the term "quarantine," derived from the Italian and Latin words for forty.[17] The first record of such restrictions in America was a law enacted by the Massachusetts Bay Colony in 1647.[18] In subsequent years, quarantine regulations were expanded and modified as situations required for the safeguarding of the population. Cholera, plague, and yellow fever were the primary concerns in the early years of the United States. Later, when people began to travel by air more than by ship, the regulations were modified and updated to meet the new challenges of air travel.

This potential for the international transmission of infectious disease is never more pronounced than in time of war. The influenza pandemic of 1918 and 1919 and the transmission of hepatitis to United Nations peacekeepers assigned to Haiti are two examples at opposite ends of the 20th century.[19-22] At the conclusion of hostilities, the fighting force is wounded, tired, parasitemic, and incubating various diseases but anxious to get back home to their loved ones at the first opportunity. In the modern age, the time frame for this return can be literally hours. Because of the modern military's ability to rapidly transport large numbers of the returning force, service members can lift off the ground half a world away and be on leave with their relatives in as little as 48 hours. Table 49-1 gives a few examples of important medical problems that have few, if any, early symptoms and have been or potentially may be important in redeploying veterans.

Political Ramifications

Another important consideration of redeployment is the political ramifications of veterans who return complaining of new medical problems. A recent example shows how public policy goals can appear to be at odds with the science of the day when considering postdeployment medical syndromes. The Clinton administration announced the day after Memorial Day 1996 that veterans who had served in or near the Republic of Vietnam during the United States' participation in the Vietnam War are presumed to have a service-connected disorder attributable to Agent Orange exposure if they develop prostate cancer or peripheral neuropathy. These conditions were additions to the list of conditions for which the Department of Veterans Affairs (VA) already compensates Vietnam veterans, including certain respiratory cancers, multiple myeloma, porphyria cutanea tarda, soft-tissue sarcoma, non-Hodgkin's lymphoma, Hodgkin's disease, and chloracne.[23] For the first time in history, the administration extended the service-connected presumption to the children of Vietnam veterans by designating spina bifida in veterans' children as being service-connected. These new designations were an outgrowth of an Institute of Medicine's report[24] that concluded there was "limited/suggestive evidence" of an association between Agent Orange exposure and these conditions. Secretary of the VA Jesse Brown pointed out that public policy as illustrated by pertinent legislation "is clear: If the evidence for an association to Agent Orange is equal to the evidence against, the veteran must be given the benefit of the doubt."[25pA20] The validity of the science, however, remains to be established when the exposure of interest becomes "stationed in the Republic of Vietnam" and not the "exposure to Agent Orange." In choosing to compensate veterans who were in or near the theater— and not necessarily exposed to the presumptive agent, the government has based its decision on factors other than epidemiologic data.[26]

The question thus becomes not if there will be redeployment medical issues but rather what type will they be, how they will present, and how they can best be detected and managed. If history is any guide, the medical aspects of redeployment will continue to be important in future operations.

THE REDEPLOYMENT MEDICAL PLAN AND ITS GOALS

To address these problems that recur after so many conflicts, the military has developed the redeployment medical plan. Its goals are to enable the military to identify and treat diseases and disability among returning service members, characterize new diseases or new presentations of old diseases

TABLE 49-1

SOME PREVENTABLE, DEPLOYMENT-ASSOCIATED HEALTH CONDITIONS WITH MINIMAL EARLY SYMPTOMS AND POTENTIALLY SERIOUS DELAYED MANIFESTATIONS

Condition	Complication	Latency	Intervention	Example
Tuberculosis	Active tuberculosis	Years	PPD/Rx	WW I,[1] Vietnam[2]
Leishmaniasis	Skin sores, espundia, kala azar	?	Skin examinations, serology	Persian Gulf War[3]
Strongyloidiasis	Dissemination	Decades	Stool examinations	WW II[4–6]
Syphilis	Tertiary syphilis	Decades	RPR	WW II,[7] Vietnam[8]
Hookworm	Anemia	Months	Stool examinations	Grenada[9]
Malaria	Malaria	Weeks/years	Terminal prophylaxis	Vietnam,[10] Korea,[11] Somalia (Operation Restore Hope)[12]
Toxoplasmosis	Dissemination	?	Stool examinations	Panama
Stress	PTSD	Months/years	Counseling	Vietnam[13]
Toxic exposure radiation	Cancer	Decades	Education	Vietnam, WW II[14,15]
HIV	Immunodeficiency	Years	Screening, counseling, treatment	Uruguayan soldiers[16]

PTSD: posttraumatic stress disorder
PPD: purified protein derivative
RPR: reactive plasma reagin

1. *Medical Aspects of Gas Warfare*. Vol 14. In: *The Medical Department of the United States Army in the World War*. Washington, DC: US Army Surgeon General; 1926: 876.
2. Greenberg JH. Public health problems relating to the Vietnam returnee. *JAMA*. 1969;207:697–702.
3. Magill AJ, Grogl M, Gasser RA Jr, Sun W, Oster CN. Visceral infection caused by *Leishmania tropica* in veterans of Operation Desert Storm. *N Engl J Med*. 1993;328:1383–1387.
4. Byard RW, Oliver NW, Rowbottom DJ. Strongyloidiasis in veterans. *JAMA*. 1987;258:3258–3259.
5. de Sa Pereira M. Persistence of strongyloidiasis. *JAMA*. 1980;244:2264.
6. Genta RM, Weesner R, Douce RW, Huitger-O'Connor T, Walzer PD. Strongyloidiasis in US veterans of the Vietnam and other wars. *JAMA*. 1987;258:49–52.
7. Sternberg TH, Howard EB, Dewey LA, Padget P. Venereal diseases. Coates JB Jr, Hoff EC, Hoff PM, eds. *Communicable Diseases Transmitted through Contact or by Unknown Means*. Vol V. In: *Preventive Medicine in World War II*. Washington, DC: Office of the Surgeon General, Dept of the Army; 1960: 183–188.
8. Minkin W. Treatment of gonorrhea by penicillin in a single large dose. *Mil Med*. 1968;133:382–386.
9. Kelley PW, Takafuji ET, Wiener H, et al. An outbreak of hookworm infection associated with military operations in Grenada. *Mil Med*. 1989;154:55–59.
10. Waterhouse BE, Riggenbach RD. Malaria: potential importance to civilian physicians. *JAMA*. 1967;202:683–685.
11. Rosemary B, Fritz RF, Hollister AC Jr. An outbreak of malaria in California, 1952-1953. *Am J Trop Med*. 1954;3:779–788.
12. Centers for Disease Control and Prevention. Malaria among U.S. military personnel returning from Somalia, 1993. *MMWR*. 1993;42:524–526.
13. Health status of Vietnam veterans, I: psychosocial characteristics. The Centers for Disease Control Vietnam experience study. *JAMA*. 1988;259:2701–2707.
14. Bullman TA, Kang HK. The effects of mustard gas, ionizing radiation, herbicides, trauma, and oil smoke on US military personnel: the results of veteran studies. *Annu Rev Public Health*. 1994;15:69–90.
15. National Research Council Committee on the Biological Effects of Ionizing Radiation. *Health Effects of Exposure to Low Levels of Ionizing Radiation: BEIR V*. Washington, DC: National Academy Press; 1990.
16. Artenstein AW, Coppola J, Brown AE, et al. Multiple introductions of HIV-1 subtype E into the western hemisphere. *Lancet*. 1995;346:1197–1198. Published erratum: *Lancet*. 1995;346:1376.

promptly, compensate fairly those with known disabilities, and safely and expeditiously return the fit to duty or home. There are generally three purposes for the medical plan for the redeployment of personnel to home or the redistribution of forces within a theater.

The first purpose of the redeployment plan is to recognize the infectious diseases present in the force and to prevent the spread of these diseases to other forces or to the civilian population. The usual way to minimize this problem is to provide some sort of medical screening in the theater of operations before the movement of personnel and then to use vector elimination procedures, such as agricultural washdowns and airline and shipboard fogging operations, to keep the disease vectors from following the forces to the new location.

Preventing or lessening the medical consequences of military occupational exposures on personnel is the second purpose of the redeployment plan. The range of potential exposures in a theater of operations can be very broad. The many common and potential exposures in a military environment are discussed in section 4 of this book and elsewhere.[27,28] The manifestations of these exposures can be quite varied and therefore require a careful plan for monitoring the consequences of these exposures in the returning force. Planning and documentation must take into account the requirement for professional-quality environmental sampling within the theater of operations. The Department of Defense (DoD) has noted this need for samples in its evolving directives on force medical protection and surveillance.[29–32] The intent is to quantify, geographically categorize, and link exposure to individuals operating in specified areas within an operations area. As a result, DoD requires not only targeted environmental sampling but also individual serum samples for certain exercises or contingency operations. The intent is to use the enhanced medical and environmental knowledge to influence current and future operations and to help guide redeployment medical care.

Another aspect of deployment occupational exposure is the acute and chronic effect of psychiatric trauma. Statistics from World War I and World War II indicate that about 25% of veterans seeking care did so for psychiatric complaints.[12] Most of the "preventive psychiatry" guidelines that have been developed since World War II are to be used in-theater, but one important aspect of the redeployment plan is not. It is how quickly personnel return home. The cohesion of mission-oriented small groups has been shown to be essential to prevent breakdowns in combat. Accordingly, the best way for service members to work out their trauma is to discuss it with others in their unit who went through the same experiences. The modern, rapid time frame for redeployment by air, as opposed to the past's slow transport on troop ships, does not allow for this necessary process. Another aspect to this problem is whether the theater commander routinely redeploys personnel as units or as individuals. Historically, units fought together and went home together. Modern personnel rotation policies, which are based on time exposed, are designed to give combat experience to more personnel, but they work against the psychological health of the individual and the unit.[12] Interestingly, the preventive medicine community may be well positioned to integrate these and similar mental health issues into routine postdeployment education, reminders, and screening because of their proximity to the commanders and their customary involvement with operational plans. Interventions provided by a preventive medicine practitioner may be more acceptable than those of a psychiatric team for the "normal" survivor of the deployment or warzone experience.

The third purpose of the redeployment medical plan is to ascertain the force's medical fitness for subsequent duty. In the modern all-volunteer force, it is very important to determine quickly who is medically fit for continued duty and who must be released from active duty.

BEFORE WRITING THE REDEPLOYMENT MEDICAL PLAN

The epidemiologic method is a useful model for approaching the challenges of developing a medical redeployment plan. This method describes the appropriate actions whenever there is suspicion of new disease in a population.[33] The first five steps of this public health method—observation, counting cases or events, relating cases or events to the population at risk, making comparisons, and developing the hypothesis—are intimately linked to the methodology employed in the medical plan for redeployment. Although there is no established format or gold standard for redeployment medical planning, focusing on this method and remembering the strengths and weaknesses of various medical screening tools (Table 49-2) provides some guidance.

As a practical matter, the medical personnel writing the medical annex of the redeployment plan must operate within constraints often beyond their control. Any measure that slows the return of the force or creates additional logistical burdens or expense is likely to be challenged. To implement the plan, the medical department will need to obtain the approval of the line commander responsible for the overall movement of personnel. Critical decisions

TABLE 49-2

STRENGTHS AND WEAKNESSES OF MEDICAL SCREENING TOOLS[*]

	Interim Medical History	Limited Physical Examination	Laboratory Procedures	Biological Monitoring
Sensitivity	+	+/−	++	++
Specificity	+	+/−	−	++
Low cost	++	++	+/−	+/−
Acceptability	++	++	+/−	+/−
Ease of performance	++	++	+/−	+/−
Accuracy	+/−	+/−	++	++
Reproducibility	+/−	+/−	++	++

[*]Assumes adequate clinical skills and state-of-the-art technology
Reprinted from: Deeter DP, Ruff JM. US Army health programs and services. In: Deter DP, Gaydos JC, eds. *Occupational Health: the Soldier, and the Industrial Base.* In: *The Textbook of Military Medicine.* Washington, DC: Dept of the Army, Office of The Surgeon General, Borden Institute; 1993: 77. Table 3-2.

will need to be made about the implementation of the plan. What portions of the medical plan must be implemented in the theater and what portions will be done after return home? What additional resources will be required in-theater and at home? Will special diagnostic tests be used to validate the threat? If so, will they be biomarkers, various environmental and zoological samples, or something else? Will specialized laboratory support be required, such as the Army's Theater Army Medical Laboratory or the Navy's Forward Deployable Laboratory?

Resistance during this phase of planning often springs from the perception that these efforts are "just research." This perception exists both in the line and the medical communities. In fact, the efforts may be "just research" or unnecessary in a "healthy" force if the disease and nonbattle injury experience is minimal. Even in the best of times, there is generally great reluctance to dedicate already sparse personnel resources to "new" medical requests. However, pointing out the three purposes listed above as the basis for the efforts, plus the growing DoD emphasis on improved redeployment care and citing pertinent directives, should help lessen resistance to the plan.

ELEMENTS OF THE REDEPLOYMENT MEDICAL PLAN

Redeployment medical plans will have to address certain broad topics. These will include at a minimum service member education, medical screening, surveillance, and establishment of priorities for data gathering. The chances of a smooth redeployment, with a minimum of unexplained or undiagnosed illnesses, increase if these issues are discussed and decided on long before anyone packs a duffel bag.

Education

The first area that the plan should address is service member education. Providing an accurate update of the nature of the medical threat that was encountered and a thorough explanation of any special countermeasures taken helps the exposed population know when something new may be happening to them. Additionally, good individual knowledge is necessary because many of these individuals will leave the military or go to new duty stations in the first few months after a deployment. Simple measures, such as educating them about how and why to continue their postdeployment medical regimen of anti-malaria prophylaxis or about any special vaccinations they may have received, can have profound effects. Future civilian or military medical providers will need to know these sorts of important points in the patient's medical history. Providing a medical summary sheet of the deployment in each individual's medical record may be the best way to do this. Listing agencies and phone numbers where subsequent questions can be directed may also be helpful.

Medical Screening

The second area that needs to be addressed in the redeployment plan is how to medically screen the returning force. There are many ways that this can be done. The simplest is to screen only those with a current complaint, but this is too easily influenced by service members' desires to return home quickly and would likely miss many prevalent conditions. A more practical but administratively burdensome method is to require personnel to fill out a standardized health screening questionnaire before deployment to verify deployability (Figure 49-1).[29,30] This has the obvious advantage of providing some documentation of medical conditions that existed before the deployment. These screening questionnaires, when coupled with the individual's record of medical care, provide a better baseline for the service member's health before and during the deployment.[34,35]

Postdeployment Surveillance

The third area of the redeployment medical plan is postdeployment surveillance for medical problems; implementation of this can become a sensitive issue. "Cradle to grave" medical surveillance is being planned by the Department of Defense.[29,30] A version of the framework envisioned is illustrated in Table 49-3 and a listing of the guidance provided for postdeployment screening of service members returning from Bosnia (Exhibit 49-1). What is available now is a patchwork of datasets, including inpatient medical datasets and operational weekly disease surveillance for large joint military operations outside the United States. Additionally, computerized casualty datasets, veteran disability datasets, active duty and VA inpatient hospitalization records, pharmacy utilization data, Composite Health Care System records, and summaries of routinely reportable diseases of interest are available through the VA and the individual services.

The ability to accumulate active, ongoing disease surveillance is crucial to understanding the medical consequences of deployment. Until the services have data that more clearly delineate the baseline rates of various medical conditions, it will be very difficult to count cases or events or to relate cases or events to the population at risk—both crucial steps in the epidemiologic method. Before active surveillance is made the norm, inpatient datasets or targeted screening of representative subpopulations will have to be used to look for diseases and conditions of interest.

Active, "real-time," weekly disease surveillance was first used successfully on a large scale by the US military during the Persian Gulf War.[36,37] The focus of the surveillance effort was to identify diseases and conditions that have effective public health intervention strategies. This weekly data summary provided the medical personnel and the line commanders with accurate information about what diseases and conditions were active in the deployed personnel throughout the theater of operations; it also made possible the rapid application of appropriate interventions to limit the impact of disease on the forces. Continuing to use this surveillance tool among elements of the redeploying force may be an interim solution to the problem of identifying new conditions or increased rates of disease among service members. Due to the recognized success of these efforts, a Joint Staff memorandum institutionalized this effort for all joint military operations outside the United States.[38] This effectively began the DoD effort to institutionalize active disease surveillance for military personnel.

Another important initiative during the Persian Gulf War was the deployment of a public health laboratory into the theater of operations. The Navy Research and Development Command deployed a forward lab to Al Jubayl, Saudi Arabia, under the control of the Navy Central Command Surgeon. This laboratory could use modern research laboratory techniques to rapidly identify infectious threats.[37,39] Medical threat information generated by the forward laboratory helped define and quantify the medical threat in the theater. This type of information is crucial to identifying the areas of concern for the redeployment medical plan. Although the command relationships of the laboratory were blurred somewhat during this deployment, a consensus has formed that this capability was critical to the medical officers advising the operational commander.[40] A forward laboratory formally tasked to support the efforts of the force preventive medicine advisors could be responsive to the mini-outbreaks of disease identified through active surveillance and provide the scientific characterization of the threat necessary to focus appropriate public health interventions, provide medical treatment recommendations, and advise the affected line commanders about the exact nature of the medical threat.

The ability to couple this in-theater disease incidence and laboratory identification information with postdeployment medical surveillance via record linkage will be crucial to future efforts to analyze deployment-related disease. This is being done by the Comprehensive Clinical Evaluation

33823

PRE-DEPLOYMENT Health Assessment

Authority: 10 U.S.C. 136 Chapter 55. 1074f, 3013, 5013, 8013 and E.O. 9397

Principal Purpose: To assess your state of health before possible deployment outside the United States in support of military operations and to assist military healthcare providers in identifying and providing present and future medical care to you.

Routine Use: To other Federal and State agencies and civilian healthcare providers, as necessary, in order to provide necessary medical care and treatment.

Disclosure: **(Military personel and DoD civilian Employees Only)** Voluntary. If not provided, healthcare WILL BE furnished, but comprehensive care may not be possible.

INSTRUCTIONS: Please read each question completely and carefully before marking your selections. Provide a response for each question. If you do not understand a question, ask the administrator.

Demographics

Last Name

Today's Date (dd/mm/yyyy)

First Name — MI

Social Security Number

Deploying Unit

DOB (dd/mm/yyyy)

Gender
- ○ Male
- ○ Female

Service Branch
- ○ Air Force
- ○ Army
- ○ Coast Guard
- ○ Marine Corps
- ○ Navy
- ○ Other

Component
- ○ Active Duty
- ○ National Guard
- ○ Reserves
- ○ Civilian Government Employee

Pay Grade
- ○ E1
- ○ E2
- ○ E3
- ○ E4
- ○ E5
- ○ E6
- ○ E7
- ○ E8
- ○ E9
- ○ O1
- ○ O2
- ○ O3
- ○ O4
- ○ O5
- ○ O6
- ○ O7
- ○ O8
- ○ O9
- ○ O10
- ○ W1
- ○ W2
- ○ W3
- ○ W4
- ○ W5
- ○ Other

Location of Operation
- ○ Europe
- ○ SW Asia
- ○ SE Asia
- ○ Asia (Other)
- ○ South America
- ○ Australia
- ○ Africa
- ○ Central America
- ○ Unknown

Deployment Location (IF KNOWN) (CITY, TOWN, or BASE):

List country (IF KNOWN):

Name of Operation:

Administrator Use Only

Indicate the status of each of the following:

Yes	No	N/A	
○	○	○	Medical threat briefing completed
○	○	○	Medical information sheet distributed
○	○	○	Serum for HIV drawn within 12 months
○	○	○	Immunizations current
○	○	○	PPD screening within 24 months

DD FORM 2795, MAY 1999

ASD (HA) APPROVED SEPTEMBER 1998 Ver 1.3

33823

(**Fig. 49-1** *continues*)

33823

PLEASE FILL IN SOCIAL SECURITY # ☐☐☐ - ☐☐ - ☐☐☐☐

Health Assessment

1. Would you say your health in general is: ○ Excellent ○ Very Good ○ Good ○ Fair ○ Poor

2. Do you have any medical or dental problems? ○ Yes ○ No

3. Are you currently on a profile, or light duty, or are you undergoing a medical board? ○ Yes ○ No

4. Are you pregnant? (FEMALES ONLY) ○ Don't Know ○ Yes ○ No

5. Do you have a 90-day supply of your prescription medication or birth control pills? ○ N/A ○ Yes ○ No

6. Do you have two pairs of prescription glasses (if worn) and any other personal medical equipment? ○ N/A ○ Yes ○ No

7. During the past year, have you sought counseling or care for your mental health? ○ Yes ○ No

8. Do you currently have any questions or concerns about your health? ○ Yes ○ No

Please list your concerns: _____

_____

Service Member Signature

I certify that responses on this form are true.

Pre-Deployment Health Provider Review (For Health Provider Use Only)

After interview/exam of patient, the following problems were noted and categorized by Review of Systems. More than one may be noted for patients with multiple problems. Further documentation of problem to be placed in medical records.

REFERRAL INDICATED

○ None
○ Cardiac
○ Combat / Operational Stress Reaction
○ Dental
○ Dermatologic
○ ENT
○ Eye
○ Family Problems
○ Fatigue, Malaise, Multisystem complaint

○ GI
○ GU
○ GYN
○ Mental Health
○ Neurologic
○ Orthopedic
○ Pregnancy
○ Pulmonary
○ Other _____

FINAL MEDICAL DISPOSITION:
○ **Deployable**   ○ **Not Deployable**

Comments: (If not deployable, explain)

_____

_____

_____

I certify that this review process has been completed.
Provider's signature and stamp:

Date (dd/mm/yyyy)
☐☐ / ☐☐ / ☐☐☐☐

End of Health Review

33823

DD FORM 2795, MAY 1999   ASD (HA) APPROVED SEPTEMBER 1998 Ver 1.3

Fig. 49-1. Predeployment Health Assessment, Department of Defense Form 2795

TABLE 49-3

COMPONENTS OF MEDICAL SURVEILLANCE BY THE PHASE OF DEPLOYMENT

Tasks	Predeployment	During Deployment	Postdeployment
Identify population at risk	Field a seamless DoD ambulatory health data system Ensure deployment readiness of individuals using automated record system	Collect data on unit strength and locations and on individuals' deployment histories	Archive deployment information related to units and individuals Disseminate findings
Assess health	Perform continuous health status surveillance and track deployability status Maintain serum bank	Do real-time disease surveillance Analyze surveillance data and report to commanders	Do scenario-specific screening and targeted medical evaluations Continue medical surveillance
Identify exposures of medical interest	Prepare and distribute threat assessments for potential AORs Identify threats during planning phase for specific contingencies	Do special assessments of occupational and environmental exposures while in theater Look for related clinical cases	Update medical threat assessment based on special assessments, ongoing intelligence collection activities, and disease surveillance data
Institute individual and unit force protection measures	Determine PM countermeasures and incorporate into OPLANS Execute predeployment countermeasures (train, equip, supply, immunize)	Reinforce or introduce added protective countermeasures based on analysis of disease surveillance data	Identify requirements for new countermeasures Incorporate measures into OPLANS

PM: preventive medicine
DoD: Department of Defense
AOR: area of operations
OPLANS: operations plans
Adapted from: US Dept of Defense. *Implementation and Application of Joint Medical Surveillance for Deployments*. Washington, DC: DoD; 1997. DoD Instruction 6490.3.

Program as it looks at the medical complaints of previously uncharacterized Persian Gulf War illnesses. Additionally, reporting of sentinel events through the DoD or the Centers for Disease Control and Prevention, when coupled to emerging, laboratory-based, automatic electronic surveillance, will allow comparisons that have been impossible in prior deployments. These comparisons will provide a better understanding of the actual health situation of redeploying personnel and help to firmly establish (or rule out) multifactorial deployment syndromes.

Final questions include: How will we assess the quality of the data gathered? What are the sensitivity and specificity of the measures to be used? Have those measures been validated on the population of concern or a similar one? These questions are important to the immediate plans for deployment,

but their answers also will form the basis for any subsequent investigation into health effects from the deployment.

Setting the Priorities

The final general area that the redeployment medical plan must address is how to establish the data points of medical interest in this population. The clinical or administrative surveys mentioned previously are one important part, but the service medical departments have the ability to collect other potentially important medical information. Will information be collected about stress and mental health? Should medical personnel collect serum samples, hair samples, or other body fluids? What type of environmental or zoological sampling should be done before leaving the theater of operations? Can

---

EXHIBIT 49-1

DEPARTMENT OF DEFENSE (HEALTH AFFAIRS) GUIDANCE FOR POSTDEPLOYMENT SCREENING FOR BOSNIA

- On departure from Bosnia or within 30 days of return to home station, personnel shall receive a redeployment medical briefing and medical evaluation and the information shall be documented on Standard Form 600, Chronological Record of Medical Care. Completed assessments shall be placed in the member's medical record, and a copy forwarded to the Bosnia Deployment Surveillance Office.

- As part of the medical evaluation, medical staff will collect serum (one 10 cc red top tube spun down) from all personnel within 30 days of return from deployment. This shall be used for diagnosis, medical surveillance, and other purposed if needed in the future. They shall not be used for any genetics related testing.

- As part of the redeployment medical assessment, all Service members shall complete a diagnostic battery to identify individuals at risk for development of mental health diagnoses known to be related to deployment.

- The Services shall ensure that members receive a medical debriefing within 30 days after arrival at their home station, or as soon as possible in the case of Guard/Reserve personnel. These briefings shall reinforce medical guidance and provide additional information. Additionally, stress management and family advocacy resources shall be made known and readily available to Service members and their families.

- A representative sample of units and personnel may be identified to receive diagnostic evaluations in order to more definitely assess overall health status and evaluate possible medical sequelae of deployment.

- The Services' epidemiologic/surveillance centers shall maintain rosters of deployed personnel to conduct active postdeployment medical surveillance.

- Deployed medical staff shall document lessons learned.

Reprinted from: Assistant Secretary of Defense. *Medical Surveillance Plan for U.S. Ground Forces Deploying to Bosnia.* Washington, DC: Department of Defense; 1996.

---

personnel records be linked to the service member's geographic location within the theater for subsequent analysis of the exposure? The answer to these questions seems to be yes. Early efforts were made to do all of these in the deployments to Haiti and Bosnia. This rational approach is in line with the recommendations of the Presidential Advisory Committee on Gulf War Veterans Illnesses and the requirements of public law.[41] But no one knows for certain which, if any, of these measures will prove truly useful for subsequent analysis. Additionally, the ability to link datasets in a rational, retrievable, relevant fashion that can be continually updated from a forward deployed force is as necessary as it is daunting. In the interim, retrospective data analysis that uses surrogate markers for exposure in place of documented exposure has yet to be validated. Also, the purely retrospective nature of the analysis is less desirable than a prospective analysis, which could look more robustly at the medical consequences of deployment.[42] Carefully designed prospective studies would be very expensive and labor intense but may be necessary in some cases, such as to look at the known relationship between deployments, combat, and stress. It may be time to study more carefully the relationship between deployment, stress, and subsequent somatic complaints since this is a question that has seemed to linger after all major deployments (Table 49-4).[43]

THE ROLE OF THE DEPARTMENT OF DEFENSE, THE DEPARTMENT OF VETERANS AFFAIRS, AND SELECTED ADVISORY PANELS

The Department of Defense

The role of the DoD regarding medical problems associated with a deployment historically has been 3-fold. First, the DoD is responsible for maintaining a fit and ready fighting force. This includes treating the sick and wounded so they can return to duty or separating them if they are no longer able to serve. Second, it is responsible to the country to implement any medical lessons learned in the plans

TABLE 49-4

SOMATIC SYMPTOMS COMMONLY ASSOCIATED WITH WAR-RELATED MEDICAL AND PSYCHOLOGICAL ILLNESSES

Symptom	War and Illness					
	US Civil War, Da Costa Syndrome	World War I, Effort Syndrome	World War II, Combat Stress Reaction	Vietnam, Agent Orange Exposure	Vietnam and Other Conflicts, Post-Traumatic Stress Disorder	Persian Gulf War, Unexplained Illnesses
Fatigue or exhaustion	+	+	+	+	+	+
Shortness of breath	+	+	+		+	+
Palpitations and tachycardia	+	+	+		+	
Precordial pain	+	+			+	+
Headache	+	+	+	+	+	+
Muscle or joint pain				+	+	+
Diarrhea	+		+	+	+	+
Excessive sweating	+	+	+			
Dizziness	+	+	+	+	+	
Fainting	+	+				
Disturbed sleep	+	+	+	+	+	+
Forgetfulness		+	+	+	+	+
Difficulty concentrating		+	+	+	+	+

Reprinted with permission from: Hyams KC, Wignall FS, Roswell R. War syndromes and their evaluation: from the U.S. Civil War to the Persian Gulf War. *Ann Intern Med*. 1996;125:399.

for future operations to lessen disease and injury. And third, it is responsible to disseminate medical information that may be of interest to military veterans and to the country from any ongoing research or intelligence activities. Administratively, the DoD usually provides lists of personnel and service history information for postservice medical claims. In this regard, the DoD role has expanded in light of its actions with the Comprehensive Clinical Evaluation Program and other database creation and linkage activities.

The DoD has undertaken several initiatives designed to expand its capacity to study deployment medical syndromes. These efforts build on the 1993 Joint Staff memorandum that instituted active disease surveillance for all joint military operations taking place outside the United States. Arguably the next major step was the participation of the Office of the Assistant Secretary of Defense (Health Affairs) in the preventive medicine guidance given by the US Commander in Chief, European Command, for the US forces involved in the peace implementation mission in Bosnia.[34,35] These memorandums were released at a time when the Office of the Assistant Secretary of Defense (Health Affairs) and other DoD agencies were extensively involved with the investigation into Persian Gulf War illnesses. It seems clear that this input was designed to collect what all involved hoped would be useful information if investigations of future syndromes were required. The DoD has since increased its efforts to study the health of military forces before, during, and after deployments. Public Law 105-85, enacted in January 1997, mandates improved medial tracking for deployments, tracking of new investigational drugs, and reports on medical tracking efforts. The DoD Instructions and Directives mentioned earlier and a policy charter designed to expand the surveillance capability and preventive medicine input into military activities have all been promulgated.

The Joint Preventive Medicine Policy Group Charter was signed in January 1997.[44] This group improves preventive medicine support in joint operations and facilitates coordination between DoD agencies by acting as a single clearinghouse for preventive medicine recommendations for those formulating DoD policy.

The Department of Veterans Affairs

In addition to the DoD, there are three civilian governmental agencies that are likely to be involved in evaluating the scientific basis of postdeployment medical problems of service members and veterans. The first of these, the VA, is the primary partner to the DoD in the treatment and investigation of postdeployment medical problems.[45] The VA provides treatment to those with service-connected injury and illness through a large network of VA hospitals and rehabilitation centers. It coordinates the large body of research on veterans' health problems. It also aids in determining benefits for veterans with service-connected conditions and associated disability.

Selected Advisory Panels

The second governmental agency involved in service member and veteran health matters is the Medical Follow-up Agency (MFUA). The MFUA began epidemiologic research on military veteran populations after World War II. It publishes periodic proceedings of ongoing and planned research, sources of data on veterans, and methodological considerations for those who are interested in the results and techniques of health research on military populations. In 1970, the Institute of Medicine was chartered as a component of the National Academy of Sciences to enlist distinguished members of appropriate professions to examine policy matters pertaining to the health of the public.[46,47] Since that time, the MFUA has been placed under the Institute of Medicine, where its expert panels continue their work analyzing the health of veterans.

The third important civilian epidemiologic oversight agency is the Armed Forces Epidemiological Board. The Board was formally chartered as a civilian scientific and medical advisory board to the Department of the Army in 1953.[47] It was first conceived of in 1940 and was the logical outgrowth of a series of commissions started before World War II to look at medical and scientific questions of interest to the Army (see Chapter 5, Conserving the Fighting Strength: Milestones of Operational Military Preventive Medicine Research and Chapter 8, The Basic Training Environment).

SUMMARY

There is no gold standard method for preparing for redeployment and postdeployment medical problems. However, using emerging computer information technology with older public health methods may enable military medical personnel to find new ways to locate and analyze disease trends and so allow a better understanding of the health effects of deployments. These efforts may uncover new syndromes, whether they be new psychological patterns of disease or new infectious diseases. But it must be remembered that preparation for redeployment begins before deployment and continues throughout the deployment. The redeployment plan is the best opportunity to institutionalize a redeployment medical process that may minimize postdeployment medical problems in the active duty and veteran populations.

REFERENCES

1. Smart C. *The Medical and Surgical History of the War of the Rebellion*. Part III. Vol 1. In: *The Medical and Surgical History of the War of the Rebellion (1861–65)*. Washington, DC: US Army Surgeon General; 1888: 989.

2. Sargent W, Slater E. Acute war neuroses. *Lancet*. 1940;2:1–2.

3. Van Putten T, Yager J. Posttraumatic stress disorder: emerging from the rhetoric. *Arch Gen Psychiatry*. 1984;141:411–413.

4. *Medical Aspects of Gas Warfare*. Vol 14. In: *The Medical Department of the United States Army in the World War*. Washington, DC: US Army Surgeon General; 1926: 876.

5. Bullman TA, Kang HK. The effects of mustard gas, ionizing radiation, herbicides, trauma, and oil smoke on US military personnel: the results of veteran studies. *Annu Rev Public Health*. 1994;15:69–90.

6. Haley RW, Kurt TL, Hom J. Is there a Gulf War Syndrome? Searching for syndromes by factor analysis of symptoms. *JAMA*. 1997;277:215–222. Published erratum: *JAMA*. 1997;278:388.

7. Haley RW, Hom J, Roland PS, et al. Evaluation of neurologic function in Gulf War veterans: a blinded case-control study. *JAMA*. 1997;277:223–230.

8. Haley RW, Kurt TL. Self-reported exposure to neurotoxic chemical combinations in the Gulf War: a cross-sectional epidemiologic study. *JAMA*. 1997;277:231–237.

9. The Iowa Persian Gulf Study Group. Self-reported illness and health status among Gulf War veterans: a population-based study. *JAMA*. 1997;277:238–245.

10. Landrigan PJ. Illness in Gulf War veterans: causes and consequences. *JAMA*. 1997;277:259–261.

11. Gillett MC. *The Army Medical Department, 1865–1917*. Washington, DC: US Army Center of Military History; 1995: 517.

12. Jones FD, Sparacino LR, Wilcox VL, Rothberg JM, Stokes JW, eds. *War Psychiatry*. Part I. In: The *Textbook of Military Medicine*. Washington, DC: Office of the Surgeon General, US Department of the Army, and Borden Institute; 1995.

13. Greenberg JH. Public health problems relating to the Vietnam returnee. *JAMA*. 1969;207:697–702.

14. Gilbert DN, Moore WL Jr, Hedberg CL, Sanford JP. Potential medical problems in personnel returning from Vietnam. *Ann Intern Med*. 1968;68:662–678.

15. Waterhouse BE, Riggenbach RD. Malaria: potential importance to civilian physicians. *JAMA*. 1967;202:683–685.

16. Gasser RA Jr, Magill AJ, Oster CN, Tramont EC. The threat of infectious disease in Americans returning from Operation Desert Storm. *N Engl J Med*. 1991;324:859–864.

17. Rosen G. *A History of Public Health*. Baltimore: Johns Hopkins University Press; 1993.

18. Williams RC. *United States Public Health Service 1798–1950*. Washington, DC: US Public Health Service; 1951.

19. Reid AH, Taubenberger JK. The 1918 flu and other influenza pandemics: "over there" and back again. *Lab Invest*. 1999;79:95–101.

20. Reid AH, Fanning TG, Hultin JV, Taubenberger JK. Origin and evolution of the 1918 "Spanish" influenza virus hemagglutinin gene. *Proc Natl Acad Sci USA*. 1999;96:1651–1656.

21. Gambel JM, Drabick JJ, Seriwatana J, Innis BL. Seroprevalence of hepatitis E virus among United Nations Mission in Haiti (UNMIH) peacekeepers, 1995. *Am J Trop Med Hyg*. 1998;58:731-736.

22. Drabick JJ, Gambel JM, Gouvea VS, et al. A cluster of acute hepatitis E infection in United Nations Bangladeshi peacekeepers in Haiti. *Am J Trop Med Hyg*. 1997;57:449–454.

23. Service connection expanded for Agent Orange exposure. *US Medicine*. 1996;32(13&14):3.

24. Institute of Medicine. *Veterans and Agent Orange: Update 1996*. Washington, DC: IOM; 1996.

25. Brown J. Letter to the editor. *Washington Post*. Washington, DC; June 12, 1996: A20.

26. A bad Agent Orange decision. *Washington Post*. Washington; May 31, 1996: A22. Editorial.

27. Walker RI, Cerveny TJ, eds. *Medical Consequences of Nuclear Warfare*. Part I, Vol 2. In: *Textbook of Military Medicine*. Washington, DC: Office of the Surgeon General, US Dept of the Army, and Borden Institute; 1989.

28. Deeter DP, Gaydos JC, eds. *Occupational Health: The Soldier and the Industrial Base.* Part III, Vol 2. In: *Textbook of Military Medicine.* Washington, DC: Office of the Surgeon General, Dept of the Army, and Borden Institute; 1993.

29. US Dept of Defense. *Implementation and Application of Joint Medical Surveillance for Deployments.* Washington, DC: DoD; 1997. DoD Instruction 6490.3.

30. US Dept of Defense. *Joint Medical Surveillance.* Washington, DC: DoD; 1997. DoD Directive 6490.2.

31. US Dept of Defense. *Combat Stress Control (CSC) Programs.* Washington, DC: DoD: 1999. DoD Directive 6490.5.

32. Joint Chiefs of Staff. *Deployment Health Surveillance and Readiness.* Washington, DC: Department of Defense; 1998. JCS Memorandum MCM-251-98.

33. Tyler CW Jr, Last JM. Epidemiology. *Maxcy-Rosenau-Last Public Health & Preventive Medicine.* 13th ed. Norwalk, Conn: Appleton & Lange; 1992: 14.

34. Assistant Secretary of Defense (Health Affairs). *Medical Surveillance for U.S. Forces Deploying in Support of NATO Peace Implementation in Bosnia.* Washington, DC: Dept of Defense; 1996. Health Affairs Policy 96-019.

35. Assistant Secretary of Defense (Health Affairs). *Policy for Post-Deployment Mental Health Screening in the Bosnia Theater.* Washington, DC: Dept of Defense; 1996. Health Affairs Policy 97-017.

36. Hanson RK. Personal communication, 1996.

37. Hyams KC, Hanson K, Wignall FS, Escamilla J, Oldfield EC 3rd. The impact of infectious diseases on the health of U.S. troops deployed to the Persian Gulf during operations Desert Shield and Desert Storm. *Clin Infect Dis.* 1995;20:1497–1504.

38. Chairman of the Joint Chiefs of Staff. *Medical Surveillance Report.* Washington, DC: Department of Defense; 1993. Joint Staff Memorandum J-4A 00106-93.

39. Hyams KC, Bourgeois AL, Escamilla J, Burans J, Woody JN. The Navy Forward Laboratory during Operations Desert Shield/Desert Storm. *Mil Med.* 1993;158:729–732.

40. Dept of the Navy. *Forward Deployable Laboratory.* Washington, DC: DN; 1995. Naval Warfare Publication 4-02.4 Part C.

41. National Defense Authorization Act for Fiscal Year 1998. Public Law 105-85; 1997.

42. Brundage JF. Military preventive medicine and medical surveillance in the post-cold war era. *Mil Med.* 1998;163:272–277.

43. Hyams KC, Wignall FS, Roswell R. War syndromes and their evaluation: from the U.S. Civil War to the Persian Gulf War. *Ann Intern Med.* 1996;125:398–405.

44. Mazzucchi JF. *Joint Preventive Medicine Policy Group Charter.* Washington, DC: Deputy Assistant Secretary of Defense (Health Affairs); 1997.

45. Gronvall JA. The VA's affiliation with academic medicine: an emergency post-war strategy becomes a permanent partnership. *Acad Med.* 1989;64:61–66.

46. Institute of Medicine. *Science.* 1971;172:635.

47. Woodward TE. *The Armed Forces Epidemiological Board: Its First Fifty Years 1940–1990.* Washington, DC: Borden Institute, Office of the Surgeon General, US Dept of the Army; 1990.

ABBREVIATIONS AND ACRONYMS

A

A/C/Y/W-135: the tetravalent vaccine
A2LA: American Association for Laboratory Accreditation
AAFMS: Army Aviation Fighter Management System
ABCA's QSTAG: American, British, Canadian, and Australian's Quadripartite Standardization Agreement
AC: active component of the US Armed Forces
AC: alternating current
AC: hydrogen cyanide (hydrocyanic acid)
ACGIH: American Conference of Governmental Industrial Hygienists
ACIP: Advisory Committee on Immunization Practices
ACLS: Advanced Cardiac Life Support
ADE: antibody-dependent enhancement
AFEB: Armed Forces Epidemiological Board
AFMIC: Armed Forces Medical Intelligence Center
AGE: arterial gas embolism
AHF: Argentine hemorrhagic fever
ALT: alanine aminotransferase
AMAL: Authorized Medical Allowance List
AMB: amphotericin B
AMS: acute mountain sickness
ANG: Air National Guard
ANSI: American National Standards Institute
AOR: area of responsibility
AR: Army regulation
ARCENT: US Army component, US Central Command
ARD: acute respiratory disease
ARNG: Army National Guard
ARS: acute radiation syndrome
ARS: anti-rabies serum
ASD(HA): Assistant Secretary of Defense (Health Affairs)
ASHRAE: American Society of Heating, Refrigerating, and Air-Conditioning Engineers
ASMB: area support medical battalion
AST: aspartate aminiotransferase
ASVAB: Armed Services Vocational Aptitude Battery
ata: atmosphere-absolute
ATC: Air Transportable Clinic
ATH: Air Transportable Hospital

B

BAL: British anti-Lewisite
BCG: bacille Calmette-Guérin
BEEF: Base Engineer Emergency Force
BHF: Bolivian hemorrhagic fever
BI: battle injury
BMI: body mass index
BOD: biochemical oxygen demand
BOD_5: biochemical oxygen demand measured after 5 days
BPG: benzathine penicillin G
BUMED: Bureau of Medicine and Surgery
BW: biological warfare
BW: biological weapon

C

C and R: Construction and Repair
CA: civil affairs
CAM: Chemical Agent Monitor
CATT: card agglutination test
CBI: China–Burma–India theater, World War II
CBIRF: Chemical Biological Incident Response Force
CCHF: Crimean-Congo hemorrhagic fever
CCP: critical control point

CDC: Centers for Disease Control and Prevention
CEE: Central European TBE
CENTAF: US Air Force component, US Central Command
CENTCOM: US Central Command
CERCLA: Comprehensive Environmental Response, Compensation, and Liability Act
CF: complement fixation
CFA: circulating filarial antigen
CFR: case fatality rate
CFR: Code of Federal Regulations
CFU: colony-forming unit
CG: phosgene (carbonyl chloride)
CHCS II: Composite Health Care System II
CHO: carbohydrate
CHO-E: carbohydrate-electrolyte
CHPPM: Center for Health Promotion and Preventive Medicine
CINC: Commander-in-Chief
CINCCENT: Commander in Chief, US Central Command
CIVD: cold-induced vasodilation
CK: cyanogen chloride
CL: confidence limits
CL: cutaneous leishmaniasis
CMR: crude mortality rate
CN: Mace
CNS: central nervous system
CO: carbon monoxide
COA: course of action
COD: chemical oxygen demand
CONPLAN: concept plan
C-P: chloroquine plus primaquine
CPAP: continuous positive airway pressure
CPE: chemical protective ensemble
CRS: congenital rubella syndrome
CS: Clinical Services
CSC: combat stress casualty
CSC: combat stress control
CSF: cerebrospinal fluid
CSF-VDRL: cerebrospinal fluid - Venereal Disease Research Laboratory
CSR: Combat Stress Reaction
CSW: commercial sex workers
CT: cholera toxin
CW: chemical warfare

D

DACOWITS: Defense Advisory Committee on Women in the Services
DALY: disability adjusted life years
DAN: Diver Alert Network
dapsone: 4,4'diaminodiphenylsulfone
DART: Disaster Assistance Response Teams
DASD: Deputy Assistant Secretary of Defense
dBP: decibel peak
DC: direct current
DCI: decompression illness
DCL: diffuse cutaneous leishmaniasis
DCS: decompression sickness
DDT: dichlorodiphenyltrichloroethane
DEET: *N,N*-diethyl-1,3-methylbenzamide
DDT: dichloro-diphenyl-trichloroethane
DEC: diethylcarbamazine citrate
DEPMEDS: deployable medical system
DHF: Dengue hemorrhagic fever
DHHS: Department of Health and Human Services

DIA: Defense Intelligence Agency
DIC: disseminated intravascular coagulation
DMAT: Disaster Medical Assistance Team
DMO: Diving Medical Officer
DMT: Diving Medical Technicians
DNA: deoxyribo-nucleic acid
DNBI: disease and nonbattle injury
DoD: Department of Defense
DODMERB: Department of Defense Medical Evaluation
  Review Board
DOEHRS-HC: Defense Occupational and Environmental
  Health Readiness System in Hearing Conservation
DP: displaced person
DPMIAC: Defense Pest Management Information Analysis
  Center
DPRK: Democratic Peoples Republic of Korea
DSM-III: American Psychiatric Associations' Diagnostic and
  Statistical Manual
DT: dye test
DTaP: diphtheria-tetanus-acellular pertussis
DTP: diphtheria-tetanus-pertussis

E

EAF: enteroadherent factor
EAST: enteroaggregative heat-stabile toxin
ECHO: European Community Humanitarian Office
ECPPC: epidemiological classification of paralytic polio-
  myelitis cases
EEE: Eastern equine encephalitis
EFMP: Exceptional Family Member Program
EHIC: enterohemorrhagic *E coli*
EIA: enzyme immunoassay
EIA: enzyme-linked immunoassay
EIEC: Enteroinvasive *E coli*
ELISA: enzyme-linked immunosorbent assay
EMJH: Tween 80-albumin
EMPCER: estimated mean per capita energy requirement
EOD: explosive ordnance disposal
EPA: US Environmental Protection Agency
EPEC: Enteropathogenic *E coli*
EPICON: Epidemiologic Consultant Service
EPW: enemy prisoner of war
ER: emergency room
ERIG: equine rabies immune globilin
ESFs: Emergency Support Functions
ETEC: Enterotoxigenic *E coli*

F

FAMA: fluorescent antibody to membrane antigen assay
FCO: Federal Coordinating Officer
FDA: Food and Drug Administration
FEMA: Federal Emergency Management Agency
FLA: front line ambulance
FNV: French Neurotropic Vaccine
FHP: Force Health Protection
FRERP: Federal Radiological Emergency Response Plan
FRP: Federal Response Plan
FSME: Fruhsommer-meningoenzephalitis
FTA-ABS: fluorescent treponemal antibody absorbed
FUOs: fevers of undetermined origin

G

G1: Personnel
G3: Operations
G4: Logistics
G6PD: glucose 6–phosphate dehydrogenase

GABHS: group A β-hemolytic streptococcus
GA: tabun
GB: sarin
GBS: Guillain–Barré syndrome
G-CSF: granulocyte colony-stimulating factor
GD: soman
GF: no expansion, no common name
GI: gastrointestinal
GLOC: G force–induced loss of consciousness
GTMO: US Naval Base at Guantanamo Bay, Cuba

H

HACCP: Hazard Analysis Critical Control Point
HACE: high altitude cerebral edema
HAPE: high altitude pulmonary edema
HARH: high altitude retinal hemorrhage
HAV: hepatitis A virus
HAZMIN: hazard minimization
HBIG: hepatitis B immune globulin
HBV: hepatitis B virus
HCA: humanitarian civic assistance
HCV: hepatitis C virus
HDAg: hepatitis D antigen
HDV: hepatitis D virus
HEV: hepatitis E virus
HGV: hepatitis G virus
HDCV: human diploid cell rabies vaccine
HDR: Humanitarian Daily Ration
heliox: helium-oxygen mixture
HEPA: high efficiency particulate air
HFRS: hemorrhagic fever with renal syndrome
HGE: human granulocytic ehrlichiosis
HIS: health information system
HIV: human immunodeficiency virus
HIV-1: human immunodeficiency virus-1
HME: human monocytic ehrlichiosis
HMMWV: High Mobility Multipurpose Wheeled Vehicle
HPM: Humanitarian Pouched Meal
HPS: hantavirus pulmonary syndrome
HRIG: human rabies immunoglobulin
HPV: human papilloma virus
HSO&R: Health Services Operations and Readiness
HTLV-I: human t-cell lympho-trophic virus type I

I

ICRC: International Committee of the Red Cross
ICU/CCU: intensive care unit/cardiac care unit
ID: immunodiffusion
IDA: Individual Dynamic Absorption
IDC: Independent Duty Corpsman
IDE: Investigational Device Exemption
IFA: immunofluorescent assay
IFA: indirect fluorescent antibody
IG: immune globulin
IgG: immunoglobulin G antibody
IgM: immunoglobulin M antibody
IM: intramuscular
IMA: Individual Mobilization Augmentee
IMB: Information, Motivation, and Behavioral Skills
IND: investigational new drug
IPP: immunoperoxidase
IPV: inactivated polio vaccine
IRR: incidence rate ratio
IRR: Individual Ready Reserve
IUD: intrauterine device
IV: intravenous

J

JCS: Joint Chiefs of Staff
JE: Japanese encephalitis
JEV: Japanese encephalitis virus
JOTC: Jungle Operations Training Center
JTF: Joint Task Force
JTF-CS: Joint Task Force-Civil Support

K

KFD: Kyasanur Forest disease

L

LCR: ligase chain reaction
LD_{50}: the dose that is lethal to 50% of those exposed
LET: leukocyte esterase test
LFA: Lead Federal Agency
LGV: lymphogranuloma venereum
LIC: low-intensity conflict
LITE: low-intensity training and exercise
LPS: lipopolysaccharide
LR: leishmaniasis recidivans
LRP II: Food Packet, Long Range Patrol II
LT: heat-labile toxin

M

MACV: Military Assistance Command, Vietnam
MAST: military anti-shock trousers
MCA: Medical Civic Action
MCLG: maximum contaminant level goal
MCRD: Marine Corps Recruit Depot
MEDCAP: Medical Civic Action Program
MEDIC: Medical Environmental Disease Intelligence and Countermeasures
MEDRETE: Medical Readiness Training Exercise
MEF: Marine Expeditionary Force
MEPCOM: US Military Entrance Processing Command
MEPS: Military Entrance Processing Stations
MEPSCAT: Military Enlistment Physical Strength Capacity Test
MFUA: Medical Follow-up Agency
MH: Mantel-Haenszel
MIC: methyl isocyanate
MHA-TP: microhemagglutination treponemal pallidum
MHS: Military Health System
ML: mucosal leishmaniasis
MMR: measles-mumps-rubella vaccine
MMRS: Metro-politan Medical Response System
MOPP: mission-oriented protective posture
MOS: Military Occupational Specialty
MOUT: military operations in urbanized terrain
MRC: major regional conflict
MRDA: Military Recommended Daily Requirement
MRE: Meal, Ready-to-Eat
MSDS: Material Safety Data Sheet
MREs: Meals Ready to Eat
MSF: Mediterranean spotted fever
MSG: Monosodium glutamate
MTFs: medical treatment facilities
MUAC: mid–upper arm circumference
MWD: military working dog

N

NAMRU: Naval Medical Research Unit
NAVCENT: US Navy component, US Central Command
NBC: nuclear, biological, and chemical

NCA: National Command Authority
NCO: noncommissioned officer
NDMS: National Disaster Medical System
NEISS: National Electronic Injury Surveillance System
NEPMU: US Navy Environmental and Preventive Medicine Unit
NER: Near East Relief
NFCI: nonfreezing cold injury
NGU: nongonococcal urethritis
nitrox: nitrogen-oxygen mixture
NOE: nap-of-the-earth
NPDES: National Pollutant Discharge Elimination System
NS: normal saline
NSC: Naval Safety Center
NSN: National Stock Number
NSU: nonspecific urethritis
NTU: nephalometric turbidity unit

O

OCHA: Office for the Coordination of Humanitarian Affairs
OCONUS: outside the continental United States
OCP: oral contraceptive pill
OCS: Officer Candidate School
OFDA: Office of Foreign Disaster Assistance
OOTW: operations other than war
OPLAN: operational plan
OPORD: operation order
OPSEC: operational security
OPV: oral polio virus
OR: odds ratio
ORS: oral rehydration solution
ORT: oral rehydration therapy
OSHA: Occupational Safety and Health Administration
otempo: operational tempo

P

P: peak
PAG: protective action guide
2-PAM Cl: pralidoxime chloride
Pap: Papanicolaou
PAR: population attributable risk
PCEC: purified chick embryo cell culture
PCR: polymerase chain reaction
PCR/RFLP: Polymerase chain reaction/restriction fragment length polymorphism
PEEP: positive end-expiratory pressure
PEL: permissible exposure limit
PFGE: pulsed-field gel electrophoresis
PFIB: perfluoroisobutylene
PH DART: Public Health Disaster Assistance Response Team
PHF: potentially hazardous food
PM: preventive medicine
PMO: Preventive Medicine Officer
PMT: Preventive Medicine Technician
PO_2: partial pressure of oxygen
POIS: pulmonary over-inflation syndrome
POW virus: Powassan encephalitis
PPM: personal protection measure
PPNG: penicillinase-producing *N gonorrhoeae*
ProMED: Program for Monitoring Emerging Diseases
PSRC: Presidential Selected Reserve call-up
PT: physical training
PTSD: post-traumatic stress disorder
PTT: partial thromboplastin time
PULHES: *p*hysical capacity, *u*pper extremities, *l*ower extremities, *h*earing, *e*yes, overall *p*sychiatric impression
PVNTMED: preventive medicine
PVOs: private voluntary organizations

R

RAD 4: Research Area Directorate, Medical, Chemical, and
  Biological Research Program
RC: reserve component of the US Armed Forces
RCRA: Resource Conservation and Recovery Act
RCW: Ration, Cold Weather
RDIC: Resuscitation Device, Individual, Chemical
RFLPs: restriction fragment length polymorphisms
rhG-CSFL recombinant human granulocyte colony-stimulating
  factor
RL: Ringer's Lactate
RMSF: Rocky Mountain spotted fever
RNA: ribonucleic acid
ROWPU: Reverse Osmosis Water Purification Unit
RR: relative risk
RTC: Navy Recruit Training Command
RPR: rapid plasma reagin
RSSE: Russian spring-summer encephalitis
RVA: rabies vaccine adsorbed
RVF: Rift Valley fever

S

SARA Title III: Superfund Amendment and Reauthorization
  Act Title III
sarin: GB; O-isopropyl methylphosphonofluoridate
SASO: Security and Support Operations
SCAP: Supreme Commander for the Allied Powers
scuba: self-contained underwater breathing apparatus
SEAL: US Navy *Sea*, *Air*, and *Land*
SEB: staphylococcal enterotoxin B
SF: US Special Forces
SFG: Special Forces Group
SFG: spotted fever group
sIgA: secretory immunoglobulin A
SIN: Sindbis
SMS: Sleep Management System
SOF: Special Operations Forces
soman: GD
SPF: sun protection factor
SPRINT: Special Psychiatric Rapid Intervention team
SRP: soldier readiness processing
SRSVs: small round structured viruses
ST: heat-stable toxin
STANAG: standardization agreement
STD: sexually transmitted diseases

T

tabun: GA
TAIHOD: Total Army Injury and Health Outcomes Database
TAML: Theater Area Medical Lab
TB: tuberculosis
TBE: tick-borne encephalitis
Td: tetanus-diphtheria
TdaP: tetanus-diphtheria-acellular pertussis
TIG: Tetanus immune globulin

TMP/SMX: trimethoprim-sulfamethoxazole
TOC: total organic carbon
TrD: Trinidad donkey
TSCA: Toxic Substances Control Act

U

UN: United Nations
UNDP: United Nations Development Program
UNHCR: United Nations Office of the High Commissioner for
  Refugees
UNICEF: United Nations Children's Fund
URI: upper respiratory infection
USACHPPM: The United States Army Center for Health
  Promotion and Preventive Medicine
USAFR: Air Force Reserve
USAFR: US Air Force Reserve
USAID: US Agency for International Development
USAMRICD: US Army Medical Research Institute of Chemi-
  cal Defense
USAMRIID: US Army Medical Research Institute of Infectious
  Diseases
USAR: US Army Reserve
USARV: US Army, Vietnam
USASOC: US Army Special Operations Command
USCGR: US Coast Guard Reserve
USDA: US Department of Agriculture
USEPA: US Environmental Protection Agency
USMCR: US Marine Corps Reserve
USNR: US Naval Reserve
USSOCOM: US Special Operations Command
UTI: urinary tract infection

V

VA: Department of Veterans Affairs
VAPP: vaccine-associated paralytic poliomyelitis
VAERS: Vaccine Adverse Events Reporting System
VECTOR: Soviet Institute of Microbiology and Virology, now
  named Russian State Research Center of Virology and
  Biotechnology
VEE: Venezuelan equine encephalitis
VHF: Venezuelan hemorrhagic fever
VL: visceral leishmaniasis
Vo_2max: maximum oxygen consumption
VtL: viscerotropic
VX: no expansion, no common name
VZIG: varicella-zoster immune globulin

W

WBC: white blood cell
WBGT: Wet Bulb Globe Temperature
WEE: Western equine encephalitis
WFP: World Food Program
WHO: World Health Organization
WNF: west Nile fever
WRAIR: Walter Reed Army Institute of Research

INDEX

A

ACIP

See Advisory Committee on Immunization Practices

Acquired immunodeficiency syndrome. *See also* Human
immunodeficiency virus infection; Sexually transmitted
diseases

  fear of, 1147, 1156

  histoplasmosis and, 1076

  nontyphoidal salmonellosis and, 1023

  toxoplasmosis and, 951–952

Acute motor axonal neuropathy

  campylobacter enteritis and, 1010

Acyclovir

  genital herpes treatment, 1167

  varicella treatment, 1226

Adenosine arabinoside

  rabies treatment, 966

Adenovirus infections

  description, 1128–1129

  epidemiology, 1129

  pathogen description, 1013

  pathogenesis and clinical findings, 1015, 1129

  vaccines, 1129–1130

Advisory Committee on Immunization Practices

  Japanese encephalitis vaccination recommendation, 843

  measles recommendations, 1216, 1217

  mumps recommendations, 1221

  pertussis recommendations, 1230

  polio vaccination recommendations, 1240

  varicella recommendations, 1226–1227

Afghan War

  malaria and, 808

Africa

  anthrax and, 976

  bancroftian filariasis and, 884

  brucellosis and, 980

  campylobacter enteritis, 1009

  chikungunya and, 827

  cholera and, 1033

  Ebola hemorrhagic fever and, 961

  epidemic typhus fever and, 875

  helminths and, 1055

  Lassa fever and, 959

  loiasis and, 888

  Lyme disease and, 863

  malaria and, 807, 808

  melioidosis and, 1079

  meningococcal disease and, 1133

  onchocerciasis and, 887

  o'nyong-nyong and, 827

  plague and, 880

  Q fever and, 953

  rabies and, 965

  Rift Valley fever and, 825–826

  sandfly fever and, 858

  schistosomiasis and, 1063

  Sindbis and Sindbis-like viral infections and, 828

  toxoplasmosis and, 949

  viral gastroenteritis and, 1013

  West Nile fever and, 830

  yellow fever and, 833, 834, 835

African sleeping sickness

  diagnosis, 900

  epidemiology, 899–900

  incidence, 900

  mortality rate, 900

  pathogen description, 899

  pathogenesis and clinical findings, 900

  therapy, 900–901

  transmission, 899–900

Age factors

  age-specific incidence rates, 758

  amebiasis, 1040, 1041

  brucellosis, 981

  Chagas' disease, 898

  death and injury from natural disasters and, 1301–1302

  enterohemorrhagic *Escherichia coli*, 1005, 1006

  feeding programs, 1386

  histoplasmosis, 1076

  human monocytic ehrlichiosis, 867

  influenza, 1128

  Japanese encephalitis, 840

  Mycoplasma pneumoniae infections, 1125

  nontyphoidal salmonellosis, 1024

  nutritional assessment, 1379–1380

  pertussis, 1228, 1229

  polio, 1238

  rubella, 1219

  sexually transmitted diseases, 1148–1149, 1154–1155

  Streptococcus pyogenes infections and, 1121

  tetanus, 1232

  varicella, 1224

  viral gastroenteritis, 1015

  viral hepatitis, 1178, 1180

  yellow fever, 835

Agent Orange exposure

  redeployment and, 1428

AHF

  See Argentine hemorrhagic fever

AIDS

  See Acquired immunodeficiency syndrome

Air National Guard

  Weapons of Mass Destruction Civil Support Teams, 1368

Airborne precautions, 1259–1260

Albendazole

  helminth infection treatment, 1059

Alcohol abuse

  See Substance abuse

Alcohol consumption

  death and injury from natural disasters and, 1301–1302

  sexually transmitted diseases and, 1148, 1154

Allergic reactions

  bancroftian filariasis and, 885

  diethylcarbamazine citrate, 889

  vaccines, 839, 843, 844

Amantadine

  influenza treatment, 1128

Amazon River basin

  malaria and, 807

  Oropouche fever and, 823–824

Amebiasis

  diagnostic approaches, 1041

  epidemiology, 1039–1040